TISSUE
ENGINEERING
INTELLIGENCE
UNIT 1

Tissue Engineering of Vascular Prosthetic Grafts

TISSUE
ENGINEERING
INTELLIGENCE
UNIT 1

Tissue Engineering of Vascular Prosthetic Grafts

Peter Zilla, M.D., Ph.D.

University of Cape Town
Cape Town, South Africa

Howard P. Greisler, M.D.

Loyola University
Maywood, Illinois, U.S.A.

R.G. LANDES
COMPANY

AUSTIN, TEXAS
U.S.A.

TISSUE ENGINEERING INTELLIGENCE UNIT

Tissue Engineering of Vascular Prosthetic Grafts

R.G. LANDES COMPANY
Austin, Texas, U.S.A.

Please address all inquiries to the Publishers:
R.G. Landes Company, 810 South Church Street, Georgetown, Texas, U.S.A. 78626
Phone: 512/ 863 7762; FAX: 512/ 863 0081

ISBN: 1-57059-549-6

Cover: *"Endocytosis" by Thomas Maciag at <www.forestreetgallery.com> 1-877-874-8084. The Editors and Publisher express their appreciation for permission to use this picture.*

The Editors and Publisher gratefully acknowledge the support of Medtronic.

Library of Congress Cataloging-in-Publication Data

Tissue engineering of prosthetic vasxcular grafts [edited by] Peter Zilla, Howard P. Greisler.
   p.   cm.--(Tissue engineering intelligence unit)
   Includes bibliographical referecnces and index.
   ISBN 1-57059-549-6 (alk. paper)
   1. Blood vessel prosthesis. 2. Vascular grafts. 3. Biomedical materials. I. Zilla, P.P. (Peter Paul) II. Greisler, Howard P. III. Series.
   [DNLM: 1. Blood Vessel Prosthesis. 2. Blood Vessels--transplantation. 3. Cell Transplantation. 4. Endothelium, Vascular--cytology. 5. Host vs Graft reaction--immunology. 6. Biocompatyible Materials. WG 170 T616 1999]
RD598.55.T57 1999
617.4'130592--dc21
DNLM/DLC
for Library of Congress
                     99-24890
                     CIP

CONTENTS

PART III
Biointeractive Prostheses: Complete Healing

PART III
Biointeractive Prostheses: Complete Healing

EDITORS

Peter Zilla, M.D., Ph.D.
Cardiovascular Research Unit
University of Cape Town Medical School
Cape Town, South Africa
Chapters 1, 13, 15, 17, 18

Howard P. Greisler, M.D.
Department of Vascular Surgery
Loyola University
Maywood, Illinois, U.S.A.
Chapters 26, 28, 45

CONTRIBUTORS

James M. Anderson, M.D., Ph.D.
Institute of Pathology
University Hospital of Cleveland
Cleveland, Ohio, U.S.A
Chapter 19

William A. Beresford
Department of Anatomy
Robert C. Byrd Health Science Center
West Virginia University
School of Medicine
Morgantown, West Virginia, U.S.A.
Chapter 37

Karin A. Blumofe
Chapter 28

Gary L. Bowlin, Ph.D.
Department of Biomedical Engineering
University of Akron
Akron, Ohio, U.S.A.
Chapter 3

Karen J.L. Burg, Ph.D.
Department of General Surgery Research
Carolinas Medical Center
Charlotte, North Carolina, U.S.A.
Chapter 46

Patrick T. Cahalan
Intelligent Biocides
Tewksbury, Massachusetts, U.S.A.
Chapters 42, 44, 49

David Cheung
University of Southern California
  School of Medicine
Childrens Hospital Los Angeles
Division of Surgical Research
Los Angeles, California, U.S.A.
Chapter 27

Richard R. Clark, M.D.
Department of Dermatology
State University of New York at Stony Brook
Stony Brook, New York, U.S.A.
Chapter 31

Alexander W. Clowes, M.D.
Department of Surgery
Division of Vascular Surgery
University of Washington Medical School
Seattle, Washington, U.S.A.
Chapters 22, 56

Monika M. Clowes
Department of Surgery
Division of Vascular Surgery
University of Washington Medical School
Seattle, Washington, U.S.A.
Chapter 56

D.J. Conway, M.Sc.
Department of Computation & Applied Mechanics
University of Cape Town
Cape Town, South Africa
Chapter 40

S.L. Cooper
Chapter 50

Fabiola Cordoba
University of Southern California
  School of Medicine
Childrens Hospital Los Angeles
Division of Surgical Research
Los Angeles, California, U.S.A.
Chapter 27

Arthur J. Coury, Ph.D.
Focal, Inc.
Lexington, Massachusetts, U.S.A.
Chapter 43

Lester Davids, M.Sc.
Cardiovascular Research Unit
University of Cape Town Medical School
Cape Town, South Africa
Chapter 1

Edwin T. Den Braber, Ph.D.
Katolieke Universiteit Nijmegen
Faculty of Medical Sciences
Dental School
Nijmegen, The Netherlands
Chapter 48

Manfred Deutsch, M.D.
Chirurgischen Abteilung
Krankenhaus Wien-Lainz
Vienna, Austria
Chapters 15, 17, 18

Dominic Dodd, M.B.Ch.B., F.R.C.S.
Chapter 9

Duane L. Donovan, M.D.
Summa Health System
Akron City Hospital
Akron, Ohio, U.S.A.
Chapter 10

A.S. Douglas
Mechanical Engineering Department
Johns Hopkins University
Baltimore, Maryland, U.S.A.
Chapter 40

Terri Dower, B.Sc.(Hons.)
Cardiovascular Research Unit
University of Cape Town Medical School
Cape Town, South Africa
Chapter 1

Ruediger C. Braun-Dullaeus
Department of Medicine
Brigham & Women's Hospital
Harvard Medical School
Boston, Massachusetts, U.S.A.
Chapter 23

Victor J. Dzau
Chairman, Department of Medicine
Brigham & Women's Hospital
Harvard Medical School
Boston, Massachusetts, U.S.A.
Chapter 23

John W Eaton, Ph.D.
Department of Pediatrics
Baylor College of Medicine
Houston, Texas, U.S.A.
Chapter 20

Teddy Fischlein, M.D.
Johann Wolfgang Goethe-Universität Frankfurt
Klinik für Thorax-, Herz und Gefäßchirurgie
Frankfurt, Germany
Chapters 8, 18

M. Fittkau
Department of Thoracic and Cardiovascular Surgery
J.W. Goethe University
Frankfurt/Main, Germany
Chapter 8

David Fox
Chapter 45

Takashi Fujiwara, Ph.D.
Laboratory Animal Center
Ehime University
School of Medicine
Shingenobu Ehime, Japan
Chapter 38

Randolph L. Geary, M.D.
Assistant Professor of Surgery
  & Comparative Medicine
Bowman Gray School of Medicine
Medical Centre Boulevard
Winston-Salem, North Carolina, U.S.A.
Chapter 56

Alberto Giudiceandrea
Vascular Unit
University Department of Surgery
Royal Free Hospital and School of Medicine
London, U.K.
Chapter 2

Werner Müller-Glauser, Ph.D.
Department of Surgery
Clinic for Cardiovascular Surgery
University Hospital Zürich
Zürich, Switzerland
Chapter 11

Anders Haegerstrand, M.D., Ph.D.
Department of Neuroscience
Karolinska Institute
Stockholm, Sweden
Chapter 14

Caroline Gillis-Haegerstrand, M.D., Ph.D.
Department of Neuroscience
Karolinska Institute
Stockholm, Sweden
Chapters 14, 16

George Hamilton, F.R.C.S.
Royal Free Hospital
London, U.K.
Chapter 2

William P. Hammond, M.D.
The Hope Heart Institute
University of Washington
School of Medicine
Seattle, Washington, U.S.A.
Chapter 35

Bo Han
University of Southern California
   School of Medicine
Childrens Hospital Los Angeles
Division of Surgical Research
Los Angeles, California, U.S.A.
Chapter 27

Timothy J. Hcilizer
Chapter 28

Lynn L.H. Huang
University of Southern California
   School of Medicine
Childrens Hospital Los Angeles
Division of Surgical Research
Los Angeles, California, U.S.A.
Chapter 27

Jeffrcy A. Hubbell, Ph.D.
Professor Of Biomedical Engineering
Institute of Biomedical Engineering
   and Department of Materials
Swiss Federal Institute of Technology (EHT) Zürich
   & University of Zürich
Zürich, Switzerland
Chapter 51

John A. Jansen, DDS., Ph.D.
Department of BioMaterials
Katolieke Universiteit Nijmegen
Faculty of Medical Sciences
Dental School
Nijmegen, The Netherlands
Chapter 48

Terry L. Kaiura
Division of Vascular Surgery
Beth Israel Hospital
Boston, Massachusetts, U.S.A.
Chapter 32

K. Craig Kent, M.D.
Division of Vascular Surgery
New York Hospital/
   Cornell University Medical Center
New York, New York, U.S.A.
Chapter 32

Alisa E. Koch, M.D.
Department of Medicine
Section of Arthritis and Connective Tissue Diseases
Northwestern University Medical School
Chicago, Illinois, U.S.A.
Chapter 25

Willie R. Koen, M.B.Ch.B., F.C.S.
Cardiovascular Research Unit
University of Cape Town Medical School
Cape Town, South Africa
Chapter 34

Kazunori Kon, Ph.D.
Laboratory Animal Center
School of Medicine
Ehime University
Shingenobu Ehime, Japan
Chapter 38

Pieter Koolwijk, Ph.D.
Gaubius Laboraroty
Leiden, The Netherlands
Chapter 29

K.H. Lam
Department of Artificial Organs
Division Biomaterials and Biocompatability
University of Groningen
Groningen, The Netherlands
Chapter 47

Nina M.K. Lamba, Ph.D.
Department of Chemical Engineering
University of Delaware
Colburn Lab
Newark, Delaware, U.S.A.
Chapter 50

Peter I. Lelkes, Ph.D.
Director, Laboratory of Cell Biology
University of Wisconsin Medical School
Milwaukee Clinical Campus
Sinai Samaritan Medical Center, Winter Research
Milwaukee, Wisconsin, USA
Chapter 5

John M. McPherson
Biotherapeutic Product Development Department
Genzyme Corporation
Framingham, Massachusetts, U.S.A.
Chapter 31

Michael J. Mann
Department of Medicine
Brigham & Women's Hospital
Harvard Medical School
Boston, Massachusetts, U.S.A.
Chapter 23

Stephen P. Massia, Ph.D.
Department Chemical, Bio, & Materials Engineering
Arizona State University
Tempe, Arizona, U.S.A.
Chapter 54

Sharon O. Meerbaum
Summa Health System
Akron City Hospital
Akron, Ohio, U.S.A.
Chapter 10

Johann Meinhart, Ph.D.
Krankenhaus Wien Lainz
Vienna, Austria
Chapters 15, 17, 18

Ira Mills
Department of Surgery
Yale University School of Medicine
New Haven, Connecticut, U.S.A.
Chapter 39

Toshitaka Nabeshima
Department of Neuropsychopharmacology
and Hospital Pharmacy
Nagoya University School of Medicine
Tsuruma-cho, Showa-ku, Nagoya, Japan
Chapter 55

Victor V. Nikolaychik
Laboratory of Cell Biology
Department of Medicine
University of Wisconsin Medical School
Milwaukee Clinical Campus
Milwaukee, Wisconsin, U.S.A.
Chapter 5

Marcel Nimni
University of Southern California
    School of Medicine
Childrens Hospital Los Angeles
Division of Surgical Research
Los Angeles, California, U.S.A.
Chapter 27

Erik L. Owens, M.D.
Department of Surgery
University of Washington Medical School
Division of Vascular Surgery
Seattle, Washington, U.S.A.
Chapter 22

Mehmet C. Oz, M.D.
Columbia University
New York, New York, U.S.A.
Chapter 36

Miralem Pasic, M.D., Ph.D.
Deutsches Herzzentrum Berlin
Klinik für Herz-Thorax und Gefäßchirurgie
Berlin, Germany
Chapter 11

Alyssa Panitch
Department of Polymer Science and Engineering
University of Massachusetts
Amherst, Massachusetts, U.S.A.
Chapter 53

Richard J. Powell, M.D.
Dartmouth-Hitchcock Medical Center
Department of Surgery
Lebanon, New Hampshire, U.S.A.
Chapter 33

Thomas Schmitz-Rixen
Zentrum fuer Chirurgie
Johann-Wolfgang Goethe Universität
Frankfurt-am-Main, Germany
Chapter 2

E. Helene Sage, Ph.D.
University of Washington
School of Medicine
Department of Biological Structure
Seattle, Washington, U.S.A.
Chapter 30

Tsunehisa Sakurai
First Department of Surgery
Nagoya University School of Medicine
Tsuruma-cho, Showa-ku, Nagoya, Japan
Chapter 55

Mark M. Samet
Department of Medicine
Laboratory of Cell Biology
University of Wisconsin Medical School
Milwaukee Clinical Campus
Milwaukee, Wisconsin, U.S.A.
Chapter 5

J.M. Schakenraad
Department of Pathology
University Hospital
Rottendam Dijkzicht, The Netherlands
Chapter 47

Ann Marie Schmidt
Columbia University
New York, New York, U.S.A.
Chapter 36

Steven P. Schmidt, PhD
Falor Centre for Vascular Studies
Akron City Hospital
Akron, Ohio, U.S.A.
Chapters 3, 10

Alexaneder M. Seifalian
Vascular Unit
University Department of Surgery
Royal Free Hospital and School of Medicine
London, U.K.
Chapter 2

S.W. Shalaby
Poly-Med, Inc.
Anderson, South Carolina, U.S.A.
Chapter 46

Paula K. Shireman, M.D.
Department of Vascular Surgery
Loyola University
Maywood, Illinois, U.S.A.
Chapters 26, 28

J.Vincent Smyth
Department of Vascular Surgery
Manchester Royal Infirmary
England
Chapters 4, 9

Talia B. Spanier, M.D.
Columbia University
New York, New York, U.S.A.
Chapter 36

Greg R. Starke, Ph.D.
Department of Computation & Applied Mechanics
University of Cape Town
Cape Town, South Africa
Chapter 40

Bauer E. Sumpio, M.D., Ph.D.
Departmenmt of Surgery
Yale University School of Medicine
New Haven, Connecticut, U.S.A.
Chapter 39

Zoltan Szekanecz, M.D., Ph.D.
Third Department of Medicine
University Medical School of Debrecen
Hungary
Chapter 25

Liping Tang
Department of Pediatrics
Baylor College of Medicine
Houston, Texas, U.S.A.
Chapter 20

David A. Tirrell, M.D.
Materials Res. Science & Engineering Center
University of Massachusetts at Amherst
Amherst, Massachusetts, U.S.A.
Chapter 53

Marko Turina, M.D.
Department of Surgery
Clinic for Cardiovascular Surgery
University Hospital Zürich
Zürich, Switzerland
Chapter 11

Victor W.M. Van Hinsbergh, Ph.D.
Gaubius Laboraroty
Leiden, The Netherlands
Chapter 29

Robert B. Vernon, Ph.D.
Department of Biological Structure
University of Washington
School of Medicine
Seattle, Washington, U.S.A.
Chapter 30

Manuela Vici, D.Sc.
Institute di Microscopica Elettronica Clinica
Universita di Bologna
Policlinico S.Orsola
Bologna, Italy
Chapter 7

David A. Vorp
University of Pittsburgh
Pittsburgh, Pennsylvania
Chapter 45

Sharon M. Wahl
Chief, Oral Infection & Immunity
National Institute of Dental Health
National Institutes of Health
Laboratory of Immunology
Bethesda, Maryland, U.S.A.
Chapter 21

Michael G. Walker, M.D.
Department of Vascular Surgery
Manchester Royal Infirmary
Manchester, U.K.
Chapters 4, 9

David F. Williams, Ph.D., D.Sc.
Department of Clinical Engineering
Faculty of Medicine
Royal Liverpool University Hospital
Liverpool, U.K.
Chapter 41

Stuart K. Williams, Ph.D.
University of Arizona
Department of Surgery
Tucson, Arizona, U.S.A.
Chapters 6, 12

Keiko Yamamura
Department of Hospital Pharmacy
Nagoya University School of Medicine
Tsuruma-cho, Showa-ku, Nagoya, Japan
Chapter 55

Ioannis V. Yannas
Department of Mechanical Engineering
Massachusetts Institute of Technology
Cambridge, Massachusetts, U.S.A.
Chapter 52

Ian Zachary
The Wolfson Institute for Biomedical Research
University College London
London, U.K.
Chapter 24

John Zagorski
Chief, Oral Infection & Immunity
National Institute of Dental Health
National Institutes of Health
Laboratory of Immunology
Bethesda, Maryland, U.S.A.
Chapter 21

PART I

Bio-Inert Prostheses: Insufficient Healing

The Lack of Healing in Conventional Vascular Grafts

Lester Davids, Terri Dower, Peter Zilla

Introduction

Seldom has any prosthetic implant become the nemesis of so many manufacturers as small diameter synthetic vascular grafts. In the era of microsphere-encapsulated cell transplants and human gene therapy it is astonishing that we still do not fully understand why the incorporation of prosthetic cardiovascular grafts does not even remotely resemble healing. Even if the postnatal organism has mostly forgotten the "restitutio ad integrum" healing of the fetal period—the complete regeneration of highly complex tissue with its original cell components—it is nevertheless capable of repairing every nonlethal injury other than chronic infection with a quiescent scar tissue. In the case of synthetic implants, however, the tissue response is a far cry from any concluded repair event. The majority of contemporary prosthetic vascular grafts are not only continually lacking typical components of a healthy native artery such as a midgraft endothelium, contractile arrangements of smooth muscle cells, functionally differentiated elastin formations and other specialized components of a vessel's extracellular matrix. Synthetic vascular grafts are also lacking the much simpler ability to restore tissue integrity through a quiescent scar formation. Even after prolonged periods of implantation, chronic inflammation dominates the interstices of these prostheses while the luminal patency is endangered by thrombotic surface appositions or the uncontrolled proliferation of a so-called "neointima".

Today's dilemma is certainly the consequence of a multitude of developments of the past three decades. When modern cardiovascular surgery first set out to replace arteries with synthetic grafts, a graft had simply to act as a nonleaking blood conduit. When it soon became obvious that the surface thrombogenicity of these prostheses was significantly higher than that of native vessels, this complication was seen as a shortcoming of imperfect materials rather than the lack of active physiological functions. This material-centered era only slowly gave way to the realization that the right cells need to be an integral part of a synthetic substitute vessel. However, a full commitment to truly "healing" grafts was further delayed by the industry's fear of disproportionate delays for new products resulting from a new dimension of complexity.

This historical retrospect makes it clear that the most consequential reason for the scanty patchwork of data available today lies in the fundamentally different concepts of graft designs in this earlier era. Instead of a holistic engineering approach which defined all biological components separately before sensibly combining them, grafts were mostly manufactured on the basis of material choices and mechanical strength. Therefore, completed products were investigated with the intention to fulfill regulatory requirements rather than learn about principal mechanisms. As a consequence, a multitude of poorly defined variants such as entirely different synthetics, a wide range of interstitial space dimensions and a variety

Tissue Engineering of Prosthetic Vascular Grafts, edited by Peter Zilla and Howard P. Greisler.

of animal models make it extremely difficult today to extract significant information from decades of prosthetic graft research. At the same time, biology has only recently provided us with the necessary diagnostic means to analyze tissue reactions with regard to the identification of cell types as well as secretion products. Thus, the emergence of basic biological tools and engineering technologies in the recent past—promising the development of implants which may eventually heal "ad integrum"—does not build on a comprehensive knowledge regarding the shortcomings of previous concepts.

Since the retrospective deduction of biological principles from data which had mostly been obtained with a different intention will not be able to create a full understanding of the apparent absence of physiological healing patterns in prosthetic vascular grafts, a systematic experimental approach will need to supplement the erratic experience of the past thirty years. For any eventual conclusions preceding serious tissue engineering approaches of the future, well planned, biologically oriented in vivo and in vitro experiments will need to be performed. In this chapter we will nevertheless attempt to retrospectively identify certain criteria which may have influenced the mitigated healing response of prosthetic vascular grafts in the past. In order to avoid dealing with an infinite number of variables, we have concentrated our efforts on those two basic graft types which have been dominating the field of synthetic vascular prostheses for the past decades: Dacron and expanded polytetrafluoroethylene.

Midgraft Healing

No other aspect of prosthetic graft research missed the point as fundamentally as did midgraft healing. In spite of a unanimous agreement with regard to the limits of transanastomotic tissue outgrowth in man, the vast major-

ity of studies of the last three decades focused unintentionally on exactly this type of healing. By choosing animal models which far exceed the human ability of transanastomotic healing, as well as graft lengths which were in average one tenth of those clinically used, midgraft healing under experimental conditions occurred predominantly through anastomotic outgrowth rather than transmural ingrowth. Considering the fact, however, that prosthetic arterial graft endothelialization in humans—mainly restricted to the anastomotic region—often involves less than one thirtieth of the entire surface, facilitated anastomotic outgrowth will most likely continue to play a limited role.

Therefore, in spite of the countless studies which investigated prosthetic arterial grafts, a description of midgraft healing—clearly distinguishable from transanastomotic events—is the exception rather than the rule. Nevertheless, by putting the sporadic observations of all these studies into a framework, a surprisingly consistent pattern of healing became apparent. A further confusion arising from the multitude of animal models used also proved to be less of a problem than expected. As with any other aspect of graft healing, by and large midgraft healing also confirmed the previous belief that it is not the healing pattern itself but its time course which distinguishes the various animal models from each other. However, there are healing aspects like the impenetrable inner fibrin capsule of Dacron grafts in humans which may well be based on principal differences between the species rather than simply on a protracted time course of common events. Nevertheless, these principal differences may again reflect differences in the time course of common sequences, as certain biological phenomena may only occur at a certain point in time. Therefore, a solution to graft healing could well lie in the facilitation of the ideal timing of crucial biological events.

Fig. 1.1. Schematic diagram depicting the histological summary of events over time for different experimental models for low porosity (< 30 μm) ePTFE. Detailed histological descriptions can be found in the text.

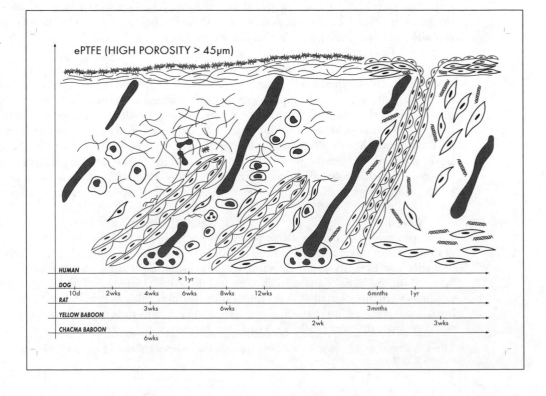

ePTFE Grafts

In spite of the wide range of internodal distances which were experimentally evaluated and the distinct characteristics of each of those grafts, a certain cut off point emerged beyond which tissue ingrowth has seemed to be principally possible. This cut off point was identified to lie somewhere between 30 μm and 45 μm of internodal distance. Therefore, it became customary to refer to grafts with an internodal distance of less than or equal to 30 μm as low porosity ePTFE grafts and to those of 45 μm or more as high porosity ePTFE grafts.

Low Porosity ePTFE Grafts
(< 30 mm Internodal Distance)

In contrast to other prosthetic grafts, low porosity ePTFE hardly shows any difference between animal models with regard to the time course of midgraft healing.

During the initial 2 weeks of implantation, a fine-fibrillar layer of a fibrin coagulum of approximately 15 μm thickness covers the graft surface.[1,2] During the following weeks the thickness of this thrombus does not further increase,[3,4] but its composition becomes more variable, reaching from acellular loosely[3,5] (Fig. 1.2) or highly compressed fibrin[4,23] to platelet carpets (Fig. 1.3) with interspersed granulocytes.[1,5] Interestingly, these dense layers of sometimes almost pure platelets often show a morphology of low grade activation (Fig. 1.3) or even nonactivation.[5] In spite of this lack of morphological signs of activation, these platelets almost seem to melt into a dense, amorphous matrix.[5] During the subsequent months[4,6,7] the blood surface still remains covered by either unorganized, compacted fibrin or a more amorphous platelet rich material, but the thickness of this layer increases to about 80-290 μm.[4,5,8] Even after prolonged observation periods of up to 3 years, midgrafts lack all forms

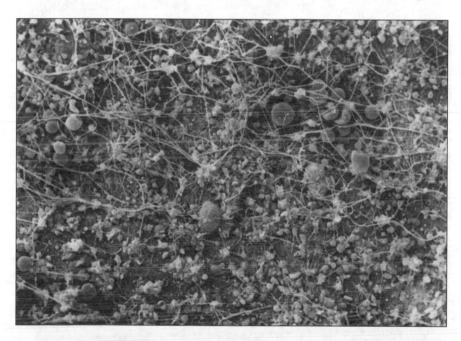

Fig. 1.2. Surface fibrin on ePTFE (30 μm internodal distance) after 4 weeks of implantation in the chacma baboon model. Loosely covering fibrin meshwork on a dense carpet of platelets adheres to a compact, more amorphous thrombus in the depth.

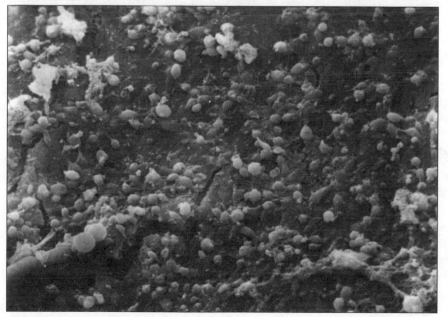

Fig. 1.3. Surface of ePTFE graft (30 μm internodal distance) after 4 weeks of implantation in the chacma baboon. One can recognize the ePTFE structure in the left lower corner. A relatively thin layer of amorphous thrombus covers the synthetic surface. Densely adherent platelets which are mostly discoid in shape seem to melt into the amorphous protein layer.

of cellular coverage.[6,9-11] However, anecdotal descriptions of multilayered cell islands in the central segments of grafts[1,5] add to the decades old controversy concerning the origin of intimal cells.[12]

Similar to surface healing, transmural tissue ingrowth remains incomplete. Until week 2 most of the interstices of the grafts are devoid of any recognizable cellular material,[1] with only scanty macrophages beginning to migrate into the micropores.[13] After 3 weeks the fibrin matrix in the graft wall has slowly become populated with inflammatory cells,[2] but there is hardly any connective tissue ingrowth into the graft.[13-17] In the chacma baboon model we find a typical triple layer picture, with macrophages invading from the blood surface and the adventitia into an otherwise almost acellular central fibrin matrix (Fig. 1.4). Apart from scanty

multinucleated giant cells[13,18,19] and macrophages[8-20] demarcating the outer graft surface against a well developed fibroelastic perigraft tissue,[1,7] no persistent inflammatory reaction is found around the graft.[7] However, there is a distinct difference between wrap-reinforced and nonreinforced grafts with regard to the tissue interaction with the outside environment. In nonwrapped grafts, relatively few foreign body giant cells (FBGC) adhere to the PTFE nodes on the outside surface, while single macrophages have infiltrated the interstices. In wrapped grafts, the narrow structure of the wrap limits the infiltration of the interstices with cells. Therefore, the almost acellular fibrin matrix usually found in the center of the prosthetic wall extends all the way to the outside surface. This outside surface, in return, borders upon a distinct layer of macrophages and FBGC (Fig. 1.4). This indi-

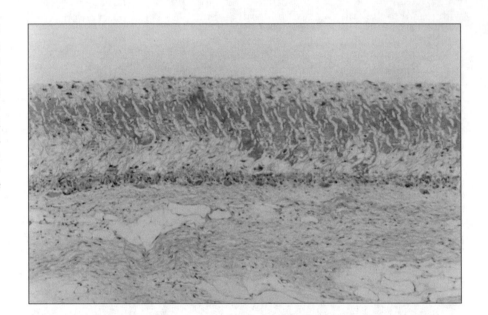

Fig. 1.4. 30 µm ePTFE graft after 6 weeks in the chacma baboon. One can clearly recognize the fine porous wrap at the outer surface. A layer of foreign body giant cells (FBGC) demarcates the ePTFE from an otherwise well-healed surrounding tissue. Loose and scanty cell infiltrates from the blood surface and the adventitial side simultaneously progress towards the acellular central fibrin matrix, filling the interstices.

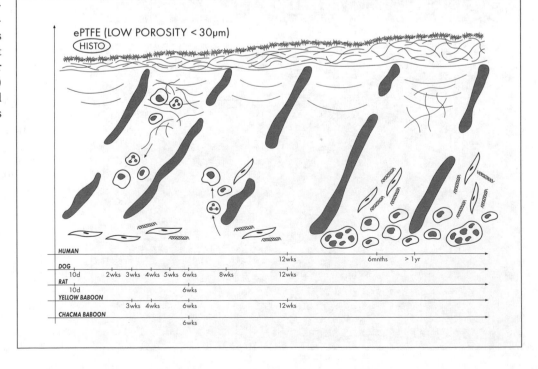

Fig. 1.5. Schematic diagram depicting the histological summary of events over time for different experimental models for high porosity (>45 µm) ePTFE. Detailed histological descriptions can be found in the text.

cates once more that the formation of FBGC may be significantly influenced by surface structures, because the material is PTFE in both instances. In the case of the ePTFE wrap it is difficult to say whether the higher density of FBGC is a result of the finer porosity and structure of the PTFE or the overall result of an impenetrable barrier plane compared to the relatively open spaced single nodes in unwrapped ePTFE. Eventually, after 6 weeks of implantation, connective tissue cells occasionally begin to grow into the interstices of unwrapped prosthesis from outside.[13,14,17,21-23] Six months after implantation, however, connective tissue ingrowth from outside still remains moderate and mostly limited to the outer part of the graft wall,[18-20,24-26] while the majority of interstitial graft spaces continue to be primarily occupied by fibrin and a mild inflammatory infiltrate in the proximity of the surfaces.[25] In contrast to the early days of implantation, however, these cells lie in a very fine fibrillar extracellular meshwork which has replaced the solid acellular fibrin. If present, this scanty and loose connective tissue contains hardly any capillaries.[113,25]

High Porosity ePTFE Grafts
(> 45 µm Internodal Distance)

In contrast to low porosity ePTFE grafts, there is a distinct difference in high porosity ePTFE grafts with regard to the time course of healing events in humans and different animal models.

Initially, the blood surface resembles that of low porosity ePTFE grafts. It is covered by a thin fibrin layer which over time develops into a variable coagulum of fibrin, platelets and erythrocytes.[27] In dogs and other more senescent animal models, this stage lacking endothelial coverage persists well into the sixth week of implantation.[27-29] In the senescent chacma baboon, for instance, we find a six week pannus ingrowth of only 7.8 ± 3.5 mm reaching onto otherwise nonendothelialized grafts (Fig. 1.6). The surface of these grafts is covered either by a relatively thin layer of smooth fibrin containing white blood cells and a few platelets or by

a more amorphous protein matrix densely covered by platelets and a few white blood cells (Fig. 1.7). Overall, the thickness of the surface thrombus is moderate, because one can recognize the nodal ePTFE structure throughout the graft (Fig. 1.8). Histologically, a homogenous fibrin layer covered by a carpet of platelets enshrouds the ePTFE surfaces. Except for very few occasional polymorphnuclear granulocytes, this fibrin layer is practically acellular (Fig. 1.7). The presence of a layer of macrophages underneath this fibrin matrix—which is demarcated for the depth of the graft by a zone of equally acellular fibrin—indicates that the surface fibrin has previously been permeable to inflammatory cells. In contrast to the senescent chacma baboon, high porosity ePTFE grafts lead to early and spontaneous endothelialization in juvenile recipients such as young yellow baboons. Patches of endothelial cells[30] and capillary orifices—approximately 100-500 µm apart[31]—appear on the blood surface as early as 1-2 weeks after implantation, leading to confluence shortly thereafter.[30-35] Since the endothelium soon rests on a well developed layer of actin positive cells[3-33,35] which contains only a few macrophages,[36] the fibrin matrix which initially covers the inner surface and provides the outgrowth substrate for the endothelium represents a very transient matrix under these circumstances. These actin positive cells appearing underneath the endothelium[9,33] also exhibit the ultrastructural characteristics of arterial smooth muscle cells.[30] Although proliferating smooth muscle cells resemble wound fibroblasts, there is currently more evidence against fibroblasts trans-differentiating into smooth muscle cells[19,37-40] than there is for it. Therefore, it is likely that these cells are derived from pericytes accompanying EC.[9,33] Over time the endothelium and its subendothelial tissue layer develop into a stable neointima[20,31,35,41,42] with a higher density of actin positive cells adjacent to the endothelium than to the graft surface.[20,26,31,40,43-49] This intimal thickening is evenly distributed along the entire graft surface and not confined to the anastomotic region as in low porosity ePTFE grafts.[30] It is

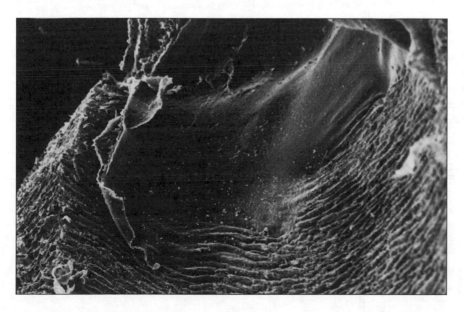

Fig. 1.6. Pannus outgrowth onto 60 µm ePTFE after 6 weeks of implantation in the chacma baboon. One can clearly see the anastomotic outgrowth of the pannus and the endothelium tapering off onto an otherwise nonendothelialized ePTFE surface.

Fig. 1.7. Platelet-rich surface coverage of the midsection of a 60 μm ePTFE graft after 6 weeks of implantation in the chacma baboon. One can faintly recognize the ePTFE surface in the central upper part of the picture. The dense carpet of platelets is again dominated by discoid shaped thrombocytes which do not resemble the typical morphology of aggregated platelets.

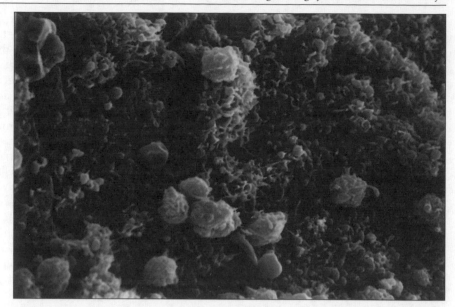

Fig. 1.8. 60 μm ePTFE after 6 weeks of implantation the chacma baboon. The surface thrombus is delicate and still allows the underlying PTFE structure to be recognized.

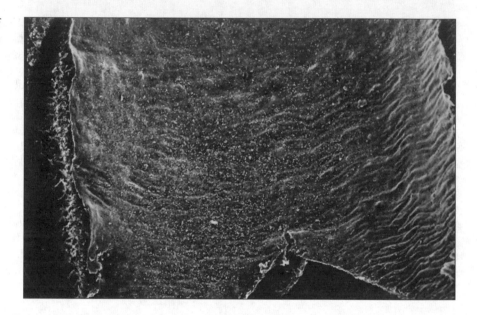

particularly noteworthy that these smooth muscle cells only started to appear in the intima and began to proliferate after endothelial cells had covered the luminal surface.[30] With SMCs multiplying in the inner one third of the intima adjacent to an endothelium[33] and without the concomitant presence of platelets[33] the situation is the opposite of traumatized arteries. Therefore, it is conceivable that endothelial cells themselves produce growth promoting substances for smooth muscle cells. This is further supported by the fact that after 3 months, SMCs are predominantly found in the subendothelial intima relatively distant from the macrophages in the interstices.[33] Apart from hinting at the involvement of endothelial cells in intimal smooth muscle cell proliferation, this observation of an increasing smooth muscle cell proliferation with increasing distance from the macrophages is inconsistent with the hypothesis that macrophages are an important source of SMC mitogens,[134,189] unless an inverse gradient applies in which low concentrations of

macrophage products stimulate SMC proliferation and high ones are inhibitory.[69] Eventually the discovery of PDGF-A mRNA in the overlying endothelial cells resolved the issue of the source of SMC mitogens.[114b] This cytokine is not only one of the strongest currently known proliferative agents for smooth muscle cells, but was previously already shown in vitro to be secreted by endothelial cells vectorially into the abluminal basal compartment.[228] Its strong presence also explains the 5-100 times higher proliferative activity of SMCs and the 10-100 times higher one of endothelial cells[50,51] in grafts than in normal arteries. Nevertheless, the presence of higher levels of PDGF and the proof of a higher mitotic activity does not indicate whether this is an adaptive response or a primary phenomenon. On the one hand one could argue that a high cycling rate may simply be the consequence of an upregulated PDGF production. On the other hand, however, it is also quite likely that a poor anchorage of endothelial cells at this stage leads to mechanical detachment and this in turn upregulates PDGF production as a reparative response. The latter explanation is supported by the morphological appearance of endothelial cells. Typical for endothelial surfaces affected by a distinct cell loss,[5] these endothelial cells lack the regular spindle shaped pattern[30] and are larger than those in arteries.[30] This sequence of a higher cell loss preceding a higher mitotic activity, rather than a higher cycling rate, being the reason for higher endothelial cell shedding would coincide with the finding for in vitro endothelialized grafts that a distinct degree of endothelial cell detachment occurs during early implantation in spite of continual endothelial integrity.[5] However, since the overall thickness of this neointima may also represent an adaptation attempt of the tissue to flow conditions in an otherwise rigid graft, the PDGF upregulation in the surface endothelium could as a third explanation also be a natural mechanism of macrovascular endothelial cell response to environmental changes such as flow. This would explain why a many-fold thicker neointima is found under low flow conditions than under high flow conditions.[54]

When surface healing occurs so early and independently of transanastomotic tissue ingrowth, the cell source for it can only be perigraft tissue which reaches the blood surface through apt transmural ingrowth. However, since complete transmural ingrowth does not readily occur in other graft types, it is particularly interesting to see whether it differs substantially in high porosity ePTFE grafts compared with other prostheses.

Comparably to other grafts, the basically acellular earliest interstitial fibrin matrix gets progressively populated with macrophages and polymorphnuclear leukocytes[28,33] during the initial period of graft implantation followed by capillary ingrowth. In the juvenile yellow baboon, these capillaries reach through the entire wall as early as after 2 weeks of implantation. Although fibroblasts from the perigraft region soon follow the capillaries,[16] the majority of the graft interstices still remain populated with macrophages.[33] In more senescent animal models like the dog or the chacma baboon, it takes 2-5 weeks and longer until sprouting capillaries begin to reach into the macrophage dominated outer one third to one half of the graft wall[27-29] (Fig. 1.9). Distinctly different from Dacron grafts, these microvessels resemble mature arterioles which are small in diameter (23.06 ± 13.11 µm; personal observation) and regularly accompanied by at least one layer of smooth muscle cells. However, in spite of this initial vascularization, the histological picture of these implants remains dominated by a triple layer appearance even after 6 weeks of implantation: While the blood and the adventitial part of the prostheses is infiltrated by inflammatory cells, the central zone of the prosthetic wall often remains filled with an almost acellular amorphous matrix (Fig. 1.10). Within this triple layered structure the cellularity of the outer third is regularly higher than that of the inner third of the graft, although it does not change much over time. Ham 56 positive macrophages continue to dominate over connective tissue cells,[55] while foreign body giant cells are conspicuously absent.[56] In spite of the scanty presence of connective tissue, the homogenous fibrin matrix initially filling the interstices gradually gets replaced by a loose transparent extracellular meshwork wherever inflammatory cell infiltrates reach into the interstices (Fig. 1.11). On the outside, high porosity ePTFE grafts are embedded into a moderately developed mature fibrous tissue which contains hardly any inflammatory cells. Only the direct interface between adventitial tissue and graft occasionally shows a few single FBGCs.

Dacron Grafts

In Dacron grafts the issue of porosity is slightly complicated through the optional combination of the grafts with a velour surface which differs from the basic texture.

Low Porosity Dacron Grafts (Woven)

Immediately after implantation a thin layer of fibrin, erythrocytes, white blood cells and platelets is deposited on the blood surface of the prosthesis.[40,57] During the first few

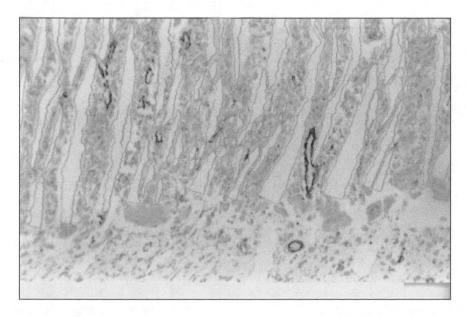

Fig. 1.9. Immunohistochemical staining of α-actin in a 60 µm ePTFE graft after 6 weeks of implantation (chacma baboon). It is obvious that those vessels which were capable of penetrating into the outer half of the graft all contain at least one layer of smooth muscle cells.

hours to days this thrombus layer slowly starts thickening until it reaches a stable equilibrium of compacted fibrin.[45] In dogs this stage is reached within 6 months,[45] whereas in humans it is observed after 1 1/2 years.[223] Exceptionally, fibrous tissue begins to organize the basis of the fibrin capsule in a few scanty areas of the graft.[40,45] This process is observed after 4-8 weeks in dogs[40,45] and after 1 1/2 years in humans.[58] Those few areas of a pseudoneointima where tissue reaches the blood surface[40,58,59] have a thickness which is comparable to that of the surrounding compacted fibrin (400-500 μm).[58] In humans these rare and localized neointimal spots extend over less than 1 mm and are collagen rich, with increasing cellularity towards the graft surface.[47] The situation is similar with regard to EC. In areas which represent true midgraft regions—unaffected by anastomotic ingrowth—no endothelial cells are found within the first 1-2 years.[40,58,59] After prolonged implantation periods of up to 11 years—which are naturally restricted to humans—small islands of endothelial cells may occasionally

appear.[58,59] These endothelial islands always rest on the compacted fibrin rather than on the scanty islands of connective tissue.

Underneath this apparently impenetrable fibrin layer, healing is most likely to take place; at least with regard to perigraft tissue ingrowth, the initial events of graft incorporation are similar to ePTFE. A fibrin matrix fills the narrow prosthetic interstices within minutes of implantation,[57] and organizing tissue begins to invade the fibrin layer surrounding the graft to form the outer fibrous tissue capsule.[45,57] In the interface between this fibrous tissue and the Dacron yarns a variable degree of foreign body giant cells begins to build up.[57] Subsequently, a few capillaries and fibroblasts start growing into the tight interstitial spaces of the woven Dacron.[40,57] This process is quite variable in its extent and time course. In dogs it can be seen as early as 2-3 weeks after implantation,[40] whereas in humans it may be observed after 5 months[11] but may also be absent after up to 18 years.[47,58,59] However, even if tissue does occasionally grow through the

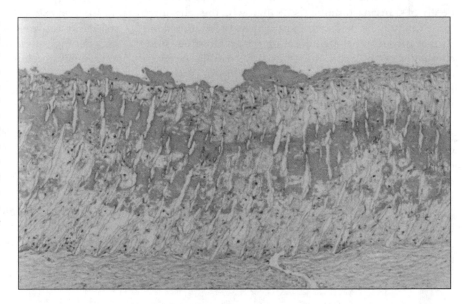

Fig. 1.10. 60 μm ePTFE graft without external wrap reinforcement. There is hardly any inflammatory tissue demarcating the graft against the surrounding, well-healed fibrous adventitial tissue. After 6 weeks the central zone of the interstitial spaces is still filled by an acellular fibrin matrix. The outer and inner third of the graft shows a loose infiltration with cells which previously degraded the acellular fibrin matrix. The blood surface is covered by a thin irregular thrombus which is practically acellular, not even containing inflammatory cells.

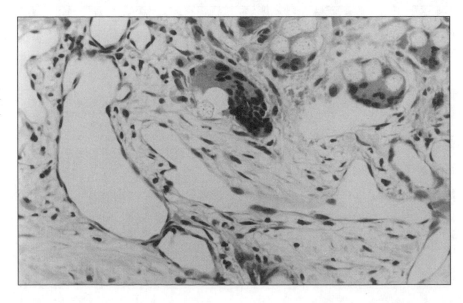

Fig. 1.11. Knitted Dacron graft (Vascutec) after 6 weeks of iliac interposition in the chacma baboon. Typically, the Dacron structure is packed with foreign body giant cells and demarcated from the surrounding adventitia by granulation tissue which contains hugely dilated capillary sinuses.

interstices of the prostheses, it does not break through the compacted fibrin of the inner capsule to reach the blood surface[43] even after decades of implantation.

High Porosity Dacron Grafts (Knitted)

There is a distinct difference regarding the healing response to variations in porosity between Dacron grafts and ePTFE grafts. In ePTFE grafts, the fibrin matrix may get rapidly replaced by inflammatory and connective tissue if the porosity is increased. In Dacron grafts, the mighty inner fibrin capsule mostly persists in both high and low porosity grafts although interstitial healing is more accelerated in the higher porosity prostheses.

In knitted dacron prostheses the initial surface net of fibrin, white blood cells, erythrocytes and platelets[48] increases during the first week of implantation to a thickness of 100-120 μm.[44,60] During the subsequent 5 weeks of implantation it appears as if the inner fibrin capsule has not yet reached an equilibrium and therefore holds a wide range of thickness: 100-500 μm in humans,[60] 30-210 μm in dogs[2,61-66] and 290-300 μm in the yellow baboon.[35,91] After a subsequent further insignificant increase,[60-62] the thickness of the internal capsule eventually reaches an equilibrium before sixth months of implantation.[61,62] Although a superficial screening of the literature suggests that it is only a matter of time until this entire layer of compacted fibrin gets organized by ingrowing tissue, deeper analysis makes it likely that this may well be a misinterpretation based on the confusion of midgraft healing with anastomotic outgrowth. It is true that the vast majority of studies describe a mature endothelium and a well developed intimal smooth muscle layer, resting directly on the graft surface,[2,67-69] but the graft length and implantation period in these studies make it almost certain that this mature neointimal tissue represents nothing but extended anastomotic outgrowth.[2,22,32,35,44,68-70] This suspicion is confirmed by descriptions of true midgraft re-

gions in particularly long grafts in which the inner fibrin capsule appears to be both impenetrable for the ingrowing interstitial graft tissue[43,44,48,59,60,71,72] and nonendothelialized.[60,72,73] This lack of surface healing occurs[43,44,48,59,60,71,72,74,75] although transmural tissue reaches the compacted fibrin of the blood surface within 3-4 weeks in the calf,[60] the yellow baboon[35] and the dog,[2,76] and 3-6 months in humans.[48,60] However, in spite of this dominant healing deficit, complete tissue replacement of the inner fibrin capsule may sporadically occur in the absence of a surface endothelium and with a poorly differentiated fibroblast matrix rather than with smooth muscle cells.[61] Occasionally, even complete endothelialization of very long prostheses is seen[46,77] comparable to those in highly porous ePTFE grafts. In the yellow baboon, for instance, knitted Dacron grafts may form complete endothelial linings, although not as readily and consistently as in 60 μm ePTFE.[32,35,78,79] They initially show small islands of endothelium after 2 weeks, and in a minority of implants even confluence after 4 weeks.[32]

However, in contrast to the case of high porosity ePTFE grafts, it remains unclear whether this endothelium is derived from transmural tissue ingrowth, facilitated transanastomotic outgrowth or fall-out healing.[12,80] The latter is a phenomenon predominantly observed in Dacron grafts where—apparently independently of transmural tissue ingrowth and with some delay—endothelial islands emerge on the surface of the compacted fibrin. These islands are well separated from the transmurally ingrowing fibrous tissue by a distinct layer of compacted fibrin.[43,48,59,60,71] They either rest directly on the fibrin[43,59,72] or on a few layers of actin positive cells with no other tissue connection,[59,71] an observation which can be made in dogs after 2-6 months[72] and in humans perhaps in every fourth graft after 1-11 years.[43,59,71] However, although sporadic endothelialization occasionally occurs in limited areas of the

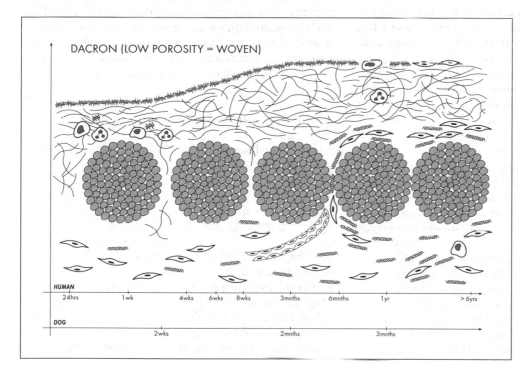

Fig. 1.12. Schematic diagram depicting the histological summary of events over time for different experimental models for woven Dacron. Detailed histological descriptions can be found in the text.

Fig. 1.13. Schematic diagram depicting the histological summary of events over time for different experimental models for knitted Dacron. Detailed histological descriptions can be found in the text.

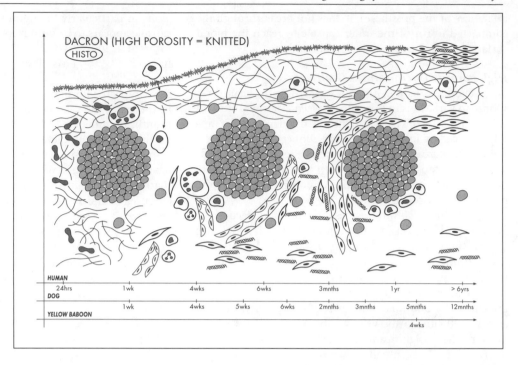

grafts, the majority of the surface remains covered by fibrin only.

If one focuses on the transmural tissue ingrowth itself, it also begins with the infiltration of the surrounding outer fibrin matrix by granulation tissue.[2,48] Initially it is primarily macrophages which begin to invade the interstitial fibrin,[14] populating the entire depth of the graft at the end of the first month of implantation.[60] Early giant cell formation surrounding the yarns and—if present—the velour fibrils commences after 7 days and increases, predominantly in the outer half of the graft wall,[62] during the following months.[61,62] The subsequent ingrowth of blood vessels and fibroblasts varies not only between the different animal models but also within one and the same recipient species. In dogs for instance, the interstitial tissue ingrowth can either reach the inner fibrin capsule as early as 2-4 weeks after implantation[2,61,63,76] or be absent as late as after 2 months.[72,81] Similarly, clinical implants in humans show all stages of ingrowth for up to three months.[179] From then onwards, ingrowing adventitial tissue reaches the internal fibrous capsule without exception in all animal species.[2,11,43,59,60,71,81,82] This tissue contains a moderate number of capillaries, fibroblasts and collagen[2,11,43,59,71,82] and eventually extends along the inside surface of the graft.[60,62,71] However, a clear, layered structure of tissue elements still dominates the histological picture. The Dacron fibers appear to demarcate themselves expressively against the surrounding tissue by a particularly distinct accumulation of foreign body giant cells (FBGC). Between this outer layer of the prosthetic wall which is packed with FBGC and the surrounding connective tissue capsule with its longitudinally aligned collagen bundles,[59,60,81] hugely dilated capillary sinuses are usually present during the early weeks of implantation. These sinuses typically consist of a single endothelial cell layer which contains no smooth muscle cells or cell types other than macrophages and FBGC, which snuggle against

its basal lamina (Fig. 1.11). Those few capillaries which sometimes reach through the entire graft wall and reach the inner capsule also remain free of smooth muscle cells.

However, in areas where transanastomotic ingrowth has resulted in a mighty neointima covering the surface, one occasionally finds true multilayered vessels with smooth muscle cells underneath the endothelium.

In summary, the porosity of knitted, and to some extent even woven, Dacron prostheses eventually allows a certain degree of tissue ingrowth from outside. At the same time, however, it seems that the compacted inner fibrin capsule on the blood surface of Dacron grafts represents an ingrowth barrier for transmural connective tissue regardless of whether the grafts are knitted or woven. Although this barrier may eventually be overcome by ingrowth of undifferentiated fibrous tissue, capillaries remain unconnected to the often poorly endothelialized blood surface.[75] The peculiar coincidence of zones which are densely packed with foreign body giant cells and hugely dilated capillary sinuses in the vicinity is particularly obvious in Dacron prostheses. Moreover, it is also interesting that the fibrin coverage on Dacron grafts seems to have a higher propensity to capture blood-borne cells than that on ePTFE grafts.[80] In this context it is also noteworthy that the resulting isolated endothelial islands often rest on equally isolated smooth muscle layers.[43,59] However, in spite of the scientific excitement arising from this observation, the rare and late occurrence of the phenomenon makes it the least typical healing characteristic of Dacron grafts.

High Porosity Dacron Velour

The rationale behind a filamentous coverage of Dacron fabric was the attempt to improve the healing between perigraft tissue and the prosthesis. Initially only used as an external cover,[60] it was soon also applied as an internal cover.[83] Interestingly, it was thought that a finer and more even porosity would cover the coarser structure of the knitted fabric underneath and thus achieve facilitated healing. As is obvious from our porosity analysis (see "Porosity") the opposite is true, and velour materials actually provide significantly wider ingrowth spaces than knitted or woven structures. This wider porosity does result in a firmer tissue integration on the outside,[15,84] but reduces platelet survival and leads to less pronounced pseudointimal development on the inside.[85] In order to study the healing pattern of entire velour structures, we have fabricated graft tubes out of pure velour material and studied the tissue reaction in the chacma baboon. Similarly to previous results,[86] the transanastomotic outgrowth of a neointima is significantly less distinct than in nonveloured knitted Dacron, even after weeks of implantation. The fibrin matrix itself often appears looser than on ePTFE and, moreover, often covered with relatively densely adherent macrophages (Fig. 1.14). The loose fibrin often

contains white blood cells in deeper layers which one can still recognize from the surface (Fig. 1.15). Nevertheless, one also finds areas of densely packed fibrin, covered with morphologically mostly unactivated platelets and white cells comparable to ePTFE (Fig. 1.16). Very rarely does one see vessel openings on the surface (Fig. 1.17). The relatively freely lying single fibers of the material are completely engulfed by conglomerates of foreign body giant cells, whereas the interstices are dominated by a loose fibrin matrix containing lymphocytes, polymorphonuclear granulocytes, macrophages and FBGCs. In spite of the wide open porosity, hardly any fibroblasts or collagen are found in the interstices. The huge and dilated capillary sinuses, which were all localized between the outer layer of the graft and the surrounding tissue in knitted prostheses, are equally present but scattered throughout the meshwork of the grafts. These often enormously dilated capillary sacs are all factor VIII positive, and

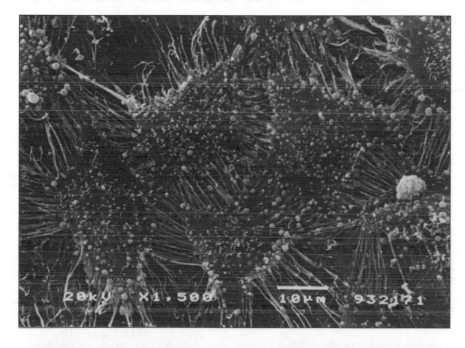

Fig. 1.14. Blood surface of the midgraft section of a Dacron velour tube (6 weeks, chacma baboon). Typically, large areas of the fibrin surface are covered with dense layers of spreading macrophages.

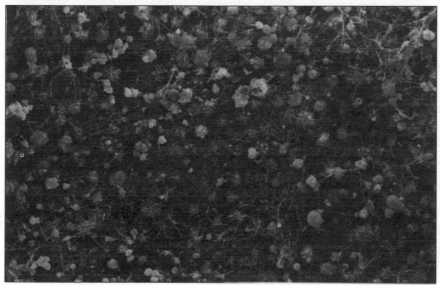

Fig. 1.15. Same graft as Figure 1.10, but showing a more loose meshwork of fibrin with inflammatory cells lying on the surface and in the depth of the structure. One can still recognize those white blood cells which are lying close to the surface.

Fig. 1.16. Midgraft section of a Dacron velour tube covered by an amorphous protein layer with an adherent carpet of disk shaped platelets. Occasionally, white blood cells lie in lacunar spaces which appear to have been excavated from the fibrin layer.

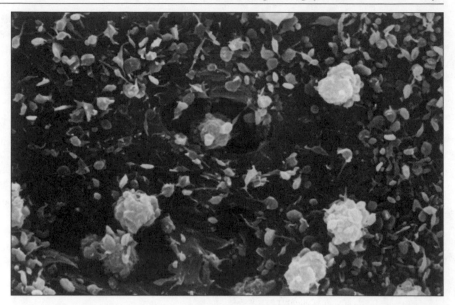

Fig. 1.17. Midgraft section of a Dacron velour tube after 6 weeks of implantation in the chacma baboon. One very rarely sees capillary openings surrounded by small islands of endothelial cells, which grow onto the otherwise endothelial-free compacted fibrin surface.

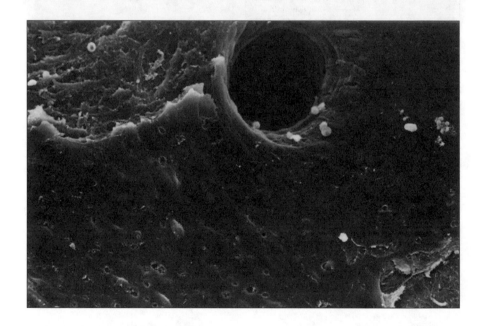

Fig. 1.18. Histological cross-section of a Dacron velour tube after 6 weeks of implantation in the chacma baboon. The loose structure allows capillary ingrowth at all levels. As a consequence the dilated capillary sinuses—which are otherwise only found in the outer half of knitted prostheses—are scattered throughout the graft wall. The capillary sinuses themselves consist of factor viii positive endothelial cell monolayers resting on basement membranes surrounded purely by inflammatory cells, which are predominantly foreign body giant cells.

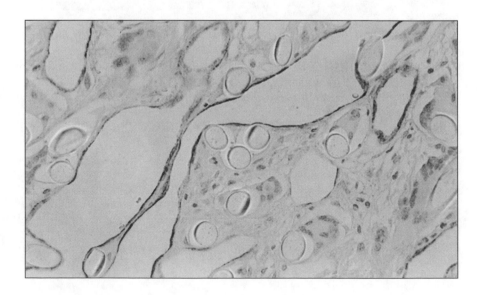

equally as devoid of smooth muscle cells as knitted prostheses (Fig. 1.18). Occasionally, the simultaneous infiltration mode from inside and outside can still be detected after 6 weeks, with a central cell free zone of fibrin wedged between the inner and outer graft thirds, the outer being dominated by foreign body giant cells.

These observations indicate that in spite of wide open interstitial spaces, there seems to be a distinct inhibition for connective tissue ingrowth in Dacron scaffolds. It is even more obvious from velour explants than from the narrower structures of knitted Dacron that capillarization is rather overshooting than underdeveloped. These widely dilated endothelial sacs, however, neither reach the blood surface nor attract concomitantly ingrowing smooth muscle cells.

Transanastomotic Healing

The assessment of anastomotic tissue ingrowth is another ambiguous task within the attempt to interpret the healing of prosthetic vascular grafts. Although surface endothelialization—which under experimental circumstances overwhelmingly happens through transanastomotic ingrowth—was indirectly the focus of almost every single study in the past, there is hardly any other aspect of prosthetic graft healing which is so vaguely described.

When all studies included in this review are taken into account, the average graft length is 10.8 ± 2.6 cm. This value includes the 11% of grafts which were longer than 10 cm. If those grafts—which were substantially longer than the others (36.6 ± 2.4 cm)—are excluded, the mean length of the remaining 89% of prostheses is only 5.5 ± 1.2 cm. With a median implantation period of 91.8 ± 17.3 days in Dacron grafts and 60.0 ± 9.36 days in PTFE grafts, it does not come as a surprise that transanastomotic ingrowth was frequently completed before the prostheses were retrieved. This often makes it impossible to determine retrospectively the point in time when the surface coverage through transanastomotic tissue ingrowth was completed. To create further uncertainty, measurements of tissue ingrowth vary widely amongst those studies where surface endothelialization was not completed prior to explantation, and which could thus be admitted to a comparative ingrowth assessment.

Another point of confusion relates to the terms "neointima" and "pannus". As we have argued under the topic "midgraft healing", prior to the use of high porosity ePTFE grafts neointimal tissue formation was mostly restricted to transanastomotic ingrowth, even if many of the investigators were not aware of it. As opposed to the mostly fibrinous "pseudoneointima" of midgraft regions, "neointima" could almost synonymously be used as the term for transanastomotically ingrowing tissue covering the blood surface of the graft. However, with truly transmurally derived neointimas observed in certain contemporary prostheses, it seems necessary to restrict the term "neointima" to surface tissue which results from transmural midgraft healing and to keep describing the anastomotic tissue ingrowth as "pannus". As necessary as this restriction of the term "neointima" is, it eliminates further bits of assumed clarity. Since the majority of studies describe prostheses in which the anastomotic pannus has already reached the midgraft

region, the widely used term "neointima" in these studies actually refers to anastomotic pannus tissue.

However, in spite of the poorly defined criteria with regard to anastomotic tissue ingrowth and the scanty data available for some of these criteria, certain trends concerning animal models, material and porosity still become apparent.

Pannus Tissue

Within less than 2 days of implantation, a straightening and disruption of the internal elastic membrane of the adjacent native artery occurs.[87] Simultaneously, the smooth muscle cells of the inner one-third of the media begin to proliferate[87] and migrate through the ruptured internal elastic membrane into the intima. It is primarily this hyperplastic intimal tissue which—together with the endothelium—migrates and proliferates onto the graft surface, thereby slowly replacing the inner fibrinous capsule from the anastomosis towards the midgraft. Typically, endothelial cells precede this outgrowth,[19,28,88] followed by connective tissue cells. This means that the foremost edge of the outgrowing endothelium initially rests on the fibrin matrix of the inner capsule[6,28,88] before a few layers of smooth muscle cells appear underneath.[14,25,27,13] This edge of outgrowing endothelium often does not resemble a solidly migrating formation of endothelial cells, but rather deeply meandered, tattered and irregularly shaped islands and tongues of endothelium (Fig. 1.19). Very often, the foremost edge consists of loosely lying endothelial cells, surrounded by platelet-covered fibrin (Fig. 1.20). Eventually, a multilayered connective tissue, which increases in thickness over time, slowly builds up between the graft and the blood surface.[19] This tissue does not consist exclusively of secretory smooth muscle cells[69] but also of fibroblasts, collagen and a few macrophages.[30,40,52,55,61,62,68] After a few months a layered structure develops with a hypercellular myofibroblast-dominated luminal aspect and a fibro-collagenous and glucosaminoglycan-rich aspect near the graft surface.[68,89] However, even at that stage this subendothelial tissue lacks features of native arteries like elastic fibers between the smooth muscle cell layers[20] and an internal elastic membrane[69] separating the endothelium from the bulk of smooth muscle cells. Altogether, the undifferentiated pannus near the anastomosis of a prosthetic graft has not much in common with the organized intimal structures of a native vessel. Thus, transanastomotic tissue outgrowth remains a far cry from a self-terminating healing process leading to true neo-artery structures on the inside of a prosthetic graft.

In spite of the undifferentiated hyperplastic nature of this pannus tissue, however, there are various circumstances which significantly affect at least its tissue composition and thickness. Anatomical position, for instance,[72,81] as well as the difference between distal and proximal anastomoses[64,81,90] are known to influence the thickness of pannus tissue. Moreover, tissue hyperplasia is also a means of compensating for the lack of compliance and contractility in prosthetic grafts. Therefore, variations in flow[8,52] and shear stress[52] result in an adaptive reduction or increase in thickness of the subendothelial tissue.

Fig. 1.19. Typically meandered edge of transanastomotically outgrowing endothelium (30 µm ePTFE; chacma baboon; 6 weeks).

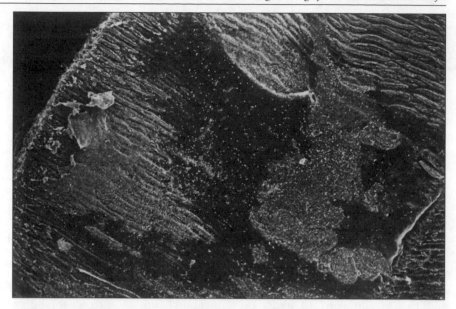

Fig. 1.20. Loosely arranged endothelial formation at the edge of transanastomotically outgrowing pannus tissue. All the cells are practically lacking contact with the neighboring endothelial cells and are surrounded by a dense carpet of blood platelets (Dacron velour, chacma baboon, 6 weeks).

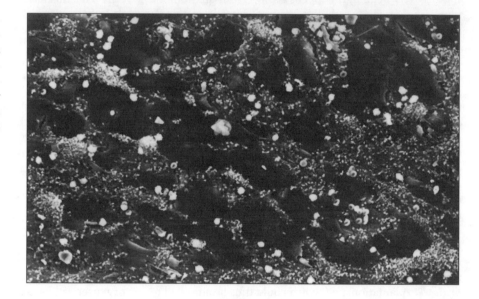

Apart from these influences, it appears as if the thickness of the anastomotic pannus is to a certain degree also predetermined by an almost template function of the initial fibrinous inner capsule. Even at an early stage when transmural tissue ingrowth has hardly reached the inner fibrinous capsule, pannus formation replicates the dimensions of the fibrin layer which it replaces. Two weeks after implantation for instance, the surface thrombus on ePTFE grafts measures about one-eighth to one-fourth of that on Dacron grafts.[1,2,44,60] Similarly, the pannus replacing this thrombus in the anastomotic region not only measures one-eighth to one-fourth on ePTFE grafts compared with Dacron prostheses,[2,35] but actually has the same thickness as the preexisting fibrin layer.[2,8,64] The alacrity, however, with which this pannus layer grows towards the midgraft region may well be accelerated by the presence of tissue underneath the inner fibrin capsule, as is the case with high porosity grafts. Although the fibrin layer on the blood surface of woven and knitted Dacron grafts is of equal thickness[2,45,58,60-62,64-66,91]

and transmural tissue ingrowth does not proceed into the inner capsule of either at this stage, pannus outgrowth onto the graft surface seems to be much faster in knitted grafts,[2,46,60,68,72,77,81] with their almost continual tissue layer underneath the fibrin capsule compared with the scanty transmural tissue ingrowth beneath the fibrin matrix of woven grafts.[40] Similarly, a significantly faster transanastomotic tissue outgrowth occurs in high porosity ePTFE grafts if interstitial tissue development is facilitated through external tissue wrapping. This facilitated outgrowth is observed before transmural tissue ingrowth could account for it.[28]

As far as the cellular and matrix composition of the pannus tissue is concerned, it appears as if the absence of a mature and confluent endothelium at the time of sub-endothelial tissue development may be one reason for its lack of differentiation. As early as 1975, Mansfield and Sauvage[92] described the prevention of undifferentiated pannus outgrowth through in vitro endothelialization of grafts in calves.

Almost 20 years later clinical in vitro endothelialization demonstrated the same phenomenon: In endothelial lined grafts in which the formation of a confluent endothelium precedes that of the subendothelial tissue,[5] smooth muscle cells rather than the occasionally observed fibroblasts[61] dominate a mature matrix which even contains an internal elastic membrane.[93] The use of purified cultured autologous endothelial cells for the in vitro lining process makes it quite unlikely that smooth muscle cell coseeding was the reason for the development of such a well differentiated subendothelial tissue rather than the interaction with the preexisting endothelium. Since a tissue which lies beneath an internal elastic membrane qualifies per definition as neo-media rather than hyperplastic neo-intima,[93] such a differentiation means a huge step towards true healing and therefore needs to be understood with regard to the underlying biological mechanisms. In another study, similar degrees of pannus maturation were observed following endothelial cell seeding with mixed microvascular cells.[61] In this case, fibroblasts were initially coseeded with other cell types at similar proportions to those normally seen in anastomotic pannus tissue. Nevertheless, the subendothelial matrix—which matured after the endothelium reached confluence—consisted of mature muscle cells and also elastin rather than the typical poorly differentiated collagen-rich pannus tissue.[61] These observations support the presumption that the early presence of an endothelium may influence the degree of differentiation of the subendothelial connective tissue of both pannus and neo-intimal tissue.

Transanastomotic Endothelialization

Endothelial outgrowth from the adjacent artery onto the surface of a prosthetic vascular graft is another enigma of prosthetic graft research. For unknown reasons, transanastomotic endothelialization stops shortly after the anastomosis in humans.[11,47,60] Yet, the experimental set-up

aiming at overcoming this limitation uses animal models which characteristically show premature and rapid surface coverage with anastomotic endothelium. In the past this rapid transanastomotic endothelialization was usually the key parameter of investigations when primarily surface endothelialization was compared between different prosthetic grafts. However, if one agrees that future grafts for clinical use will require transmural tissue ingrowth as a main cell source for surface endothelialization because of their extraordinary length, a better understanding of transanastomotic endothelialization is indeed necessary, but for a different reason than before: To be able to clearly define for each animal model a biological phenomenon which would otherwise continue to blur the distinction line between transmural and transanastomotic tissue ingrowth.

Differences Between Animal Models

Alerted by the human situation of complete ingrowth stoppage, we can hardly assume that transanastomotic endothelialization is a linearly progressing event in animal models. Therefore, extrapolation of pointwise observations to a long term situation, or even to a constant daily outgrowth distance,[2,94] seems obsolete, although it would have provided valuable additional data for an ingrowth curve. Even in the yellow baboon with its vigorous angiogenic capacity, a similar trend of ingrowth stoppage as in humans can be observed: On 30 μm ePTFE prostheses—which do not allow transmural endothelialization—transanastomotic endothelial ingrowth progressively slows down, to stop approximately 2 cm from the anastomosis.[95-97] Furthermore, high porosity ePTFE grafts, as well as a few knitted Dacron grafts, cannot be admitted into this comparison because of complete transmural surface endothelialization. Considering these exemptions and the fact that only a minority of studies describe ingrowth margins rather than percentages of surface coverage, it is difficult to compare accurately the various animal

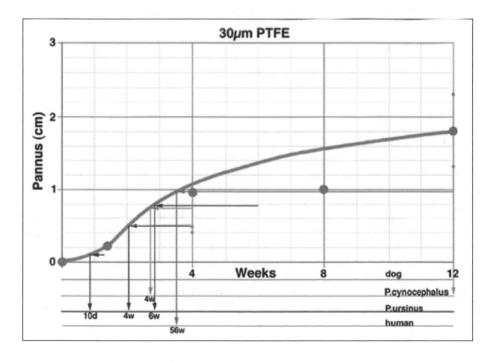

Fig. 1.21. Transanastomotic endothelial outgrowth on 30 μm expanded polytetrafluoroethylene (ePTFE) grafts in four experimental animal models. The curve was plotted using pannus outgrowth values in the dog model (top curve). Points read off the main curve correspond to humans, *Papio ursinus*/chacma baboons, and *Papio cynocephalus*/yellow baboons, as indicated by connecting arrows. The curve was drawn using Deltagraph (for Macintosh).

models with regard to transanastomotic endothelial cell outgrowth. Nevertheless, since most of the experiments in the past were based on the canine model, a relatively complete chronology can be estimated for standard grafts in the dog. Single data obtained in other animal models can then be related to the time course of surface healing in dogs. However, the accuracy of even this narrowed appraisal decreases rapidly after the 12th week of implantation when grafts in most of the studies were fully endothelialized and thus can not be used for the assessment of further transanastomotic endothelial cell outgrowth.

During the first 3 months of implantation transanastomotic endothelialization in dogs consecutively covers a distance of approximately 2 cm in ePTFE grafts[1-3,10,21,86,98-102] and more than 3 cm in Dacron prostheses.[2,60,62-64,66,72,76] These ingrowth distances also apply to the second most commonly used animal model, the yellow baboon (*Papio cynocephalus*).[9,19,32,35,52,55,91] Taking into account that the ingrowth margin of endothelium is often very irregular with endothelial tongues reaching far into the graft, a minimal length of 15 cm in all animal models therefore seems a reasonable choice for future 3 month studies.

In spite of this general guideline, there is still a distinct difference between the respective animal models with regard to transanastomotic ingrowth behavior. However, since the in vitro proliferative capacity of endothelial cells from humans and experimental animals hardly differs,[103] the distinctly prostrate transanastomotic outgrowth potential of human endothelial cells must be a consequence of the complex overall situation of the human model rather than a principal mitotic sluggishness of human endothelial cells. Therefore, one should not downplay the importance of differences between animal models. If one animal model comes significantly closer to the human situation than another, it may well hold the key to understanding the biological reasons for the human failure of graft healing. If transanastomotic ingrowth values of different species on standard ePTFE grafts are related to those of the dog, the coverage which is reached in humans after 56 weeks occurs in dogs after 3.5 weeks,[1,2,21,98,86,100] in the yellow baboon after 5.6 weeks and in the chacma baboon after 7.6 weeks. Thus, the transanastomotic outgrowth is 2.1 times slower in the chacma baboon than in the dog. The difference between the two primate species may well be due to the fact that the chacma baboon represents a senescent model with a body mass of up to 40 kg, whereas the yellow baboon is a juvenile model which is on average 2 years old and weighs 10 kg. In this context, it is interesting to note that the difference between the two kinds of baboons is much more pronounced in transmural than transanastomotic ingrowth. Transmural capillarization leads to surface endothelialization of high porosity ePTFE grafts after 2 weeks in the yellow baboon, whereas perigraft tissue has usually not even grown into the outer two-thirds of these prostheses in the chacma baboon (personal observation).

Other animal models like rats, calves[104] and pigs[105] are either too different or not sufficiently documented. However, pigs are usually large enough for vascular implants at a young age, but dog puppies are too small. Therefore, dogs

are usually also senescent at implantation,[74] whereas pigs and calves can be expected to be juvenile. In the rat model, the issue of dimensions complicates interpretation. A transanastomotic endothelial outgrowth of approximately 2.2 mm after 6 weeks[13,16,17,88] in 30 μm ePTFE makes it impossible to relate these data to the 7.8-13.6 mm of other large animal models.

In summary, transanastomotic endothelialization is at least 7.5 times more pronounced in any animal model than in man. Within the experimental set-up, however, the senescent primate model of the chacma baboon at least promises to eventually reveal certain biological principles which make the human healing pattern of prosthetic grafts so unique.

Differences Between Grafts

Since the endothelial margin represents the frontier of transanastomotically ingrowing tissue,[19] it may well be a key player in a synergistic interaction with sub-fibrinous tissue. If one compares the two low porosity prostheses (30 μm ePTFE and woven Dacron), endothelial outgrowth seems to be twice as high on ePTFE[1-3,10,21,78,86,98-102] than on Dacron.[40,43] This difference is not too surprising, because the mighty inner fibrinous capsule of Dacron seems to have features of an ingrowth barrier for transmural capillaries.[43,44,48,59,60,71,72] One can imagine that the same biological reasons which inhibit capillary ingrowth from outside may inhibit endothelial outgrowth from the anastomosis. However, although this fibrin matrix seems to be similar in high porosity[2,35,44,60-66,91] and low porosity grafts,[45,58] it allows better transanastomotic endothelial ingrowth under high porosity[40,46,47,60,68,72,81] than low porosity conditions.[1,2,21,40,43,86,98-102] Since this observation only relates to grafts in which the transmural tissue ingrowth did not traverse the fibrinous capsule and the time would have been too short for fallout endothelialization, the endothelium can be assumed to be of transanastomotic origin. If however, a main difference for transanastomotic endothelial ingrowth on an otherwise not ideal surface seems to be a well developed tissue layer underneath the fibrin capsule, it is reasonable to speculate that this distant tissue layer may somehow affect surface endothelialization.

Porosity

Porosity was long known to be a determining factor behind the fate of prosthetic vascular grafts. Initial attempts to replace arteries with solid tubes of synthetic material soon demonstrated that porosity is a prerequisite for graft patency.[45,49] Subsequently, pioneers of prosthetic vascular grafts[60,71,74] unsuccessfully tried to achieve complete graft healing through porosity. However, only with the advent of highly porous ePTFE grafts did it become apparent that complete surface healing of arterial prostheses was theoretically possible beyond a certain porosity, and this only in a very juvenile animal model. In the endothelium-centered 1980s, excitement arose primarily from the fact that higher porosity may allow surface endothelialization.[30,32] However, if tissue engineering of prosthetic vascular grafts ever intends to truly emulate functional arteries, the tandem of deep-seated suspicion of the presence of smooth muscle cells and the narrow focus on endothelial cells will need to give way to a more comprehensive mode of tissue ingrowth. Nevertheless, our current biological understanding validates the view that the ability of a prosthetic graft to allow capillary ingrowth still holds the key to today's grander picture.

Researchers were long puzzled as to why interstitial graft spaces of particular prostheses were sufficient to allow macrophages and other inflammatory cells to immigrate, whereas connective tissue cells of similar dimensions were often conspicuously absent.[2,18,22,24] Today we understand that certain of these connective tissue cells, like smooth muscle cells, mainly follow the ingrowing endothelial cells.[106,107] Therefore, one important determining dimension for complete graft healing is that which mechanically allows capillaries to sprout into the meshwork of a synthetic graft and still leave some space for accompanying cells. Since the average diameter of a capillary is ~10 µm,[108-110] it would seem as if the minimum area required for ingrowth of capillaries is at least 20-80 µm.[2] The diameter of a functional vessel, i.e., an endothelium and at least one layer of smooth muscle cells, is approximately 23.06 ± 13.11 µm in diameter (personal observations).

The attempt to determine porosity requirements for graft healing is no doubt complicated by material specific characteristics and structural uniqueness. The complex three dimensional structure of contemporary grafts results in a wide range of voids between the synthetic surfaces, which hardly allows a precise definition of ingrowth spaces. For manufacturers, a way out of this dilemma was the introduction of water permeability as a means of defining porosity. With this method, materials could be separated on the basis of low and high porosity. For example, materials such as Dacron were distinguished not only on the basis of being knitted and woven, but further characterized as being of high porosity (1500 to 4000 ml/cm^2/min) or low porosity (200-1000 ml/cm^2/min).[111] The same principle applied to ePTFE on the basis of distances between the nodes of the expanded material. However, although these values served as useful parameters in characterizing the materials, they were not helpful with regard to healing. The poorly defined space dimensions made it impossible to come to a conclusive answer concerning the role porosity plays in the mitigation of tissue ingrowth into prosthetic vascular grafts. If one attempts to gain a better understanding of the relationship of porosity and healing, one needs to make a clear distinction between porosity and permeability in order to avoid a confusion of terminology. It is important to understand that these terms are not synonymous, because a highly porous material may have a low permeability and vice versa.

Permeability

The permeability of a material can be defined as its ability to allow other substances (either gaseous, liquid or solid) to pass through its pores or interstices. The customary method for measuring permeability is using water and measuring the area and the applied hydrostatic pressure gradient across a porous membrane. The permeability value is therefore directly proportional to the measured volume of water that passes through the material per unit time, assuming that the thickness of the membrane remains constant. The resultant measurement has been misleadingly called "water porosity" by surgeons and manufacturers alike.

Porosity

Porosity, in contrast, refers to the void spaces (pores) within the boundaries of a solid material, compared to its total volume. Although one could argue that the voids within a material will allow water to flow through them, numerous pores may well be cul-de-sacs and thus fail to provide an open corridor from one side of the graft to the other. Moreover, vascular prostheses are not designed to be rigid structures. They are compressible for ease of handling and can be readily deformed by radial and longitudinal tensions as well as by internal pressures, even in the relatively noncompliant contemporary grafts. Such stresses not only change the dimensions of the prostheses, but also lead to a redistribution of the yarns and fibers within the material. Naturally, the change in textile structure by both circulatory stress and compression by ingrowing tissue itself affects the distribution, size and tortuosity of the channels that run from one side of the graft to the other. Since the limiting factor for tissue ingrowth is the bottleneck of the narrowest part of a transmural space, it is further important to look at interstitial spaces throughout their three dimensional course.

Unfortunately, hardly any information is available regarding the dimensions of porous structures in vascular grafts. In order to get a better insight into this critical parameter for tissue incorporation, we have evaluated interstitial space dimensions in a few typical contemporary grafts, both before and after implantation. Moreover, we have investigated these prostheses regarding their true maximum interstitial ingrowth spaces and their resulting theoretical ability to accommodate transmural microvessels. Microvessels were decided to be the dimension against which measurements were compared, based on their central role in a variety of healing aspects from surface endothelialization to neo-media formation.

Theoretical Considerations for Healing of Vascular Grafts

Although the process of expanding teflon material to the typical nodes-and-fiber structure of ePTFE grafts (Fig. 1.22A) allows for a wide range of internodal distances, the resulting changes in ingrowth spaces are moderate. With well-defined anchor points and a rigid material like teflon, the distensibility of the fibrils is limited (Fig. 1.22B), thus making disproportional increases in internodal distance necessary to achieve increases in fibril length and hence an increase of ingrowth dimensions of a few micrometers. To try to correlate true ingrowth spaces with internodal distances as defined by the manufacturers of ePTFE grafts is insufficient, therefore, if not combined with the assessment of fibril dimensions. Furthermore, in order to accurately determine ingrowth spaces, one needs to assess these structures throughout the entire thickness of the graft wall. In a similar way, one needs to measure more than just bundle densities and fiber diameters in knitted (Fig. 1.24) and woven

Fig. 1.22. Scanning electron micrograph of a 30 μm expanded
polytetrafluoroethylene (ePTFE) graft
(Impra Inc., USA) showing the typical nodes-and-fibril structure. x750,
(top) inner surface and (bottom) outer
surface.

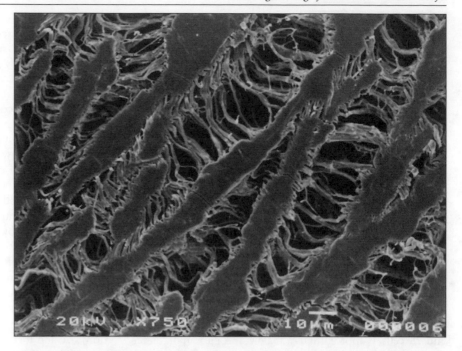

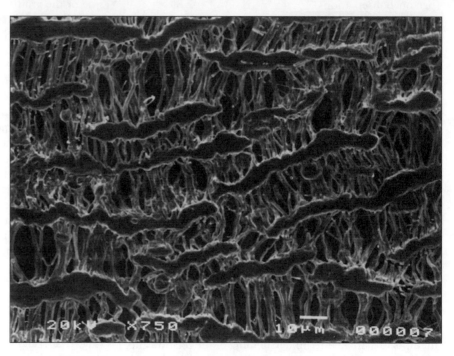

Dacron materials (Fig. 1.25) to obtain an accurate measurement of cell ingrowth spaces. These assessments are further
complicated by the introduction of externally wrapped PTFE
grafts (Fig. 1.23) and veloured Dacron surfaces (Fig. 1.26).[60]
These coverings are intended to prevent the grafts from aneurysmal dilatations and to increase the tissue bond between
graft and perigraft tissues, with a subsequent better healing
response.[111]

Taking all these factors into account, our approach
toward the assessment of true ingrowth spaces in commercially obtained both low porosity (< 30 μm) and high porosity (60 μm) ePTFE, Dacron velour and knitted Dacron

grafts was based on the combined image analyses of histological cross-sections and scanning electron microscopy
(SEM) of surface structures (see figure legends). Based on
these measurements (Table 1.1), we attempted to reconstruct
the maximum ingrowth space dimensions throughout the
graft wall and draw conclusions about whether the graft
materials would sufficiently allow transmural ingrowth for
microvessels invading from the adventitia. In order to calculate ingrowth spaces, we measured a number of parameters related to the material characteristics (Table 1.1).

Scanning electron microscopic examination of the two
different porosities of ePTFE used in this study gave a good

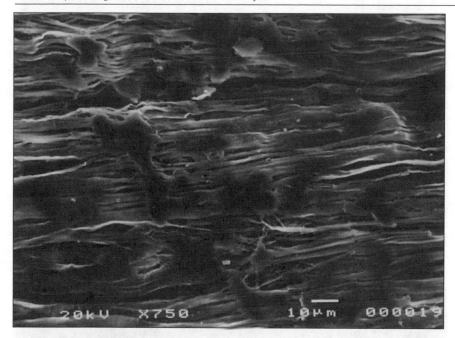

Fig. 1.23. Scanning electron micrograph of a 30 μm expanded polytetrafluoroethylene (ePTFE) graft (Impra Inc., USA) showing external circumferential wrap. The nodes-and-fibril structures can be seen through the wrap. x750, outer surface.

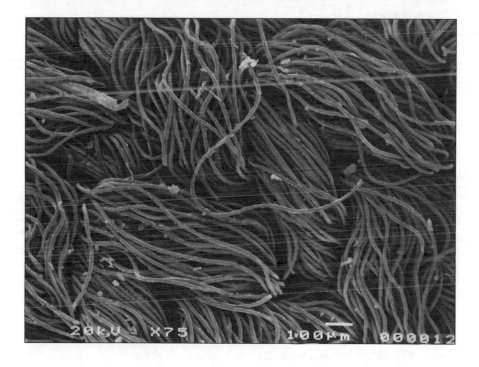

Fig. 1.24. Scanning electron micrograph of a knitted Dacron prosthesis (Vascutek; water porosity = 1350 ml/cm^2/min), showing reasonably tightly knitted bundles of fibers, x75.

indication of surface dimensions with respect to internodal distances, internodal spaces, mean fibril lengths and mean interfibril space (Table 1.1). Internodal distance was measured from the center of one node to the center of another, whereas internodal space width was defined as the actual space between the margins of two adjacent nodes. No significant difference was found between the inside and outside surfaces for each respective graft. However, the internodal distance stated by the manufacturers did not precisely match the internodal distance we measured.

It could be argued that the internal diameter of ePTFE grafts may influence the manufacturing process and thus

the node-to-fibril structure and dimensions. Based on this, we measured internodal fibril lengths in 6 contemporary 30 μm ePTFE grafts with varying internal diameters (Table 1.2). Only the inner surface was measured, as all the grafts contained dense outer circumferential wraps sometimes additionally reinforced with rings. The results showed a reasonably consistent fibril length irrespective of internal diameter (Table 1.2). The values of 24.28 ± 3.48 μm and 20.69 ± 2.35 μm for the 6 and 10 mm I.D. grafts (W.L. Gore and Associates, Flagstaff, Ariz.) respectively, are in agreement with earlier studies.[1] However, although there were hardly any differences in internodal distance between grafts of

Fig. 1.25. Scanning electron micrograph of a woven Dacron prosthesis (DeBakey; water porosity = 232 ml/cm^2/min), showing tightly woven, well-defined bundles of fibers, x75.

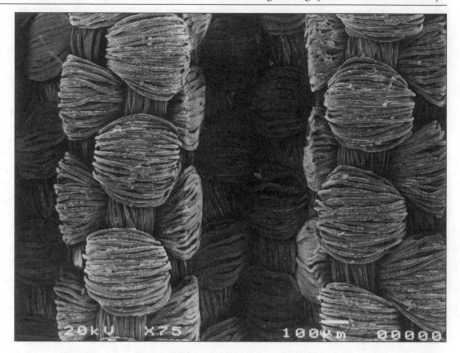

Fig. 1.26. Scanning electron micrograph of the double veloured Dacron prosthesis (Cooley; water porosity = 1660 ml/cm^2/min), showing a completely wide open, random array of fibers. Inset: Dacron felt (USCI) used in our study, x75.

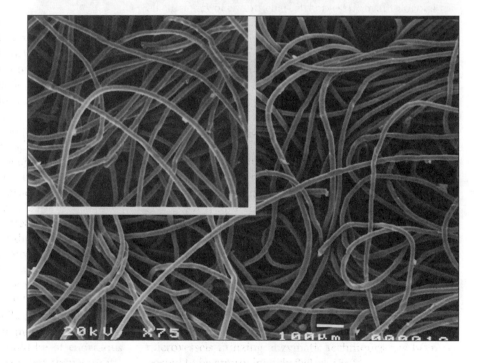

different inner diameter from the same manufacturer, there were distinct differences in internodal distance between comparable grafts of different manufacturers. In 30 µm ePTFE grafts from Impra (Table 1.1), a mean inner fibril length of 17.79 ± 5.62 µm was opposed by 23.57 ± 6.21 µm measured in W.L. Gore products (Table 1.2).

In order to calculate the minimum continual transmural ingrowth channels through the wall of both ePTFE grafts (Figs. 1.27 and 1.28), a mathematical approach was chosen relating three dimensional structures of nodes and fibers to factors such as the obstruction caused by internodal fibrils from one layer to the next. The underlying assumption of a worst scenario was that, beginning at the adventitial surface, each successive layer of fibrils lies in the center of the preceding layer, thereby creating the greatest possible obstruction. Therefore, this approach provides the narrowest possible channel spaces for continual tissue ingrowth from outside to inside.

Figures 1.27 and 1.28 illustrate the theoretical comparison between the minimum continual transmural ingrowth channel and the maximum available ingrowth space of a given layer throughout the walls of the 30 and 60 µm PTFE grafts. The reason for the discrepancy between the two curves in the 30 µm PTFE (Fig. 1.27) is the fact that the

Table 1.1. Material characteristics of 5 mm internal diameter ePTFE grafts (Impra, Inc.)

Internodal Distance as stated by the manufacturer (mm)	Mean Internodal Distance (peak to	Mean Internodal Space Width (mm)	Mean Fibril Lengths (mm)	Mean Interfibril Space (mm)
30:INSIDE	24.12 ± 6.47	16.88 ± 5.49 95% CI: 15.78-19.80	17.79 ± 5.62 95% CI: 14.92-18.84	ND*
30:OUTSIDE	27.27 ± 13.19	14.49 ± 6.21 95% CI: 12.27-16.72	15.14 ± 6.12 95% CI: 12.95-17.33	5.11 ± 2.39
60:INSIDE	53.01 ± 20.44	42.41 ± 15.39 95% CI: 37.23-47.58	45.72 ± 16.22 95% CI: 40.27-51.17	ND*
60:OUTSIDE	47.94 ± 9.90	28.14 ± 6.36 95% CI: 25.99-30.28	30.80 ± 7.03 95% CI: 28.43-33.16	4.53 ± 0.76

Material characteristics of both low (30 μm) and high (60 μm) porosity 5 μm internal diameter (ID) ePTFE grafts (Impra, Inc.) as measured by SEM anaylses. Counts were done over 5 random fields using a calibrated NIH image analyses system. Results are presented as mean ±SD with 95% confidence intervals calculated around each mean vaule. n = 60. ND* = Not determined beacause cell ingrowth occurs through the fibrils from the outside surface only.

Table 1.2. Comparative values of contemporary 30μm ePTFE grafts (W.L. Gore and Associates)

30mm ePTFE Internal Diameter (mm)	Mean Internodal Fibril Length ± SD (mm) (Inner Surface)
3	21.12±5.56
5	23.57±6.21
6	24.28±3.48
10	20.69±2.35
15	32.09±5.10
22	26.17±2.43

Counts were done on 5 random fields on the inner surface of all the grafts using calibrated NIH image analysis software. The outer surface of all the grafts was covered with a circumferentially dense wrap. The 5 and 15mm ID grafts were further reinforced with external rings. Results are presented as mean±SD. A clear discrepancy exists between the 5mm ID internodal fibril lengths of the two manufactured grafts.

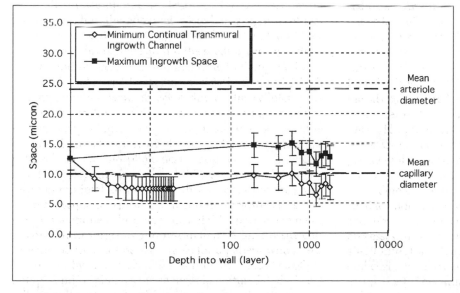

Fig. 1.27. Comparison of mean ingrowth space and the theoretically predicted minimum continual transmural ingrowth channels for 30 μm ePTFE. The ingrowth spaces (■) were determined by image analysis on histological cross-sections (n = 2) which were subdivided into 10 consecutive layers extending from the lumen to the adventitia. In each layer, internodal measurements were done in 8 random fields using a Leica Q500MC image analyzing system. Mean ingrowth spaces are expressed as graphic points for each measured layer (μm). Vertical lines denote ±1 S.D. For the theoretically calculated continual transmural ingrowth channels (–◇–), internodal spaces, fibril lengths and mean interfibril spaces were measured using scanning electron microscopy. The results were plotted on a logarithmic scale representing full wall thickness (2000 layers). Vertical lines denote ±1 S.D.

Fig. 1.28. Comparison of mean ingrowth space and the theoretical prediction of the minimum continual transmural ingrowth channel for 60 μm ePTFE. The identical protocol was followed as in Figure 1.27.

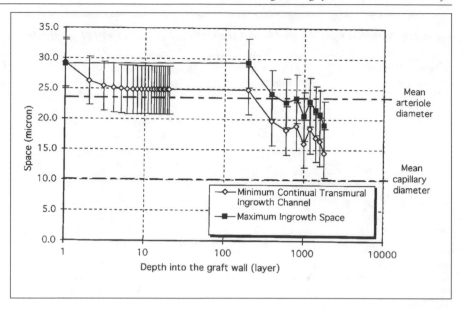

maximum space (Fig. 1.27, line marked with solid squares) has been worked out on the basis of the maximum ingrowth space available between two fibrils without taking the interaction of the neighboring fibrils into account. These spaces are therefore ingrowth spaces in isolation. If one compares the maximum ingrowth space available through the graft (assuming that each histological layer equals 200 true layers as previously established by SEM, resulting in a total of 2000 layers throughout the entire wall thickness) to the theoretically available transmural ingrowth channel (Fig. 1.27, lined marked by open diamonds), it becomes obvious that the available space is in fact much less than it appears initially on the basis of isolated layers of nodes and fibrils. Interestingly, the minimal ingrowth channel from outside for 30 μm PTFE grafts progressively diminishes in size over the first 10 layers, as a result of the obstruction caused by the successive layers of fibrils. Thereafter, the values remain consistent before increasing again till layer 200. Throughout the rest of the graft, the predicted channel size would not accommodate capillaries, although the ingrowth space of each isolated layer of nodes and fibrils would remain theoretically sufficient for capillary ingrowth. This calculation corresponds with the histological observation that only a few capillaries are found in the wall of nonwrapped 30 μm PTFE grafts, and those few are restricted to the outer third.

In 60 μm PTFE grafts (Fig. 1.28), the minimum dimension of transmural ingrowth channels from outside also progressively diminishes in size in the first 20 layers, after which the values become consistent throughout the rest of the graft wall till layer 200. From then onwards the maximum diameter of a continual transmural ingrowth channel decreases again as a consequence of the narrowing of the internodal space. Despite the fact that the calculated channel size represents the "worst" scenario in terms of ingrowth dimensions, as it nears the lumen it still provides sufficient space for ingrowing arterioles within the 5% confidence interval. Therefore, complete transmural vascularization would still be possible in these grafts. Transmural capillarization,

in contrast, would be permitted by 100% of the transmural spaces.

Assessment of Ingrowth Spaces in Dacron Grafts

If the task of assessing interstitial graft spaces is considered difficult in ePTFE, it gets even more challenging when Dacron prostheses are concerned. In the era prior to protein pretreatment of vascular prostheses, porosity was directly proportional to bleeding. Therefore, textured grafts made of polyester braids aimed at providing surgeons with an instantly hemostatic alternative. In contrast to ePTFE, however, high or low porosity is not primarily achieved through a variation of the same manufacturing process, but rather through the different procedures of knitting and weaving. Moreover, an additional variable is introduced by the needle density used in the knitting process and by optional combination with a velour surface, which further influences the size of the open spaces between the braids.

Woven Dacron

Commercially, woven fabrics consist of two sets of yarns, the warp and the weft, which are interlaced at right angles to each other (Fig. 1.25). Woven material is often preferred by surgeons, as it is known for its high bursting strengths, low permeability to liquids, minimal tendency to deform under stress and less proneness to kinking. However, the woven structure also has poor compliance, limited elongation, a tendency to fray and, above all, a very low porosity. In spite of this low porosity, tissue ingrowth into the tight interstitial spaces of the fabric is occasionally observed.[40,57]

However, since the available space does not appear to allow for cell infiltration in the manufactured configuration, one must assume that cellular ingrowth is a consequence of a rearrangement of the relatively loosely lying interstitial fibers. Theoretically, therefore, the number of fibers, fiber diameter and bundle area could be measured to obtain a reasonable measurement of ingrowth spaces. This information would then be used to determine a packing factor for the material. The main shortfall of this approach, however, is that although the native graft material seems flexible and reorganization of fibers seems theoretically feasible, the interstices of the graft upon implantation are soon filled with a fibrin matrix which polymerizes into a fairly rigid structure, thus embedding the fibers and bundles and allowing very little room for movement. It seems likely that the proteolytic process required for this rearrangement needs a critical tissue presence with its associated degrading capacity, which in turn would need a higher initial porosity. This may explain why single cells such as macrophages and fibroblasts are found near the surface of woven prostheses, but only very occasionally capillaries.[40,57]

Knitted Dacron

According to the manufacturers,[112] knitted constructions contain a set of yarns which are interlooped around each other as opposed to interlaced (Fig. 1.24). The specific type and the compliance behavior of knitted fabrics depends on the direction in which the yarns are interlooped. If the yarns lie predominantly in the lengthwise direction then the fabric is "warp knit" whereas if they lie in the transverse direction, the fabric is "weft knit". A significant difference between these two types of knit is that weft knit fabrics will unravel, whereas warp knits will not. This is an important consideration for the surgeon, as the grafts are often cut at preimplantation for perfect abutting to the anastomoses. Undoubtedly, once implanted, the difference is negligible.

Due to the difference in structure of Dacron grafts as opposed to PTFE, a slightly different approach was adopted to calculate ingrowth spaces. Surface measurements made by SEM, and the histological assessment of wall thickness and ingrowth space dimensions, are the same as in ePTFE. However, while fibrils cause the main spatial limitation in PTFE, fiber orientation and the arrangement of fiber bundles throughout the graft thickness limit the spaces in knitted

Dacron. We therefore analyzed explanted histological sections for knitted as well as pure velour prostheses (Fig. 1.26) through ten layered areas from the adventitial surface to the lumen. The details of the measurements are described in the figure legends. The commercial knitted graft (Vascutek) used in this study had a water porosity of 1350 ml/cm^2/min, falling into the lower range of porosities for knitted materials.[15] On the basis of interfiber measurements through the graft wall, a graphical representation showing the mean values for maximum ingrowth spaces could be obtained (Fig. 1.29). In spite of the fact that this material lies in the lower range of porosity within knitted grafts, it was still surprising to see how narrow the maximum ingrowth spaces through the knitted graft were. When one compares the percentage distribution of spaces theoretically permissive for capillaries and/or arterioles (Fig. 1.29B,C), however, the mean size of spaces within the first third of the graft wall (14.44 ± 3.74 μm, layers 7-10) would accommodate capillaries. In addition, albeit at a low percentage (5.16 ± 0.56%), the mean ingrowth space of 24.64 ± 1.75 μm would also allow a few arterioles to surpass this zone (Fig. 1.29C). Towards the middle of the graft (layers 4-6) the restriction for capillaries becomes less pronounced (13.92 ± 2.68 μm), defying the common sense expectation that cells would encounter more tightly packed bundles in this midzone of the prosthesis. The luminal third of the graft (layers 1-3) has consistently narrow spacing, allowing capillary ingrowth only in 30.4 ± 0.38% with a mean ingrowth space of 12.34 ± 2.50 μm. None of the spaces in this zone allow arteriole ingrowth (Fig. 1.29C).

Velour Surfaces

The term "velour" in a textile context refers to a thick-bodied fabric, either woven, knitted or nonwoven, that has a smooth, soft surface by virtue of additional yarns. All commercial velours, however, are knitted designs. They may be distinguished from the earlier knitted prostheses by their

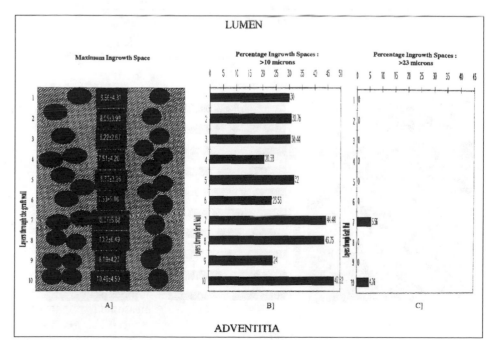

Fig. 1.29. Graphic representation of maximum ingrowth spaces for knitted Dacron. Histological cross-sections of explanted samples were subdivided into 10 consecutive layers extending over the full thickness of the wall from lumen to adventitia. Interfiber spaces were measured in 8 randomly selected fields in each zone. Results in (A) are expressed as mean + SD. A frequency distribution histogram was applied to the results from (A) to obtain percentages of ingrowth spaces of > 10 μm and > 23 μm (B, C).

thicker fabric and greater porosity, as well as lower fabric density and packing factor. To assess ingrowth space within velour graft types has been very difficult, and most researchers have relied on methods such as water porosity. However, a few authors[113] have attempted to measure its true dimensions by looking at pile height and the amount of piles in the veloured knit. The impetus for using velours stemmed from a conviction that a rougher and more porous surface both externally and internally would facilitate the development of neointimal and perigraft tissue.

In order to assess the qualities of pure velour structures, we manufactured velour tubes made of Dacron velour felt (Fig. 1.26, inset). In sharp contrast to the seemingly restrictive interfiber spaces of the knitted material, the Dacron velour showed mean ingrowth spaces ranging from $30.02 \pm 2.95\,\mu m$ at the adventitia, to $36.88 \pm 20.06\,\mu m$ at the lumen, with an overall mean ingrowth space of $27.97 \pm 4.80\,\mu m$ (Fig. 1.30A). These mean ingrowth spaces, as in the case of the knitted grafts, were assessed on the basis of histological measurements of interfiber distances through ten consecutive areas of explanted samples (see figure legend). Interestingly, although the mean space seems sufficient for arteriole ingrowth, the wall profile (Fig. 1.30A) shows that the space becomes narrowed towards the central part of the graft and may have a restrictive effect on ingrowth. The reason for this central restriction is the presence of numerous bundles in this area causing an overall smaller interfiber space. Despite this restriction, the calculated maximum spaces would still allow the ingrowth of capillaries and arterioles at all levels. Percentage distribution profiles for both the capillaries and arterioles (Fig. 1.30B,C) show a similar distribution pattern as the mean ingrowth space profile (Fig. 1.30A), with the majority of spaces of more than 23 μm (Fig. 1.30C) being in the outer and inner one-third of the graft.

Taking all these results into account, it seems that the dimensions of graft porosity may have been overestimated for most of the contemporary vascular prostheses. It becomes clear that, although surface measurements of graft materials give a good indication of ingrowth characteristics, additional information such as interfiber distances and theoretically predicted channel spaces throughout the graft wall are critical for assessing the degree of pure mechanical restrictions for tissue ingrowth into prosthetic vascular grafts.

Fibrin

Prior to implantation, conventional nonpretreated grafts represent simply synthetic scaffolds. Therefore, all biological components which eventually fill the interstices of these scaffolds are host derived. Within this process of host incorporation, proteinaceous ingrowth matrices naturally precede infiltration with cellular components. Since the implantation of a vascular prostheses inflicts a surgical wound, this proteinaceous matrix is fibrinous. In low porosity grafts, the surrounding fibrin coagulum derives entirely from iatrogenically injured vessels. The cut ends of these vessels constrict within a few minutes and get sealed with aggregating blood platelets. As a result, the hematoma around the graft usually remains moderate. Within a few minutes tissue thromboplastin generates thrombin, which, together with platelet factor 3 (PF 3) released by the few entrapped platelets, leads to the transformation of fibrinogen into fibrin. Particularly in nonpretreated porous grafts, blood may also extravasate from the graft lumen to the outside. In this case the activation of the clotting cascade occurs through contact of factors XII, prekallikrein, XI and high molecular weight kinogen[114] and, again, through released platelet PF 3. Although blood does not seep through the wall of less porous grafts, plasma still clots within the synthetic meshwork through a similar mechanism. Therefore, one can assume that the entire fibrinous matrix initially surrounding the graft and filling its interstices is representative of typical wound fibrin, which distinctly favors tissue ingrowth.

Fig. 1.30. Graphic representation of ingrowth spaces for Dacron velour. An identical protocol was followed as for Figure 1.29. Results are expressed as mean ± SD.

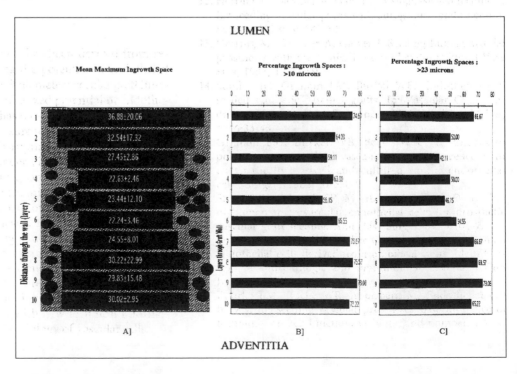

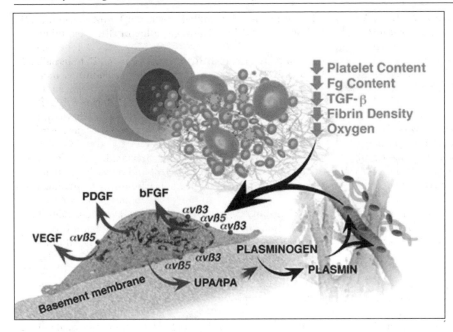

Fig. 1.31. Hypothetical sequence of cellular ingrowth events in native fibrin. The normal hemostatic process of clot formation leads to a relatively low platelet number, fibrinogen and TGF-β content. The resulting low density of thick fibrin fibers together with mild hypoxia has a pro-angiogenic effect as it causes an immediate upregulation within the endothelial cell of integrins $\alpha_V\beta3$ and $\alpha_V\beta5$, which facilitate adhesion to the extracellular matrix, and the release of proliferative and pro-migratory cytokines such as vascular endothelial growth factor (VEGF), platelet-derived growth factor (PDGF) and basic fibroblast growth factor (bFGF). The upregulation of the endothelial cell-specific integrins causes the release of serine proteases, urokinase and tissue plasminogen activator (u/tPA). These proteases in turn convert surrounding plasminogen to plasmin, which acts on the neighboring extracellular matrix to expose attachment sites for the cell-specific integrins. This whole process eventually leads to revascularization and the maintenance of vessel integrity at the wound site.

In contrast to this loose initial fibrin matrix, an entirely different fibrin clot may be continually generated on the blood surface. While the interstitial and external clotting environment is characterized by a small blood pool with limited availability of coagulation factors and platelets, undiminishing amounts of fibrinogen and platelets are present at the blood-contacting surface of the prosthesis. Therefore, this consecutively increasing inner layer of thrombus obviously differs in both its mode of generation and its composition.

Outer Fibrin Matrix

Since tissue ingrowth into prosthetic grafts occurs primarily from outside, the outer fibrin clot surrounding the grafts serves as a provisional matrix for cell migration from the adjacent tissue. However, in order to understand possible adverse qualities of the inner fibrin matrix, one needs to understand the principal interactions occurring between cells and the more natural wound-type fibrin on the outside of the graft. This blood clot filling the adventitial wound space consists mainly of crosslinked fibrin, plasma fibronectin, vitronectin and thrombospondin (TSP),[115] containing low levels of platelet derived cytokines like TGF-β and PDGF. This fibronectin-rich fibrin matrix offers binding sites for integrins of ingrowing cells. For macrophages it is primarily $\alpha_5\beta_1$,[116] whereas it is $\alpha_V\beta_3$ for new blood vessels.[117] The integrin $\alpha_V\beta_5$ has also been implicated in the formation of new blood vessels.[118] However, whether invasion of endothelial cells into a fibrin matrix is $\alpha_V\beta_5$-dependent remains to be established, as the role of this integrin points to it interacting selectively with a vitronectin-rich matrix.[119]

The interaction between integrins and the matrix also influences other regulatory mechanisms. For instance, a "stressed" fibrin matrix as a result of contraction increases the responsiveness of cells to PDGF.[120] This is an important aspect of the triggering of angiogenesis at such an early stage. Furthermore, TGF-β—which is a chemotactically highly potent cytokine for macrophages—is potentially active in fibrin,[121] whereas it is inactivated in collagen matrices by decorin.[120] The relatively low platelet concentration in wound fibrin makes it likely that TGF-β augments macrophage infiltration without inhibiting vessel ingrowth. This can be explained by the concentration dependence of TGF-β which is only inhibitory for angiogenesis at high concentrations[108] but chemotactic for macrophages in trace amounts.[122] This early fibrin matrix also facilitates protease upregulation and the resulting degradation of the fibrin clot to enable tissue ingrowth. The initial events in this process are again regulated through an integrin-ligand mechanism. Ingrowing endothelial cells for instance, induce their protease secretion through the binding of $\alpha_5\beta_1$ to fibronectin and fibronectin fragments in the fibrin matrix.[117,120] The relatively low number of platelets contributing to this initial clot also makes it likely that the concentration of platelet-derived thrombospondin (TSP1)—a potent inhibitor of proteases[145]—does not result in a mitigation of tissue ingrowth.

Inner Fibrin Matrix

Although the mechanism of ingrowth inhibition into prosthetic vascular grafts may well be a multifactorial event, it is conspicuous that the most impenetrable part of the graft wall in humans seems to be the inner fibrinous capsule. This phenomenon has been reported for more than 20 years in porous Dacron grafts.[43,44,48,59,60,71,72,74,75] We have also observed it in 60 μm ePTFE prostheses in the chacma baboon where the impenetrability of the inner fibrin layer even applies to inflammatory cells. After a few weeks of implantation, we found the fibrin coverage of the blood surface to be

Fig. 1.32. Hypothetical sequence of events in the inner fibrin capsule on prosthetic grafts. Fibrin is continually deposited due to platelet and macrophage accumulation and their subsequent degranulation. Platelets and red blood cells become entrapped in a constantly increasing, compacted fibrin layer. Degranulation of the α-granules of the platelets causes a microenvironmental increase of inactive transformting growth factor-beta which becomes sequestered into the extracellular matrix in a latent form. Endothelial cells at the outer surface of the graft material upregulate u/tPA through an integrin-extracellular matrix mediated effect. These serine proteases convert blood-borne plasminogen to plasmin, which in turn activates the latent TGF-β. TGF-β acts on the endothelial cells to initiate dif-

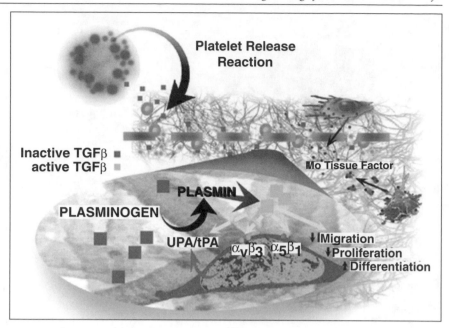

ferentiation with a concomitant decrease in migration and proliferation. This mechanism may therefore cause a premature cessation of angiogenesis and a reduction in transmural vascularization. Additionally, blood-borne macrophages express tissue factor following adherence to biomaterials. This transmembrane protein initiates further fibrin deposition. Macrophages in the depth may shed vesicles containing tissue factor activity which could further facilitate fibrin deposition on the surface.

almost completely acellular (Fig. 1.10). It is therefore tempting to ask whether it is possible to recognize obvious differences in the composition or structure of the inner fibrin capsule which may be responsible for this distinct ingrowth inhibition. In pursuing this question it seems as if the mode of fibrin generation on the inside of grafts already provides significant clues with regard to growth inhibitory properties. First of all, there is a uniqueness about this particular fibrin clot: Both clotting factors and platelets are not consumed from a predefined quantity as is the case in a hematoma, but rather replenished on an ongoing basis. On the one hand, a process of platelet-enrichment through surface adherence results in an disproportionate density of thrombocytes which undergo activation through surface contact and shear stress. As a consequence of this augmented platelet release reaction, high concentrations of α-granule products like platelet factor 3, fibrinogen and von Willebrand factor, as well as dense granule contents such as calcium, continually sustain the coagulation process.[123-125] On the other hand, the rapid replenishment of blood plasma next to the platelet carpet on the graft surface further guarantees undiminishing concentrations of fibrinogen and other clotting factors. Thus, one can assume that the fibrin generated on the inner surface of vascular prostheses has a high content of fibrinogen. Since TGF-β is also liberated from α-granules, and its incorporation into fibrin matrices correlates with its preexisting concentration, this fibrinogen rich fibrin matrix can also be expected to be particularly rich in TGF-β. Based on these considerations, one needs to ask the initial question differently: Can high fibrinogen concentrations as well as other α-granule release products like TGF-β and thrombospondin and dense granule products like calcium

affect the structure and/or composition of fibrin in such a way that it becomes hostile to tissue ingrowth?

Fibrin Structure

It is a relatively recent discovery that fibrin structure influences cell growth. At lower fiber density a fibrin matrix strongly stimulates capillary morphogenesis,[126] whereas it only stimulates endothelial migration without three dimensional capillary formation at higher fiber density. On an ultrastructural level, a similar inverse correlation between cell growth and fiber density was found.[127] The higher the density of fibrin fibers and the lower the average thickness of these fiber bundles, the lower the penetrability for cells.[127] Since in vascular grafts cellular ingrowth seems more inhibited in the inner than the outer fibrin matrix, it is therefore of interest whether inside circumstances favor the generation of a denser fibrin matrix with lower fiber bundle thickness. It was recently demonstrated that an increase in fibrinogen concentration by a factor of 3 resulted in a decrease in fiber bundle thickness and an increase in fiber bundle density, also by a factor of 3.[127] Considering the high platelet density on the blood surface of grafts and the undiminishing pool of clotting factors, one can assume that the fibrinogen concentration inside this surface clot is higher than outside, thus resulting in a fibrin matrix of higher fiber density and lower fiber diameter. The suspicion that higher fibrinogen contents inhibit cellular ingrowth was further substantiated by other studies using fibroblasts[128] and endothelial cells.[61,129]

Cytokine Content

The high density of platelets adherent to the blood surface, as well as their ongoing activation,[5,130] suggest a high concentration of platelet α-granule contents at the time of coagulation. Amongst other substances, the α-granules of platelets contain platelet derived growth factor (PDGF) and transformting growth factor-beta (TGF-β).[5] PDGF is a dimeric growth factor which is mitogenic for endothelial cells and smooth muscle cells. TGF-β, in contrast, is a potent inhibitor of cell proliferation, migration and proteinase production in vascular endothelial cells.[131] In view of the suspected inhibitory effect of the inner fibrin matrix on angiogenesis it is reasonable to hypothesize that particularly high levels of TGF-β contribute to the mitigated vessel outgrowth. However, the TGF-β content of human platelet α-granules exists exclusively in the β1 isoform, stored in a latent form in which the precursor peptide (the latency-associated peptide LAP) remains noncovalently associated with the mature 25 kDa TGF-β1 dimer.[132] In addition, the latent TGF-β complex from platelets has an additional protein, the latent TGF-β binding protein (LTB-P) which is linked with a disulphide bond to the LAP.[133] Since the activation of TGF-β only occurs when the mature 25 kDa dimer is released from the LAP[121] and the entire complex is incorporated into the fibrin structure, fibrin degradation is a prerequisite for liberating inhibitory TGF-β concentrations from the matrix. Coincidentally, the release of the active 25 kDa TGF-β dimer needs the same proteases, such as plasmin, which are needed to degrade the fibrin matrix.[134] Therefore, a likely explanation for the late inhibition of capillarization through TGF-β would be the following scenario: Initially, endothelial cells from the adventitial region of the vascular prosthesis are attracted into its interstices by the PDGF and VEGF released by platelets and polymorphnuclear granulocytes.[135,136] Since the fibrin matrix represents a more or less normal wound matrix at this stage, cell receptors involved in initial migration and proliferation, such as the integrins $\alpha_v\beta_3$ and $\alpha_v\beta_5$, are expressed together with the upregulation of serine proteases (uPA, tPA), enabling the matrix degradation required for migration. Moreover, the interstices of the prostheses contain a mixture of macrophages and foreign body giant cells (FBGC) which are generators of large amounts of pro-angiogenic cytokines such as bFGF (predominantly under hypoxic conditions), and only minor amounts of inhibitory TGF-β.[56] Under those favorable circumstances, capillary ingrowth slowly proceeds towards the inner fibrin layer with its higher fibrinogen and TGF-β content, as well as its denser fibrin structure. With increasing TGF-β concentrations as well as changing fibrin composition, angiogenesis slows down. The increase of TGF-β may be further augmented by macrophages, which degrade fibrin matrices through the upregulation of endogenous serine proteases without concomitant release of plasminogen activator inhibitor (PAI-1). Therefore, matrix degradation by macrophages is much less controlled than degradation by endothelial cells, where a balanced, focalized proteolysis of the pericellular matrix through the up or downregulation of proteases and PAI-1 occurs.[137,138] Eventually, both fibrin structure and liberated and activated TGF-β amounts may be sufficient to bring ingrowing capillaries to a complete halt. A main challenge in substantiating this scenario will be the detection of high TGF-β amounts in the inner fibrous capsule, because the incorporation into the LAP-LTBP-TGF-β complex may well make it immunohistochemically unrecognizable.

Inhibition of Matrix Degradation

Apart from directly inhibiting ingrowing endothelial cells, capillarization and tissue ingrowth into the inner fibrin layer may also be indirectly inhibited through a particularly high PAI-1 concentration in the matrix. Fibrinolysis of the fibrin matrix in normal wound healing is primarily due to plasmin activation from its precursor molecule, plasminogen. In vivo, this conversion to plasmin is mediated by tissue plasminogen activator (tPA) and urokinase plasminogen activator (uPA), both of which are derived from endothelial cells, macrophages and giant cells. The action of these proteases is inhibited by PAI-1, secreted by endothelial cells and platelets. If one assumes that platelets play an disproportionate role in fibrin generation on the inside of the graft, one must also reckon with an disproportionately high level of platelet-derived PAI-1.[139]

Angiogenesis Inhibitors

Another platelet-derived protein which may detrimentally affect capillarization of the inner fibrin capsule is the extracellular matrix molecule thrombospondin (TSP1). TSP1 is a large, multi-functional ECM glycoprotein that can influence endothelial cell function in vitro[140] and angiogenesis both in vitro and in vivo.[141,142] The role of TSP1 in modulating endothelial cell function has been widely investigated. TSP1 was initially identified and characterized as a protein released from the α-granules of platelets upon activation by thrombin. TSP1 is now known to also be produced by many other cell types such as endothelial cells, fibroblasts, smooth muscle cells and monocytes/macrophages.

Thrombospondin occurs in two forms—soluble and matrix-bound. The effect of the matrix-bound TSP1 is often different from that of the soluble form. Soluble TSP1, for instance, has been demonstrated to inhibit the proliferation of endothelial cells[143] while matrix-bound TSP1 appears to be a permissive substrate for endothelial cell proliferation. Migratory, invading endothelial cells adhere to insoluble, matrix-bound TSP1 while soluble TSP1 may saturate surface receptors and produce an anti-adhesive effect.[144] The anti-adhesive activity of soluble TSP1 may interfere with the angiogenic process by preventing the cell-to-substrate or cell-to-cell interactions necessary for endothelial cell migration and capillary formation. Furthermore, recent reports have revealed that TSP1 can also function as a protease inhibitor.[145] These findings suggest that, apart from its direct effect on cells, soluble TSP1 may also influence angiogenesis by affecting ECM turnover and composition. There is further evidence that TSP1 may inhibit the proteolytic enzymes of the fibrinolytic pathway, including plasmin and urokinase plasminogen activator.[146] The modulation of protease activity therefore provides a potentially crucial role for TSP1 in regulating angiogenesis, as it seems to be a factor in correcting the balance of protease activity, which is essential for angiogenesis.

Another important interaction of TSP1, particularly with respect to capillarization of vascular prostheses, is its interaction with transformting growth factor-beta (TGF-β). TSP1 has been shown to bind and activate secreted and ECM-sequested transformting growth factor-b.[147] It follows therefore that the interaction between soluble TSP1 and TGF-β may prove to be crucial in inhibiting cell growth and proliferation. Even more interesting is the fact that TGF-β and TSP1 are both found in the α-granules of platelets,[148,149] increasing their presence in equal proportions in an environment characterized by a significant platelet release reaction. Since thrombospondin released by platelets is not incorporated into a secreted extracellular matrix, it would provide another explanation for the inhibitory effect of a platelet-rich fibrin matrix, since the anti-proliferative effect of TSP1 is determined by the soluble form of this secreted protein.

The one paradox that remains unresolved is the finding that macrophages in wounds, as well as in other inflammatory settings, actively produce TSP1. The finding that the macrophages are releasing a molecule that inhibits angiogenesis is at first surprising. However, TSP1 release from macrophages may represent a "direct" control of angiogenesis, instead of an "indirect" control of angiogenesis through the protease activation of latent TGF-β.

Fibrinogenic Effect of Macrophages

One of the most puzzling questions is why the inner fibrin capsule of Dacron grafts differs from that of ePTFE grafts although the blood exposure of the material itself is only a transient initial event. From the first thin layer of fibrin which covers the synthetic material, one would expect no further difference between the surfaces with regards to the thrombus formation. This, however, is not the case. If the exposed surfaces themselves do not differ because of the capping effect of the fibrin, what are the most likely differences which could be responsible for the qualitative and quantitative composition of the inner fibrin capsule? One such difference may well be the surface structure. Prior to any cell accumulation, the relatively coarse surface of knitted Dacron is covered by a thrombus of more than 100 μm,[44,60] whereas the fine-structured surface of ePTFE lies under a thin fibrin coagulum of only 15 μm.[1,2] However, the fate of crimped surfaces demonstrates that fibrin tends to equalize surface unevenness. As a consequence, all graft surfaces will eventually have the same smooth fibrin coverage, irrespective of their structure. If there are no differences between the initial surface fibrin, and the material itself is hidden underneath, the most likely explanation for an ongoing difference in thrombogenicity would be the active participation of cellular components in the coagulation process. Since the predominant cell type at the time of the most significant difference in fibrin buildup between the Dacron and ePTFE are inflammatory cells, and later on specifically the macrophages, one needs to answer the question of whether macrophages may be key players in the formation of the inner fibrin capsule. In this context, it is interesting to note that macrophages are able to express procoagulant activities (PCA) through their adherence to surfaces.[150] Adhesion of macrophages to biomaterials causes activation and induction of this procoagulant activity by inducing the expression of tissue factor, a transmembrane protein.[151] This factor is capable of initiating the extrinsic pathway of coagulation,[152] leading to fibrin generation.[153] In vitro studies have shown that, in particular, the adherence to Dacron initiates more procoagulant activity than adherence to ePTFE. This seems to relate to the ability of Dacron to adhere more monocytes than ePTFE,[154] rather than to its surface characteristics. Hence, the increased deposition of fibrin onto the luminal surface of Dacron grafts over time, as opposed to ePTFE, may relate to the initially higher adherence of monocytes to Dacron. In addition, macrophages are known to secrete both Il-1β and TNF-α following adherence to synthetic materials. These cytokines also enhance tissue factor expression,[155] leading to a further induction of PCA and further fibrin deposition. Since Dacron induces higher levels of secretion of these cytokines than ePTFE, this may further facilitate fibrin deposition on the Dacron surface. It would appear, therefore, that differences in the ability to mediate monocyte adhesion and activation and so differentially upregulate procoagulant activity could partially explain the observed differences between the luminal fibrin layer of Dacron and ePTFE. In addition, tissue factor activity has been associated with membrane vesicles that apparently are shed concomitantly with procoagulant activity.[156,157] Macrophages in the depth, therefore, could theoretically influence fibrin deposition on the surface by shedding vesicles containing transmembrane tissue factor. The higher number of macrophages present in the depth of Dacron grafts as opposed to ePTFE grafts would, therefore, augment coagulation.

In summary, although fibrin forms a pro-angiogenic matrix and seems to be an "ideal" scaffold for wound healing, it may also present its Janus face under different circumstances. It seems likely that the unusual situation of ongoing surface thrombogenicity within the blood stream also produces an unusual fibrin matrix which is rich in fibrinogen and ingrowth inhibitory cytokines.

Macrophages

Macrophages dominate the tissue reaction against prosthetic vascular implants more persistently than any other cell type. The deviation from a normal healing process, however, is not their early presence but the tenacity with which they reside in the graft structure even after years of implantation. Their physiological role in early phases of wound healing is opposed by the perseverance of a chronic inflammatory reaction to which they significantly contribute in later stages. Although it is difficult to answer the often recurring question of whether macrophages are friends or foes in prosthetic graft healing, it seems that they are both: friends at the beginning and foes at the end. Their active secretion of cytokines may act as a key chemotactic and mitogenic factor for capillary and connective tissue ingrowth in the early phases of wound healing. Their continual presence, however, may increasingly derail the delicate chronology of cytokines required for the successful accomplishment of healing and also result in material degradation. The difficulty in identifying the key events responsible for this adverse development lies in the multitude of contributing factors. On the prosthetic side the different materials, structures and microstructures of the graft are all capable of separately influencing the foreign body reaction against the implant. From the biological standpoint, distinctly different environments characterize the luminal and the outer aspect of grafts.

The dynamics of macrophage infiltration can best be studied on ePTFE grafts, with their fairly even wall structure. In the first weeks of implantation one can typically observe a sandwich structure of macrophage populations in the graft wall with a relatively distinct accumulation of Ham 56 and CD68 positive cells at the inside and outside surface, separated by a cell-free fibrin matrix in between.[13,18,54,28,33] This triple layered infiltration pattern clearly proves that recruitment occurs from both sides. At the luminal surface the extravasation of blood-borne cells into the porosity of the material occurs simultaneously with insudation of blood proteins immediately following implantation. At the adventitial surface, however, only a few monocytes may extravasate during the initial bleeding phase prior to hemostasis. Subsequently, macrophages have to get there by adhering to capillary endothelial cells and transmigrating through basement membranes via the sequential action of a number of adhesion molecules on both the monocyte (leukocyte specific β2 integrins)[158] and the endothelial cell surface (ICAMs).[159]

It follows, therefore, that macrophages, irrespective of whether they originate from the blood or from transmigration into the adventitial tissue, are faced with a similar task to begin with, namely, to infiltrate a provisional fibrin matrix probably not much different from that found in a normal wound. During infiltration, macrophage migration is facilitated by a low level of basic uPA activity. This should also be sufficient to liberate and activate platelet derived TGF-β from the fibrin matrix[160] which was previously incorporated during hemostasis-related fibrinogenesis.[139] Since TGF-β upregulates the expression of integrins on the surface of the blood monocytes thereby promoting adhesion and migration,[161] it acts as a strong chemotactic agent to recruit macrophages to the inflammatory site.[122] Moreover, it also upregulates the uPA activity of macrophages[162] to further facilitate migration. Macrophages are also capable of binding and internalizing fibrin through the Mac-1 receptor, which augments fibrinolysis by a plasmin-independent mechanism.[163] The degradation products of fibrinolysis, in return, also act as chemoattractants, recruiting still more macrophages into the implant site.[164] In addition, trafficking of monocytes to inflammatory sites also involves the superfamily of chemoattractant cytokines (chemokines) and their receptors.[165] Specifically, the C-C chemokine MCP-1 has been demonstrated immunohistochemically to be expressed by macrophages residing at the implant site as early as 48 h postimplantation.[166] This sequence of events illustrates how this initial phase of healing is dominated by self-augmentation of macrophage chemotaxis. Until the macrophage actually contacts the material surface, the recruitment into the wound fibrin of the prosthetic graft does not deviate from that taking place in normal wound healing.

Following material contact, one of the most important determinants in the chronic inflammatory reaction against synthetic vascular grafts is the biomaterial itself. Adherence, spreading and the secretion of inflammatory mediators like TNF-α,[167-171] IL-1β[154,163,167,172-177] and IL-6[167-169,171] have been extensively investigated on all major biosynthetics. Dacron, for instance, was shown to lead to a higher density of cells with a morphology indicative of activation than ePTFE,[154] as well as to higher TNF-α,[178] IL-6[168] and Il-1β secretion.[168,179] Not only does Dacron induce a greater response, but it seems to induce an earlier response as well, with the IL-1 peak occurring on day 4 on Dacron but only on day 7 on all other biomaterials.[177] Furthermore, material differences influence not only the ability of macrophages to secrete cytokines but also the expression of other markers of activation, for example, MHC-II,[180] Cd11b[181] or TGF-β.[29] Expanded PTFE and Dacron also differentially induce alteration of expression of subunits of the β2 integrins,[182] which mediate both cell-substratum and cell-cell interactions.

However, there is mounting evidence that these effects are indirect, rather than directly material-mediated. The different abilities of the various materials to adsorb plasma proteins, in particular, appear to be a main determinant behind the distinct macrophage reaction against certain biomaterials.[183-185] On materials such as polyethylene terephthalate (PET), polytetrafluoroethylene (PTFE) and polyurethanes, the major blood proteins albumin, fibrinogen and IgG are the predominant proteins adsorbed onto the material surface, with other blood proteins adsorbed to a lesser extent.[183-185] Protein adsorption is not dependent, however, on relative protein concentrations in the blood,[184] but is determined primarily by the nature of hydrophobic interactions between the material surface and hydrophobic domains of the protein. Since most proteins have a net negative charge, secondary electrostatic interactions are also important in protein-material interactions and are governed by the chemical nature of the material. The overall combination of hydrophobic and electrostatic interactions will have several effects on the process of protein adsorption. Firstly, different biomaterials adsorb different types and relative concentrations of proteins, with more hydrophobic materials adsorbing more protein. It has also been shown that the nature of the adsorbed proteins changes over time with varying rates of adsorption versus desorption on different materials.[183] Finally, material-dependent conformational changes as a result of these interactions can be detected by differences in elutability of proteins on different chemical structures.[186,187] These changes in conformation differentially expose hydrophilic domains to the aqueous environment, which may or may not contain sites capable of mediating cell adhesion. When comparing two hydrophobic surfaces of different chemical structure, therefore, although a nonpolar hydrophobic material may adsorb more protein, the influence that interactions with polar groups on a chemically different surface will have on the conformation of these adsorbed proteins will ultimately determine the differences in cellular interaction. This may explain why PTFE which, with a surface tension of 18.5 dynes/cm^2,[188] is certainly more hydrophobic than Dacron (43 dynes/cm²)[188] and should thus adsorb more protein,[189,190] mediates less cell adhesion. One can imagine that the increased polarity of the carboxyl groups of PET compared to the apolar fluorine groups of PTFE affects the conformation of the adsorbed proteins to the extent that Dacron binds more macrophages than PTFE.[154]

Of the predominant proteins absorbed, fibrinogen has been shown to be a primary mediator of this adhesion as conformational changes on adsorption expose the P1 epitope which is recognized by the Mac-1 receptor (Cd11b/cd18, $\alpha_m\beta_2$) of the macrophage.[191-194] This receptor also binds to adsorbed fragments of the complement component C3 (C3bi),[195] but studies in complement—depleted mice indicate that this is not a major mechanism of monocyte adherence.[191-193] As we have previously noted, the luminal surface of a vascular prosthesis is exposed to a practically unlimited pool of fibrinogen derived from the circulating blood and released by platelets on activation. The insudation of this fibrinogen into the depth of the graft structure facilitates macrophage adhesion to the material. Thus, the superior healing pattern of identical implants in the subcutaneous position, with limited exposure to circulating or platelet fibrinogen, may well be partly explained by this phenomenon.

Apart from the material effects on adhesion, the structure of grafts certainly plays another important role with regard to the macrophage response. Increasing diameters of synthetic fibers, for instance, result in increasing numbers of adherent, nonspreading macrophages—a morphology indicative of nonactivated cells.[196] This effect may be due to the associated changes in curvature. In addition to microstructure, the overall porosity of the material will also have important implications. Ultimately this will be constrained by two factors: high enough porosity to allow tissue ingrowth, yet low enough to limit continuous insudation of fibrinogen. It seems reasonable to expect a diminished chronic macrophage response in grafts where a temporarily sealing ingrowth matrix limits the ongoing insudation of plasma and hence limits monocyte adhesion to the material through fibrinogen adsorption.

As the deposition of fibrin onto the graft surface continues, the inner macrophage zone increasingly becomes wedged between two almost acellular fibrin matrices, one in the graft center and one on the blood surface.[2-4,7,60,66,72,82] As discussed under "Fibrin", the most likely explanation for this mitigated macrophage recruitment from the blood seems to be the changing physical nature of the fibrin matrix of the inner capsule due to different fiber structure and concentrations of fibrinogen. In the outer wall of the graft, however, a macrophage-dominated cell infiltrate continues to populate the outer one third to one half of the prosthetic structure within 1-3 months.[27,28] As the macrophage population migrates into the depth of the graft structure, it must eventually overstep the maximum distance of a cell from a capillary and thus get into a mild hypoxic state. Macrophages exposed to hypoxia, however, are synthesizing and releasing increased amounts of PDGF as well as aFGF and bFGF.[197] Medium conditioned by hypoxic macrophages in culture is

mitogenic for hypoxic endothelial cells through the release of the FGFs. This suggests a paracrine mechanism in which hypoxia stimulates macrophages to release mitogenic factors for hypoxically preconditioned endothelial cells, thereby promoting angiogenesis. Additionally, TNF-α, which is also upregulated in macrophages by hypoxia,[198] is known to play a role in macrophage mediated angiogenesis, presumably through the activation and recruitment of further monocytes.[199] The role of TNF-α in angiogenesis is, however, controversial and seems to depend on the biological context.[200,201] These effects are further potentiated by upregulation of MIP-1, a potent macrophage chemoattractant, during oxygen deprivation.[198] Therefore, macrophages residing in the outer half of synthetic grafts together with VEGF-releasing infiltrating neutrophils[136] are likely to continue to contribute to a pro-angiogenic milieu at this stage. The low concentration of TGF-β released with migration-associated degradation of the provisional wound fibrin should not be inhibitory for endothelial cell proliferation at this stage.[137]

As the organization of the macrophages within the graft wall changes and transmural endothelial cell ingrowth begins, the situation where the outer wall of the graft is dominated by single macrophages also slowly begins to change by the increasing appearance of foreign body giant cells.[13,19,52,55,64] These may persist for the lifetime of the implant. As macrophage adhesion is determined by material characteristics, so is macrophage fusion to form giant cells dependent on material surface as well as on structure. It has been shown that relatively hydrophilic material surfaces induce more fusion than relatively hydrophobic surfaces.[202-206] Theoretical analyses show that the time-dependent foreign body giant cell formation is also influenced by the initial density of adherent macrophages.[203,204] Therefore, any surface characteristic which influences the number of adherent cells will also influence the extent of giant cell formation. Most conspicuous is the absence of foreign body giant cells (FBGCs) inside the wall structure of ePTFE grafts, compared to Dacron and polyurethane. Although a rim of giant cells often demarcates these prostheses against the surrounding tissue[19] and the interstices are sometimes packed with single macrophages, no fusion occurs. We have regularly observed this phenomenon in both high porosity and low porosity ePTFE in the primate. Although the internodal distances of a 60 μm ePTFE graft provide both wide localized ingrowth spaces of approximately 47.94 ± 9.90 μm and a significant adhesion area on the stretched fibrils, macrophages prefer a solitary existence under these circumstances. Similarly, the PTFE nodes—which are the adhesion site for foreign body giant cells on their smooth end on the exterior of the grafts— remain free of giant cells inside the graft wall where numerous fibrils subdivide their surface. The absence of giant cells on the nodal surface subdivided by numerous fibrils indicates that giant cell formation may be suppressed by geometrical space limitations. However, given the in vitro evidence that fewer monocytes adhere to ePTFE and it is less inflammatory than Dacron,[168,178,179,182] and that a more hydrophobic surface decreases the propensity of single macrophages to fuse,[202-204,206] the inflammatory potential of the surface may also play a role in giant cell formation where a more chemically inert, more hydrophobic ePTFE surface reduces fusion.

Not only do mononuclear cells gradually fuse to form more giant cells in a material-dependent manner, but further complexity is added by the changing nature of the mononuclear macrophage population over time. Macrophages found in intimate contact with synthetic materials in situ were ED1 and MHCII positive, whereas ED2 positive macrophages were observed lying behind the ED1 positive cells.[169] This indicates a pattern of distribution of not only mono—versus multinuclear macrophages, but also immature (ED1 positive) versus mature (ED2 positive), and activated (MHCII positive) versus nonactivated macrophages within the implant site. Theoretical analysis shows that up to 5 weeks of implantation, FBGCs are in fact formed from the fusion of a small percentage of the adherent macrophages which are already present on the third day of implantation.[203,204] This raises the issue of fusogenic potential of different subsets of cells. Expression of cell surface receptors may be a prerequisite. For example, inhibitors of mannose receptor activity have been shown to inhibit IL-4 induced fusion in vitro, suggesting that this receptor may play a role in giant cell formation.[207] Elaboration of certain cell surface markers in a material or environment dependent manner may be required for a higher propensity for giant cell formation.

If it is difficult to decide whether macrophages are beneficial for graft healing or not, it is even more difficult to decide whether the presence of foreign body giant cells represents a state of pacification or a particularly detrimental variant of chronic inflammation. One indication for the FBGCs role as a mediator of pacification of inflammation arises from the fact that their fusion can be induced by IL-4.[99,208] IL-4 is secreted by Th2 lymphocytes and is known to downregulate several macrophage inflammatory functions, for example, the release of certain inflammatory mediators,[209] the secretion of reactive oxygen intermediates[210] and collagenase production,[211] to mention a few. In this context it has been proposed that giant cells may represent a attempt to "mop-up" the deleterious effect of persistent chronic foreign body reaction. In contrast, a detrimental role for the giant cell is suggested by the fact that material surface cracking occurs directly beneath adherent foreign body giant cells, implicating the secretory products of these cells in the degradation of biosynthetics.[212] The presence of actin-containing adhesive structures[202] indicates that the adhesion of the giant cell to the biomaterial forms a sealed compartment with a high local concentration of degradative enzymes. It is also peculiar that the accumulation of giant cells in Dacron regularly coincides with the development of huge convolutes of capillary sinuses in the vicinity. These widely dilated and irregularly shaped endothelial sacs are principally devoid of any second cell layer (Figs. 1.11, 1.18). In contrast, 60 μm ePTFE, with its scanty presence of foreign body giant cells, shows arterioles in its outer interstitial spaces with one or more layers of smooth muscle cells. This histological observation, where the lack of giant cells correlates with the absence of malformed vessels in the form of

capillary sinuses and the presence of smooth muscle cells, seems to indicate that the giant cell contributes to the misdirecting of the process of transmural capillary ingrowth. In situ hybridization of human explants has demonstrated that interstitial macrophages and foreign body giant cells are still secreting Il-1β even after numbers of years.[213] Although Il-1β is known to stimulate both smooth muscle cell proliferation and fibronectin deposition in atherosclerotic plaque formation,[214] it has been suggested that this interleukin can also inhibit vascular smooth muscle proliferation in an autocrine fashion through nitric oxide upregulation.[215] The giant cells, therefore, may be responsible for not only affecting capillarization but also inhibiting smooth muscle cell ingrowth through persistent Il-1β secretion. In summary, the true character of the FBGC remains elusive. On the one hand, their persistence at the implant site and their destructive role in biodegradation, as well as their possible role in the mitigation of vessel formation, seem to label them as villains in incomplete graft healing. Yet, the evidence supporting a role for a typically anti-inflammatory cytokine—IL-4—in stimulating giant cell formation is fairly convincing both in vitro and in vivo.[99,208] Given that inflammation associated with normal wound healing is resolved because of the transient nature of the macrophage response, it would appear that the inability to remove the inflammatory stimulus (a nondegradable biomaterial) confounds even the best intentions of these cells to mediate healing. The consequence is a chronic ongoing inflammation and the derailing of the normal sequence of healing events.

In summary, two distinct zones develop in prosthetic vascular grafts over time: one close to the blood surface which becomes increasingly uninhabitable for macrophages, and one in the outer portion of the graft which is densely packed with macrophages and later on with foreign body giant cells. It is well documented that macrophages infiltrating a wound environment stimulate the proliferation of endothelial cells and, hence, angiogenesis. However, the apparent lack of correlation between the number of resident macrophages in the interstices of grafts and the extent of transmurally ingrowing vessels indicates that macrophages are not alone in affecting endothelial ingrowth, but that other factors, for example, the nature of the ingrowth matrix, may affect the overall extent of capillarization. Aside from an often impenetrable fibrin matrix, the protracted ingrowth of connective tissue, specifically smooth muscle cells from outside, may well have to do with ongoing macrophage activation in the presence of persistent material stimulus. The secretion of inhibitory cytokines like Il-1β by both macrophages and foreign body giant cells may be partly responsible. What is becoming increasingly obvious is that a macrophage is not always a macrophage and that the contribution of each of these subsets of macrophage populations to the lack of healing of the vascular graft remains to be investigated. Overall, the macrophage remains the Jekyll and Hyde of graft healing, but as our insight into the mechanisms of healing grows so does our understanding of which critical questions remain to be answered in the elucidation of the role of this enigmatous cell, namely:

1. If monocyte adhesion to biomaterials is prevented completely, do we compromise healing in any way;

2. To what extent does engineering tissue ingrowth modulate the deleterious effect of the inflammatory cell by promoting selective cellular infiltration before the development of chronic inflammation; and

3. Can we identify secretory products of macrophages or giant cells which specifically mediate the mitigation of tissue ingrowth, either endothelial sprouts or smooth muscle cells?

Prosthetic Wall Vascularization

The "restitutio ad integrum" healing of a vascular prosthesis—the formation of a neo-artery in place of a removed segment—would necessitate the formation of vasa vasorum in the graft wall, accompanied by the growth of a fully functional medium in an inflammation-free environment. The second best solution—the formation of granulation tissue with the resulting conclusion of the healing process through scar tissue—would at one stage also require extensive capillarization. Even if conventional synthetic grafts are lacking the sophisticated biological information necessary for "ad integrum" healing, their porosity would in many cases at least allow the ingrowth of granulation tissue. From our daily surgical practice we are all familiar with the alacrity with which the formation of such granulation tissue and the subsequent stabilization through scar tissue is usually accomplished. The tissue gap in technically the best of all surgical wound closures is often more than one millimeter wide, but capillarization is not only complete, but scar tissue formation is already beginning, as early as after seven days. It is therefore surprising that an equally short distance in the case of the wall of prosthetic vascular grafts does not accomplish the same degree of full thickness capillarization even after years of implantation. In order to further elucidate this major shortcoming in graft healing. one needs to ask two key questions:

1. Why does adventitial capillary sprouting into the outer fibrinous capsule and later on into the interstices of the prosthetic graft occur at such a slow pace and eventually come to a halt; and

2. Why is anastomotic endothelial cell outgrowth so futile concerning both surface endothelialization and capillary sprouting into the depth?

The initial angiogenic response of the surrounding tissue to a freshly implanted vascular prosthesis does not seem to differ from any other wound repair. This early phase is typically characterized by infiltration into the wound fibrin of a relatively high proportion of polymorphonuclear granulocytes, but also lymphocytes and a few macrophages. Capillaries within the adventitia sprout into the freshly formed fibrin matrix within days of injury.[2,13,48,62,63,76,94] During this formation of early granulation tissue, the matrix is probably inconspicuous with regard to fibrinogen concentration, fiber constitution and cytokine content and, as such, is naturally pro-angiogenic. The sprouting endothelial cells bind via $\alpha_v\beta_3$ to the RGD site of the fibrin α-chain and migrate into the pores of the graft. This also promotes survival of the angiogenic sprout by sustaining an anti-apoptotic response through inhibition of p53 activation.[216]

Apart from the favorable matrix environment, white blood cells provide various pro-angiogenic stimuli at this stage. Infiltrating neutrophils are a source of VEGF,[136] and macrophages migrating into a presumably mildly hypoxic environment secrete acidic and basic FGF as well as PDGF.[197] These cytokines are both chemotactic and mitogenic for endothelial cells. Once again, integrin mediated binding to the wound matrix is central to these responses, with both $\alpha_v\beta_3$ and $\alpha_v\beta_5$ involved in growth factor-stimulated angiogenesis, although via different mechanisms:[59] bFGF-induced angiogenesis is mediated by the $\alpha_v\beta_3$ integrin, whereas $\alpha_v\beta_5$ integrin is crucial in VEGF-stimulated angiogenesis.

Although the initial phase of vascularization resembles normal wound healing, the subsequent phase of centripetal vessel ingrowth through the interstices of the graft is already substantially slowed and often only reaches the outer half of the graft wall.[60,78] Considering the fact that capillarization of several millimeters of wound fibrin is normally accomplished in humans within days, the time period of several months required for achieving this ingrowth can only be explained by a significant deviation from normal wound healing. One obvious difference between normal and graft healing is the nature of the chronic inflammatory response. Specifically, the macrophage-derived giant cells which gradually build up in the outer parts of the graft[27,28,33,60,62] are only formed in response to a foreign body. In high porosity Dacron grafts, this foreign body reaction is not only associated with mitigated ingrowth but also the formation of hugely dilated capillary sacs as opposed to regular vessels (Figs. 1.11, 1.18). Moreover, in some models, the conspicuous lack of smooth muscle cells, and therefore of vessels other than capillaries, indicates that not only angiogenesis but also musculogenesis is inhibited. Given these unique circumstances, it should be possible to describe biological interactions, which at this stage of graft healing, may be responsible for the gradual mitigation of transmural ingrowth. Histological analysis suggests that probably both matrix- and cell-mediated phenomena are responsible for the inhibition of angio- and musculogenesis.

As far as the matrix is concerned, we have already discussed the possibility of a gradual transition in the nature of the fibrin from the outer wound to a fibrinogen-rich blood surface which may gradually slow down the capillarization from outside to inside. In this regard, it is interesting that studies on matrix control of angiogenesis[217,218] have observed that it is specifically capillary morphogenesis that depends on extracellular matrix (ECM).[219] Especially, the ability of endothelial cells to exert mechanical forces on the surrounding matrix,[217] and the subsequent development of matrix networks[218] to guide capillary sprout formation, are matrix determined. Physical and/or biochemical aspects of fibrin formation will, therefore, affect the malleability of the matrix and hence the susceptibility to cell mediated traction and the realignment of matrix fibers. Hence, the significance of the qualitative change in the matrix towards the lumen may be inhibition of capillary ingrowth.

In addition to matrix mediated effects, two histological observations hint at cellular events playing a role in the mitigation of vascularization. Firstly, there is the fact that capillary sprouting increasingly comes to a halt towards the acellular inner fibrinous capsule, while the macrophage-dominated chronic inflammatory tissue, which is limited to the outer half of the graft, reaches a state of sufficient vascularization.[2,11,27-29,60] It would appear that, although hypoxic macrophages may initially be responsible for a pro-angiogenic stimulus, the vascularization which has taken place in the meantime in the outer half of the graft re-establishes a normoxic environment. With an increasing oxygen tension in the tissue, one would expect a downregulation of the secretion of certain endothelial cell mitogens[220,221] and hence a downregulation of the angiogenesis. Moreover, the short-lived neutrophil response may further deprive angiogenesis of a potent stimulator—VEGF.[56,136,222]

The second and perhaps most unique observation is not that angiogenesis gradually slows down, but the fact that vessel formation is so derailed that the endothelial cells form sinuses as opposed to tubes. It seems likely that this sinus formation may be due to the lack of appropriate intercellular alignment and adhesion events, which are as critical to the process of angiogenesis as the migration and proliferation of endothelial cells.[218] One hint of what the mechanism may be comes from an in vitro model of bFGF-induced angiogenesis. It was observed that, in fibrin gels, stimulation of endothelial cells with bFGF alone resulted in large lumen sinuses similar to those seen in grafts, whereas the addition of TGF-β at picogram concentrations reduced the lumen dimensions.[223] Addition of nanograms of TGF-β mitigated lumen formation completely. Given these in vitro observations, it would appear that ultimately the 3-dimensional organization of capillary sprouts depends on a balance of proliferating versus differentiating stimuli, where an overriding mitogenic stimulus (in this model, bFGF) results in large sinuses but increasing concentrations of a differentiating stimulus (TGF-β) arrests proliferation and so facilitates tube formation. Driven to the other extreme, an overriding differentiating stimulus arrests both proliferation and tube formation. If one concludes that the sinuses are the result of overriding mitogenic signals in the outer zone of the graft wall, where could these signals originate? As previously mentioned, histologically we observe that sinus formation is associated with the gradual buildup of giant cells. The obvious association of these cells with the capillary sinuses indicates that they may be secreting an abundance of endothelial cell mitogens. Although macrophages themselves are known to stimulate endothelial proliferation,[197,220] the limited information available on the nature of secretory products of the foreign body giant cell makes it difficult to define exactly what paracrine mechanism may be involved.

To further complicate the situation, the success of graft wall vascularization appears to depend not only on the interaction of these pro- and anti-angiogenic influences of inflammatory cells and matrix, but also on the interplay of these two factors with the angiogenic vigor of host endothelial cells. The example of 60 μm ePTFE grafts in different animal models illustrates best that there seems to be a net effect between the endothelial cell's inherent ability to rapidly proliferate and migrate on the one hand and the gradual build up of an environment which inhibits angiogenesis on the other. In the juvenile animal model of the yellow baboon, for instance, capillary outgrowth is rapid and thus completed before a changing environment can inhibit it.[30,32,34] Under senescent circumstances as in humans[78] and the chacma baboon, however, the protracted angiogenic potential of endothelial cells does not allow completion of capillary ingrowth prior to the change in the biological environment. This seems to explain why the same graft leads to rapid spontaneous endothelialization in the one model but disproportionately fails to achieve this goal in another.

While unfavorable matrix characteristics, continual macrophage presence and host specific endothelial cell characteristics offer a possible explanation for the slowing down of capillary ingrowth, the lack of musculogenesis within the graft wall is more challenging to explain. With potent tools of tissue engineering available, one needs to overcome the deep seated suspicion of the presence of smooth muscle cells based on their role in intimal hyperplasia. This suspicion prevails despite reports that smooth muscle cell proliferation reaches an equilibrium on prosthetic vascular grafts,[61,93] depending partly on functional interactions with physiological regulators like blood flow.[54] However, the goal of eventually emulating functional arteries through "smart" engineered scaffolds will necessarily need to assign the significant role of creating a "healthy" neo-media to smooth muscle cells. It is therefore paramount to try to understand mechanisms of ingrowth inhibitions for smooth muscle cells also and not only for endothelial cells. Therefore, one must see two peculiar observations in prosthetic midgraft healing in this context: the absence of smooth muscle cells in most parts of the graft wall[2,16,26,27,94,224] and at the same time the presence of smooth muscle cells underneath luminal endothelial cells,[2,14,30-33,35,59,67,77,81] sometimes separated by acellular fibrin[59] from transmurally ingrowing connective tissue.

With transdifferentiation of fibroblasts being only a remote possibility, the presence of smooth muscle cells seems to be dependent on the differentiation of mural/mesenchymal cells in the wake of angiogenesis.[106,107] Embryonic data suggests that endothelial tube structures form first and direct the subsequent recruitment of the surrounding cells—pericytes in small vessels and smooth muscle cells (SMC) in larger vessels. This promotion of mural cell proliferation and migration is primarily achieved through the synthesis and secretion of platelet derived growth factor-BB (PDGF-BB) by endothelial cells, which upregulates smooth muscle cell expression of collagenase, $\alpha_v\beta3$ and PDGF-receptors. The upregulation of these factors allows the mural cells to move toward the endothelial cell, eventually establishing intercellular contact through adherens junctions. This intimate contact between the two cell types drives the expression and activation of TGF-β, resulting in a local high concentration sufficient to inhibit endothelial cell migration and proliferation[225] as well as to promote differentiation of the pericytes/smooth muscle cells. This delicate cytokine balance between endothelial cells and smooth muscle cells reflects the interdependence of these two cell types, further emphasizing that smooth muscle cells require the presence of endothelial cells for migrating into tissue.

If, on the one hand, capillaries eventually reach the inner fibrinous capsule of prosthetic grafts and, on the other hand, mesenchymal cell differentiation into smooth muscle cells normally "follows" the outgrowing endothelial sprouts, why are capillaries often found in abundance but without accompanying smooth muscle cells? Similarly to the inhibition of capillarization, both cell-matrix and cell-cell interactions seem to play a role in the inhibition of musculogenesis. As discussed under "Fibrin", platelet activation at the blood surface may result in relatively high TGF-β concentrations in the nonfavorable fibrin matrix. Should migration-associated degradation liberate this TGF-β, it may indeed prematurely inhibit proliferative responses of smooth muscle cells and switch the phenotype of these cells to a resting one. In this way, the biological signals encoding the maturation and eventually the arrest of a proliferative event may be prematurely transmitted to the smooth muscle cells as a result of the changing fibrin environment over time. However, as tempting as TGF-β may be as an explanation for the mitigation of further capillary ingrowth into the inner fibrinous capsule, it does not explain the absence of smooth muscle cells in areas of dilated endothelial sinuses towards the adventitial surface where the fibrin is assumed to be closer to normal wound fibrin both in structure and cytokine content. Because these sinuses are associated with macrophages and giant cell formation, one explanation may be the immunohistochemical observation that macrophages and giant cells are secreting Il-1β even after years of implantation.[213] This cytokine has been show to upregulate smooth muscle cell nitric oxide production[215] and could, as such, negatively regulate smooth muscle cell mitogenesis in areas of macrophage infiltration, in contrast to its role in the pathogenesis of atherosclerosis.[214] More likely, however, is an absence of PDGF-BB secretion by the endothelial cells, because they never reach maturation associated with vessel formation.

In addition, we have already discussed the role of a slowly changing matrix on the mitigation of full thickness wall capillarization. Such arrested endothelial cells may cease to send out chemotactic signals to smooth muscle cells in form of PDGF. Interestingly, although ingrowing capillaries in high porosity Dacron grafts were completely devoid of smooth muscle cells in the chacma baboon model, 60 μm ePTFE grafts in chacma and yellow baboons showed arterioles with layers of actin positive smooth muscle cells (Fig. 1.9). This indicates that in those grafts in which capillarization was able to overcome ingrowth inhibition at an early stage and proliferation of the endothelial cells was not arrested, the smooth muscle cell component is normally developed.[2,30-33,35,46,77,81] This supports the hypothesis that mitigation of capillarization influences smooth muscle cell migration. Moreover, it is noticeable that the combination of high porosity ePTFE with a juvenile and vigorously endothelializing animal model achieves the most differentiated layers of smooth muscle cells.[30-33,35] These smooth muscle cells are observed in immediate proximity to endothelial cells within the initial 2-3 weeks of implantation when biological circumstances seem to be more in favor of angiogenesis, and hence smooth muscle cell recruitment, than at a later stage. Therefore, if the fibrinogenic potential of a graft is relatively low, the angiogenic vigor of endothelial cells of

a species high and the porosity favorable to allow ingrowth together with early sealing of the interstices against continual fibrin/fibrinogen insudation, capillaries may reach across the entire distance before the biological environment changes. As a consequence, no premature maturation event would prevent the endothelial cells from chemotactically attracting mural cells to trail them. This scenario seems to explain best why 60 μm ePTFE grafts in the juvenile yellow baboon show such a distinctly different healing pattern with regard to smooth muscle cell ingrowth compared to other grafts and species. However, if the fibrinogenic potential of a graft is relatively high and the angiogenic potential of the host endothelial cell low, it is reasonable to imagine that the slowly changing biological environment allows the first part of a chronological sequence but prevents the second one. As the circumstances deteriorate to a point where the entire process begins to halt, the first step—in this case, capillary sprouting—has already materialized while the subsequent step—the site-directed migration of mural cells—has not even commenced yet.

When both endothelial cells and smooth muscle cells do reach the blood surface, additional large vessel signals appear to play a role in their relationship. Flow conditions and compliance mismatch may result in an overriding stimulus for smooth muscle cell proliferation[229] despite their direct contact with endothelial cells, which would normally terminate smooth muscle cell mitogenesis through the effect of TGF-β. It is well established that the endothelium transduces flow-related signals and directs smooth muscle cell proliferation when required. It is not surprising, therefore, that expression of the smooth muscle cell mitogen PDGF-AA has been detected in the endothelial cells of the well developed intima of grafts implanted in the yellow baboon,[52,226] while very little PDGF-B chain is detected. Considering the complexity of, for example, PDGF signaling where PDGF is a homo- or heterodimer of two different chains with three resulting isoforms, not to mention two different receptors selectively binding all or only one of these isoforms, it is possible that these factors may combine to generate a wide variety of results and afford the cell a relatively tight control of the outcome.[227,229] This would explain why PDGF-AA is present during intimal proliferation although PDGF-BB normally directs smooth muscle cell migration and proliferation during angiogenesis.

If premature maturation signals are the reason for the stoppage of transmural ingrowth of capillaries at the inside of the inner fibrinous capsule, is it possible to apply the same interpretation to the ingrowth stoppage of anastomotic surface endothelium? At first thought, events only partially resemble those occurring in the graft wall. Since angiogenesis is a complex process including matrix degradation, migration and proliferation, the earlier termination of endothelial outgrowth in the wall matrix may be due to the inhibition of either of these three. Since surface migration does not require matrix degradation to the same extent, it must be either proliferation or migration which is primarily affected under these circumstances. Extrapolation of the number of population doublings[230] required to cover the trans-anastomotic ingrowth area clarifies that it is not the dividing potential of the endothelial cell which is the limiting factor of endothelial outgrowth. Therefore, inhibitory factors other than an exhausted mitotic capacity must play a role. One explanation could be activated platelets that accumulate in and on the pseudointimal layer throughout the length of the graft. The complex signaling arising from platelet degranulation and the high local TGF-β concentration which results could affect endothelial cell proliferation at the surface. However, there must be an additional explanation for transanastomotic ingrowth stoppage, because it is also seen in grafts with minimal surface fibrin or platelet coverage. The possible involvement of an additional factor becomes apparent in Dacron grafts, where the outgrowth of endothelium is more pronounced in a high porosity (knitted) Dacron[40,46,47,60,68,81,107] than in a low porosity (woven) one.[40,43] The difference between the two types of Dacron grafts obviously lies not in the composition of the fibrinous pseudointima but in the ingrown tissue underlying this fibrin matrix. Could this ingrowing tissue in some way be facilitating endothelial ingrowth from the anastomosis so that the gradual cessation of transmural ingrowth becomes reflected in a similar mitigation of outgrowth from the anastomoses? Paracrine signaling over such distances is known to occur during embryogenesis, so it is not beyond probability that ingrowing tissue directs transanastomotic outgrowth but the underlying mechanism has yet to be determined.

In summary, the most striking shortcomings of prosthetic wall vascularization, namely, the failure of the capillaries to reach the luminal surface as well as the absence of mature smooth muscle cells and hence arterioles, could be partly attributed to both the surrounding matrix and the surrounding inflammatory cells. Graft healing therefore seems to be a race between the endothelial cell's angiogenic potential and the buildup of inhibitory influences. Since the endothelial cell remains a relative constant in human implants it makes sense that graft designs should aim at, firstly, preventing the deposition of unfavorable, compacted fibrin and, secondly, attenuating the chronic inflammatory response. This could well be achieved by incorporating an ingrowth matrix which not only temporarily seals the porosity of the graft wall to protein insudation but at the same time selectively promotes vascular cell infiltration while inhibiting the buildup of a prolonged macrophage response.

Conclusion

Healing of prosthetic vascular grafts implies transmural tissue ingrowth. During the past three decades, however, the focus of research was almost entirely on transanastomotic rather than transmural ingrowth. In spite of this one-sided approach, an analytic effort combining historical data and personal experience with biological principles helped to clarify some main issues involved in the mitigation of the entire healing process of contemporary arterial prostheses.

The complete surface endothelialization through transanastomotic ingrowth in animal models under shorter term experimental conditions often suggested that these models differ in principle from the human situation with its stoppage of endothelial ingrowth. In contrast to this

widely held opinion, it would appear that in fact transanastomotic endothelialization progressively slows down in all models, although at different rates. One can therefore not extrapolate short term observations to a long term situation. Since the cessation of tissue outgrowth cannot be due to an exhausted mitotic potential of endothelial cells, migration and proliferation appear to get actively arrested by changing biological circumstances. The fibrinogen and platelet-rich environment at the blood surface makes the buildup of a dense and fine fibrillar fibrin capsule likely, containing unusually high concentrations of TGF-β. Such a matrix seems theoretically capable of prematurely turning the outgrowing endothelium into a noncycling, resting intimal tissue.

Porosity has always been regarded as a crucial determinant for tissue ingrowth. However, porosity alone is not sufficient to quantify the available space for ingrowth. Even in so-called high porosity ePTFE grafts for instance, full-thickness transmural ingrowth of microarterioles is only possible in a marginal percentage of interstitial spaces. The graft wall structure may provide the simplest level of inhibition, and therefore this factor needs to be considered. The dimensions of the available ingrowth space in ePTFE grafts have not previously been assessed in order to determine the dimensions of a transmural channel. The mathematical calculations presented for these grafts in this chapter reveal that porosity was previously overestimated as a sole determinant for tissue ingrowth. Similarly, the measurements of interfiber spaces in Dacron grafts revealed a maximum space sufficient for capillaries, and limited access to arteriolar ingrowth.

On the biological level, a continual buildup of seemingly adverse conditions eventually prevents the completion of transmural tissue ingrowth in most of the cases. In those instances in which microvessels successfully reach the blood surface, it appears that tissue ingrowth is completed more rapidly and hence before the environment turns inhibitory. When identifying inhibitory structures, the compact inner fibrin capsule and the outer zone, with massive accumulation of foreign body giant cells, appear to be the primary culprits. The special composition of the internal fibrinous capsule provides a reasonable explanation for the fact that it is almost impenetrable for capillaries. In contrast, the outer graft zone which is packed with foreign body giant cells seems rather to affect the quality of angiogenesis by derailing the delicate process of endothelial—and smooth muscle cell—sprouting. While unrivaled endothelial proliferation leads to the formation of hugely dilated capillary sacs as opposed to vessels, no smooth muscle cells follow the angiogenic efforts of the endothelial cells. This lack of musculogenesis occurring in the graft wall corresponds conspicuously with the presence of foreign body giant cells. The presence of giant cells is in turn a consequence of a pronounced macrophage attraction by the synthetic materials. This macrophage infiltration is augmented by fibrinogen insudation from the blood stream.

If one tries to draw any conclusions from these observations for the tissue engineering of future grafts the following main guidelines appear to be crucial:

- In order to design future experiments with a view towards transmural rather than transanastomotic ingrowth, minimal graft lengths of 15 cm should be observed;
- Any structural design of a graft scaffold should make provision for continual transmural ingrowth spaces capable of accommodating at least arterioles in order to theoretically allow the ingrowth of both endothelial cells and smooth muscle cells;
- Considering that tissue ingrowth faces an increasingly adverse microenvironment, a key issue to successful healing will be to facilitate rapid completion of vascularization;
- Since fibrinogen immobilization to the biomaterial is a main mediator of macrophage recruitment, a temporarily sealing ingrowth matrix may prevent this event and thus reduce the macrophage presence.

In summary, we eventually begin to understand key aspects of the aborted healing events in yesterday's prostheses. This does not only prepare us better for the de novo design of tomorrow's tissue engineered grafts, but also helps us to change the angle from which we approach graft design: The main emphasis will need to be on the delicate manipulation of biological chronologies in the context of an accurately modeled synthetic scaffold designed to limit inflammatory responses to material contact.

References

1. Graham LM, Burkel W E, Ford JW, Vinter DW, Kahn RH, Stanley JC. Expanded polytetrafluoroethylene vascular prostheses seeded with enzymatically derived and cultured canine endothelial cells. Surgery 1982; 91:550-559.
2. Herring MB, Baughman S, Glover J, Kesler K, Jesseph J, Campbell J, Dilley R, Evan A, Gardner A. Endothelial seeding of dacron and polytetrafluoroethylene grafts: The cellular events of healing. Surgery 1984; 96:745-754.
3. Boyd KL, Schmidt SP, Pippert TR, Sharp WV. Endothelial cell seeding of ULTI carbon-coated small diameter PTFE vascular grafts. ASAIO Transactions 1987; 33:631-635.
4. Kao WJ, McNally AK, Hiltner A, Anderson JM. Role for IL-4 in FBGC formation on a poly(etherurethane urea) in vivo. J Biomat Res 1995; 29:1267-1275.
5. Zilla P, Preiss P, Groscurth P, Rösemeier F, Deutsch M, Odell J, Heidinger C, Fasol R, von Oppell U. In vitro-lined endothelium: Initial integrity and ultrastructural events. Surgery 1994; 116:524-534.
6. Friedman EW, Hamilton AJ. Polytetrafluoroethylene grafts in the peripheral venous circulation of rabbits. The American J Surg 1983; 146:355-359.
7. Zamora JL, Navarro LT, Ives CL, Weilbaecher DG, Gao ZR, Noon GP. Seeding of arteriovenous prostheses with homologous endothelium. J Vasc Surg 1986; 3:860-866.
8. Binns RL, Ku DN, Stewart MT, Ansley JP, Coyle KA. Optimal graft diameter: Effect of wall shear stress on vascular healing. J Vasc Surg 1989;10:326-337.
9. Golden MA, Hanson SR, Kirkman TR, Schneider PA, Clowes AW. Healing of polytetrafluoroethylene arterial grafts is influenced by graft porosity. Journal of Vascular Surgery 1990;11:838-845.
10. Lewis DA, Lowell RC, Cambria RA, Roche PC, Gloviczki P, Miller VM. Production of endothelium-derived factors from sodden expanded polytetrafluorethylene grafts. J Vasc Surg 1997; 25:187-197.
11. Sottiurai VS, Yao JST, Flinn WR, Batson RC. Intimal hyperplasia and neointima: An ultrastructural analysis of thrombosed grafts in humans. Surgery 1983; 93: 809-817.
12. Stumb MM, Jordan GL, DeBakey ME. Endothelium growth from circulating blood on isolated intravascular Dacron hub. Amer J Path 1963; 43:361-368.
13. van der Lei B, Wildevuur RH. Microvascular polytetrafluorethylene prostheses: The cellular events of healing and prostacyclin production. Plastic and Reconstructive Surgery 1988; 81:735-741.
14. Bartels HL, van der Lei B, Robinson PH. Prosthetic microvenous grafting in the rat femoral vein. Laboratory Animals 1993; 27:47-54.
15. Guidoin RG, King M, Marois M, Martin L, Marceau D. New polyester arterial prostheses from Great Britain: An in vitro and in vivo evaluation. Ann Biom Engin 1986; 14:351-367.
16. Stronck JWS, van der Lei B, Wildevuur CRH. Improved healing of small-caliber polytetrafluoroethylene vascular prostheses by increased hydrophilicity and by enlarged fibril length. An experimental study in rats. J Thorac Cardiovasc Surg 1992; 103:146-152.
17. Van Der Lei B, Stronck JW, Wildevuur RH. Enhanced healing of 30 µm Gore-tex PTFE microarterial prostheses by alcohol-pretreatment. British Journal of Plastic Surgery 1991; 44:428-433.
18. Bellón JM, Buján J, Contreras LA, Jurado F. Similarity in behaviour of polytetrafluoroethylene (ePTFE) prostheses implanted into different interfaces. J Biomed Mat Res 1996; 31:1-9.
19. Clowes AW, Gown AM, Hanson SR, Reidy MA. Mechanisms of arterial graft failure: I. Role of cellular proliferation in early healing of PTFE prostheses. Amer J of Path 1985; 118:43-54.
20. Florian A, Cohn LH, Dammin GJ, Collins JJ. Small vessel replacement with Gore-tex (expanded polytetrafluoroethylene). Arch Surg 1976; 111:267-270.
21. Hanel KC, McCabe C, Abbott WM, Fallon J, Megerman J. A biomechanical, scanning electron, and light microscopic evaluation Ann Surg 1982; 195:456-463.
22. Mathisen SR, Wu H, Sauvage LR, Usui Y, Walker MW. An experimental study of eight current arterial prostheses. J Vasc Surg 1986; 4:33-41.
23. Sterpetti AV, Lepidi S, Cucina A, Patrizi AL, Palumbo R, Taranta A, Stipa F, Cavallaro A, Santoro-D'Angelo L, Stipa S. Growth factor production after polytetrafluoroethylene and vein arterial grafting: An experimental study. J Vasc Surg 1996; 23:453-460.
24. Campbell CD, Goldfarb D, Roe R. A small arterial substitute: Expanded microporous polytetrafluoroethylene: Patency versus porosity. Ann Surg 1975; 182:138-143.
25. Kenney DA, Tu R, Peterson RC. Evaluation of compliant and noncompliant PTFE vascular prostheses. ASAIO Transactions 1988; 34:661-663.
26. Matsumoto H, Hasegawa T, Fuse MD, Yamamoto M, Saigusa M. A new vascular prosthesis for a small caliber artery. Surgery 1973; 74:519-523.
27. Douville EC, Kempczinski RF, Birinyi LK, Ramalanjaona GR. Impact of endothelial cell seeding on long-term patency and subendothelial proliferation in a small-caliber highly porous polytetrafluoroethylene graft. J Vasc Surg 1987; 5:544-550.

28. Bull DA, Hunter GC, Holubec H, Aguirre ML, Rappaport WD, Putnam CW. Cellular origin and rate of endothelial cell coverage of PTFE grafts. J Surg Res 1995; 58:58-68.

29. Greisler HP, Petsikas D, Cziperle DJ, Murchan PM, Henderson SC, Lam TM. Dacron stimulation of macrophage transformting growth factor-beta release. Cardiovascular Surgery 1996; 4: 169-173.

30. Clowes AW, Kirkman TR, Clowes MM. Mechanisms of arterial graft failure. II. Chronic endothelial and smooth muscle cell proliferation in healing polytetrafluorethylene prostheses. J Vasc Surg 1986; 3:877-884.

31. Kohler TR, Kirkman TR, Kraiss LW, Zierler BK, Clowes, AW. Increased blood flow inhibits neointimal hyperplasia in endothelialized vascular grafts. Circulation Research 1991; 69:1557-1565.

32. Clowes AW, Zacharias RK, Kirkman TR. Early endothelial coverage of synthetic arterial grafts: Porosity revisited. The Amer J Surg 1987; 153:501-504.

33. Golden MA, Au YPT, Kirkman TR, Wilcox JN, Raines EW, Ross R, Clowes AW. Platelet-derived growth factor activity and mRNA expression in healing vascular grafts in baboons. J Clin Invest 1991; 87:406-414.

34. Lado MD, Knighton DR, Cavallini M, Fiegel,VD, Murray C, Phillips GD. Induction of neointima formation by plataelet derived angiogenesis fraction in a small diameter, wide pore, PTFE graft. Int J Artif Organs 1992; 15:727-736.

35. Zacharias RK, Kirkman TR, Clowes AW. Mechanisms of healing in synthetic grafts. J Vasc Surg 1987; 6:429-436.

36. Golden MA, Au YPT, Kenagy RD, Clowes AW. Growth factor gene expression by intimal cells in healing polytetrafluoroethylene grafts. J Vasc Surg 1990; 11:580-585.

37. Florey HW, Greer SJ, Poole JCF, Werthessen NT. The pseudointima lining fabric grafts of the aorta. Br J Exp Pathol 1961; 42:236-246.

38. Ghidoni JJ, Liotta D, Hall CW, Adams JG, Lechter A, Barrionueva M, O'Neal RM, DeBakey ME. Healing of pseudointimas in velour-lined, impermeable arterial prostheses. Am J Pathol 1968; 53:375-390.

39. Lo Gerfo FW, Quist WC, Nowak MD, Crawshaw HM, Haudenschild CC. Downstream anastomotic hyperplasia: A mechanism of failure in Dacron arterial grafts. Ann Surg 1983; 197:479-483.

40. Stewart GJ, Essa N, Chang KHY, Reichle FA. A scanning and transmission electron microscope study of the liminal coating on dacron prostheses in the canine thoracic aorta. J Lab Clin Med 1975; 85:208-226.

41. Branson DF, Picha GJ, Desprez J. Expanded polytetrafluoroethylene as a microvascular graft: A study of four fibril lengths. Plastic and Reconstructive Surgery 1985; 76:754-763.

42. Kogel H, Amselgruber W, Frösch D, Mohr W, Cyba-Altunbay S. New techniques of analyzing the healing process of artifical vascularization and endothelialization. Res Exp Med 1989; 189:61-68.

43. Berger K, Sauvage LR, Rao AM, Wood SJ. Healing of arterial prostheses in man: Its incompleteness. Ann Surg 1972; 175: 118-127.

44. Berkowitz HD, Perloff JL, Roberts B. Pseudointimal development on microporous polyurethane lattices. Surgery 1972; 14:888-896.

45. Harrison HJ. Synthetic materials as vascular prostheses. Ia. A comparative study in small vessels of nylon, dacron, orlon, ivalon sponge and teflon. Amer J Surg 1958; 95:3-15.

46. Noishiki Y. Pattern of arrangement of smooth muscle cells in neointimae of synthetic vascular prostheses. J Thor and Cardiovasc Surg 1978; 75:894-901.

47. Szilagyi DE, Smith RF, Elliott JP, Allen HM. Long-term behaviour of a dacron arterial substitute: Clinical roentgenologic and histologic correlations. Ann Surg 1965; 162:453-475.

48. Wesolowski SA, Fries CC, Gennigar G, Fox LM, Sawyer PN, Sauvagae LR. Factors contributing to long-term failures in human vascular prosthetic grafts. Cardiovas Surg 1964; 38:544-567.

49. Wesolowski SA, Fries CC, Karlson K E, De Bakey M, Sawyer PN. Porosity: Primary determinant of ultimate fate of synthetic vascular grafts. Surgery 1961; 50:91-96.

50. Martinet Y, Bitterman PB, Morne JF, Grotendorst GR, Martin GR, Crystal RG. Activated human monocytes express the c-sis proto-oncogene and release a mediator showing PDGF-like activity. Nature (Lond) 1986; 319:158-160.

51. Shimokado K, Raines EW, Madtes DK, Barrett TB, Benditt EP, Ross R. A significant part of macrophage-derived growth factor consists of at least two forms of PDGF. Cell 1985; 43:277-286.

52. Kraiss LW, Geary RL, Mattson, EJR, Vergel S, Au YPT, Clowes AW. Acute reductions in blood flow and shear stress induce platelet-derived growth factor—A expression in baboon prosthetic grafts Circ Res 1996; 79:45-53.

53. Zerwes H, Risau W. Polarized secretion of a platelet-derived growth factor-like chemotactic factor by endothelial cells in vitro. J Cell Biol 1987; 105:2037-2041.

54. Bellón JM, Buján J, Hernando A, Honduvilla NG, Jurado F. Arterial autografts and PTFE vascular microprostheses: Similarities in the healing process. Eur J Vasc Surg 1994; 8:694-702.

55. Kraiss LW, Raines EW, Wilcox JN, Seifert RA, Barrett BT, Kirkman TR, Hart CE, Bowen-Pope DF, Ross R, Clowes AW. Regional expression of the platelet-derived growth factor and its receptors in a primate graft model of vessel wall assembly. J Clin Invest 1993; 92:338-348.

56. Anderson JM, Miller KM. Biomaterial biocompatability and the macrophage.Biomaterials 1984; 5:5-10.

57. Weselow A. Biological behaviour of tissue and prosthetic grafts. In Haimovici, ed. Vascular Surgery: Principles and Techniques. New York: Appleton-Century-Crofts. 1984:93-118.

58. Wu MH, Shi Q, Wecheak AR, Clowes AW, Gordon IL, Sauvage LR. Definitive proof of endothelialisation of a dacron arterial prosthesis in a human being. J Vasc Surg 1995; 21:862-867.

59. Shi Q, Hong M, Onuki Y, Ghali R, Hunter GC, Johansen KH, Sauvage LR. Endothelium on the flow surface of human aortic dacron vascular grafts. J Vasc Surg 1997; 25:736-742.

60. Sauvage LR, Berger K, Wood SJ, Nakagawa Y, Mansfield PB. An external velour surface for porous arterial prostheses. Surgery 1971; 70:940-953.

61. Baitella-Erberle G, Groscurth P, Zilla P, Lachat M, Muller-Glauser W, Schneider J et al. Long term results of tissue development and cell differentiation on Dacron prostheses seeded with microvascular cells in dogs. J Vasc Surg 1993; 18:1019-1028

62. Burkel WE, Ford JW, Vinter DW, Kahn RH, Graham LM, Stanley JC. Fate of knitted dacron velour avascular grafts seeded with enzymatically derived autologous canine endothelium. ASAIO Transactions 1982; 28:178-184.

63. Graham LM, Vinter DW, Ford JW, Kahn RH, Burkel WE, Stanley JC. Endothelial cell seeding of prosthetic vascular grafts. Early experimental studies with cultured autologous canine endothelium. Arch Surg 1980; 115:929-933.

64. Margolin DA, Kaufman BR, DeLuca DJ, Fox PL, Graham LM. Increased platelet-derived growth factor production and intimal thickening during healing of dacron grafts in a canine model. J Vasc Surg 1993; 17:858-867.

65. Schmidt SP, Hunter TJ, Hirko M, Belden TA, Evancho MM, Sharp WV, Donovan DL. Small diameter vascular prostheses: Two designs of PTFE and endothelial cell-seeded and nonseeded dacron. J Vasc Surg 1985; 2:292-297.

66. Schmidt SP, Monajjem N, Evancho MM, Pippert TR, Sharp WV. Microvascular endothelial cell seeding of small diameter dacron vascular grafts. J Invest Surg 1988; 1:35-44.

67. Criado E, Marston WA, Reddick R, Woosley JT. Endothelial coverage of endovascular dacron grafts in dogs. J Vasc Surg 1996; 2:736-737.

68. Sottiurai VS, Sue SL, Rau DJ, Tran AB. Comparative analysis of pseudointima biogenesis in gelseal coated dacron knitted graft versus crimped and noncrimped graft. J Cardiovasc Surg 1989; 30:902-909.

69. Nomura Y. The ultra-structure of the pseudointima lining synthetic arterial grafts in the canine aorta with special reference to the origin of the endothelial cell. Cardiovasc Surg 1970; 22:282-29.

70. Mesh CL, Majors A, Mistele D, Graham LM, Ehrhart LA. Graft smooth muscle cells specifically synthesise increased collagen. J Vasc Surg 1995; 22:142-149.

71. De Bakey ME, Jordan Jr GL, Abbott JP, Halbert B, O'Neal R. The fate of dacron vascular grafts. Arch Surg 1964; 89:757-782.

72. Hertzer NR. Regeneration of endothelium in knitted and velour dacron vascular grafts in dogs. J Cardiovas Surg 1981; 22:223-230.

73. Rosenfeld JC, Savarese R, McCombs PR, DeLaurentis DA. Endothelial infiltration and lining of knitted dacron arterial grafts. Surgical Forum 1981.

74. De Bakey ME, Jordan GL Jr, Beall AC, O'Neal RM, Abbott JP, Halpert B. Basic biologic reactions to vascular grafts and prostheses. Surg Clin North Am 1965;45:477.

75. Herring MB, Dilley R, Jersild RA Jr, Boxer L, Gardner A, Glover J. Seeding arterial prostheses with vascular endothelium. Ann Surg 1979; 190:84-90.

76. Burkel WE, Vinter DW, Ford JW, Kahn RH, Graham LM, Stanley JC. Sequential studies of healing in endothelial seeded vascular prostheses: Histologic and ultrastructure characteristics of graft incorporation. J Surg Res 1981; 30:305-324.

77. Shi Q, Wu MH, Hayashida N, Wechezak AR, Clowes AW, Sauvage LR. Proof of fallout endothelialization of impervious dacron grafts in the aorta and inferior vena cava of the dog. J Vasc Surg 1994; 20:546-557.

78. Kohler TR, Stratton JR, Kirkman TR, Johansen KH, Zierler BK, Clowes AW. Conventional versus high-porosity polytetrafluoroethylene grafts: Clinical evaluation. Surgery 1992; 112:901-907.

79. Sauvage LR, Berger KE, Wood SJ, Smith JC, Mansfield PD. Interspecies healing of porous arterial prostheses. Arch Surg 1974; 109:698-705.

80. Hammond W. Surface population with blood-borne cells. In: Zilla P, Greisler H, eds. Tissue Engineering of Prosthetic Vascular Grafts. Austin: Landes Bioscience, 1998.

81. Qu MH, Shi Q, Kouchi Y, Onuki Y, Ghali R, Yoshida H, Kaplan S, Sauvage LR. Implant site influence on arterial prosthesis healing: A comparative study with a triple implantation model in the same dog. J Vasc Surg 1997; 25:528-536.

82. Gouny P, Hocquet-Cheynel C, Martin-Mondiere C, Bensenane J, Bonneau M, Nussaume O. Incorporation of fibronectin-impregnated vascular prostheses in the pig. Microscope study. J Cardiovasc Surg 1995; 36:573-580.

83. Sauvage LR, Berger K, Mansfield PB. Future directions in the development of arterial prostheses for small and medium caliber arteries. Surgery 1974; 54:213-228.

84. Liudenauer SM, Weber TR, Miller TA. Velour vascular prostheses. Trans Am Soc Artif Intern Org 1974; 20:314-319.

85. Clagett PC. In vivo evaluation of platelet reactivity with vascular prostheses. In: Stanley JC, ed. Biologic and Synthetic Vascular Prostheses. New York: Grune & Stratton, 1982:131-152.

86. Köveker GB, Burkel WE, Graham LM, Wakefield TW, Stanley JC. Endothelial cell seeding of expanded polytetrafluoroethylene vena cava conduits: Effects on luminal production of prostacyclin, platelet adherence, and fibrinogen accumulation. J Vasc Surg 1988; 7:600-605.

87. Hamdan AD, Misare B, Contreras M, LoGerfo FW, Quist WC. Evaluation of anastomotic hyperplasia progression using the cyclin specific antibody MIB-1. Am J Surg 1996; 172:168-171.

88. van der Lei B, Wildevuur RH. Improved healing of microvascular PTFE prostheses by induction of a clot layer: An experimental study in rats. Plastic and Reconstructive Surgery 1989; 84:960-968.

89. Chen C, Ku DN, Kikeri D, Lumsden AB. Tenascin: A potential role in human arteriovenous PTFE graft failure. J Surg Res 1996; 60:409-416.

90. Wu MH, Kouchi Y, Onuki Y, Shi Q, Ghali R, Sauvage LR. Effect of differential shear stress on platelet aggregation, surface thrombisis, and endothelialization of bilateral carotid-femoral grafts in the dog. J Vasc Surg 1995; 22:382-392.

91. Shepard AD, Eldrup-Jorgensen J, Keough EM, Foxall TF, Ramberg K, Connolly RJ, Mackey WC, Gravis V, Auger KR, Libby P, O'Donnell TF, Callow AD. Endothelial cell seeding of small-caliber synthetic grafts in the baboon. Surgery 1986; 99:318-325.

92. Mansfield PB, Wechezak AR, Sauvage LR. Preventing thrombus on artificial vascular surfaces: True endothelial cell linings. ASAIO Transactions 1975; 21:264-271.

93. Deutsch M, Meinhart J, Vesely M, Fischlein T, Groscurth P, von Oppell U, Zilla P. In vitro endothelialization of expanded polytetrafluorethylene grafts: A clinical case report after 41 months of implantation. J Vasc Surg 1977; 25:757-763.

94. Zhang H, Williams GM. Capillary and venule proliferation in the healing process of dacron venous grafts in rats. Surgery 1992; 111:409-415.

95. Goldman MA, Norcott HC, Hawker RJ, Drolc Z, McColum CN. Platelet accumulation on mature Dacron grafts in man. Br J Surg 1982; 69:S38-S40.

96. Stratton JR, Thiele BL, Ritchie JL. Platelet desposition on dacron aortic bifurcation grafts in man: Quantitation with indium-III platelet imaging. Circulation 1982; 66:287-1293.

97. McCollum CN, Kester R, Rajah SM, Learoyd P, Pepper M. Arterial graft maturation: The duration of thrombotic

activity in Dacron aortobifemoral grafts measured by platelet and fibrinogen kinetics. Br J Surg 1981; 68:61-64.

98. Hussain S, Glover JL, Augelli N, Bendick PJ, Daupin D, McKain M. Host response to autologous endothelial seeding. J Vasc Surg 1989; 9:656-664.

99. Kaufman BR, DeLuca DJ, Folsom DL, Mansell SL, Gorman ML, Fox PL, Graham LM. Elevated platelet-derived growth factor production by aortic grafts implanted on a long-term basis in a canine model. J Vasc Surg 1992; 15:806-816.

100. Ombrellaro MP, Stevens SL, Kerstetter K, Freeman MB, Goldman MH. Healing characteristics of intraarterial stented grafts: Effect of intraluminal position on prosthetic graft healing. Surgery 1996; 120:60-70.

101. Plate G, Hollier LH, Fowl RJ, Sande JR, Kaye MP. Endothelial seeding of venous prostheses. Surgery 1984; 96:929-936.

102. Seeger JM, Klingman, N. Improved in vivo endothelialization of prosthetic grafts by surface modification with fibronectin. J Vasc Surg 1988; 8:476-482.

103. Zilla P, Fasol R, Dudeck U, Kadletz M, Siedler S, Preiss P et al. In situ cannulation, microgrid follow-up and low density plating provide first passage endothelial cell mass cultures for in vitro lining. J Vasc Surg 1990; 12:180-189.

104. Zilla P, Fasol R, Grimm M, Fischlein T, Eberl T, Preiss P, Krupicka O, von Oppell U, Deutsch M. Growth properties of cultured human endothelial cells on differently coated artificial heart materials. J Thorac and Cardiovasc Surg 1991; 101:671-680.

105. Hollier LH, Fowl RJ, Pennell RC, Heck CF, Winter KA, Fass DN, Kaye MP. Are seeded endothelial cells the origin of neointima on prosthetic vascular grafts? J Vasc Surg 1986; 3:65-73.

106. Beck L Jnr, D'Amore PA. Vascular development: Cellular and molecular regulation. FASEB Journal 1997; 11:365-373.

107. Hirschi KK, Rohosky SA, D'Amore PA. Cell-cell interactions in vessel assembly: A model for the fundamentals of vascular remodelling. Thrombosis and Haemostasis 1997; 77:894-900

108. Cheresh DA, Berliner SA, Vicente V, Ruggeri ZM. Recognition of distinct adhesive sites on fibrinogen by related integrins on platelets and endothelial cells. Cell 1989; 58:945-53.

109. Dvorak HF, Nagy JA, Berse B, Brown LF, Yeo KT, Yeo TK, Dvorak AM, Van De Water L, Sioussat TM, Senger GR. Vascular permeability factor, fibrin, and the pathogenesis of tumor stoma formation. Ann NY Acad Sci 1992; 667:101-111.

110. Gamble JR, Matthias LJ, MeyerG, Kaur P, Russ G, Faull R, Berndt MC, Vadas MA. Regulation of in vitro capillary tube formation by anti-integrin antibodies. J Cell Biol 1993; 121:931-943.

111. Tabbara M, White RA. Biologic and prosthetic materials for vascular conduits. In: Veith FJ, Hobson RW, Williams RA and Wilson SE, eds. Vascular Surgery: Principles and Practice. USA: McGraw-Hill, Inc., 1994:523-535.

112. King M, Blais P, Guidoin R, Prowse E, Marcois M, Gosselin C, Noel HP. Polyethylene terephthalate (Dacron®) vascular prostheses—material and fabric construction aspects. Biocompatibility of Clinical Implant Materials, 1981;Vol II:177-207.

113. Herring M, Gardner A and Glover J. Endothelial seeding on vascular prostheses. Arch Surg 1979; 114:679.

114. Colman RW, Scott CF, Schmaier AH, Wachtfogel YT, Pixley RA, Edmunds LH Jr. Initiation of blood coagulation at artificial surfaces. Ann NY Acad Sci 1987; 516:253-267.

115. Clark RAF.Mechanisms of cutaneous wound repair. Dermatology in General Medicine 1993; 473-486.

116. Albelda SM, Buck CA. Integrins and other cell adhesion molecules. FASEB Journal 1990; 4:2868-2880.

117. Luscinkas FW, Lawler J. Integrins as dynamic regulators of vascular function. FASEB Journal 1994; 8:929-938.

118. Brooks PC, Clark RAF, Cheresh DA. Requirement for vascular integrin $\alpha_v\beta_3$ for angiogenesis. Science 1994; 264:569.

119. Friedlander M, Brooks PC, Shaffer RW, Kincaid CM, Varner JA, Cheresh DA. Definition of two angiogenic pathways by distinct α_v integrins. Science 1995; 270:1500-1502.

120. Gailit J, Clark RAF. Wound repair in the context of the extracellular matrix. Cur Opin Cell Biol 1994; 6:717-725.

121. Grainger DJ, Wakefield L, Bethell HW, Farndale RW, Metcalfe JC. Release and activation of platelet latent TGF-β in blood clots during dissolution with plasmin. Nature Medicine 1995; 1:932-937.

122. Pierce GF, Mustoe TA Lingelbach C, Masakowski VR, Griffin GL, Senior RM, Deuel TF. Platelet-derived growth factor and transformting growth factor-b enhance tissue repair activities by unique mechanisms. J Cell Biol 1989; 109:429-440.

123. Marcus AJ. Platelet function. N Engl J Med 1969; 280:1213-1220, 1278-1284, 1330-1335.

124. Marcus AJ. The role of lipids in platelet function: With particular reference to the arachiodonic acid pathway. J Lipid Res 1978; 19:793.

125. Walsh PN. Platelet coagulant activities and hemostasis: A hypothesis. Blood 1974; 43:597.

126. Nehls V, Herrmann R. The configuration of fibrin clots determines capillary morphogenesis and endothelial cell migration. Microvascular Research 1996; 51(3):347-364.

127. Herbert CD, Nagaswami C, Bittner GD, Hubble JA, Weisel JW. Effects of fibrin micromorphology on neurite growth from dorsal root ganglia cultured within 3-dimensional fibrin gels. J Biomed Mat Res 1998 (in press).

128. Henke CA, Roongta U, Mickelson DJ, Knutson JR, McCarthy JB. CD44-related chondroitin sulphate proteoglycan, a cell surface receptor implicated with tumour cell invasion, mediates endothelial cell migration on fibrinogen and invasion into the fibrin matrix. J Clin Invest 1996; 97:2541-2552.

129. Dejana E, Lampugnani MG, Giorgi M et al. Fibrinogen induces endothelial cell adhesion and spreading via the release of endogenous matrix proteins and the recruitment of more than one integrin receptor. Blood 1990; 75:1509-1517.

130. Zilla P, Deutsch M, Meinhart, Puschmann R, Eberl T, Minar E, Dudczak R, Lugmaier H, Schmidt P, Noszian I, Fischlein T. Clinical in vitro endotheliaization of femoropopliteal bypass grafts: An acturial follow-up over three years. J Vasc Surg 1994; 19:540-548.

131. Rifkin DB, Kojima S, Abe M and Harpel JG. TGF-β: Structure, function and formation. Thrombosis and Haemostasis 1993; 70:177-179.

132. Wakefield LM, Smith DM, Flanders KC, Sporn MB. Latent transformting growth factor-b from human platelets. J Biol Chem 1988; 263:7646-7654.

133. Miyazono K, Hollman U, Wornstadt C, Heldin C-H. Latent high molecular weight complex of transforming growth factor β1: Purification from human platelets and structural characterisation. J Biol Chem 1988; 263:6407-6417.

134. Harpel JG, Metz CN, Kojima S, Rifkin DB. Control of transformting growth factor-b activity: Latency vs. activation. Progress in Growth Factor Research 1992; 4:321-335.

135. Mohle R, Green D, Moore MAS, Nachman RL, Rafii S. Constitutive production and thrombin-induced release of vascular endothelial growth factor by human megakaryocytes and platelets. Proc Natl Acad Sci USA, 1997; 94:663-668.

136. Taichman NS, Young S, Cruchley AT, Taylor P, Paleolog E. Human neutrophils secrete vascular endothelial growth factor. J Leukoc Biol 1997; 62:397-400.

137. Pepper MS, Vassalli JD, Orci L, Montesano R. Biphasic effect of transformting growth factor–b1 on in vitro angiogenesis. Exp Cell Res 1993; 204(2):356-363.

138. Pepper MS, Vassalli JD, Wilks JW, Schweigerer L, Orci L and Montesano R. Modulation of bovine microvascular endothelial cell proteolytic properties by inhibitors of angiogenesis. J Cell Biochem 1994; 55(4):419-434.

139. Devine DV, Carter CJ. Profibrinolytic and antifibrinolytic effects of platelets. Cor Art Dis 1995; 6:915-922.

140. Murphy-Ullrich JE, Mosher DF. Interactions of thrombospondin with cells in culture: Rapid degradation of both soluble and matrix thrombospondin. Seminars in Thrombosis and Haemostasis 1987; 13(3):343-351.

141. Good DJ, Polverini PJ, Rastinejad F, LeBeau MM, Lemons RS, Frazier WA and Bouck NP. A tumour suppressor-dependent inhibitor of angiogenesis is immunologically and functionally indistinguishable from a fragment of thrombospondin. PNAS 1990; 87:6624-6628.

142. Iruela-Arispe ML, Bornstein P, Sage H. Thrombospondin exerts an antiangiogenic effect on cord formation by enothelial cells in vitro. PNAS 1991; 88:5026-5030.

143. Bagavandross P, Wilks JW. Specific inhibition of endothelial cell proliferation by thrombospondin. Biochem Biophys Res Comm 1990; 170:867-872.

144. Murphy-Ullrich JE, Hook M. Thrombospondin modulates focal adhesions in endothelial cells. J Cell Biol 1989; 109:1309-1319.

145. Hogg PJ. Thrombospondin 1 as an enzyme inhibitor. Thrombosis and Haemostasis 1994; 72: 787-792.

146. Mosher DF, Misenheimer TM, Stenflo J, Hogg PJ. Modulation of fibrinolysis by thrombospondin. Ann N Y Acd Sci 1992; 667:64-9.

147. Schultz-Cherry S, Ribeiro S, Gentry L, Murphy-Ullrich JE. Thrombospondin binds and activates the small and large forms of latent transformting growth factor–β in a chemically defined system. JBC 1994; 269(43):26775-26782.

148. Assoian RK, Fleurdelys BE, Stevenson HC, Miller PJ, Madtes DK, Raines EW, Ross R and Sporn MB. Expression and secretion of type 1 transforming growth factor by activated human macrophages. Proc Natl Acad Sci 1987; 84:6020-6024.

149. DiPietro LA, Polverini PJ. Angiogenic macrophages producc the angiogenic inhibitor thrombospondin-1. Amer J Pathol 1993; 143:678-684.

150. Van Ginkel CJW, Van Aken WG, Oh JIH, Vreeken J. Stimulation of monocyte procoagulant activity by adherence to different surfaces. Brit J Haemot 1997; 37:35-45.

151. Kalman PG, Rotstein OD, Niven J, Glynn MFX, Romaschin AD. Differential stimulation of macrophage procoagulant activity by vascular grafts. J Vasc Surg 1993; 17:531-537.

152. Bach RR. Initiation of coagulation by tissue factor. CRC Crit Rev Biochem 1988; 23:339-368

153. Nemerson Y. Tissue factor and haemostasis. Blood 1988; 71:1-8.

154. Miller KM, Huskey RA, Bigby LF, Anderson JM. Characterisation of biomedical polymer-adherent macrophages: IL-1 generation and SEM studies. Biomaterials 1989; 10:187-196.

155. Schwager I, Jungi TW. Effect of human recombinant cytokines on the induction of macrophages procoagulant activity. Blood 1994; 83(1):152-160.

156. Bastida E, Ordinas A, Escolar G, Jamieson GA. Tissue factor in microvesicles shed from U87MG human glioblastoma cells induces coagulation, platelet aggregation and thrombogenesis. Blood 1984; 64:177-184.

157. Lewis JC, Bennett-Cain AL, DeMars CS, Doellgast GJ, Grant KW, Jones NL, Gupter M. Procoagulant activity after exposure of monocyte-derived macrophages to minimally oxidized low density lipoprotien. Colocalization of tissue factor antigen and nascent fibrin fibers at the cell surface. Amer J Path 1995; 147:1029-1040.

158. Hogg N, Berlin C. Structure and function of adhesion receptors in leukocyte trafficking. Immunology Today 1995; 16:327-330.

159. Mantovani A, Dejana E. Cytokines as cummunication signals between leukocytes and endothelial cells. Immunology Today 1989; 10;370-375.

160. Nunes I, Shapiro RL, Rifkin DB. Characterization of latent TGF-beta activation by murine peritoneal macrophages. J Immunol 1995; 155:1450-9.

161. Wahl SM, Allen JB, Weeks BS, Wong HL, Klotman PE.Transforming growth factor beta enhances integrin expression and type IV collagenase secretion in human monocytes. Proc Natl Acad Sci USA 1993; 90:4577-81.

162. Garcia M. Transformting growth factor-beta 1 stimulates macrophage urokinase expression and release of matrix-bound basic fibroblast growth factor. J Cell Physiol 1993; 155:595-605.

163. Loscalzo J. The macrophage and fibrinolysis. Semin Thromb Hemost 1996; 22:503-6.

164. Gross TJ, Leavell KJ, Peterson MW. Cd11b/cd18 mediates the neutrophil chemotactic activity of fibrin degradation product D domain. Thromb Haemost 1997; 5:894-900.

165. Premack BA, Schall TJ. Chemokine receptors: Gateways to inflammation and infection. Nature Medicine 1996; 2:1174-1178.

166. Rhodes NP, Hunt JA, Williams DF. Macrophage subpopulation differentiation by stimulation with biomaterials. J Biomat Res 1997; 37:481-488.

167. Azeez A, Yun J, DeFife K, Colton E, Cahallan L, Verhoeven M, Cahallan P, Anderson JM, Hiltner A. In vitro monocyte adhesion and activation on modified FEP copolymer surfaces. J Appl Poly Sci 1995; 58:1741-1749.

168. Bonfield TL, Colton E, Marchant RE, Anderson JM. Cytokine and growth factor production by monocytes/macrophages on protein preadsorbed polymers. J Biomat Res 1992; 26:837-850.

169. Hunt JA, Meijs G, Williams DF. Hydrophillicty of polymers and soft tissue responses; a quantitative analysis. J Biomat Res 1997; 36:542-549.

170. Hunt JA, Flanagan, BF, McLaughlin PJ, Strickland I, Williams DF. Effect of biomaterial surface charge on the inflammatory response: Evaluation of cellular infiltration and TNF-β production. J Biomat Res 1996; 31:139-144.

171. Yun JK, DeFife, K, Colton E, Stack S, Azeez A, Cahalan L, Verhoeven M, Cahalan P, Anderson JM. Human monocyte/macrophage adhesion and cytokine production on surface modified poly(tetrafluoroethylene/hexafluoropropylene) polymers with and without protein preadsorption. J Biomat Res 1995; 29:257-268.

172. Bonfield TL, Colton E, Anderson JM. Plasma protein adsorbed biomedical polymers: Activation of human monocytes and induction of IL-1. J Biomat Res 1989; 23:535-548.

173. Bonfield TL, Anderson JM. Functional versus quantitative comparison of Il-1β from monocytes/macrophages on biomedical polymers. J Biomat Res 1993; 27:1195-1199.

174. Krause TJ, Robertson FM, Liesch JB, Wasserman AJ, Greco RS. Differential production interleukin 1 on the surface of biomaterials. Arch Surg 1990; 125:1158-1160.

175. Miller KM, Anderson JM. Human monocyte/macrophage activation and IL-1 generation by biomedical polymers. J Biomat Res 1988; 22:713-731.

176. Miller KM, Anderson JM. In vitro stimulation of fibroblast activity by factors generated from human monocytes activated by biomedical polymers. J Biomat Res 1989; 23:911-930.

177. Miller KM, Rose-Caprara V, Anderson JM. Generation of IL-1 like activity in response to biomedical polymer implants: A comparison of in vitro and in vivo models. J Biomat Res 1989; 23:1007-1026.

178. Swartbol P, Truedsson L, Pärsson, Norgren L. Tumor necrosis factor-α and interleukin-6 release from white blood cells induced by different graft maerials in vitro are affected by pentoxifylline and iloprost. J Biomed Mater Res 1997; 36:400-406.

179. Bonfield TL, Colton E, Anderson JM. Protein adsorption of biomedical polymers influences activated monocytes to produce fibroblast stimulating factors. J Biomat Res 1992; 26:457-465.

180. Petillo O, Peluso G, Ambrosio, L, Nicolais L, Kao WJ, Anderson JM. In vivo induction of macrophage Ia antigen (MHC class II) expression by biomedical polymers in the cage implant system. J Biomat Res 1994; 28:635-646.

181. Gemmell CH, Black JP, Yeo EL, Sefton MV. Material induced up-regulation of leukocyte Cd11b during whole blood contact: Material differences and a role for complement. J Biomat Res 1996; 32:29-35.

182. Swartbol P, Truedsson L, Pärsson, Norgren L. Surface adhesion molecule expression on human blood cells induced by vascular graft materials in vitro. J Biomat Res 1996; 32:669-676.

183. Anderson JM, Ziats NP, Azeez A, Brunstedt MR, Stack S, Bonfield TL. Protein adsorption and macrophage activation on PDMS and silicone rubber. J of Biomat Sci Polymer Edition 1995; 7:159-169.

184. Anderson JM, Bonfield TL, Ziats NP.Protein adsorption and cellular adhesion and activation on biomedical polymers. Biomaterials 1990; 13:375-382.

185. Ziats NP, Pankowsky DA, Tierney BP, Ratnoff OD, Anderson JM. Absorption of Hageman factor and other human plasma proteins to biomedical polymers. J Lab Clin Med 1990; 116:687-96.

186. Rapoza RJ, Horbett TA. Postadsorptive transitions in fibrinogen: Influence of polymer properties. J Biomat Res 1990; 24(10):1263-1287.

187. Slack SM, Horbett TA. Changes in fibrinogen adsorbed to segmented polyurethanes and hydroxyethylmethacrylate-ethylmethacrylate copolymers. J Biomat Res 1992; 26(12):1633-1649.

188. Zisman WA. Ind Eng Chem 1963; 55:18-25.

189. Boffa GA, Lucien N, Faure A, Boffa MC. J Biomat Res 1977; 11:3-17.

190. Noishiki Y. Application of immunoperoxidase method to electron microscopic observation of plasma protein on polymer surface. J Biomed Mater Res 1982; 16:359-67.

191. Tang L, Eaton JW. Fibrin(ogen) mediates acute inflammatory responses to biomaterials. J Exper Med 1993; 178:2147-2156.

192. Tang L, Lucas AH, Eaton JW. Inflammatory responses to implanted polymeric biomaterials: Role of surface-absorbed IgG. J Lab Clin Med 1993; 122:292-300.

193. Tang L, Eaton JW. Inflammatory responses to biomaterials. Amer J Clin Path 1995; 103:466-471.

194. Tang L, Ugarova TP, Plow EF, Eaton JW. Molecular determinants of acute inflammatory responses to biomaterials. J Clin Invest 1996; 97: 1329-1334.

195. McNally AK, Anderson JM. Complement C3 participation in monocyte adhesion to different surfaces. PNAS 1994; 91:10119-10123.

196. Bernatchez SF, Parks PJ, Gibbons DF. Interaction of macrophages with fibrous materials in vitro. Biomaterials 1996; 17:2077-2086.

197. Kuwabara K, Ogawa S, Matsumoto M, Koga S, Clauss M, Pinsky DJ, Lyn P, Leavy J, Witte L, Joseph-Silverstein J, Furies MB, Torcia G, Cozzolino F, Kamada T, Stern DM. Hypoxia-mediated induction of acidic/basic fibroblast growth factor and platelet-derived growth factor in mononuclear phagocytes stimulates growth of hypoxic endothelial cells. Proc Nat Acad Sci 1995; 92:4606-4610.

198. Van Otteren GM, Standiford TJ, Kunkel SL, Danforth JM, Stricter RM. Alterations of ambient oxygen tension modulate the expression of tumour necrosis factor and macrophage inflammatory protein-1 from murine alveolar macrophages. Amer J Respir Cell Mol Biol 1995; 13(4):399-409.

199. Leibovich SJ, Polverini PJ, Shepard HM, Wiseman DM, Shively V, Nuseir N. Macrophage-induced angiogenesis is mediated by tumour necrosis factor-α. Nature 1987; 329:630-632.

200. Patterson C, Perrella MA, Endege WO, Yoshizumi M, Lee M, Haber E. Downregulation of vascular endothelial growth factor receptors by tumour necrosis factor-α in cultured human vascular cells. Journal of Clinical Investigation 1996; 98(2):490-496.

201. Spyridopoulos I, Brogi E, Kearney M, Sullivan AB, Cetrulo C, Isner JM, Losordo DW. Vascular enothelial growth factor inhibits endothelial cell apoptosis induced by tumour necrosis factor-α: Balance between growth and death signals. J Mol Cell Cardiol 1997; 29:1321-1330.

202. Defife KM, Jenney CR, Colton E, Anderson JM. Confocal and light microscopic evaluation of silane surface-dependent macrophage development and IL-4 induced foreign body giant cell formation. Fifth World Biomaterials Congress 1996.

203. Kao WJ, Zhao QH, Hiltner A, Anderson JM. Theoretical analysis of in vivo macrophage adhesion and FBGC formation on PDMS, low density polyethylene and PEUs. J Biomat Res 1994; 28:73-79.

204. Kao WJ, Hiltner A, Anderson JM, Lodoen GA. Theoretical analysis of in vivo macrophage adhesion and FBGC formation on strained poly(etherurethane urea) elastomers. J Biomat Res 1994; 28:819-829.

205. Mathur A, Collier TO, Kao WJ, Wiggins M, Schubert MA, Hiltner A, Anderson JM. In vivo biocompatabiity and biostability of modified polyurethanes. J Biomater Res 1997; 36:246-257.

206. McNally AK, Anderson JM. The lymphokine IL-4 induces very large FBGC and syncytia from human macs in a material surface property dependent manner in vitro. Fifth World Biomaterials Congress 1996.

207. McNally AK, DeFife KM, Anderson JM. IL-4 induced macrophage fusion is prevented by inhibitors of mannose receptor activity. Am J of Pathol 1997; 149:975.

208. McNally AK, Anderson JM. IL-4 induces foreign body giant cells from human monocytes/macrophages. Amer J Pathol 1995; 47:1487-1499.

209. Essner R, Rhoades K, McBride WH, Morton DL, Economou JS. IL-4 downregulates IL-1 and TNF gene expression in human monocytes. J Immunol 1989; 142:3857-3861.

210. Lehn M, Weiser WY, Engelhor S, Gillis S, Remold HG. IL-4 inhibits H_2O_2 production and antileishmanial capacity of human culture monocytes mediated by fn-γ. J Immunol 1989; 143:3020-3024.

211. Lacraz S, Nicod L, Galve-de Rochemonteix B, Bauberger C, Dayer J-M, Welgus HG. Supression of metalloproteinase biosynthesis in human macrophages by interleukin-4. J Clin Invest 1992; 90:382-388.

212. Zhao Q, Topham N, Anderson JM, Hiltner A, Lodoen G, Payet CR. Foreign-body giant cells and polyurethane biostability: In vivo correlation of cell adhesion and surface cracking. J Biomat Res 1991; 35:177-183.

213. Anderson J. Inflammatory reaction: The nemesis of implants. In: Zilla P and Greisler H, eds. Tissue Engineering of Prosthetic Vascular Grafts. Austin: Landes Bioscience, 1998.

214. Forsyth EA, Hamdy MA, Neville RF, Sidawy AN. Proliferation and extracellular matrix production by human infragenicular smooth muscle cells in response to interleukin-1β. J Vasc Surg 1997; 26:1002-1008.

215. Makita S, Nakamura M, Yoshida H, Hiramori K. Autocrine growth inhibition of IL-1 beta-treated cultured human aortic smooth muscle cells: Possible role of nitric oxide. Heart Vessels 1996; 11:223-8.

216. Meredith JE Jr, Schwartz MA. Integrins, adhesion and apoptosis. Trends in Cell Biol 1997; 7:146-150.

217. Davis GE, Camarillo CW. Regulation of endothelial cell morphogenesis by integrins, mechanical forces and matrix guidance pathways. Exper Cell Res 1995; 216:113-123.

218. Vernon RB, Sage EH. Between molecules and morphology: Extracellular matrix and creation of vascular form. Amer J Pathol 1995; 147(4):873-883.

219. Polverini PJ. Cellular adhesion molecules: Newly identified mediators of angiogenesis. Amer J Pathol 1996; 148(4):1023-1029.

220. Iijima K, Yoshikawa N, Connolly DT, Nakamura H. Human mesangial cells and peripheral blood mononuclear cells produce vascular permeability factor. Kidney International 1993; 44:959-966.

221. Polverini PJ, Contran RS, Gimbrone MA Jr, Unanue ER. Activated macrophages induce vascular proliferation. Nature 1977; 269:804-806.

222. Anderson JM. Mechanisms of inflammation and infection with implanted devices. Cardiovasc Pathol 1993; 2:33S-41S.

223. Pepper MS, Belin D, Montesano L, Orci L and Vassalli JD. Transforming growth factor-b1 modulates basic fibroblast growth factor-induced proteolytic and angiogenic properties of endothelial cells in vitro. J Cell Biol 1990; 111:743-755.

224. van der Lei B, Dijk F, Bartels H, Jongebloed WL, Robinson PH. Healing of microvenous PTFE prostheses implanted into the rat femoral vein. Brit J Plastic Surg 1993; 46:110-115.

225. Sato Y, Rifkin DB. Inhibition of endothelial cell movement by pericytes and smooth muscle cells: Activation of a latent transforming growth factor—β1-like molecule by plasmin during coculture. J Cell Biol 1989; 109:309-315.

226. Clowes AW. Platelet-derived growth factor activity and mRNA expression in healing vascular grafts in baboons. J Clin Invest 1991; 87:406-414.

227. Jiang B, Yamamura S, Nelson PR, Mureebe L, Kent KC. Differential effects of platelet-derived growth factor isotypes on human smooth muscle cell proliferation and migration are mediated by distinct signaling pathways. Surgery 1996; 120:427-432.

228. Koyama N, Hart CE, Clowes AW. Different functions of the platelet-derived growth factor-α and—β receptors for the migration and proliferation of cultured baboon smooth muscle cells. Circ Res 1994; 75:682-691.

229. Sterpetti AV, Cucina A, D'Angelo LS, Cardillo B, Carvallaro A. Shear stress modulates the proliferation rate, protein synthesis, and mitogenic activity of arterial smooth muscle cells. Surgery 1993; 113:691-699.

230. Watkins MT, Sharefkin JB, Zajtchuk R, Maciag TM, D'Amore PA, Ryan US, Van Wart H, Rich NM. Adult human saphenous vein endothelial cells: Assessment of their reproductive capacity for use in endothelial seedingof vascular prostheses. J Surg Res 1984; 36:588-96.

CHAPTER 2

Noncompliance: The Silent Acceptance of a Villain

Alexander M. Seifalian, Alberto Giudiceandrea,
Thomas Schmitz-Rixen, George Hamilton

Introduction

Arterial occlusive disease is a problem of epidemic proportions in our aging society with increasing need for vascular reconstructive surgery.[1] The best results are achieved with autologous vein, but because this is often not available, historically there has been extensive research into production of a suitable substitute graft material.[2] At present there are a handful of such vascular grafts that are either commercially available or under development, but unfortunately no graft material has yet performed satisfactorily.[3,4] Baird and Abbott's hypothesis of 1976 that a difference in circumferential compliance of a vascular graft and the host artery is detrimental to graft performance was eventually experimentally verified in 1987.[5,6] The nature of compliance mismatch is complex, as it is determined by the compliance differences of the host artery, the anastomosis, and the graft itself. The hemodynamic consequences of mismatch include increased impedance and decreased distal perfusion as well as disturbed flow, turbulence and low shear stress rates,[5] These changes could lead to the development of myointimal hyperplasia around the anastomosis, finally resulting in graft failure, particularly in small diameter vessels.[7,8] Some efforts have been made over the years to engineer prosthetic grafts with compliance similar to that found in human artery.[9,10] To date these attempts have failed due to a variety of reasons, explaining our current acceptance of highly noncompliant and inferior graft materials. This chapter will give an overview of the history of compliance in vascular grafting, a discussion of the nature of compliance and its measurement as a means of understanding the most recent attempts to engineer a more compliant graft.

Historical Overview

Cardiovascular physiology started in 1628 with Harvey's "De motu cordis et Sanguinis in Animalibus" in which he describes the circulation.[11] Fifty years later in 1676 Robert Hook described the proportionality between stress and strain ("Ut Tensio Sic Vis" or, as the extension so the force) and the concept of elasticity of materials. Isaac Newton and his "Principia Matematica" was the first to relate elasticity (hence compliance) to wave velocity. His formula (equation 1) showed that velocity in a medium c is equal to the product of elasticity K and the density of the flowing medium ρ.

$$c = \sqrt{(K / \rho)} \qquad (1)$$

Thomas Young (1773-1829) investigated this principle in detail, both theoretically and experimentally, and gave his name to the elastic modulus. The Reverend Stephen Halea

Tissue Engineering of Prosthetic Vascular Grafts, edited by Peter Zilla and Howard P. Greisler.
©1999 R.G. Landes Company.

in 1733 analyzed the role of a compliant vessel in maintaining a continuous blood flow throughout the pulsation of a cardiac cycle.[12] The German translation of his work "Hemostatic", introduced the important analogy in understanding the physiological role of distensibility in arteries, namely the W*indkessel.* This is an air reservoir which was fitted to fire engines of the 18th century in order to smoothen out the oscillations in flow of water due to intermittent pumping, thus ensuring a constant flow to quench the fire.

Otto Frank in 1899 introduced a theoretical approach to explain the *Windkessel* effect on pressure waves.[13] But it was not until 1950 through the work of Wormersley and McDonald that a rational mathematical approach to pulse flow and change in diameter over the cardiac cycle was reached which allowed comprehensive understanding of the hemodynamics of arterial flow.[14,15]

Parallel to these physiological understandings, vascular surgery evolved. The first great step which led to the foundation of vascular surgery was the pioneering work of Alexis Carrel in developing a technique for suturing blood vessels.[16] This work published in 1902 lead to his Nobel Laureate in 1912. The first use of a graft to replace an excised segment of artery was reported by Goanes in Spain in 1906 when he bridged the defect with the popliteal vein of the patient.[17] Later, homologous grafts were used but these attempts were frustrated by early graft degeneration and infections. In 1952 appeared the first report of a synthetic graft made from Vinyon-N, a new synthetic cloth used to manufacture ladies undergarments.[18] In 1954 Vinyon-N was formally introduced to clinical practice. Since then many different materials have been introduced, with only Darcon and Teflon performing acceptably, such that virtually all modern prosthetic grafts are made from these materials.[19] It was not until 1976 that Baird and Abbott postulated compliance mismatch as a major factor affecting graft patency.[5,6] Since then a considerable amount of research has elucidated the nature of compliance mismatch, but as yet has not led to production of a more compliant graft.[9,10,20]

Physical Properties of the Vessel Wall

Knowledge of the elastic properties of the arterial wall is essential to study the dynamics of the arterial system. During systole, with an increase in pressure the arterial wall circumference increases, with return during diastole to its previous dimension. This function of the vascular wall is of crucial physiological importance and due to a combination of elastic and viscous components inherent to arterial tissue.

Solid materials have elasticity to varying extents as an inherent mechanical feature and this is defined as the ratio of applied stress to resultant strain. Young's modulus expresses this quality of elasticity and is measured in units of dyne/cm². Solid materials which regain their original dimensions when the stress is withdrawn are perfectly elastic, while those which retain the entire deformation are plastic. The property of viscosity distinguishes a fluid from a solid. When stress is applied to a fluid it will undergo viscous flow. The vessel wall exhibits properties of both an elastic solid and a viscous fluid and thus can be most properly described as being visco-elastic.

The deformation undergone by this class of material depends on the magnitude of the stress and on the rate at which it is applied. Vessel compliance, the reciprocal value of Young's elastic modulus, is generally defined as the ratio of change in diameter over change in blood pressure (%/mm Hg x 10⁻²).[20] It is defined by equation (2) where D and P are diameter and pressure, and the d and s subscripts denote diastole and systole respectively.

$$Compliance = \frac{(D_s - D_d)}{(P_s - P_d) x (D_d)} x 10^4 \qquad (2)$$

For convenience in comparing different vessels a standard reporting mean pressure of 100 mm Hg has been adopted. When thickness is a major fraction of the diameter of the vessel the distinction between inner and outer diameter becomes important. It must, therefore, be specified which diameter is used in calculating compliance. To compute the absolute compliance the pressure should be recorded at the exact point of diameter measurement, but this is not always the case, especially when calculating compliance in a clinical setting.[21,22]

Assessment of Compliance

There are several strategies used to assess the elastic properties of vascular tissues. Classification of these methods is to some extent arbitrary and these so-called different methods share certain common principles. Two distinct methods are commonly used, namely longitudinal compliance, which assesses elasticity of a selected length of the vascular system, and circumferential compliance. This latter method is the most frequently used and assesses the compliance of the cross sectional area of interest of the vessel or graft.

Longitudinal Compliance

This technique is based on monitoring of pulse wave velocity (PWV) of blood down a given arterial pathway.[23,24] The elastic component of the wall plays an important role in determining the velocity of propagation of a pulse wave. The Moert-Kortensweg equation (3) describes this relationship. In this equation E is Elastic module, h is wall thickness, R is radius and ρ is density of blood.

$$PWV = \sqrt{(Eh / 2R\rho)} \qquad (3)$$

The compliance C can be computed from the above principle in equation 4.

$$C = (PWV^2 / 2\rho) \qquad (4)$$

This approach is based on the assumption that ($1/2R$) is small and that the vessel or grafts are filled with viscous liquid. Experimental evaluation of this methodology reveals an error of 16-24% in computation of compliance, thus requiring a correction factor.[25]

Since the pulse pressure and flow pulse propagates along a vessel with the same velocity, arterial compliance can therefore be indirectly measured by observing the flow pulse with Doppler ultrasound. Values for the time taken for this pulse to travel a unit length of the arterial pathway, in the absence of reflection from the periphery, can then be applied to equation 4 to give the average arterial compliance of a section of artery over which the pulse was measured. This technique requires a simultaneous use of two Doppler devices.[26] To further complicate this method, increased PWV due to generalized stiffening of an artery or local plaque formation cannot be distinguished and accounted for. As a result, this approach has now been overtaken by recent noninvasive accurate assessments of cross-sectional compliance.

Circumferential Compliance

The most popular and acceptable method of computing compliance is from measurement of changes in diameter over a cardiac cycle.

The first approach for assessment of elasticity, and so compliance, is based on measurement of pressure and diameter curves over the cardiac cycle. In quasistatic compliance slow inflation and deflation of the blood vessels generate a pressure diameter curve. The arterial wall, being an anisotropic material, has a nonlinear elastic behavior. The incremental elastic modulus is calculated using equation 5.

$$E_{inc} = \frac{2(1-\sigma^2)R_i^2 R_o \Delta P_i}{(R_o^2 - R_i^2)\Delta R_o} \qquad (5)$$

E_{inc} is the incremental elastic module, R is radius, o and i subscripts denote inner and outer radius respectively, σ is Poisson ratio, ΔR and ΔP are change in radius and pressure respectively.

The second approach is based on assessment of excursions of diameter and pressure during a cardiac cycle and is known as dynamic compliance. Since strain relates not only to the magnitude of stress but also to the rate at which it is applied, it is logical to look at the elastic property in the physiological setting of pulsatile flow. A potential problem in simultaneous recordings of changes in diameter and pressure is the phase lag between the pressure and diameter curves, which is caused by the viscous component of the vascular wall. A complex elastic modulus has therefore been defined to formulate this concept.

$$E = \sqrt{(E_{dyn} + \mu w^2)} \qquad (6)$$

Where $E_{dyn} = \frac{\Delta P}{\Delta l} \frac{l_m}{q_m} \cos\phi$ is the elastic component and $\mu w = \frac{\Delta P}{\Delta l} \frac{l_m}{q_m} \sin\phi$ is the viscous component. l_m is the average circumference and q_m the average cross section area, P is the amplitude of the applied stress and Dl/l is the strain, w is the angular frequency, m is viscosity and f phase lag between the pressure and diameter curves.

Changes in diameter and pressure over cardiac cycle can be measured at selected points on the vessel of interest, giving a more complete picture of the viscoelastic properties of the arterial wall. Recording of the pressure in vivo, however, requires insertion of an arterial catheter with its attendant possible complications. In the clinical setting, quasistatic compliance is more widely used. This technique

requires recording of systolic and diastolic pressures as well as noninvasively recording diameter over cardiac cycle.

A wide spectrum of techniques have been used to measure the circumferential compliance in vitro as well as in the clinical setting, although less successfully. These methodologies include electrical, optical, ultrasound, magnetic resonance imaging and digital angiography.

Assessment of Compliance Using Electrical Techniques

Measurement of changes in diameter by placement of electrical resistance probes on blood vessels was first reported in 1960.[27] The principle of this technique is based on placement of transducers on the arterial wall with continuous changes in diameter being electrically produced. The device which utilizes a miniature differential transformer measures changes in external diameter of blood vessels and was used in particular to map the mechanical properties at several sites along the aorta and some of its major branches.[28] This methodology is highly invasive and effectively could only be used intraoperatively. In addition, the use of the device imposes mechanical restraint on the vessel because of the need to apply calipers or coils. Since a typical change in diameter of a blood vessel is in the order of about 5%, the degree of distortion and frictional force caused by these instruments led to acceptably high errors in measurements on small blood vessels. Furthermore these instruments measure external diameter only, giving no information about internal diameter movement, and all of this is can further be compounded by problems in identifying exactly the limit of the external wall in a native artery.

Optical Techniques

The main principle of this technique is application of light to measure diameter of the vessel. The vessel of interest is placed in a laser scanning system; this consists of a laser light and photocell detectors. In operation the laser tube emits a light source which after passing through appropriate objects sweeps along a particular axis at a known velocity. The presence of an artery in the beam path prevents light from reaching a photocell during a particular time. Knowing this time and sweep velocity calculations are made to compute the outside diameter of then artery in continuous mode.[29] This system has been applied to assess the compliance of canine carotid artery, femoral artery and prosthetic grafts in vitro by placing the vessels in pulsatile flow circuits.[30] The technique has reported accuracy of detection in the order of 13 μm changes in outer diameter of the artery.[29] The disadvantage of this system is that it is restricted to experimental use only. In addition, it detects only changes in outer diameter and gives no information regarding inner wall movement, which may be different, particularly in thickened vessels.

Ultrasonic Techniques

Ultrasound has been the favored method of compliance measurement over the past two decades. There are two ways in which ultrasound has been applied to assess the compliance of blood vessels. The first measures the PWV along a segment while the other is based on the local distention wave form of a local artery (local compliance).[20] This latter method requires assessment of diameter of the artery under investigation at the onset of a cardiac cycle, and thus distention during the cardiac cycle under local pulse pressure. A radio frequency data acquisition system linked to a computer is required and M-mode echo images of the blood vessel will be displayed. The anterior and posterior walls are identified manually or automatically. The radio frequency signals from the ultrasound M-mode output over a cardiac cycle are digitized and relayed to a wall tracking system[31] (see Fig. 2.1). From these signals end-diastolic and end-systolic intraluminal diameters can be easily determined and thus the maximum changes in diameter or distention for each beat. Blood pressure can be detected noninvasively and compliance computed.

Ultrasound has inherent inaccuracies relating mainly to problems in recognizing the exact inner or outer diameter of the blood vessel.[32,33] In vivo studies of the inter- and intraobserver variability reveal errors of 5% in measuring static diameter, and 10-15% in measuring pulsatile diameter changes.[34] Increased angle of insonation by the transducer in the longitudinal axis will falsely increase diameter and its changes. Due to the tortuous nature of some vessels in vivo it is difficult to be exactly perpendicular to the vessel axis. The variability introduced by this problem in measuring diameter can affect the quality of results especially in looking at small caliber vessels and consequently small changes over the cardiac cycle. This uncertainly is partially overcome by the use of intravascular ultrasound, which has the major drawback, however, of being invasive.[35]

Magnetic Resonance Imaging Techniques

Magnetic resonance imaging (MRI) is a noninvasive imaging modality that is rapidly gaining clinical acceptance, although widespread introduction has been delayed by its expense. MRI has been used directly to measure regional aortic compliance as well as total cardiac aortic compliance.[36]

This technique is applicable clinically as well as experimentally for assessment of compliance. The disadvantage of MRI is that in vascular diseases such as atherosclerosis, focal lesions are formed; thus the compliance at one site may be very different from that at another. Further problems may occur in follow up studies to monitor the course of the disease or response to therapy, since relocation of the original site of measurement is very difficult. MRI, therefore, while useful in demonstrating accurately pathological disease, has limitations in these measurements.

Digital X-ray Techniques

Angiography, or radiographic imaging of blood vessels, has a well established role as the gold standard in the diagnosis of vascular disease and is widely used in clinical practice for obtaining high quality vessel images.[37,38] Digital X-ray angiography has the necessary temporal and spatial resolution for volume blood flow measurement and estimation of diameter over cardiac cycles. Diameter estimates are either based on accurate vessel edge location or by densitometry, i.e., by integrating image brightness perpendicular to the axis of the vessel.[39-41] The latter technique and principle yield a number proportional to the vessel's area independent of lumen shape, in both healthy and diseased vessels. This technique has been used for estimation of compliance as well as blood flow in the vessel of interest.[42,43] Measurement of vascular diameter and volume blood flow in vessels which are tortuous and which do not lie parallel to the imaging plane relies on accurate computation of the 3-dimensional (3D) path length of the vessel, X-ray magnification and the angle between the vessel axis and the X-ray beam. These factors can be computed from accurate 3D reconstruction of vascular geometry.[42,44,45] The authors and collaborators have described a novel technique of measurement of vessel cross sectional area, and hence diameter, using densitometric methods applied to standard intraarterial digital subtraction angiograms.[41,43] The technique is based

Fig. 2.1. Displacement curves of the anterior (ant) and posterior (pos) walls of the common carotid artery in healthy young male (age 25 years). The bottom trace is the difference between the displacements of both arterial walls and represents the change in arterial diameter during the cardiac cycle. The first sign on the distention tracing refers to the trigger of the R-wave of the ECG (I), after which detection of end diastole and peak systole (I) starts. Abbreviation: b, heart beat; dist, distention; cca, common carotid artery. The data is obtained using a wall tracking system (Pie Medical, Masstricht, The Netherlands).

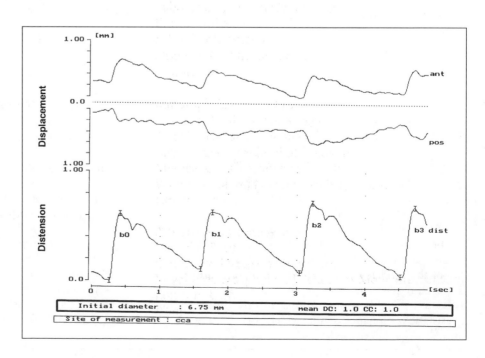

on image densitometry in which the integral intensity of the contrast bolus is computed along a profile perpendicular to the projection of the vessel axis. As illustrated in Figure 2.2, the true cross-section A is related to the densitometric measure a by:

$$A = a\left[\left(\frac{\cos\theta}{M}\right)\left(\frac{1}{K}\right)\right] \quad (7)$$

The X-ray magnification factor M and angle θ between the vessel axis and the X-ray axis are computed from the 3D reconstruction of the vascular configuration from two views. The densitometric calibration constant K relates the image gray value to the mass of iodine integrated along the X-ray path from X-ray focus to image. These were obtained from data generated from 3D reconstructions of biplanar X-ray angiographic data.[42] Although it requires vascular catheter-

ization, X-ray angiography is still the modality of choice for critical morphological vascular studies. That X-ray angiography has not been widely used for measuring blood flow is due in part, we believe, to the use of inappropriate algorithms for processing the imaging digital data.[46,47] The method does, however, have great potential, especially when combined with lower dose digital subtraction angiography and the new nonionic contrast agents.[48] Mini-puncture needles and catheters have led to increased safety of the technique and the equipment and expertise is available in most centres.[49]

Synthetic and Biological Grafts

Prosthetic grafts fare well when used in the aortic or aortofemoral position, but are much less successful for

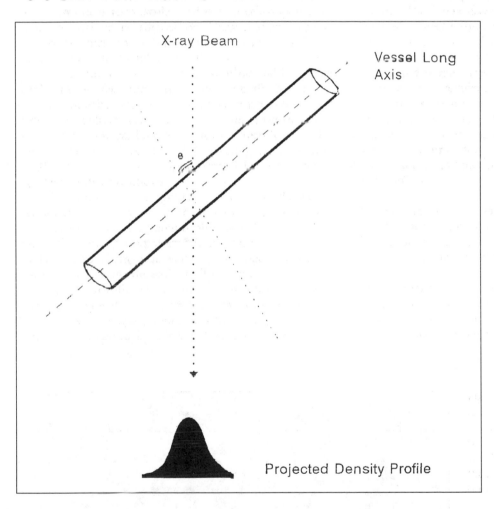

Fig. 2.2. The true cross-section is related to the integral of image intensity along a profile perpendicular to the projection of the vessel axis. See text for details.

Table 2.1. Summary of results from literature for five years cumulative patency rates of infrainguinal reconstruction with autogenous vein study

Research Workers	No of limbs	Operative mortality	Primary graft patency (%)	Secondary graft patency (%)	Limb salvage (%)	Patient survival (%)
Taylor et al 1990[51]	516	1	75	80	90	28
Berganini et al 1991[52]	361	3	63	81	86	57
Donaldson et al 1992[53]	440	2	72	83	84	66

bypasses below the inguinal ligament, with the patient's own saphenous vein giving the best long term patency rates.[2,50] Because of dismal patency rates, prosthetics are not used in coronary bypass grafting. Primary 5 year patency rates for autogenous vein bypasses range between 63-75%, and secondary patency rates between 80-83%, leading to limb salvage rates which range from 84-92% (Table 2.1).[51-53] These are good clinical results but, unfortunately, in up to 40% of patients autogenous vein may not be available or be inadequate because of coexisting disease such as varicose veins or previous venous thrombosis.

In these circumstances a prosthetic graft is the only possible option.[3] Since 1950, prosthetic grafts have been used in a variety of locations for arterial reconstruction. Knitted and woven Dacron grafts provided favorable results in high flow large caliber, vessels but performed poorly in more challenging small caliber low flow conditions characteristic of infrainguinal bypasses, particularly to the below knee arteries. To date the most successful prosthetic grafts in this situation have been expanded polytetrafluoroethlylene (PTFE) and the Dardik biograft or human umbilical vein tanned with glutaraldehyde.[54,55] The human umbilical vein graft was introduced at roughly the same time as PTFE but never gained broad acceptance, primarily because of a propensity for dilatation and aneurysm formation as early as 2 years after implantation, occurring in up to 57% of the grafts.[54,56,57] This phenomenon of graft dilatation is common to all biografts and is attributed to a combination of deterioration of collagen crosslinks with time, and proteolytic digestion by host enzymes almost certainly mediated by an immune response.[58] In vitro testing of 2 types of biografts, a bovine carotid and the human umbilical vein graft, with long term perfusion with proteolytic enzymes, demonstrated changes in the structural integrity of the graft. This was detected by a degree in compliance, thus providing experimental data for the role of proteolytic digestion in these grafts failures.[59] Despite this, clinical experience with the human umbilical vein gives a 5 year patency with approximately 60% for femoral popliteal grafting with up to 80% in the above knee location.[60,61] Thus these grafts perform clinically well in the short term and have been recommended for use in patients with a short life expectancy.

Results achieved with PTFE bypass grafting are less satisfactory particularly so onto the below knee tibial vessels. On average the long term patency rates (> 3 years) in infrapopliteal reconstructions is dismal.[62,63] PTFE grafting into the popliteal artery at the knee shows a slightly better 5 year patency rate of 40%.[61-63] Recently, better patency rates, even to the tibial level, have been reported with the use of PTFE bypass grafting onto an interposition vein collar or patch which is placed onto the distal artery. In part this may be due to improvement of the compliance match between the host artery and the graft.[64]

Compliance mismatch has an important role in graft failure. Various research workers have shown that compliance of biological conduit is significantly greater than that of prosthetic material; this compares well with patency rates for the two different graft materials (Table 2.2).[51,54,63] It appears that as compliance mismatch increases, patency decreases; linear regression analysis of this data shows a highly significant correlation for this association, as shown in Figure 2.3. The patency data for the different grafting materials used in the femoro-popliteal position used in this study were obtained from several recent large studies and compliance data from a study performed by Abbot et al in Boston.[51,54,55,63] Finally, prosthetic grafts have poor dynamic compliance profiles in comparison to arteries with no increase in compliance occurring at low pressure, an important physiological response to shock (Fig 2.4).[20]

Causes of Graft Failure

Causes of graft failure are complex and include technical failure, poor selection, compliance mismatch, primary thrombotic failure related to low flow environments, devel-

Table 2.2. Summary of results from literature relationship between compliance vs. patency rate.[51,54,63]

Graft type	Compliance (%mm Hg x 10⁻²)	Patency %
Host artery	5.9 ± 0.5	
Saphenous vein	4.4 ± 0.8	75
Umbilical vein	3.7 ± 0.5	60
Bovine heterograft	2.6 ± 0.3	59
Dacron	1.9 ± 0.3	50
PTFE	1.6 ± 0.2	40

Fig. 2.3. Data reported from compliance of the various biological and prosthetic grafts vs. patency rate.

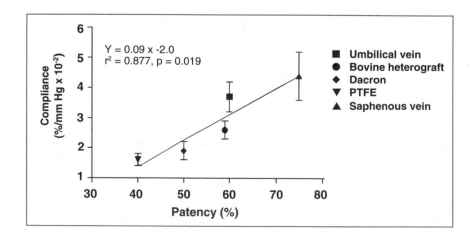

$Y = 0.09 x - 2.0$
$r^2 = 0.877$, $p = 0.019$

■ Umbilical vein
● Bovine heterograft
◆ Dacron
▼ PTFE
▲ Saphenous vein

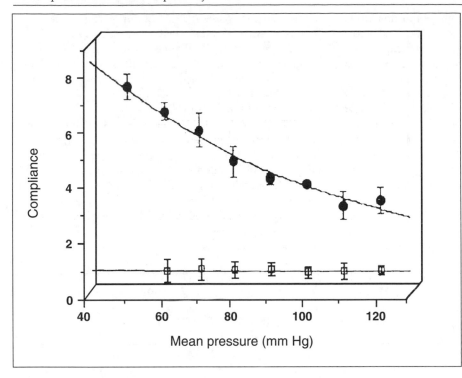

Fig. 2.4. Compliance-pressure curve comparing human superficial femoral artery (●) with PTFE 6 mm graft (□). Note that an important feature of human vessel is the increased compliance found at lower physiological pressures. This has the important benefit of preserving pulsatile energy in situations of shock, thus optimizing flow. This dynamic change in compliance is totally absent in PTFE and Dacron grafts, and may be a further reason for prosthetic graft thrombosis occurring during hypotensive states.

opment of intimal hyperplasia, late failure due to graft generation and late failure due to progression of native vessel arterial sclerosis. More than one of these factors may be implicated in graft failure. Much research has been focused on these various factors, with particular emphasis on reducing the thrombogenicity of grafts either by modifying the luminal surface or by endothelial cell seeding. Much less effort has been directed into the role of compliance in graft failure. Possibly, this is because of limitations in materials and material technology. There is much clinical data which emphasizes the importance of compliance mismatch and certainly it is established experimentally that current noncompliant grafts owe their inferior performance to lack of distensibility when compared to native arteries.[6] It is most important to consider compliance mismatch as composed of two major parts, namely tubular and anastomotic.

Tubular Compliance

Tubular compliance mismatch refers to the imparity of elasticity between the prosthetic conduit and the native artery. Essentially this results in an adverse hemodynamic effect and reduced distal perfusion, as was previously discussed. A compliant wall acts as an elastic reservoir absorbing energy during systole, which is released during diastole. A rigid vessel wall consequently diminishes the pulsatile component of the diastolic recoil, thus reducing the energy available for distal perfusion.

Impedance is the term given to resistance to pulsatile flow. Change in impedance occurs at the interface between a compliant artery and noncompliant graft, and this results in propagation of less than 60% of the pulsatile energy.[65] Optimal organ perfusion depends on pulsatile flow, and it has been shown that change from pulsatile to steady state flow causes peripheral resistance to increase by 10%.[66] Wave

reflection of the graft artery interface also leads to increased velocity gradients and turbulence. As a consequence of these mechanical effects, vibratory weakening of the arterial wall has been postulated as a cause of endothelial damage, intimal hyperplasia and even anastomotic aneurysm formation.

Anastomotic Compliance Mismatch

Anastomotic compliance mismatch refers to the variation in compliance occurring specifically at the anastomotic site. The change in compliance from native artery and prosthetic material is not monotonic because the creation of an anastomosis always generates a focal decrease in diameter and a drop in compliance. This is partially determined by the elasticity, or rather rigidity, of the suture material, and partly by the surgical technique, depending on whether a continuous or interrupted anastomosis is used. Interrupted anastomotic suture techniques give more compliant anastomoses. There is also a paradoxical increase in compliance of about 50% which occurs within a few millimeters on either side of the suture line (Fig. 2.5). This characteristic is known as the para-anastomotic hypercompliance zone (PHZ).[20,67,68] It has been hypothesized that PHZ may be responsible for the intimal hyperplasia which characteristically develops at the same area as this hyper-compliance. Thus mismatch of elastic properties around the anastomosis may act to promote intimal hyperplasia in at least 3 different ways:

1. Compliance mismatch between the artery and graft may lead to a region of excessive mechanical stress, possibly resulting in wall injury, a major event in the initiation of intimal hyperplasia;[6,69,70]
2. Cyclic stretching has a positive influence on replication of vascular smooth muscle cells and production of extracellular matrix.[70,71] Experimentally, it has

Fig. 2.5. Para-anastomotic hyper-compliant zone (PHZ). Typical compliance profile of a continuous anastomosis: Compliance vs. distance. Anastomosis is at 0 mm.

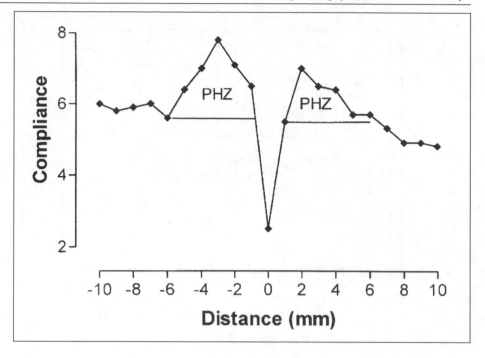

been demonstrated that vascular smooth muscle cell start to produce extracellular matrix and to replicate when they are subjected to high levels of distension.[72] Also, animal studies have confirmed that intimal thickening is associated with increased tangential stress;[73]

3. Flow studies show that a sudden increase in compliance is associated with enhanced particle residence time, flow separation and stasis leading to low shear stress conditions.[74,75] Also, from animal studies it is known that high levels of shear stress have a deleterious effect on endothelial cells but, most importantly, there is also mounting evidence that intimal thickening occurs in areas of low shear rate. An example of this phenomenon in humans is of the sudden increase in compliance found in the carotid bulb where the above hemodynamic changes occur. Since this is a site with predilection for the occurrence of atherosclerosis, one could postulate that increased compliance with prolonged particle residence time, flow separation and low shear stress conditions can cause damage, allowing initiation of arteriosclerosis in man.

Signal Transduction Pathways and Flow

Flow is an important modulator of vascular structure and function, probably mediated through the effects of the function on the endothelial cell.[76,77] Pathways by which flow acts on the vessel wall are poorly defined, but an essential role is attributed to the endothelial cell.[78-80] Nitric oxide (NO) plays an important role in this pathway, and it has been shown that specific potassium channel antagonists can block flow mediated vasodilatation and nitric oxide release, suggesting that the signal transduction pathway underlying flow-mediated vasodilatation may be the activation of the

potassium channel on the endothelial cell membrane.[73] The finding of free calcium concentrations proportional to the shear rate suggests an important role of calcium in the signal transduction pathway.[81] Shear rate dependent release of growth factor is reflected by a varying expression of multiple growth factor-related genes when wall shear rates are changed.[82] A possible mechanism underlying the increased expression of growth factor genes may be a recently described shear rate-induced transcription factor which may not only regulate the expression of platelet derived growth factor (PDGF) genes but also of tissue plasminogen activator (tPA), intracellular adhesion molecule 1 (ICAM-1) and transforming growth factor-b1 (TGF-β1).[83] A shear stress dependent release of PDGE-β mRNA has also been observed in cultured human umbilical vein cells.[84] These findings begin to illuminate the link between mechanical effects and changes and the development of intimal hyperplasia in human vessels and bypass grafts.

Development of a Graft with Better Compliance

The ideal characteristics of a graft are biocompatability, a nonthrombogenic surface, physical durability, elastic or compliant properties similar to those of a native artery, resistance to infection and ease of implantation. Advances in manufacture of biomaterials and tissue engineering are leading to developments in the manufacture of more compliant grafts. What is not known, however, is the range of compliance required to give the ideal match between the graft and the host artery. Arteries change with age with loss of elastin and consequent reduction of elasticity and thus compliance. When the ravages of arteriosclerosis with medial calcification occurring as a result of age are added to these effects, the compliance of the host artery in a patient requiring a bypass may be dramatically reduced (Fig. 2.6).[20]

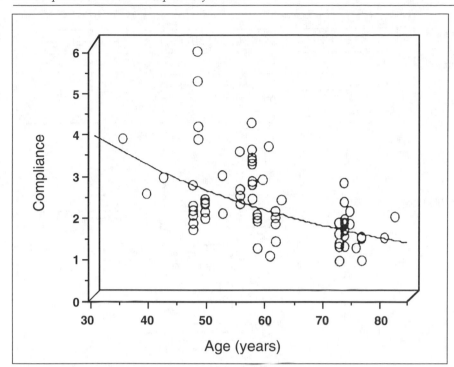

Fig. 2.6. Tendency of correlation of compliance at mean pressure 100 mm Hg with increasing age on human pathology without calcification and major plaque formation.

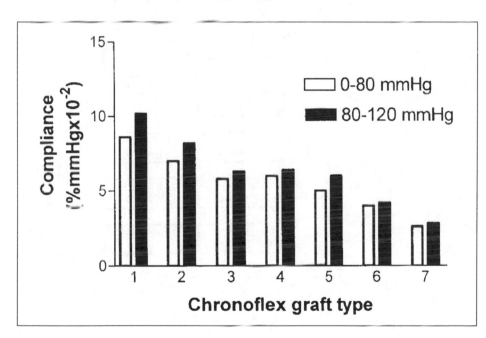

Fig. 2.7. Compliance versus pressure excursion of different CronoFlex graft types (1-7).

Thus the aim should be to develop a graft which is pulsatile, but it may even be detrimental to have a graft which is too compliant. Study of typical compliances in aged and diseased human arteries, coronary, femoral, popliteal and tibial, is required before the ideal graft can be designed.

Development of more compliant grafts is currently occurring, either using biomaterials or by tissue engineering of vascular grafts. An example of developments in biomaterials is the manufacture of grafts using polyurethane. Grafts have been made from this material for quite some time and the major problem has been biodegradability and subsequent aneurysm formation. A novel formulation of a polyurethane graft, namely CronoFlex (Poly Medica Indus-

tries, Tarvin, Cheshire, UK) has recently allowed production of artificial blood vessels with specific compliance characteristics (Fig. 2.7).[10] In this process the graft material is made using either a single shot method (Fig. 2.8)[9] or a prepolymer technique (Fig. 2.9).[9] In a single shot method, all reactants are added simultaneously and the final structure is thus dependent on the relative reactivity of the formulation. In the prepolymer method the ingredients are added sequentially, allowing close engineering and design of the final structure. Using a coagulation precipitation technique, porosity of the graft can be varied to form either micro- or macroporous structures. By varying the quantity and type of chemical groupings within the polyurethane polymer,

Fig. 2.8. Production of polyurethane graft using single shot polymerization method. See text for details.

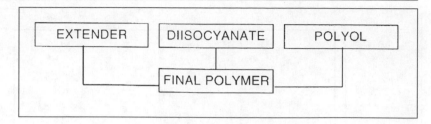

Fig. 2.9. Production of polyurethane graft using prepolymer polymerization method.

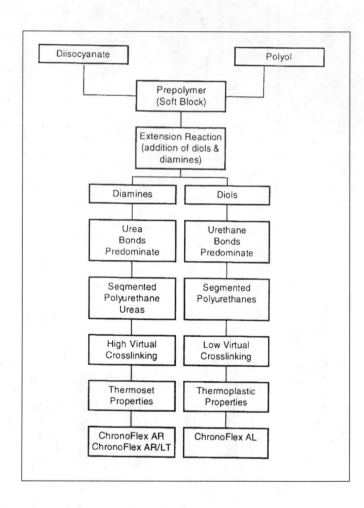

it is possible to manipulate the level of crosslinking and thus control mechanical properties. Thus a graft can be designed and modulated, varying not only the characteristics of the polymer but also the degree of "sponginess" of the graft wall by modulating the size of the pores or bubbles in the wall of the graft. This allows design of a graft to a specific compliance. This particular formulation of polyurethane grafts, known colloquially as the "bubble graft," has demonstrably higher compliance characteristics than others (Fig. 2.10).[10] By modulation of the outer wall of the graft using various strategies to strengthen it, kinking as the graft crosses the knee joint can be avoided. Extensive animal studies have shown no tendency for the CronoFlex graft to develop aneurysms.

A further important area in design of such a biomaterial is in selection of optimal luminal characteristics. It is possible to design the lumen of the graft so that it is inherently nonthrombogenic by incorporation, for example, of heparin or nonthrombogenic polymers. The alternative approach is to make the lumen more attractive for endothelial cell adhesion and seeding. A simple example of such a methodology is the CronoFlex graft lumen, which is constituted of many pits and valleys. Experimental evidence suggests that endothelial cells adhere better and are more resistant to the effects of flow shear stress because they can shelter within the pits, and proliferate upwards to endothelialize the graft (Fig. 2.11).[85]

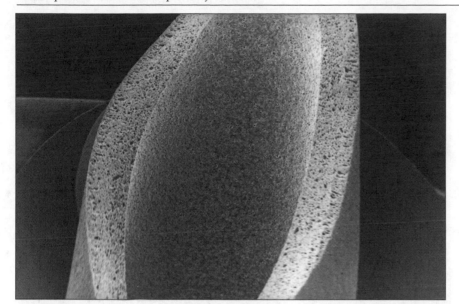

Fig. 2.10. Scanning electrom microscopy cross-section of ChronoFlex graft. (A) Nonreinforced (original magnification x12.4).

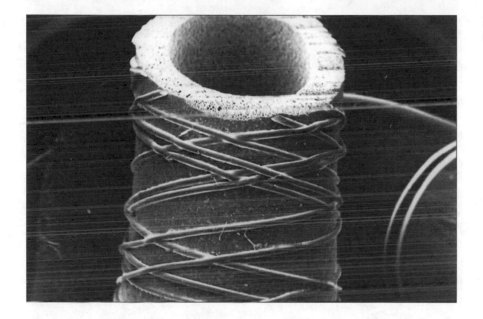

Fig. 2.10.(B) Externally reinforced (original magnification x110.5).

Tissue engineering holds much promise for the development of more compliant grafts. The relative roles of collagen, elastin and smooth muscles in the mechanical characteristics of an artery are now well understood. Experimentally, the development of arterial grafts using combinations of smooth muscle cells, collagen and endothelial cells is possible. Major problems persist in terms of the source of these cells. Ideally these should be from the patient, but certainly in peripheral vascular grafting the time and logistics involved would mitigate against the widespread use of this new technology. The important role of the immune response in eventual biodegradability means that such tissue engineered grafts made from nonautologus cells would require the use of either immunosuppressive therapy, or cells of fetal origin, which are said to be nonimmunogenic. Little data is available as yet on the compliance characteristics of these materials. Certainly this approach would hold the greatest promise of developing a graft with the necessary visco-elastic properties comparable to those of human arteries.

The Future

In the very near future it will be possible to move away from the use of the rigid materials, mostly Daron and PTFE, which are currently used in bypass grafting. Initially, prosthetic biomaterials with suitably designed and compatible compliance characteristics will be used, with clinical trials expected to begin within 2 years. The further addition of endothelial cell seeding to these more compliant grafts holds

Fig. 2.11. Scanning electron microscopy (original magnification x660) of fibronection coated PTFE (A, top) and CPU (B, bottom) grafts after exposure to flow for 6 h.

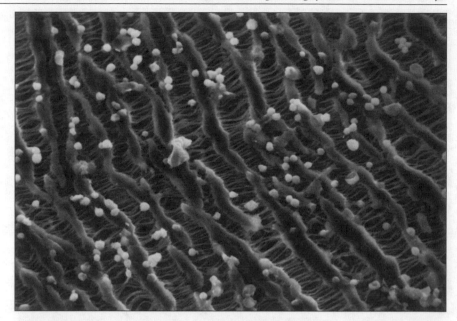

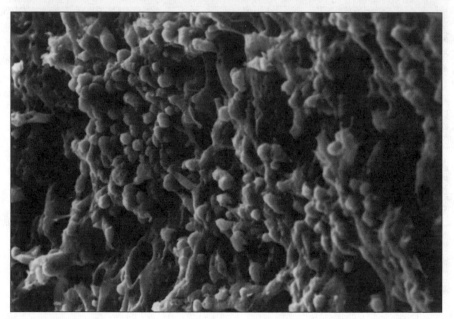

the promise of providing an off the shelf vascular conduit with performance approximating that of the human saphenous vein. In the longer term, perhaps 5-10 years from now the problems of designing tissue engineered grafts, perhaps from the patient's own cells, will have been conquered, with the exciting probability that cardiac and vascular surgeons will have available a conduit as good as a human artery to rescue failing hearts, organs and limbs.

Acknowledgments

We wish to thank Mr. Alan Edwards, Poly Medica Industries, Tarvin, Cheshire, UK for providing us with polyurethane graft figures.

References

1. Dormandy JA, Stock G. European consensus document on critical limb ischaemia. Berlin: Springer, 1990:XXIX-XXXV.
2. Michaels J. Choice of material for above-knee femoropopliteal bypass graft. Br J Surg 1989; 76:7-14.
3. Brewster DC, Rutherford RB. Prosthetic Grafts. In: Vascular Surgery. 4th ed. Philadelphia: Saunders W.B., 1995:492-521.
4. Quinones-Baldrich WJ, Busuttil RW, Baker JD et al. Is the preferential use of polytetrafluoroethylene grafts for femoropopliteal bypass justified? J Vas Surg 1988; 8:219-28.
5. Baird RN, Abbott WM. Pulsatile blood-flow in arterial grafts. The Lancet 1976; 30:948-9.
6. Abbott WM, Megerman JM, Hasson JE et al. Effect of compliance mismatch upon vascular graft patency. J Vasc Surg 1987; 5:376-82.

7. Kinley CE, Paasche PE, MacDonald AS. Stress at vascular anastomosis in relation to host artery: Synthetic graft diameter. Surgery 1974; 75(1):28-30.

8. Madras P, Ward C, Johnson W, Singh P. Anastomotic hyperplasia. Surgery 1981; 90(5):992-3.

9. Reed AM, Potter J, Szycher M. A solution grade biostable polyurethane elastomer: CronoFlex AR. Journal of Biomaterials Applications 1994; 8:210-36.

10. Edwards A, Carson RJ, Bowald S, Quist WC. Development of a microporous compliant small bore vascular graft. Journal of Biomaterials Applications 1995; 10:171-87.

11. Harvey W. (1628) De Motu Cordis, Frankfurt: William Fitzer. Translated as movement of the heart and blood in animals by Franklin, K.J. (1957). Oxford: Blackwell Scientific Publications.

12. Hales S. (1733) Statical essays: containing haemastaticks, reprinted 1964, No. 22, History of Medicine Series, Library of New York Academy of Medicine. New York: Hafner Publishing.

13. Frank O. Die Theorie der Pulswelle. Z Biol 1927; 85:91-130.

14. Womersley JR. Oscillatory flow in arteries: The constrained elastic tube as a model of arterial flow and pulse transmission. Phys Med Biol 1957; 2:313-23.

15. McDonald DA. The realtion of pulsatile pressure to flow in arteries. J Phsysiol 1955; 127:533-52.

16. Carrel A. La technique operatoire des anastomoses vasculaires et la transplantation des visceres. Lyon Med 1902; 98:859-64.

17. Goyanes J. Nuevos trabajos de cirugia vascular, substitucion plastica de las arterias por las venas or arterioplastia venosa, aplicada, como nuevo metodo, al tratamiento de los aneurismas. Siglo Med 1906; 53:546-9.

18. Voorhees AB, Jaretzke AL, Blakemore AH. The use of tubes constructed from Vinyon-N cloth in briding arterial defects. Ann Surg 1952; 135:332-6.

19. Turner RJ, Sawyer PN. Modern Vascular Grafts. In: Vascular Graft Development: An Industrial Perspective. New York; McGraw-Hill, 1985.75-105.

20. Schmitz-Rixen T, Hamilton G. Compliance: A critical parameter for maintenance of arterial reconstruction? In: Greenhalgh RM, Hollier LH, eds. The maintenance of arterial reconstruction. London: WB Saunders, 1991:23-43.

21. Murgo JP, Westerhof N, Giolma JP, Altobelli SA. Aortic input impedance in normal man: Relationship to pressure wave forms. Circulation 1980; 62:105-16.

22. O'Rourke MF. Systolic blood pressure: Arterial compliance and early wave reflection and their modification by antihypertensive therapy. J Hum Hypertens 1989; 3:47-52.

23. O'Rourke M. Arterial compliance and wave reflection. Arch Mal Coeur 1991; 84(III):45-8.

24. Lehmann ED. Elastic properties of the aorta. The Lancet 1993; 342:1417.

25. Bergel, DH. The visco-elastic properties of the arterial wall. Ph.D. Thesis, London University, 1960.

26. Bertram CD. Ultrasonic transit-time measurement for arterial diameter measurement. Med Biol Eng Comp 1977; 15:489-99.

27. Patel DJ, Mallos AJ, Fry DL. Aortic mechanics in the living dog. J App Physiology 1961; 16:283-99.

28. Peterson LH, Jenesen RE, Parnell J. Mechanical properties of arteries in vivo. Circulation Research 1960; 8:622-39.

29. Brant AM, Rodgers VGJ, Borovetz HS. Measurement in vitro of pulsatile arterial diameter using a helium-neon laser. J Appl Physiol 1987; 62:679-83.

30. Megermann JM, Hasson JE, Warnock D, L'Italien GJ, Abbott WM. Noninvasive measurments of nonlinear arterial elasticity. American Journal of Physiology 1986; 250:H181-8.

31. Hoeks APG, Brands PJ, Smeets FAM, Reneman RS. Assessment of the distensibility of superficial arteries. Ultrasound Med Biol 1990; 16(2):121-8.

32. Jaffe CC. Doppler applications and limit of the method. Clin Diagn Ultrasound 1984; 13:1-10.

33. Beach KW. The evaluation of velocity and frequency accuracy in ultrasound duplex scanners. Journal of Vascular Technology 1990; 14(5):214-20.

34. Hansen D, Bergqvist D, Mangell P et al. Non-invasive measurement of pulsatile vessel diameter change and elastic properties in human arteries—a methodological study. Clin Physiol 1993; 13:631-43.

35. Hansen ME, Yual EK, Megerman J. et al. In vivo determination of human arterial compliance: Preliminary investigation of a new technique. Cardiovascular & Interventional Radiology 1994; 17(1):22-6.

36. Mohiaddin RH, Longmore SR. MRI studies of atherosclerotic vascular disease: Structural evaluation and physiological measurements. Brit Med Bull 1989; 45.968-90.

37. Pond GD, Osborne RW, Capp MP et al. Digital subtraction angiography of peripheral vascular bypass procedures. AJR 1982; 2:279-81.

38. Guthaner DF, Wexler L, Enzmann DR et al. Evaluation of peripheral vascular discase using digital subtraction angiography. Radiology 1983; 147(2):393-8.

39. Brown BG, Bolson E, Bolson E, Frimer M, Dodge HT. Quantitative coronary arteriography. Estimation of dimensions hemodynamic resistance and atheroma mass of coronary artery lesions using the arteriogram and digital computation. Circulation 1977; 55:329-37.

40. Reiber JHC, Kooijman CJ, Slager CJ. Computer assisted analysis of the severity of obstructions from coronary cineangiograms: A methodological review. Automedica 1984; 5:219-38.

41. Hawkes DJ, Colchester ACF, de Belder MA et al. The measurement of absolute lumen cross sectional area and lumen geometry in quantitative angiography. In: Todd-Pokropek AE, Viergever MA, eds. Medical images: Formation, Handling and Evaluation. Nato ASI Series. Heidelburg: Springer-Verlag, 1992:609-26.

42. Hawkes DJ, Seifalian AM, Colchester ACF, Iqbal N, Hardingham CR, Bladin CF, Hobbs KEF. Validation of volume blood flow measurements using three-dimensional distance-concentration functions derived from digital x-ray angiograms. Investigative Radiology 1994; 29:434-42.

43. Seifalian AM, Hawkes DJ, Giudiceandra A. et al. A novel technique of blood flow and compliance measurement using digital subtraction angiography. In: Greenhalgh RM, ed. Vascular imaging for surgeons. London: W.B.Saunders Company Ltd, 1995:51-70.

44. Hawkes DJ, Hardingham CR, Seifalian AM et al. Recent advances in extracting quantitative information from x-ray angiographic data. Innov Tech Biol Med 1992; 13:99-107.

45. Hawkes DJ, Mol CB, Colchester ACF. The accurate 3-D reconstruction of the geometric configuration of vascular trees from x-ray recordings. In: Guzzardi R, ed. Physics

and engineering of medical imaging. NATO ASI. Holland: Martinus Nijhoff Publications, 1987:250-258.

46. Seifalian AM, Hawkes DJ, Colchester ACF, Hobbs KEF. A new algorithm for deriving pulsatile blood flow waveforms tested using simulated dynamic angiographic data. Neuroradiology 1989; 31:263-9.

47. Du Boulay GH, Brunt J, Colchester A et al. Volume flow measurement of pulsatile flow by digitised cine angiography. Acta Radiologica 1987;Suppl 13:59-62.

48. Bettman MA, Morris TW. Recent advances in contrast agents. RCNA 1986; 24(3):347-57.

49. Cope C. Minipuncture angiography. RCNA 1986; 24(3):359-67.

50. Crawford ES, Bomberger RA, Glaeser DH et al. Aortoiliac occlusive disease: Factors influencing survival and function following reconstructive operation 0ver a twenty-five year period. Surgery 1981; 90(6):1055-67.

51. Taylor LM, Edwards JM, Porter JM. Present status of of reversed vein bypass grafting: Five years result of a modern series. J Vasc Surg 1990; 11(2):193-205.

52. Bergamini TM, Towne JB, Bandyk DF. Experience with in situ saphenous vein bypasses during 1981 to 1989: Determinant factors of long term patency. J Vasc Surg 1991; 13(1):137-47.

53. Donaldson MC, Mannick JA, Whittemore AD. Causes of primary graft failure after in situ saphenous vein bypass grafting. J Vasc Surg 1992; 15(1):113-8.

54. Dardik H, Ibrahim IM, Dardik I. Evaluation of glutaraldehyde tanned human umbilical cord vein as a vascular prosthesisfor bypass to the popliteal, tibial and peroneal arteries. Surgery 1978; 83(5):577-88.

55. Walden R, L'Italien G, Megerman J. Matched elastic properties and successful arterial grafting. Arch Surg 1980; 115:1166-1169.

56. Dardik H, Ibrahim IM, Sussman B. Biodegradation and aneurysm formation in umbilical vein grafts: Observations and a realistic strategy. Ann Surg 1984; 199:61-8.

57. Hasson JE, Newton WD, Waltman MD et al. Mural degenaration in the glutaraldehyde-tanned umbilical vein graft: incidence and implications. J Vasc Surg 1986; 4:243-50.

58. Mattila SP, Fogarty TJ. Antigenicity of vascular heterograft. J Surg Res 1973; 15:81-90.

59. Hamilton G, Megerman J, L'Italien GJ et al. Prediction of aneurysm formation in vascular grafts of biologic origin. J Vasc Surg 1988; 7(3):400-8.

60. McCollum C, Kenchington G, Alexander C. PTFE or HUV for femoro-popliteal bypass: A mnulti-center trial. Eur J Vasc Surg 1991; 5(4):435-43.

61. Aalders GJ, van Vroonhoven TJM. PTFE versus HUV in above knee femoro-popliteal bypass. Six year results of a randomized clinical trial. J Vasc Surg 1992; 16:816-23.

62. Witthermore AD, Kent KC, Donaldson MC. What is the proper role of polytretrafluoroethlene grafts in infrainguinal reconstruction? J Vasc Surg 1998; 10(3):299-305.

63. Veith FJ, Gupte SK, Ascer E et al. Six-year prospective muticenter randomized comparison of autologous saphenous vein and expanded polytetrafluoroethylene graft in infrainguinal arterial reconstruction. J Vasc Surg 1986; 3(1):104-14.

64. Beard JD, Benveniste GL, Miller JH, Baird RN, Hoskins PR. Haemodynamics of the interposition vein cuff. Br J Surg 1986; 73:823-5.

65. Strandness DE, Summer DS. Hemodynamics for Surgeon. New York: Grune &Stratton, Inc. Pub., 1975.

66. Giron F, Birtwell WS, Soroff HS, Deterling RA. Hemodynamic effects of pulsatile and nopulsatile flow. Arch Surg 1966; 93(5):802-10.

67. Abbott WM, Megermann JM. Adaptives responses of arteries to grafting. Journal of Vascular Surgery 1989; 9:377-9.

68. Hasson JE, Megermann JM, Abbott WM. Increased compliance near vascular anastomosis. Journal of Vascular Surgery 1985; 2:419-23.

69. Bassiouny HS, White S, Glagov S et al. Anastomotic intimal hyperplasia: Mechanical injury or flow induced. Journal of Vascular Surgery 1992; 15:708-17.

70. Clowes AW, Clowes MM, Fingerle J, Reidy MA. Kinetics of cellular proliferation after arterial injury. Laboratory Investigation 1989; 60:360-4.

71. Sottiurai VS, Sue SL, Feinberg EL II et al. Distal anastomotic intimal hyperplasia: Biogenesis and etiology. Eur J Vasc Endovasc Surg 1988; 2:245-56.

72. Predel HG, Yang Z, von Segesser L et al. Implication of pulsatile stretch on growth of saphenous vein and mammary artery smooth muscle. Lancet 1992; 340:878-9.

73. Cooke JP, Rossitch E, Andon NA et al. Flow activates a endothelial potassium channel to relaese an endogenous nitrovasodilator. Journal of Clinical Investigation 1991; 88:1663-71.

74. Stewart S, Lyman DJ. Effects of vascular graft/natural artery compliance mismatch on pulsatile flow. J Biomech 1992; 25:297-310.

75. Ojha M, Cobbold RS, Johnston KW. Haemodynamics of a side to end proximal arterial anastomosis model. Journal of Vascular Surgery 1993; 17:646-55.

76. Kamiya A, Ando J, Shibata M, Masuda H. Roles of fluid shear stress in physiological regulation of vascular structure and function. Biorheology 1988; 25(1-2):271-8.

77. Hofstra L, Bergmans DC, Leunissen KM, Hoeks AP, Kitslaar PJ, Tordoir JH. Prosthetic arteriovenous fistulas and venous anastomotic stenosis: influence of a high flow velocity on the development of intimal hyperplasia. Blood Purif 1996; 14(5):345-9.

78. Luscher TF. Endothelial control of vascular tone and growth. Clin Exp Hypertens 1990; 12:897-902.

79. Luscher TF. Imbalance of endothelium-derived relaxing and contracting factors. A new concept in hypertension. Am J Hypertens 1990; 3:317-30.

80. Koo E, Gotlieb AI. Endothelial stimulation of intimal cell proliferation in a porcine aortic organ culture. American Journal of Pathology 1989; 134:497-503.

81. Shen J, Luscinskas FW, Conolly A et al. Fluid shear stress modulates cytosolic free calcium in vascular endothelial cells. American Journal of Physiology 1992; 31:c384-c390

82. Taubmann MB, Rollins BJ, Poon M et al. JE mRNA accunulates rapidly in aortic injury and in platelet-derived growth factor-stimulated vascular smooth muscle cells. Circulation Research 1992; 70:314-25.

83. Resnick N, Collins T, Aktinson W et al. Platelet-derived growth factor beta chain contains a cis-acting fluid shear-stress-responsive element. Proc Natl Acad Sci USA 1993; 90:4591-5.

84. Hsieh HJ, Li NQ, Frangos JA. Shear stress increases endothelial-platelet-derived growth factor mRNA levels. American Journal of Physiology 1991; 260:H642-H646.

85. Giudiceandra A, Seifalian AM, Krijgsman B, Hamilton G. Effect of prolonged pulsatile shear stress in vitro on endothelial cell seeded PTFE and compliant polyurethane vascular grafts. Eur J Vasc Endovasc Surg 1998; 15:147-154.

PART II

Biolized Prostheses: Surface Healing

Endothelial Cell Seeding: A Review

Steven P. Schmidt, Gary L. Bowlin

Introduction

The field of Tissue Engineering offers the promise of further elucidating and clarifying the interactions between endothelial cells and smooth muscle cells. This understanding is central to the creation of a successful small diameter vascular graft—a goal which has heretofore eluded researchers. Small diameter vascular grafts are defined as being less than 6 mm in internal diameter. These grafts fail in patients from thrombosis and intimal hyperplasia, processes which may, at least in part, originate from aberrant endothelial and smooth muscle cell interactions. Clarification of the biology of these two cell types and their interactions is critical in order to develop therapeutic solutions to the problems of small vessel prosthetic grafting. These solutions will also undoubtedly involve further elucidation of the roles of extracellular matrix in endothelial cell and smooth muscle cell biology, as well as of the responsiveness of these cells to a variety of cytokines.

An endothelial cell lining does not naturally develop on the luminal surfaces of prosthetic vascular grafts in humans.[1,2] This is in contrast to other animal species that have been studied in which neoendothelialization of graft luminal surfaces occurs by endothelial cell proliferation from perianastomotic artery, the microvessels of graft interstices, or circulating progenitor endothelial cells.[3] Because endothelial cells release molecules that modulate coagulation, platelet aggregation, leukocyte adhesion and vascular tone, the absence of these cells lining prosthetic grafts, in combination with the inherent hostility of the biomaterial/blood contacting surface, predisposes these grafts to platelet deposition leading to thrombosis. Although the precise mechanisms of the genesis of anastomotic intimal hyperplasia are still being defined, endothelial cell/smooth muscle cell dysfunctions are thought to be involved.

Early investigators in the field of small-diameter graft development sought to promote graft endothelialization by transplantation of autologous endothelial cells onto vascular grafts prior to their implantation—a process that became known as endothelial cell seeding. The hypothesis underlying this research effort was really quite simple—that is, by promoting the establishment of the patient's own endothelial cells on the blood-contacting surface of a vascular prosthesis, a "normal" endothelium-lined neointima would form on the graft whose biology would counteract rheologic, physiologic, and biomaterial forces promoting graft failure. In retrospect this simple hypothesis seems deceptively naive.

A review of the history of endothelial cell seeding research has been published which details early animal and clinical studies.[4] The results of these early animal studies were really quite promising. This early optimism has been tempered, however, by clinical results that have often been disappointing. It is clear that modifications of traditional methodologies to

Tissue Engineering of Prosthetic Vascular Grafts, edited by Peter Zilla and Howard P. Greisler.
©1999 R.G. Landes Company.

promote endothelialization of vascular grafts are needed if endothelial cell transplantation is to be technically successful. What is even more important, however, is that academicians and physician researchers and investigators have grown to appreciate the complex biology of the cells forming the vascular wall, and that technically successful transplantation of endothelial cells does not necessarily presume a positive outcome clinically in terms of vascular graft performance. The simple hypotheses of early endothelial cell seeding studies have led to investigations providing enormous insights into the biology of vascular wall cells, as well as stimulating suggestions for alternative therapeutic avenues that may utilize concepts and techniques of endothelial cell seeding.

The purpose of this chapter is to summarize the historic context and current base of knowledge regarding many of the technical issues relevant to endothelial cell seeding. Special reference will be made to recent exciting research methodologies designed to promote endothelial cell attachment to prosthetic graft materials—a technology known as electrostatic endothelial cell seeding. The wealth of animal studies has been reviewed elsewhere[4] and will not be detailed here. Subsequent chapters in this text will summarize clinical outcomes.

Historic Context

The origin of the concept for the vascular prosthesis is credited to Voorhees, Jaretski, and Blakemore, who presented the first published hypothesis on synthetic tubes as replacements for natural blood vessel deficits in 1952.[5] The first clinical applications of this hypothesis were published in 1954 and showed that the prosthetic tubes could be used in the arterial setting.[6] This publication prompted a race to develop the best material for use as a prosthetic vascular graft. The two designs of large diameter vascular grafts (> 6 mm I.D.) which are used successfully today clinically are made of Dacron or expanded polytetrafluoroethylene (ePTFE). Patency rates for small diameter (< 6 mm I.D.) vascular prostheses configured from these same materials are unacceptable when utilized clinically, however, due to acute thrombus formation[7,8] and chronic anastomotic hyperplasia[9-11] which consequently prevent clinical usage. Malcolm Herring, M.D., introduced the hypothesis underlying the technology of endothelial cell seeding in 1978 in an attempt to increase the patency rate of small caliber prosthetic grafts. Herring proposed that if these small diameter vascular grafts could be utilized successfully, they could be of enormous clinical importance in peripheral and coronary bypass grafting procedures.[12]

Endothelial cell seeding since its inception has been largely experimental, with significant technical success in animal models. The technology has not been translated successfully to any extent thus far published in human vascular surgery. Surgeons have long expressed concerns about many of the technical issues which must be overcome in order to transplant endothelial cells successfully in a relevant time frame for human surgery. Moreover, the long term benefits of a transplanted endothelial cell lining on graft patency in patients has not been demonstrated.

Many research efforts have focused upon methodologic issues in an effort to maximize cell harvest-ing and transplantation efficiencies in an appropriate time frame for clinical practicality. We will review briefly the history of these studies and then describe the novel technology of electrostatic cell seeding, which we feel offers a solution to many of the deficiencies of other approaches for transplanting cells onto vascular prostheses.

Autologous Endothelial Cell Harvesting

Before endothelial cell seeding or transplantation can occur, autologous endothelial cells must be harvested from an "appropriate, autologous" source. Sources of endothelial cells most often reported have been:

1. Nonessential vessels (i.e., saphenous vein); and
2. Omental or subcutaneous adipose tissue (i.e., microvascular endothelial cells).

From the nonessential vessels, endothelial cells have been harvested by two techniques:

1. Mechanical scraping;[13] and
2. Enzymatic digestion.[14,15]

Mechanical scraping uses an abrasive action to remove the endothelial cells from the vascular wall, which leads to endothelial cell damage as well as the potential for significant contamination with smooth muscle cells.[12,13] The overall efficiency of endothelial cell harvest from autologous vessels by mechanical methods is < 75%.[14] Enzymatic harvesting of cells from the vascular tissue requires collagenase or trypsin digestion to remove the endothelium.[16-18] This enzymatic digestion process can create damage to cellular proteins, which in turn affects cell viability and attachment potential to a vascular prosthetic surface.[19,20] The overall efficiency of endothelial cell harvest from autologous vessels using the enzymatic harvesting technique varies between 80-100% of the available endothelial cells.[14]

Due to the limited availability of nonessential autologous vessels in patients, the ready supply of endothelial cells harvested by either of the previously mentioned techniques is necessarily limited. This limitation has prompted investigators to seek alternative sources which could supply a greater number of endothelial cells. The alternative sources which have been most intensively studied include the mesothelium and the microvasculature, each of which offers the potential for derivation of large cell numbers. Microvascular endothelial cells can be harvested from microvessels (arterioles, capillaries, and venules) found in adipose tissue.[16,21,22] The overall efficiency of isolation of endothelial cells from microvessels utilizing enzymatic techniques has been reported to be approximately 84% ± 5%.[23]

Tissue culture of endothelial cells offers an alternative approach to derive large numbers of cells for transplantation from a small inoculum of harvested cells. The tissue culture approach was first reported by Graham et al.[24] Jaffee et al[17] initially reported that 92 h were required for an endothelial cell culture to double in number. However, improvements in cell culturing techniques have reduced that time to approximately 24 h using commercially available media (Clonetics Corporation. Unpublished data). Thus, relatively large numbers of endothelial cells can be obtained from low derived inocula of cells in a time span of days to weeks in culture. A number of valid issues with tissue culture have been voiced, however. The exposure of endothelial cells in culture to an undefined serum (e.g., fetal bovine serum) as a part of the tissue culturing media presents the opportunity for both genotypic and phenotypic modulation.[25] In addition, multiple passages of cells in culture and media changes create vulnerability to cultures becoming contaminated.

Endothelial Cell Seeding Techniques

Numerous methodologies for endothelial cell transplantation onto prosthetic surfaces have been reported in the literature. These investigations can be differentiated and summarized by virtue of the unique physical force utilized in each transplantation process to seed endothelial cells to a vascular prosthetic blood-contacting surface:

1. Gravitational;[12,26-29]
2. Hydrostatic;[30,31] and
3. More recently, electrostatic.[32]

The hypothesis for each of these approaches has been that the transplantation of endothelial cells (initially low surface density, cells/area) on a graft luminal surface will promote, through time, the development of a mature, physiologically appropriate, confluent graft luminal endothelial cell-lined neointima.

The most basic of the three seeding techniques that have been tested utilizes gravitational forces to deliver endothelial cells to a vascular prosthetic luminal surface. The basic concept has been to fill the graft with the harvested endothelial cells resuspended in tissue culture medium or blood plasma. The filled graft is maintained horizontally and rotated periodically or continuously over a prolonged seeding time period. Biological glues have commonly been used with this technique to promote endothelial cell attachment to the prosthetic material. One disadvantage of using a glue is that any nonendothelialized surface becomes more thrombogenic due to the exposure of blood cells to the glue.[8]

A significant disadvantage of these early attempts at gravitational endothelial cell seeding was that the transplanted endothelial cells were in a spheroid morphology on the graft surface upon completion of the transplantation procedure. Thus, the potential existed for a significant loss of endothelial cells from the graft surface when blood flow was restored through the graft if the seeding time was short (< 2 h) and the cells had minimal time to flatten and mature. Endothelial cell losses up to 95% in the initial 24 h postimplantation were observed due to this cellular morphologic immaturity.[33] To overcome this limitation of immature morphology, attempts were made to endothelialize the graft luminal surface by allowing adhesion to the graft with subsequent morphological maturation in tissue culture (7-14 days in vitro).[27,28,34-37] These efforts did in fact result in minimal losses of endothelial cells from the grafts upon subsequent exposure to blood flow. However, as previously mentioned, the practicality of this approach remains of concern to surgeons and researchers. A long tissue culture period may not be acceptable for a patient who needs emergency bypass surgery. In addition, the questions of genotypic and/or phenotypic changes in cultured endothelial cells as well as the potential for infection (cell culture contamination) have been of major concern to investigators in this field.

Hydrostatic seeding techniques use a pressure differential (internal pressure[26,30] or external vacuum[31]) to force harvested endothelial cells resuspended in aliquots of heparinized autologous blood onto the luminal surface of microporous graft materials. Experience has revealed at least three major limitations of the hydrostatic seeding techniques. The first is that this technique is not adequate for fully heparinized patients due to the graft porosity. In heparinized patients, heparin interacts with the antithrombin III molecule which inhibits the action of thrombin to form subsequent clots within the graft pores, which is necessary to maintain hemostasis.[38] Secondly, immediately following the preclotting technique, the surface may be rough and thrombogenic.[26] The third limitation of this seeding technique is that, as previously mentioned, the endothelial cells adhere to the graft surface in a spheroid morphology (100% spheroid shaped) directly from the seeding suspension; thus an incubation period should be employed (> 2 h) for adhesion maturation prior to implantation.[31]

As described above, many investigators have attempted to increase the number of endothelial cells adhered to grafts as well as the magnitude of surface adhesion (flattening) by placing adhesive proteins such as fibronectin on the graft blood contacting surface to act as a "glue".[39-48] Significant research efforts have focused on glue formulations including fibronectin, extracellular matrix, collagen, laminin, fibrin, fibroblast matrix, and plasma.[27,40,41,43,45-50] The most commonly investigated "glue" has been fibronectin. Fibronectin is an adhesive glycoprotein which is found in the basement membrane to which the endothelial cells are attached in natural blood vessels. This glycoprotein is required to attach the endothelial cells to culture flasks in vitro and it has thus made sense to try it as the primary "glue" to enhance endothelial cell adhesion to other artificial surfaces. The problem associated with using fibronectin or any other "glue" arises from the minimal number of endothelial cells which can be harvested relative to the total graft surface area to be covered, as well as the inefficiency of the seeding procedures.[51] Any nonendothelialized graft surface or subsequent loss of endothelial cells from the surface upon implantation renders the exposed, fibronectin-treated graft surface attractive to platelets, thus potentially promoting thrombotic events that could lead to graft failure.[8] Ramalanjaona et al[40,52] showed that the number of endothelial cells adhered was increased and the loss of cells upon exposure to shear stress was reduced using a fibronectin "glue". The problem these investigators encountered was that the areas not endothelialized were thrombogenic, and experimental subjects required anticoagulant therapy to reduce the complications due to thrombus formation.

One of the most difficult of the technical issues related to endothelial cell derivation from autologous sources and subsequent transplantation is the time required for these processes. It has been our experience that a minimum of 45-60 minutes is required for "immediate" seeding of endothelial cells onto a prosthetic graft being directly implanted in a patient. This minimum time frame does not allow for cell flattening and maturation onto the graft prior to restoration of blood flow through the graft. Some investigators have suggested that a time greater than two hours from harvest to transplantation would most definitely not be acceptable clinically, due to the chance of genotypic and/or phenotypic changes to the endothelial cells which may occur while they are exposed to media containing undefined serum.[25] In addition, it is obvious that longer time periods required for endothelial cell seeding of the vascular prostheses equates to longer periods of time for patients under anesthesia, and thus the potential for complications. The length of time and dosage of anesthesia and its safety are difficult to generalize due to the fact that exposure complication encompasses multiple drugs, techniques, anesthetists, and patients.[53,54]

The necessity for an incubation period for attachment and morphological maturation of transplanted endothelial cells is related to the nature of the electrostatic interactions between the endothelial cells and the prosthetic graft materials. Endothelial cells are negatively charged.[55,56] The clinically successful vascular prosthetics (i.e., ePTFE) are highly negatively charged. This negativity repels platelets which are also negatively charged.[57-61] Thus, the initial adherence of transplanted endothelial cells must overcome this negative-negative charge repulsive force (long range) between cells and graft material in order for the seeding procedure to be successful. Experiments using platelets have demonstrated that the cellular adhesion of platelets on a negatively charged substrate is one order of magnitude less (ten times) than expected by gravitational settling alone due to this electrostatic, repulsive, interaction which must be overcome by a stochastic process.[62-64] Similar short range repulsive interactions alter cellular morphologies by preventing or slowing morphological maturation even when cells overcome the repulsive interactions with the material and attach to the surface. This reality is further demonstrated by endothelial cell and fibroblast studies that have shown the dependence of cell adherence on the substrate surface charge.[65-70] These studies used varying substrates with varying surface charges to study cell adhesion, spreading, and contact regions between the cells and the substrates. The overall results from these studies indicated that an increasingly positively charged surface leads to enhanced adhesion, spreading, and magnitude of contact regions. The results on increasingly negatively charged substrates indicated the inverse, with inhibited adhesion, reduced spreading, and reduced contact regions.

Electrostatic Endothelial Cell Seeding

The only conclusion that can be drawn from evaluating 15 years of research efforts related to cell seeding techniques is that few concrete technical advancements have been made. We have recently proposed and tested a novel device that we feel will be of significant value in improving the efficiency of transplanted cell attachment, as well as minimizing cellular losses upon implantation.[32] The technique is called electrostatic endothelial cell seeding. The electrostatic seeding technique has been evaluated in vitro using the prototype apparatus shown in Figure 3.1. The key to this technique is that it enhances endothelial cell adhesion by inducing a temporary positive surface charge or a "temporary glue" on the negatively charged ePTFE graft luminal surface. Following cell transplantation the ePTFE graft luminal surface reverts to its original highly negatively charged surface. Thus, any nonendothelialized graft surfaces or any exposed graft surfaces resultant from endothelial cell losses upon restoration of blood flow remain nonthrombogenic due to the restored high negative surface charge of the graft material itself.

The basic issue underlying electrostatic endothelial cell seeding is: "How can the surface potential of the graft be altered to attract endothelial cells without rendering the surface thrombogenic?" The electrostatic endothelial cell seeding technique takes advantage of graft material properties (dielectric material). When a dielectric material is placed within a capacitor (electrostatic seeding apparatus), the electrons of the atoms and ions which make up the dielectric material (near surface) are attracted to the capacitor surface which has accumulated the positive charge. The nuclei of the dielectric material (near surface) are attracted to the

Fig. 3.1. Prototype electrostatic endothelial cell seeding apparatus. Features include: (a) external conductor, (b) internal conductor, (c) electric motor drive/pulley system, (d) filling apparatus, (e) voltage source, (f) pillow blocks, and (g) internal conductor end supports.

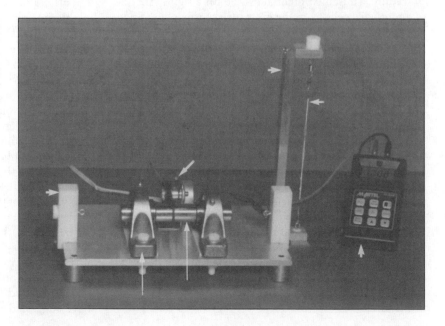

negatively charged surface. These small displacements, or polarizations, are what induce the surface charge on the graft luminal surface. It should be noted that the electrons in a dielectric material are not free and the displacements of the electrons are very slight. Also, the interior volume of the graft material, dielectric, remains unchanged, thus leaving a net charge of zero over the dielectric material.[71,72]

Several in vitro studies have been performed utilizing this electrostatic seeding technique. When human umbilical vein endothelial cells were transplanted onto 4 mm I.D. ePTFE using the electrostatic cell seeding technique, a complete nodal area coverage of morphologically mature (completely flattened) endothelial cells (73,540 cells/cm^2) was obtained in 16 minutes (+1.0 Volt applied to apparatus) with minimal cellular membrane damage or effect on endothelial cell viability.[32] A section of electrostatically seeded ePTFE is illustrated in the scanning electron micrograph in Figure 3.2. These in vitro evaluations of the electrostatic seeding technique revealed no significant losses of endothelial cells upon exposure of the graft to a wall shear stress of 15 dynes/cm^2 for up to 120 minutes immediately after seeding. The majority of endothelial cell loss (up to 30%) occurs within the first 30 minutes of implantation using traditional techniques.[33,40] Thus, the electrostatic seeding procedure is superior to the gravitational and hydrostatic seeding procedures in terms of the seeding time required, magnitude of endothelial cell adhesion (attachment), and cellular retention. It is also speculated that the actin microfilaments which make up the endothelial cell cytoskeleton and possess an electrostatic potential will also be rearranged by the electrostatic endothelial cell seeding technique to assist in the maintenance of endothelial cell adhesion (act as an anchoring system), although this has not yet been demonstrated in our experiments.[73,74] It is also hoped that the enhanced cell attachment resultant from electrostatic endothelial cell seeding may allow the seeded endothelial cells to synthesize the

necessary fibronectin (< 3 days) and basement membrane collagen (< 1 week) to maintain cellular adhesion on the graft for the long term.[75-77] Preliminary in vivo studies (unpublished) using a canine femoral artery implantation model suggests thromboresistance of the electrostatically seeded grafts.

Genetically Engineering Endothelial Cells for Seeding Vascular Prostheses

It has recently been suggested that genetically engineered endothelial cells could be transplanted, which might promote the reduction/prevention of anastomotic hyperplasia and enhance thromboresistance of small diameter vascular prostheses. Additional theoretical therapeutic applications using manipulated endothelial cells include the possibilities of gene replacement, correction, or augmentation which may be effective in the treatment of atherosclerosis. Localized drug delivery may also be feasible due to the direct contact of transplanted endothelial cells within the blood stream.[78,79]

The initial use of transplanted, genetically modified endothelial cells is credited to Zweibel et al.[80,81] Since that time, the study of endothelial cell transfection (incorporation of foreign DNA) using retroviral and electroporation methodologies has demonstrated long term cell viability as well as stable transfection using the reporter genes β-galactosidase, chloramphenicol acetyltransferase, luciferase and human tissue plasminogen activator (tPA), growth hormone, urokinase, and nitric oxide synthase genes.[82-93] The efficiencies of retroviral and electroporation transfection of endothelial cells are 1-2% and 10%, respectively.[85,89] Adenovirus-mediated gene transfer is highly dose dependent and produces only transient transfection.[87] Transfection and endothelial cell seeding are procedures each of which requires long time periods of laboratory work, which again raises a red flag among the pragmatists concerned with

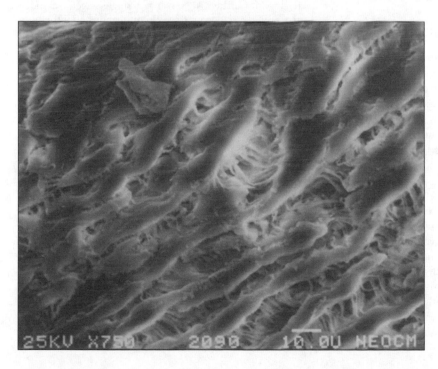

Fig. 3.2. Scanning electron micrograph immediately after the electrostatic seeding of human umbilical vein endothelial cells (+1.0 Volt applied for 16 minutes) on ePTFE (GORE-TEX®; 30 μm internodal distance) illustrating the complete, morphologically mature coverage of the nodal areas (Magnification x750).

additional genotypic (other than desired alteration) or phenotypic changes and infections. Transplantation of transfected endothelial cells does not appear to affect initial seeding densities.[82] However, retention of endothelial cells is significantly reduced due to retroviral transfection (no data available for electroporated cells). This decrease in retention is in addition to the already expected loss using a gravitational seeding procedure. Thus, further refinement of all of these techniques is imperative in order for them to be embraced clinically.

It is speculated that the electrostatic endothelial cell seeding device previously described may be used to successfully seed/transfect endothelial cells simultaneously in 16 minutes. The concept is being evaluated by applying high voltage pulses (> 200 Volts) while performing the low voltage, +1.0 Volt, seeding procedure. The high voltage pulses (100 μs duration) are either a single pulse or multiple (i.e., 4) pulses at set time intervals (4-5 seconds). It is expected that the electroporation pulses will be applied midway through the seeding procedure when the endothelial cells and DNA will be in close proximity at the graft luminal surface. It is expected that the small electric field used for seeding (and maintained continuously) will allow increased cellular transfection by maintaining the cellular membrane pores created for a slightly longer time period. This speculation is based on the theory that the cell membrane pores are created by protrusions of cellular membrane structures (and/or underlying cortical layer) induced by application of an electric field.[94] This, in conjunction with the electrophoretic motion of the DNA towards the graft luminal surface and the endothelial cells, is expected to contribute to an increased transfection efficiency. Currently, electroporation techniques have a maximum overall transfection efficiency of 10-20%.[95,96] Along with the increase in transfection efficiency, the electrostatic seeding/transfection procedure may also contribute to increased or maintained cellular retentions upon implantation when compared to currently available techniques.

Conclusion

A wealth of information has been derived from research protocols investigating the potential of endothelial cell seeding in improving small diameter vascular graft function. Realization of the hypothesized potential of endothelial cell seeding for patients has remained heretofore elusive. This may be due in large measure to the complex biology of the vascular wall and the disruption created by the transplantation process. One wonders, however, whether or not that potential has yet been adequately tested, as various traditional methodologies and techniques for endothelial cell transplantation have all been, to one extent or another, inadequate when applied clinically. The technique of electrostatic endothelial cell seeding which we have described in this chapter in the historic context of endothelial cell seeding offers the potential to circumvent or alleviate many of those technical issues. It is with renewed enthusiasm then that we are revisiting the technology of endothelial cell seeding of vascular grafts armed with new technical information and new insights into the biology of vascular cells.

References

1. Berger K, Sauvage LR, Rao AA, Wood S. Healing of arterial prostheses in man: Its incompleteness. Ann Surg 1972; 175:119-27.
2. Sauvage LR, Berger KE, Wood SJ et al. Interspecies heal of porous arterial prostheses. Arch Surg 1974; 109:698-706.
3. Clowes AW, Kirkman TR, Reidy MA. Mechanisms of arterial graft healing. Rapid transmural capillary ingrowth provides a source of intimal endothelium and smooth muscle in porous PTFE prostheses. Am J Pathol 1986; 123:221-9.
4. Schmidt SP, Meerbaum SO, Sharp WV. Endothelial-lined vascular prostheses. In: Wise DL, Trantolo DJ, Altobelli DE et al., eds. Encyclopedic handbook of biomaterials and bioengineering, Part B: Applications. New York: Marcel Dekker, Inc., 1995:1089-1110.
5. Voorhees AB, Jaretski A, Blakemore AH. Use of tubes constructed from vinyon 'n' cloth in bridging arterial deficits. Ann Surg 1952; 135:332-8.
6. Blakemore A, Voorhees AB. The use of tubes constructed of vinyon 'n' cloth in bridging arterial deficits: Experimental and clinical. Ann Surg 1954; 140:324-30.
7. Clagett GP, Burkel WE, Sharefkin JB et al. Platelet activity in vivo in dogs with arterial prostheses seeded with endothelial cells. Circulation 1984; 69:632-9.
8. Kempczinski RF, Ramalanjaona GR, Douville C et al. Thrombogenicity of a fibronectin-coated, experimental polytetrafluoroethylene graft. Surgery 1987; 101:439-44.
9. Clowes AW, Reidy MA. Mechanisms of arterial graft failure: The role of cellular proliferation. Ann NY Acad Sci 1987; 516:673-8.
10. Clowes AW, Kirkman TR, Clowes MM. Mechanisms of arterial graft failure. II. Chronic endothelial cell and smooth muscle cell proliferation in healing polytetrafluoroethylene prostheses. J Vasc Surg 1986; 3:877-84.
11. Clowes AW, Gown AM, Hanson SR et al. Mechanism of arterial graft failure I: Role of cellular proliferation in early healing of PTFE grafts. Am J Path 1985; 118:43-54.
12. Herring M, Gardner A, Glover J. A single-staged technique for seeding vascular grafts with autogenous endothelium. Surgery 1978; 84:848-54.
13. Herring M, Gardner A, Glover J. Seeding human arterial prostheses with mechanically derived endothelium. J Vasc Surg 1984; 1:279-89.
14. Stanley JC, Graham LM, Burkel WE. Endothelial cell seeded synthetic vascular grafts. In: Vascular Graft Update: Safety and Performance. Philadelphia: ASTM, 1986:33-43.
15. Graham LM, Burkel WE, Ford JW et al. Expanded polytetrafluoroethylene vascular prostheses seeded with enzymatically derived and cultured canine endothelial cells. Surgery 1982; 91:550-9.
16. Sharp WV, Schmidt SP, Meerbaum SO et al. Derivation of human microvascular endothelial cells for prosthetic vascular graft seeding. Ann Vasc Surg 1989; 3:104-7.
17. Jaffe EA, Nachman R, Becker C et al. Culture of human endothelial cells derived from umbilical veins. Identification by morphologic and immunologic criteria. J Clin Invest 1973; 52:2745-56.
18. Bourke BM, Roche WR, Appleberg M. Endothelial cell harvest for seeding vascular prostheses: The influence of technique on cell function, viability, and number. J Vasc Surg 1986; 4:257-63.

19. Gimbrone MA, Cotran RS, Folkman J. Human vascular endothelial cells in culture. Growth and DNA synthesis. J Cell Biol 1974; 60:673-84.

20. Sharefkin JB, Van Wart HE, Cruess DF et al. Adult human endothelial cell enzymatic harvesting. Estimates of efficiency and comparisons of crude and partially purified bacterial collagenase preparations by replicate microwell culture and fibronectin degradation measured by enzyme-linked immunosorbent assay. J Vasc Surg 1986; 4:567-77.

21. Jarrell BE, Williams SK, Stokes G et al. Use of freshly isolated capillary endothelial cells for the immediate establishment of a monolayer on a vascular graft at surgery. Surgery 1986; 100:392-9.

22. Williams SK, Wang TF, Castrillo R et al. Liposuction-derived human fat used for vascular graft sodding contains endothelial cells and not mesothelial cells as the major cell type. J Vasc Surg 1994; 19:916-23.

23. Rupnick MA, Hubbard FA, Pratt K et al. Endothelialization of vascular prosthetic surfaces after seeding or sodding with human microvascular endothelial cells. J Vasc Surg 1989; 9:788-95.

24. Graham LM, Vinter DW, Ford JW et al. Endothelial cell seeding of prosthetic vascular grafts. Early experimental studies with cultured autologous canine endothelium. Arch Surg 1980; 115:929-33.

25. Schmidt SP, Sharp WV, Evancho MM et al. Endothelial cell seeding of prosthetic vascular grafts-current status. In: Szycher M, ed. High Performance Biomaterials. Lancaster; Technomic Publishing Co., 1991:483-96.

26. Yates SG, Barros AAB, Berger K et al. The preclotting of porous arterial prostheses. Ann Surg 1978; 188:611-22.

27. Anderson JS, Price TM, Hanson SR et al. In vitro endothelialization of small-caliber vascular grafts. Surgery 1987; 101:577-86.

28. Foxall TL, Auger KR, Callow AD et al. Adult human endothelial cell coverage of small-caliber dacron and polytetrafluoroethylene vascular prostheses in vitro. J Surg Res 1986; 41:158-72.

29. Mazzucotelli JP, Roudiere JL, Bernex F et al. A new device for endothelial cell seeding of a small-caliber vascular prosthesis. Artif Organs 1993; 17:787-90.

30. Kempczinski RF, Rosenman JE, Pearce WH et al. Endothelial cell seeding of a new PTFE vascular prosthesis. J Vasc Surg 1985; 2:424-9.

31. Van Wachem PB, Stronck JWS, Koers-Zuideveld R et al. Vacuum cell seeding: A new method for the fast application of an evenly distributed cell layer on porous vascular grafts. Biomaterials 1990; 11:602-6.

32. Bowlin GL. Electrostatic endothelial cell seeding of vascular prostheses. Doctoral Dissertation, The University of Akron, 1996:1-354.

33. Rosenman JE, Kempczinski RF, Pearce WH et al. Kinetics of endothelial cell seeding. J Vasc Surg 1985; 2:778-84.

34. Shindo S, Takagi A, Whittemore AD. Improved patency of collagen-impregnated grafts after in vitro autogenous endothelial cell seeding. J Vasc Surg 1987; 6:325-32.

35. Prendiville EJ, Coleman JE, Callow AD et al. Increased in vitro incubation time of endothelial cells on fibronectin-treated ePTFE increases cell retention in blood flow. Eur J Vasc Surg 1991; 5:311-9.

36. Sentissi JM, Ramberg K, O'Donnell K et al. The effect of flow on vascular endothelial cells grown in tissue culture on polytetrafluoroethylene grafts. Surgery 1986; 99:337-43.

37. Budd JS, Allen KE, Hartley G et al. The effect of preformed confluent endothelial cell monolayers on the patency and thrombogenicity of small calibre vascular grafts. Eur J Vasc Surg 1991; 5:397-405.

38. Turgeon ML. Clinical Hematology: Theory and Procedure. Boston: Little, Brown, and Co., 1988:279-86.

39. Kesler KA, Herring MB, Arnold MP et al. Enhanced strength of endothelial attachment on polyester elastomer and polytetrafluoroethylene graft surfaces with fibronectin substrate. J Vasc Surg 1986; 3:58-64.

40. Ramalanjaona G, Kempczinski RF, Rosenman JE et al. The effect of fibronectin coating on endothelial cell kinetics on polytetrafluoroethylene grafts. J Vasc Surg 1986; 3:264-72.

41. Seeger JM, Klingman N. Improved in vivo endothelialization of prosthetic grafts by surface modification with fibronectin. J Vasc Surg 1988; 8:476-82.

42. Pratt KJ, Jarrell BE, Williams SK et al. Kinetics of endothelial cell-surface attachment forces. J Vasc Surg 1988; 7:591-9.

43. Van Wachem PB, Vreriks CM, Beugeling T et al. The influence of protein adsorption on interactions of cultured human endothelial cells with polymers. J Biomed Mater Res 1987; 21:701-18.

44. Van Wachem PB, Beugeling T, Mallens BW et al. Deposition of endothelial fibronectin on polymeric surfaces. Biomaterials 1988; 9:121-3.

45. Schneider A, Melmed RN, Schwalb H et al. An improved method for endothelial cell seeding on polytetrafluoroethylene small caliber vascular grafts. J Vasc Surg 1992; 15:649-56.

46. Lee YS, Park DK, Kim YB et al. Endothelial cell seeding onto the extracellular matrix of fibroblasts for the development of a small diameter polyurethane vessel. ASAIO J 1993; 39: M740-5.

47. Bellon JM, Bujan J, Honduvilla NG et al. Endothelial cell seeding of polytetrafluoroethylene vascular prostheses coated with a fibroblastic matrix. Ann Vasc Surg 1993; 7:549-55.

48. Gosselin C, Vorp DA, Warty V et al. ePTFE coating with fibrin glue, FGF-1, and heparin: Effect on retention of seeded endothelial cells. J Surg Res 1996; 60:327-332.

49. Williams SK, Jarrell BE, Friend L et al. Adult human endothelial cell compatibility with prosthetic graft material. J Surg Res 1985; 38:618-29.

50. Kaehler J, Zilla P, Fasol R et al. Precoating substrate and surface configuration determine adherence and spreading of seeded endothelial cells on polytetrafluoroethylene grafts. J Vasc Surg 1989; 9:535-41.

51. Lindblad B, Burkel WE, Wakefield TW et al. Endothelial cell seeding efficiency onto expanded polytetrafluoroethylene grafts with different coatings. ACTA Chir Scand 1986; 152:653-6.

52. Ramalanjaona GR, Kempczinski RF, Ogle JD et al. Fibronectin coating of an experimental PTFE vascular prosthesis. J Surg Res 1986; 41:479-83.

53. Longnecker DE, Murphy FL. Introduction to anesthesia. 8th ed., Philadelphia: W.B. Saunders Co., Harcourt Brace Jovanovich, Inc., 1992:419-27.

54. Guyton AC. Textbook of medical physiology. 8th ed. Philadelphia: W.B. Saunders Co., Harcourt Brace Jovanovich, Inc., 1991:269-71.

55. Sawyer PN, Harshaw DH. Electroosmotic characteristics of canine aorta and vena cava walls. Biophy J 1966; 6:653-63.

56. Srinivasan S, Sawyer PN. Role of surface charge of the blood vessel wall, blood cells, and prosthetic material in intravascular thrombosis. J Colloid Sci 1970; 32:456-63.

57. Sawyer PN, Srinivasan S. Studies on the biophysics of intravascular thrombosis. Am J Surg 967; 114:42-59.

58. Lowell J. The electrification of polymers by metals. J Phys D: Appl Phys 1976; 9:1571-85.

59. Yu ZZ, Watson PK, Facci JS. The contact charging of PTFE by mercury: The effect of a thiophene monolayer on charge exchange. J Phys D: Appl Phys 1990; 23:1207-11.

60. Yu ZZ, Keith PK. Contact charge accumulation and reversal on polystyrene and PTFE films upon repeated contacts with mercury. J Phys D: Appl Phys 1989; 22:798-801.

61. Abramson HA. The electrophoresis of the blood platelets of the horse with the reference to their origin and to thrombus formation. J Exp Med 1928; 47:677-83.

62. Marmur A, Gill WN, Ruckenstein E. Kinetics of cell deposition under action of an external force. Bull Math Biol 1976; 38:713-21.

63. Ruckenstein E, Prieve DC. Dynamics of cell deposition on surfaces. J Theor Biol 1975; 51:429-38.

64. Ruckenstein E, Marmur A, Rakower SR. Sedimentation and adhesion of platelets onto horizontal glass surface. Thrombus Haemostas 1976; 36:334-42.

65. Van Wachem PB, Hogt AH, Beugeling T et al. Adhesion of cultured human endothelial cells onto methacrylate polymers with varying surface wettability and charge. Biomaterials 1987; 8:322-9.

66. Macarak EJ, Howard PS. Adhesion of endothelial cells to extracellular matrix proteins. J Cell Phys 1983; 116:76-86.

67. Sugimoto Y. Effects on the adhesion and locomotion of mouse fibroblasts by their interacting with differently charged substrates. Exp Cell Res 1981; 135:39-45.

68. Schakenraad JM, Arends J, Busscher HJ et al. Kinetics of cell spreading on protein precoated substrata: A study of interfacial aspects. Biomaterials 1989; 10:43-50.

69. Niu S, Matsuda T, Oka T. Endothelialization on various segmented polyurethanes: Cellular behavior and its substrate dependency. ASAIO Trans 1990; 36: M164-8.

70. Van Wachem PB, Schakenraad JM, Feijen J et al. Adhesion and spreading of cultured endothelial cells on modified and unmodified poly(ethyleneterephthalate): A morphological study. Biomaterials 1989; 10:532-9.

71. Fink DG, Christiansen D, eds. Electronics engineers' handbook. 3rd ed. New York: McGraw-Hill Book Co., 1989:6:29-64.

72. Halliday D, Resnick R. Fundamentals of physics. 2nd ed. New York: John Wiley & Sons, Inc., 1981:484-502.

73. Ando T, Kobayashi N, Munekata E. Electrostatic potential around actin. In: Sugi H, Pollack GH, eds. Mechanism of myofilament sliding in muscle contraction. New York: Plenum Press, 1993:361-76.

74. Gottlieb AI, Langille BL, Wong MKK et al. Biology of disease: Structure and function of the endothelial cytoskelaton. Lab Invest 1991; 65:123-37.

75. Jaffe EA, Mosher DF. Synthesis of fibronectin by cultured human endothelial cells. J Exp Med 1978; 147:1779-91.

76. Jaffe EA, Minick CR, Adelman B et al. Synthesis of basement membrane collagen by cultured human endothelial cells. J Exp Med 1976; 144:209-25.

77. Howard BV, Macarak EJ, Gunson D et al. Characterization of the collagen synthesized by endothelial cells in culture. Proc Natl Acad Sci USA 1976; 73:2361-4.

78. Nabel EG, Plautz G, Nabel GJ. Gene transfer into vascular cells. JACC 1991; 17:189B-94B.

79. Callow AD. The vascular endothelial cell as a vehicle for gene therapy. J Vasc Surg 1990; 11:793-8.

80. Zweibel JA, Freeman SM, Kantoff PW et al. High-level recombinant gene expression in rabbit endothelial cells transduced by retroviral vectors. Science 1989; 243:220-2.

81. Ryan US, Hayes BA, Maxwell G et al. Endothelial cells as vehicles for continuous release of recombinant gene products. In: Zilla P, Fasol R, Callow A, eds. Applied cardiovascular biology. Basel: S. Karger, 1990:22-9.

82. Sackman JE, Freeman MB, Petersen MG et al. Synthetic vascular grafts seeded with genetically modified endothelium in the dog: Evaluation of the effect of seeding technique and retroviral vector on cell persistence in vivo. Cell Trans 1995; 4:219-35.

83. Huber TS, Welling TH, Sarkar R et al. Effects of retroviral-mediated tissue plasminogen activator gene transfer and expression on adherence and proliferation of canine endothelial cells seeded onto expanded polytetrafluoroethylene. J Vasc Surg 1995; 22:795-803.

84. Powell JT, Klaasse Bos JM, Van Mourik JA. The uptake and expression of the factor VIII and reporter genes by vascular cells. FEBES 1992; 303:173-7.

85. Kahn ML, Lee SW, Dichek DA. Optimization of retroviral vector-mediated gene transfer into endothelial cells in vitro. Circ Res 1992; 71:1508-17.

86. Hong Z, Guangbin Z, Xiaojun Z et al. Enhanced adeno-associated virus vector expression by adenovirus protein-cationic liposome complex. Chinese Med J 1995; 108:332-7.

87. Hong Z, Guangbin Z, Airu Z et al. Adenovirus mediated gene transfer of vascular smooth muscle cells and endothelial cells in vitro. Chinese Med J 1995; 108:493-6.

88. Von der Leyen HE, Gibbons GH, Morishita R et al. Gene therapy inhibiting neointimal vascular lesions: In vivo transfer of endothelial cell nitric oxide synthase gene. Proc Natl Acad Sci 1995; 92:1137-41.

89. Kotnis RA, Thompson MM, Eady SL et al. Attachment, replication and thrombogenecity of genetically modified endothelial cells. Eur J Vasc Endovasc Surg 1995; 9:335-40.

90. Wilson JM, Birinyi LK, Salomon RN et al. Implantation of vascular grafts lined with genetically modified endothelial cells. Science 1989; 244:1344-6.

91. Dunn PF, Newman KD, Jones M et al. Seeding of vascular grafts with genetically modified endothelial cells: Secretion of recombinant TPA results in decreased seeded cell retention in vitro and in vivo. Circulation 1996; 93:1439-46.

92. Schwachtgen JL, Ferreira V, Meyer D et al. Optimization of the transfection of human endothelial cells by electroporation. Biotechiques 1994; 5:882-7.

93. Kotnis RA, Thompson MM, Eady SL et al. Optimisation of gene transfer into vascular endothelial cells using electroporation. Eur J Vasc Endovasc Surg 1995; 9:71-9

94. Popov SV, Margolis LB. Formation of cell outgrowths by external force: A model study. J Cell Sci 1988; 90:379-89.

95. Spencer SC. Electroporation technique of DNA transfection. In: Murray EJ, ed. Methods in molecular biology. Clifton: The Humana Press, Inc., 1991:45-52.

96. Davis LG, Dibner MD, Battey JF. Basic methods in molecular biology. Norwalk: Appleton & Lange, 1986:293-95.

CHAPTER 4

Surface Precoating in the 1980s:
A First Taste of Cell-Matrix Interactions

J. Vincent Smyth, Michael G. Walker

Technical difficulties and the frequent lack of available saphenous vein for peripheral arterial reconstruction resulted in the development of a variety of prosthetic materials from which grafts could be constructed. Of these, polyester elastomer (Dacron) and expanded polytetrafluoroethylene (ePTFE) emerged as the most successful in clinical practice, and remain leaders in the field today. However, small caliber prosthetic grafts have consistently shown lower patency rates, especially when passing across the knee joint, when compared with autologous vein conduits. The understanding that the endothelial lining of vein grafts was responsible for the improved patency rates achieved in peripheral bypass naturally led to attempts to create such a lining on prosthetic grafts, when explants showed that no significant endothelialization of such grafts occurs naturally in humans, contrary to the results seen in animals where virtually complete endothelial linings develop on prosthetic grafts in a matter of weeks.

Almost all of the work performed up to 1980 utilized animal tissue models such as bovine, canine or murine endothelium, and extremely promising results had been repeatedly achieved both in vivo and in vitro in terms of reduction in graft thrombogenicity, resistance to infection, accelerated re-endothelialization and improved patency.[1-6] In order to make the transition to clinical practice, however, it was clear that human cell lines would be required, and human umbilical vein endothelial cells (Huvecs) were used as the principal experimental model until Jarrell showed that human adult endothelial cells (HAECs) could be harvested from saphenous veins and cultured.[7] This work has now advanced so that the acute enzymatic harvesting of autologous vein can be routinely achieved, with virtually complete denudation of the donor vein segment and a large proportion of harvested cells remaining viable for culture. There is now extensive experience with both cell lines toward the desired end point of successful graft seeding to the rapid development of an endothelial monolayer that resists the shear stress of flow.[8]

Almost as soon as the successful culture of Huvecs on prosthetic graft material was first reported, it was clear that human cell lines were more fragile and fastidious in their requirements than the canine or bovine endothelial cultures that had principally been used up to this point. The establishment of a culture was slower even under optimal conditions, and when achieved these were less hardy and prone to failure from infection. Even so, successful culture was reported on all the common graft materials, with typical appearances of cobblestone morphology and cells expressing endothelium-specific markers such as vWF. Although human cell lines showed slower cell division and spreading across the culture surfaces than animal cell lines, even under the optimal experimental conditions of tissue culture, the main reason for the delayed development of the monolayer was found to be low cell attachment to the graft.

Endothelial Cell Attachment to Prosthetic Grafts

The first seeding experiments were carried out in what we would now classify as a static system, where the cells were introduced to the graft surface in a suspension of culture medium and allowed to settle on the graft over a period of time, then cultured in situ. Early work relied on qualitative phase contrast microscopy of the seeded surface at intervals after seeding to assess degree of coverage. Later, the work of Sharefkin led to the use of the radio-isotope [111]Indium as an endothelial cell label,[9] and attachment to grafts could be accurately quantified. It was discovered that prosthetic grafts exhibit a uniformly poor surface for retention of seeded cells, typically around 4% for ePTFE,[10,11] while cell adherence to plain Dacron was negligible because of its porosity, resulting in leakage of the seeding solution.[12,13] Three approaches to the problem of rapidly developing a monolayer were explored.

The proportion of seeded cells that remained attached to the graft could be increased by increasing the length of time that the seeding suspension was exposed to the graft material.[10,14-16] However, the seeding kinetics indicated that the rate of increase fell off after around 30 minutes, and that even with exposure times of over 60 minutes, the development of a confluent monolayer was not significantly accelerated. Additionally, prolonged incubation times are incompatible with the constraints of the operating room.

Using more endothelial cells per graft area in the seeding solution, a higher seeding density, produced a greater number of cells attaching to the graft, but only in the same proportion and consequently with an enormous waste of seeded cells.[15,17] At established attachment rates to plain

grafts, up to 20 times as many cells as were required to form a monolayer would be needed for seeding, thus greatly increasing the required cell numbers. Although this could be accommodated by the use of preculture in the laboratory,[18] this method is not compatible with routine surgical practice and would necessitate a preliminary operation for vein harvest and carry risks of disease transmission or graft infection. To overcome the problem of limited cell harvests, the use of microvascular (capillary) endothelium[19] and mesothelial[20] cells have been proposed, but these only offer a partial solution in terms of available cell numbers, as they share many of the attachment and adhesion difficulties experienced with Huvecs and HAECs, and raise additional problems with tissue availability. As a consequence, to achieve rapid development of confluence in the clinical arena where such large cell numbers could not be obtained acutely using established methods, either new sources of endothelial cells would be required or cell attachment significantly improved to permit successful seeding at subconfluent densities.

It had been noticed that the results of human cell seeding work did not parallel those seen in the animal in vivo models of prosthetic graft seeding. Significantly better attachment was seen in the latter, and it was realized that the preclot typically used for the endothelial cell suspension acted as a graft coating, improving cell adherence. By using preclot or serum to coat the graft prior to seeding the endothelial cells, attachment rates could be dramatically improved to over 60% of seeded cells in a range of models.[10,21]

As a result, investigators began precoating the culture dishes and seeding surfaces with a variety of matrices before the cells were exposed, and similar improvements in cell attachment were seen[11,22-27] (Figs. 4.1-4.3). Comparative studies of a range of potential graft surface coatings were made. Because of Dacron's inherent porosity, gelatin or collagen-sealed grafts were frequently used, and this not surprisingly

Fig. 4.1. Cell attachment to prosthetic grafts as a function of graft coating.

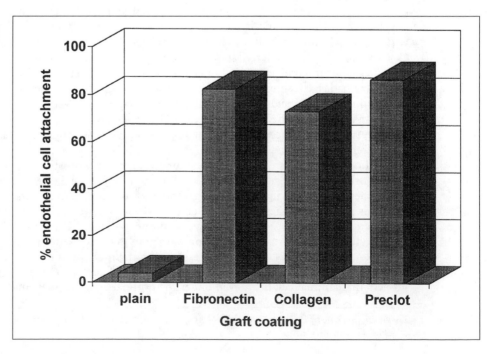

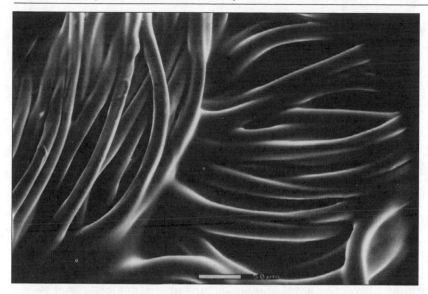

Fig. 4.2. Electron micrograph of uncoated prosthetic graft.

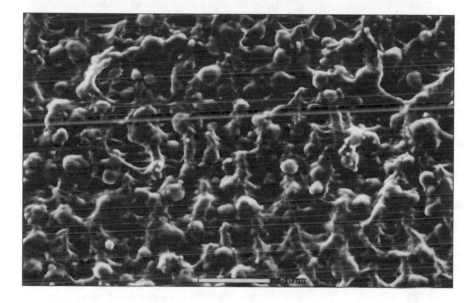

Fig. 4.3. Electron micrograph of fibronectin-coated graft after endothelial seeding.

improved initial cell adherence accordingly, as did all graft coating matrices compared to the plain graft materials.

Histological examination of the vascular endothelium indicated that in the body it was supported by a protein-rich basement membrane layer, and that this layer was produced actively at least in part by the endothelium. Examination of endothelial cells in culture showed that the adherent cells secreted a similar layer on artificial surfaces[28,29] and that a principal component of the basement membrane was fibronectin (FN).

Following the work of Ramalanjoana[21] and others,[30-32] FN has become the most commonly used seeding matrix because of efficacy and availability, giving consistently high cell adherences in experiments using a variety of graft types, including ePTFE and Dacron. Preclot, serum, plasma, laminin, gelatin, collagen and fibrin glue have also been investigated,[10,27,33-36] the first three because they are readily available in the clinical situation, and the remainder because they, along with fibronectin, are found as native constituents of extracellular matrix. Although preclot, serum and plasma show good rates of endothelial attachment, this is thought to be due to their high FN content. Laminin and collagens I, III and IV have not proved as effective as FN in facilitating endothelial cell attachment. Gelatin-sealed Dacron grafts show good initial cell adherence, but the stability of the gelatin crosslinking under physiological conditions is uncertain, as it degrades and may not provide a suitable matrix for long enough to allow the cells to establish their own FN-rich basement membrane layer on the graft. Fibrin glue has been used successfully in some seeding work, but requires fibrinolytic inhibition prior to use without offering any advantages in terms of cell retention. In the laboratory model, however, almost equivalent results to those with FN have been achieved and, in retrospect, it is clear that one reason for the success of the early animal seeding experiments using prosthetic grafts had been the serendipitous use of FN-rich preclot as a readily available cell suspension to seed the graft, sealing the porous Dacron used in this work.

Many workers have investigated the attachment kinetics of endothelial cells to FN-coated graft surfaces.[10,15,27,37] In the laboratory, the optimum incubation time for cell attachment to a coating matrix appears to be 30 minutes with no significant benefit evident beyond this, though some workers have found as little as 15 minutes adequate. As with uncoated grafts, improved cell attachment is also seen with increasing the seeding density, up to a point whereafter the proportion of seeded cells attaching falls off, though the absolute number continues to increase. The kinetics of improved cell adherence to FN-coated graft surfaces implied some specific binding mechanism, and this was confirmed by the finding that endothelial cells express specific FN receptors on their cell membrane.

Comparative studies of different grafts seem to suggest that ePTFE is a better surface for matrix coating than Dacron, although there is some disagreement between individual studies. This may be related to the nature of the graft surface at the fiber level, with a flatter surface being offered by the multinodal fibrillary construction than the woven or knitted Dacron. Minor refinements in terms of graft composition, pore size, internodal distances or woven vs. knitted Dacron, do not seem to affect the cell seeding kinetics significantly. On precoated grafts, the differences in endothelial cell adherence between graft materials is not striking once the porosity of the Dacron is reduced by sealing the graft with the surface coating, and this can be explained by the production of essentially similar attachment characteristics at the molecular level on the surfaces to which the seeded endothelial cells are exposed.

With the establishment of a FN-rich coating as the optimal seeding surface, several workers have investigated the adsorption kinetics of FN onto prosthetic grafts,[38,39] showing that the development of FN-graft binding is proportional to the FN concentration and the duration of incubation, though there may be minor differences between graft materials. The optimum concentration of FN to use as the seeding matrix has been investigated,[40] and the relationship between the concentration of FN graft coating and rates of endothelial cell adherence approximates first order kinetics to 50 μg/ml, with no benefit obtained by increasing this to 250 μg/ml, further evidence for specific FN-binding sites on the cell surface.

Cell Migration

It had been noted that following seeding, cells initially attached to the graft in a rounded morphology, later developing a more flattened phenotype responsible for the 'cobblestone' appearance of the mature endothelial monolayer.[32] Increased duration of incubation was associated with progression of the cell morphology from rounded and poorly attached, to flattened and adherent, and this was generally accepted to indicate the acclimatization of the seeded cell to the seeding surface. The speedier development of an adherent monolayer following seeding onto prepared graft and culture surfaces was thought to correspond with the more rapid establishment of the flattened phenotype, as noted microscopically.[16,33]

Following flattening, where incomplete confluence results from seeding, the endothelial cells then migrate across the seeding surface to produce a monolayer. By some elegant work using removable discs, the migration of saphenous vein endothelial cells following establishment of healthy cultures was measured on a variety of culture surfaces.[41] These showed that surface precoating not only improves initial adherence, but also promotes cell migration and development of confluence. Again, fibronectin was the most effective coating agent, with gelatin and extracellular matrix showing some advantage over uncoated culture flasks. Interestingly, laminin, despite being a constituent of the cell substratum in vivo, did not improve cell migration, implying that its role in the body is not primarily concerned with maintenance of endothelial monolayer integrity. In addition to enhancement of cell-surface adhesion, seeded cells also proliferate more rapidly on precoated surfaces,[22] and some groups developed variations of the surface coatings specifically designed to improve graft endothelialization by promoting cell migration and proliferation.[42] Coatings enriched with growth factors such as FGF have been shown to enhance ingrowth through the graft interstices[43] and the development of an endothelial lining with a minimum of smooth muscle hyperplasia.[44] The ability of small diameter vascular prostheses to adsorb and retain ECGF under flow conditions has been clearly demonstrated[45] though in the rabbit model used, no differences in graft re-endothelialization was seen at 1 month. Although the combination of growth factor-enhanced graft coatings and human endothelial cell seeding would appear to be a promising avenue of investigation, there have been no reports of such work.

Endothelial Cell Retention Under Flow Conditions

The advantages of precoated over plain grafts also extend to dynamic seeding systems, in which the seeded grafts are exposed to the shear stress of flow, though different groups have achieved wide variation in results. A range of levels of flow, and thus shear stresses, have been used, including systems that approximate rates of flow seen in grafts.[46,47] Electron microscopy of seeded grafts exposed to pulsatile flow systems show that a proportion of endothelial loss occurs in areas where the underlying graft is exposed by loss of surface coating,[48] and that this is more marked with FN-coating than with preclot, which may account for the differences some workers have seen in levels of cell retention. The monolayer's resistance to denudation under flow is a combination of the strength of the endothelial cell attachment to the matrix, and of the matrix to the graft. With regard to the former, factors previously observed to improve cell adherence such as duration of incubation, and also degree of confluence and interval prior to commencement of flow, are also relevant to resisting denudation under flow. Established endothelial monolayers formed by culture on the graft resist flow better than acutely attached cells,[46,49,50] although previously noted problems with duration of incubation or graft preculture apply in terms of clinical applicability. Cell loss appears to occur in a biphasic pattern,[47,51] with an initial rapid rate presumably corresponding to loosely attached cells or areas of coating, which settles after a few minutes to a slower, more steady rate of loss (Fig. 4.4). However, we have noted that within a flow system sudden changes in the level of pulsatile shear stress result in a further period of rapid loss which then returns to the slower rate.

The bond between coating and graft has been less thoroughly investigated, but seems to depend on the nature of the graft, with gelatin-coated Dacron performing significantly less well than ePTFE.[38,40] Whether the FN-gelatin or the gelatin-Dacron interface is the important one is as yet uncertain, but clinically may not be particularly important, as ePTFE is the usual graft of choice in the infrainguinal region where it is expected that seeding will be most applicable. Up to 75% of applied matrix may be lost in the first 15 minutes after restoration of flow, but thereafter the graft-matrix bond appears stable within the time scale of the laboratory model. Electron microscopy of coated grafts after exposure to flow shows clearly that this early loss occurs at least partly by detachment of regions of matrix from the graft, presumably where the matrix-graft bond is less established, with matrix solubility probably contributing more towards the later, slow rate of matrix loss.

Seeding of Native Vascular Surfaces

The difficulties in achieving an endothelial monolayer on prosthetic grafts immediately after seeding, given the almost inevitable shortfall in numbers of seeded cells, ethical and technical problems with cell or graft preculture, and the high losses from even FN-coated graft surfaces under flow, have prompted workers to examine the seeding potential of native arterial surfaces. The use of autologous cells and native conduits avoids any potential immune or foreign body reaction which might result in cell loss, and seeding following angioplasty or endarterectomy have both been considered. The advantages of seeding such regions are that the area for seeding is lower due to shorter segments being involved, thus increasing the seeding density without needing an increase in the numbers of seeded cells, and that cell attachment and retention on autologous native surfaces might be expected to be optimal.

Seeding after endothelial denudation by angioplasty balloon has been assessed in a rabbit iliac vein model[52] using a double balloon catheter-based system and has shown that acute seeding with autologous cells on a relatively short time scale can restore a monolayer,[53] which is maintained on restoration of flow. This monolayer retains functional integrity[54] and may reduce neointimal hyperplasia.[55] However, the relevance of these results to chronic arterial disease in humans remains uncertain, especially with previous experience of promising animal seeding studies. Endothelial cell seeding following endarterectomy in animals has also given hope, demonstrating most of the advantages seen in seeded prosthetic grafts.[56-60]

Work using human cell lines has demonstrated excellent cell attachment to both endarterectomy and vein angioplasty surfaces,[61-63] and in the latter model flow studies have suggested cell retention kinetics similar to coated grafts. Following endarterectomy the exposed surface is very similar to that on which the endothelium normally rests and is high in FN, which probably accounts for the optimal attachment rates seen, and HAECs seeded onto endarterectomized vessels have been shown to be capable of forming a monolayer,[61] again retaining functional integrity.[64]

Mechanism of Cell Adherence

As a result of the improvements in seeding efficiency produced by surface coatings, increasing interest has developed in the interactions between endothelial cells and the matrix. The attachment and migration characteristics of the endothelial cell are due to the presence of a wide range of adhesion molecules and ligand-specific receptors on the cell membrane.[65] Many of the receptors have multiple, overlapping roles in different pathways, or respond to more than one signal molecule. Variation in ligand affinity and patterns of receptor activation are common and the degree of complexity of the intracellular responses to the extracellular environment is only now becoming more fully

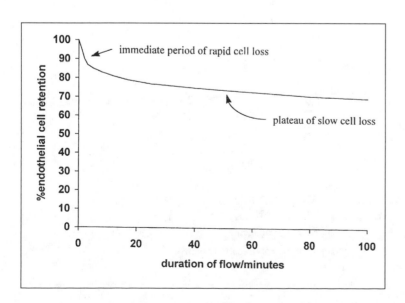

Fig. 4.4. Cell retention on seeded grafts under flow.

appreciated. Some receptors are endothelial cell specific, some are shared with other vascular cells such as platelets or leukocytes, and some also occur on other vessel wall cell types including smooth muscle cells and fibroblasts. Because of their differential actions, different classes of adhesion molecules are frequently asymmetrically arranged between the luminal and abluminal cell membrane (Fig. 4.5).

There are three main families of adhesion molecules present on endothelial cells, though classification is amended from time to time as new members are continually being identified and characterized, and many are known by more than one name. The three major adhesion molecules families consist of the selectins or leukocyte adhesion molecules (ELAMs), responsible for initial capture of circulating leukocytes in response to inflammatory mediators; the immunoglobulin superfamily, also implicated in cell-cell interactions; and the integrins, involved in both cell-substratum and cell-cell interactions.

The selectins present on endothelial cells comprise two major groups; E-selectin or ELAM-1, and P-selectin or granule membrane protein-140 (GMP-140). These are induced by inflammatory mediators and promote the adherence of leukocytes to affected regions of endothelium via leukocyte surface ligands such as fucose groups. They are located on the luminal membrane surface and play little part in endothelium-substratum interactions. The immunoglobulin superfamily contains several classes, differing in the length and composition of a string of immunoglobulin domains which lie on the luminal side of the endothelial cell membrane, attached to a peptide chain that extends through this to a cytoplasmic terminal carboxyl group. They include the intercellular adhesion molecules (ICAMs) -1, -2, and -3; vascular cell adhesion molecule-1 (VCAM-1); and platelet endothelial cell adhesion molecule-1 (PECAM-1). ICAM-1 and VCAM-1 are inducible in response to circulating inflamma-

tory mediators, ICAM-2 and ICAM-3 are constitutively produced, but all bind to circulating leukocytes. PECAM-1 is constitutively produced and binds platelets in addition. Again, these molecules are principally involved in the endothelial response to inflammation, and these groups are therefore not further considered.

Cell-substratum interactions such as the endothelial cell adherence to prosthetic grafts and coatings are mediated by the integrin family of adhesion molecules,[66] which are 10- to 100-fold more common on the cell membrane than selectins or immunoglobulin-like adhesion molecules, and are present principally on the abluminal surface. Integrins are heterodimeric molecules, each subtype being composed of a noncovalently bonded pair of α and β subunits, each of which has multiple variants. There are several subclasses, distinguished by their β subunit, though their specific ligand is to a large extent determined by the α subunit. They bind with relatively low affinity to their ligands, made up for in large part by their frequency of expression, allowing multiple weak bonds to the substratum rather than a few strong links, and thus facilitating cell spread and migration without loss of firm adhesion, the 'Velcro' theory of cell attachment. Ligand binding is cation dependent, Ca^{2+} or Mg^{2+} depending on the integrin, bound to specific sites on the α subunit.

The VLA group, identified by a β_1 subunit, includes specific receptors found on the abluminal endothelial cell membrane for fibronectin, laminin and collagen. A β_2 subunit identifies the leucam group which are found on circulating inflammatory cells and bind to ICAMs on endothelial cells. The cytoadhesin group of integrins, with a β_3 subunit, includes low specificity, multiligand receptors binding fibrinogen, fibronectin, vitronectin, thrombospondin, laminin and vWF. Individual moieties with β_4-β_8 subunits binding a variety of basement membrane proteins, including those mentioned previously, have also been identified.

Fig. 4.5. Vascular endothelial cell adhesion molecules.

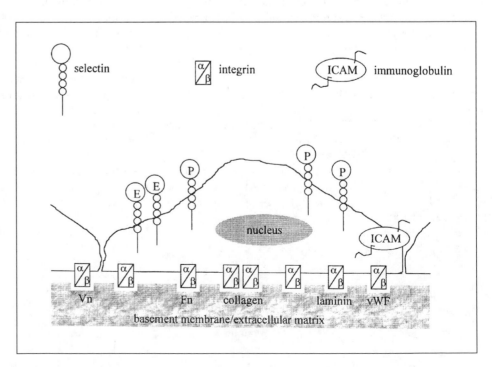

The action of the integrins is a transmembrane link between the outside of the cell and the internal cytoskeleton. On ligand binding, the intracellular end of the β moiety binds to α actin, which stimulates assembly of attachment constructs, preventing the integrin from being pulled out of the cell. In addition to allowing motility and morphological changes by the endothelial cell, integrins can propagate extracellular matrix molecule orientation by the alignment of the resulting cytoskeletal elements, and by giving direction to the matrix molecules being laid down by the cell; this organization can be passed on to adjacent cells.

Nonendothelial Cell Lines

Although most work has concentrated on the interactions between the seeding surface and the endothelial cells, the nature of the graft coating also has important effects on other cell types that come into contact. The ability of myofibroblasts and circulating macrophages to produce mitogens and growth factors that influence endothelial cells has been well documented,[67] and these cell species can respond to stimulation by graft materials and coatings.[68] This has been clearly shown in work on both polygalactin bioresorbable prostheses and Dacron, where macrophage activation from graft interaction results in release of FGF and the stimulation of endothelial ingrowth. Bioresorbable prostheses differ from Dacron in their ability to promote mitogenesis in the macrophages in addition to cytokine release,[69] indicating differences between graft materials.

Future Directions

Results from work on endothelial cell responses to stimuli have shown that the monolayer is subject, and responds, to a wide range of physical and biological factors. Both expansile stress from arterial pulsatility[70,71] and the shear stress of flow[46,72] elicit functional changes in the expression of biologically important factors by the endothelium. The cells are also subject to circulating agents, and locally produced paracrine factors deriving from leukocytes, platelets and macrophages.[73-78] In addition, the nature of the underlying layer on which the monolayer is developed affects the endothelial cell function, a feature of both apparently passive basement membrane components,[79-81] as well as other cell types in the supporting layers.[82,83]

Where the 1970s were the decade of developing viable cell culture, and the 1980s were primarily concerned with the kinetics of seeded cells' interactions with the graft surface, the 1990s have so far shown an explosion in understanding of the molecular biology of the adhesion mechanisms of the endothelial cell and of the responses and relationships between viable seeded cells and the environment within which they are placed. Powerful research laboratory tools such as the polymerase chain reaction and advances in genetic manipulation techniques are proving important in the growing appreciation of the complexity of the largest organ in the body, and making sense of the active biological role of what was once thought to be a passive nonthrombogenic layer.

References

1. Claggett GP, Burkel WE, Sharefkin JB et al. Platelet reactivity in vivo in dogs with arterial prostheses seeded with endothelial cells. Circ 1984; 69:632-636.
2. Ramberg K, Keough E, Callow AD et al. Indium-111 labeled platelet imaging of endothelial-cell-seeded small-calibre synthetic grafts in the baboon. ASAIO J 1985; 8:95-98.
3. Birinyi LK, Douville EC, Lewis SA et al. Increased resistance to bacteraemic graft infection after endothelial cell seeding. J Vasc Surg 1987; 5:193-197.
4. Sharefkin JB, Latker C, Smith M et al. Early normalisation of platelet survival by endothelial cell seeding of dacron arterial prostheses in dogs. Surgery 1982; 92:385-393.
5. Budd JS, Allen KE, Hartley G et al. The effect of preformed confluent endothelial cell monolayers on the patency and thrombogenicity of small calibre vascular grafts. Eur J Vasc Surg 1991; 5:397-405.
6. Hess F, Steeghs S, Jerusalem R et al. Patency and morphology of fibrous polyurethane vascular prostheses implanted in the femoral artery of dogs after seeding with subcultivated endothelial cells. Eur J Vasc Surg 1993; 7:402-408.
7. Jarrell BE, Levine E, Shapiro S et al. Human adult endothelial cell growth in culture. J Vasc Surg 1984; 1:757-764.
8. Welch M, Durrans D, Carr HMH et al. Endothelial cell seeding; a review. Ann Vasc Surg 1992; 6(4):473-484.
9. Sharefkin JB, Lather C, Smith M et al. Endothelial cell labelling with indium-111 oxine as a marker of cell attachment to bioprosthetic surfaces. J Biomed Mater Res 1983; 17:345-357.
10. Vohra R, Thomson GJL, Carr HMH et al. Comparison of different vascular prostheses and matrices in relation to endothelial cell seeding. Br J Surg 1991; 78:417-420.
11. Williams SK, Jarrell BE, Friend L et al. Adult human endothelial cell compatibility with prosthetic graft material. J Surg Res 1985; 38:618-629.
12. Campbell JB, Lundgren C, Herring MB et al. Attachment and retention of Indium-111-labeled endothelial cells onto polyester elastomer. ASAIO J 1985; 8:113-117.
13. Radomski JS, Jarrell BE, Williams SK et al. Initial adherence of human capillary endothelial cells to Dacron. J Surg Res 1987; 42:133-140.
14. Budd JS, Allen KE, Bell PRF. Effects of two methods of endothelial cell seeding on cell retention during blood flow. Br J Surg 1991; 78:878-882.
15. Kent KC, Oshima A, Whittemore AD. Optimal seeding conditions for human endothelial cells. Ann Vasc Surg 1992; 6(3):258-264.
16. Jarrell BE, Williams SK, Solomon L et al. Use of an endothelial monolayer on a vascular graft prior to implantation: Temporal dynamics and compatibility with the operating room. Ann Surg 1986; 203:671-678.
17. Tannenbaum G, Ahlborn T, Benvenisty A et al. High density seeding of cultured endothelial cells leads to rapid coverage of polytetrafluoroethylene grafts. Curr Surg 1987:318-321.
18. Watkins MT, Sharefkin JB, Zajtchuk R et al. Adult human saphenous vein endothelial cells: Assessment of their reproductive capacity for use in endothelial seeding of vascular prostheses. J Surg Res 1984; 36:588-596.
19. Jarrell BE, Williams SK, Stokes G et al. Use of freshly isolated capillary endothelial cells for the immediate establishment of a monolayer on a vascular graft at surgery. Surgery 1986; 100:392-399.

20. Nicholson LJ, Clarke JM, Pittilo RM et al. The mesothelial cell as a non-thrombogenic flow surface. Thromb Haemost 1984; 52(2):102-104.

21. Ramalanjoana G, Kempczinski RF, Rosenman JE et al. The effect of fibronectin coating on endothelial cell kinetics in polytetrafluoroethylene grafts. J Vasc Surg 1986; 3:264-272.

22. Sank A, Rostami K, Weaver F et al. New evidence and new hope concerning endothelial seeding of vascular grafts. Am J Surg 1992; 164:199-204.

23. Stansby G, Shukla N, Fuller B et al. Seeding of human microvascular endothelial cells onto PTFE graft material. Br J Surg 1991; 78:1189-1192.

24. Thomson GJL, Vohra R, Walker MG. Cell seeding for small diameter ePTFE grafts: A comparison between adult human endothelial and mesothelial cells. Ann Vasc Surg 1989; 3(2):140-145.

25. Vohra R, Thomson GJL, Carr HMH et al. In vitro adherence and kinetics studies of adult human endothelial cell seeded polytetrafluoroethylene and gelatin-impregnated Dacron grafts. Eur J Vasc Surg 1991; 5:93-103.

26. Thomson GJL, Vohra RK, Carr HMH et al. Adult human endothelial cell seeding using expanded polytetrafluoroethylene vascular grafts: A comparison of four substrates. Surgery 1991; 109:20-27.

27. Pratt KJ, Jarrell BE, Williams SK et al. Kinetics of endothelial cell surface attachment forces. J Vasc Surg 1988; 7:591-599.

28. van Wachem PB, Beugeling T, Mallens BW et al. Deposition of endothelial fibronectin on polymeric surfaces. Biomaterials 1988; 9:121-123.

29. van Wachem PB, Mallens BW, Dekker A et al. Adsorption of fibronectin derived from serum and from human endothelial cells on to tissue culture polystyrene. J Biomed Mater Res 1987; 21:1317-1327.

30. Seeger JM, Klingman N. Improved endothelial cell seeding with cultured cells and fibronectin-coated grafts. J Surg Res 1985; 38:641-647.

31. Kesler KA, Herring MB, Arnold MP et al. Enhanced strength of endothelial attachment on polyester elastomer and polytetrafluoroethylene graft surfaces with fibronectin substrate. J Vasc Surg 1986; 3:58-64.

32. Curti T, Pasquinelli G, Preda P et al. An ultrastructural and immunocytochemical analysis of human endothelial cell adhesion on coated vascular grafts. Ann Vasc Surg 1989; 3(4):351-363.

33. Kaehler J, Zilla P, Fasol R et al. Precoating substrate and surface configuration determine adherence and spreading of seeded endothelial cells on PTFE grafts. J Vasc Surg 1989; 9:535-541.

34. Baker KS, Williams SK, Jarrell BE et al. Endothelialization of human collagen surfaces with human adult endothelial cells. Am J Surg 1985; 150:197-200.

35. Dalsing MC, Kevorkian M, Raper B et al. An experimental collagen-impregnated Dacron graft: Potential for endothelial seeding. Ann Vasc Surg 1989; 3(2):127-133.

36. Zilla P, Fasol R, Preiss P et al. Use of fibrin glue as a substrate for in vitro endothelialization of PTFE vascular grafts. Surgery 1989; 105:515-522.

37. Mosquera DA, Goldman M. Endothelial cell seeding. Br J Surg 1991; 78:656-660.

38. Carr HMH, Vohra R, Welch M et al. Fibronectin binding to gelatin-impregnated Dacron (Gelseal) prostheses. Artif Organs 1992; 16:342-345.

39. Budd JS, Allen KE, Bell PRF et al. The effect of varying fibronectin concentration on the attachment of endothelial cells to polytetrafluoroethylene grafts. J Vasc Surg 1990; 12:126-130.

40. Vohra RK, Thompson GJL, Sharma H et al. Fibronectin coating of expanded polytetrafluoroethylene (ePTFE) grafts and its rôle in endothelial seeding. Artif Organs 1990; 14:41-45.

41. Hasson JE, Wiebe DH, Sharefkin JB et al. Migration of adult human vascular endothelial cells: Effect of extracellular matrix proteins. Surgery 1986; 100:384-390.

42. Lalka SG, Oelker LM, Malone JM et al. Acellular vascular matrix: A natural endothelial cell substrate. Ann Vasc Surg 1989; 3(2):108-117.

43. Greisler HP, Cziperle DJ, Kim DU et al. Enhanced endothelialization of ePTFE grafts by fibroblast growth factor type 1 pretreatment. Surgery 1992; 112:244-254.

44. Gray JL, Kang SS, Zenni GC et al. FGF-1 affixation stimulates ePTFE endothelialization without intimal hyperplasia. J Surg Res 1994; 57:596-612.

45. Greisler HP, Klosak JJ, Dennis JW et al. Biomaterial pretreatment with ECGF to augment endothelial cell proliferation. J Vasc Surg 1987; 5:393-399.

46. Sentissi JM, Ramberg K, O'Donnell TFJ et al. The effect of flow on vascular endothelial cells grown in tissue culture on polytetrafluoroethylene grafts. Surgery 1986; 99:337-342.

47. Vohra RK, Thomson GJL, Sharma H et al. Effects of shear stress on endothelial cell monolayers on expanded polytetrafluoroethylene (ePTFE) grafts using preclot and fibronectin matrices. Eur J Vasc Surg 1990; 4:33-41.

48. James NL, Schindhelm K, Slowiaczek P et al. Endothelial cell seeding of small diameter vascular grafts. Artif Organs 1990; 14:355-360.

49. Miyata T, Conte MS, Trudell LA et al. Delayed exposure to pulsatile shear stress improves retention of human saphenous vein endothelial cells on seeded ePTFE grafts. J Surg Res 1991; 50:485-493.

50. Schneider PA, Hanson SR, Price TM et al. Durability of confluent endothelial cell monolayers on small calibre vascular prostheses in vitro. Surgery 1988; 103:456-462.

51. Rosenman JE, Kempczinski RF, Pearce WH et al. Kinetics of endothelial cell seeding. J Vasc Surg 1985; 2:778-784.

52. Thompson MM, Budd JS, Eady SL et al. A method to transluminally seed angioplasty sites with endothelial cells using a double balloon catheter. Eur J Vasc Surg 1993; 7:113-121.

53. Thompson MM, Budd JS, Eady SL et al. Platelet deposition after angioplasty is abolished by restoration of the endothelial cell monolayer. J Vasc Surg 1994; 19:478-486.

54. Thompson MM, Budd JS, Eady SL et al. Endothelial cell seeding of damaged native vascular surfaces: Prostacyclin production. Eur J Vasc Surg 1992; 6:487-493.

55. Thompson MM, Budd JS, Eady SL et al. The effect of transluminal endothelial seeding on myointimal hyperplasia following angioplasty. Eur J Vasc Surg 1994; 8:423-434.

56. Bush HL, Jakubowski JA, Curl GR et al. Luminal healing of arterial endarterectomy: Role of autogenous endothelial cell seeding. Surg Forum 1985; 36:446-450.

57. Bush HL, Jakubowski JA, Sentissi JM et al. Neointimal hyperplasia occurring after carotid endarterectomy in a canine model: Effect of endothelial cell seeding vs perioperative aspirin. J Vasc Surg 1987; 5:118-125.

58. Schneider PA, Hanson SR, Price TM et al. Confluent durable endothelialisation of endarterectomised baboon aorta

by early attachment of cultured endothelial cells. J Vasc Surg 1990; 11:365-372.

59. Krupski WC, Bass A, Anderson JS et al. Aspirin-independent antithrombotic effects of acutely attached cultured endothelial cells on endarterectomised arteries. Surgery 1990; 108:283-291.

60. Sterpetti AV, Schultz RD, Bailey RT. Endothelial cell seeding after carotid endarterectomy in a canine model reduces platelet uptake. Eur J Vasc Surg 1992; 6:390-394.

61. Smyth JV, Rooney OB, Dodd PDF et al. Culture of human endothelial cells on endarterectomy surfaces. Eur J Vasc Endovasc Surg 1995; 10:308-315.

62. Walluscheck KP, Steinhoff G, Haverich A. Endothelial cell seeding of native vascular surfaces. Eur J Vasc Endovasc Surg 1996; 11:290-303.

63. Thompson MM, Budd JS, Eady SL et al. Effect of seeding time and density on endothelial cell attachment to damaged vascular surfaces. Br J Surg 1993; 80:359-362.

64. Smyth JV, Rooney OB, Dodd PD et al. Production of plasminogen activator inhibitor-1 by human saphenous vein endothelial cells seeded onto endarterectomy specimens in vitro. J Vasc Surg 1997; 25:722-725.

65. Mousa SA, Cheresh DA. Recent advances in cell adhesion molecules and extracellular matrix proteins: Potential clinical implications. DDT 1997; 2:187-199.

66. Extracellular matrix receptors on animal cells: The integrins. In: Alberts B, Bray D, Lewis J et al. Molecular biology of the cell. 3rd ed. New York: Garland Publishing, Inc, 1994:995-1000.

67. Sterpetti AV, Crucina A, Napoli P et al. Growth factor release by smooth muscle cells is dependent on haemodynamic factors. Eur J Vasc Surg 1992; 6:636-638.

68. Greisler HP, Henderson SC, Lam TM. Basic fibroblast growth factor production in vitro by macrophages exposed to Dacron and polyglactin 910. J Biomater Sci Polym Ed 1993; 4:415-430.

69. Greisler HP, Dennis JW, Endean ED et al. Macrophage/biomaterial interactions: The stimulation of endothelialization. J Vasc Surg 1989; 9:588-593.

70. Sumpio BE, Widmann MD, Ricotta J et al. Increased ambient pressure stimulates proliferation and morphological changes in cultured endothelial cells. J Cell Physiol 1994; 158:133-139.

71. Iba T, Sumpio BE. Tissue plasminogen activator expression in endothelial cells exposed to cyclic strain in vivo. Cell Transpl 1992; 1:43-50.

72. Eskin SG, Ives CL, Frangos JA et al. Cultured endothelium: The response to flow. ASAIO J 1985; 8:109-112.

73. Kugiyama K, Sakamoto T, Misumi I et al. Transferable lipids in oxidized low-density lipoprotein stimulate plasminogen activator inhibitor-1 and inhibit tissue-type plasminogen activator release from endothelial cells. Circ Res 1993; 73:335-343.

74. Yamamoto C, Kaji T, Sakamoto M et al. Effect of endothelin on the release of tissue plasminogen activator and plasminogen activator inhibitor-1 from cultured human endothelial cells and interaction with thrombin. Thromb Res 1992; 67:619-624.

75. Loskutoff DJ, Ny T, Sawdey M et al. Fibrinolytic system of cultured endothelial cells; regulation by plasminogen activator inhibitor. J Cell Biochem 1986; 32:273-280.

76. van Hinsbergh VWM, Bertina RM, van Wijngaarden A et al. Activated protein c decreases plasminogen activator inhibitor activity in endothelial cell-conditioned medium. Blood 1985; 65:444-451.

77. van Hinsbergh VWM, Kooistra T, van den Berg EA et al. Tumor necrosis factor increases the production of plasminogen activator inhibitor in human endothelial cells in vitro and in rats in vivo. Blood 1988; 72:1467-1473.

78. Hanss M, Collen D. Secretion of tissue-type plasminogen activator and plasminogen activator inhibitor by cultured human endothelial cells: Modulation by thrombin, endotoxin and histamine. J Lab Clin Med 1987; 109:97-104.

79. Lundgren CH, Herring MB, Arnold MP et al. Fluid shear disruption of cultured endothelium: The effect of cell species, fibronectin crosslinking and supporting polymer. ASAIO Trans 1986; 32:334-338.

80. Ives CL, Eskin SG, McIntire LV et al. The importance of cell origin and substrate in the kinetics of endothelial cell alignment in response to steady flow. ASAIO Trans 1983; 29:269-274.

81. Li JM, Menconi MJ, Wheeler HB et al. Precoating ePTFE grafts alters production of endothelial cell derived thrombomodulators. J Vasc Surg 1992; 15:1010-1017.

82. Christ G, Seiffert D, Hufnagl P et al. Type 1 plasminogen activator inhibitor synthesis of endothelial cells is downregulated by smooth muscle cells. Blood 1993; 81:1277-1283.

83. Scott-Burden T, Vanhoutte PM. Regulation of smooth muscle cell growth by endothelium-derived growth factors. Tex Heart Inst J 1994; 21:91-97.

─────────────── CHAPTER 5 ───────────────

Surface Precoating in the 1990s:
The Fine Tuning of Endothelial Cell Transplantation

Mark M. Samet, Victor V. Nikolaychik, Peter I. Lelkes

Introduction

Each year 900,000 people in the USA alone suffer from arterial disorders requiring some form of surgical intervention. Over half of these procedures involve peripheral reconstruction using vascular grafts to bypass an occluded vessel segment. However, 60% of the patients undergoing vascular surgery do not have a suitable vessel for grafting and, therefore, need synthetic grafts.[1] In this realm, about 350,000 artificial vascular grafts are implanted annually, and the numbers are expected to rise rapidly in the future. In spite of the increasing demand for vascular prostheses, the long term success of their use as arterial substitutes is, at best, mixed.[2,3] In artery bypasses, with bore sizes $\geq$ 5 mm in diameter Dacron® and ePTFE grafts demonstrate cumulative patency rates similar to those of the natural grafts.[1] But, as small artery substitutes, these prostheses have performed poorly and, to date, no vascular prosthesis of $\leq$ 4 mm in diameter remains patent for more than a couple of months.[1] The high failure rates of small diameter prosthetic grafts are believed to be intimately associated with the poor healing and rejection process of the implanted conduit.[3-7] One of the key determinants in this "cause and effect" relationship is the problem of insufficient hemocompatibility of the polymeric graft material.[8]

Insufficient hemocompatibility of the biomaterials is also a pressing issue in the field of cardiac prostheses. Each year, end-stage heart diseases claim some 75,000 victims in the USA alone. Although 28,000 of these patients qualify for heart transplants, the supply of donated hearts is limited to approximately 2,000 hearts per year.[9,10] Thus, the majority of these patients has no realistic hope of long term survival, unless permanent total artificial hearts (TAH) or ventricular assist devices (VAD) become available.

The vision of developing a permanent cardiac prosthesis is more than a half century old. The first practical implementation of this idea was achieved in the 1950s by W.J. Kolff and his collaborators, who kept a dog alive for 90 min after successfully replacing the native heart with an artificial device.[11] By the mid-1970s, the first generation of TAHs and VADs was undergoing advanced clinical trials.[11-14] These units were activated externally by pneumatic drivers and connected trough transcutaneous pressure lines. Besides restricting the patient's postoperative quality of life, these lines served as a major source for bacterial infection and initiated thromboembolic complications. The newest generation of cardiac prostheses, designed to be totally implantable, are powered by a compact electrical source.[14] In spite of significant mechanical and electronic improvements in the new designs, the permanent or even temporary clinical use of cardiac prostheses as a bridge to recovery[15] is still thwarted by serious obstacles such as infections and thromboembolic complications which are manifested in stroke and multiple organ failures.[16,17] As in the case of artificial vascular grafts, many of the complications with cardiac prostheses can be traced back to the problem of inadequate hemocompatibility of the blood-contacting biomaterials in these devices. Thus, it follows that if we can successfully overcome the blood compatibility barrier, we shall markedly improve the clinical prospects of both artificial hearts and small diameter prosthetic grafts.

Endothelialization: Past and Current Approaches

The interaction of blood with "medical-grade" biomaterials commonly results in thrombus formation and/or thromboembolic complications. After decades of disappointing attempts to passivate the synthetic blood-contacting surfaces by chemical modifications or by generation of a pseudoneointima,[15,18] the focus has turned towards establishing on the synthetic blood-contacting surfaces "nature's own blood-compatible container",[19] i.e., reconstructing the endothelial cell (EC) lining of the vascular wall. The rationale for covering the prosthetic luminal surface with a viable layer of ECs, i.e., endothelialization, is rather simple: in vivo, ECs present under normal physiologic conditions an anti-thrombogenic surface which is pivotal to the prevention of fibrin deposition and inhibition of platelet adhesion on the vessel wall. Thus, it has been reasoned that endothelialization of cardiovascular prostheses would reduce the thrombogenicity of these devices. In addition, adverse immunogenic responses from the host would be avoided by transplanting autologous cells. Indeed, these principles were successfully demonstrated more than two decades ago in artificial grafts.[20] However, in 1975, the art of procuring and culturing endothelial cells was in its infancy, and very little was known about EC-biomaterial compatibility. Since then, together with significant advances in endothelial cell biology, molecular biology, and biotechnology,[21,22] a fairly thorough understanding has been gained of the basic requirements for successfully growing endothelial cells on the biomaterials used in cardiovascular prostheses: PTFE, ePTFE, Dacron®, and various brands of polyurethanes (PUs).[23-26] In recent years, endothelialization of vascular graft surfaces with autologous ECs may have solved several important problems in cardiovascular surgery[27-31] and paved the way for the development of new areas, such as biohybrid organs[32] and gene therapy.[33-36] Thus, at present, the question is no longer whether or not endothelialization is feasible, but, rather, how it can be optimized.

Optimization, or fine tuning of endothelialization is a multifaceted task. It involves, but is not limited to, improvement of endothelial cell attachment and growth on the synthetic surface, enhancement of cell adaptation to and subsequent endurance in a hemodynamic environment, and finally, promotion of the anti-coagulant repertoire of the entire EC lining. Several researchers have used genetically modified ECs as a vehicle for achieving these goals,[23,33] while others focused on increasing the hydrophilicity of the synthetic scaffold[37] or preconditioning the cultured endothelium by mechanical forces.[38,39] Many investigators, however, turned to surface treatment with select extracellular matrix (ECM) proteins or blood plasma proteins ("fibrin glue"), with or without supplements, as a means for improving cellular performance in grafts.[40,41] Our ongoing studies focus on surface coating as a means for optimizing endothelialization.[42,43] Specifically, our motivation is to form a multifunctional protein complex that will perform as a biointegrator between the living cells and the underlying polymeric scaffold in cardiac prostheses.

Fine Tuning of Endothelialization via Surface Coating

The best biointegrating interface for ECs is their native basement membrane which, in vivo, contributes to the maintenance of the architectural and functional integrity of the endothelium.[44] This basement membrane is comprised of structural proteins such as collagens, as well as adhesive proteins such as laminin (LM) and fibronectin (FN). These and several other ECM proteins regulate, via RGD (arginine-glycine-aspartic acid)-based integrin-mediated reception, cell adhesion and spreading.[45] In addition, many of these ECM molecules are also actively synthesized during cell proliferation/migration.[46] Using ECM-contained adhesive proteins, various researchers have employed FN, LM, or collagen iv (Col IV), or a combination thereof, as a surface coating to facilitate endothelialization of biomaterials.[40,47,48] Similarly, short RGD peptides, or their mimics, have been covalently coupled to the PU backbone to achieve the same goal.[49]

We revisited the effectiveness of select ECM-contained adhesive monoproteins to promote cells growth on PUs. For this purpose we seeded bovine aortic ECs (BAEC) at a density of 25,000 cells/cm^2 onto PU substrates and monitored their growth for several days. As a control, we cultured BAECs on tissue culture grade polystyrene (TC) in 24 well plates (Costar, Cambridge, MA). The PU samples were made of Chronoflex, and fitted into the wells of 24 well plates as previously described.[50] The surface of the PUs was either left uncoated or was coated by passive adsorption for 1 h with FN (20 μg/ml, pH=7.4) or Col IV (300 μg/ml, pH=3.0) prior to cell seeding. The results of this study are summarized in Figure 5.1a. Each data point (mean ± standard deviation) represents the number of cells per cm^2 from 3 independent experiments (6 wells per case). As expected, the cells grew poorly on plain (uncoated) PU, and their number by day nine was significantly lower than in controls ($0.92 \pm 0.1 \times 10^5$ vs. $1.96 \pm 0.8 \times 10^5$, p < 0.05). Proliferation of BAEC improved significantly upon coating the PUs with either FN or Col IV, but it did not match the rate of growth on TC. Interestingly, there was no substantial difference in the rate of growth between cells cultured on FN or Col IV coatings. In fact, on day 9, the number of cells in both cases was almost equal ($1.77 \pm 0.87 \times 10^5$ on FN vs. $1.69 \pm 0.11 \times 10^5$ on Col IV, p=0.425). Thus, our data confirm the findings of others that biomaterials coated with ECM proteins are more cytocompatible than their untreated counterparts.[40,51,52] Moreover, our results also imply that in coating the polymeric scaffold with only one kind of ECM adhesive protein, the particular type of this protein is of secondary importance for ECs grown in a static environment.

Subsequently, we examined whether the effectiveness of a particular surface coating in promoting cell growth may depend on the method of protein immobilization onto the polymeric surface. To this end, we seeded BAEC at a density of 25,000 cells/cm^2 onto PUs coated by different means with ECM proteins, and monitored their growth for several days. The PU samples consisted of 4 separate groups:

Group #1: PU coated with FN by adsorption. The starting concentration of FN was 20 µg/ml (pH=7.4). After 1 h of incubation at 37°C, the final concentration on the surface, as determined by the sulforhodamine B assay,[53] was 20 ng/cm^2.

Group #2: PU coated with FN by photoimmobilization using the method of Clapper et al.[54] The final concentration of FN on the surface was as in group #1.

Group #3: PU coated with Col IV by adsorption. The starting concentration was 300 µg/ml at pH = 3.0. After 1 h of incubation at 37°C, the final concentration on the surface was 50 ng/cm^2.

Group #4: PU coated with Col IV by photoimmobilization. The final concentration of Col IV on the surface was as in group #3.

As shown in Figure 5.1b, the cells grew equally well on FN substrates, whether adsorbed or photoimmobilized. On the other hand, when Col IV-based substrates were used, cell growth was significantly better on PU coated by adsorption than by photoimmobilization ($1.69 \pm 0.11 \times 10^5$ vs. $1.33 \pm 0.11 \times 10^5$, $p < 0.05$). Thus, for select proteins some methods of immobilization may indeed result in better substrates for cell growth than others. However, in our hands, no ECM-derived, monoprotein coating of PU can match the conditions offered by a tissue culture-grade polystyrene. Clearly, a substrate comprised of two dimensionally assembled, ECM adhesive monoproteins does not provide for an adequate surface coating that can be used as a vehicle for optimizing endothelialization of cardiovascular prostheses. Hence, more sophisticated approaches are required to generate a biointegrated proteinaceous meshwork at the PU surface which would structurally mimic the topology of the subendothelial basement membrane and also provide space for the incorporation of the endogenous, EC-derived extracellular proteins. Such a provisional ECM meshwork might be found in fibrin glue, the reaction product of fibrinogen and thrombin.

In the past, fibrin glue was shown to be beneficial in supporting both EC attachment and growth on synthetic materials[40,42,43,55-57] and for establishing a stable, shear-resistant monolayer on ePTFE grafts.[58] To improve this coating we substituted purified fibrinogen with plasma cryoprecipitate. Indeed, the results of those studies were encouraging: After 4 days in culture the number of cells on fibrin-based coating was higher by almost 45% than on TC. Cell coverage was even higher when the fibrin-based coating was supplemented with heparin and insulin.[42] Based on these findings, we assessed the efficacy of the fibrin-based coating to promote EC growth on the luminal surface of PU-covered "ersatz" ventricles, (T-25 tissue culture flasks[61]). For comparison purposes we also used "ersatz" ventricles covered with either plain or FN-coated PU. In all cases the luminal surface of the PUs used (Biospan™)[50] was smooth and the coatings were prepared without supplements such as growth factors, heparin, or insulin.

The study was conducted in two sequential steps to realistically mimic a full scale endothelialization of the blood sac of a VAD. First, the cells (BAECs) were seeded with rotation for 3 h onto either precoated or plain PU surfaces.[61] Thereafter, the "ersatz" ventricles were removed from the rotator and kept in an upright position, and the adherent ECs were allowed to spread and proliferate for several days. We monitored cell growth every other day by Alamar Blue assay.[50] The results obtained are presented in Figure 5.2a. As expected, the lowest rate of growth was obtained on plain PU. On FN-coated PU the cells grew somewhat better, presumably because there were more cells attached immediately after seeding and so they could interact more effectively with one another. In the past, several studies had already shown that such interactions play an important role

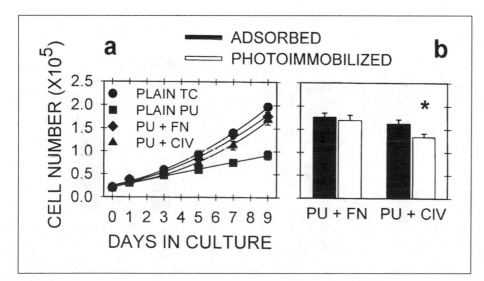

Fig. 5.1. Cell growth on various substrates under static conditions: (a) Effect of select surface treatments on cell proliferation. FN or Col IV were immobilized onto PU samples by adsorption as detailed in the text. (b) Effect of protein immobilization methods on cell densities. FN or Col IV were immobilized onto PU samples either by adsorption or photoimmobilization as detailed in the text. Cell number was quantitated every other day by Alamar Blue assay.

in cell proliferation in vitro.[62,63] By contrast, cells seeded on plasma cryoprecipitate-made fibrin substrate (CRY) grew rapidly and reached confluence by the seventh day in culture. Importantly, purified fibrinogen-made fibrin substrate (FBG) was not as effective as CRY in promoting cell growth; even on the ninth day in culture the number of cells on FBG was still significantly lower than on CRY ($2.86 \pm 0.28 \times 10^5$ vs. $3.41 \pm 0.25 \times 10^5$, $p < 0.05$). Since both coatings are comprised of a fibrin-based matrix, it is likely that some of the intrinsic plasma proteins contained in CRY may have contributed to the enhanced rate of cell growth on this substrate.

Smooth-surface PUs have been used in cardiac prostheses as a means of preventing platelet aggregation and thrombus formation on the blood-contacting surfaces. However, notwithstanding the improvements in PU manufacturing and surface processing, the microscopic appearance of the luminal surface in these devices has never been completely smooth, and also the hemocompatibility of the smooth surfaces has not met the initial expectations. On the other hand, textured PU surfaces have been advocated as a scaffold of choice for enhancing pseudoneointima formation[64,65] and for promoting endothelial cell attachment onto the luminal surface of cardiovascular devices.[29,66,67] In adopting the latter concept for the endothelialization of VAD blood sacs, we evaluated CRY enhancement of cell growth on textured PU. The experiments were conducted in the same manner as above with smooth, uncoated PUs serving as controls. Figure 5.2b exemplifies our findings for plain and CRY-coated PUs after seven days in culture. BAECs proliferated much faster on the uncoated, textured PU than on its smooth counterpart, ($2.17 \pm 0.21 \times 10^5$ vs. $1.49 \pm 0.21 \times 10^5$, $p < 0.05$). Again, the significant difference in the number of cells covering the surfaces may have resulted, in part, from more efficient attachment of cells on textured surface than on smooth PU. Application of CRY coating masked the topological difference between the two types of surfaces and enhanced cell growth with the same effectiveness. Thus, the number of cells on both PUs was virtually the same at all times; for example, on the seventh day in culture (Fig. 5.2b) we measured $3.24 \pm 0.23 \times 10^5$ cells/cm^2 on smooth PU+CRY vs. $3.56 \pm 0.23 \times 10^5$ cells/cm^2 on textured PU+CRY

($p = 0.24$). On both CRY-coated PUs, the number of cells was about 1.5 times higher than on plain, textured PUs. These data suggest that fibrin-based coating is indeed a preferred substrate for optimizing EC growth on the luminal surface of cardiovascular prostheses.

In addition to enhancing cell growth, increasing the initial efficiency of cell attachment onto biomaterials is pivotal for successfully establishing an EC monolayer in prosthetic devices. In the past, we and others have explored various ways for increasing the affinity of synthetic surfaces to cells, for example, by glow discharge treatment,[68] coating with substrates composed of select proteins,[40,69,70] or both.[61] Indeed, when BAECs were seeded under static conditions onto various PU substrates, we saw a substantial improvement in attachment efficiency on treated surfaces vs. plain PU (Fig. 5.3a). Our study also indicated that the most suitable surface for cell attachment was TC; CRY-coated PU was second to the best ($94.1 \pm 3.23\%$, $p < 0.05$). In our hands, the performance of CRY (and FBG) coatings was dependent upon the concentration of fibrinogen employed. As demonstrated in Table 5.1, cell attachment efficacy of purified fibrinogen varied in a bell-shaped manner between concentration levels of 0-30 mg/ml. The best performance was obtained at 5 mg/ml but, for preparing a coating of controllable thickness on a textured surface, we used only 3.5 mg/ml.

Optimal adherence of endothelial cells under static conditions onto flat PU substrates or a TC surface does not necessarily translate into efficient attachment of cells during endothelialization under rotation of a complex geometric structure such as a cardiovascular prosthesis. In our hands, there are four equally important factors that determine the efficiency of cell attachment under these unique conditions: number of cells in the inoculum, speed of rotation, duration of seeding and surface treatment by coating.

By fine tuning these parameters we were able to improve the homogeneity of surface coverage, optimize the time of residence/contact of cells with the substrate, and thus promote cell attachment. We established the following as optimal for lining our artificial ventricles: speed at 10 rotations/h, duration of seeding at 3 h, and inoculation density at 6.0×10^4 cells/cm^2. Utilizing these settings, we examined the efficiency of attachment of cells that were seeded onto

Fig. 5.2. Cell growth on various substrates in PU-covered "ersatz" ventricles after seeding with rotation: (a) Effect of select surface coatings on cell proliferation. (b) Cell densities in cultures grown on smooth and textured PUs, with or without CRY coating. "ersatz" ventricles, consisting of PU-covered T-25 flasks, were seeded with rotation for 3 h at an inoculation density of 60,000 cells/cm^2. After stopping the seeding, the adherent BAECs were allowed to spread and proliferate under static conditions. Cell number was assessed every other day by Alamar Blue assay, and the cultures were refed after completion of the assay.

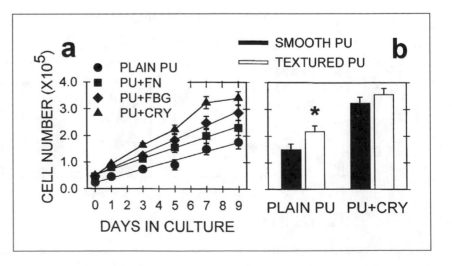

various substrates in smooth PU-covered "ersatz" ventricles. Plain TC served as controls. The results obtained are shown in Figure 5.3b. In contrast to the findings under static conditions, plain TC was the least suitable substrate for cell attachment under rotation, whereas CRY ranked the best (553.1 ± 21% over TC). FBG ranked second to the best (328.2 ± 13% over TC) and FN-based substrate was the third with a considerably lower efficiency (257.3 ± 11% over TC).

The topography of the luminal surface in most vascular grafts is primarily rough.[71,72] Also, some of the TAHs and VADs that are currently tested or developed, including the Heartmate® and the Milwaukee Heart™, have a rough luminal surface. To gain a more factual representation of the attachment efficiencies during endothelialization of artificial devices, we repeated the above experiments using "ersatz" ventricles covered with textured PU. Figure 5.4a presents a typical SEM photomicrograph of a textured surface that was prepared, as previously reported,[43] by sprinkling NaCl crystals (in this case the mean diameter was 32 μm) over a wet PU cast. The entire surface appears corrugated by

abundant, randomly dispersed cavities of varying dimensions, ranging in size from 30-120 μm in diameter. Figure 5.4b exemplifies attachment efficiencies on plain and CRY-coated PUs. It is apparent from panel A that cell attachment onto an uncoated, textured surface was significantly better than onto plain smooth PU (134.8 ± 8% and 108.2 ± 6%, respectively, compared to TC controls, $p < 0.05$). This improvement was likely due to the increase in cell residence time at the site of contact and isolation from fluid currents, rather than resulting from enhancement in surface affinity. In the case of CRY-coated PUs, the fibrin meshwork completely filled the pores in the textured PU and masked the topological differences between rough and smooth surfaces (Figs. 5.4 c,d). The resulting substrates had a finely patterned luminal surface that was enriched in numerous RGD binding sites inherent to the component proteins. As shown in panel B of Figure 5.4b, cells adhered readily onto both these substrates, leading to similar attachment efficiencies of more than 500% above control level. Thus, by using CRY coating, we completely eliminated the difference in attachment efficiencies between smooth and rough PUs.

Having optimized cell attachment and growth on PUs, we determined whether the CRY coating could also enhance the retention of ECs in a monolayer that is exposed to dynamic conditions. For these in vitro studies, we used VAD blood sacs which were fabricated from a commercially available PU (Biospan™) by the lost wax technique.[43] For cell seeding, the lumina of fully assembled VADs were filled with 125 ml of Air/CO_2-presaturated culture medium containing 4.0×10^7 BAECs, mounted onto the rotating arm of the seeding apparatus[61] and rotated at 10 rotations/h for 3 h. Following seeding, the VADs were placed, in an upright position, in a standard CO_2 incubator. Cell proliferation was measured every other day, and the cultures were refed after conclusion of each Alamar Blue assay.[50] Two days after seeding, the monolayers in the blood sacs had reached confluence. We then maintained them for eight additional

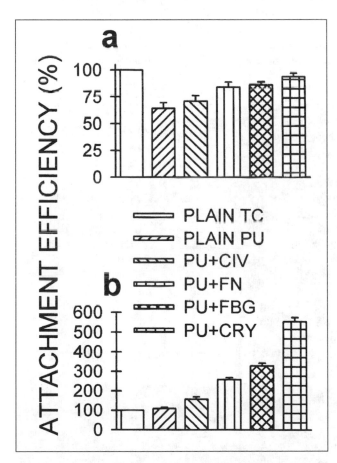

Fig. 5.3. Efficiency of cell attachment onto various substrates: (a) under static conditions, and (b) after seeding with rotation of "ersatz" ventricles. BAECs were inoculated at a density of 60,000 cells/cm². After 3 h of seeding, the cultures were washed gently with medium to remove nonadherent cells, and assayed by Alamar Blue assay to determine the number of cells attached to the surface. The resulting numbers were normalized to data obtained on TC surface.

Table 5.1 Efficiency of cell attachment as a function of fibrinogen concentration

Concentration of Fibrinogen (mg/ml)	Efficiency of Cell Attachment (%) [a]
0.0	61.48 ± 4.87
0.5	72.13 ± 1.87
1.0	76.28 ± 3.14
2.0	83.56 ± 3.14
5.0	84.01 ± 2.91
10.0	83.72 ± 3.47
15.0	79.56 ± 2.43
20.0	76.44 ± 2.05
30.0	72.11 ± 1.52

[a]The study was conducted under static conditions and the number of cells recorded at each fibrinogen concentration was normalized to the number of cells obtained on plain TC. The fibrinogen used in this particular study was purified in the Hemostasis Research Laboratory at Sinai Samaritan Medical Center, Milwaukee, WI, and was kindly donated by its director, Dr. M. Mosesson.

days under static conditions to allow the cells to synthesize, assemble, and mature their ECM on the underlying scaffold.[73] Following a total of eleven days in a static environment, the monolayers were exposed for 24 h to one of the following dynamic conditions:

1. Flexing of the blood sac wall at 1 Hz between systole and diastole positions, with minimal flow of medium inside the blood sac;
2. Perfusion of the blood sac in an assembled VAD with pulsatile flow at the mean rate of 500 ml/min (blood sac wall was maintained motionless during the whole period); and
3. Pumping action of the VAD at 1 Hz, mean flow rate of 3.2 l/min, and ejection pressure of 150 mm Hg.

For all tests, the VADs were connected aseptically to a mock loop consisting of a PVC venous reservoir, as previously described.[43] The status of the monolayer lining the blood sacs was evaluated by the Alamar Blue assay before and after each run. Our findings for FN and CRY-based coatings are presented in Table 5.2. It is apparent that 24 h of flexing did not dislodge cells from the scaffolds. In fact, the rhythmic movement of the wall even increased cell density markedly in all cultures by more than 13%. This observation is in line with the findings previously reported by others.[74] On the other hand, exposure of ECs grown on FN coat-

ing to pulsatile flow resulted in denudation of the monolayers by more than 30%, but did not compromise the monolayers established on CRY coating. In fact, our results indicate that on CRY coating there was minimal, if any, cell loss due to exposure to the hemodynamic forces encountered in a pumping artificial ventricle.

Morphological Aspects of the Endothelialized Surfaces

It has long been recognized that the morphology and function of vascular ECs, as well as the architecture of the subendothelial matrix, are modulated by hemodynamic forces and by the tissue-specific microenvironment. In most

Table 5.2. Cell retention under dynamic conditions in EC monolayers established on either FN or CRY coating

Dynamic Condition	% of cells remaining on FN coating[a]	% of cells remaining on CRY coating[a]
Flexing	120.7 ± 7.6 *	113.1 ± 3.3 *
Perfusion	69.0 ± 7.1 *	91.6 ± 13.2
Pumping	65.0 ± 16.0 *	95.2 ± 6.3

[a]The data were normalized to the number of cells measured before the test; * indicates significant difference, p<0.05.

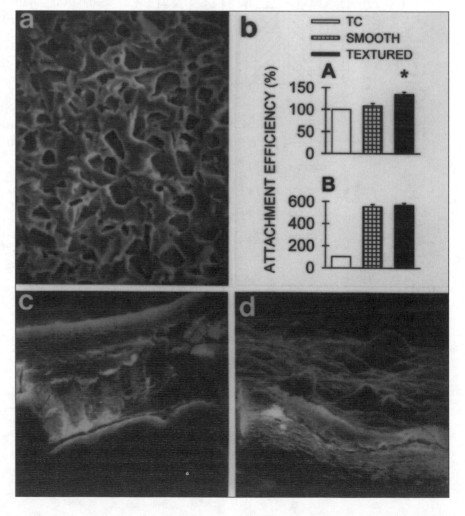

Fig. 5.4. (a) A typical electron microscopic (SEM) appearance of uncoated, textured PU (magnification x160). The average pore area, evaluated by computer-aided image analysis was 9370 ± 12 μm². (b) Efficiency of cell attachment onto: A. uncoated PU, and B. CRY-coated PU after seeding with rotation of "ersatz" ventricles. Cell enumeration was performed by Alamar Blue assay and the resulting data were normalized to values obtained for TC. (c,d) Typical SEM views of CRY-coated, textured and smooth PU surfaces, respectively. The specimens were cut at a 30° inclination to reveal both the coating and the underlying PU scaffold (magnification x650).

studies, these characteristics have primarily been addressed in the context of cellular response to mechanical forces.[74-79] To gain a better insight into adaptation of the cells on different surfaces, we focused on morphological aspects of the EC monolayer and the subendothelial region on plain and coated PUs in postconfluent, static cultures. After seven days in culture, the cells were removed by treatment with detergent and the surface was examined by scanning electron microscopy.

A typical electron microscopic view of the subendothelial region of cells grown on uncoated, smooth PU is presented in Figure 5.5a. The ECM, made of isolated regions of fibers that were interlaced by short fibrils, formed thin sheets of web-like structures of variable density. These regions only partially covered the PU surface and were connected to one another by wider filamentous bands. The subendothelial region on uncoated, textured PU (Fig. 5.5b) appeared similar to the ECM on smooth PU, except that oftentimes the long fibrillar structures bridged across cavities and recesses within the surface. On both PUs, however, a large fraction of the surface area appeared devoid of any matrix-related material. Whether this was due to nonuniform deposition

and/or assembly of the EC-derived ECM, or if it was an artifact of specimen preparation, is unclear. In any event, the subendothelial matrix in either case did not appear to provide sufficient mechanical stability and sturdiness for supporting the cells during exposure to the dynamic conditions inside a beating ventricle. By contrast to the scanty ECM on plain PUs, the subendothelial regions assembled on FN and CRY coatings were more substantial, oftentimes spanning the entire viewing areas (Figs. 5.5c and d, respectively). On FN coated PU, (Fig. 5.5c), the network appeared planar and in many sites it was much denser than on uncoated PUs. CRY alone formed a 3-dimensional and continuous meshwork atop the PU, composed of crosslinked fibrin and other highly organized adhesive plasma proteins such as fibronectin and vitronectin (Fig. 5.5d). When the cells grown on top this structure were removed, the remaining ECM was comprised of thick bands of extremely dense structures, closely apposed to the CRY meshwork, resembling the amorphous, natural basement membrane. Apparently the architectural differences between the two coatings, as manifested in their improved scaffolding capabilities and, ultimately, in their potential to minimize cell loss during

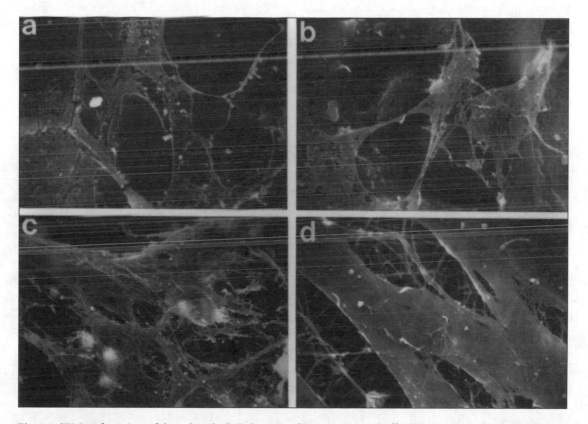

Fig. 5.5. SEM en face view of the subendothelial region after seven days of cell culturing under static conditions on: (a) uncoated, smooth PU, (b) uncoated, textured PU, (c) FN-coated textured PU, and (d) CRY-coated textured PU. BAECs were grown in blood sacs as described in the text. On seventh day, select samples of 1 x 1 cm^2 were excised from the blood sacs and rinsed with PBS. The cells were removed from the surface by treatment with 0.1% Triton X-100 and subsequent wash with 0.025 M NH$_4$OH. The samples were rinsed with 0.1 M Na-cacodylate buffer and, consecutively, with ddH$_2$O. Following serial dehydration (30 sec each) by ethanol and critical point drying, specimens from each sample were sputter coated with gold-palladium (~210 Å in thickness) and viewed by Philips PW-6700 microscope (Eindhoven, The Netherlands) at a magnification of x2500).

exposure of the endothelialized surfaces to flow-induced forces, played a considerable role in enhancing interactions with EC-derived matrices.

One of the conceivable advantages of the CRY coating over any other factitious substrates is its 3-dimensional meshwork architecture. Before endothelialization, and while still naive, this unique structure consists of an array of criss-crossed fibers which evenly cover the entire area (Fig. 5.6a). The distance between adjacent fibers is not constant, and it can be manipulated, as already reported elsewhere,[42] in order to optimize its ability to support the overlying cells. Indeed, on a finely patterned meshwork, endothelial cells propagate readily across the entire surface and form a confluent monolayer within 48 h after seeding. Seven days after seeding, the underlying ECM appears matured and well integrated into the CRY meshwork (Fig. 5.6c). A subendothelial "basement membrane" on top of the fibrillar, "provisional matrix" is clearly visible through a shrinkage gap which was artificially created during sample preparation. When grown atop this subendothelial complex, the cells seem well differentiated and closely apposed next to each other (Fig. 5.6b). In a transverse view, the densely packed ECs appear as a continuous chain, which relative to the thickness of the CRY coating, looks very thin (Fig. 5.7a). Along the EC chain, cell to cell contact between neighboring cells is well established (Fig. 5.7b).

Concluding Remarks

Endothelialization of cardiovascular prostheses, as a means of overcoming their inadequate hemocompatibility, is a multifaceted task. It involves numerous aspects, notably:

1. Procurement of autologous endothelial cells from the prospective donor and their propagation into large quantities;
2. Preparation of the biomaterial surface for cell seeding and establishment of a stable, shear resistant monolayer atop the synthetic material; and
3. Manipulation of the ECs to express their athrombogenic and fibrinolytic repertoires during static culturing and after implantation into the host.

Each of these aspects is complex and encompasses critical issues that require attention from a wide spectrum of disciplines, such as biology, chemistry, bioengineering and medicine. In many instances the solutions to these problems are not straightforward and call for additional research and for the development of novel technologies. However, more often than not, genuine progress is achieved through innovative approaches. Indeed, in recent years we have witnessed promising developments with the use of genetically engineered endothelial cells[23,33] and bioabsorbable materials[6] in vascular prostheses. Also, the reconstitution of hierarchically structured walls by ECs, smooth muscle cells, and fibroblasts[80-82] provides a reason for cautious optimism. Yet another promising approach, explored by us and others,[40-42] is to precoat the biomaterial surface with a three dimen-

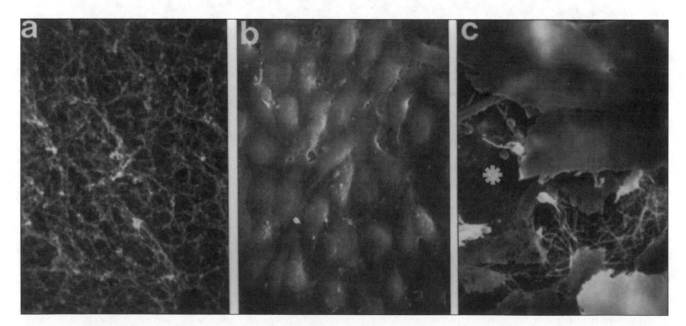

Fig. 5.6. Scanning electron microscopic view of: (a) CRY-meshwork before cell seeding (magnification x2500), (b) Confluent and well-differentiated BAEC monolayer after 7 days in static culture (magnification x650), and (c) Shrinkage gap in the BAEC monolayer which was formed during specimen processing in order to provide a detailed insight into the subendothelial region; * indicates a section of the extracellular matrix deposited and organized by BAEC (magnification x2500). On the seventh day, select samples of 1 x 1 cm^2 were excised from the blood sacs and rinsed with PBS. The samples were fixed for 30 min at room temperature with 1% glutaraldehyde in 0.1 M Na-cacodylate buffer and postfixed with OsO$_4$ for 25 min. Further processing followed the procedure described in Figure 5.5.

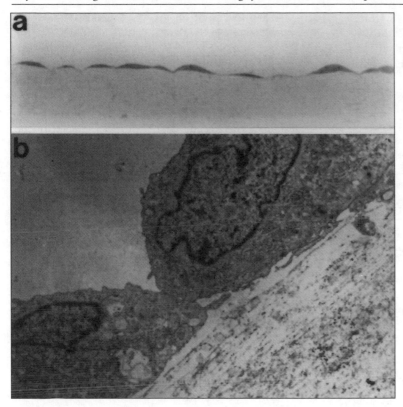

Fig. 5.7. A transverse view of an endothelialized, cryoprecipitate coated surface seven days after seeding. BAEC monolayer and CRY-coating were gently peeled off from PU surface, and immediately immersed in Karnovsky's fixative for 30 min at room temperature. The specimens were subsequently postfixed in a 1% OsO_4 solution for 40 min, dehydrated by using graded ethanol and, finally, embedded in SPURR. (a) Semithin sections of 1 µm were cut from the specimens and stained with toluidine blue for observation by light microscopy (magnification x100). (b) Ultrathin sections of 60-90 nm were mounted on copper grid and examined in a Philips 400, electron microscope (Eindhoven, The Netherlands) at a magnification of x3000.

sional meshwork of cryoprecipitate-derived plasma proteins that serves as a biointegrator between the endothelial cell monolayer and the underlying synthetic scaffold. In this chapter we have presented our experience with the plasma cryoprecipitate-produced fibrin meshwork as it relates to optimizing endothelial cell attachment and growth, and to increasing resistance to denudation of the cellular monolayer upon exposure to the dynamic conditions inside a beating cardiac prosthesis.

Our in vitro studies establish that denudation of endothelialized prostheses can be minimized by culturing ECs on a 3-dimensional meshwork, rich in both structural and adhesive proteins, as well as by allowing the confluent monolayer time for maturation. All these factors, viz, seeding of endothelial cells on the three dimensional "provisional matrix" and subsequent establishment of the subendothelial ECM, as well as the functional maturation of the EC monolayer, will likely play vital roles in averting denudation of ECs by mechanical forces. Fine tuning of the surface coating will confer added physical stability to the neobasement membrane ("shock absorber effect") and promote functional contacts between the cells in the monolayer. However, once in contact with blood/plasma, other factors may also be of importance for the maintenance of an intact EC monolayer. For example, monolayer integrity may be challenged by various proteases, activated plasma proteins and/or circulating blood cells when the cell culture media is replaced by plasma or citrated blood during mock loop tests in vitro. Similar, and even more demanding, challenges should also be expected during in vivo trials.

Currently, the focus of our work and that of others is to further optimize the hemocompatibility of the blood-contacting surfaces in cardiac prostheses by broadening the concept of "endothelialization". Over the years, progress in this area has been made largely by extending the idea of a "passive endothelial cell lining", as applied in the 1980s and before, to the concept of biointegration of the textured polymeric scaffold, the 3-dimensional matrix and the "active" interaction between the cells and their matrix. This integral approach requires the coordinated input of a multidisciplinary team of scientists, and is only one of the many steps needed for the recreation of the entire vascular wall structure lined by a nonthrombogenic cellular lining. In the past it has been assumed that this cellular lining should be comprised only of endothelial cells, but recently there is some evidence that other cell types, either native or genetically modified, can also be rendered nonthrombogenic when exposed to pulsatile blood flow.

Reconstruction of the cardiac/vascular wall in vitro requires a thorough understanding of how to coculture the diverse cell types comprising the entire vascular wall, e.g., smooth muscle cells, fibroblasts and endothelial cells, in order to achieve a hierarchic, structural and functional organization resembling that of the adventitia, media and intima. Interestingly, preliminary data suggest that exposure of such cocultures to hemodynamic forces such as cyclic strain and pulsatile flow will sort out the cells and initiate their hierarchic arrangement. Unanswered, as yet, is the question of whether the cells lining the blood-contacting surfaces are indeed functional, viz., whether the cellular lining will indeed reduce the thrombogenicity of the devices. An exciting approach is to use genetically modified cells, which would accelerate the hierarchic organization within the vessel wall and/or overexpress specific molecules that characterize the anticoagulant/nonthrombogenic endothelial cells' surface.

Finally, in our opinion, the ultimate cardiovascular "prosthesis" will be a man-made, tissue-engineered replacement organ. In the not too distant future we envisage that dramatic progress in cell and molecular biology, in concert with novel approaches to 3-dimensional tissue culturing, will yield functional replacement tissue equivalents and, perhaps, even entire organs. Some of these exciting procedures, as futuristic as they may sound, are currently being explored by us and several other groups. Hence, the dream of generating ex vivo autologous replacement "spare parts", has materialized during the past few years and appears to be achievable. We truly believe that our current struggle to optimize the design and hemocompatibility of cardiovascular bioprostheses will soon be surpassed by a new area of "as good as new" tissue-engineered replacement organs, recreated from the patients' own cells.

Acknowledgments

The present study was supported by the Milwaukee Heart™ Research Foundation. We thank the entire engineering group of the Milwaukee Heart™ Project for providing the polyurethane sheets, blood sacs and VADs for this study. We are also grateful to Mrs. D. M. Wankowski for her skillful technical assistance in performing the experiments, to Mrs. I. Hernandez for her technical expertise in conducting the SEM studies, and to Mr. M. D. Silverman for his helpful technical suggestions and critical comments.

References

1. Moneta GL, Porter JM. Arterial substitutes in peripheral vascular surgery: A review. J Long-Term Effects of Medical Implants 1995; 5:47-67.
2. Noishiki Y. Progress and problems in the development of vascular prostheses. Artif Organs 1995; 19:3-6.
3. Greisler HP. Currently available vascular prostheses. In: Greisler HP, ed. New biologic and synthetic vascular prostheses. Austin: R.G. Landes Co., 1991:20-32.
4. Jarrell BE. Vascular and endothelial cell technology. In: Skalak R, Fox CF, eds. Tissue engineering. New York: Alan R. Liss, Inc., 1988:1-3.
5. Choi ET, Callow AD. The effect of biomaterials on the host. In: Greco RS, ed. Implantation biology: The host response and biomedical devices. Boca Raton: CRC Press, 1994:39-53.
6. Yeager A, Callow AD. New graft materials and current approaches to an acceptable small diameter vascular graft. Trans Am Soc Artif Intern Organs 1988; 34:88-94.
7. Noishiki Y, Tomizawa Y, Yamane Y, Matsumoto A. The vicious cycle of nonhealing neointima in fabric vascular prostheses. Artif Organs 1995; 19:7-16.
8. Sheppeck RA, LoGrefo FW. Blood and biomaterials. In: Greco RS, ed. Implantation biology: The host response and biomedical devices. Boca Raton: CRC Press, 1994:55-65.
9. Funk M. Epidemiology of end-stage heart disease. In: Hognes JR, VanAntwerp M, eds. The artificial heart: Prototypes, policies, and patients. Washington DC: National Academy Press, 1991:251-261.
10. Marshall E. Artificial heart: The beat goes on. Science 1991; 253:500-502.
11. Kolff WJ. Experiences and practical considerations for the future of artificial hearts and of mankind. Artif Organs 1988; 12:89-111.
12. Joyce LD, DeVries WC, Hastings WL et al. Response of the human body to the first permanent implant of the Jarvik-7 total artificial heart. Trans Am Soc Artif Intern Organs 1983; 29:81-87.
13. Bernhard WF. A fibrillar blood-prosthetic interface for both temporary and permanent ventricular assist devices: Experimental and clinical observations. Artif Organs 1989; 13:255-271.
14. Nose Y. My life with the National Institutes of Health Artificial Heart program. Artif Organs 1990; 14:174-190.
15. Westaby S. The need for artificial hearts. Heart 1996; 76:200-206.
16. Ward RA, Wellhausen SR, Dobbins JJ et al. Thromboembolic and infectious complications of total artificial heart implantation. Ann N Y Acad Sci 1987; 516:638-650.
17. Green K, Liska J, Egberg N et al. Hemostatic disturbances associated with implantation of an artificial heart. Thromb Res 1987; 48:349-362.
18. Yozu R, Golding LA, Jacobs G et al. Preclinical evaluation of a biolized temporary ventricular assist device. Trans Am Soc Artif Intern Organs 1989; 35:556-558.
19. Gimbrone MA Jr. Vascular endothelium: Nature's blood-compatible container. Ann N Y Acad Sci 1987; 516:5-11.
20. Mansfield PB, Wechezak AR, Sauvage LR. Preventing thrombus on artificial vascular surfaces: True endothelial cell linings. Trans Am Soc Artif Intern Organs 1975; 21:264-272.
21. In: Simionescu N, Simionescu M, eds. Endothelial cell dysfunctions. New York: Plenum Press, 1992:1-565.
22. In: Simionescu N, Simionescu M, eds. Endothelial cell biology in health and disease. New York: Plenum Press, 1988:1-458.
23. Dunn PF, Newman KD, Jones M et al. Seeding of vascular grafts with genetically modified endothelial cells: Secretion of recombinant TPA results in decreased seeded cell retention in vitro and in vivo. Circulation 1996; 93:1439-1446.
24. Williams SK, Rose DG, Jarrell BE. Microvascular endothelial cell sodding of ePTFE vascular grafts: Improved patency and stability of the cellular lining. J Biomed Mater Res 1996; 28:203-212.
25. Urayama H, Kasashima F, Kawakami T et al. An immunohistochemical analysis of implanted woven Dacron and expanded polytetrafluoroethylene grafts in humans. Artif Organs 1996; 20:24-29.
26. Brunstedt MR, Ziats NP, Rose-Caprara V et al. Attachment and proliferation of bovine aortic endothelial cells onto additive modified poly(ether urethane ureas). J Biomed Mater Res 1993; 27:483-492.
27. Park PK, Jarrell BE, Williams SK et al. Thrombus-free, human endothelial surface in the midregion of a Dacron vascular graft in the splanchnic venous circuit: Observations after nine months of implantation. J Vasc Surg 1990; 11:468-475.
28. Schneider PA, Hanson SR, Price TM, Harker LA. Confluent durable endothelialization of endarterectomized baboon aorta by early attachment of cultured endothelial cells. J Vasc Surg 1990; 11:365-372.

29. Okoshi T, Soldani G, Goddard M, Galletti PM. Very small-diameter polyurethane vascular prostheses with rapid endothelialization for coronary artery by pass grafting. Thorac Cardiovasc Surgeon 1993; 105:791-795.

30. Baitella-Eberle G, Groscurth P, Zilla P et al. Long-term results of tissue development and cell differentiation on Dacron prostheses seeded with microvascular cells in dogs. J Vasc Surg 1993; 18:1019-1028.

31. Van Belle E, Tio FO, Couffinhall T et al. Stent endothelialization: Time course, impact of local catheter delivery, feasibility of recombinant protein administration, and response to cytokine expedition. Circulation 1997; 95:438-448.

32. Langer R, Vacanti JP. Artificial organs. Sci Am 1995; 273:130-133.

33. Wilson JM, Birinyi LK, Salomon RN et al. Implantation of vascular grafts lined with genetically modified endothelial cells. Science 1989; 244:1344-1346.

34. Callow AD. The vascular endothelial cell as a vehicle for gene therapy. J Vasc Surg 1990; 11:793-798.

35. Nabel EG, Plautz G, Nabel GJ. Transduction of a foreign histocompatibility gene into the arterial wall induces vasculitis. Proc Natl Acad Sci USA 1992; 89:5157-5161.

36. Koh GY, Kim S-J, Klug MG et al. Targeted expression of transforming growth factor-β in intracardiac grafts promotes vascular endothelial cell DNA synthesis. J Clin Invest 1995; 95:114-121.

37. Kottke-Marchant K, Veenstra AA, Marchant RE. Human endothelial cell growth and coagulant function varies with respect to interfacial properties of polymeric substrates. J Biomed Mater Res 1996; 30:209-220.

38. Ott MJ, Ballermann BJ. Shear stress-conditioned, endothelial cell-seeded vascular grafts: Improved cell adherence in response to in vitro shear stress. Surgery 1995; 117:334-339.

39. Ballermann BJ, Ott MJ. Adhesion and differentiation of endothelial cells by exposure to chronic shear stress: A vascular graft model. Blood Purif 1995; 13:125-134.

40. Kaehler J, Zilla P, Fasol R et al. Precoating substrate and surface configuration determine adherence and spreading of seeded endothelial cells on polytetrafluoroethylene grafts. J Vasc Surg 1989; 9:535-541.

41. Gosselin C, Ren D, Ellinger J, Greisler HP. In vivo platelet deposition on polytetrafluoroethylene coated with fibrin glue containing fibroblast growth factor 1 and heparin in a canine model. Am J Surgery 1995; 170:126-130.

42. Nikolaychik VV, Samet MM, Lelkes PI. A new, cryoprecipitate based coating for improved endothelial cell attachment and growth on medical grade artificial surfaces. ASAIO J 1994; 40: M846-M852.

43. Nikolaychik VV, Wankowski DM, Samet MM, Lelkes PI. In vitro testing of endothelial cell monolayers under dynamic conditions inside a beating ventricular prosthesis. ASAIO J 1996; 42: M487-M494.

44. Horwitz AF, Thiery JP. Cell-to-cell contact and extracellular matrix. Curr Opin Cell Biol 1994; 6:645-647.

45. Ruoslahti E. RGD and other recognition sequences for integrins. Annu Rev Cell Dev Biol 1996; 12:697-715.

46. In: Hay ED, ed. Cell biology of extracellular matrix. 2nd Edn. New York: Plenum Press, 1991:1-468.

47. Fasol R, Zilla P. Endothelialization of artificial heart materials. In: Unger F, ed. Assisted Circulation 3. Berlin: Springer-Verlag, 1989:580-598.

48. Sipehia R, Martucci G, Lipscombe J. Transplantation of human endothelial cell monolayer on artificial vascular prosthesis: The effect of growth-support surface chemistry, cell seeding density, ECM protein coating, and growth factors. Art Cells Blood Subs and Immob Biotech 1996; 24:51-63.

49. Lin H-B, Sun W, Mosher DF et al. Synthesis, surface, and cell-adhesion properties of polyurethanes containing covalently grafted RGD-peptides. J Biomed Mater Res 1994; 28:329-342.

50. Nikolaychik VV, Samet MM, Lelkes PI. A new method for continual quantitation of viable cells on endothelialized polyurethanes. J Biomater Sci Polymer Edn 1996; 7:881-891.

51. Nichols WK, Gospodarowicz D, Kessler TR, Olsen DB. Increased adherence of vascular endothelial cells to Biomer precoated with extracellular matrix. Trans Am Soc Artif Intern Organs 1981; 27:208-212.

52. Seeger JM, Klingman N. Improved in vivo endothelialization of prosthetic grafts by surface modification with fibronectin. J Vasc Surg 1988; 8:476-482.

53. Skehan P, Storeng R, Scudiero D et al. New colorimetric cytotoxicity assay for anticancer-drug screening. J Natl Cancer Inst 1990; 13:1107-1112.

54. Clapper DL, Daws KM, Guire PE. Photoimmobilized ECM peptides promote cell attachment and growth on biomaterials. 20th Annual Meeting of the Society for Biomaterials 1994; 345 (Abstract).

55. Zilla P, Fasol R, Preiss P et al. Use of fibrin glue as a substrate for in vitro endothelialization of PTFE vascular grafts. Surgery 1989; 105:515-522.

56. Sirois E, Côte MF, Doillon CJ. Growth factors and biological supports for endothelial cell lining: In vitro study. Int J Artif Organs 1993; 16:609-619.

57. Gosselin C, Vorp DA, Warty VS et al. ePTFE coating with fibrin glue, FGF-1, and heparin: Effect on retention of seeded endothelial cells. J Surg Res 1996; 60:327-332.

58. Muller-Glauser W, Zilla P, Lachat M et al. Immediate shear stress resistance of endothelial cell monolayers seeded in vitro on fibrin glue-coated ePTFE prostheses. Eur J Vasc Surg 1993; 7:324-328.

59. DePalma L, Criss VR, Luban NLC. The preparation of fibrinogen concentrate for use as fibrin glue by four different methods. Transfusion 1993; 33:717-720.

60. In: Harris JR, ed. Blood separation and plasma fractionation. New York: John Wiley & Sons, 1991:1-497.

61. Wankowski DM, Samet MM, Nikolaychik VV, Lelkes PI. Endothelial cell seeding with rotation of a ventricular blood sac. ASAIO J 1994; 40: M319-M324.

62. Gimbrone MA, Jr., Cotran RS, Folkman J. Human vascular endothelial cells in culture. J Cell Biol 1974; 60:673-684.

63. Schor AM, Schor SL, Allen TD. Effects of culture conditions on the proliferation, morphology and migration of bovine aortic endothelial cells. J Cell Sci 1983; 62:267-285.

64. Dasse KA, Chipman SD, Sherman CN et al. Clinical experience with textured blood contacting surfaces in ventricular assist devices. ASAIO J 1987; 10:418-425.

65. Graham TR, Dasse K, Coumbe A et al. Neo-intimal development on textured biomaterial surfaces during clinical use of an implantable left ventricular assist device. Eur J Cardiothorac Surg 1990; 4:182-190.

66. Okoshi T. New concept of microporous structure in small diameter vascular prostheses. Artif Organs 1995; 19:27-31.

67. Okoshi T, Soldani G, Goddard M, Galletti PM. Microporous polyurethane inhibits critical mural thrombosis and enhances endothelialization at blood-contacting

surface. In: Akutsu T, Koyanagi H, eds. Heart replacement: Artificial heart 5. Tokyo: Springer-Verlag, 1996:47-52.

68. Patterson RB, Messier A, Valentini RF. Effects of radiofrequency glow discharge and oligopeptides on the attachment of human endothelial cells to polyurethane. ASAIO J 1995; 41: M625-M629.

69. Greisler HP. Endothelial cell transplantation onto synthetic vascular grafts: Panacea, poison or placebo. In: Greisler HP, ed. New biologic and synthetic vascular prostheses. Austin: R.G. Landes Co., 1991:47-64.

70. Thomson GJL, Vohra RK, Carr MH, Walker MG. Adult human endothelial cell seeding using expanded polytetrafluoroethylene vascular grafts: A comparison of four substrates. Surgery 1991; 109:20-27.

71. Marchant RE, Wang I-W. Physical and chemical aspects of biomaterials used in humans. In: Greco RS, ed. Implantation biology: The host response and biomedical devices. Boca Raton: CRC Press, 1994:13-38.

72. Frazier OH, Kadipasaoglu KA, Parnis SM, Radovancevic B. Biomaterials used in cardiac surgery. In: Greco RS, ed. Implantation biology: The host response and biomedical devices. Boca Raton: CRC Press, 1994:165-178.

73. Lelkes PI, Samet MM. Endothelialization of the luminal sac in artificial cardiac prostheses: A challenge for both biologists and engineers. J Biomech Eng 1991; 113:132-142.

74. Iba T, Sumpio BE. Morphological response of human endothelial cells subjected to cyclic strain in vitro. Microvasc Res 1991; 42:245-254.

75. Sumpio BE, Banes AJ, Buckley M, Johnson G Jr. Alterations in aortic endothelial cell morphology and cytoskeletal protein synthesis during cyclic tensional deformation. J Vasc Surg 1988; 7:130-138.

76. Barbee KA, Davies PF, Lal R. Shear stress-induced reorganization of the surface topography of living endothelial cells imaged by atomic force microscopy. Circ Res 1994; 74:163-171.

77. Nerem RM, Levesque MJ, Sato M. Vascular dynamics and the endothelium. In: Schmid-Schonbein GW, Woo SL-Y, Zweifach BW, eds. Frontiers in biomechanics. New York: Springer-Verlag, 1986:324-341.

78. Girard PR, Helmlinger G, Nerem RM. Shear stress effects on the morphology and cytomatrix of cultured vascular endothelial cells. In: Frangos JA, ed. Physical forces and the mammalian cell. San Diego: Academic Press, Inc., 1993:193-222.

79. Thoumine O, Nerem RM, Girard PR. Changes in organization and composition of the extracellular matrix underlying cultured endothelial cells exposed to laminar steady shear stress. Lab Invest 1995; 73:565-576.

80. Hirai J, Kanda K, Oka T, Matsuda T. Highly oriented, tubular hybrid vascular tissue for a low pressure circulatory system. ASAIO J 1994; 40: M383-M388.

81. Matsuda T, Takaichi S, Kitamura T et al. A reconstituted vessel's wall model on microporous substrates as a small-caliber artificial graft. In: Akutsu T, Koyanagi H, Takatani S et al., eds. Artificial heart 2. Tokyo: Springer-Verlag, 1988:65-73.

82. Hirai J, Matsuda T. Self-organized, tubular hybrid vascular tissue composed of vascular cells and collagen for low-pressure-loaded venous system. Cell Transplantation 1995; 4:597-608.

PART II

Biolized Prostheses: Surface Healing

Microvascular Endothelial Cell Transplantation

CHAPTER 6

Microvascular Endothelial Cell Transplantation: A Review

Stuart K. Williams

Early Development of Endothelial Cell Transplantation Technology

The development of an endothelial cell lining on the lumenal surface of vascular implants (e.g., peripheral vascular grafts, arteriovenous fistulas, coronary artery bypass grafts) has been realized only with the understanding of the complex physiology of these cells. The development and first clinical experiences with polymeric vascular grafts provided the initial evidence of the importance of a functional endothelium on the lumenal surface of blood vessels. These synthetic blood vessels perform adequately in large diameter (> 6 mm) positions (e.g., abdominal aortic replacements); however, as the diameter of the synthetic grafts needed became smaller, long term function was compromised. The best evidence for the need of a lumenal endothelial cell lining is provided by the poor patency observed when synthetic grafts with diameters less then 6 mm are used. These grafts exhibit extremely poor, clinically unacceptable, long term patency, due predominantly to the formation of blood clots, resulting in lost patency.

The bypass of occluded native vessels with diameters less then 6 mm has been limited to the use of autologous native blood vessels. While these vessels have provided acceptable long term patency, clinicians have realized the importance of maintaining the integrity of the lumenal lining of endothelial cells.[1-4] Autologous vessels provide superior long term patency as compared to synthetic grafts, due not only to their compliant natural tissue characteristics, but also to the antithrombogenic nature of the endothelial cell lining. Procedures which disrupt the endothelium, such as angioplasty and atherectomy, provide additional evidence for the need to maintain a functional endothelium.

The first report of the successful isolation and transplantation of endothelial cells was a report by Dr. Malcolm Herring in 1978.[5] His methods involved the use of a large vessel-derived endothelium obtained by scraping the lumenal surface of vein segments. These cells were subsequently transplanted onto the lumenal surface of polymeric graft materials, a process which was termed seeding. The methods used for seeding include mixing the isolated cells with autologous blood and subsequently using this blood-cell inoculum to preclot porous grafts. The lumenal blood-contacting surface was observed to be predominantly fibrin and red cells, with endothelial cells present predominantly within the resulting clot. The hypothesis behind these studies was that seeded endothelial cells would migrate from within the clot to the lumenal blood flow surface, proliferate and finally form a continuous monolayer through the formation of typical interendothelial cell junctions. Subsequent work by a large number of investigators, including work from the laboratories of Schmidt,[6] Stanley[7] and Graham,[8] established the ability to accelerate the formation of monolayers on prosthetic grafts using large vessel endothelial cells as a source of cells for seeding.

Tissue Engineering of Prosthetic Vascular Grafts, edited by Peter Zilla and Howard P. Greisler.
©1999 R.G. Landes Company.

Publication of these studies established the feasibility of performing endothelial cell transplantation and resulted in extensive work to optimize seeding technology. Numerous questions were identified which needed to be addressed before endothelial cell transplantation was expected to be found clinically acceptable. These questions identified numerous issues related to the source of tissue for subsequent endothelial cell transplantation, the function of immediately isolated endothelium and methods to improve the interaction of endothelium with prosthetic graft surfaces. Subsequent laboratory work has established the efficacy of intraoperative methods for endothelial cell isolation and deposition onto the lumenal surface of vascular grafts.

Sources of Endothelium for Transplantation

As described above, Herring first reported the use of venous-derived endothelium for subsequent transplantation. The yield of cells from a suitable piece of vein segment was approximately 1×10^4 cells.[9] Thus, based on the largest piece of vein which could be obtained from a patient, only 10,000 endothelial cells could be obtained. Under even the most ideal conditions, this cell number would provide a relatively sparse coating of cells, requiring extensive cell proliferation to achieve a monolayer. Kempzinski et al[10] reported that even if cells could be isolated and deposited on the surface of polymeric grafts with optimal efficiency, a large number of these cells would be lost from the lumenal surface of the graft due to the effects of blood flow-induced shear on the lumenal surface. Endothelial cells seeded onto grafts with this technology would be required to undergo even more extensive proliferation or, alternatively, a new source of endothelial cells obtained in large numbers must be found.

Cultured Endothelium for Transplantation

Methods for the isolation and culture of nonhuman endothelial cells were first reported in the 1920s, providing methods for the expansion of endothelial cell numbers by in vitro proliferation.[11] However, the same methods used for nonhuman endothelial cell proliferation had no stimulatory effect on human endothelial cell proliferation. During the 1970s a method for human endothelial cell isolation, based on the pioneering work of Lewis in 1922, provided human endothelial cells in culture; however, these cells exhibited minimal proliferative capacity. A number of endothelial cell growth factors were discovered that slightly stimulated human endothelial cell proliferation. The major breakthrough in human endothelial cell growth in culture was work performed by Dr. Susan Thornton, working with Dr. Elliot Levine, which identified heparin as an integral cofactor with endothelial cell growth factor for the stimulation of human umbilical vein endothelial cell growth in culture.[12] Jarrell and coworkers[13] subsequently reported that heparin and ECGF would stimulate human adult endothelial cell growth in culture. For the first time, cells from human artery and vein segments from numerous anatomical positions could be grown in large quantities. Large numbers of human endothelia could be produced from single endothelial cells, providing nearly unlimited supplies of human adult endothelium. These breakthroughs in culture

methods provided a means to produce large quantities of autologous endothelial cells by obtaining a small segment of a patient's blood vessel, isolating and culturing the endothelium in heparin and endothelial cell growth supplement (ECGS) and transplanting these cells at very high seeding densities onto prosthetic grafts.

Large vessel-derived endothelial cell seeding at high density was achieved in vitro; however, additional questions have been raised, delaying wide spread clinical utilization of this technique. Concerns related to the use of cultured endothelium for cell transplantations are surmountable. Dr. Peter Zilla has performed a careful series of studies to address the major concerns raised about using cultured cells, as well as providing evidence of the efficacy of this form of tissue engineering.[14-16] Some of these questions included concerns relating to the derivation of cells from large vessel sources, which requires a separate surgical procedure, most likely from patients with an already compromised circulatory system. This increased risk of a separate vascular complication had to be weighed against the need for endothelial cell transplantation. If cultured cells were used for transplantation, the conditions of culture must be evaluated to determine the effect on subsequent cell function. Bovine derived serum components such as viruses, and growth factors such as heparin and ECGS, would be carried with transplanted cells into patients, requiring characterization of their effects. Considering that endothelial cells have an extremely low mitotic index, the stimulation of endothelial cell growth must be considered to determine how cell growth may alter endothelial cell function. Finally, little data is available concerning the appropriateness of transplanting vein-derived endothelial cells into an arterial circulation with respect to the ability of these cells to differentiate and function under arterial conditions. Nonetheless, this technique has been successfully implemented in a series of patients undergoing peripheral bypass surgery. Initial results indicate both the safety and efficacy of large vessel endothelial cell transplantation.[16]

Current Considerations in Endothelial Cell Transplantation

Use of Microvessel Endothelium for Tissue Engineering of Vascular Grafts

Given the small numbers of cells available if autologous vein-derived endothelium are used without culture, and concerns about culturing effects, investigators have been considering alternate sources of endothelial cells for transplantation. In 1986 Jarrell and Williams[17] reported methods for the isolation of autologous microvessel endothelial cells from adipose tissue for use in cell transplantation. The source of fat for this EC isolation was initially fat deposits associated with omentum. This fat is well vascularized, with a density of endothelial cells in excess of 10^6 endothelial cells per gram of fat isolated. The need to place cells in culture to increase cell number is obviated by the large amounts of endothelium available per gram of omental associated fat. However, access to omental-associated fat still would necessitate a separate surgical procedure, with related complications.

The use of omental-associated fat-derived endothelial cells was questioned by Visser et al,[18] who reported that omental tissue derived from humans contains predominantly mesothelial cells and not endothelium. This report raised a significant controversy concerning the use of omental-associated fat as a source of endothelial cells for transplantation. Since this initial report by Visser et al, subsequent reports have clarified the controversy and provided additional options for obtaining microvessel endothelial cells.[19] First it was established that investigators have erroneously used the terms omentum and omental fat interchangeably. These two tissues are histologically and anatomically distinct. While omentum as used by Visser et al is a vascularized tissue with an extensive number of mesothelial cells present, omental-associated fat, as used by Jarrell and Williams, is composed of predominantly endothelial cells and adipocytes. This is not to say that use of omental-associated fat avoids the possibility of mesothelial cells in the primary cell isolate. Omental fat deposits are covered by a thin layer of mesothelium, and a single cell population isolated from omental-associated fat will contain a small number of mesothelial cells in addition to endothelium. Careful isolation of omental-associated fat away from omentum will reduce contamination by mesothelium.

Alternate anatomic sources for microvascularized autologous human fat for endothelial cell transplantation have been reported since these original reports using omentum-associated fat. A significant improvement was the identification of subcutaneous fat as a source of endothelial cells and the use of liposuction to derive this fat from patients.[20] A patient undergoing endothelial cell transplantation therefore does not need to undergo a laparotomy to remove omental fat or undergo a separate vascular procedure to remove a segment of vein. A small amount (50 cc) of fat can be removed using a hand held syringe cannula device. This procedure requires less then five minutes and requires a small skin incision or trocar puncture to insert the liposuction cannula. The liposuction cannulas used for this procedure have been continuously improved for plastic and cosmetic surgical applications.

The use of liposuction fat is also advantageous since the tissue is effectively minced during the liposuction removal process. Scanning electron microscopic evaluation of liposuction fat (Fig. 6.1) illustrates the morphological characteristics of this tissue. The predominant cell type present at this magnification is adipocytes. Recently, a complete characterization of cells present in liposuction-derived fat was reported and established that the major cell type, other than adipocytes, present in this tissue is endothelium.[19] Prior to any cell dissociation procedures, human subcutaneous fat contains in excess of 85% endothelium based on the total cells present per unit volume of fat. Adipocytes account for approximately 12% of the cell population, again before any tissue dissociation and cell isolation techniques are used. Therefore, following tissue dissociation and cell isolation, endothelial cells must account for at least 85% of the cells in the final inoculum.

Markers for Isolated Endothelial Cells

One significant difficulty in establishing the identity of cells present in the primary isolate following tissue digestion has been the relative lack of a dependable marker of endothelial cells. While antibodies directed against von Willebrand factor or factor VIII-related antigen (FVIIIrAg) have been used somewhat routinely for endothelial cell identification, these markers do not unfailingly react with freshly isolated microvascular endothelial cells. First, upon primary isolation and due in part to the action of proteolytic enzymes, endothelial cells will release these proteins from cytoplasmic granules, thus resulting in cells which exhibit negative staining properties.[21] Also confounding is the relative lack of Weibel-palade bodies in fat-derived microvessel endothelial cells. The cytoplasmic inclusions contain extremely high concentrations of vWF, which subsequently stain

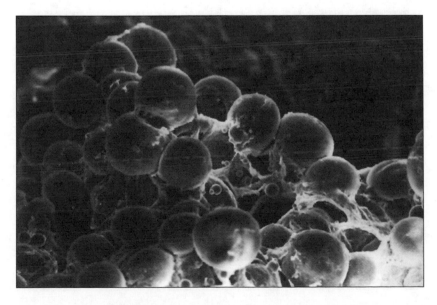

Fig. 6.1. Scanning electron micrograph of human liposuction-derived subcutaneous fat, illustrating the predominance of adipocytes.

extremely well in cell types such as vein-derived endothelium. Venous endothelial cells contain a significant number of Weibel-palade bodies, such that investigators who observe vWF staining in microvessel endothelial cells correctly assess cells with limited reaction product as compared to venous endothelium. Often investigators will suggest that since the bright punctate staining common with Weibel-palade bodies is not observed in microvascular endothelial cells, these cells must not be endothelium. On the contrary, microvascular endothelium is phenotypically distinct from venous or arterial endothelial cells and shows appropriate differences in markers such as vWF and FVIIIrAg. Upon primary culture of microvessel endothelial cells, the morphology often takes on a fibroblastic appearance and, in concert with the relatively minimal reaction with vWF antibodies, investigators will often conclude that the predominant cell type in fat is fibroblasts. What is actually being observed is the ability of endothelial cells to phenotypically differentiate under different in vitro and or in vivo conditions. Interestingly, a recent report suggests that fibroblasts can differentiate in vivo into endothelial cells. This phenotypic drift may be a common characteristic of pluripotent mesenchymal cells, with possible utilization in future cell transplantation technologies.

The methods for the isolation of endothelial cells from fat are essentially modifications of the methods first reported by Wagner in 1972 for the isolation of endothelial cells from rat epididymal fat pads.[22] Human fat microvessel endothelial cells are isolated by first digesting the fat with a proteolytic enzyme mixture composed predominantly of collagenase and trypsin. The characteristics of this enzyme are critical for successful isolation of endothelial cells from fat.[23] Following collagenase digestion the slurry is centrifuged, resulting in the separation of buoyant adipocytes from more dense endothelium. The endothelial cell rich pellet is then used for cell transplantation procedures.

Cell Deposition on Graft Surfaces: Seeding vs. Sodding

The availability of large quantities of autologous endothelial cells does not necessarily overcome another major concern related to endothelial cell transplantation. The deposition of endothelial cells onto the lumenal (blood flow) surface of vascular grafts is a critical step in the transplantation process. Once placed as an interpositional graft, cells on the lumenal surface must resist the flow of blood and remain adherent to the polymeric surface during the maturation of an endothelial cell monolayer. The original methods used to transplant endothelial cells onto graft surfaces were termed seeding procedures, since relatively low concentrations of cells were placed in suspension in either whole blood or plasma, and this suspension transferred to the inner lining of vascular grafts. The endothelial cells in this inoculum were subsequently expected to proliferate and migrate to the blood flow surface, creating a contiguous lining of cells. An alternate form of transplantation, described using the term sodding, was subsequently suggested and evaluated in vitro as well as in preclinical animal and human studies.[24] Sodding describes a method of endothelial cell deposition wherein a concentration of cells which would provide a confluent density of cells on the lumenal graft surface is forcibly deposited onto the graft lumenal surface. This forced deposition is most easily carried out by establishing a pressure gradient across the flow surface of the graft whereby the cells are essentially filtered onto the surface of the graft. While previous methods used gravity to allow cell deposition, sodding of cells using pressure deposition results in near immediate association of cells with the lumenal surface. The time to prepare a tissue engineered vascular graft for implantation, a period inclusive of tissue isolation, cell isolation and cell deposition, has effectively been reduced to less than 60 minutes.[20]

Fig. 6.2. Endothelial cell monolayer established on an ePTFE graft using autologous microvascular endothelial cell transplantation. The graft was implanted as an interpositional device in the carotid artery in a canine model and explanted after 5 weeks.

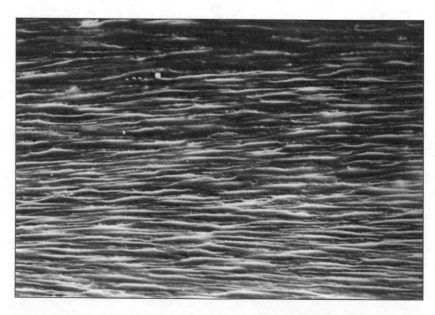

Animal Models of Endothelial Cell Transplantation

The availability of methods for endothelial cell isolation and culture, as well as methods to deposit cells onto graft surfaces, has resulted in numerous investigations to evaluate the efficacy of endothelial cell transplantation.[25-33] The earliest animal models were developed to evaluate the ability to accelerate the formation of endothelial cell linings on polymeric grafts. Most of these studies have been performed in the canine model, due primarily to the acceptance of this animal model as a predictor of graft function in humans. Earliest studies established the ability to accelerate the formation of a continuous monolayer of endothelial cells on the lumenal surface of vascular grafts (Fig. 6.2). In general, monolayer formation is highly dependent on the density of cells used to treat the graft surface. When cells are transplanted at confluent densities or greater, monolayer formation appears to be complete in under three weeks. Subconfluent densities require more extended periods of time.

Mechanisms Underlying the Formation of a Neointima in Tissue Engineered Vascular Grafts Using Microvascular Endothelial Cell Transplantation

A number of preclinical animal studies have established that, following the transplantation of microvessel endothelial cells onto synthetic grafts, the accelerated formation of an endothelial cell monolayer on the lumenal flow surface is observed. The earliest time point evaluated is 4 days in a rat aortic graft model of microvessel endothelial cell transplantation.[34] At this time a confluent layer of endothelial cells is observed. Studies in dogs have established that the endothelial cell lining observed in microvessel endothelial cell sodded grafts remains stable for periods of up to one year, the longest published animal implant data.[33] Figure 6.3 illustrates the lining on a microvascular endothelial cell sodded ePTFE graft explanted after one year. This morphologic data establishes the ability to accelerate the formation of an endothelial cell lining, but questions have been raised regarding whether the cells present on the lumenal surface of microvessel sodded grafts represent the same cells transplanted during the initial sodding procedure. This question has been addressed using a method to trace the fate of transplanted endothelial cells using a fluorescent tagging method.[35] A fluorescent dye is permanently incorporated into the membranes of microvessel endothelial cells at the time they are transplanted onto the lumenal surface of vascular grafts. This dye has unique characteristics in that it is long lived and provides a marker of the fate of transplanted cells. If, however, fluorescently labeled cells duplicate, each daughter cell receives one half the fluorescence of the initial cell. For cells which undergo multiple duplication, a process which could occur following cell transplantation, the subsequent progeny would contain undetectable amounts of fluorescence. Use of this technique in a canine model of microvessel endothelial cell sodding revealed that after 5 weeks the monolayer of endothelial cells on the flow surface exhibited extensive fluorescence, establishing their identity as cells present in the original cell inoculum used for sodding. Thus, following sodding, the microvessel endothelial cells need simply adhere to the polymer surface and to each other to form a confluent monolayer without the need to undergo extensive cell proliferation.

Preclinical Animal Trials of Endothelial Cell Transplantation

With the development of methods for the isolation of endothelial cells from numerous tissue sources, including macro- and microvascular sources, numerous animal studies have been performed to evaluate the effects of endothelial cell transplantation on small diameter vascular graft patency. These studies use small diameter grafts (< 6 mm), most often in the canine species. The predominance of canine models for these preclinical evaluations is based on the general acceptance of this model as being similar to humans with respect to graft healing. While the canine species is commonly used, techniques for graft placement (e.g., end to end,

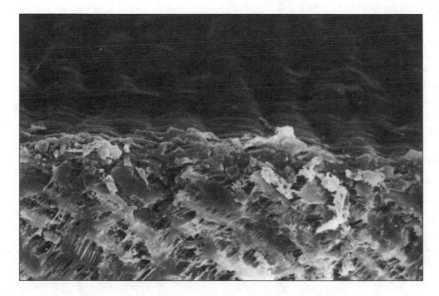

Fig. 6.3. Scanning electron micrograph of a sodded ePTFE carotid artery after one year.

end to side anastomoses) site of placement (e.g., femoral, carotid, aortofemoral), use and duration of antiplatelet/anticoagulant drugs (e.g., asprinin, persantine) and the type and use of control grafts (e.g., paired vs. nonpaired grafts) varies significantly among investigators. The rationale for the choice of each variable is often based on the goals of individual studies. Quite often decisions are based on the need to evaluate healing characteristics of grafts as compared to evaluation of patency. The use of paired grafts (e.g., carotid or femoral interpositional grafts) is most common, since cell transplanted grafts can be compared to control grafts in the same animal. Variability in animal to animal thrombotic state is partially accounted for in paired graft models.

Due to the variability in animal models previously used by investigators, comparison of data is complicated. Table 6.1 illustrates a compilation of the results of published animal trials using 4 mm inner diameter polymer grafts in preclinical studies of endothelial cell transplantation. These studies were chosen for the ability to evaluate patency using nonpaired statistical analysis within each study. The significance of endothelial cell transplantation can be evaluated first by assessing the fractional increase in patency between cell transplanted and control grafts. In this column a positive fractional increase in patency indicates a benefit of cell transplantation, a zero increase indicates no benefit and a negative fractional increase indicates cell transplantation has a negative influence on graft patency. The 95% confidence limits have been provided for each study to indicate variability. The major conclusion from this table is the consistently observed positive benefit of endothelial cell transplantation with respect to graft patency. Although not all studies presented in this table demonstrated a statistically significant improvement in patency with cell transplantation, treatment of grafts with endothelial cells was the most common predictor of improved patency. Most significantly, only two reports provide evidence of statistically significant improvement in graft patency as a direct result of endothelial cell transplantation.[25-33] Both of these reports are unique in that they treated the lumenal surface of grafts with a confluent density of endothelial cells using the method known as sodding. One of these two reports used autologous microvessel endothelial cells as the source of cells for sodding. Thus, preclinical animal studies of endothelial cell transplantation have, until recently, not provided evidence of statistically significant improvement in graft patency following endothelial cell transplantation. On the other hand, deposition of endothelial cells at high densities and the use of microvessel endothelial cell sodding has provided statistically significant improvement in patency in preclinical animal studies.

Microvascular Endothelial Cell Transplantation for Arteriovenous Fistulas and Coronary Artery Bypass Grafts

Arteriovenous Fistulas for Dialysis

The initial preclinical animal studies of endothelial cell transplantation were consistently performed in models which sought to duplicate the environment typical of pe-

Table 6.1. Endothelial cell-seeded graft versus control graft canine studies using paired 4 mm diameter grafts

Investigator	Site	Graft	Duration	Antiplatelet Therapy	Endothelial Cell-Seeded Grafts Patent	Clotted	Control Grafts Patent	Clotted	Fractional Increase in Patency for Seeded Grafts	95% Lower and Upper Confidence Intervals	Chi-Square *
Allen[25]	Femoral and carotid	Dacron	28 wk	2 wk	27	1	8	20	0.68	0.50,0.86	24.7
Belden[26]	Carotid	Dacron	4 wk	None	30	7	26	11	0.11	-0.09,0.30	0.7
Douville[27]	Carotid	ePTFE	12 wk	6 wk	12	7	6	13	0.36	0.02,0.62	2.64
Kempczinski[10]	Carotid	ePTFE	13 wk	4 wk	32	9	25	16	0.17	0.03,0.37	2.07
Schmidt[28]	Carotid	Dacron	4 wk	None	7	2	5	4	0.22	-0.20,0.65	0.25
Shindo[30]	Femoral	Dacron	4 wk	None	8	4	1	11	0.58	0.27,0.89	6.4
Stanley[31]	Iliofemoral	Dacron	16 wk	2 wk	11	3	6	8	0.32	0.01,0.62	2.64
Tannenbaum[32]	Carotid	ePTFE	10 wk	None	14	1	11	4	0.2	0.06,0.46	0.96
Williams[33]	Carotid	ePTFE	12 wk	4 wk	9	2	1	10	0.73	0.44,1.00	8.98

*For chi-square >3.84 for 1 degree of freedom, P<0.05.

ripheral arterial interpositional grafts. The development of a synthetic peripheral arterial graft is clearly of clinical importance; however, new designs in synthetic grafts for use in other anatomical positions are also of great interest. In the USA, prosthetic grafts are presently the most common vascular access created for hemodialysis.[36] These grafts exhibit a failure rate requiring intervention to restore patency at a mean of nine months after patency.[37] The estimated annual cost to the USA health care system to maintain vascular access for hemodialysis is believed to be in excess of $900 million.[37] The reason for the failure of these grafts is common to all synthetic grafts and includes the development of predominantly distal anastomotic neointimal thickening and thrombosis due to the inherent thrombogenicity of polymer materials. Recent studies have begun to evaluate the use of microvascular endothelial cell transplantation to improve AV graft function.[38] These initial studies have demonstrated that the healing of microvessel endothelial cell sodded grafts is quite different, depending on the site of anatomic placement. While arterial interpositional grafts sodded with endothelial cells exhibit a relatively thin neointimal lining, sodded grafts placed in the AV position in dogs have been reported to exhibit a dramatic thickening in the neointima throughout the length of the graft. These results suggest that the high flow characteristics of AV fistulas create an environment which may stimulate neointimal thickening.

Tissue Engineered Coronary Artery Bypass Grafts

While synthetic grafts have been used extensively for revascularization in the peripheral arterial position, the use of synthetic, nonautologous vessels for coronary artery bypass grafting has routinely led to failure. The need for an antithrombogenic endothelial cell lining on synthetic CABG is clearly indicated. The development of tissue engineered CABG using microvessel endothelial cell transplantation has used two designs of synthetic grafts. Phillips and coworkers report the use of the Possis Perma-Flow CABG as a synthetic conduit for coronary bypass and have evaluated the use of microvessel endothelial cell sodding to create an endothelial cell lining on these grafts.[39] Arzoumann and coworkers have developed an alternative synthetic CABG using microvessel endothelial cell sodding.[40] This unique model involves the initial sodding of ePTFE grafts with placement and maturation in an AV fistula position first, followed by conversion to the coronary position. The maturation in the AV position was reported to be necessary for the creation of a maximally antithrombogenic lining of endothelial cells on the lumenal flow surface prior to conversion to the CABG position. These reports suggest that use of tissue engineered CABG in humans is on the horizon.

Future of Microvessel Endothelial Cell Transplantation

While the original goal of endothelial cell transplantation studies has focused on small diameter vascular grafts, the availability of operating room compatible methods for endothelial cell transplantation has expanded the possible application of these cells. The development of gene therapy methodologies has begun to target the endothelial cell as a cellular vehicle for gene therapy.[41] Endothelial cells reside at the interface between blood and tissue and therefore maintain a strategic position for the production and release of therapeutic materials. Molecular biologists have begun to take advantage of the extensive methodology established for endothelial cell transplantation. Reports of genetic modification of endothelial cells have exploded recently as the attractiveness of this cell is realized. The use of genetically modified microvascular endothelial cells has moved beyond prosthetic devices, and studies are ongoing to establish the use of these cells in almost every anatomic site under consideration for gene therapies. Again, the availability of methods to easily isolate and transplant endothelial cells, especially subcutaneous fat-derived microvessel endothelial cells, provides an exciting new use for endothelial cell transplantation.

References

1. Quist WC, Haudenshield CC, Logerfo FW. Qualitative microscopy of implanted vein grafts: Effects of graft integrity on morphological fate. J Thorac Cardiovasc Surg 1992; 103:671-677.
2. Richardson JV, Wright CB, Hiratzka LF. The role of endothelium in the patency of small venous substitutes. J Surg Res 1980; 28:556-562.
3. Cambria RP, Megerman J, Abbot WM. Endothelial preservation in reversed and in situ autogenous vein grafts. Ann Surg 1985; 202(1):50-55.
4. Angelini GD, Breckenridge IA, Psaila JV, Williams HM, Henderson AH, Newby AC. Preparation of human saphenous vein for coronary artery bypass grafting impairs its capacity to produce prostacyclin. Cardiovasc Res 1987; 21:28-33.
5. Herring M, Gardner A, Glover J. A single staged technique for seeding vascular grafts with autogenous endothelium. Surg 1978; 84:498-504.
6. Schmidt SP, Hunter TJ, Sharp WV, Malindzak GS, Evancho MM. Endothelial cell seeded four millimeter Dacron vascular grafts. J Vasc Surg 1984; 1:434-441.
7. Stanley JC, Burkel WE, Ford JW. Enanced patency of small diameter, externally supported Dacron iliofemoral grafts seeded with endothelial cells. Surg 1982; 92:994.
8. Graham LM, Vinter DW, Ford JW. Immediate seeding of enzymatically derived endothelium in Dacron vascular grafts. Early studies with autologous canine cells. Arch Surg 1980; 115:1289-1294.
9. Kesler KA, Herring MB, Arnold MP, Glover JL, Park HM, Helmus MN, Bendick PJ. Enhanced strength of endothelial attachment on polyester elastomer and polytetrafluoroethylene graft surfaces with fibronectin substrate. J Vasc Surg 1986; 3:58-64.
10. Kempczinski RF, Rosenman JE, Pearce WH, Rodersheimer LR, Berlatzky Y, Ramalanjaona GR. Endothelial cell seeding of new PTFE vascular prostheses. J Vasc Surg 1985; 2:424-429.
11. Lewis WH. Endothelium in tissue culture. Am J Anat 1922; 30:39-59.
12. Thornton SC, Mueller SN, Levine EM. Human endothelial cells: Cloning and long term serial cultivation employing heparin. Science 1983; 222:623-624.
13. Jarrell BE, Levine EM, Shapiro SS, Williams SK, Carabasi RA, Mueller SN, Thornton SC. Human adult endothelial cell growth in culture. J Vasc Surg 1984; 1:757-764.

14. Zilla P, Fasol R, Preiss P, Kadletz M, Deutsch M, Schima H, Tsangaris S, Groscurth P. Use of fibrin glue as a substrate for in vitro endothelialization of ePTFE vascular grafts. Surgery 1989; 105(4):515-522.

15. Zilla P, Preiss P, Groscurth P, Rosemeier F, Deutsch M, Odell J, Heidinger C, Fasol R, von Oppel U. In vitro-lined endothelium: Initial integrity and ultrastructural events. Surgery 1994; 116(3):524-534.

16. Zilla P, Deutsch M, Meinhart J, Puschmann R, Eberl T, Minar E, Dudczak R, Lugmaier H, Schmidt P, Noszian I. Clinical in vitro endothelialization of femoropopliteal bypass grafts: An actuarial follow-up over three years. J Vascular Surgery 1994; 19(3):540-548.

17. Jarrell BE, Williams SK, Stokes G, Hubbard FA, Carabasi RA, Koolpe E, Greener D, Pratt K, Moritz MJ, Radomski J, Speicher L. Use of freshly isolated capillary endothelial cells for the immediate establishment of a monolayer on a vascular graft at surgery. Surg 1986; 100(2):392-399.

18. Visser MJP, van Bockel JJ, van Muijen GNP, van Hinsbergh VWM. Cells derived from omental fat tissue and used for seeding vascular prostheses are not endothelial in origin: A study on the origin of epitheloid cells derived from human omentum. J Vasc Surg 1991; 13:373-381.

19. Williams SK, Wang TF, Castrillo R, Jarrell BE. Liposuction derived human fat used for vascular graft sodding contains endothelial cells and not mesothelial cells as the major cell type. J Vasc Surg 1994; 19:916-923.

20. Williams SK, Jarrell BE, Rose DG, Pontell J, Kapelan BA, Park PK, Carter TL. Human microvessel endothelial cell isolation and vascular graft sodding in the operating room. Ann Vasc Surg 1989; 3(2):146-152.

21. Lenzi R, Alpinin G, Liu MH, Rand JH, Tavoloni N. Von willebrand factor antigen is not an accurate marker of rat and guinea pig liver endothelial cells. Liver 1990; 10:372-379.

22. Wagner RC, Matthews MA. The isolation and culture of capillary endothelium from epididymal fat. Microvasc Res 1975; 10:286-297.

23. Williams SK, McKenney S, Jarrell BE. Collagenase lot selection and purification for adipose tissue digestion. Cell Transplantation. 1995; 4:281-289.

24. Williams SK, Carter T, Park PK, Rose DG, Schneider T, Jarrell BE. Formation of a multilayer cellular lining on a polyurethane vascular graft following endothelial cell sodding. J Biomed Mat Res 1992; 26:103-117.

25. Allen BT, Long JA, Clark RE, Sicard GA, Hopkins KY, Welch MJ. Influence of endothelial cell seeding on platelet deposition and patency in small-diameter Dacron arterial grafts. J Vasc Surg 1984; 1:224-232.

26. Belden TA, Schmidt SP, Falkow LJ, Sharp WV. Endothelial cell seeding of small-diameter vascular grafts. Trans Am Soc Artif Intern Organs 1982; 28:173.

27. Douville EC, Kempczinski RF, Birinyi LK, Ramalanjaona GR. Impact of endothelial cell seeding on long term patency and subendothelial proliferation in a small-caliber highly porous polytetrafluoroethylene graft. J Vasc Surg 1987; 5:544.

28. Schmidt SP, Hunter TJ, Hirko M. Small diameter vascular prostheses: Two designs of PTFE and endothelial cell seeded and nonseeded Dacron. J Vasc Surg 1985; 2:292-297.

29. Shepard AD, Eldrup-Jorgensen J, Keough EM. Endothelial cell seeding of small caliber synthetic grafts in the baboon. Surg 1986; 99:318.

30. Shindo S, Takagi A, Whittemore AD. Improved patency of collagen impregnated grafts after in vitro autogenous endothelial cell seeding. J Vasc Surg 1987; 6:325.

31. Stanley JC, Burkel WE, Linbald B. Endothelial cell seeding of synthetic vascular prostheses. Acta Chir Scand Suppl 1985; 529:17-27.

32. Tannenbaum G, Ahlborn T, Benvenisty A, Reemstma K, Nowygrod R. High density seeding of cultured endothelial cells leads to rapid coverage of PTFE grafts. Curr Surg 1983; 222:623.

33. Williams SK, Rose DG, Jarrell BE. Microvascular endothelial cell sodding of ePTFE vascular grafts: Improved patency and stability of the cellular lining. J Biomed Mater Res 1994; 28:203-212.

34. Ahlswede KM, Williams SK. Microvascular endothelial cell sodding of 1-mm expanded polytetrafluoroethylene vascular grafts. Arteriosclerosis and Thrombosis 1994; 14:25-31.

35. Williams SK, Kleinert LB, Rose D, McKenney S. Origin of endothelial cells that line expanded polytetrafluoroethylene vascular grafts sodded with cells from microvascularized fat. J Vasc Surg 1994; 19:594-604.

36. Palder SB, Kirkman RL, Whittemore AD. Vascular access for hemodialysis. Ann Surg 1986; 202:235-239.

37. Windus DW. Permanent vascular access: A nephrologist's view. Am J Kid Dis 1993; 21(5):457-471.

38. Williams SK, Jarrell BE, Kleinert LB. Endothelial cell transplantation onto polymeric arteriovenous grafts evaluated using a canine model. J Invest Surg 1994; 7:503-517.

39. Phillips M, Yamaguchi H, Miller V, Williams SK, Morris JJ, Shaff HJ. Endothelial cell sodding of the Permaflow prosthetic coronary artery bypass conduit. Annals of Thor Surg 1998; in press.

40. Arzouman D, Kleinert LB, Patula VB, Phillips M, Williams SK, Copeland JG. Endothelial cell sodding of ePTFE coronary artery bypass grafts. Abstract. American Heart Association 70th Scientific Session.

41. Stopeck AT, Vahedian M, Williams SK. Transfer and expression of the interferon gamma gene in human endothelial cells inhibits vascular smooth muscle cell growth in vitro. Cell Transplant 1997; 6(1):1-8.

Morphological Aspects of Microvascular Cell Isolates

Manuela Vici

Introduction

The lack of spontaneous endothelialization after implantation of small caliber vascular grafts in humans has made the lining of the prosthetic surface with endothelial cells advisable in order to reduce thrombogenicity and promote hemocompatibility. This has added a promising new field to tissue engineering.

Numerous research areas are critical for the success of tissue engineering. Some are related to the biological side, others to the engineering side. With regard to the former, issues such as cellular differentiation and growth, as well as the influence of biological components (extracellular matrix, growth factors etc.) on cell functions or the establishing of cell sources and of cell preservation are likely to be crucial for the future of tissue engineering.[1]

Morphology is one of the aspects that can effectively contribute to adding information about cell biology related to tissue engineering. It is well established that the level of compatibility of a certain cell type with a particular substratum can be evidenced by studying the morphological changes which occur when the cell surface interacts with the material examined. Of course, the use of transmission and scanning electron microscopy permits the collection of very detailed information. A clear example comes from the study of cell adhesion to lenses in ophthalmology, where correlated transmission and scanning electron microscopy investigations have permitted the description of different steps in cellular adhesion onto a particular substratum.[2]

Briefly, rounded cells always indicate the initial attachment to the substratum. This initial interaction depends mostly on the ability of cells to form cytoplasmic extensions which bring the cell close enough to the substratum to allow adhesion. This surface behavior corresponds inside the cell to a reorganization of cytoskeletal elements, which produces a flattening effect, first of the periphery and then, while adhesion is proceeding, of the cell body. Filaments develop into a network, eventually forming specialized contacts between the cell surface and the substratum. This surface and cytoskeletal modification continues until the cell is completely spread over the substratum. On the other hand, a negative response in cell adhesion can be described by a permanent rounded cellular shape with no cytoskeletal modifications and consequently no interaction with the surface.

Other examples can describe the correlation between morphological aspects and cell functionality. Nucleus morphology can always give information about cell viability. Cultured or seeded cells with pyknotic nuclei testify that the environment in which they are placed is totally unsuitable. Moreover, nuclei together with the organelle apparatus can inform about phenotypical changes, for example the change from a quiescent phenotype toward a synthetic phenotype is always characterized by a remarkable increase of rough endoplasmic reticulum cisternae.

Tissue Engineering of Prosthetic Vascular Grafts, edited by Peter Zilla and Howard P. Greisler.
©1999 R.G. Landes Company.

For all these reasons we believe morphological information to be very important for studies involved in the tissue engineering of vascular grafts. Moreover, when identification or localization of certain cell types is also requested, they can successfully be supplied by immunocytochemical investigations.

Microvascular Cells

Microvessels are considered the alternative to vein as a source of endothelial cells for cell transplantation. There are many tissues in humans which are abundant in capillaries and promptly available either surgically or by noninvasive methods. During years of experiments the protocols of the isolation of microvascular endothelial cells have become increasingly fast and efficient—normally a large number of viable endothelial cells is easily obtainable per gram of tissue.

Sources of Microvascular Endothelial Cells

Jarrel and Williams first started to harvest microvascular endothelial cells enzymatically for cell transplantation.[3] Initially they reported on methods established for the isolation and culture of human adult microvessel endothelial cells from different sources of human fat such as omental, perirenal and subcutaneous fat. Then they focused on human subcutaneous fat tissue as the most suitable source of endothelial cells, as it is composed mainly of adipocytes richly perfused with microvascular endothelium and pericytes.

Human subcutaneous fat is easily obtainable either surgically by patients undergoing abdominal surgery, (this is what has been mainly experienced in our lab), or by liposuction of fat deposits on the abdominal wall.[4]

Omentum and omentum-associated fat has also been utilized as a rich source of microvascular endothelial cells, but recently it has been proved by Williams et al that because of its anatomical location, the primary isolate from omentum often comprises not pure endothelium but a mixture of cells including endothelium, smooth muscle cells and mesothelium.[5]

Microvascular endothelial cells can also be harvested from other sources. Hewett et al developed a method for the isolation and long term culture of human microvessel endothelial cells from mammary adipose tissue obtained at breast reduction.[6] Robinson et al reported on the seeding of immortalized human dermal microvascular endothelial cells.[7] Procedures for the isolation and culture of microvascular endothelium from neonatal foreskins have also been previously described by Sherer et al, Marks et al, and Karasak et al.[8-10] Hewett et al isolated and cultured microvessel endothelial cells from lung tissue obtained from lung transplant recipients.[11] Haraldsen et al established a method for the isolation and culture of intestinal microvascular endothelial cells.[12] Kacemi et al devised a method of isolation and culture of endothelial cells from villous microvessels from human placenta.[13] Masek et al and Schweitzer et al described two simple methods for the isolation and culture of endothelial cells from human bone marrow.[14,15] McDouall et al isolated and cultured microvascular endothelial cells from the human heart.[16] Finally, Grimwood et al developed a novel method for the isolation of microvascular endothelium from first trimester decidua.[17]

Isolation of Microvascular Endothelial Cells

Jarrel and Williams first documented how microvascular endothelial cells can easily be recovered from enzymatically disrupted fat tissue.[3]

In our lab we developed a modification of the Jarrel method starting from human subcutaneous fat tissue excised from the abdominal wall of patients undergoing surgery for abdominal aneurysms.[18] The fat tissue is carefully minced and mixed with a 0.2% collagenase solution in an Erlenmayer flask and incubated under constant agitation for 30 minutes at 37°C. After digestion, the floating adipocytes are discharged and the suspension centrifuged. The pellet is first washed in PBS-BSA and then filtered through a 120 µm nylon filter; the suspension is gently layered onto 45% sterile Percoll and endothelial cells are recovered from the milky layer formed after centrifugation. Normally a variable number of viable cells ranging from 2.5-8 x 10^5 is obtained per g of tissue. Recently we proposed an alternative method of microvascular endothelial cell isolation based on the use of magnetic polystyrene beads (Dynabeads M-450) coated with anti-CD34 monoclonal antibody.[19] After the mincing and collagenase digestion of the subcutaneous fat tissue, the cells filtered and suspended in PBS-BSA as previously described are incubated with anti-CD34 coated Dynabeads (Dynabeads M-450 CD34, Dynal) at a ratio of 10 beads to 1 endothelial cell for 30 minutes at 4°C under gentle mixing. Rosetted cells are positively collected by means of three wash cycles performed with a Dynal Magnetic particle concentrator (MPC). Rosetted cells are then resuspended in M199 plus 20% FCS containing 10 µl DetachaBead (Dynal) per 1 x 10^7 Dynabeads used for rosetting, and incubated for 1 h at room temperature with constant agitation. After incubation cells are negatively recovered using the Dynal MPC. Usually approximately 0.8 x 10^5 cells per g of fat tissue are obtained.

Recently, Chen et al proposed a simple new method for the isolation of microvascular endothelial cells avoiding both chemical and mechanical injuries.[20] They indicated that when small pieces of lung or muscles of the chest wall of rats are placed into a flask, erythrocytes and leukocytes leave the tissues first, followed by vascular endothelial cells. Fibroblasts and other mixed cells grow after 72 hours of culture. When the tissues are discarded within 60 hours the flask contains only microvascular endothelial cells and blood cells. The latter can be cleared out after the cells are subcultured.

Microvascular Cell Isolates

The purity of a microvascular isolate has always been a major concern when microvessel-derived endothelial cells are chosen for cell transplantation. The attempt to characterize the cell population of a microvascular primary isolate from human fat tissue has lead to controversies. This is a consequence of the fact that the type of cells involved in a microvascular primary isolate correlates directly with the source of microvessels chosen.

Omentum and omentum fat are rich in mesothelial cells; consequently the primary isolate comprises a heterogeneous cell population including endothelial cells, pericytes, fibroblasts and mesothelial cells. Human subcutaneous fat is composed predominantly of adipocytes, pericytes and microvascular endothelial cells (Fig. 7.1a,b), and thus the primary isolate is expected to be more homogeneous. Recent studies are focusing on the fact that mesothelial cells can also be utilized for the seeding of vascular prostheses, behaving very much like endothelial cells derived from large vessels when seeded.[21]

Thus, depending on the aim of the study, the characterization of the cell population of a microvascular primary isolate can be very important. To do this we focused on morphological studies. Our conviction (derived from expe-

rience) is that the possibility of collecting information such as the appearance of subcellular components, or the presence of intercellular connections, from a primary isolate, can give a realistic description of the biological status of the cells analyzed and can add an indispensable contribution when an accurate characterization of the cell types involved is necessary.

For example, as already mentioned, the morphological changes in rough endoplasmic reticulum, Golgi apparatus and mitochondria are correlated to the level of metabolic activity of the cell; Weibel-palade bodies are undoubtedly considered a morphological marker for endothelial cells, while "fibronexus" is the morphological marker for myofibroblasts. Moreover, the fact that cells start to develop intercellular junctions when placed in culture or when seeded, often gives positive information about growth and stability. Furthermore, the localization of molecules specifically present in certain cells by immunohistochemistry is definitely helpful for the characterization of the different cell types involved in a primary isolate and can also contribute to the definition of molecular pathways signaling, when present, metabolic alterations.

Electron Microscopic and Immunocytochemical Profiles of Microvascular Cell Isolates

To characterize the phenotype of the microvascular cells recovered from human subcutaneous fat tissue precisely, cell samples obtained at different steps in the isolation procedure have been studied by means of electron microscopy as well as by immunohistochemical and immunoelectron microscopic techniques using a wide variety of antibodies.

Transmission Electron Microscopy

All the samples processed for transmission electron microscopy (TEM) analysis were first fixed in 2.5% cacodylate-buffered glutaraldehyde, then postfixed with 1% OsO_4, dehydrated in a graded series of alcohols, and embedded in araldite. Thin sections were obtained with a Reichert Omu3 ultramicrotome, counterstained with uranyl acetate and lead citrate and examined under a Philips 400T transmission electron microscope.

With TEM, enzymatically harvested microvascular endothelial cells (MECs) appear both as single cells and multicell aggregates (Fig. 7.2). Generally MECs show oval to round nuclei with clumps of condensed chromatin at the nuclear periphery. Occasional nucleoli are also seen. Nuclear irregularity is present in some cells. In particular, invagination of the nuclear envelope and deep clefts appear to be responsible for the presence of cleaved and convoluted endothelial nuclei. The bulky cytoplasm contains a small Golgi apparatus, mitochondria, short strands of rough endoplasmic reticulum, and many intermediate filaments (Fig. 7.3A), occasionally arranged to form characteristic fibrous bodies. Moreover, small to moderate quantities of microcystic lacunae, which appear as the remains of the primitive vascular lumen and of micropinocytotic vesicles, can be clearly seen (Fig. 7.3A). Sometimes, clustered microvascular endothelial cells present tight junctions (Fig. 7.2), which appear

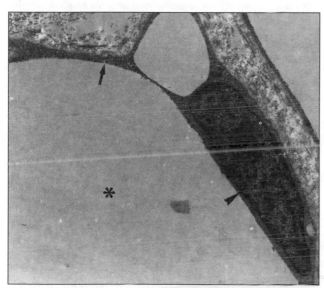

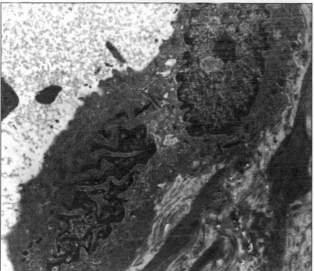

Fig. 7.1. Human subcutaneous fat tissue from abdominal wall. (A), top. Characteristic appearance of an adipocyte. Lipid droplet (asterisk); cytoplasm (arrow); nucleus (arrowhead). (TEM; x11,600). (B), bottom. Microvascular endothelial cells. Weibel-palade bodies are visible (arrows). (TEM; x9,000).

as sites of membrane fusion with adjacent electron-dense "fuzzy" cytoplasm. Specific rod-shaped microtubulated bodies (the so-called Weibel-palade bodies) are occasionally seen but are evident in less than 5% of the cells examined, particularly in the clustered elements (Fig. 7.2). Weibel-palade bodies are specifically found in the endothelium (Fig. 7.3B); their typical rod shape is contoured by a membrane containing numerous parallel cylindrical tubules embedded in an electron-dense matrix. Immunological studies have shown that Weibel-palade bodies are sites of storage of the von Willebrand protein.

MECs isolated with the help of CD34-coated Dynabeads appear, prior to DetachaBeads application, with 1-6 beads bound to the plasma membrane (Fig. 7.4). After bead detachment, MECs are present mainly as single cells, morphologically homogeneous and well preserved. Weibel-palade bodies are occasionally observed in the cytoplasm together with other typical endothelial features previously mentioned (intermediate filaments, micropinocytotic vescicles and microcystic lacunae).[19]

When other sources of microvascular cells are chosen, the primary isolate can be more heterogeneous and other cell types can be described. Mesothelial cells are characteristically identified by their numerous microvilli at the apical surface; they are heterogeneous in nature and measure up to 3 μm in length and 0.1 μm in diameter. In the cytoplasm there are some pinocytotic vesicles, very few Golgi membranes, scanty granular endoplasmic reticulum and many mitochondria. Junctions of all types can be found in situ. Intermediate filaments are present, sometimes prominent and often arranged in a perinuclear, circumferential distribution.[22]

Smooth muscle cells (SMCs) are delimited by a basal lamina and present elongated and lobated nuclei with characteristic symmetrical clefts. The cytoplasm is rich in intermediate filaments and microfilaments and very few organelles are found. Microfilaments are usually disposed parallel to the long axis of the cell, among which are interspersed numerous focal densities. These are electron dense structures scattered in the cytoplasm which are part, together with the contractile filaments, of the contractile apparatus. Precisely three different kinds of filaments can be described: myosin filaments (18 nm in diameter); actin filaments (6-8 nm in diameter) and vimentin and desmin intermediate filaments. In the subplasmalemmal site there are many micropinocytotic vescicles and plasmalemmal introflexions called "caveolae" which increase the plasmalemmal surface by about 25%. SMCs can form gap junctions and under specific conditions can change into a "synthetic" phenotype and become myofibroblasts.

Myofibroblasts are characterized by nuclear polymorphism, cytoplasmic extensions and abundant rough endoplasmic reticulum, Golgi apparatus and mitochondria. They are connected to the extracellular matrix by the so-called "fibronexus", which are transmembrane complexes of intracellular microfilaments in apparent continuity with extracellular fibronectin fibers. These cell to stroma attachment sites are more developed and numerous than in smooth muscle cells, and three types of fibronexus can be described: plaquelike, tracklike and tandem associations. Within the cytoplasm there are numerous bundles of microfilaments (stress fibers) arranged parallel to the long axis of the cell, with interspersed numerous dense bodies.

Fibroblasts have no basal lamina and display a slender fusiform and smoothly contoured nucleus; in the cytoplasm microfilaments are sometimes arranged in bundles beneath the plasma membrane and there is a well developed Golgi area and abundant dilated cisternae of rough endo-

Fig. 7.2. Multicell aggregate of isolated microvascular endothelial cells after Percoll step. Weibel-palade bodies (arrows). Tight junctions (arrowheads). (TEM; x6,500).

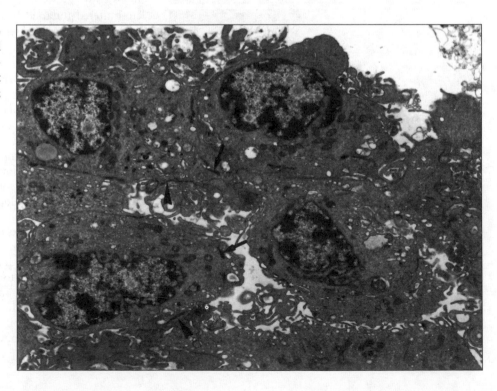

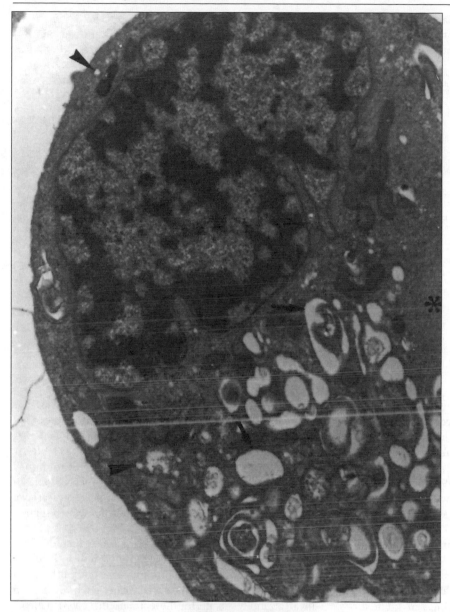

Fig. 7.3. Percoll isolated microvascular endothelial cells. (A), top. The predominant cytotype is characterized by microcystic lacunae (arrow), micropinocytotic vesicles (arrowheads) and extensive intermediate filaments (asterisk). (TEM; x20,000). (B), bottom left. Weibel-palade bodies at higher magnification. (TEM; x26,000). With permission from: Vici M, Pasquinelli G, Preda P et al. Electron microscopic and immunocytochemical profiles of human subcutaneous fat tissue microvascular endothelial cells. Ann Vasc Surg, 1993; 7:541-548. (C), bottom right. Numerous gold particles (arrowheads) bind CD34 antigen on the cell surface (TEM; x12,000). With permission from: Vici M, Pasquinelli G, Preda P et al. Electron microscopic and immunocytochemical profiles of human subcutaneous fat tissue microvascular endothelial cells. Ann Vasc Surg, 1993; 7:541-548.

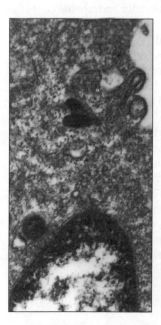
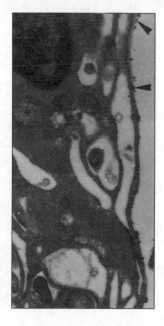

plasmic reticulum. Cell contours are generally smooth or display a few short cytoplasmic extensions.

Pericytes that are embedded within the basement membrane of microvessels share with vascular SMCs the α-smooth muscle actin content and also intermediate filament proteins. In fact, both cell types express vimentin or vimentin and desmin. Pericytes form an integral part of the microvascular wall.[23]

A few adipocytes can also be found in a primary microvascular isolate from enzymatically treated adipose fat tissue. Mature adipocytes have characteristic features (Fig. 7.1A): The nucleus is flattened against the cytoplasmic membrane by a large lipid droplet, with only a thin, tenuous rim of cytoplasm surrounding it. Adjacent to the cell membrane are deposits of basement membrane. In situ capillaries are closely opposed to the adipocyte membrane.[24]

Fig. 7.4. Dynabeads isolated microvascular endothelial cells. Immunomagnetic beads are closely adherent to the plasma membrane. (TEM; x3,400).

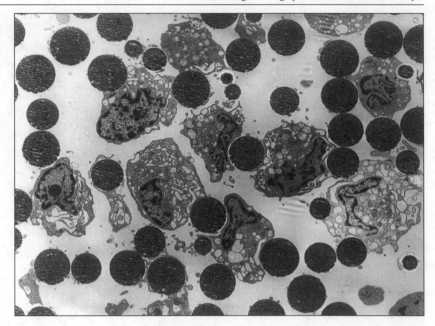

Scanning Electron Microscopy

Isolated MECs were seeded at a density of 1 x 10^5/cm^2 on both uncoated and coated glass coverslips. As coating materials we used poly-L-lysine and fibronectin; briefly, glass coverslips were incubated with 1 mg/ml poly-L-lysine diluted in PBS at room temperature for 1 hour, or with 5 μg/cm^2 fibronectin suspended in M199 and kept at 37°C for 2 h. The seeded coverslips were fixed with 2.5% glutaraldehyde in 0.1 M cacodylate buffer, postfixed with 1% OsO$_4$, dehydrated in a graded series of alcohol and critical point dried. Mounted samples were coated with gold and examined in a Philips 505.

Most of the MECs show many slender microvilli, bulbous protrusions and membrane folds, the overall impression being a flower-like appearance (Fig. 7.5A). The surface specializations probably begin at the original luminal aspect of the cell membrane. At the same site the extracellular space appears by TEM to be compartmentalized into microcystic lacunae by interdigiting cytoplasmic flaps. On the contrary, other elements exhibit a smoother surface morphology, and scanning electron microscopy (SEM) occasionally reveals microvillus-like projections and irregular surface corrugations.

Exposure of MECs to nonvascular surfaces induces rapid morphological changes. Isolated MECs lose their convoluted appearance and become relatively spherical, extending long, slender filopodia making tenuous contact with the substrate. As the endothelial attachment proceeds, the interaction appears more tenacious. Endothelial cells seem to sink into the surface and indent it with peripheral cytoplasmic flaps (skirted cells) (Fig. 7.6A). In the late stage MECs completely spread over the substrate, resulting in a fried egg appearance. At the same time, round to stellate, as well as elongated, spreading endothelial cells begin to appear (Fig. 7.6B).

Immunophenotyping

The immunophenotype of a primary microvascular isolate can be studied using a wide variety of antibodies. One of the most commonly employed, when endothelial cells need to be identified, is the FVIII RA antibody. FVIII RA is specifically expressed by endothelial cells. With immunohistochemistry a positive staining gives a typical cytoplasm granularity, while at the immunoelectron microscopical level FVIII RA specifically stains Weibel-palade bodies and slightly stains the cell membrane.

Other typical endothelial cell markers include: *Ulex europaeus* type i lectin, which selectively binds to L-fucose residues of the endothelial membrane—the binding between the lectin and the endothelial surface can then be evidenced with an antibody specific for the lectin itself;[25] CD31, a membrane glycoprotein that is the platelet endothelial cells adhesion molecule PECAM 1;[26] CD34, a surface glycophosphoprotein expressed on hemopoietic stem and progenitor cells, small-vessel endothelial cells, and embryonic fibroblasts. The function of CD34 is not yet clear. Recent studies on the functions of this molecule indicate that CD34 expressed on endothelial cells may play a role in leukocyte adhesion and "homing" during the inflammatory process. A role for CD34 in adhesion has been theorized because, like other known adhesion molecules, CD34 is a heavily glycosylated surface sialomucin.[27]

PAL-E is a monoclonal antibody specific for endothelial cells. It markedly stains endothelium of capillaries, medium size and small veins, and venules. The antigenic determinant recognized by PAL-E is associated with endothelial vesicles.[28]

EN4 was originally described as a monoclonal antibody that reacts specifically with human endothelial cells and the reagent has not been assigned to any of the presently known CD. Recently, Burgio et al have demonstrated

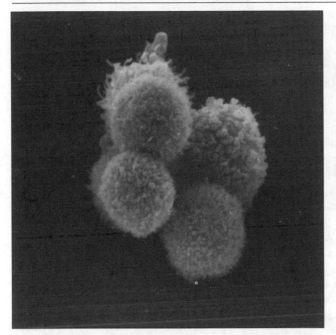 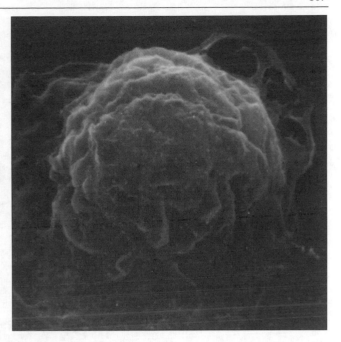

Fig. 7.5. Percoll isolated microvascular endothelial cells. (A), left. SEM of a multicell aggregate. (SEM; x4,200). With permission from: Curti T, Pasquinelli G, Preda P et al. An ultrastructural and immunocytochemical analysis of human endothelial cell adhesion on coated vascular grafts. Ann Vasc Surg, 1989; 3:351-363. (B), right. Immunoelectron microscopic demonstration of FVIII RA. SEM reveals strong positivity at cell surface. (SEM; x8.500). With permission from: Curti T, Pasquinelli G, Preda P et al. An ultrastructural and immunocytochemical analysis of human endothelial cell adhesion on coated vascular grafts. Ann Vasc Surg, 1989; 3:351 363.

that EN4 and CD31 monoclonal antibody recognize the same 130 kDa antigen.[29]

Since a primary microvascular isolate can be composed of a mixture of cell types, it might also be useful to characterize most of them. Vascular smooth muscle cells specifically express vimentin and smooth muscle actin, while a low percentage is desmin positive. Cytokeratins such as CK8 and CK18 can be found in some SMCs. Pericytes also express smooth muscle-specific actin. Nonproliferating mesothelial cells express both vimentin and a variety of cytokeratins (CK7, CK8, CK18, CK19).[22] Adipocytes express S 100 protein, while monocytes and macrophages can be detected using antibodies against specific antigens such as 150.95 protein and MAC 387.

We studied the immunophenotype of microvascular isolates from human subcutaneous fat tissue at different steps in the isolation procedure with the help of different immunocytochemical techniques using monoclonal and polyclonal antibodies. Immunofluorescence was performed by first seeding the isolate onto fibronectin-coated coverslips for 1 hour at 37°C, and then fixing the cells with cold acetone and incubating them with the primary antisera. A second incubation with a fluorescein-conjugated anti-rabbit or anti-mouse Ig followed. Coverslips were then mounted and observed under a photomicroscope equipped with an epifluorescent condenser.

Immunoenzymatic labeling was also performed on MECs cells using the alkaline phosphatase monoclonal antialkaline phosphatase (APAAP) procedure.[30] The APAAP technique is particularly suitable for clear and specific staining of cytoplasmic and surface membrane antigens on cell smears at optical level. Cells seeded onto fibronectin-coated coverslips were fixed in acetone-metanol (7:3 at -20°C for 10 minutes) and incubated in the primary antibody, then in anti-mouse immunoglobulin and finally in APAAP complexes. The reaction was revealed by adding the substrate containing naphtol AS phosphate and new fuchsin. For polyclonal antibodies, samples were treated with a bridge antibody.

Protein a-gold technique was performed on MECs seeded on fibronectin-coated coverslips by incubating cells, after the primary antibody, with 18 nm protein a-gold particles.[31,32] The reaction was then silver enhanced. For monoclonal antibodies a secondary antibody was employed.

For immunoelectron microscopy, suspensions of MECs were fixed in 3% paraformaldehyde, then incubated with the primary antibody and afterwards with an appropriate dilution of 18 nm protein a-gold complexes. Finally, MECs were postfixed in 1.7% glutaraldehyde and embedded in araldite. Immunolabeling specificity was always checked by omitting the incubation with the specific primary antibody or replacing the primary antibody with an unrelated antibody.

Our investigation was performed employing the following antibodies. As endothelial cell markers we used: a polyclonal antibody against Factor viii RA; a polyclonal antibody specific for the *Ulex europaeus* type i lectin previously bound to the endothelial membrane; a monoclonal antibody against CD31 antigen and QB-End 10, a monoclonal antibody specific for the CD34 antigen. Antibodies

Fig. 7.6. Microvascular endothelial cells—substrate interaction. (A), top. SEM reveals different stages of adhesion. Round, surface convoluted cell (arrow); skirted-cell (arrowhead). (SEM; x2,300). With permission from: Curti T, Pasquinelli G, Preda P et al. An ultrastructural and immunocytochemical analysis of human endothelial cell adhesion on coated vascular grafts. Ann Vasc Surg 1989; 3:351-363. (B), bottom. Different stages of adhesion on fibronectin-coated glass. (SEM; x600). With permission from: Curti T, Pasquinelli G, Preda P et al. An ultrastructural and immunocytochemical analysis of human endothelial cell adhesion on coated vascular grafts. Ann Vasc Surg 1989; 3:351-363.

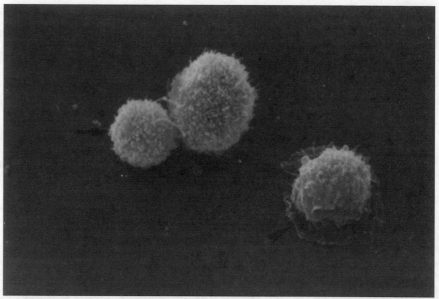

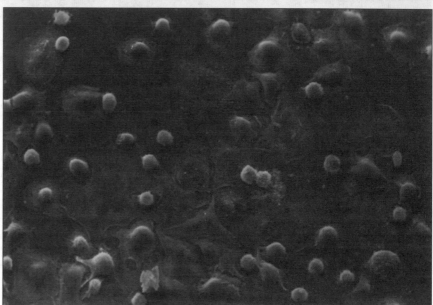

directed against cytoskeletal proteins (actin, smooth muscle actin, desmin and vimentin), monocyte-macrophage specific antigens (MAC 387, anti-protein 150.95) and S-100 protein, which is present in adipocytes, were also used.

Following collagenase digestion approximately 90% of MECs stained for factor VIII, as well as for CD31, CD34, and *Ulex*. After the Percoll step, cell isolate weakly expressed factor VIII (5%) (Fig. 7.7A). Furthermore, 18% of the isolated cells stained for CD31 (Fig. 7.7B) and 5% were labeled with *Ulex europaeus*. Remarkably these endothelial-specific antigens were found mostly in cell clumps. Interestingly, CD34 was detected in 90% of the harvested cells comprising the primary isolate irrespective of the separation step (Figs. 7.7C and 7.3C). Only 1-2% of cells expressed monocyte-macrophage specific antigens, 150.95 protein and MAC 387. Immunostaining for desmin and S-100 protein was almost negative. Smooth muscle actin was expressed in few cells.

With immunohistochemistry we concluded that enzymatically harvested MECs did not contain adipocytes and pericytes, since immunostaining showed protein S-100 and desmin to be virtually nonexistent. Furthermore, the presence of pericytes was ruled out by a negative response for smooth muscle-specific actin. As demonstrated by immunostaining for monocyte-macrophage specific antigen (150.95 protein and MAC387), the presence of mononuclear blood cells was negligible (1-2%).

On the other hand, our results on MECs harvested from human abdominal subcutaneous fat tissue (which as previously demonstrated show ultrastructural features typical of endothelium), using common endothelial cell markers (FVIII RA, *Ulex europaeus*, CD31) have apparently led to some discrepancies that we related to factor VIII release and surface antigen rearrangements occurring in vitro during procedures of cell isolation, mainly at the Percoll step. Interestingly, immunoelectron microscopic demonstration

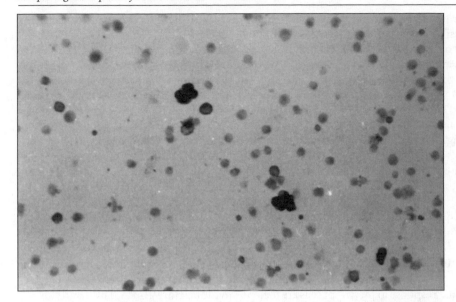

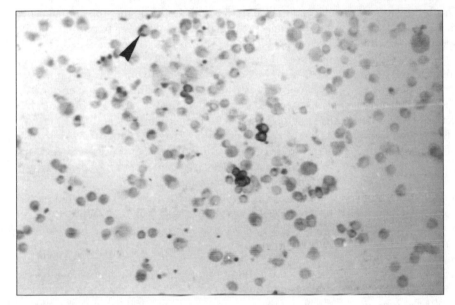

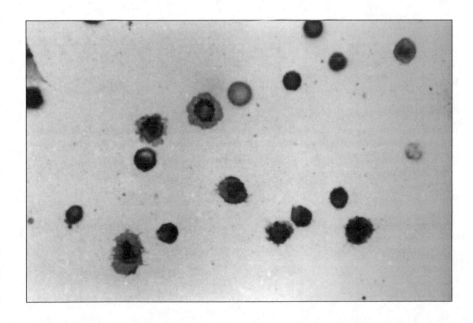

Fig. 7.7. Immunophototyping of isolated microvascular endothelial cells. (A), top. Percoll isolated microvascular endothelial cells. Factor VIII is expressed only in clustered cells. (APAAP technique; x170). With permission from: Vici M, Pasquinelli G, Preda P et al. Electron microscopic and immunocytochemical profiles of human subcutaneous fat tissue microvascular endothelial cells. Ann Vasc Surg 1993; 7:541-548. (B), center. Percoll isolated microvascular endothelial cells. CD31 antigen is expressed by clustered endothelial cells and occasional single elements (arrowhead). (APAAP techniques; x170). With permission from: Vici M, Pasquinelli G, Preda P et al. Electron microscopic and immunocytochemical profiles of human subcutaneous fat tissue microvascular endothelial cells. Ann Vasc Surg 1993; 7:541-548. (C), bottom. Percoll isolated microvascular endothelial cells. CD34 antigen is present on approximately 90% of cells. (Protein a-gold-silver stain; x350). With permission from: Vici M, Pasquinelli G, Preda P et al. Electron microscopic and immunocytochemial profiles of human subcutaneous fat tissue microvascular endothelial cells. Ann Vasc Surg 1993; 7:541-548.

of factor VIII RA by SEM reveals a moderate to strong positivity at the cell surface (Fig. 7.5B). A possible adverse effect of Percoll on cell function has also been observed by DOT immunoassay. Precisely, DOT immunoassay documented an intense factor VIII delivery in the washing solutions following Percoll density gradient, while CD34 was always negative. Notably, in MECs obtained with the Dynabeads procedure, where the Percoll step was omitted, factor VIII RA was expressed by the vast majority of cells (Fig. 7.7D) and DOT immunoassay of the washing buffers collected after Dynabeads application was virtually negative excluding any loss of factor VIII during the isolation steps. Only CD34 was constantly expressed by MECs during and after the isolation by Percoll density gradient. We concluded that QB-End/10 monoclonal antibody, which recognizes the highly resistant CD34 molecule on the surface of endothelial cells, is particularly well suited for characterizing enzymatically harvested MECs.[33]

Also, Williams et al observed a cellular response to the isolation procedure. They studied the cell population of liposuction-derived human fat before and after collagenase dispersion with the help of immunocytochemistry and scanning electron microscopy.[5] Samples of liposuction-derived human fat have been processed for the presence of FVIII RA-von Willebrand factor, α-smooth muscle cell actin, cytokeratin (CK18) and EN4. The same study was performed on the cells recovered after collagenase dispersion of the liposuction fat. 86.1% of the cells in intact liposuction-derived fat expressed vWF, 5.7% were positive for α-smooth muscle cell actin, 1% expressed the mesothelial cell-related antigen cytokeratine peptide 18 and 89.6% of the cells in intact fat resulted positive for EN4. After collagenase digestion of the fat and centrifugal separation of adipocytes from vascular and stromal cells, the expression of vWF, α-smooth muscle cell actin, and cytokeratin was 77.5%, 5.8%, and 2.1% respectively. 74.6% of the isolated cells expressed EN4.

This study demonstrated that the major cell component present in liposuction-derived fat, before and after collagenase digestion, has been characterized as endothelium, while only a minor fraction is composed of cells common to mesodermally derived tissue. The fact that after collagenase isolation the cells expressing vWF and EN4 were fewer than those observed in intact fat suggests that a portion of cells lose vWF and EN4 during the isolation procedure.

Stansby et al attempted to characterize microvascular endothelial cells from human omental tissue using both endothelial-specific markers, (namely anti-factor VIII, EN4, PAL-E and QB-End/40) and monoclonals against antigens specific of cells of connective tissue origin (Thy-1 and CDw44).[34] The authors found that the microvascular cells they harvested from omentum are extremely heterogeneous with respect to their antigenic expression and are probably initially a mixture of several different cell types: only occasional cells are positive for factor VIII RA, Thy-1 and CDw44 glycoprotein. No positivity for EN4, PAL-E and QB-End/40 was reported. After culture it seems likely that one cell type predominates, as the cultures are then homogeneous both morphologically and immunophenotypically. The majority of cells are then positive for factor VIII RA, Thy-1 and Cdw44 glycoprotein. A small proportion (< 5%) is also positive for the endothelial markers EN4, PAL-E and QB-End/40. The authors suggest that Thy-1 and CDw44 glycoprotein positive cells, which were shown to take up acetylated ldl and produce prostacyclin, might be pericytes.

Also, Meerbaum et al performed an immunohistochemical investigation on the primary isolate enzymatically harvested from subcutaneous fat tissue obtained by liposuction and used for limited clinical trials.[35] They found 55.8% of cells positive for factor VIII while 42.5% were reactive to muscle-specific actin. 9.4% of cells reacted with monocyte-macrophage specific markers. They speculated on the possibility that contaminating cells might have been pericytes. They also observed that Percoll separation negatively affects cell attachment and growth in culture.

Discussion

Since our unit was founded in 1962, it has been devoted to the elaboration of a subcellular approach to clinical manifestation. As soon as the Vascular Surgery unit of the hospital where we were placed decided to start looking

Fig. 7.7. Immunophototyping of isolated microvascular endothelial cells. (D). Dynabeads isolated microvascular endothelial cells. Almost all the cells are positive for factor VIII. (APAAP technique; x500).

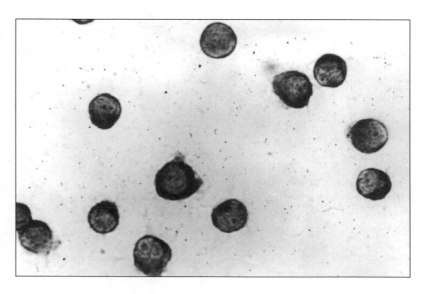

into the endothelial cell seeding of vascular grafts, it asked for our participation, finding our experience immediately important to initiate this challenging new task.

Undoubtedly a successful morphological approach correlates well with experience, both for technical skill, which is always a guarantee for precision and efficiency, and for the ability to collect and interpret the results obtained. For example, each lab which focuses on ultrastructure has elaborated its own protocols, and it is always very important to learn, when observing samples, how to distinguish artifacts from the "real" structure.

Although the optimization of these aspects could appear time consuming, the study of the morphology of single cells or of a tissue can give important information about their biology and function. Electron microscopy techniques represent powerful tools which provide very accurate information about cell ultrastructure and, thanks to combined immunocytochemistry, about cell biology (related to antigen expression, synthesis of specific molecules, etc.). We believe that, for all these reasons, morphology can make an important contribution to the development of the tissue engineering of vascular grafts.

As already reported, submicroscopic studies have been very important in defining the processes involved in the adhesion of cells to a surface. This information can successfully be applied to the study of vascular cell seeding onto prosthetic grafts. With the scanning electron microscope we can easily follow the different steps of adhesion of the endothelial cells seeded on the vascular substratum that we are testing. First of all, we can perceive a qualitative response: No interaction with the substratum, as revealed by a steady, rounded cellular shape, is informative of an unsuitable surface—cells do not like that substratum. At an intermediate level the endothelial cell has already started to interact with the vascular graft and the cell surface is modifying; endothelial cells now appear as skirted cells. If the interaction proceeds, meaning that the vascular substratum is particularly suitable for the cells, their surface modifies further, becoming completely flattened. Depending on the number of cells seeded, they can eventually reach each other and, by forming intercellular junctions, start to initiate a monolayer. We can explain all these surface modifications by TEM as cytoskeletal rearrangements.

TEM has been very helpful for the characterization of microvascular primary isolates. We already know that the cell types involved in a primary microvascular isolate vary with the source chosen. Different sources placed in anatomically different sites, clearly comprise, besides microvessels, other cell types. Whether a microvascular isolate contains pure endothelium or not can be of primary importance during clinical trials. TEM with the help of immunocytochemistry can give a very accurate description of the cell types involved in a microvascular isolate. Ultrastructurally there are morphological markers that can, without doubt, allow different cell types to be recognized. This is supported by immunocytochemistry which localizes molecules specifically synthetized by certain cells or groups of cells. Moreover, together they can also permit the identification of alterations of the biological status.

One example comes from our own experience. Our attempt to characterize microvascular endothelial cells immunohistochemically yielded some discrepancies. After Percoll density gradient isolation, we found that typical markers (factor VIII, *Ulex europaeus*, and CD31) were expressed by only a small percentage of cells. Immunohistochemically we concluded that microvascular endothelial cells harvested from human subcutaneous fat tissue did not contain contaminating stromal cells such as adipocytes and pericytes, and the presence of mononuclear blood cells was negligible. Moreover, harvested cells showed ultrastructural features typical of endothelium. Subcellular criteria included residual lumina, loosely textured intermediate filaments, micropinocytotic vesicles, and Weibel-palade bodies. Interestingly, factor VIII, CD31 and *Ulex europaeus* almost exclusively stained cell aggregates. Likewise, TEM demonstrated Weibel-palade bodies in clustered endothelial cells only, whereas single cells, which also showed the subcellular features of endothelium, lacked these highly specific endothelial organelles.

We hypothesized an adverse effect of Percoll on endothelial cell function. Our hypothesis was supported by the finding of factor VIII in the washing solutions after Percoll separation, documented by DOT immunoassay and by the detection of factor VIII by immunoSEM on the surface of some of the cells, which could represent a possible step in the delivery of factor VIII in the washing solutions following the Percoll treatment. Interestingly, when using alternative methods where the Percoll step is omitted the majority of the harvested endothelial cells stain for factor VIII.[19] Accordingly, the decreased expression of CD31 and other membrane glycoproteins, or part of them, could be a consequence of surface antigen rearrangements also induced by the Percoll step.

Here we have reported on other authors who also performed correlated morphological and immunohistochemical studies in order to determine the cellular composition of a microvascular primary isolate; in some cases these studies have also led to evaluation of the influences of the isolation procedures chosen over the cell function.

Being correlated to the potential of technological apparatus, the "limits" of morphological studies are subject to constant modification. Computer science, together with innovative technology, has permitted the development of very elaborate microscopes, adding a new perspective to the study of morphology. Confocal microscopy is an advanced technique used to produce multidimensional cellular and subcellular structural images. It provides high resolution images and its optical sectioning ability allows images to be obtained from different depths within a thick tissue specimen, avoiding processing and sectioning procedures. For this reason, confocal microscopy has made it possible to view biological tissues under more physiological conditions than was previously possible. Commonly, its biological application addresses the localization of immunofluorescently labeled proteins in cell culture or within excised blocks of tissue. Because of its noninvasive optical sectioning capability, it is also ideally suited to the study of living cells in situ and of tissue in intact living animals.[36]

Confocal microscopy immunofluorescence staining allows a better resolution than that with traditional immunofluorescence. It would therefore be possible to perform very detailed in situ or in vivo studies of adhesion molecules or other cell products in cultures or, in the near future, in implanted grafts. The scanning resolution of the confocal microscope has also remarkably improved on that of the traditional SEM. More precise evaluations about surface information such as cell lining, for example, can be simultaneously supported, thanks to the optical sectioning ability, by "deeper" information regarding thickenings and their biological compounds. Understandably, confocal microscopy is considered to be one of the techniques that in the near future will enormously improve the understanding of biological events.

The constant development of technologies for the quantitative analysis of images has made image analysis the most suitable tool for quantitative studies on cell seeding, or whenever a precise definition of the number of cells (or part of stained cells) is necessary. Supported by microanalysis, quantitative multielemental analysis in small sections of samples can be performed routinely. X-ray microanalysis is being widely employed in evaluating the biocompatibility and biostability of alternative biomaterials. Precisely, studies have been performed in order to describe the influence of biomaterials on organic matrix synthesis and the calcification process by using X-ray microanalysis coupled with TEM[37] or high resolution electron microscopy.[38] The vascular graft field has already gained from this technique. It has allowed the testing of biocompatibility of new polymers to be employed in new synthetic grafts.[39] It has also made it possible to assess whether chemical degradation of ePTFE occurs when such arterial substitutes are implanted in humans.[40]

Lately, techniques have been developed to understand the state of specific gene expression at cellular and/or subcellular levels. In situ hybridization is a powerful and well established light microscopic technique used to localize mRNA, and recent advances have been made with the help of transmission electron microscopy.[41] It is already possible to detect, using properly chosen nucleic acid probes (radioactive or biotinylated), genes or products of genes in the cell examined.

Recently, genetic manipulation has been introduced in order to ameliorate vascular graft implantation. For example seeding of small diameter vascular grafts with endothelial cells genetically engineered to secrete fibrinolytic or antithrombotic proteins has been performed to improve graft patency rates.[42] Another example concerns the attempt to improve the biomaterial-blood compatibility by inducing, with genetical manipulation, the inhibition of SMC proliferation.[43] TEM-in situ hybridization, with the help of specific probes, could theoretically permit the visualization of genetically engineered cells so that we can obtain information regarding the quantification of seeded genetically engineered cells, their proliferation and metabolic activity, and more besides.

All of these techniques briefly listed are usually presented in manuals as "innovative microscopy". They are supported by very sophisticated machines and, as a consequence, their potential is continuously improving. As we have seen, they have already been successfully employed in the tissue engineering of prosthetic vascular grafts, and it is becoming clearer that their future development will be of great value in the evolution of this field.

Acknowledgments

I would like to thank Prof. Massimo Derenzini for supporting me and giving me the free run of the archives of the Institute, and Prof. Massimo D'Addato of the Vascular Surgery Unit, Director of the Center for the Study of Vascular Prostheses, and his staff for their collaboration. I am also extremely grateful to Dr. Paola Preda and Dr. Gianandrea Pasquinelli for their invaluable assistance and to Mr. Walther Mantovani for his indispensable technical skill. Finally, thanks to Patrizia and Lorenzo for their patience.

References

1. Langer R, Vacanti JP. Tissue engineering. Science 1993; 260:920-926.
2. Versura P, Maltarello MC, Fontana L et al. Ultrastructural investigation demonstrating reduced cell adhesion on heparin-surface-modified intraocular lenses. Ophtalmic Res 1991; 23:1-11.
3. Williams SK, Jarrel BE, Rose DG. Isolation of human fat-derived microvessel endothelial cells for use in vascular graft endothelialization. In: Zilla PP, Fasol RD, Deutsch M eds. Endothelialization of Vascular Grafts. Basel: Karger 1987:211-217.
4. Jarrel BE, Williams SK. Microvessel derived endothelial cell isolation, adherence, and monolayer formation for vascular grafts. J Vasc Surg 1991; 13:733-734 (special communication).
5. Williams SK, Wang TF, Castrillo R et al. Liposuction-derived fat used for vascular graft sodding contains endothelial cells and not mesothelial cells as the major cell type. J Vasc Surg 1994; 19:916-923.
6. Hewett PW, Murray JC, Price EA et al. Isolation and characterization of microvessel endothelial cells from human mammary adipose tissue. In Vitro Cell Dev Biol Anim 1993; 29A: 325-331.
7. Robinson KA, Candal FJ, Scott NA et al. Seeding of vascular grafts with an immortalized human dermal microvascular endothelial cell line. Angiology 1995; 46:107-112.
8. Sherer GK, Fitzharris TP, Faulk WP et al. Cultivation of microvascular endothelial cells from human preputial skin. In Vitro 1980; 16:675-684.
9. Marks RM, Czerniecki M, Penny R. Human dermal microvascular endothelial cells: an improved method for tissue culture and a description of some singular properties in culture. In Vitro Cell Dev Biol 1985; 21:627-635.
10. Karasek MA. Microvascular cell culture. J Invest Dermatol 1989; 93:33S-38S.
11. Hewett PW, Murray JC. Human lung microvessel endothelial cells: Isolation, culture, and characterization. Microvasc Res 1993; 46:89-102.
12. Haraldsen G, Rugveit J, Kvale D et al. Isolation and long term culture of human intestinal microvascular endothelial cells. Gut 1995; 37:225-234.

13. Kacemi A, Challier JC, Galtier M et al. Culture of endothelial cells from human placental microvessels. Cell Tissue Res 1996; 283:183-190.

14. Masek LC, Sweetenham JW. Isolation and culture of endothelial cells from human bone marrow. Br J Hematol 1994; 88:855-865.

15. Schweitzer CM, van der Schoot CE, Drager AM et al. Isolation and culture of human bone marrow endothelial cells. Exp Hematol 1995; 23:41-48.

16. McDouall RM, Yacoub M, Rose ML. Isolation, culture, and characterization of MHC class II-positive microvascular endothelial cells from the human heart. Microvasc Res 1996; 51:137-152.

17. Grimwood J, Bicknell R, Rees MC. The isolation, characterization and culture of human decidual endothelium. Hum Reprod 1995; 10:2142-2148.

18. Curti T, Pasquinelli G, Preda P et al. An ultrastructural and immunocytochemical analysis of human endothelial cell adhesion on coated vascular grafts. Ann Vasc Surg 1989; 3:351-363.

19. Preda P, Pasquinelli G, Vici M et al. Isolation of human microvascular endothelial cells using monoclonal anti-CD34 coated dynabeads. VIII International symposium on the biology of vascular cells. August 30-September 4 1994; Heidelberg, Germany.

20. Chen SF, Fei X, Li SH. A new simple method for isolation of microvascular endothelial cells avoiding both chemical and mechanical injuries. Microvasc Res 1995; 50:119-128.

21. Hernando A, Garcìa-Honduvilla N, Bellòn JM et al. Coatings for vascular prostheses: Mesothelial cells express specific markers for muscle cells and have biological activity similar to that of endothelial cells. Eur J Vasc Surg 1994; 8:531-536.

22. Carter D, True L, Otis CN. Serous membranes. In: Sternberg SS ed. Histology for pathologists. New York: Raven Press 1992:499 514.

23. Schurch W, Seemayer TA, Gabbiani G. Myofibroblast. In: Sternberg SS ed. Histology for pathologists. New York: Raven Press 1992:109-144.

24. Brooks JJ, Perosio PM. Adipose tissue. In: Sternberg SS ed. Histology for pathologists. New York: Raven Press 1992:33-60.

25. Holthofer H, Virtanen I, Kariniemi AL et al. Ulex europaeus 1 lectin as a marker for vascular endothelium in human tissues. Lab Invest 1982; 47:60-66.

26. Newman PJ, Albelda SM. Cellular and molecular aspects of PECAM-1. Nouv Rev Fr Hematol 1992; 34: S9-S13.

27. Krause DS, Fackler MJ, Civin CI et al. CD34: Structure, biology, and clinical utility. Blood 1996; 87:1-13.

28. Schlingemann RO, Dingjan GM, Emeis JJ et al. Monoclonal antibody PAL-E specific for endothelium. Lab Invest 1985; 52:71-76.

29. Burgio VL, Zupo S, Roncella S et al. Characterization of EN4 monoclonal antibody: A reagent with CD31 specificity. Clin Exp Immunol 1994; 96:170-176.

30. Cordell JL, Falini B, Erber WN et al. Immuno-enzymatic labeling of monoclonal antibodies using immune complexes of alkaline phosphatase and monoclonal antialkaline phosphatase (APAAP complexes). J Histochem Cytochem 1984; 32:219-229.

31. Frens G. Controlled nucleation for the regulation of the particle size in monodisperse gold solution. Nature Phys Sci 1973; 241:20-22.

32. Roth J, Bendayan M, Orci L. Ultrastructural localization of intracellular antigens by the use of protein a-gold complexes. J Histochem Cytochem 1978; 26:1077-1081.

33. Vici M, Pasquinelli G, Preda P et al. Electron microscopic and immunocytochemical profiles of human subcutaneous fat tissue microvascular endothelial cells. Ann Vasc Surg 1993; 7:541-548.

34. Stansby G, Fuller B, Hamilton G. Human omental microvascular endothelial cells: Are they endothelial? In: Zilla PP, Fasol RD, Callow A eds. Applied Cardiovascular biology. Basel: Karger 1992:120-123.

35. Meerbaum SO, Sharp Wv, Schmidt SP. Lower extremity revascularization with polytetrafluoroethylene grafts seeded with microvascular endothelial cells. In: Zilla PP, Fasol RD, Callow A eds. Applied Cardiovascular biology. Basel: Karger 1992:107-119.

36. Petroll WM, Jester JV, Cavanagh HD. In vivo confocal imaging: General principles and application. Scanning 1994; 16:131-149.

37. Serre CM, Papillard M, Chavassieux P et al. In vitro induction of a calcifying matrix by biomaterials constituted of collagen and/or hydroxyapatite: An ultrastructural comparison of three types of biomaterials. Biomaterials 1993; 14:97-106.

38. Lee YS. Morphogenesis of calcification in porcine bioprosthesis: Insight from high resolution electron microscopic investigation at molecular and atomic resolution. J Electron Microsc (Tokyo) 1993; 42:156-165.

39. Zhang Z, King M, Guidoin R et al. In vitro exposure of a novel polyesterurethane graft to enzymes: A study of the biostability of the Vascugraft arterial prosthesis. Biomaterials 1994; 15:1129-1144.

40. Guidoin R, Maurel S, Chakfé N et al. Expanded polytetrafluoroethylene arterial prostheses in humans: Chemical analysis of 79 explanted specimens. Biomaterials 1993; 14:694-704.

41. Cenacchi G, Musiani M, Gentilomi G et al. In situ hybridization at the ultrastructural level: Localization of cytomegalovirus DNA using digoxigenin labelled probes. J Submicros Cytol Pathol 1993; 25:341-345.

42. Scott-Burden T, Tock CL, Schwarz et al. Genetically engineered smooth muscle cells as linings to improve the biocompatibility of cardiovascular prostheses. Circulation 1996; 94: II235-II238.

CHAPTER 8

Functional Aspects of Microvascular Cell Isolates

M. Fittkau, Teddy Fischlein

Because of the limited availability of autologous venous endothelium for transplantation onto vascular implants, microvascular cells from human subcutaneous fat tissue were first used for the coating of synthetic vascular prostheses in 1986.[1,2] Subcutaneous fat tissue is easily accessible, usually available in sufficient amounts and very well vascularized.[3] In comparison to the method used for macrovascular endothelial cell harvest, however, the isolation of microvascular endothelium from adipose tissue represents a fundamentally different approach because the enzymatic detachment of endothelial cells cannot be achieved by perfusion of the vascular system. It requires a complete dissociation of the tissue, followed by gradual separation of capillary segments and endothelial cells from lipids and cellular and noncellular connective tissue components. In particular, the complete removal of other, rapidly proliferating cells such as fibroblasts and pericytes represents a core problem when isolating microvascular endothelial cells.

In cooperation with the Physiological Institute of the University of Munich (LMU) we developed a method for the isolation of pure microvascular endothelial cells (Fig. 8.1). Following enzymatic detachment, the endothelial cells are centrifuged over a density gradient and thus separated from other cell types. Approximately one week after seeding, the remaining contaminating cells are eliminated using a combination of specific antibodies and complement.[4] In this procedure mixed cell cultures are incubated with diluted human serum and polyclonal antibodes. The latter are intednded to eliminate alcalic phosphatase positive contaminating cell types (i.e., pericytes). After 2 h the contaminating cells are rinsed off the cultures with ECs remaining in the flask. Subsequently, microvascular endothelial cells can be examined under the phase contrast and fluorescent microscope after incorporation of 3,3'-dioctodecylindocarbocyamine (DiI) acetyl-LDL (Fig. 8.2). Like macrophages, ECs internalize Ac-LDL via a specific receptor, in contrast to fibroblasts and smooth muscle cells.

For the purpose of transplantation onto synthetic vascular prostheses, the question of to what extent microvascular endothelium differs from its macrovascular counterpart with regard to its significant metabolic functions remains of fundamental importance. In this context, priority is placed on the antiaggregatory (release of NO and prostacyclin, loss of adenine nucleotide), anticoagulative (release of antithrombin III and protein S, activation of protein C), profribrinolytic (release of plasminogen activator) and antifibrinolytic activity (plasminogen activator inhibitor) as shown in Figure 8.3.

Tissue Engineering of Prosthetic Vascular Grafts, edited by Peter Zilla and Howard P. Greisler.
©1999 R.G. Landes Company.

Fig. 8.1. Primary mixed microvascular culture with central endothelial clone surrounded by pericytes.

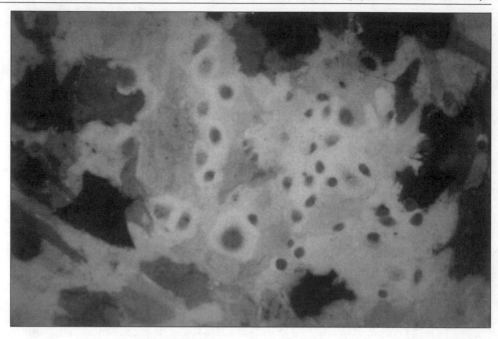

Antiaggregatory Properties of Microvascular Endothelial cells

Prostacyclin (PGI₂)

PGI$_2$ activates the thrombocytes' adenylate cyclase by adhesion to their guanosine-nucleotide receptors. The resulting increase of intracellular cyclic adenosine monophosphate (cAMP) causes platelet inhibition.[5] While this takes place, prostacyclin signals a relaxation of the vascular smooth muscle cells and blocks interaction between the endothelial cells and the monocytes. Among the stimulants of PGI$_2$ synthesis are thrombin, histamine, bradykinin and—possibly to an even higher degree—shear stress.[5] In microvascular endothelial cells of various tissue types in both humans and animals, comparable values of basal PGI$_2$ release were found to those in macrovascular endothelial cells.[5-9] However, significant differences were found in terms of the secretion capacity and responsiveness in relation to various stimulants. Histamine and thrombin for instance—when applied to microvascular endothelial cells—resulted in a weaker increase in PGI$_2$ production[6,7] than found in venous endothelial cells, whereas bradykinin caused a stronger PGI$_2$ stimulation in microvascular than in macrovascular EC.[8] Arachidonic acid as a nonspecific precursor in the prostaglandin synthesis caused a significant increase in the prostacyclin release in all cases.[6-9] After transplantation onto cardiovascular implants such as synthetic ePTE-vascular prostheses[7,8] or detoxified biological cardiac valve protheses,[9] this centrally important antiaggregatory function was fully retained.

Nitric Oxide (NO)

NO diffuses into thrombocytes and causes an increase of cyclic guanosine monophosphate (cGMP). This leads to an inhibition of platelet activation, adhesion and aggregation. With respect to the inhibition of adherence and aggregation of thrombocytes as well as the dissolution of primary aggregates, NO and PGI$_2$ exert a significant synergetic ef-

fect.[10] In addition, NO functions as a strong vasodilator, immunomodulator and neurotransmitter. The release of NO is locally continued and triggered by activated thrombocytes and various mediators (thrombin, adenine nucleotides, bradykinin, thromboxane, histamine, etc.). In comparison to macrovascular cells, cardiac microvascular endothelial cells (rat) showed a low basic release of NO. However, when stimulated with a combination of inflammation mediators, a significant increase of NO release could be detected within 24 h through induction of NO synthetase II.[12]

Adenine Nucleotide Metabolism

An enzyme expressed on the endothelial cell surface dephosphorylates the strongly proaggregatory platelet release product adenosine diphosphate (ADP) to adenosine monophosphate (AMP). Subsequently, AMP is further catabolized to adenosine, an endothelium-independent vasodilator. Intracellularly, yet another degradation takes place, the final product of which is uric acid in the case of microvascular cells, while macrovascular cells—due to their lack of xanthine dehydrogenases—catabolize no further than to hypoxanthine.[12]

Anticoagulative Properties

Thrombomodulin

Endothelial cells express the membrane protein thrombomodulin, which catalyzes the thrombin activation of protein C. The anticoagulative effect of the thus activated protein C is a result of the neutralization of the activated factors V and VIII, as well as of the inhibition of plasminogen-activator inhibitor (PAI). Thrombomodulin is expressed by endothelial cells throughout the vasculature. However, it reaches a particular high density in microvascular cells of the lung.[13] In vitro measurements in omental microvascular endothelial cells showed thrombomodulin activity with the transformation of protein C in homogenized cells to be

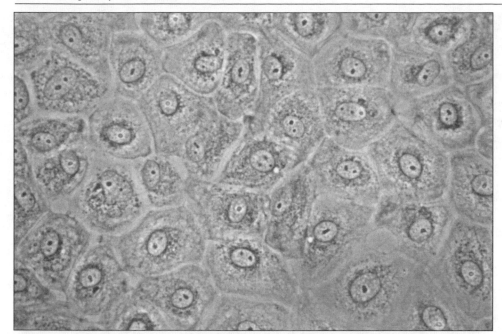

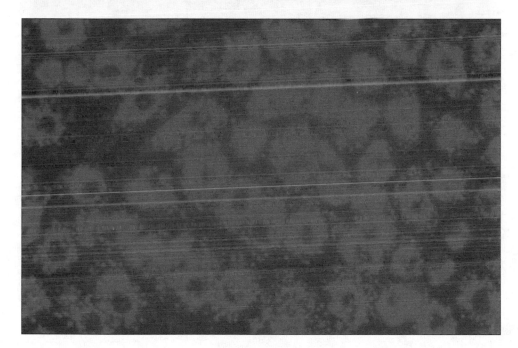

Fig. 8.2. Light-microscopy photographs of microvascular endothelial cell isolates from human fat tissue: (A, top) Phase contrast print, (B, bottom). After incorporation of Dil-marked Ac-LDL. (Prof. S. Nees, Phys. Inst. Univ. of Munich.)

approximately 6-fold higher than in confluent cell cultures.[14] In human macrovascular endothelial cells (saphenous vein), thrombomodulin activation was seen even after transplantation onto ePTFE vascular prostheses.[15]

Heaprin Sulfate

Heaprin sulfate, which is also expressed on the cell's surface, inactivates thrombin as a cofactor of antithrombin III as well as the activated forms of the coagulation factors IX, X and XII. By quantifying the acceleration of the thrombin-antithrombin complex formation, a significant production of heaprin sulfate by microvascular endothelial cells from fat tissue (epididymal fat pads, mouse) was shown.[16] Enzymatic treatment, for instance trypsinization

for passaging of cultured cells, causes the destruction of those proteoglycans.

Profibrinolytic and Antifibrinolytic Properties

Plasminogen Activators (PA, Tissue Type PA and Urokinase Type PA) and Plasminogen Activator Inhibitor (PAI)

The endothelium represents the most important site of production for tissue-type plasminogen activator (tPA). In combination with plasminogen activator inhibitor (PAI type I), which is also synthetisized by endothelial cells, the endothelium significantly contributes to the intravasal fibrinolytic activity, which requires, however, a finely tuned regulating control mechanism.

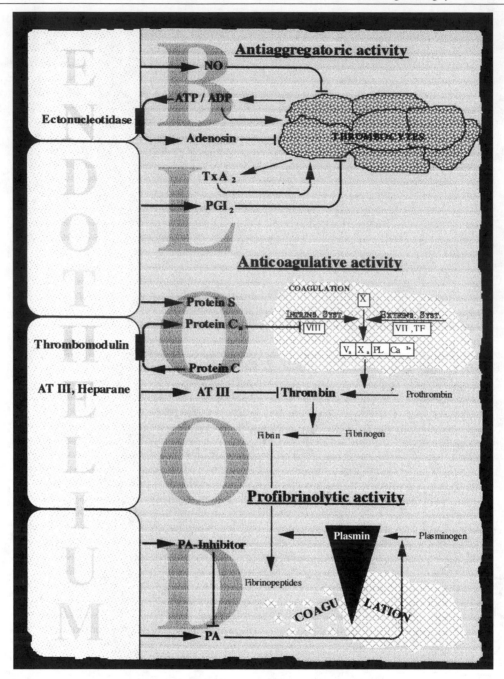

Fig. 8.3. Antithrombotic properties of the endothelium.

tPA

Thrombin and shear stress are the most important physiological stimuli for synthesis and release of tPA. In vitro, endothelial cells from different blood vessels and flow areas show significant differences with regard to their fibrinolytic potential. The largest production of tPA was measured in endothelial cells from the vena cava. When compared to microvascular (foreskin) as well as macrovascular aortic and umbilical endothelial cells, the tPA production in vena cava endothelial cells was 4- and 20-fold higher, respectively.[17-21]

In contrast to microvascular endothelial cells from foreskin, endothelial cells from the omentum (human) showed inconsistent results. When the tPA production of omental endothelial cells was compared with that of human umbilical vein endothelial cells, it was three times higher in one study[17] but 100 times higher in another.[21]

uPA

In primary cultures of human endothelial cells, the presence of urokinase type plasminogen activator (uPA) could not be proven. uPA activity could, however, be proven in subcultures of human endothelial cells of various macrovascular and microvascular sites.[17]

Plasminogen Activator Inhibitor (PAI)

PAI is the physiological inhibitor of the plasminogen activator. Among the stimuli for its release are inflammation, hormones and cytokines. Its molar concentration in plasma is higher than that of tPA. As a potent regulator of the fibrinolytic endothelial function, PAI is produced by both macrovascular and microvascular endothelial cells.[21-30]

Conclusion

In summary, the metabolic functional performance of microvascular endothelial cells corresponds to that of their macrovascular counterparts. Differences are mainly found in the quantity of the synthetic activities. However, it appears that following transplantation of microvascular endothelial cells, a certain adaptation to the new environment will be necessary. Even when mixed cultures were seeded in the course of animal experiments (dog), a regulation and adaptation to the physiological requirements could be observed.[31] Whether the same observations will apply to humans is questionable. Due to the lack of systematic examination following clinical studies, relevant results cannot as yet be supplied.

References

1. Jarell BE, Williams SK, Stokes G et al. Use of freshly isolated capillary endothelial cells for the immediate establishment of a monolayer on a vascular graft at surgery. Surgery 1986; 100:392-399.
2. Radomski JS, Jarrel BE, Williams SK et al. Initial adherence of human capillary endothelial cells to Dacron. J Surg Res 1987; 42:133-140.
3. Weiss. Cell tissue biology New York: Urban & Schwarzenberg. 1988:191-205.
4. Fittkau M, Fischlein T, Reichart B, Juchem G, Nees S. Autologe Endothelialisierung menschlicher Gefäß–prothesen. Z Kard 1994; 83, Supp:1:38.
5. Wu KK, Thiagarajan P. Role of endothelium in thrombosis and hemostasis. Annu Rev Med 1996; 47:315-331.
6. Stansby G, Shukla N, Hamilton G, Jeremy J. Comparison of prostanoid synthesis in cultured human vascular endothelial cells derived from omentum and umbilical vein. Eur J Vasc Surg 1991; 5:501-506.
7. Budd JS, Allen K, Hartley J, Walsh A et al. Prostacyclin production from seeded prosthetic vascular grafts. Br J Surg 1992; 79:1151-1153.
8. Sterpetti AV, Schultz RD, Hunter WJ et al. Comparison of two techniques to isolate microvascular endothelial cells from the omentum. J Surg Res 1990; 48:101-106.
9. Fischlein T, Lehner G, Lante W, Fittkau M et al. Endothelialization of cardiac valve bioprotheses. Artif Organs 1994; 17 No 6:345-352.
10. Radomski MW, Palmer PMJ, Moncada S. The anti-aggregating properties of vascular endothelium interactions between prostacyclin and nitric oxide. Br J Pharmacol 1987; 92:639-642.
11. Ungureanu-Longrois D, Balligand JL, Okada I et al. Contractile responsiveness of ventricular myocytes to isoproterenol is regulated by induction of nitric oxide synthase activity in cardiac microvascular endothelial cells in heterotypic primary culture. Circ Res 1995; 77 No 3:486-493.
12. Des Rosiers C, Nees S, Gerlach E. Purine metabolism in cultured aortic and coronary endothelial cells. Biochem Cell Biol 1989; 67:8-15.
13. Carley WW, Niedbala MJ, Gerritsen ME. Isolation, cultivation and partial charaterization of microvascular endothelium derived from human lung. Am J Respir Cell Mol Biol 1992; 7:620-630.
14. Anders E, Alles J, Delvos U, Pötzsch B et al. Microvascular endothelial cells from human omentum tissue. Modified method for long-term cultivation and new aspects of characterization. Microvasc Res 1987; 34:239-249.
15. Gillis-Haegerstrand C, Frebelius S, Haegerstrand A, Swedenborg J. Cultured human endothelial cells seeded on expanded polytetrafluoroethylene support thrombin-mediated activation of protein C. J Vasc Surg 1996; 24(2):226-234.
16. Marcum JA, Rosenberg RD. Heparinlike molecules with anticoagulant activity are synthesized by cultured endothelial cells. Biochemical and Biophysical Research Communications 1985; 126 No 1:365-372.
17. Van Hinsbergh VWM. Regulation of the synthesis and secretion of plasminogen activators by endothelial cells. Haemostasis 1988; 18:307-327.
18. Rijken DC, Van Hinsbergh VWM, Sens EHC. Quantitation of tissue-type plasminogen activator in human endothelial cell cultures by use of an enzyme immunoassay. Thromb Res 1984; 33:145-153.
19. Van Hinsbergh VWM, Binnema D, Scheffer MA, Sprengers ED et al. Production of plasminogen activators and inhibitor by serially propagated endothelial cells from adult human blood vessels. Arteriosclerosis 1987; 7:389-400.
20. Van Hinsbergh VWM, Sprengers ED, Kooistra T. Effect of thrombin on the production of plasminogen activators and PA inhibitor-1 by human foreskin microvascular endothelial cells. Thromb. Haemostasis 1987; 57:148-153.
21. Speiser W, Anders E, Preissner KT, Wagner O et al. Differences in coagulant and fibrinolytic activities of cultured human endothelial cells derived from omental tissue microvessels and umbilical veins. Blood 1987; 69:964-967.
22. Booyse FM, Osikowicz G, Feder S, Scheinbuks J. Isolation and characterization of a urokinase-type plasminogen activator (M$_r$ = 54,000) from cultured human endothelial cells indistinguishable from urokinase. J Biol Chem 1984; 259:7198-7205.
23. Booyse FM, Scheinbuks J, Radek J, Osikowicz G et al. Immunological identification and comparison of plasminogen activator forms in cultured normal human endothelial cells and smooth muscle cells. Thromb Res 1981; 24:495-504.
24. Loskutoff DJ, Van Mourik JA, Erickson LA, Lawrence D. Detection of an unusually stable fibrinolytic inhibitor produced by bovine endothelial cells. Proc Natn Acad Sci USA 1983; 80:2956-2960.
25. Emeis JJ, Van Hinsbergh VWM, Verheijen JH, Wijngaards G. Inhibition of tissue-type plasminogen activator by conditioned medium from cultured human and porcine vascular endothelial cells. Biochem Biophys Res Commun 1983; 110:392-398.
26. Philips M, Juul A, Thorsen S. Human endothelial cells produce a plasminogen activator inhibitor and a tissue-type plasminogen activator-inhibitor complex. Biochem Biophys Acta 1984; 802:99-110.

27. Van Hinsbergh VWM, Bertina RM, Van Wijngaarden A, Van Tilburg NH et al. Activated protein C decreases plasminogen activator-inhibitor activity in endothelial cell-conditioned medium. Blood 1985; 65:444-451.

28. Van Mourik JA, Lawrence DA, Loskutoff DJ. Purification of an inhibitor of plasminogen activator (antiactivator) synthesized by endothelial cells. J Biol Chem 1984; 259:14914-14921.

29. Dosne AM, Dupuy E, Bodevin E. Production of a fibrinolytic inhibitor by cultured endothelial cells derived from human umbilical vein. Thromb Res 1978; 12:377-387.

30. Sprengers ED, Verheijen JH, Van Hinsbergh VWM, Emeis JJ. Evidence for the presence of two different fibrinolytic inhibitors in human endothelial cells conditioned medium. Biochem Biophys Acta 1984; 801:163-170.

31. Baitella-Eberle G, Groscurth P, Zilla P, Lachat M et al. Long-term results of tissue development and cell differentiation on Dacron prostheses seeded with microvascular cells in dogs. J Vasc Surg 1993; 18 (6):1019-1028.

CHAPTER 9

Automated Seeding Devices

Dominic Dodd, J. Vincent Smyth, Michael G. Walker

Introduction

Almost as soon as the application of endothelial seeding to enhance graft patency was recognized, groups started to develop techniques and equipment to facilitate the process. The requirements of an ideal seeding system for clinical work include simplicity, efficiency and speed. These considerations must be applied to the delivery of a high yield of viable endothelial cells using a readily available tissue source. The maintenance of sterility to avoid introduction of infective agents; effective seeding onto the graft while retaining the functional integrity of seeded cells; and the rapid development of monolayer within a time-frame suitable for operating room use are also fundamental. The search for a reproducible, inexpensive, low-tech, high efficacy technique has been a tortuous and convoluted one in which the solution to each problem has led to further questions.

In the design of a fully automated seeding device, several key steps must be considered. The automated seeding process commences with tissue reception. A closed system in which sterility is maintained is essential. The tissue receiver may be combined with a mechanical homogenization process to speed subsequent cell separation by enzymatic digestion. The aim of this stage is to acquire large numbers of endothelial cells (ECs) with relatively few contaminating cell types. Subcutaneous adipose tissue is a ready source of microvascular endothelial cells and is easily harvested in sufficient quantities from all but the thinnest of patients. Once ECs have been isolated, maximal graft-cell attachment is needed. The constraints of the operating room mean that this must be achieved in a relatively short time. Graft surface coatings clearly have a major role in determining the efficiency of this stage. Finally, the seeded graft must be presented to the operating team in a package that will maintain its sterility and preserve the viability of the seeded EC lining. Ideally, a fully automated system should optimize cell harvest and seeding efficiency; however, a compromise between these aims and the duration of the procedure must be met. Completion of the seeding process in approximately one hour is a realistic time scale in a busy operating room. Much of this time will be taken by cell digestion and separation, leaving little time for cell attachment or final rinsing.

If vascular graft seeding is to be widely adopted in clinical practice, a reliable, easily used system is required that can be accommodated in a conventional operating room. It should be recognized that surgeons' enthusiasm for the introduction of a complex and time consuming process into the operating room is limited. Unless the process is automated, vascular graft seeding will remain a "laboratory" technique, confined to very few surgical centers. Therefore, in addition to the development of graft materials and coatings for optimal seeding performance, automation of the seeding process must be achieved. This aspect

Tissue Engineering of Prosthetic Vascular Grafts, edited by Peter Zilla and Howard P. Greisler.

of seeding technology is both a biological and engineering challenge. Perhaps the difficulties in successfully achieving this goal are reflected in the relatively small number of publications of techniques and designs investigated.

Early Seeding Techniques

At the beginning of the 1980s, seeding methodology relied on mechanical harvesting of the endothelial cells by metal pledget from vein segments.[1] As well as being laborious, the yield of viable cells was relatively low due to harvest trauma. In addition, the low specificity of mechanical harvesting resulted in frequent contamination of the endothelial culture with fibroblasts and smooth muscle cells. This technique sufficed for laboratory work and was successful using animal cell lines, but a major step forward was made with the adoption of enzymatic harvesting, leading to the now routine collagenase incubation-based method.[2] This rapidly superseded mechanical harvesting as a straightforward method which allowed rapid procurement of pure endothelial cells, and the promise of seeding prosthetic grafts in terms of patency, resistance to infection and reduced neointimal hyperplasia began to be realized in a range of experimental laboratory and in vivo models. However, only animal cell lines had as yet been used extensively and the next step was clearly to extend this work to clinical practice.

Up to the early 1980s, work with human cell lines had been restricted to umbilical vein endothelium, HUVECs, because of difficulties with maintaining adult endothelial cell lines, HAECs, in culture. The next breakthrough in endothelial seeding was the successful culture of HAECs by Jarrell, with the recognition of the need for EDGF and heparin in the culture medium.[3] Despite significant problems with the more fragile human cell cultures and the disappointing results of cell attachment studies detailed in an earlier chapter, initial protocols using harvest, culture and seeding stages demonstrated that at least some benefit might be realized. In clinical practice, however, the time constraints of the operating room meant that cell harvesting would need to be carried out as a preliminary step, or a more rapid technique of producing an endothelial monolayer was needed, or clinical seeding would be carried out at subconfluent densities. Subconfluent seeding, whilst effective in the laboratory, has been shown to be less able to resist the shear stress of flow than an intact monolayer,[4] and has been largely abandoned. In those clinical studies that have been carried out, the seeding densities achieved were probably subconfluent, and did not result in measurable reduction in thrombogenicity measured by labeled platelet scintigraphy,[5] though there was some indirect evidence from serum markers of a reduction in platelet adhesion and activation.[6]

Optimal Conditions for Seeding

Cellular Considerations

In order to achieve the maximum coverage from a limited source of cells for seeding, optimal conditions for seeding were extensively investigated. Work with both expanded polytetrafluoroethylene (ePTFE) and polyester graft materials suggests the use of at least 150,000 cells/cm^2, seeded onto a fibronectin precoated graft and incubated for at least 30 minutes.[7] To produce a complete monolayer on a graft would thus require an initial harvest of 1.5 x $10^5 \cdot \pi \cdot d \cdot l \cdot$ (% Seeding Efficiency) cells, where d=inside diameter and l = length, of the graft. Our own work with immediately harvested saphenous vein endothelial cells has demonstrated that a seeding efficiency of 30% can be reliably achieved,[8] and thus for a standard 30 cm, 6 mm internal diameter graft suitable for a femoropopliteal graft, an initial harvest of 28 x 10^6 cells is required. A 60 cm long, 4 mm internal diameter graft such as might be used for femorotibial bypass would require 38 x 10^6 cells. This quantity of endothelial cells can not be derived from autologous saphenous vein, since such cell harvest would require a vein segment of equivalent size, which would normally be used as the preferred conduit. Microvascular endothelial cells have been proposed as an alternative cell type,[9,10] with harvests from both omentum and subcutaneous adipose tissue being used for seeding experimentally. However, considerably more experimental data have been gained with macrovascular endothelial cells to suggest inhibition of smooth muscle cell proliferation in vivo, and acceptable results of retention under arterial levels of shear stress.

Graft Material Considerations

The large majority of EC seeding studies have been carried out using commercially available graft materials that were not specifically designed for cell attachment. Indeed, considerable materials technology has been applied to make the luminal surface of these graft materials hydrophobic by negatively-charged fluoropolymer lining and consequently unsuitable for direct seeding.

There has been continued interest over the last decade on choice of graft coating materials for optimal cell attachment. It is now recognized that the extracellular matrix plays an integral role in cellular function and the choice of graft coating material will influence not only cell attachment but also cellular activity. Soluble components of the extracellular matrix such as fibronectin, collagen and laminin have all been used to achieve comparable cell attachment rates.[11,12] Recently, synthetic EC binding site peptides containing arginine-glycine-aspartic acid (RGD) have been used to precoat ePTFE, with a significant increase in EC attachment and retention compared with fibronectin.[13] The use of RGD peptides is attractive commercially, as they are simple to produce and cheaper to use than more complex protein coatings. EC attachment through focal adhesions is RGD dependent; if no RGD sequences are detected in extracellular matrix, apoptosis occurs.

In contrast, Sipehia reported the use of gaseous "plasma" surface modification to enhance cellular attachment and replication.[14] He reported the addition of amino groups to the surface of a PTFE membrane by anhydrous ammonia in a gaseous plasma increased bovine arterial EC attachment from 36 to 92% after 96 h in culture.

This suggests that appropriate surface engineering of the prosthetic material to be seeded may have as large an influence on the rapid development of a healthy neointima as cell delivery and modification itself.

Cell Delivery Considerations

In addition to selection of optimal seeding cell isolates and graft surface characteristics, the delivery of the seeding population to the graft has been investigated. Several approaches to achieve rapid, even coating of the graft lumen have been reported. These include graft rotation,[15] vacuum[16] or pressure seeding.[17] These latter two are similar in concept and rely on the use of a porous graft material to facilitate pressure gradient filtering of cells, either singly or in clumps. This latter technique is described as graft sodding.[18]

Rotational systems represent basic automated seeding devices. In those designs previously described the graft is held horizontally in a scaffold and filled with EC suspended in culture medium or heparinized blood.[19] The graft is clamped at its ends and rotated in its longitudinal axis so that gravity assists even seeding.

The duration allowed for cell attachment has also been studied. Increased resistance to shear stress has been demonstrated by Budd et al.[20] However, we found that initial cell attachment did not increase significantly on coated grafts after 30 minutes[8] and, given the time constraints in clinical practice, do not feel prolonged seeding time is justified.

Choice of Seeding Technique

Single Stage Seeding

This approach is the most attractive form of automated graft seeding. In a single operative session the patient's endothelial cells are retrieved and seeded onto the graft, which is then implanted. This avoids the need for cell culture, and reduces operative time overall. It is, however, probably the most technically demanding. To adopt this approach, adequate cell numbers must be harvested to cover the graft surface. The most simple devices include the development of harvesting kits to provide endothelial cell suspensions for seeding commercially available grafts, vein holding chambers to facilitate enzymatic harvest and graft chambers for culture in which the seeded graft can be maintained in a culture cabinet and rotated mechanically to allow even coating of the graft surface with endothelial cells.

Two Stage Seeding

Cultured two stage seeding is an alternative approach that has been successfully applied in clinical trials by Leseche et al[21] and Zilla et al.[22] This approach follows more closely the standard laboratory practice of harvesting ECs from autologous vein, which are then grown to confluence and passaged in standard tissue culture flasks until adequate cell numbers are available for seeding. Cultured ECs are then seeded onto the graft, which is maintained in a specifically constructed culture flask in which culture medium can be circulated through the lumen of the graft. The graft is incubated until confluence is deemed to have been reached on the luminal surface, at which time the graft is then implanted. This period of incubation allows basement membrane to be laid down, which significantly enhances shear stress resistance, but prolonged culture and repeated passage may produce an adverse effect on phenotype.

Although this approach allows the use of macrovascular endothelial cells with only modest requirements for initial cell number, the patient is required to undergo two surgical procedures, which means it is not compatible with revascularization in cases of critical ischemia, arguably those most in need of endothelialized grafts. Furthermore, the use of cell culture may increase the risk of pathogen transmission, both to and from the patient, unless strict safety controls are applied.

Microvascular Cells and Graft Sodding

Adipose tissue contains large numbers of microvascular endothelial cells lining its capillaries. Jarrell et al first proposed its use a an alternative EC source in 1986.[23] In particular the greater omentum offers a readily available source of adipose tissue. The use of omentum as a cell source led to some debate as to the true nature of the cells harvested, some workers demonstrating the presence of mesothelial cells[24] and others microvascular EC[25,26] as the primary cell isolate. In reality the exact harvest conditions are likely to influence predominant cell population. In any case, peritoneal mesothelial cells (PMC) have been shown to form confluent monolayers on vascular graft material in culture[27] and have demonstrated anti-thrombotic activity, producing prostacyclin,[28] and as such may be considered as an alternative to EC for seeding.

Liposuction

Williams and Jarrell, having championed the use of adipose microvascular cells, most recently advocated the use of liposuction to harvest subcutaneous tissue.[29] They have shown that before cell isolation 77% of cells harvested were of microvascular origin.

Vein Fragment Sodding

Noishiki et al first reported the use of diced fragments of canine venous tissue seeded into a porous Dacron graft.[30] They used a sodding technique to force cell clumps under pressure into the graft interstices. By this technique they sealed the graft with a heterogeneous cell population, but demonstrated in culture the development of an endothelial intimal lining.

Autoseeding

In our own laboratory, we use a single stage, highly automated seeding machine similar in concept to the technique devised by Jarrell and Williams, and to the heterogeneous sodding technique of Noishiki. This machine is a development prototype similar to that proposed by Pasic et al[31,32] and built by Sulzer AG (Winterthur, Switzerland) (Fig. 9.1). By using this method, the initial porosity of our graft is reduced to such an extent that there is no need for preclotting prior to implantation, and we use surgically excised wound margin adipose tissue as a source of tissue. In the technique originally described by Noishiki,[17] the tissue was finely diced prior to sodding, but we have incorporated an enzymatic digestion phase into our process to try to optimize viable cell numbers by reducing mechanical cell damage.

Fig. 9.1. Schematic diagram of automated seeding device incorporating a cell separation phase.

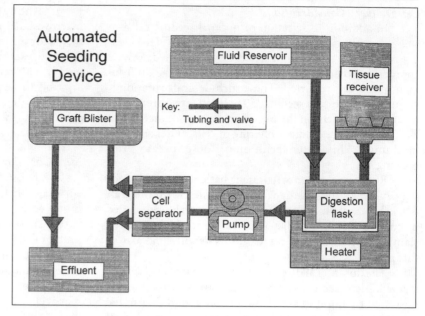

To seed a typical peripheral vascular graft using our device, the operator introduces 100-300 g adipose tissue into a tissue receiver and starts the seeding program, which is controlled by the machine's central processing unit. The adipose tissue is minced and forced through a metallic mesh by an air-driven piston into a tissue digestion flask containing 300 ml of buffered saline at 37°C. Into this is added 1,000 IU collagenase II per gram of adipose tissue and digestion continues with constant agitation for 40 minutes. After this time the digested fat forms a slurry which is coarsely filtered and seeded under pressure into the interstices of a specially prepared woven polyester graft. The graft has been precoated with bovine gelatin and retains a porosity of approximately 1500 ml/cm^2/min. After seeding, this porosity is reduced to almost zero at arterial pressure levels. The process takes 50 to 55 minutes to complete and the graft can be removed from the machine and handed to the operating team in a sterile blister pack. This device allows for a fully automated seeding process to be undertaken in the operating room without excessively prolonging the surgical procedure, or requiring on-site laboratory facilities or highly skilled cell culture technicians. Its secondary advantages are the reduction in risk of pathogen transfer and the avoidance of preliminary cell harvesting surgery. The main disadvantage with our particular machine is that a heterogeneous cell population is initially seeded onto the graft surface. This population is difficult to fully characterize, but is anticipated to include vascular smooth muscle cells, fibroblasts, adipocytes, and pericytes. If omentum is used, then PMC may also be present, although the digestion conditions in the machine are considerably more rigorous than those normally used for PMC harvest from omentum and it is likely that most PMC would be digested.

In vitro experiments using human subcutaneous adipose tissue and omentum and subsequent graft culture in our laboratory have confirmed the rapid development of a cell monolayer of typical endothelial appearance (Figs. 9.2A,B). Full characterization of the monolayer has been complicated by the apparent loss of many cell surface immunomarkers with the digestion process. Indeed, we have been unable to demonstrate the presence of tPA, vWF, CD34, CD31, eNOS or bFGF in our specimens.

We have used the seeding system for in vivo experimentation using a porcine model. Subcutaneous adipose tissue was harvested from immature Yucatan miniswine and a segment of 6 mm internal diameter graft implanted immediately after processing into the infrarenal aorta. After four weeks, the graft was explanted and compared with nonseeded control grafts, also implanted for four weeks. In our study there was no detectable loss in early patency following seeding with a mixed cell population. The presence of potentially thrombogenic tissue debris in the graft interstices did not have a detrimental effect in the immediate postimplantation phase. However, at four weeks the seeded samples, whilst remaining patent, demonstrated neointimal hyperplasia, with marked SMC proliferation. We surmise that, despite endothelial cover, neointimal hyperplasia occurs and that this may be due to seeding of SMC which are stimulated in the process. To overcome this problem we proposed the introduction of a cell separation process to minimize the seeding of nonendothelial cells. The most promising way to include EC purification in an automated seeding device would be to use immunomagnetic bead separation.[33] Beads coated with antibodies to the EC surface antigen CD34 are already commercially available and are approved for clinical use in hemopoietic stem cell separation (Baxter Healthcare Ltd, Thetford, UK). However, there is a time penalty incurred with this approach. To offset this, work is in progress to determine the feasibility of replacing enzymatic tissue digestion with a mechanical homogenization process to reduce the overall procedure time. We estimate that a highly selected EC suspension can be seeded onto a pros-

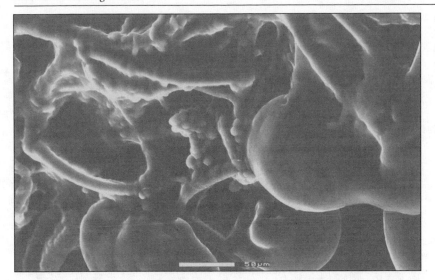

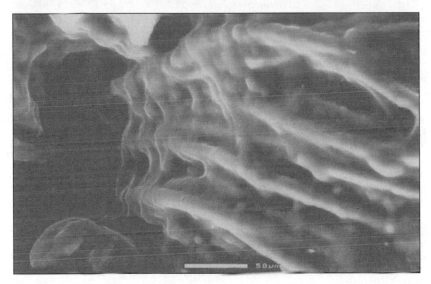

Fig. 9.2. (A, top) Environmental scanning electron micrograph of a porous polyester graft, immediately after human omental tissue seeding. Original magnification x340. (B, bottom) A similar graft after 24 h of in vitro culture. Original magnification x390.

thesis in under two hours. While this time scale may be unattractive to some vascular surgeons, we feel that the group of patients for whom this technology is required are worth the extra time spent in their treatment.

Summary

Although our understanding of vascular biology, and in particular the elucidation of many cell-matrix signaling interactions, have led to dramatic breakthroughs in the laboratory, endothelial cell seeding of vascular prosthetic grafts is not widely regarded as clinically useful. Until an automated harvesting and delivery system is fully developed, it remains unlikely that this will change.

It is hoped that the development of new surface treatments will lead to greatly increased rates of seeded cell adherence, retention and replication. In addition the role of genetically modified EC with enhanced antithrombotic activity is just now being recognized. It is possible that immunomodulated, cryopreserved bioprosthetic grafts will represent the next generation of small diameter arterial bypass prostheses.

References

1. Herring MB, Gardner AL, Glover J. A single staged technique for seeding vascular grafts with autogenous endothelium. Surgery 1978; 84:498-504.
2. Jaffe EA, Nachman RL, Becker CG, Minick CR. Culture of human endothelial cells derived from umbilical veins. J Clin Invest 1973; 52:2745-56.
3. Jarrell BE, Levine E, Shapiro S, Williams SK, Carabasi RA, Mueller S, Thornton S. Human adult endothelial cell growth in culture. J Vasc Surg 1984; 1:757-64.
4. Miyata T, Conte MS, Trudell LA, Mason D, Whittemore AD, Birinyi LK. Delayed exposure to pulsatile shearstress improves retention of human saphenous vein endothelial cells on seeded ePTFE grafts. J Surg Res 1991; 50:485-93.
5. Jensen N, Lindblad B, Bergqvist D. Endothelial cell seeded dacron aortobifurcated grafts: Platelet deposition and long-term follow-up. J Cardiovasc Surg 1994; 35:425-9.
6. Ortenwall P, Wadenvik H, Kutti J, Risberg B. Endothelial cell seeding reduces thrombogenicity of Dacron grafts in humans. J Vasc Surg 1990; 11:403-410.
7. Vohra R, Thomson GJL, Carr HMH, Sharma, Walker MG. Comparison of different vascular prostheses and matrices in realtion to endothelial seeding. Br J Surg 1991; 78:417-20.

8. Carr HMH, Vohra R, Sharma H, Smyth JV, Rooney OB, Dodd PD, Walker MG. Endothelial cell seeding kinetics under chronic flow in prosthetic grafts. Ann Vasc Surg 1996; 10:469-75.

9. Stansby G, Shukla N, Fuller B, Hamilton G. Seeding of human microvascular endothelial cells onto polytetrafluoroethylene graft material. Br J Surg 1991; 78:1189-92.

10. Schmidt SP, Monajjem N, Evancho MM, Pippert TR, Sharp WV. Microvascular endothelial cell seeding of small-diameter Dacron vascular grafts. J Invest Surg 1988; 1:35-44.

11. Thomson GJ, Vohra RK, Carr HMH, Walker MG. Adult human endothelial cell seeding using expanded poltyetrafluoroethylene vascular grafts: A comparison of four substrates. Surgery 1991; 109:20-7.

12. Koveker GB, Graham LM, Burkel WE, Sell R, Wakefield TW, Dietrich K, Stanley JC. Extracellular matrix preparation of expanded polytetrafluoroethylene grafts seeded with endothelial cells: Influence on early platelet deposition, cellular growth and luminal prostacyclin release. Surgery 1991; 109:313-9.

13. Walluscheck KP, Steinhoff G, Kelm S, Haverich A. Improved endothelial cell attachment on ePTFE vascular grafts pretreated with synthetic RGD-containing peptides. Eur J Vasc Endovasc Surg 1996; 12:321-30.

14. Sipehia R. The enhanced attachment and growth of endothelial cells on anhydrous ammonia gaseous plasma modified surfaces of polystyrene and poly(tetrafluoroethylene). Biomater Artif Cells Artif Organs 1990; 18:437-46.

15. Gerlach J, Kreusel KM, Schauwecker HH, Bucherl ES. Endothelial cell seeding on PTFE vascular prostheses using a standardized seeding technique. Artif Organs 1989; 12:270-5.

16. van Wachem PB, Stronck JW, Koers-Zuideveld R, Dijk F, Wildevuur CR. Vacuum cell seeding: A new method for the fast application of an evenly distributed cell layer on porous vascular grafts. Biomaterials 1990; 11:602-6.

17. Nosihiki Y, Yamane Y, Tomizawa Y. Sealing of highly porous fabric vascular prostheses by adipose connective tissue fragments instead of preclotting with fresh blood. J Invest Surg 1993; 6:231-40.

18. Williams SK, Jarrell BE, Rose DG, Pontell J, Kapelan BA, Park PK, Carter TL. Human microvessel endothelial cell isolation and vascular graft sodding in the operating room. Ann Vasc Surg 1989; 3:146-52.

19. Mazzutocelli JP, Roudiere JL, Bernex F, Bertrand P, Leandri J, Loisance D. A new device for endothelial cell seeding of a small-caliber vascular prosthesis. Artif Organs 1993; 17:787-90.

20. Budd JS, Allen KE, Bell PRF. Effects of two methods of endothelial cell seeding on cell retention during blood flow. Br J Surg 1991; 78:878-82.

21. Leseche G, Ohan J, Bouttier S, Palombi T, Bertrand P, Andreassian B. Above-knee femoropopliteal bypass grafting using endothelial cell seeded PTFE grafts: Five-year clinical experience. Ann Vasc Surg 1995; 9:S15-23.

22. Zilla P, Deutsch M, Meinhart J, Puschmann R, Eberl T, Minar E, Dudczak R, Lugmaier H, Schmidt P, Noszian I, Fischlein T. Clinical in vitro endothelialization of femoropopliteal bypass grafts: An actuarial follow-up over three years. J Vasc Surg 1994; 19:540-8.

23. Jarrell BE, Williams SK, Stokes G, Hubbard FA, Carabasi RA, Koolpe E, Greene D, Pratt K, Moritz MJ, Radomski J, Speicher L. Use of freshly isolated capillary endothelial cells for the immediate establishment of a monolayer on a vascular graft at surgery. Surgery 1986; 100:392-9.

24. Visser MJ, van Bockel JH, van Muijen GN, van Hinsbergh VW. Cells derived from omental fat tissue are not endothelial in origin. A study on the origin of epitheloid cells deirved from omentum. J Vasc Surg 1991; 13:373-81.

25. Williams SK, Kleinert LB, Rose D, McKenney S. Origin of endothelial cells that line expanded polytetrafluoroethylene vascular grafts sodded with cells from microvascularized fat. J Vasc Surg 1994; 19:594-604.

26. Vici M, Pasquinelli G, Preda P, Martinelli GN, Gibellini D, Freyrie A, Curti T, D'Addato M. Electron microscopic and immunocytochemical profiles of human subcutaneous fat tissue microvascular endothelial cells. Ann Vasc Surg 1993; 7:541-8.

27. Pronk A, Hoynck van Papendrecht AAGM, Leguit P, Verbrugh HA, Verkooyen RPAJ, van Vroonhoven TJMV. Mesothelial cell adherence to vascular prostheses and their subsequent growth in vitro. Cell Transplantation 1994; 3:41-8.

28. Nicholson LJ, Clarke JMF, Pittilo RM, Machin SJ, Woolf N. The mesothelial cell as a non-thrombogenic surface. Thromb Haemostas 1984; 52:102-4.

29. Williams SK, Wang TF, Castrillo R, Jarrell BE. Liposuction-derived human fat used for vascular graft sodding contains endothelial and not mesothelial cells as the main cell type. J Vasc Surg 1994; 19:916-23.

30. Noishiki Y, Yamane Y, Tomizawa Y, Okoshi T, Satoh S, Wildevuur CR. Endothelialization of vascular prostheses by transplantation of venous tissue fragments. ASAIO Trans 1990; 36:346-8.

31. Pasic M, Muller-Glauser W, von Segesser LK, Lachat M, Mihaljevic T, Turina M. Superior late patency of small-diameter Dacron grafts seeded with omental microvascular cells: An experimental study. Ann Thorac Surg 1994; 58:677-83.

32. Pasic M, Muller-Glauser W, Odermatt B, Lachat M, Siefert B, Turina M. Seeding with omental cells prevents late neointimal hyperplasia in small-diameter Dacron grafts. Circulation 1995; 92:2605-16.

33. Jackson CJ, Garbett PK, Nissen B, Schrieber L. Binding of human endothelium to Ulex europaeus I-coated Dynabeads: Application to the isolation of microvascular endothelium. J Cell Sci 1990; 96:257-62.

CHAPTER 10

Healing Patterns Following Microvascular Seeding—
A Clinical Evaluation of Microvascular-Seeded
A-V Access Grafts

Steven P. Schmidt, Sharon O. Meerbaum, Duane L. Donovan

Introduction

The need for a more successful artificial bypass graft to replace small and medium-diam eter blood vessels remains an important issue in vascular surgery. Approximately 600,000 patients require arterial reconstructive surgeries in the United States annually, including 20,000 femoropopliteal bypasses. In addition, each year approximately 90,000 new patients with end stage renal disease (ESRD) present to vascular surgeons for access-related surgeries for chronic hemodialysis. Surgeons prefer to use autologous native vessels as bypass conduits. For peripheral revascularizations, the collective experiences of vascular surgeons have been that long term performances of bypass grafts constructed from native veins are superior to those using other biologic or synthetic alternatives. Likewise, autogenous arteriovenous (AV) fistulas of the Brescia-Ciminio type are the hemodialysis access procedures that theoretically provide the longest term trouble-free patency compared to synthetic graft alternatives. Nevertheless, limitations of the use of native veins as bypass grafts have been described. Less than 15% of the entire dialysis population have well-functioning native AV fistulas. Eighty percent of dialysis patients receive polytetrafluoroethylene (PTFE) vascular grafts for access, which is accompanied by the morbidity attendant with implantation of these grafts. When used as peripheral vascular replacements, one-quarter to one-third of saphenous vein bypass grafts deteriorate, as assessed by histology, in the relatively higher flows and pressures of the arterial circulation. It is common, therefore, for patients with no usable native veins available for grafting (or remaining veins of poor quality) to present to vascular surgeons for repeated revascularization procedures. The use of synthetic vascular grafts is imperative in these patients.

The long term performances of commercially available synthetic vascular prosthetics are poor. Primary patency of PTFE grafts used for AV access is approximately one year;[1] the patency rate for PTFE grafts implanted for femorodistal reconstruction is approximately 20% at three years.[2] Failure of vascular grafts at short times postoperatively has been generally attributed to the combination of low flow hemodynamics plus the inherent thrombogenicities of the graft materials. Late graft failure most frequently occurs from anastomotic neointimal hyperplasia (NIH) and consequent narrowings at the outflow tract. In synthetic grafts used for hemodialysis access, midgraft hyperplasia adjacent to frequently used needle puncture sites may also cause failure. The etiology of NIH remains to be clarified.

Tissue Engineering of Prosthetic Vascular Grafts, edited by Peter Zilla and Howard P. Greisler.
©1999 R.G. Landes Company.

One of the early assumptions for the superiority of autogenous vascular grafts compared to synthetic grafts was the presence of an intact endothelium on the luminal surfaces of the native grafts. Under in vivo conditions of normal circulatory physiology, endothelial cells (ECs) are the most nonthrombogenic cells known. The blood-contacting (luminal) surfaces of synthetic vascular grafts implanted in animals endothelialize, in time, along their entire lengths and typically achieve long term patencies. This endothelialization occurs, however, only in the anastomotic regions of human vascular grafts and is limited at most to 2-3 cm of ingrowth.

Although the issues remain debatable, it has generally been accepted that humans do not heal synthetic bypass grafts with an endothelial cell lining as other animals do. As a consequence of this failure to heal, in addition to other clinical issues, it is generally regarded as not feasible to utilize small caliber vascular grafts (< 6 mm I.D.) clinically in patients, as these grafts fail quickly from accumulated thrombus and/or neointimal hyperplasia.

The logical assumption of many researchers has been that synthetic graft performances in humans may be enhanced and patencies extended by promoting endothelialization of the luminal surfaces of these synthetic grafts. One method of creating such an endothelialized surface is transplantation of autogenous ECs onto the blood-contacting graft surface. A new research technology has thus evolved called "endothelial cell seeding (ECS)" to investigate this possibility. The underlying logic supporting ECS investigations is that the presence of transplanted endothelium mimics the anti-thrombogenic intima of native vessels. In addition, it has been suggested that rapid endothelialization in anastomotic regions may normalize aberrant flow patterns, which are thought to contribute to the genesis of intimal hyperplastic lesions.[3]

Animal studies have shown that endothelialization of prosthetic grafts can be encouraged by transplanting endothelial cells into or onto the graft at the time of implantation. These endothelial cell-seeded grafts typically have improved patencies versus nonseeded controls when evaluated in animals. To date, however, the prospect from animal studies of successful long term performances of endothelial cell-seeded grafts in humans has not been realized in the clinical trials that have been reported, which are few in number when compared with the numbers of reported animal studies.

The first true clinical trial of endothelial cell seeding in patients was reported by Herring et al.[4] Seeded endothelial cells were derived by mechanical methods from autologous veins and transplanted onto Dacron grafts, which were subsequently implanted in patients as femoropopliteal reconstructions. Analyses revealed no differences in patencies between seeded and nonseeded grafts; smokers had especially poor graft patencies. Herring and his colleagues[5] were able to confirm endothelialization of the luminal graft surface from a seeded graft retrieved from a patient via histological analysis. Zilla et al[6] also reported early clinical data from a series of patients who underwent femoropopliteal bypass using endothelial cell-seeded expanded polytetrafluoroethylene (ePTFE) grafts. There were no dif-

ferences between seeded and nonseeded graft patencies in this study and the extent of endothelialization of seeded grafts was minimal. Ortenwall et al[7,8] reported reduced platelet deposition on both seeded Dacron and polytetrafluoroethylene grafts implanted in patients. Kadletz et al[9] also observed little or no platelet accumulation on PTFE prostheses that had been endothelialized in vitro prior to implantation in patients. Herring et al[10] compared the performances of 66 seeded PTFE grafts with 53 autologous vein grafts and concluded that at 30 months vein graft patency was superior and that seeding did not improve patency in below the knee bypasses. In contrast, Leseche and his colleagues[11] reported good clinical results when endothelial cell-seeded PTFE grafts were implanted as above-knee femoropopliteal bypass grafts. These investigators utilized a two stage seeding technique in which a period of in vitro incubation was utilized to increase the number of available autologous endothelial cells for transplantation onto the graft.

The bottom line in this discussion is that the efficacy of endothelial cell seeding in improving prosthetic graft patency has not been resolved. In fact, proving that graft performance is indeed enhanced as a result of endothelial cell seeding is complicated in and of itself. Among investigators there has been minimal consensus related to many technical issues. One such issue has been the definition of the specific tissue source of endothelial cells for transplantation. Our laboratory program of endothelial cell transplantation has focused upon the use of microvascular endothelial cells (MVEC) derived from enzymatic processing of subcutaneous fat. We have been impressed with the relative numbers of endothelial cells that can be derived from fat sources compared with the limited endothelial cell harvests typically available from autologous blood vessels. Because subcutaneous fat from which MVEC can be derived is available in virtually all patients presenting for vascular surgery, we initiated a clinical trial of endothelial cell seeding in patients requiring PTFE grafts for A-V access. The study compared the histological appearances of biopsies derived from MVEC-seeded and nonseeded ePTFE arteriovenous fistulas implanted in patients for blood access for renal dialysis.

Materials and Methods

AV Fistula Study

Following informed consent, 9 patients (3 males and 6 females; mean age 59.8 years) enrolled in the AV fistula study. All of these patients had renal disease requiring long term hemodialysis. In this study patients were randomized to receive either microvessel cell "seeded" ePTFE grafts or "nonseeded" ePTFE grafts as AV fistulas. The purpose of the study was to compare the histological appearances of biopsy samples of each type of graft at scheduled postimplantation times including 1 month, 3 months and 1 year after surgery. The details of the experimental methologies are reported elsewhere.[12] An average of 1.1×10^7 microvessel cells were transplanted onto the seeded grafts. Records of the length of graft implanted were not kept, so it is impossible to estimate the density of the cells which were transplanted onto the graft.

Results

There were no operative complications attendant upon derivation of subcutaneous fat. The patients tolerated all operative procedures well. Harvesting the microvessel cells added one hour to the total operative time for each patient.

A complicating issue in this study was the refusal of patients to comply with the biopsy schedule. One patient agreed to a one month biopsy only. One additional patient agreed to biopsies at one and three months. A third patient presented for biopsies at one month and 16 months. And one patient was biopsied at one month, three months, 20 months and 24 months. Only two patients agreed to one year postimplantation biopsies. Therefore, the data from this study must be interpreted in light of only limited postimplantation biopsy samples.

The seeded grafts from biopsied patients at one month postimplantation revealed few red blood cells and no accumulating thrombus. The intimal lining consisted of areas of single cells in thickness to areas with beginning organization of fibrinous material. factor VIII analysis confirmed that the neointima was lined by endothelial cells.

Interestingly, the neointimas of seeded grafts obtained at subsequent postimplantation periods were thicker than the neointimas at one month. The thickening consisted of concentric intimal fibrous material, which appeared as a mixture of myofibroblasts and fibroblasts with prominent collagen deposition. No significant inflammatory cells were found. These thickened intimas were also lined by factor VIII positive endothelial cells. At 20 months the biopsied seeded graft revealed significant concentric intimal thickening, with the beginning of calcification of the intimal plaque. There were no accumulations of foamy macrophages or cholesterol clefts. The luminal surface was smooth and no thrombi were observed. At 24 months, the biopsy sample from a seeded graft showed significant concentric fibrous plaque formation with a high level of collagenation in the region of the thickening closest to the lumen. Large vessels could be seen within the fibrous thickening (Fig. 10.1).

The nonseeded graft which was biopsied at one month postimplantation revealed a luminal surface with exposed graft material and some adherant red blood cells. No endothelial cells were seen or identified by factor VIII staining on the luminal surface of the nonseeded grafts. At 16 months a biopsied section of a nonseeded graft revealed irregular areas of intimal fibrous thickening; however, there was no inflammatory response or calcification, and the flow-contacting surface of the nonseeded graft remained thin.

Discussion

Ten years of research efforts have investigated the potential efficacy of ECS in enhancing vascular graft performances in in vitro benchtop laboratory models of seeding, animal implants, and preliminary clinical studies. In our opinion, however, the definitive studies have yet to be performed and reported that support or refute ECS as a modality of clinical significance to the vascular surgeon. The research described in this report was intended to accomplish that goal. The research was performed in patients requiring placement of synthetic PTFE grafts for access for hemodialysis. We felt that data derived from the analysis of endothelial cell-seeded grafts in hemodialysis patients would offer insight into the potential efficacy of endothelial cell seeding for other synthetic vascular graft applications as well.

Unfortunately patient compliance with this protocol and the post operative biopsy schedule was minimal, at best, which was disappointing. This was especially disappointing because in the seeded samples that were analyzed the intima was greatly thickened compared to the nonseeded grafts. This would be an important observation if it could be repeated in a relatively large number of patients.

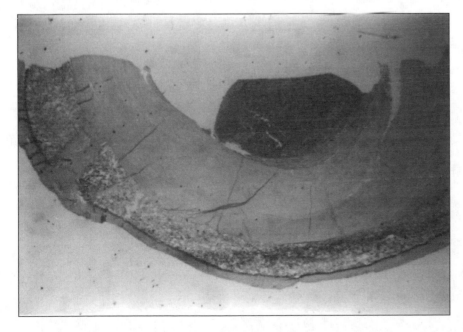

Fig. 10.1. Neointima of microvessel cell-seeded ePTFE graft, biopsy at 24 months postimplantation. See text for description.

It is interesting to speculate on the etiology of the intimal thickening of the seeded grafts analyzed in this study. Certainly the AV fistula is an aberrant hemodynamic environment, in which high wall shear stresses may continually perturb transplanted endothelial cells, resulting in a continual state of activation. If this is in fact the case, then endothelial cell seeding will not enhance graft performance—it will only exacerbate the inevitable failure due to intimal hyperplasia. However, one must caution again that the results described herein are from only a limited number of patients in the unusual hemodynamic environment of the AV fistula, and may not be representative of the fate of seeded grafts implanted elsewhere within the vascular tree.

In summary, we recommend that a well-orchestrated study of endothelial cell seeding in AV fistulas be conducted to clarify this issue, with sufficient numbers of patients such that the impact of endothelial cell seeding on the performance of synthetic AV fistula can be clarified. Transplantation of microvessel-derived endothelial cells resulted in factor VIII positive graft sections, but "graft healing" resulted in thickened neointimas which jeopardized blood flow through the graft.

References

1. Bell D, Rosenthal J. Arteriovenous graft life in chronic hemodialysis. Arch Surg 1988; 123:1169.
2. Bergen J, Veith F, Bernhard V et al. Randomization of autogenous vein and polytetrafluoroethylene grafts in femoro-distal reconstructions. Surg 1982; 92:921.
3. Eguchi H, Okadome K, Mii S et al. Significance of the endothelial lining in prevention of intimal thickening of autogenous vein grafts in dogs. J Surg Res 1991; 50:179.
4. Herring M, Gardner A, Glover J. Seeding human arterial prostheses with mechanically derived endothelium. The detrimental effect of smoking. J Vasc Sur 1984; 1:279-89.
5. Herring M, Baughman S, Glover J. Endothelium develops on seeded human arterial prosthesis: A brief clinical note. J Vasc Surg 1985; 2:727-30.
6. Zilla P, Fasol R, Deutsch M et al. Endothelial seeding of PTFE vascular grafts in humans: A preliminary report. J Vasc Surg 1987; 6:535-41.
7. Ortenwall P, Wadenvik H, Risberg B. Reduced platelet deposition on seeded versus unseeded segments of expanded polytetrafluoroethylene grafts: Clinical observations after a 6-month follow-up. J Vasc Surg 1989; 10:374-380.
8. Ortenwall P, Wadenvik H, Kutti J et al. Endothelial cell seeding reduces thrombogenicity of Dacron grafts in humans. J Vasc Surg 1990; 11:403-410.
9. Kadletz M, Magometschnigg H, Minar E et al. Implantation of in vitro endothelialized polytetrafluoroethylene grafts in human beings. A preliminary report. J Thorac Cardio Surg 1992; 104:736-742.
10. Herring M, Smith J, Dalsing M et al. Endothelial seeding of polytetrafluoroethylene femoral popliteal bypasses: The failure of low-density seeding to improve patency. J Vasc Surg 1994; 20:650-655.
11. Meerbaum S, Sharp W, Schmidt S. Lower extremity revascularization with polytetrafluoroethylene grafts seeded with microvascular endothelial cells. In: Zilla P, Fasol R, Callow A, eds. Applied Cardiovascular Biology 1990-91. Int Soc Appl Cardiovasc Biol. Basel: Karger, 1992; 2:107-119.
12. Schmidt S, Meerbaum S, Anderson J et al. Evaluation of expanded polytetrafluoroethylene arteriovenous access grafts onto which microvessel-derived cells were transplanted to "improve" graft performace: Preliminary results. Ann Vasc Surg 1998; 12:405-411.

Neointimal Hyperplasia in Small Diameter Prosthetic Vascular Grafts: Influence of Endothelial Cell Seeding with Microvascular Omental Cells in a Canine Model

Miralem Pasic, Werner Müller-Glauser, Marko Turina

Introduction

Ideal Vascular Graft

The ideal vascular graft should be biocompatible, resistant to infection, nonthrombogenic, easy to suture, and most important, durable. Unfortunately, none of the existing prosthetic vascular grafts lives up to all of these criteria. Therefore, the early patency of prosthetic grafts depends on a multitude of secondary factors such as the creation of a technically satisfactory anastomosis, the degree of interaction of blood components with the vessel wall, and an adequate distal run-off. Long-term patency is mainly dependent on the progression of proximal and distal arterial disease, and the healing of the anastomosis. The interaction between blood components, mostly platelets and leukocytes, and the vessel wall is particularly complex in areas of injury or at suture lines. Overall, the lack of an endothelial surface is one of the most important variables causing the relatively poor patency of small diameter synthetic bypass grafts when compared to autologous saphenous veins, although other factors such as length, caliber, flow, and kink resistance may also affect the patency of small diameter arterial prostheses.[1]

Intimal Hyperplasia

Intimal hyperplasia is a characteristic fibromuscular cellular response to vascular injury during vascular reconstruction[2,3] and represents—apart from surface thrombogenicity—the second most important reason for prosthetic graft failure. All forms of vascular reconstruction cause both injury and a wound healing response,[4] resulting in different degrees of intimal or neointimal proliferation after reconstruction. Neointimal hyperplasia, particularly pronounced in the area of distal anastomoses, accounts for more than 20% of late failures of infrainguinal prosthetic graft revascularizations.[5-8,13] On gross examination, intimal hyperplasia is a white, firm, fibrous lesion.[9,10] Histologically, it is characterized by cellular proliferation and accumulation of extracellular matrix material, occurring as a result of excessive proliferation and accumulation of smooth muscle cells.[11] The formation of neointimal hyperplasia occurring after implantation of prosthetic vascular grafts is, however, not identical to intimal proliferation after endarterectomy or angioplasty, in that it is primarily due to chronic inflammatory responses associated with implanted synthetic grafts.[12]

Tissue Engineering of Prosthetic Vascular Grafts, edited by Peter Zilla and Howard P. Greisler.
©1999 R.G. Landes Company.

In contrast to occlusions after angioplasty or atherectomy, which tend to appear in the first 6 months,[14,15] the stenosing intimal lesions of autologous or prosthetic grafts usually appear later.[5,13]

Pathogenesis of Anastomotic Hyperplasia

The pathogenesis of anastomotic hyperplasia, which includes the interaction of the various cells and the mitogens and cytokines they produce, and regulation of cellular growth is not fully understood. Cell migration and proliferation during intimal thickening appear to be regulated by factors from the blood, particularly platelets and leukocytes, as well as by interaction with adjacent vascular wall cells.[16] Operative manipulation and hemodynamic factors such as high and low flow velocities, high and low wall shear stress,[17] and mechanical compliance mismatch[18] also influence smooth muscle cell proliferation and intimal thickening. A possible explanation for the smooth muscle cell proliferation beneath the pannus endothelium in prosthetic grafts is the production of smooth muscle cell mitogens by perturbed anastomotic endothelial cells.[19] These endothelial cells are known to produce platelet-derived growth factor (PDGF) and other mitogens.[20,21] Furthermore, endothelial cells are not only actively involved in the regulation of smooth muscle cell migration and proliferation during pathologic changes such as intimal hyperplasia, but also during normal processes such as vessel development, depending on their state of activation. It is unknown whether endothelial cells on implanted prosthetic grafts become permanently activated or if they return to the "normal" inactive state.[19] It is, however, known that a recovered endothelial layer after arterial injury or after endothelial cell lining of a prosthetic graft only decreases or slows the process of intimal proliferation, without preventing it completely.

Endothelial Cells and Neointimal Hyperplasia

Endothelial cells possess both inhibitional and proliferative properties with regard to smooth muscle cell proliferation. On the one hand, the degree of myointimal hyperplasia caused by arterial damage is less in areas which are covered by regenerating endothelium.[22,23] This may be due to synthesis of heparin proteoglycans.[24] Neointimal smooth muscle cells may even become nonproliferative when the overlying endothelial layer is re-established. Therefore, the confluent endothelial cells in a seeded graft may synthesize active substances which inhibit proliferation of smooth muscle cells by releasing inhibitors of smooth muscle cells such as heparan sulfate,[24,26] endothelium-derived relaxing factor (EDRF),[27-30] and prostacyclin.[31,32] Grafts, whether seeded or nonseeded, produce prostacyclin (PGI$_2$) in small amounts,[28,30,33] but seeded grafts have a significantly higher production of prostacyclin than the nonseeded ones; it is, nevertheless, lower than that of the native arteries.[27-30] In an in vitro model of vascular injury, endothelial cell seeding significantly increases both basal and stimulated PGI$_2$ release from damaged vein segments.[34] On the other hand, incomplete late suppression of smooth muscle cell proliferation may cause late intimal and medial thickening at anastomotic areas despite regeneration of a morphologically intact endothelium. One explanatory finding is that PDGF is also produced in endothelialized grafts.[25] For weeks after graft insertion in dogs, PDGF production of ePTFE grafts seeded with autologous venous endothelial cells is even greater than in nonseeded controls; it correlates positively with endothelial cell coverage and inversely with platelet deposition.[25]

Although endothelial cells play an important role in preventing or inhibiting neointimal hyperplasia by releasing inhibitors of smooth muscle cells,[35-37] incomplete endothelialization seen at the anastomotic areas in nonseeded grafts may induce smooth muscle cell proliferation beneath the endothelium[38,39] due to platelet-derived growth factor, and other mitogen production by perturbed endothelial cells.[40-42] In contrast to a vein graft, in a seeded prosthesis there is only a subendothelial layer, without the medial layer. This might be a reason for early suppression of smooth muscle cell proliferation after completion of the endothelial layer, which does not occur in vein bypass. The influence of complete endothelialization of a prosthetic graft on the development of late neointimal hyperplasia is unknown.

The complexity of the pathways leading to formation of neointimal hyperplasia suggests that one agent alone will likely not be entirely effective in its prevention. This multifactorial cause seems to be responsible for failed single medical therapies aiming at the prevention of anastomotic hyperplasia. By achieving a confluent endothelium in a seeded graft, however, one possible factor for neointimal anastomotic hyperplasia—the nonendothelialized luminal surface of the graft—might be excluded, or might be converted into an active factor for prevention of late neointimal hyperplasia.

Experimental Studies with Endothelial Cell Seeding at the University Hospital Zurich

At the University Hospital Zurich we performed several studies whose main aim was to test whether complete endothelial-like cell coverage of a small vascular graft—seeded with omentally derived cells—is capable of reducing or even preventing late neointimal proliferation and anastomotic hyperplasia.[43-46] In one study[44] we performed long-term tests for up to 1 year in 24 mongrel dogs (weight 20-30 kg; age 1-4 years). The dogs were cared for according to the European Convention on Animal Care. All experiments were reviewed and approved by the Ethics Committee of the University Hospital Zurich. Anesthesia was induced with sodium thiopental (20 mg/kg IV); the dogs were intubated and ventilated with an oxygen, nitrous oxide and halothane mixture. Intraoperatively the animals received an infusion of lactated Ringer's solution at the rate of 10 ml/kg per h during the operation.

Surgical Technique

A small supraumbilical laparotomy was made, and as much of the omentum as possible was removed and placed in a sterile 150 ml plate containing 60 ml of HEPES buffered saline. The omentum was further processed in the cell laboratory by the cell-laboratory staff, while the surgical staff closed the abdominal incision and performed exposure of the arteries for the implantation. Starch-free gloves were used throughout the study to avoid the cytotoxic effect of glove powder.[47] A midline neck incision was made and both common carotid arteries were dissected free. A 6 cm segment of each artery was isolated between the vascular bulldog clamps and excised, and then both ends were beveled to approximately 45 degrees. A 4 mm internal diameter uncrimped Dacron graft (Sulzer Brother, Ltd., Winterthur, Switzerland) with an average water porosity of 700 ml/min per cm^2 at 120 mmHg was simultaneously preclotted with autologous blood and seeded. Immediately thereafter they were implanted into the right carotid artery. The oblique end-to-end anastomoses were performed with a continuous 7-0 polypropylene suture. Paired anatomic sites (the common carotid arteries) were used throughout the study; each dog received one seeded (inserted into the right carotid artery) and one nonseeded graft (inserted into the left carotid artery).

Medication

All animals received prophylactic cephalosporine antibiotics (cefalexinum monohydratum, 1200 mg/day) and analgesics (buprenorphine chloride 0.9 mg/day) for 4 days postoperatively, as well as dipyridamole (Dip, 75 mg/day) and acetylsalicylic acid (ASA, 325 mg/day) orally, beginning on 1 and 4 days before surgery, respectively. The antiplatelet medication (ASA) was continued for 4 weeks postoperatively.

Microvascular Endothelial Cell Harvesting

The cell harvesting procedure followed the modified method of Schmidt et al.[48] The omentum (28.8 g ± 7.3 g SD) was rinsed with HBS-2, trimmed, minced with two scalpels into very small pieces, and aspirated into a 10 ml pipette; the tissue was then transferred into a 50 ml Erlenmayer flask containing 1500 U/ml collagenase type II (Sigma Chemical Co., St. Louis, MO, USA). The ratio was 1 g of omental tissue to 2 ml of collagenase. The suspension of omental tissue and collagenase was incubated for 40 minutes in a 37°C shaking water bath at 100 rotations per minute. The digested tissue was homogenized by repetitive pipetting, transferred into 15 ml tube, and centrifuged twice at 100G for 5 minutes. The supernatant contained mainly adipocytes and the collagenase solution. The cell pellet was resuspended in 10 ml PBS, filtered through a 250 micron pore size polyester mesh (Bolting Cloth Weaving, Zurich, Switzerland) to remove nondigested large tissue fragments, and then washed twice with HBS-2. Finally, a suspension of the endothelial cells (2 ml) was added to 15 ml of autologous plasma and centrifuged at 45G for 20 minutes onto the prosthesis using a rotation device (Sulzer Brothers, Ltd., Winterthur, Switzerland). After implantation, the seeded grafts demonstrated clusters of cells adhering to the Dacron fibers on the prosthetic lumen embedded in red thrombus, preventing the wash-out and subsequent loss of the seeded cells.[49] Cell seeding density was 1.75 (0.77 to 2.72, 95% confidence intervals) x 10^6 cells per square centimeter of graft surface, ranging from 0.37 x 10^6 to 4.54 x 10^6 cells.

Cell Identification

An aliquot of approximately 0.5 ml of the cell suspension was removed for quantification of harvested cells. Cell numbers were assessed by fluorometric deoxyribonucleic acid measurements of cell pellets.[50] Cell identification relied on specific perinuclear uptake of acetylated low density lipoprotein,[51] immunohistochemical staining for von Willebrand factor[52] and the determination of cell viability in culture.[53,54] Viability was defined as the number of attached cells counted after 18 h in the cell culture, and was attributed to those cells which resisted rinsing with PBS. After washing, the cell culture was trypsinized and the number of cells was calculated by fluorometric deoxyribonucleic acid measurements on cell pellets.[50] The density of viable cells per cm^2 of a seeded graft was estimated by the ratio of the number of viable cells to the seeded graft surface.

Graft Surveillance and Explantation

Graft patency was assessed by angiography at 1, 5, 12, 26, and 52 weeks after surgery. The angiographic catheter was introduced through the common femoral artery and than forwarded into the common carotid artery. The angiographic examination was performed by manual injection of 10 ml of diluted (1:1 with 0.9% sodium chloride) nonionic angiographic dye (Iopromidum Ultravist 370, Schering, Berlin, Germany).

The prostheses were explanted after 5 weeks (n=6 dogs), 12 weeks (n=6 dogs), 26 weeks (n=6 dogs) and 52 weeks (n=6 dogs). After transfemoral angiography, the grafts were dissected free and then removed with the adjacent 3 cm of proximal and distal carotid artery. Grafts were histologically investigated with light microscopy after staining with hematoxylin-eosin. For scanning electron microscopy, grafts were processed according to the method of Schrotter.[55] Immunohistochemical staining for von Willebrand factor was performed on formalin-fixed paraffin embedded tissue. Sections were predigested for 10 min with 0.1% pronase E (Merck, Dreieich, Germany) at 37°C. After blocking endogenous endoperoxidase with methanol-H$_2$O$_2$, rabbit antiserum against von Willebrand factor (factor VIII-related antigen) was applied. Rabbit antibodies were detected using the ABC/peroxidase method with diaminobenzidine as a substrate of the color reaction.[52] Sections were counterstained with hemalum. (All immunological reagents were from DAKOA/S, Glostrup, Denmark). The maximum thickness of the neointimal tissue within 10 mm of the suture lines, as well as of the central part of the graft, were measured on hematoxylin-eosin stained cross section by means of a computer-assisted automated image analysis system (Video planimeter, Zeiss Inc., Switzerland).

Late neointimal hyperplasia was assumed if a significant difference in neointimal thickness was found when comparing:

1. The mean neointimal thickness of certain parts of the grafts with the mean neointimal thicknesses of the other parts at the same time point (e.g., the mean value of the neointimal thicknesses of all the distal parts of all grafts explanted at three months after

implantation vs. the mean value of the proximal or central parts of the same group of grafts, etc.); or

2. The difference between the mean neointimal thicknesses of the same parts of the grafts at different time points (e.g., the mean value of the neointimal thicknesses of all the distal parts of all grafts explanted at three months after implantation vs. the mean value of the neointimal thicknesses of all the distal parts of all grafts explanted at six months after implantation, etc.).

Statistics

Patency data determined by serial angiographic studies were tabulated and presented in the life table format by the method of Cutler and Ederer.[56] Event-free proportions at 1, 5, 12, 26, and 52 weeks postoperatively are reported with 95% confidence limits. The data are presented as means with 95% nonparametric confidence intervals. Differences in mean values for neointimal thicknesses at different time points and between different locations were assessed by repeated ANOVA measures; simple regression was used to evaluate the development of the neointimal thickness during the time at the same location. A value of $p < 0.05$ was considered to be significant.

Endothelial Cells Reduce Late Neointimal Proliferation

Based on the combination of three highly conclusive parameters (patency rate, angiographic findings, histological examinations), our study strongly supported the hypothesis that complete coverage with endothelial-like cells of the luminal side of a small vascular graft seeded with omentally-derived cells reduces or even prevents late neointimal proliferation and anastomotic hyperplasia.

Improved Patency of Seeded Grafts

The actuarial patency rates at 1, 5, 12, 26, and 52 weeks were 100%, 95%, 95%, 95%, and 95% for seeded grafts, and 100%, 86%, 49%, 40%, and 13% for nonseeded grafts, respectively (Fig. 11.1).

Angiographic Differences of Seeded and Nonseeded Grafts

We found obvious angiographic and histological differences between the seeded and the nonseeded grafts with regard to neointimal hyperplasia, except when the nonseeded grafts were also completely covered with endothelial-like cells. According to the fine structural details of the grafts seen on angiography and later confirmed by histological examination, thrombotic processes and neointimal hyperplasia were confirmed as the two main causes of graft occlusion. Early graft occlusions were obviously caused by thrombotic processes, because these grafts showed smooth anastomotic regions with intraluminal clots on angiography. Contrary to these early findings, progression of late neointimal proliferation, predominantly in the anastomotic regions, was the dominant finding in grafts with late occlusion. The first changes in terms of neointimal hyperplasia were noted by angiographic studies performed at 3 months after graft insertion, with a trend to progression with time. However, this anastomotic stenosis was not observed in the two nonseeded grafts which were totally covered with endothelial-like cells.

Histological Findings

Histological studies of the seeded grafts revealed a neointima with luminal endothelial-like lining and highly organized subendothelial layers in the absence of anastomotic neointimal hyperplasia (Fig. 11.2). The subintimal tissue was covered by a luminal monolayer of coherent epithelial-like, flat cells expressing von Willebrand factor (Fig. 11.3). Microscopic examinations confirmed that neointimal hyperplasia had caused the anastomotic stenosis seen by angiography. Furthermore, histological examinations revealed that the stenotic lesions seen on angiography in the central parts were predominantly caused by a thrombotic process, although it was difficult to distinguish

Fig. 11.1. Actuarial patency rate of seeded and nonseeded grafts. All experimental animals received antiplatelet medication for 4 weeks postoperatively. C.L., Confidence limits.

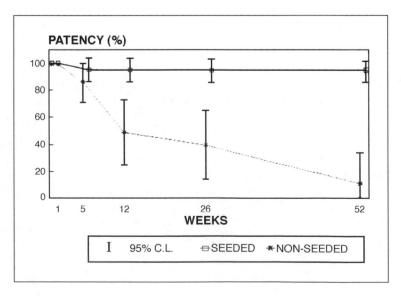

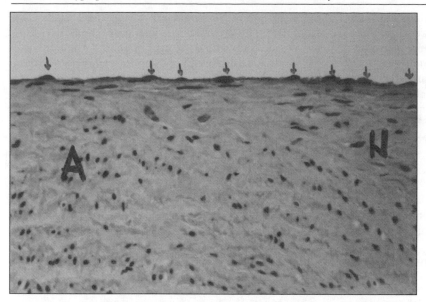

Fig. 11.2. Immunohistochemical staining for von Willebrand factor of the proximal anastomotic region of a seeded Dacron graft explanted at 1 year showing the monolayer nature of the cells covering the graft (arrowheads indicate the black-stained nuclei) (magnification x700). A=the common carotid artery, N=neointima.

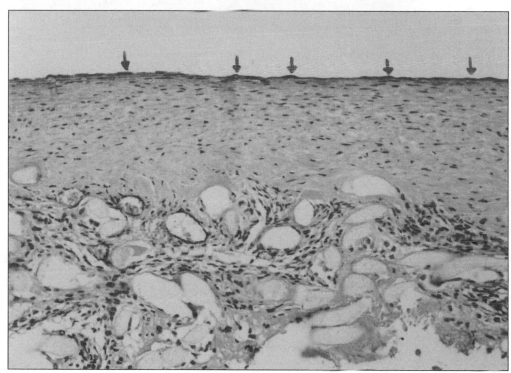

Fig. 11.3. Immunohistochemical staining for von Willebrand factor of the longitudinal sections of the central region of a seeded graft 6 months after implantation (magnification x1000). The highly organized intima is covered by a luminal monolayer of coherent, flat epithelial-like cells (arrowheads indicate the black-stained nuclei) expressing von Willebrand factor (brown reaction product).

hyperplasia from organized thrombus in some specimens of the occluded nonseeded grafts.

Spontaneous Endothelialization

In contrast to the confluent endothelial lining of seeded grafts, the nonseeded grafts showed a varying degree of spontaneous coverage with endothelial-like cells (Fig. 11.4). The extent of this process was time dependent; two patent nonseeded grafts, for instance, were completely covered by endothelial-like cells after one year. However, these grafts did not show any neointimal hyperplasia, and in that resembled seeded grafts. In the other patent nonseeded grafts, scanning electron microscopy revealed

large areas covered with coagulum consisting of fibrin, platelets, and occasional leukocytes interspersed with regions of spontaneous coverage by endothelial-like cells.

Neointimal Tissue Thicknesses

In endothelial seeded grafts, the measurements of the maximum thicknesses of the neointimal tissue at the anastomoses as well as in the central parts of the seeded small diameter Dacron grafts showed neither late neointimal proliferation nor anastomotic hyperplasia. The mean neointimal tissue thickness of the seeded grafts increased during the initial 26 weeks and then stabilized or slightly regressed after this period (Fig. 11.5). Simple regression analysis showed progressive reduction of the mean neointimal thickness (-0.5 mm per week). However, this tissue regression was statistically not significant. There was no difference when comparing any specific part among the different grafts at any time point, nor in comparison with two nonseeded grafts which were totally covered with endothelial-like cells. Repeated ANOVA measures revealed no significant difference among mean neointimal thicknesses of seeded grafts at different time points (p=0.51) or different locations (Greenhouse-Geisser corrected p=0.16).

Graft Occlusion

In summary, both the angiographic studies and histological examinations revealed that neointimal proliferation and anastomotic hyperplasia were the main factors leading to late occlusion of the nonseeded grafts. To obtain fine assessment of our implants, we used conventional angiog-

raphy for routine long-term surveillance, because this type of angiography provided fine anatomical details enabling us to identify structural changes in grafts.[5] Angiograms of the seeded grafts showed a smooth intimal surface without luminal narrowing, whereas angiographic examinations of most nonseeded grafts demonstrated different degrees of luminal stenosis at the anastomotic regions in the late phase of implantation.

Thus, the main factors for occlusion of prosthetic small diameter vascular grafts are increased graft surface thrombogenicity and technical error in the early postoperative course, and progression of the atherosclerotic disease and neointimal hyperplasia in the late phase.[57] In our comparative study, technical errors such as incorrectly performed anastomoses were excluded by postoperative angiography; atherosclerotic process as a possible cause for late occlusion was also excluded by the use of young animals. Therefore,

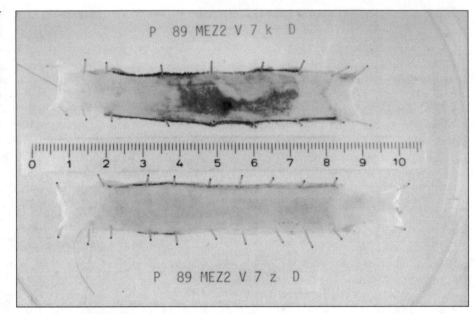

Fig. 11.4. Macroscopic appearance of the luminal surface of a nonseeded graft (upper position) and a seeded graft (lower position) explanted 6 months after surgery. The nonseeded graft exhibits spontaneous endothelialization in the central portion and anastomotic neointimal ingrowth. The seeded graft is thrombus free.

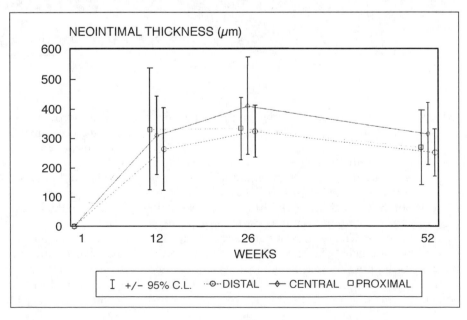

Fig. 11.5. Neointimal tissue thickness of seeded 4 mm I.D. uncrimped Dacron grafts explanted between 5 and 52 weeks after implantation. C.L., Confidence limits.

thrombotic graft occlusion was found to be the main cause of early failure. In all explants, the cause of occlusion was determined after considering the results of all diagnostic methods (angiographic, histological and macroscopic findings), never relying on one single method only. Since grafts were explanted at the dates assigned by preoperative randomization and not immediately after occlusion was noted, it was sometimes difficult to distinguish hyperplasia from organized thrombus in occluded control grafts. Once thrombosis of a graft has occurred, the thrombus rapidly becomes organized and fibrotic, such that it is difficult to distinguish from pre-existing hyperplasia. The technique of quantitative histologic analysis of neointimal hyperplasia used in our study permits accurate measurement only in grafts that are patent, so that progression can be observed. However, the progressive course of hyperplasia can only be compared between different animals. Therefore, we performed the two types of comparisons described above: firstly, simultaneous measurements and comparisons of the different locations at the same time point and secondly, measurement and comparisons of the same locations on different specimens at different times.

The Role of Complete Endothelial Coverage

The second important observation of our study is that complete coverage of the prosthetic surface with endothelial-like cells per se, regardless of by which method this has been achieved, was the single most important factor for prevention of late neointimal hyperplasia and the subsequent improvement of graft patency. This conclusion is further supported by the fact that late neointimal hyperplasia was found in nonseeded grafts which were only partly covered by endothelial-like cells, but not found in the nonseeded grafts which were totally covered with endothelial-like cells through spontaneous outgrowth.

We further conclude that an omental seeding technique may reduce or prevent late neointimal hyperplasia via the mechanism of complete luminal coverage with endothelial-like cells. However, it should be emphasized that the improved overall patency rate of the seeded grafts can only be partly attributed to the reduction or prevention of late neointimal hyperplasia, while other mechanisms such as reduced thrombogenicity due to luminal surface coverage with endothelial-like cells also contribute substantially.

The third important observation of our study is that we found no scanning electron microscopic differences between seeded grafts and the regions of the nonseeded grafts which were covered with endothelial-like cells. Although spontaneous endothelialization of nonseeded grafts is usually seen in animals, the precise origin of luminal endothelial-like cells in both endothelialized seeded and nonseeded grafts remains unclear. The findings of endothelialized anastomotic regions as well as islands of endothelium throughout the grafts indicate that spontaneous endothelialization can occur by several mechanisms, such as migration of endothelial cells from the host artery towards the prosthesis, endothelial cell ingrowth from capillaries originating outside the graft and passing through the interstices of the fabric, or from circulating blood cells.[58] However, coverage with

endothelial-like cells of a synthetic vascular graft following seeding with pure endothelial cells or with a mixture of different cells from omentum is an unknown process, too. It probably requires cell duplication, although it has been shown that endothelial cells remain on the graft surface after cell transplantation.[59] Due to the similarity of the scanning microscopic findings between the seeded grafts and the spontaneously endothelialized regions in nonseeded grafts, it can be speculated that these two different processes probably involve similar mechanisms leading to surface coverage with endothelial-like cells and ultimately to a thrombogenicity of the graft surface.

Intimal and Neointimal Hyperplasia

It should be emphasized that the term "late neointimal hyperplasia" does not refer to the absence of any neointimal tissue on the luminal side of a seeded prosthetic vascular graft. It is a well established fact that seeding with omental cells produces a neointima on these grafts. Therefore, we defined the term "late neointimal hyperplasia" in our study as a significant increase of the neointimal thickness in certain parts of the seeded grafts (proximal, central, distal) as compared with the other parts at the same time point, or the difference between the neointimal thicknesses of the same parts of the grafts at different points in time.

Neointimal hyperplasia in a nonseeded graft is a process of smooth muscle cell proliferation which occurs at both the proximal and distal anastomoses between a prosthetic nonseeded graft and the adjacent artery. However, it occurs to a significantly greater degree at the distal anastomosis than the proximal one.[60] In our study, we found no difference in neointimal thickness between any parts (proximal, distal, or central) of the seeded grafts at any time point. This makes late neointimal hyperplasia an unlikely event in seeded prostheses because one would expect:

1. Changing intimal thickness in predefined graft areas over time; and
2. Differences in intimal thickness within one and the same graft at the same time point, particularly when comparing anastomotic regions with midgraft areas.

The regular angiographic follow-up and microscopic examination revealed that there was a significant difference between the seeded and the nonseeded grafts with reference to neointimal hyperplasia. The fact that no difference between the neointimal thicknesses was found when comparing the two nonseeded grafts which were patent at 1 year (and were *totally* covered with endothelial-like cells) and the seeded grafts does not speak against the hypothesis but rather sheds more light on the impact of complete endothelialization on neointimal proliferation.

Intimal hyperplasia (intimal changes in a venous or arterial graft or native artery) and neointimal hyperplasia (de novo generation of an intima on a synthetic graft surface which was previously lacking an intima) are a characteristic fibromuscular cellular response to vascular injury during vascular reconstruction.[61] It is characterized by cellular proliferation and accumulation of extracellular matrix material which occur as a result of excessive proliferation of smooth muscle cells.[62] All forms of vascular reconstruction cause injury and a wound healing response,[4] leading to intimal or neointimal proliferation after reconstruction with vein or prosthetic grafts[63,64] as well as in a host artery after endarterectomy, atherectomy, or coronary angioplasty.[65-68] However, formation of neointimal hyperplasia occurring after implantation of prosthetic vascular grafts is not identical to intimal proliferation after endarterectomy or angioplasty, largely due to chronic inflammatory responses associated with implanted synthetic grafts. Early after implantation of a prosthetic graft, leukocytes adhere to the graft surface, followed by monocyte infiltration and formation of foreign body giant cells. The latter characterize the chronic inflammatory or foreign body response to vascular prostheses.[69] Neointimal hyperplasia in a synthetic graft had already been recognized in the early phase of peripheral vascular surgery.[8,70] It occurs both in Dacron and polytetrafluoroethylene grafts[71,72] as early as 3 months and as late as 1 year after implantation.[7,8,70] In contrast to occlusions after angioplasty or atherectomy, which tend to appear in the first 6 months,[73] the stenosing intimal lesions of autologous or prosthetic grafts usually appear later after surgery.[5,6] Anastomotic hyperplasia involves both the proximal and distal anastomoses but it has a predilection for the distal anastomosis, with a tendency to progress with time.[72] Neointimal hyperplasia in the area of the distal anastomoses accounts for 20%-50% of late lower extremity bypass graft failures.[6-8]

The regulation of cell migration, proliferation, and growth during intimal thickening appear to be regulated by factors from the blood, particularly platelets and leukocytes, and the interaction of vascular wall cells and grafts themselves.[16] Operative manipulation and hemodynamic factors such as high and low flow velocities, high and low wall shear stress,[17] as well as compliance and diameter mismatch between graft and host artery,[18] also influence smooth muscle cell proliferation and intimal thickening.

It has been proposed that growth factors such as platelet-derived growth factor and basic fibroblast growth factor released from activated platelets, leukocytes, altered smooth muscle cells and endothelial cells may be involved in the smooth muscle cell migration and proliferation after vascular injury.[74,75] Basic fibroblast growth factor is a prototype of the family of heparin-binding growth factors that regulate a variety of cellular responses including cell growth, morphogenesis and differentiation of various cell types, including smooth muscle cells.[76] Fibroblast growth factors deliver their signals to cells by binding to a dual receptor system which activates the bound growth factor before its delivery to the signal-transducer receptors.[77,78] Signaling of growth and differentiation involves multiple pathways.[79] At least two families of receptors bind basic fibroblast growth factor and mediate its response: tyrosine kinase-containing fibroblast growth factor receptors,[77] and heparan sulfate proteoglycans.[80] Both are known to undergo internalization by different pathways.[79] Heparan sulfate proteoglycans are obligate partners in binding of basic fibroblast growth factors to their receptors; fibroblast growth factors do not bind to fibroblast growth factor receptors unless heparan sulfate or its analog, heparin, is present.[81] The activation of intrinsic tyrosine kinase function of receptor tyrosine kinases upon binding of growth factors can trigger cytoplasmic signal transduction pathways.[77] These regulatory mechanisms of specific cell behavior are not well understood. Thus, analysis of biological activity of growth factors on smooth muscle cell growth might be useful for antagonizing pathological smooth muscle cell migration and proliferation.[75,76,82]

The complexity of the pathways leading to formation of neointimal hyperplasia suggests that one agent alone will likely not be entirely effective for its prevention. This multifactorial cause is responsible for failed single medical therapies for preventing anastomotic hyperplasia. Since growth factors are the main stimuli for smooth muscle cell migration and proliferation, several pharmacological approaches to smooth muscle cell hyperplasia might be useful.[83] Different agents, such as anti-inflammatories,[84] antihypertensive drugs,[85,86] fish oil,[87] prostaglandin analogues,[88] α_1-adrenergic blocking agents,[89] and anticoagulants[90] have been shown to suppress the process of intimal hyperplasia in animal studies. The role of anti-platelet therapy in the prevention of intimal hyperplasia after arterial reconstruction remains controversial.[91,92] Human trials have demonstrated that aspirin and dipyridamole significantly improve patency of prosthetic, but not saphenous vein, femoropopliteal bypasses;[93,94] they are particularly beneficial when started before operation[94] or within 24 h of operation.[95] However, clinical trials of anti-platelet agents suggest that platelet inhibition alone does not prevent anastomotic intimal hyperplasia.[96]

The present study showed that establishing an endothelial-like cell coverage on the luminal surface of small diameter prosthetic grafts plays an important role in reduction or prevention of late neointimal and anastomotic hyperplasia. Anastomotic neointimal hyperplasia was suppressed in those grafts that were totally covered with endothelial-like cells, regardless of whether they had been seeded or not. In contrast, occluded control grafts showed clearly visible anastomotic tissue ingrowth in the late phase. Therefore, seeding with omental cells may play an important role in preventing or inhibiting late smooth muscle cell proliferation by total coverage of the prosthetic luminal surface with endothelial-like cells. The characteristic of endothelial cells to possess both inhibitory and proliferative properties on smooth muscle cells may thus play an important role in pathogenesis of neointimal hyperplasia.[97,98] A possible explanation for the smooth muscle cell proliferation beneath endothelium in the nonseeded grafts is the production of smooth muscle cell mitogens by perturbed endothelial cells.[69] By reaching early luminal confluence of endothelial-like cells in a seeded graft, one possible factor for neointimal anastomotic hyperplasia, namely nonendothelialized luminal surface of the graft, might be excluded, or might be converted into an active factor for prevention of late neointimal hyperplasia. Although endothelialized surfaces will not alter all factors potentially contributing to anastomotic intimal hyperplasia, they seem to reduce the deposition and activation of circulating blood elements, including platelets, leukocytes, and components of the coagulation and complement system. They furthermore seem to decrease the release of mitogen factors for smooth muscle cells and prevent thrombus formation by generation of prostacyclin, antithrombotic factors and plasminogen activators.

Omental Microvascular Cells

A large number of cells can be harvested from the omentum. The cells derived from omental suspension comprise a mixture of microvascular endothelial cells and mesothelial cells, with a few other cell types.[48,99] Overall, the contamination of a seeding suspension with nonendothelial cells depends on the harvesting method. A purer endothelial cell yield can be achieved by lowering the separation density during the harvesting procedure, but this leads to a reduced number of all cells available for seeding. Wang et al[100] estimated that 10% or less of the total cell number of harvested omentum cells were nonendothelial in origin. Kern et al[101] obtained a completely pure microvascular endothelial cell population harvested from omental tissue with no growth of other cell types in serially passaged cultures, but the endothelial cell yield was greatly reduced, at only 10^3 endothelial cells per gram of omental tissue.

Origin of the Omental Cells

The identification of the cells derived from omentum poses a problem and there is no consensus in the literature regarding their identity and origin.[102,103] It is sometimes difficult to establish the identity of isolated endothelial cells, especially their distinction from mesothelial cells,[104] because both types of cells are present in omental tissue. Like endothelial cells, mesothelial cells produce prostacyclin[105,106] and possess fibrinolytic activity. These cells produce large amounts of tissue-type plasminogen activator in vitro, together with type 1 and 2 plasminogen activator inhibitor.[107] Moreover, when seeded onto vascular prostheses these cells acquire a confluent monolayer lining with no adherent platelets or amorphous material within one month after surgery.[108,109] In tissue culture, both types of cells show similar growth patterns under light microscopy.[102,104,105] However, it has been shown that in a culture of mixed cells derived from omentum, endothelial cells were rapidly displaced by mesothelial cells, resulting in a pure culture of mesothelial cells.[103] Similarly, in a tissue culture of endothelial cells and fibroblasts, endothelial cells are suppressed by fibroblasts that proliferate to form a confluent layer.[110] In our study, we did not seed the grafts either with omentum cells immediately after harvesting or with cultured cells. In this way, the suppressive effect of mesothelial cells on endothelial cells in culture could be excluded in our study.

Although the origin of the omentally derived cells has remained controversial, its endothelial nature has usually been proven by morphological and functional criteria. The most widely methods used for identification of endothelial cells are the demonstration of von Willebrand factor by immunofluorescence staining,[111] and the uptake of diacetylated low-density lipoprotein.[51] The incorporation of [^{35}S]methionine into von Willebrand factor demonstrates the ability of the cultured microvascular endothelial cells from human omental tissue to synthesize von Willebrand factor,[112] proving the identity of the cultured cells as endothelial. However, it could be speculated that the extensive

immunostaining seen in some of our specimens in the upper layers of the intima could be caused by previous platelet deposition and therefore previous thrombosis, which was supposedly prevented by the seeding with omental cells. The other methods for identification of these cells, and their differentiation from mesothelial cells, are the use of endothelial cell-specific monoclonal antibodies, such as antibody BMA 120,[113] and the characterization of different biological functions typical for these cells.[112] Moreover, endothelial cells express thrombomodulin, a cofactor for activation of protein c, intracellularly; thus they stimulate the activation of protein c by thrombin.[114,115] Furthermore, thrombomodulin has been identified immunologically on endothelial cells of veins, arteries, and capillaries as well as on the endothelium of lymphatics and on syncytiotrophoblasts.[116]

Comparing cells derived from human omental fat tissue with those of human umbilical vein endothelial cells, Visser et al[103] concluded that the cells from omental tissue were not endothelial but mesothelial in nature. Their statement was based on the observations that cells isolated from human omental tissue did not stain with endothelial specific antibodies EN4 and PAL-E; these cells contained abundant cytokeratins 8 and 18, which were absent in endothelial cells.[107] The presence of cytokeratins 8 and 18, as determined with the monoclonal antibodies M20 and M9, was abundant in the cells derived from omentum but not in the human umbilical vein endothelial cells.[103] Vimenten could be detected (monoclonal antibody V9) in both types of cells, whereas desmin (monoclonal antibody D33) was present only in omentally derived cells. A faint and diffuse staining of von Willebrand factor was seen in cells from omentum, whereas microvascular endothelial cells from subcutaneous fat displayed this factor as indistinct granular structures.[107] In contrast to the human umbilical vein endothelial cells, which stained with both anti-von Willebrand factor antibodies, omentally derived cells stained for von Willebrand factor only if the antibodies were polyclonal. Moreover, scanning electron microscopy revealed that cultured cells derived from omentum contain numerous surface microvilli, whereas human umbilical vein endothelial cells did not. All of these findings suggest that the cells derived from omentum were a mixture of predominantly mesothelial cells and a low number of microvascular endothelial cells.[103] In contrast to these findings, Stansby et al[117] were not able to prove that the omental cells were mesothelial in origin. They concluded that human omental microvascular endothelial cells were pericytic in nature.[117] Hernando et al[105] proved the nonendothelial origin of the cells derived from human omentum, demonstrating that these cells showed positivity for monoclonal antibodies specific for endothelial cells (anti-CD34 QBEND10), antibodies to intermediate filaments (anti-vimentin and anti-desmin) and anti-smooth muscle cell antibodies (anti-actin and anti-total actin).

Endothelial cells from different organs show various differences in tissue culture and in vivo; human endothelial cells harvested from saphenous or umbilical vein, for instance, exhibit distinctive features in transmission electron microscopic examination if cultivated on precoated PTFE grafts.[118] Microvascular endothelial cells migrate more slowly than their large vessel counterparts.[119] In contrast, production of prostacyclin,[120] factor VIII, angiotensin-converting enzyme and a heparin-like molecule by microvascular endothelial cells is similar in amount to that produced by large vessel endothelium.[119] Human omental microvascular endothelial cells demonstrate a lower amount of von Willebrand factor than human umbilical vein endothelial cells,[121] with weaker fluorescence in the cytoplasm than large vessel endothelial cells, as determined by immunofluorescence staining of von Willebrand factor.[111] In contrast to endothelial cells from umbilical vein, saphenous vein cells typically show tight junctions at the marginal flaps. Umbilical venous cells regularly present dense condensations of microfibrillar networks at the apical and luminal side, whereas saphenous vein cells show higher amounts of basal vesicles but rarely show basal and luminal condensations of the cytoskeleton.[118] The presence or absence of Weibel-palade bodies in transmission electron microscopy is one of the important morphologic features which distinguishes large vessel from microvascular endothelial cells. Weibel-palade bodies are endothelium-specific cytoplasmatic organelles found in abundance in large vessel endothelium,[122] but they are either absent or present to a lesser extent in microvascular endothelial cells.[101] Transmission electron microscopy of Dacron grafts seeded with omental microvascular cells reveals luminal lining cells with morphologic features of an endothelial phenotype, including numerous pinocytotic vesicles within the cytoplasm on both basal and apical sides, closely interdigitated junctions with adjacent lining cells, large nuclei, and attenuated cytoplasmatic extension, but typically without Weibel-palade bodies.[36] However, macrovascular endothelial cells always exhibit the presence of Weibel-palade bodies.[122]

Limitations of Experimental Studies

Our experimental model, using optimal conditions (high blood flow, short segment of a graft segment, both anastomoses end to end), enabled us to achieve a convincing result regarding the prevention of neointimal hyperplasia by the presence of a confluent endothelium. However, further studies under less optimal conditions (low flow, end to side anastomoses, longer grafts, other locations of implantation, etc.) are needed to fully determine the efficacy of seeding with omental cells on neointimal hyperplasia and the patency of small diameter grafts. Moreover, human trials are needed to determine the exact mechanisms of the endothelialization and to assess the clinical benefit of seeding, because animal data are not directly applicable to the clinical setting. Nevertheless, our present study optimized the procedure and eliminated safety concerns for future clinical studies.

Acknowledgments

The study was supported by the Kommision zur Förderung der wissenschaftlichen Forschung, Bern, Switzerland, Project No. 1576, 1724.1, and 2178.1. and by Sulzer Medical Technology, Ltd., Winterthur, Switzerland.

References

1. Jones DN, Rutherford RB, Ikezawa T, Nishikimi N, Ishibashi H, Whitehill TA. Factors affecting the patency of small-caliber prostheses: Observations in suitable canine model. J Vasc Surg 1991; 14:441-451.
2. Chervu A, Moore WS. An overview of intimal hyperplasia. Surg Gynecol Obstet 1990; 171:433-447.
3. Allaire E, Clowes AW. Endothelial cell injury in cardiovascular surgery: the intimal hyperplastic response. Ann Thorac Surg 1997; 63:582-591.
4. Clowes AW, Clowes MM, Reidy MA. Kinetics of cellular proliferation after arterial injury. III. Endothelial and smooth muscle growth in chronically denuded vessels. Lab Invest 1986; 54:295-303.
5. Idu MM, Truyen E, Buth J. Surveillance of lower extremity vein grafts. Eur J Vasc Surg 1992; 6:456-462.
6. Quiñones-Baldrich WJ, Alfredo AP, Ahn SS, Baker JD, Machleder HI, Moore WS. Long-term results of infrainguinal revascularization with polytetrarfluoroethylene: A ten-year experience. J Vasc Surg 1992; 16:209-217.
7. Echave V, Koornick AR, Haimov M, Jacobson JH II. Intimal hyperplasia as a complication of the use of the polytetrafluoroethylene graft for femoral-popliteal bypass. Surgery. 1979; 86:791-798.
8. Imparato AM, Bracco A, Kim GE, Zeff R. Intimal and neointimal fibrous proliferation causing failure of arterial reconstructions. Surgery 1972; 72:1007-1017.
9. Clagett GP. Morphogenesis and clinicopathologic characteristics of recurrent carotid disease. J Vasc Surg 1986; 3:10-23.
10. Colburn MD, Moore WS, Gelabert HA, Quinones-Baldrich WJ. Dose responsive suppression of myointimal hyperplasia by dexamethasone. J Vasc Surg 1992; 15:510-518.
11. Birinyi LK, Warner SJC, Salomon RN, Calow AD, Libby P. Observations on human smooth muscle cell cultured from hyperplastic lesions of prosthetic bypass grafts: Production of a platelet-derived growth factor-like mitogen and expression of a gene for a platelet-derived growth factor receptor—a preliminary study. J Vasc Surg 1989; 10:157-167.
12. Stanley JC. Discussion. J Vas Surg 1987; 5:118-125.
13. Quiñones-Baldrich WJ, Ziomek S, Henderson T, Moore WS. Patency and intimal hyperplasia: The effect of aspirin on small arterial anastomosis. Ann Vasc Surg 1988; 2:50-56.
14. Block PC, Myler RK, Stertzer S, Fallon JT. Morphology after transluminal angioplasty in human beings. N Engl J Med 1981; 305:382-385.
15. Zarins CK, Gewertz BL, Lyon RT, Rush DS, Glagov S. Arterial disruption and remodelling following ballon dilatation. Surgery 1982; 92:1086-1094.
16. Clowes AW, Reidy MA. Prevention of stenosis after vascular reconstruction: Pharmacologic control of intimal hyperplasia—a review. J Vasc Surg 1991; 13:886-891.
17. Morinaga K, Okadome K, Kuroki M, Miyazaki T, Muto Y, Inokuchi K. Effect of wall shear stress on intimal thickening of arterially transplanted autogenous veins in dogs. J Vasc Surg 1985; 2:430-433.
18. Lyon RT, Runyon-Hass A, Davais HR, Glagov S, Zarins CK. Protection from atherosclerotic lesion formation by reduction of artery wall motion. J Vasc Surg 1987; 5:59-67.
19. Graham LM, Fox PL. Growth factor production following prosthetic graft implantation. J Vasc Surg 1991; 13:742-744.

20. DiCorleto PE, Bowen-Pope DF. Cultured endothelial cells produce a platelet-derived growth factor-like protein. Proc Natl Acad Sci USA 1983; 80:1919-1923.

21. Miossec P, Cavender D, Ziff M. Production of interleukin 1 by human endothelial cells. J Immunol 1986; 136:2486-2491.

22. Bjorkerud S, Bondjers G. Arterial repair and atherosclerosis after mechanical injury. Part 5. Tissue response after induction of a large superfitial transverse injury. Atherosclerosis 1973; 18:235-255.

23. Handenschild CC, Schwartz SM. Endothelial regeneration II. Restoration of endothelial continuity. Lab Invest 1979; 41:407-418.

24. Castellot JJ, Addonizio ML, Rosenberg R, Karnovsky MJ. Cultured endothelial cells produce heparinlike inhibitor of smooth muscle cell growth. J Cell Bil 1981; 90:372-378.

25. Kaufman BR, Fox PL, Graham LM. Platelet-derived growth factor production by canine aortic grafts seeded with endothelial cells. J Vasc Surg 1992; 15:699-707.

26. Fritze LMS, Reilly CF, Rosenberg RD. An antiproliferative heparan sulfate species produced by postconfluent smooth muscle cells. J Cell Biol 1985; 100:1041-1049.

27. Schmidt SP, Hunter TJ, Falkow LJ, Evancho MM, Sharp WV. Effects of antiplatelet agent on PGI_2 production by endothelial-cell-seeded small diameter Dacron® grafts. ASAIOJ 1985; 8:99-103.

28. Boyd KL, Schmidt S, Pippert T, Hite S, Sharp W. The effects of pore size and endothelial cell seeding upon performance of small-diameter ePTFE vascular grafts under controlled flow conditions. J Biomed Mater Res 1988; 22:163-177.

29. Sterpetti AV, Hunter WJ, Schultz RD, Sugimoto JT, Blair EA, Hacker K, Chasan P, Valentine J. Seeding with endothelial cells derived from the microvessels of the omentum and from the jugular vein: A comparative study. J Vasc Surg 1988; 7:677-684.

30. Jensen N, Brunkwall J, Fält K, Lindblat B, Bergquist D. Prostacyclin is produced from endothelial cell-seeded grafts: An experimental study in sheep. Eur J Vasc Surg 1992; 6:499-504.

31. Whitehouse WM Jr, Wakefield TW, Vinter DW, Ford JW, Swanson DP, Thrall JH, Froelich JW, Brown LE, Burkel WE, Graham LM, Stanley JC. Indium-111-oxine labeled platelet imaging of endothelial seeded Dacron thoracoabdominal vascular prostheses in a canine model. Trans Am Soc Artif Intern Organs 1983; 29:183-187.

32. Clagett GP, Burkel WE, Sharefkin JB, Ford JW, Hufnagel H, Vinter DW, Kahn RH, Graham LM, Stanley JC, Ramwell PM. Platelet reactivity in vivo in dogs with arterial prostheses seeded with endothelial cells. Circulation 1984; 69:632-639.

33. Köveker GB, Burkel WE, Graham LM, Wakefield TW, Stanley JC. Endothelial cell seeding of expanded polytetrafluoroethylene vena cava conduits: Effects on luminal production of prostacyclin, platelet adherence, and fibrinogen accumulation. J Vasc Surg 1988; 7:600-605.

34. Thompson MM, Budd JS, Eady SL, Allen KE, James M, James RFL, Bell PRF. Endothelial cell seeding of damaged native vascular surfaces: Prostacyclin production. Eur J Vasc Surg 1992; 6:487-493.

35. Fritze LMS, Reilly CF, Rosenberg RD. An antiproliferative heparan sulfate species produced by postconfluent smooth muscle cells. J Cell Biol 1985; 100:1041-1049.

36. Castellot JJ, Addonizio ML, Rosenberg R, Karnovsky MJ. Cultured endothelial cells produce heparinlike inhibitor

37. Jensen N, Brunkwall J, Fält K, Lindblat B, Bergquist D. Prostacyclin is produced from endothelial cell-seeded grafts: An experimental study in sheep. Eur J Vasc Surg 1992; 6:499-504.

38. Angelini GD, Christie MI, Bryan AJ, Lewis MJ. Surgical preparation impairs release of endothelium derived relaxing factor from human saphenous vein. Ann Thorac Surg 1989; 48:417-420.

39. Graham LM, Fox PL. Growth factor production following prosthetic graft implantation. J Vasc Surg 1991; 13:742-744.

40. Miossec P, Cavender D, Ziff M. Production of interleukin 1 by human endothelial cells. J Immunol 1986; 136:2486-2491.

41. DiCorleto PE, Bowen-Pope DF. Cultured endothelial cells produce a platelet-derived growth factor-like protein. Proc Natl Acad Sci USA 1983; 80:1919-1923.

42. Kaufman BR, Fox PL, Graham LM. Platelet-derived growth factor production by canine aortic grafts seeded with endothelial cells. J Vasc Surg 1992; 15:699-707.

43. Pasic M, W. Müller-Glauser, Lachat M, Bittmann P, von Segesser L, Turina M. Langzeitresultate in der Hunderkarotis mit kleinlumigen Gefässprothesen mit mikrovaskulären Endothelzellen. Helv chir Acta 1993; 60:381-385.

44. Pasic M, Müller-Glauser W, Odermatt B, Lachat M, Seifert B, Turina M. Superior late patency of small-diameter Dacron grafts seeding with omental cells prevents late neointimal hyperplasia in small-diameter dacron grafts. Circulation 1995; 92:2605-2616.

45. Pasic M, Müller-Glauser W, von Segesser L, Odermatt B, Lachat M, Turina M. Endothelial cell seeding improves patency of synthetic vascular grafts: Manual versus automatized method. Eur J Cardio-thorac Surg 1996; 10:372-379.

46. Pasic M, Müller-Glauser W, von Segesser L, Lachat M, Mihaljevic T, Turina M. Superior late patency of small-diameter Dacron grafts seeded with omental microvascular cells: An experimental study. Ann Thorac Surg 1994; 58:677-684.

47. Sharefkin JB, Fairchild KD, Albus RA, Cruess DF, Rich NM. The cytotoxic effect of surgical glove powder particles on adult human vascular endothelial cell cultures: implications for clinical uses of tissue culture techniques. J Surg Res 1986; 41:463-472.

48. Schmidt SP, Monajjem N, Evancho MM, Pippert TR, Sharp WV. Microvascular endothelial cell seeding of small-diameter Dacron vascular grafts. J Invest Surg 1988; 1:35-44.

49. Pasic M. Endothelial-cell seeding with microvascular omental cells onto small-diameter prosthetic vascular grafts in a canine model. Habilitation. Zurich, Switzerland: The University of Zurich; 1994:79-82.

50. Anderson JS, Price TM, Hanson SR, Harker LA. In vitro endothelialization of small-caliber vascular grafts. Surgery 1987; 101:577-586.

51. Vojta JC, Via DP, Butterfield CE, Zetter BR. Identification and isolation of endothelial cells based on their increased uptake of acetylated-low density lipoprotein. J Cell Biol 1984; 99:2034-2040.

52. Hsu SU, Raine L, Fanger H. Use of avidin-biotin-peroxidase complex (ABC) in immunoperoxidase techniques: A

comparison between ABC and unlabeled antibody (PAP) procedures. J Histochem Cytochem 1981; 29:577-580.

53. Müller-Glauser W, Bay U, Lehmann KH, Turina M. An improved procedure for enzymatic harvesting of highly purified canine venous endothelial cells for experimental small diameter vascular prostheses. Ann Vasc Surg 1989; 3:134-139.

54. Zilla P, Siedler S, Fasol R, Sharefkin JB. Reduced reproductive capacity of freshly harvested endothelial cells in smokers: A possible shortcoming in the success of seeding. J Vasc Surg 1989; 10:143-148.

55. Schrötter D, Spiess E, Paweletz N, Benker R. A procedure for rupture free preparation of confluently grown monolayer cells for scanning electron microscopy. J Electr Microsc Techn 1984; 1:219-225.

56. Cutler SJ, Ederer F. Minimum utilization of the life table method in analyzing survival. J Chron Dis 1958; 8:699-712.

57. Rutherford RM, Nishikimi N. "Graft Thrombosis and Thormboembolic complications", 501-510, in Rutherford RB, ed., Vascular Surgery, third edition, WB Saunders Company 1989, Philadelphia.

58. Scott SM, Barth MG, Gaddy LR, Ahl Jr ET. The role of circulating cells in the healing of vascular prostheses. J Vasc Surg 1994; 19:585-593.

59. Williams SK, Kleinert LB, Rose D, McKenney S. Origin of endothelial cells that line expanded polytetrafluoroethylene vascular grafts sodded with cells from microvascularized fat. J Vasc Surg 1994; 19:594-604.

60. Cantelmo NL, Quist WC, Lo Gerfo FW, Quantitative analysis of anastomotic intimal hyperplasia in paired Dacron and PTFE grafts. J Cardiovasc Surg 1989; 30:910-915.

61. Chervu A, Moore WS. An overview of intimal hyperplasia. Surg Gynecol Obstet 1990; 171:433-447.

62. Angelini GD, Bryan AJ, Williams HMJ, Soyombo AA, Williams A, Tovey J, Newby AC. Time-course of medial and intimal thickening in pig venous arterial grafts: Relationship to endothelial injury and cholesterol accumulation. J Thorac Cardiovasc Surg 1992; 103:1093-1103.

63. Imparato AM, Bracco A, Geun EK, Zeff R. Intimal and neointimal fibrous proliferation causing failure of arterial reconstruction. Surgery 1972; 72:1007-1017.

64. Ip JH, Fuster V, Badimon L, Badimon J, Taubman MB, Chesebro JH. Syndromes of accelerated atherosclerosis: Role of vascular injury and smooth muscle cell proliferation. J Am Coll Cardiol 1990; 15:1667-1687.

65. Clagett GP. Morphogenesis and clinicopathologic characteristics of recurrent carotid disease. J Vasc Surg 1986; 3:10-23.

66. Healy DA, Zierler RE, Nicholls SC et al. Long-term follow-up and clinical outcome of carotid restenosis. J Vasc Surg 1989; 10:662-669.

67. Vroegindeweij D, Kemper FJ, Tielbeek AV, Buth J, Landman G. Recurrence of stenoses following balloon angioplasty and Simpson atherectomy of the femoro-popliteal segment. A randomised comparative 1-year follow-up study using colour flow duplex. Eur J Vasc Surg 1992; 6:164-171.

68. Kuntz RE, Safian RD, Levine MJ, Reis GJ, Diver DJ, Baim DS. Novel appproach to the analysis of restenosis after the use of three new coronary devices. J Am Coll Cardiol 1992; 19:1493-1499.

69. Graham LM, Brothers TE, Vincent CK, Burkel WE, Stanley JC. The role of an endothelial cell lining in limiting distal anastomotic intimal hyperplasia of 4-mm-I.D. Dacron grafts in a canine model. J Biomed Mater Res 1991; 25:525-533.

70. Szilagyi DE, Smith RF, Elliott JP, Allen HM. Long-term behavior of a dacron arterial substitute: Clinical, roentgenologic and histologic correlations. Ann Surg 1965; 162:453-477.

71. Selman SH, Rhodes RS, Anderson JM, DePalma RG, Clowes AW. Atheromatous changes in expanded polytetrafluoroethylene grafts. Surgery 1980; 87:630-637.

72. Lo Gerfo FW, Quist WC, Nowak MD, Crawshaw HM, Haudenschild CC. Downstream anastomotic hyperplasia. A mechanism of failure in dacron arterial grafts. Ann Surg 1983; 197:479-483.

73. Block PC, Myler RK, Stertzer S, Fallon JT. Morphology after transluminal angioplasty in human beings. N Engl J Med 1981; 305:382-385.

74. Ferns GAA, Raines EW, Sprugel KH, Motani AY, Reidy MA, Ross R. Inhibition of neointimal smooth muscle cell accumulation after angioplasty by an antibody to PDGF. Science 1991; 253:1129-1132.

75. Olson NE, Chao S, Lindner V, Reidy M. Intimal smooth muscle cell proliferation after balloon catheter injury. The role of basic fibroblast growth factor. Am J Path 1992; 140:1017-1023.

76. Burgess WH, Maciag T. The heparin-binding (fibroblast) growth factor family of proteins. Annu Rev Biochem 1989; 58:576-606.

77. Ullrich A, Schlessinger J. Signal tranduction by receptors with tyrosine kinase activity. Cell 1990; 61:203-212.

78. Turnbull JE, Gallagher JT. Heparan sulfate: Functional role as a modulator of fibroblast growth factor activity. Biochem Soc Trans 1993; 21:477-482.

79. Reiland J, Rapraeger AC. Heparan sulphate proteoglycan and FGF receptor target basic FGF to different intracellular destination. J Cell Sci 1993; 105:1085-1093.

80. David G. Integral membrane heparan sulfate proteoglcans. FASEB J 1993; 7:1023-1030.

81. Kan M, Wang F, Xu J, Crabb WC, Hou J, McKeehen WL. An essential heparin-binding domain in the fibroblast growth factor receptor kinase. Science 1993; 259:1918-1921.

82. Lindner V, Reidy MA. Proliferation of smooth muscle cells after vascular injury is inhibited by an antibody against fibroblast growth factor. Proc Natl Acad Sci USA 1991; 88:3739-3743.

83. Schoen FJ, Castellot JJ Jr. Vascular graft intimal fibrous hyperplasia: Prospects for pharmacological inhibition. J Vasc Surg 1991; 13:758-761.

84. Chervu A, Moore WS, Quinones-Baldrich WJ, Henderson T. Efficacy of corticosteriods in suppression of intimal hyperplasia. J Vasc Surg 1989; 10:129-134.

85. O'Malley MK, McDermott EW, Mehigan D, O'Higgins NJ. Role for prazosin in reducing the development of rabbit intimal hyperplasia after endothelial denudation. Br J Surg 1989; 76:936-938.

86. El-Sanadiki MN, Cross KS, Murray JJ, Schuman RW, Mikat E, McCann RL, Hagen P-O. Reduction of intimal hyperplasia and enhanced reactivity of experimantal vein bypass grafts with verapamil. Ann Surg 1990; 212:87-96.

87. Fanelli C, Arnoff R. Restenosis following coronary angioplasty. Am Heart J 1990; 119:357-368.

88. Kouchi Y, Esato K, O-Hara M, Zempo N. Effect of prostaglandin I$_2$ analogue TRK-100 on the suppression of intimal fibrous proliferation. J Vasc Surg 1992; 16:232-238.

———————————— CHAPTER 12 ————————————

Human Clinical Trials of Microvascular Endothelial Cell Sodding

Stuart K. Williams

History of EC Transplantation

While advances in clinical vascular surgery have resulted in significant progress in the treatment of vascular diseases, a significant frustration has been the inability to sustain the patency of small diameter (< 6 mm) synthetic vascular grafts. A specific example of the poor performance of small diameter synthetic grafts is in peripheral bypass procedures. When compared to saphenous vein autologous grafts, synthetic grafts constructed of either ePTFE or Dacron exhibit clinically poor outcomes. The clinical experience with synthetic grafts for coronary artery bypass grafting is even more disappointing, with only rare examples of successful use of synthetic grafts for coronary revascularization.

The importance of a stable endothelial cell lining on natural blood vessels toward maintenance of an anti-thrombogenic, metabolically active surface, and as a barrier controlling the selective transport of cellular and plasma protein constituents of blood, has been well established.[1,2] The importance of establishing an endothelial cell lining on synthetic grafts has also been recognized by numerous research laboratories.[3,4] Numerous techniques have been proposed toward the accelerated formation of an endothelial cell lining on synthetic grafts. These techniques generally fall into the two categories of either accelerated spontaneous endothelialization or accelerated endothelialization through cell transplantation. Spontaneous endothelialization has been explored through several mechanisms, including accelerated pannus ingrowth and stimulated migration of vascular elements directly though the wall of the graft.[5] The efficiency of spontaneous endothelialization is highly variable, with significant species to species variation. More extensive work has been performed evaluating the use of endothelial cell transplantation toward accelerated endothelialization of synthetic vascular grafts.[6]

Numerous variables have been explored during the development of techniques for endothelial cell transplantation, including source of endothelial cells for transplantation, the need to culture cells prior to transplantation, methods for cell deposition and graft surface modifications to improve cell-polymer interactions. Each of these variables has been shown to be critical to the development of operating room compatible methods for endothelial cell transplantation. Prior to the initiation of human clinical trials, endothelial cell transplantation methods were evaluated in several preclinical animal models where both the safety of the methods was established and, finally, the effects of endothelial cell transplantation on graft patency were confirmed. This latter point has been critical to support the hypothesis that the accelerated formation of an endothelial cell monolayer on synthetic vascular grafts following endothelial cell transplantation will improve graft patency.

Tissue Engineering of Prosthetic Vascular Grafts, edited by Peter Zilla and Howard P. Greisler.
©1999 R.G. Landes Company.

Following extensive evaluation of different variables for endothelial cell transplantation, our laboratory established methods for the use of autologous endothelial cell transplantation using adipose tissue-derived microvascular endothelial cells. Preclinical animal studies established that endothelial cells could be isolated from fat and transplanted rapidly onto the lumenal surface of synthetic grafts (both ePTFE and Dacron), and that this form of graft treatment resulted in a statistically significant improvement in graft patency. The development of these methods was not without controversy. Several investigators questioned whether adipose tissue even contained endothelium, suggesting the cells isolated from fat were mesothelium and not endothelium.[7] Extensive evaluation of the cellular components isolated from adipose tissue following its dissociation using collagenase established the major contribution of endothelium to the total cellular makeup of adipose tissue.[8] But more important was the fact that microvascular endothelium could be rapidly transplanted onto synthetic vascular grafts, resulting in the accelerated formation of an endothelial cell monolayer and improved patency in the grafts once implanted. A complete discussion of the results of endothelial cell transplantation studies in preclinical animal models is discussed in an accompanying chapter.

Human Trial of Microvascular Endothelial Cell Transplantation

Based on the success of preclinical animal studies, an evaluation of endothelial cell transplantation in patients requiring peripheral bypass grafts was planned. We used the term sodding to describe our method of endothelial cell transplantation, since it involved the placement of large numbers of endothelial cells directly onto the lumenal surface of synthetic grafts. Several variables were considered and evaluated prior to establishment of the final human sodding trial protocol.

Trial Variables

Source of Endothelial Cells

During previous studies we evaluated methods for isolating endothelial cells from both large vessel (vein) and microvascular sources (fat). Several sources of fat were considered, including omental-associated fat, perirenal fat and abdominal wall fat, as well as methods to remove the fat, including direct surgical excision and liposuction removal. Following extensive evaluation we identified liposuction-derived fat from the abdominal wall as having the most optimal cellular characteristics for subsequent sodding. While these cells could be subsequently cultured, we determined the cell yield from patients was more than sufficient ($>1 \times 10^6$ cells/g fat) to produce enough cells for our sodding methods.

Graft Type and Pretreatment

Clinically used ePTFE vascular grafts with nominal 30 micron internodal distance were used for all implants. To improve cell deposition all grafts were prewet with a solution containing 1 part serum (autologous) and 6 parts tissue culture medium type 199E. This solution was pushed through the interstices of the graft using a pressure gradient equal to 5 psi. Grafts were prewet for at least 30 minutes.

Cell Deposition

A suspension of endothelial cells was prepared in medium 199E at a density to provide 2×10^5 cells/cm^2 graft lumenal surface area. The solution was placed into the graft and a pressure gradient created across the wall of the graft of 5 psi, resulting in the flow of fluid through the graft and concomitant deposition of endothelial cells. We term this process pressure sodding of cells.

Time to Graft Implantation

Immediately after pressure sodding the grafts were brought to the operating field and implanted.

As part of this clinical evaluation of endothelial cell transplantation using autologous microvessel endothelial cells, a specialized endothelial cell isolation and cell deposition kit was developed. This kit and its use is diagrammed in Figure 12.1. The performance of this kit was modeled after the endothelial cell sodding procedure first developed and used during preclinical animal trails and subsequently used during human trials (Fig. 12.2).

Patients and Methods

The protocol for this study received approval from the Human Subjects Committee/Institutional Review Board of Thomas Jefferson University, Philadelphia, PA and the University of Arizona Health Sciences Center, Tucson AZ. Patients in need of a peripheral bypass graft were eligible for inclusion in the study based on the inclusion/exclusion criteria outlined in Table 12.1. Just prior to surgery all patients were phlebotomized of 150 cc of blood to obtain serum for sodding the prosthesis.

The abdomen and the site of graft placement was prepped and draped. To obtain adipose tissue for microvessel endothelial cell isolation, liposuction of subcutaneous fat

---

Table 12.1. Microvascular endothelial cell sodding trial: inclusion and exclusion criteria

Inclusion Criteria:

Patients with atherosclerotic peripheral vascular disease resulting in tissue loss. Patients with claudication alone are not included in study.
>18 years of age
Adequate fat for liposuction
No acceptable vein
Life expectancy >1 year
Informed consent

Exclusion Criteria:

Serious heart or pulmonary disease
Serious coagulopathy
Uncontrolled hypertension
Detection of positive serology for viral infection

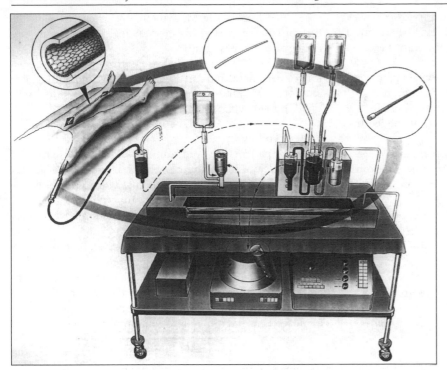

Fig. 12.1. Endothelial cell isolation and transplantation kit design.

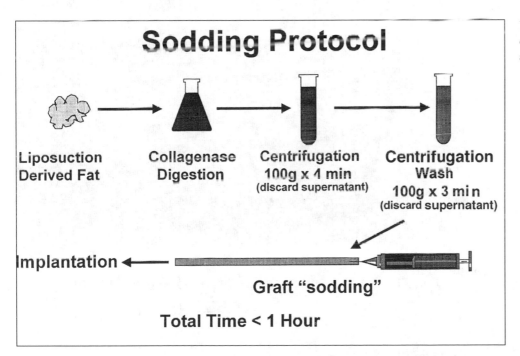

Fig. 12.2. Process of endothelial cell isolation and transplantation.

from the abdominal wall was performed with a liposuction cannula and specially designed 60 cc syringe. Approximately 50 g of fat was removed from each patient and processed for MVEC isolation. The completely assembled kit, being used during a human endothelial cell sodding procedure, is shown in Figure 12.3. The isolation procedure as outlined above resulted in ePTFE grafts with approximately 2×10^5 cells/cm^2 graft lumenal surface area. Grafts were immediately implanted in patients.

Overview of Patients

All patients were referred to participating vascular surgeons for amputation.

Pt. 01. 52 yr old M, diabetic, coronary artery and renal artery disease, rest pain, severe left lower ischemia, history of failed bypass graft in leg to receive sodded graft. Received ileo-peroneal sodded bypass graft.

Pt. 02. 82 yr old M, history of failed bypass grafts in study leg. Rest pain. Received ileo-peroneal sodded bypass graft.

Pt. 03. 71 yr old F, diabetic with history of coronary artery and peripheral vascular disease. Previously received several bypass grafts including in situ vein graft. Received femoral-tibial sodded bypass graft.

Pt. 04 69 yr old F, history of failed bypass grafts and angioplasty. Received ileo-tibial sodded bypass graft.

Pt. 05. 75 yr old F, diabetic with hypertension. History of failed bypass grafts. Received femoral-tibial sodded bypass graft.

Pt. 06. 74 yr old M. History of cardiovascular disease including CABG, peripheral vascular, renal artery procedures. Presented with intermittent claudication. Received femoral-popliteal sodded bypass graft.

Pt. 07. 72 yr old F, diabetic with hypertension. History of failed bypass grafts including previous posterior tibial in situ bypass graft in study leg which failed after 7 months. Received femoral-posterior tibial sodded bypass graft.

Pt. 08. 74 yr old M, history of peripheral and cardiac disease. Received ilio-peroneal sodded bypass graft.

Pt. 09. 75 yr old M, received ilio-tibioperoneal sodded bypass graft.

Pt. 10. 83 yr old M, diabetic, hypertensive with history of failed bypass grafts in study leg. Received femoral-tibial sodded bypass graft.

Pt. 11. 57 yr old M diabetic with hypertension. History of peripheral and cardiac bypass grafts including failed autologous peripheral graft in study leg. Received femoral-tibial sodded bypass graft.

Patient Follow Up

All patients received routine follow up evaluation of graft function, including color flow Doppler and duplex imaging. Of the original 11 patients, seven were available for follow up at four years while four expired prior to this time due to nongraft related causes. The cumulative patency of the study grafts is illustrated in Figure 12.4. As expected of the patient population in this trial, several patients have experienced other vascular complications including cardiac arrhythmias, myocardial infarctions, nonstudy leg peripheral vascular disease progression, renal disease and pulmonary embolism. Several patients have also undergone treatment for cancer. Follow up evaluation of patients did not

Fig. 12.3. Assembled endothelial cell isolation and sodding device in use in the operating room.

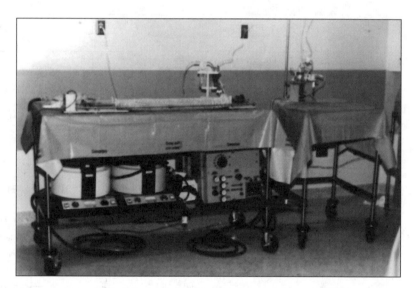

Fig. 12.4. Cumulative patency of microvascular endothelial cell sodded grafts in human peripheral vascular graft trial.

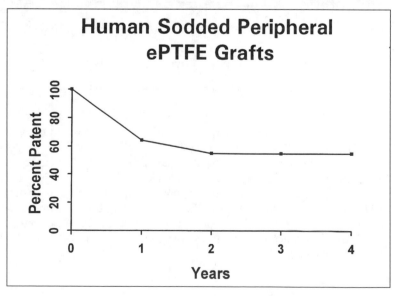

provide information predictive of subsequent graft failure. One patient exhibited a mid-graft concentric intimal thickening just below the knee approximately 9 months after graft implantation. This thickening had disappeared at subsequent graft follow-up.

Conclusions

This trial was designed as an initial safety study to evaluate the ability to isolate endothelial cells from liposuction fat and transplant these cells onto ePTFE grafts. The initial four year follow up data is quite encouraging and suggests endothelial cell transplantation can be performed using an automated kit. The patient population selected for this trial represents individuals with significant vascular disease. The lack of significant limb loss in this patient population during the first three years follow up is equally encouraging. We conclude that an expanded trial of endothelial cell transplantation using autologous endothelial cells derived from liposuction derived fat is warranted.

References

1. Quist WC, Haudenshield CC, Logerfo FW. Qualitative microscopy of implanted vein grafts: Effects of graft integrity on morphological fate. J Thorac Cardiovasc Surg 1992; 103:671-677.

2. Richardson JV, Wright CB, Hiratzka LF. The role of endothelium in the patency of small venous substitutes. J Surg Res 1980; 28:556-562.

3. Zilla P, Preiss P, Groscurth P, Rosemeier F, Deutsch M, Odell J, Heidinger C, Fasol R, von Oppel U. In vitro-lined endothelium: Initial integrity and ultrastructural events. Surg 1994; 116(3):524-534.

4. Zilla P, Deutsch M, Meinhart J, Puschmann R, Eberl T, Minar E, Dudczak R, Lugmaier H, Schmidt P, Noszian I. Clinical in vitro endothelialization of femoropopliteal bypass grafts: An actuarial follow-up over three years. J Vasc Surg 1994; 19(3):540-548.

5. Clowes AW. Graft endothelialization: The role of angiogenic mechanisms. J Vasc Surg. 1991; 13:734-736.

6. Williams SK. Endothelial cell transplantation. Cell Trans 1995; 4:401-410.

7. Visser MJP, van Bockel JJ, van Muijen GNP, van Hinsbergh VWM. Cells derived fromomental fat tissue and used for seeding vascular prostheses are not endothelial in origin: A study on the origin of epitheloid cells derived from human omentum. J Vasc Surg 1991; 13:373-381.

8. Williams SK, Wang TF, Castrillo R, Jarrell BE. Liposuction derived human fat used for vascular graft sodding contains endothelial cells and notmesothelial cells as the major cell type. J Vasc Surg 1994; 19:916-923.

Macrovascular Endothelial Cell Transplantation

──────────────── CHAPTER 13 ────────────────

In Vitro Endothelialization: Its Contribution Towards an Ideal Vascular Replacement

Peter Zilla

Every era in medicine has been driven by one particular discipline which recognized an exciting new development occurring outside its own sphere as an opportunity for a quantum leap. Although this initial phase of integrating an unfamiliar dimension into a traditional medical dominion was seldom blessed with clinical success, retrospectively this era is always perceived as the grand epoch of the particular discipline. For instance, the integration of technical achievements into a discipline like surgery, previously considered to be more a skillful art than anything else, made cardiac surgery possible. Those pioneering cardiac surgeons who dared to let a mechanical pump take over the heart's function, thus allowing procedures on the open heart, were initially viewed with suspicion by their peers. Typically, it was not a single technical aspect which was absorbed into this young discipline but rather a basic openness towards the integration of mechanical and electrical contraptions into the circulatory system, a part of the body which was considered to be untouchable since the days of Theodor Billroth. It seems also typical that the enthusiasm of such a pioneering phase eventually draws the newly discovered, unrelated support discipline further into its sphere of influence. It was not a coincidence that Earl Bakken developed the first pacemaker in Minneapolis in the wake of the emerging new discipline of cardiac surgery, which was plagued by postoperative rhythm problems in this early phase. Retrospectively, the quantum leap which this pinnacle of cardiac surgery initiated for other medical professions remains unchallenged.

In vascular surgery, the late 1970s and early 1980s may well, retrospectively, turn out to have been a similarly fateful period for medicine. However, in contrast to cardiac surgery twenty years before, it was not the world of sophisticated mechanical devices and electronics which were integrated into medicine but the amazing world of biology. Symptomatically, naive amateurism and polarization characterize the early days of this era. Amateurism, because the first to test the water were surgeons and not biologists. This is the trademark of all developments of this kind in medicine: Brave and alert medical doctors initially apply discoveries from an alien field to medicine themselves. On the one hand, this effervescent breed with their urge for knowledge has all the ingredients to overcome initial thresholds and obstacles. On the other hand, it is often a surgical discipline within the medical profession, with its desire for clear cut and simple solutions, which drives such initiatives. As a consequence, this surgical mentality may endanger its own achievements when necessary complexity falls victim to impatience. In the case of the awaking biological awareness of the late 1970s, it was indeed surgeons again who were behind it. Almost predictably, they caused their own setback as they had in previous years with heart transplantation by not handing the newborn over to scientists in time. In the case of heart transplantation, immune and

Tissue Engineering of Prosthetic Vascular Grafts, edited by Peter Zilla and Howard P. Greisler.
©1999 R.G. Landes Company.

drug research rather than the fury of an ongoing surgical push could have saved 10 years. The eventual breakthrough of the cyclosporin era fought an uphill battle against the prejudices arising from the surgical desire for a quick fix during the preceding 13 years. In the case of the incorporation of biology into prosthetic vascular surgery, it was the endless striving of surgeons to succeed with a simple and instantly applicable, single-staged procedure right from the beginning which almost meant the death knell for the entire idea 10 years later. A further tragedy which repeats itself in the early phases of "quantum leap" eras lies in the typical negative feedback amongst the alien partners which soon follows the initial enthusiasm. Surgeons often feel intimidated by the thought of scientific complexity and scientists shy away from the "gung-ho" approach of surgeons. As contradictory as it may sound, in the end it is often the perseverance of a few dedicated surgeons who continue their mission regardless, accepting a higher level of complexity. This perseverance allows an idea to survive long enough for its final breakthrough. In heart transplantation, Norman Shumway fulfilled this role. In the attempt to incorporate biological principles into prosthetic vascular surgery, in vitro endothelialization may, in retrospect, have played a similar role. If the next decade of research succeeds with tissue engineering of physiologically functional vascular prostheses, the credit for opening a new era in medicine will undoubtedly be deserved by the early pioneers of single staged endothelial cell seeding. However, the role which Norman Shumway played in heart transplantation—to prevent the flickering flame from being extinguished—may well be granted to those who continuously propagated the complex but eventually successful variant of in vitro endothelialization, to clinically prove the benefit of a principle and thus provide sufficient incentive for today's efforts towards a broadly acceptable breakthrough.

Historical Perspective

If the amateurism of the pioneering years of endothelial seeding, with its lack of involvement of basic scientists, contributed to a delay of today's drive towards an integrated approach to cardiovascular tissue engineering, one can at least explain this shortcoming by the fundamental difference between the worlds of surgeons and biologists. This does not apply to the polarization which plagued all of us who were involved in efforts to "biolize" prosthetic grafts from within our own discipline. This polarization was twofold: On the one hand, each different approach to endothelial seeding was almost religiously upheld by the respective groups which stood for it. On the other hand, a fiercely fought confrontation of principal values led to a schism which continues to divide the surgical community today. Both polarizations may be explained in terms of the previous quantum leap era, under whose spell the majority of cardiovascular surgeons still stood. One aspect of the preceding grand era of cardiovascular pioneering was that it created heroes as never before. Each facet of the overall quantum leap was associated with a big name, whether it was Lillihei, Kirklin, De Bakey, Barnard or Cooley. Even if not

openly admitted, each champion of a particular approach towards graft endothelialization therefore hoped for comparable fame. Another aspect of those days in the 1960s was that their pioneers demonstrated that almost everything which previously seemed unresolvable became feasible through the application of new materials and mechanically determined technologies. Naturally, the emergence of a new dimension like biology caused friction. As a result, at all conferences in the 1980s, the believers in existing technologies asked angrily after each talk on endothelial seeding whether the speakers were aware that graft patencies depended primarily on surgical skills. Therefore, they recommended that the presenter spend his time improving those skills rather than wasting it in the laboratory. The fact that this latter group of surgeons still represents the majority within our ranks proves how successful the previous quantum leap was in getting its new standards generally accepted. In his book *The Structure of Scientific Revolutions*, Thomas Kuhn[1] explains the mechanisms involved in such paradigm shifts. Stephen Hawking[2] brought it to the point by arguing that people are very reluctant to give up a theory in which they have invested a lot of time and effort. This theory defining concepts and procedures is the accepted paradigm, which is recognized by all scientists working in that field. If, however, unexpected developments result in increasing inconsistency with the prevailing paradigm, a tense situation ensues amongst the scientists. At that stage the majority initially questions the accuracy of the observations. If that fails, they try to modify the existing theory in an ad hoc manner. Eventually, the old paradigm becomes creaking and ugly and a new one is accepted which explains all the awkward observations in an elegant and natural manner. Quantum leaps in medicine are certainly not such revolutionary shifts in scientific paradigms, but their principles and their consequences are similar. The angry discussant, for instance, questioning the purpose of merging vascular prosthetic research with biology, is not an isolated phenomenon but rather a typical veteran who may have actively contributed to yesterday's paradigm shift. This again has many parallels in truly revolutionary paradigm shifts in science. Albert Einstein, for instance, who caused a paradigm shift in physics with his special theory of relativity in 1905 was himself, many years later, one of the major antagonists to the next paradigm shift by resisting the acceptance of quantum mechanics. Surgeons are thus in good company with regard to the resistance to paradigm shifts. However, the 13 year delay in achieving this goal in heart transplantation, and the 20 year delay in accepting biology in cardiovascular surgery, makes it clear that we are dealing with a particularly conservative discipline.

Having tried to understand the driving forces behind the twofold polarization which characterized the past 20 years of attempts to create a biologically functional vascular prosthesis, it seems easier to explain the concrete developments of those two decades as well as today's situation. The internally dividing question, for instance, regarding the principal approach to the endothelialization of a prosthetic surface, namely the acceptance of initial complexity versus a priori simplicity, was not an issue at the beginning when no pressure of expectation was exerted by the surgical community. In the early to mid 1970s, the entire initiative to surface endothelialization was driven by attempts to culture endothelial cells on synthetic surfaces prior to implantation.[3,4] Pioneers of endothelial seeding, like the groups of Jim Stanley and Linda Graham were among those who first cultured autologous endothelial cells on vascular graft surfaces.[5,6] Only subsequently in the mid-1980s, when surgeons saw the opportunity of implementing their discoveries through main commercial players, did the focus shift almost entirely to single stage procedures. Ironically, when the greatest enthusiasm for endothelial seeding seized the surgical community at the beginning of the second half of the 1980s, the death sentence was already sealed through both premature clinical trials[7-11] and "commercial kits" for clinical single staged procedures. What happened after the majority of disappointed vascular surgeons turned away from this idea really resembled the above mentioned late developments in heart transplantation. With the hype of the early 1980s over, those who continued were prepared to accept both a long and arduous route of homework prior to implementation and the knowledge that their contribution would be a quiet one.

Attitude-wise back to square one, the remaining groups focused on the main weakness of graft endothelialization, the low cellular inoculum. Mass harvest methods for microvascular cells,[12-16] as well as mass culture procedures for macrovascular endothelial cells,[17-19] were scientifically refined. One of the main reasons for a more relaxed approach in this second half of the 1980s was the conviction that a principle rather than a particular solution needed to be proven. At the onset of the era of vascular biology, nobody challenges that a biologically functional prosthesis would eventually come as a product from the shelf, integrating all encoded signals for spontaneous healing. Nevertheless, such an undertaking needs a critical mass which can more easily be achieved on the basis of at least one proven principle. Although important principles of today like intramural contractility, compliance and cellular quiescence could not yet be tackled, we all focused on the proof that graft endothelialization alone can already dramatically improve synthetic graft performance, even if the old prosthetic scaffolds of yesterday are used. In a step by step approach, adherence and shear stress resistance of cultured endothelial cells on various protein matrices were ascertained[20-37] prior to in vivo experiments ranging from canine implants[20] to primate experiments[38,39] and preclinical primate studies.[40] The success of those implants was convincing enough to apply the principle to very small diameter grafts[41] as well as to bioprosthetic surfaces[42-47] and to heart valves.[48-51] Eventually, the step into clinical trials had to be taken. However, in contrast to the clinical studies with single staged endothelial seeding, the situation regarding clinical trials with in vitro lining was distinctly different: By having accepted the disadvantages of a complex procedure, we had eliminated most of the uncertainties prior to commencing the trials.

Current and Future Perspective

Today's cumulative experience with clinical endothelial cell lining covers almost a decade and comprises more than 200 patients.[52-60] It has clearly demonstrated that in vitro endothelialized synthetic prostheses are equal or better than saphenous vein grafts with regard to patency in all anatomical positions and any clinical stage other than stage IV.[52-60]

Although ePTFE grafts with 30 μm internodal distance, which are noncompliant and do not allow transmural tissue ingrowth, were used for these studies, the autologous surface endothelium alone was not only sufficient to significantly improve patency rates, but also led to the development of a neomedia between an internal elastic membrane underneath the endothelium and the ePTFE surface.[59] This observation indicates that the previous fear of "contaminating" smooth muscle cells was unfounded. Furthermore, it not only supports the current holistic approach towards tissue engineered prosthetic vascular grafts which aim at fully functional neoarteries, but also removes the last remnants of the previous polarization between mixed microvascular mass seeding and macrovascular in vitro lining.

The tools which biology offers today often seem like a dream to those of us who believed in the idea of integrating biology into prosthetic grafts, long before vascular biology had entered its maturity. At the same time we also see that these tools require a commitment of all parties to a manyfold higher level of complexity than the one from which most of us had shied away in the early days of endothelial seeding. Last but not least, we as surgeons are still the majority shareholders in this venture, although the scientists will soon take over the supervisory board. This is a necessary and correct development which should have happened many years ago. However, even if the scientists do take over the lead, in the end there will still be three partners: the industry, the surgeons and the scientists. The industry will need strongly convincing data to voluntarily accept the replacement of a simple and profitable product by a complex and expensive one. The surgeons will need the final painful push to accept the shift of a paradigm and the biologists will need both the true commitment of the other two parties and a strong motivation with regard to the broad application of their discoveries before they will wholeheartedly join hands. This may well be the last challenge for the veteran surgeons on board. Convincing clinical studies with a method which significantly improves graft performance will eventually break the resistance against a paradigm shift amongst our peers and thus prepare the way for the acceptance of tissue engineering. Acceptance of a complex approach by surgeons will mellow the scientists who still see us as "gung-ho" cowboys. And finally, a joint front of scientists and surgeons will eventually force the industry to see beyond today's profits. Last but not least, one needs to keep in mind that even a "Los Alamos" approach to tissue engineering will take many years for the development and many years for clinical trials. This consideration certainly upgrades clinical in vitro endothelialization to a procedure which could benefit an uncountable number of patients over many years to come.

References

1. Kuhn T, Hoyningen P. The structure of scientific revolutions. Translation by A.T. Levine. Chicago: University of Chicago Press, 1993.

2. Hawking, S. Black holes and baby universes and other essays. London: Bantam Press, 1993.

3. Adachi M, Suzuki M, Kennedy JH. Neointimas cultured in vitro for circulatory assist devices. I. Comparison of cultured cells derived from autologous tissues of various organs. J Surg Res 1971; 11:483-491.

4. Mansfield PB, Wechezak AR, Sauvage LR. Preventing thrombus on artifical vascular surfaces: True endothelial cell linings. Trans Am Soc Artif Intern Organs, 1975; 21:264-272.

5. Burkel WB, Ford JW, Kahn RH. Derivation of adult venous endothelium. In Vitro 1979; 15:215.

6. Graham LM, Burkel WE, Ford JW, Vinter DW, Kahn RH, Stanley JC. Expanded polytetrafluorethylene vascular prostheses seeded with enzymatically derived and cultured canine endothelial cells. Surgery 1982; 91:550-559.

7. Zilla P, Fasol R, Deutsch M et al. Endothelial cell seeding of polytetrafluoroethylene vascular grafts in humans: A preliminary report. J Vasc Surg 1987; 6:535-541.

8. Fasol R, Zilla P, Deutsch M et al. Human endothelial cell seeding: Evaluation of its effectiveness by platelet parameters after one year. J Vasc Surg 1989; 9:432-436.

9. Walker MG, Thomson GJL, Shaw JW. Endothelial cell seeded versus non-seeded ePTFE graafts in patients with severe peripheral vascular disease. In: Zilla P, Fasol R, Deutsch M. eds. Endothelialization of Vascular Grafts. Basel: S. Karger AG, 1987:245-248.

10. Örtenwal P, Wadenvik H, Kutti J et al. Endothelial cell seeding reduces thrombogenicity of Dacron grafts in humans. J Vasc Surg 1990; 11:403-410.

11. Herring M, Smith J, Dalsing M, Glover J, Compton R, Etchberger K, Zollinger T. Endothelial seeding of polytetrafluoroethylene femoral popliteal bypasses: The failure of low-density seeding to improve patency. J Vasc Surg 1994; 20:650-655.

12. Visser MJT, Bockel H, VanMuijen GNOP et al. Cells derived from omental tissue used for seeding vascular prostheses are not endothelial in origin. J Vasc Surg, 1991; 13:373-381.

13. Vici M, Pasquinelli G, Preda P et al. Electron microscopic and immunotytochemical profiles of human subcutaneous fat tissue microvascular endothelial cells. Ann Vasc Surg, 1993; 7:541-548.

14. Jarrell B, Williams S, Stokes G et al. Use of freshly isolated capillary endothelial cells for the immediate establishment of a monolayer on a vascular graft at surgery. Surgery 1986; 7:392-399.

15. Vici M. Morphological aspects of microvascular cell isolates. In: Tissue Engineering of prosthetic vascular grafts. Zilla P, Greisler H, eds. Austin: R.G. Landes Co., 1998.

16. Fischlein T. Functional aspects of microvascular cell isolates. In: Tissue Engineering of prosthetic vascular grafts. Zilla P, Greisler H, eds. R.G. Landes Co., 1998.

17. Zilla P, Fasol R, Dudeck U, Siedler S, Priess P, Fischlein T, Müller-Glauser W, Baitella G, Sanan D, Odell J, Reichart B. In situ cannulation, microgrid follow-up and low-density plating provide first passage endothelial cell masscultures for in vitro lining. J Vasc Surg 1990; 12:180-189.

18. Haegerstrand A, Gillis C, Bengtsson L. Serial cultivation of adult human endothelium from the great saphenous vein. J Vasc Surg 1992; 16:280-285

19. Zilla P, Siedler S, Fasol R, Sharefkin JB. Reduced reproductive capacity of freshly harvested endothelial cells in smokers: A possible shortcoming in the success of seeding? J Vasc Surg 1989; 10:143-148.

20. Seeger JM, Klingman N. Improved in vivo endothelialization of prosthetic grafts by surface modification with fibronectin. J Vasc Surg 1988; 8:476-482.

21. Prendiville EJ, Coleman JE, Callow AD, Gould KE, Laliberte-Verdon S, Ramberg K, Connolly RJ. Increased in-vitro incubation time of endothelial cells on fibronectin-treated ePTFE increases cell retention in blood flow Eur J Vasc Surg 1991; 5:311-319.

22. Zilla P, Fasol R, Grimm M, Fischlein T, Eberl T, Preiss P, Krupicka O, Von Oppell U, Deutsch M. Growth properties of cultured human endothelial cells on differently coated artifical heart materials. J Thorac Cardiovasc Surg 1991; 101:671-680.

23. Shindo S, Takagi A, Whittemore AD. Improved patency of collagen-impregnated grafts after in vitro autogenous endothelial seeding. J Vasc Surg 1987; 6:325-332.

24. Kadletz M, Moser R, Preiss P et al. In vitro lining of fibronectin coated PTFE grafts with cryopreserved saphenous vein endothelial cells. Thorac Cardiovasc Surg 1987; 35:143-147.

25. Schneider PA, Hanson BR, Price TM et al. Preformed confluent endothelial cell monolayers prevent early platelet deposition on vascular prostheses in baboons. J Vasc Surg 1988; 8:229-235.

26. Anderson JS, Price TM, Hanson SR et al. In vitro endothelialization of small-caliber vascular grafts. Surgery 1987; 101:577-586.

27. Schneider A, Hanson SR, Price TM et al. Durability of confluent endothelial cell monolayers on small-caliber vascular prostheses in vitro. Surgery 1988; 103:456-462.

28. Sentissi JM, Ramberg KJ, O'Donnell TF, Connoly TF, Callow AD. The effect of flow on vascular endothelial cells grown in tissue culture on polytetra-fluoro-ethylene grafts. Surgery 1986; 99:337-342.

29. Foxall TL, Auger KR, Callow AD, Libby P. Adult human endothelial cell coverge of small-caliber Dacron and polytetrafluoroethylene vascular prostheses in vitro. J Surg Res 1986; 41:158-172.

30. Vohra RK, Thomson GJL, Sharma H, Carr HMH, Walker MG. Effects of shear stress on endothelial cell monolayers on expanded polytetrafluoroethylene (ePTFE) grafts using preclot and fibronectin matrices. Eur J Vasc Surg 1990; 4:33-41.

31. Zilla P, Fasol R, Preiss P, Kadletz M, Deutsch M, Schima H, Tsangaris S, Groscurth P. Use of fibrin glue as a substrate for in vitro endothelialization of PTFE vascular grafts. Surgery 1989; 105:515-522.

32. Ives CL, Eskin SG, McIntire LV, De Bakey ME. The importance of cell origin and substrate in the kinetics of endothelial cell alignment in response to steady flow. Trans Am Soc Artif Intern Organs 1983; 24:269-274.

33. Bengtsson LA, Radegran K, Haegerstrand A. A new and simple technique to achieve a confluent and flow resistant endothelium on vascular ePTFE-grafts using human serum. Eur J Vasc Surg 1994; 8:182-187.

34. Gillis C, Bengtsson L, Wilman B, Haegerstrand A. Secretion of prostacyclin, tissue plasminogen activator and its inhibitor by cultured adult human endothelial cells grown

on different matrices. Eur J Vasc Endovasc Surg 1996; 11:127-133.

35. Gillis-Haegerstrand C, Frebelius S, Haegerstrand A, Swedenborg J. Cultured human endothelial cells seeded on expanded polytetrafluoroethylene support thrombin-mediated activation of protein C. J Vasc Surg 1996; 24:226-234

36. Haegerstrand A, Bengtsson L, Gillis C. Serum proteins provide a matrix for cultured endothelial cells on expanded polytetrafluoroethylene vascular grafts. Scand J Thorac Cardiovasc Surg 1993; 27:21-26.

37. Leseche G, Bikfalvi A, Dupuy E, Tobelem G, Andreassian B, Caen J. Prelining of polytetrafluoroethylene grafts with cultured human endothelial cells isolated from varicose veins. Surgery 1989; 105:36-45.

38. Schneider PA, Hanson SR, Todd M, Price BA, Harker LA. Confluent durable endothelialization of endarterectomized baboon aorta by early attchment of cultured endothelial cells. J Vasc Surg 1990; 11:365-372.

39. Krupski WC, Bass A, Anderson JS, Kelly AB, Harker LA. Aspirin-independent antithrombotic effects of acutely attached cultured endothelial cells on endarterectomized arteries. Surgery 1990; 108:283-291.

40. Zilla P, Preiss P, Groscurth P, Rösemeier F, Deutsch M, Odell J, Heidinger C, Fasol R, von Oppell U. In vitro-lined endothelium: Initial inegrity and ultrastructural events. Surgery 1994; 116:524-534.

41. Gherardini G, Haegerstrand A, Matarasso A, Gurlek A, Evans GR, Lundeberg T. Cell adhesion and short-term patency in human endothelium preseeded 1.5mm polytetrafluoroethylene vascular grafts: An experimental study. Plast Reconstr Surg 1977; 99:472-478.

42. Hoch J, Dryjski M, Jarrell BE, Carabasi RA, Williams SK. In vitro endothelializaton of an aldehyde-stabilized native vessel. J Surg Res 1988; 44:545-554.

43. Bengtsson LA, Phillips R, Haegerstrand AN. In vitro endothelialization of photo-oxidatively stabilized xenogeneic pericardium. Ann Thorac Surg 1995; 60:S365-S368.

44. Bengtsson L, Ragnarson B, Haegerstrand A. Lining of viable and non-viable allogeneic and xenogeneic cardiovascular tisue with cultured adult human venous endothelium. J Thorac Cardiovasc Surg 1993; 106:434-443.

45. Leukauf C, Szeles C, Salaymeh L, Grimm M, Grabenwoger M, Moritz A, Wolner E. In vitro and in vivo endothelialization of glutaraldehyde treated bovine pericardium. J Heart Valve Dis 1993; 2:230-235.

46. Eybl E, Grimm M, Grabenwoger M, Bock P, Muller MM, Wolner E. Endothelial cell lining of bioprosthetic heart valve materials. J Thorac Cardiovasc Surg 1992; 104:763-769.

47. Grabenwoger M, Grimm M, Eybl E, Moritz A, Muller MM, Bock P, Wolner E. Endothelial cell lining of bioprosthetic heart valve material. J Card Surg 1992; 7:79-84.

48. Bengtsson LA, Haegerstrand AN. Endotheliaization of mechanical heart valves in vitro with cultured adult human cells. J Heart Valve Dis 1993; 2:352-356.

49. Bengtsson L, Radegran K, Haegerstrand A. In vitro endothelialization of commercially available heart valve bioprostheses with cultured adult human cells. Eur J Cardiothorac Surg 1993; 7:383-398.

50. Lehner G, Fischlein T, Baretton G, Murphy JG, Reichart B. Endothelialized biological heart valve prostheses in the non-human primate model. Eur J Cardiothorac Surg 1997; 11:498-504.

51. Fischlein T, Lehner G, Lante W, Fittkau M, Murphy JG, Weinhold C, Reichart B. Endothelialization of cardiac valve bioprostheses [published erratum appears in Int J Artif Organs 1994 Jul; 17(7):412].

52. Kadletz M, Magometschnigg H, Minar E, Konig G, Grabenwoger M, Grimm M, Wolner E. Implantation of in vitro endothelialized polytetrafluoroethylene grafts in human beings. A preliminary report. J Thorac Cardiovasc Surg 1992; 104:736-742.

53. Magometschnigg H, Kadletz M, Vodrazka M, Grabenwoger M, Grimm M, Bock P, Leukauf C, Trubel W, Wolner E. Changes following in vitro endothelial cell lining of ePTFE prostheses: Late morphologic evaluation of six failed grafts. Eur J Vasc Surg 1994; 8:502-507.

54. Zilla P, Deutsch M, Meinhart J, Puschmann R, Eberl T, Minar E, Dudczak R, Lugmaier H, Schmidt P, Noszian I, Fischlein T. Clinical in vitro endothelialization of femoropopliteal bypass grafts: An actuarial follow-up over three years. J Vasc Surg 1994; 19:540-548.

55. Magometschnigg H, Kadletz M, Vodrazka M, Dock W, Grimm M, Minar E, Staudacher M, Fenzl G, Wolner E. Prospective clinical study with in vitro endothelial cell lining of expanded polytetrafluoroethylene grafts in crural repeat reconstruction. J Vasc Surg 1992; 15:527-535.

56. Fischlein T, Zilla P, Meinhart J, Puschmann R, Vesely M, Eberl T, Balon R, Deutsch M. In vitro endothelializaation of mesosystemic shunt: A clinical case report. J Vasc Surg 1994; 19:549-554.

57. Leseche G, Ohan J, Boutlier S, Palombi S, Bertrand P, Andreassian B. Above-knee femoropopliteal bypass grafting using endothelial cell seeded PTFE grafts: Five year clincial experience. Ann Vasc Surg 1995; 9:S15-S23.

58. Laub HR, Duwe J, Claus M. Autologous endothelial cell seeded PTFE vascular grafts for coronary artery bypass: First clinical results. 15th Intern Cardiovasc Surg. Symposium, Zurs, Austria

59. Deutsch M, Meinhart J, Vesely M, Fischlein T, Groscurth P, von Oppell U, Zilla P. In vitro endothelialization of expanded polytetrafluoroethylene grafts; A clinical case report after 41 months of implantaton. J Vasc Surg 1997; 25:757-763.

60. Meinhart J, Deutsch M, Zilla P. Eight years of clinical endothelial cell transplantation. Closing the gap between prosthetic grafts and vein grafts. ASAIO Journal 1997; 43:M515-M521.

CHAPTER 14

Serial Cultivation of Human Endothelial Cells

Caroline Gillis-Hægerstrand, Anders Hægerstrand

Introduction

Understanding of the tremendous capabilities of the endothelial cell has grown considerably during the last decades. The use of cell culture techniques has been instrumental in this development. The single most important breakthrough for endothelial cell (EC) culture, and still probably the most used technique, was published by Jaffe and coworkers in 1973. They described how to isolate and propagate human umbilical vein endothelial cells (HUVECs).[1] Since then several modifications and improvements have been published,[2,3] with the fundamental principle remaining unchanged, i.e., the incubation of a vessel, ideally clamped at both ends, with a collagenase containing solution, and the subsequent plating and cultivation in a protein-coated tissue culture flask, the cells being fed with a medium enriched by relatively large amounts of serum and/or growth factors. Some basic ideas about the fundamental functions of ECs, e.g., the production of arachidonic acid derivatives, the expression of adhesion molecules, the tight interactions with leukocyte or smooth muscle cells and the synthesis of nitric oxide (NO), have been derived from the use of cultured ECs, mainly HUVECs. It should be remembered that ECs in culture are something very different than ECs in their natural environment. Compared to many, if not most, other cell types, it is harder to mimic in vitro what the natural circumstances are under which the ECs operate. This must be remembered when interpretations of EC functions are made. The in vivo correlate remains the only true measure of the predictive value of in vitro findings.

The idea of culturing endothelial cells for clinical purposes is not new, but only a limited number of studies have actually been performed. In this review we will discuss some basic techniques and principles for the culture of human endothelial cells and some of the future possibilities.

Characteristics of the Endothelium

The total area of ECs in a human body is indeed huge, approximately 5000 m^2.[4] The ECs *in situ* are known to have a relatively low frequency of mitotic figures. The replication rate of ECs ranges from one EC per 10^2-10^4 cells/24 h[5] to one EC per 10 cells/24 h depending on in which part of the body the endothelium is located. In areas with increased hemodynamic force, the replication rate is higher.[6] This phenomenon seems to have an in vitro correlate in that cells cultured under pressure higher than ambient, e.g., 40-100 mm Hg, show a higher frequency of divisions.[7] ECs in vitro act similarly to ECs in vivo in that they proliferate to form a monolayer and their growth is restricted by contact inhibition.[8] However, even a seemingly confluent layer of ECs with established physical contacts can become more densely populated under the right conditions, but one EC does not seem to grow on top of another EC.

Tissue Engineering of Prosthetic Vascular Grafts, edited by Peter Zilla and Howard P. Greisler.

There are differences in morphology, growth rate and protein synthesis between cultured arterial and venous ECs,[9] as well as between ECs derived from capillaries, arterioles and venules.[10] Venous ECs are larger, thinner and more pleomorphic than ECs deriving from aorta. ECs derived from veins are considered more difficult to establish in culture and they grow at a lower growth rate.[9] These differences are believed to be due to the different requirements by the hemodynamic environment. Whether this has an impact on utility for transplantation purposes is not known.

ECs from different sizes and types of blood vessels show well known differences in metabolic properties, especially in their response to vasoactive mediators.[11] The physiological significance of this heterogeneity is not clear, but may be related to local variations in the function the ECs serve, for example in arterial versus venous circulation.[12] When ECs from one source are compared, there is also a vast difference in basal secretion of, e.g., PGI_2 and plasminogen/plasminogen inhibitors in cultures of ECs from different patients.[13-15]

A characteristic that is unique for endothelial cells, regardless of their origin, is the presence of Weibel-palade bodies.[16] In granules inside the Weibel-palade bodies, P-selectin and von Willebrand factor (vWF) are colocalized. Other characteristics of the ECs, though not unique, are prostacyclin production (PGI_2),[17] angiotensin converting enzyme (ACE) activity and positive staining for the surface antigen PECAM (CD31).[18] In most cases, investigators characterize the ECs by staining with vWF, by showing the presence of Weibel-palade bodies or by showing uptake of acetylated low density lipoprotein (LDL), the latter being another characteristic not restricted to ECs.

Sources of Endothelial Cells

Several sources for isolating ECs during an operation to immediately seed a vascular graft have been demonstrated, including freshly isolated cells from veins and fat.[19-25] Techniques for isolation and culture of ECs from human tissues other than large vessels or fatty tissue have been described.[26-29] Others have successfully isolated ECs from omental tissue,[30] although it has been questioned whether they are truly endothelial.[31] It is known that mesothelial cells share several properties with ECs, especially those related to antithrombotic and fibrinolytic functions.[32-34] Subcutaneous fat is probably a better source of true ECs as compared to omental fat.[25] Sources of ECs for effective and reproducible cultivation are fewer, especially when the cells are intended for clinical purposes. Typically, veins such as the great saphenous, basilic, cephalic and external jugular have been used.[35-38] Cultured arterial ECs have not yet been used for clinical purposes to our knowledge, although that may potentially be beneficial, since the purpose is most often to replace nude or denuded tissue in an arterial position.

In spite of an increasing number of techniques, EC research is often hampered by the lack of sufficient numbers of ECs of an adequate origin. Even if vessels or tissue rich in ECs become available, the isolation and cultivation is not easy. The quality and short term storage of the tissue derived from the patient, the contamination of other cell types during culture, e.g., fibroblasts, and the long term cultivation itself to reach the desired amount of cells make EC culture for clinical purposes a complicated task.

Culture Techniques for Human ECs

A lot can be said about general requirements for culture of human cells. Some relatively general components used during culture of human ECs are summarized in Figure 14.1.

ECs are continuously exposed to blood, which is known to contain growth stimulating factors, although many at low concentrations. In our work we have been focusing on human serum as a source for stimulating growth and attachment on the prosthetic material, whereas most investigators have used serum containing medium supplemented with growth factors and heparin. Serum free alternatives are commercially available, but these are often quite expensive. Such media are typically better to introduce after an initial culture period using medium which contains serum. The basal medium in most compositions, irrespective of serum dependence or independence, normally contains a relatively high concentration of glucose, and basal media such as M199 and MEM are often used. It is generally accepted that some matrix component precoated on the tissue culture treated plastic is beneficial. Most often, as also originally described by Jaffe et al, denatured bovine collagen, i.e., gelatin, can be used. The method by which it is prepared also seems to fit with current guidelines on the use of bovine/xenogeneic material for tissue culture. Fibronectin in concentrations of approximately 1-10 µg per square centimeter is often recommended, but it should be remembered that concentration dependent functional alterations can be expected. Laminin, collagen type I or IV and extracellular matrix (ECM) have also been used. Shortly after seeding, within 6 h, ECs deposit matrix components, e.g., laminin and collagen type IV, on the plastic, and thereby influence their own attachment.

Addition of Serum and Growth Factors

Human serum (HS) and fetal calf serum (FCS) prepared for cell culture purposes contain growth factors from plasma and growth factors released from platelets upon their aggregation. It should be remembered that ECs grow considerably more slowly in blood plasma without platelets or coagulation factors, which is quite often referred to as serum. Cell culture serum must be prepared according to specific protocols. Serum contains several factors which promote proliferation, platelet derived growth factor (PDGF), epidermal growth factor (EGF), transforming growth factor β (TGF-β) and insulin-like growth factors (IGFs).[39] Fibroblast growth factors (FGFs) play many roles in cell growth, differentiation and survival,[40] and are well established growth factors for ECs. Both basic FGF and acidic FGF are often used in recombinant form to stimulate EC growth. Endothelial cell growth factor (ECGF), a precursor form of acidic FGF (AFGF), is a potent mitogen for most ECs.[39,40] A rat brain extract, known as endothelial cell growth supplement (ECGS), containing different forms of FGFs, is also commonly used[42,43] to improve cell proliferation, and was the most frequent additive to EC culture a decade ago, before purified and recombinant factors were made commercially available at reasonable prices.

Heparin and Endothelial Proliferation

The fact that heparin enhances the stimulatory effect of ECGF on cell proliferation in vitro is well established.[43,44] Both heparan sulfate and heparin act by stabilizing growth factor activity, partly by preventing proteolytic degradation of the growth factor.[45,46] The binding and mitogenic activity of bFGF are to some degree dependent on heparin-like molecules on the cell surface, or in their absence, on exogenously added heparin-like molecules.[47] It has recently been shown that heparin is an FGF-independent activating ligand for FGF receptor 4 (FGFR4) on cultured transfected myoblasts, fibroblasts and lymphoid cells.[48] In our work it was shown that heparin alone increased growth of adult human ECs when heparin was added to a medium containing as much as 40% HS. An explanation for these results in combination with 40% serum[49] is that they may be due to the presence of FGFR4 on ECs or that heparin stabilizes growth factors in serum. Different growth factors may act differently on cultured ECs from various vascular beds. While bFGF stimulates proliferation of most ECs, afgf and PDGF have been shown to have no effect on large vessel endothelium but to stimulate microvascular cell growth.[50] Bovine microvascular ECs have been shown to express a different set of growth factor receptors than bovine arterial ECs.[51] Interestingly, ECs are known to synthesize both bFGF and PDGF, which may act as autocrine and paracrine growth factors.[52-54]

Cyclic AMP and Endothelial Cell Proliferation

The addition of purified cholera toxin (CT) to the EC culture medium leads to an increase in intracellular cyclic adenosine monophosphate (cAMP) synthesis. The phosphodiesterase inhibitor IBMX decreases cAMP degradation, and both thereby act to increase the intracellular cAMP level. Cyclic AMP is an ubiquitous messenger which is involved in many cellular processes, including changes in morphology, proliferation[55,56] and release of vasoactive substances in response to stimulation.[57] When the membrane-bound adenylyl cyclase is activated, ATP is enzymatically converted to cyclic AMP, which leads to activation of protein kinase A (PKA). These events have been shown to influence cell proliferation,[55] and the role of cyclic AMP as a regulator of cell proliferation has been studied extensively. Negative control was demonstrated as early as in the 1970s. Today, however, accumulating data have shown that increase in cAMP levels is also associated with stimulatory effects on several cell types, including epithelial cells.[55,58,59] It has also been shown that activation of cAMP may enhance receptor binding of growth factors and progression of the resultant signals.[60]

Db-cAMP is a synthetic cAMP analog which can penetrate cell membranes. In our studies cholera toxin, IBMX and db-cAMP have all been shown to increase the proliferation of ECs derived from the great saphenous vein (HSVECs).[14,49] Karasek and coworkers have shown that combinations of HS and cAMP stimulation are beneficial for both growth and maintenance of the epitheloid morphology in human microvascular ECs.[26,59,61,62] HUVECs have also been shown to increase in cell number after stimulation with CT and endogenous peptides which stimulate cAMP formation.[63] Using a medium without cAMP-stimulatory compounds, Watkins and coworkers have described aberrant cell morphologies after repeated passages using trypsin.[64] In our experience using cAMP-stimulatory factors in the medium, the number of cells appearing aberrant, e.g., large and multinuclear, constitutes no more than onefiftieth of the cells even after 8-9 passages. This may be due to continuous cAMP stimulation or to the high proportion of serum. Cyclic AMP formation has also been shown to modulate EC migration,[65,66] inhibit hypoxia-induced increase in EC permeability,[67] enhance EC thromboresistance[68] and to amplify agonist-induced release of EDRF.[69] Both protective and indirect mechanisms may thus be of importance for the growth promoting effects of CT/IBMX and db-cAMP.

We have shown that HS is more efficient than FCS in stimulating growth of HSVECs and that heparin, bFGF and cAMP-elevating compounds, together with relatively high concentrations of serum, are efficient in increasing the number of HSVECs in culture.[49] The differences in ability of the different sera and other factors to enhance cell proliferation may depend on the cell type being studied. In our case, it may be speculated that HS contains factors which are especially suited for human cells and especially ECs. Human serum carries the advantage of potential autologous use, which may increase safety for the patient if the purpose of the culture is for transplantation.

Does the Culture Technique Matter from a Clinical Perspective?

Zilla and coworkers have demonstrated a cell culture technique where low density seeding of first passage ECs can yield 14×10^6 ECs in 26 days.[36] The method involves in situ administration of collagenase and basically no passaging of the cells. This may have the advantage of increasing the total yield and avoidance of exposing the cells to trypsin or EDTA, which may have negative effects on the cells. In addition to possible morphological changes, functional changes of the cells after passaging using trypsin, e.g., altered pattern of receptor expression, have also been indicated.[70]

In the study which has been used for clinical purposes, the medium contained serum, ECGS and heparin. Interestingly, heparin and ECGS have been shown to supress prostacyclin production.[44]

The choice of culture technique may actually lead to selection of a selectivley responsive subpopulation of ECs that will then constitute the majority of the cells available for transplantation. Direct comparisons of cells from one single donor cultured using different methods have not been performed. Partly differing functions of the cells on the graft, and thus the clinical result, may become a result of the choice of culture technique. On the other hand, one may speculate that the ECs will become functionally normalized once brought back a more natural environment. Nothing but large controlled studies will reveal whether the culture technique will affect the clinical results. Other aspects, e.g., safety and

Fig. 14.1. Illustration of typical/possible media and components used for serial cultivations of human ECs. PDGFs: platelet-derived growth factors, IGFs: insulin like growth factors, bFGF: basic fibroblast growth factor, ECGF/S: endothelial cell growth factor/supplement, CT: cholera toxin, IBMX: isobutyl methylxanthine, ECM: extracellular matrix.

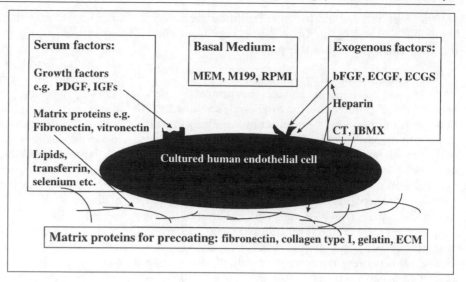

rate of successful cultures using a specific technique, will probably override such speculations.

Future Possibilities of Cultured ECS

Transfer of genes for transient or prolonged production of factors which would promote healing of denuded vessels, e.g., bFGF or VEGF, is intriguing. Nonspecific transfer to the cells of the vessel wall seems feasible in animals. The use of cultured ECs as recipients of retroviral vectors expressing secretory enzymes or hormones over long times has been studied already.[71-74] The possibility of transplanting genetically manipulated ECs expressing a substance which is lacking in patients, such as tPA or insulin, may thus be within reach. However, retroviral vectors are not considered ideal from a safety perspective. Adeno, lenti or herpes viruses often carry the same connotation, and most likely such will be used when the disease addressed with the gene therapy is lethal. Since the percentage of successfully transfected cells is often limited with the techniques not involving parts of a viral genome, the genetic manipulation would require an efficient culture method and optimal graft adherence to be of practical use. One possibility is to immortalize ECs without using retro- or adenoviral components with oncogenes such as the SV-40 Large T construct; this has already been investigated.[75] Furthermore, conditionally immortalized ECs can potentially be developed, i.e., ECs that proliferate under the control of a regulatable gene such as the tetracyclin-regulated expression of Large T antigen. At the end of the culture period, the oncogene could then be switched, which would increase safety and minimize the risk of transformation of the cells in situ. These latter more speculative opportunities remain to be investigated and deserve further efforts.

References

1. Jaffe EA, Nachman RL, Becker CG, Minick CR. Culture of human endothelial cells derived from umbilical veins. Identification by morphologic and immunologic criteria. J Clin Invest 1973; 52:2745-2756.

2. Gimbrone M, Cotran R, Folkman J. Human vascular endothelial cells in culture. Growth and DNA synthesis. J Cell Biol 1974; 60:673-684.

3. Maciag T, Hoover G, Stemerman M, Weinstein R. Serial propagation of human endothelial cells in vitro. J Cell Biol 1981; 91:420-426.

4. Jaffe E. Cell biology of endothelial cells. Hum Pathol 1987; 18(3):234-239.

5. Schwartz S. Dynamic maintenance of the endothelium. In: Freshney, e.d. The endothelial cell—a pluripotent control of the vessel wall. Basel: Karger, 1983:113-125.

6. Schwartz S, Gajdusek C, Reidy M, Selden S, Haudenschild C. Maintenance of integrity in aortic endothelium. Federation Proc 1980; 39:2618-2625.

7. Sumpio BE, Widmann MD, Ricotta J, Awolesi MA, Watase M, Increased ambient pressure stimulates proliferation and morphologic changes in cultured endothelial cells. J Cell Physiol 1994; 158(1:133-139.

8. Haudenschild C, Zahniser D, Folkman J, Klagsbrun M. Human vascular endothelial cells in culture: Lack of response to serum growth factors. Exp Cell Res 1976; 98:175-183.

9. Wagner W, Henderssin R, Hicks H, Banes A, Johnson G. Differences in morphology, growth rate and protein synthesis between cultured arterial and venous endothelial cells. J Vasc Surg 1988; 8(4):509-519.

10. Williams S, Jarrel B, Rose D. Isolation of human fat derived microvessel endothelial cells for use in vascular graft endothelialization. In: Zilla P, Fasol R, Deutsch M, eds. Endothelialization of vascular grafts. Basel: Karger, 1987.

11. Shepro D, Dunham B. Endothelial cell metabolism of biogenic amines. Annu Rev Physiol 1986; 48:335-345.

12. Manolopolos VG, Lelkes PI. Cyclic strain and forskolin differentially induce cAMP production in phenotypically diverse endothelial cells. Biochem Biophys Res Comm 1993; 191(3):1379-1385.

13. Li J, Menconi MJ, Wheeler B, Rohrer MJ, Klassen VA, Ansell JE, Appel MC. Precoating expanded polytetrafluoroethylene grafts alter production of endothelial cell-derived thrombomodulators. J Vasc Surg 1992; 15(6): 1010-1017.

14. Hægerstrand A, Gillis C, Bengtsson L. Serial cultivation of adult human endothelium from the great saphenous vein. J Vasc Surg 1992; 16(2):280-285.

15. Gillis C, Bengtsson L, Wiman B, Hægerstrand A. Release of prostacyclin and tissue plasminogen activator and its inhibitor by cultured adult human endothelial cells grown on different matrices. J Eur Vasc Surg, 1996; 11(2):127-133.

16. Weibel E, Palade G. New cytoplasmic components in arterial endothelia. J Cell Biol 1964; 23:101-112.

17. Weksler BB, Ley CW, Jaffe EA. Stimulation of endothelial cell prostacyclin production by thrombin, trypsin and ionophore A 23187. J Clin Invest 1978; 62:923-930.

18. Newman PJ, Berndt MC, Gorski J. PECAM-1 (CD-31) cloning and relation to adhesion molecules of the immunoglobulin gene superfamily. Science 1990; 247:1219-1222.

19. Herring M, Gardner A, Glover J. A single stage technique for seeding vascular grafts with autogeneous endothelium. Surgery 1978; 84(4):498-504.

20. Herring MB, Gardner AL, Glover JL. Seeding human arterial prostheses with mechanically derived endothelium. The detrimental effect of smoking. J Vasc Surg 1984; 1: 279-289.

21. Herring MB, Compton RS, LeGrand DR, Gardner AL, Madison DL, Glover JL. Endothelial seeding of polytetrafluoroethylene poplitetal bypasses: A preliminary report. J Vasc Surg 1987; 6.114-118.

22. Jarrell B, Levine E, Shapiro S, Williams S, Carabasi A, Mueller S, Thornton S. Human adult endothelial growth in culture. J Vasc Surg 1984; 1:757 64.

23. Jarrell B, Williams S, Stokes G, Hubbard A, Carabasi A, Koolpe E, Greener D, Pratt K, Moritz M, Radomski J, Speicher L. Use of freshly isolated capillary endothelial cells for immediate establishment of a monolayer on vascular graft at surgery. Surgery 1986; 100:392-99.

24. Jarrell BE, Williams SK, Carabasi RA, Hubbard FA. Immediate vascular graft monolayers using microvessel endothelial cells. In: Herring, ed. Endothelial seeding in vascular surgery. Orlando: Grune & Stratton 1987;37-55

25. Williams SK, Wang TF, Castrillo R, Jarrell BE. Liposuction-derived human fat used for vascular graft sodding contains endothelial cells and not mesothelial cells as the major cell type. J Vasc Surg 1994; 19(5).916-923.

26. Davison PM, Bensch K, Karasek MA. Isolation and growth of endothelial cells from the microvessels of the newborn foreskin in cell culture. J Invest Dermatol 1980; 75(4):316-321.

27. Grafe M, Auch-Schwelk W, Graf K, Terbeek D, Hertel H, Unkelbach M, Hildebrandt A.E.F. Isolation and characterization of macrovascular and microvascular endothelial cells from human hearts. Am J Physiol 1994; 267:2138-2148.

28. Grafe M, Graf K, Auch-Schwelk W, Terbeek D, Hertel H, Fleck E. Cultivation and characterization of micro- and macrovascular endothelial cells from the human heart. Eur Heart J 1993; 14:74-81.

29. Hewett PW, Murray JC. Immunomagnetic purification of human endothelial cells using dynabeads coated with monoclonal antibodies to PECAM-1. Eur J Cell Biol 1993; 62(2):451-454.

30. Williams SK, Jarrell BE. Cells derived from omental fat tissue and used for seeding vascular prostheses are not endothelial in origin: (Letter; Comment). J Vasc Surg 1992; 15(3):583-5.

31. Stansby G, Shukla N, Fuller B, Hamilton G. Mesothelial or endothelial? (Letter; Comment) Eur J Vasc Endovasc 1995; 10(3):387-388.

32. Pötzsch B, Grulich HJ, Rössing R, Wille D, Müller BG. Close similarity between cultured human omental mesothelial cells and endothelial cells in cytochemical markers and plasminogen activator production. In Vitro Cell Dev Biol 1991.

33. van Hinsbergh V, Koistra T, Scheffer M, van Bockel J, van Muijen G. Characterization and fibrinolytic properties of human omental mesothelial cells. Blood 1990; 75:1490-97.

34. Coene M-C, Solheid C, Claeys M, Herman AG. Prostaglandin production by cultured mesothelial cells. Arch Int Pharmacodyn 1981; 249:316-318.

35. Zilla P, Fasol R, Deutsch M, Fischlein T, Minar E, Hammarle A, Krapicka O, Kadketz M. Endothelial cell seeding of polytetrafluoroethylene vascular grafts in humans: A preliminary report. J Vasc Surg 1987; 6:535-541.

36. Zilla P, Fasol R, Dudeck U, Siedler S, Preiss P, Fischlein T, Müller-Glauser W, Baitella G, Sanan D, Odell J, Reichart B. In situ cannulation, microgrid follow-up and low-density plating provide first passage endothelial cell mass cultures for in vitro lining. J Vasc Surg 1990; 12:180-89.

37. Zilla P, Deutsch M, Meinhart J, Puschmann R, Eberl T, Minar E, Dudczak R, Lugmaier H, Schmidt P, Noszian I, Fischlein T. Clinical in vitro endothelialization of femoropopliteal bypass grafts: An actuarial follow-up over three years. J Vasc Surg 1994; 19(3):540-548.

38. Swedenborg J, Bengtsson L, Clyne N, Gillis C, Rosfors S. Haegerstrand A. In vitro endothelialization of arteriovenous loop grafts for hemodialysis. Eur J Vasc Endovasc Surg 1997; 13(3):272-277.

39. Miyazono K, Takaku F. Platelet-derived growth factors, Blood Rev 1989; 3(4):269-276.

40. Burgess W, Maciag T. The heparin-binding (fibroblast) growth factor family of proteins. Annu Rev Biochem 1989; 50.575-606.

41. Partanen J, Vainikka JK, Armstrong E, Alitalo K. Diverse receptors for fibroblast growth factors. Prog Growth Factor Res 1992; 4:69-83.

42. Schreiber AB, Kenney J, Kowalski WJ. Interaction of endothelial cell growth factor with heparin: Characterization by receptor and antibody recognition. Proc Natl Acad Sci (USA) 1985; 82(18):6138-6142.

43. Thornton S, Mueller S, Levine E. Human umbilical cells: Use of heparin in cloning and long-term serial cultivation. Science 1983; 222:623-625.

44. Minter AJ, Dawes J, Chesterman CN. Effects of heparin and endothelial cell growth supplement on haemostatic functions of vascular endothelium. Thromb Haemost 1992; 67(6):718-723.

45. Saksela O, Moscatelli D, Sommer A, Rifkin DB. Endothelial cell-derived heparan sulphate binds basic fibroblast growth factor and protects it from proteolytic degradation. J Cell Biol 1988; 107(2):743-751.

46. Sommer A, Rifkin DB. Interaction of heparin with human basic fibroblast growth factor: Protection of the angiogenic protein from proteolytic degradation by a glycosaminoglycan. J Cell Physiol 1989; 138:215-220.

47. Klagsbrun M, Baird A. A dual receptor system is required for basic fibroblast growth factor activity. Cell 1991; 67:229-231.

48. Gao G, Goldfarb M. Heparin can activate a receptor tyrosine kinase. EMBO J 1995; 14(10):2183-2190.

49. Gillis C, Jonzon B, Haegerstrand A. Effects of sera, bFGF, heparin and cyclic AMP stimulation on proliferation of human umbilical and saphenous vein endothelial cells. Cell Mol Biol 1995; 41:1131-1138.

50. D'Amore PA. Mechanisms of endothelial growth control. Am J Respir Cell Mol Biol 1992; 6(1):1-8.

51. Boes M, Dake BL, Bar RS. Interactions of cultured endothelial cells with TGF-beta, bFGF, PDGF and IGF-I. Life Sci 1991; 48(8):811-21.

52. Schweigerer L, Neufeld G, Friedman J. Capillary endothelial cells express basic fibroblast growth factor, a mitogen that promotes their own growth. Nature 1987; 325:257-259.

53. DiCorleto PE, Bowen-Pope DF. Cultured endothelial cells produce a platelet-derived factor-like protein. Proc Natl Acad Sci (USA) 1983; 80:1919-1923.

54. Vlodavsky I, Friedman R, Sullivan R, Sasse J, Klagsbrun M. Aortic endothelial cells synthesize basic fibroblast growth factor which remains cell associated and platelet-derived growth factor-like protein which is secreted. J Cell Physiol 1987; 131(3):402-408.

55. Boynton AL, Whitfeld JF. The role of cAMP in cell proliferation: A critical assessment of the evidence. Adv Cyclic Nucleotide Res 1983; 15:193-294.

56. Dumont J, Jauniaux J-C, Roger P. The cyclic AMP-mediated stimulation of cell proliferation. TIBS 1989; 14:67-71.

57. Moncada S, Vane JR. Pharmacology and endogenous roles of prostaglandin endoperoxides, thromboxane A2 and prostacyclin. Pharmacol Rev 1979; 30:292-331.

58. Green H. Cyclic AMP in relation to proliferation of the epidermal cell: A new view. Cell 1978; 15:801-811.

59. Davison P, Karasek M. Human dermal microvascular endothelial cells in vitro: Effect of cyclic AMP on cellular morphology and proliferation rate. J Cell Physiol 1981; 106:253-58.

60. Olashaw NE, Pledger WJ. Cellular mechanisms regulating proliferation. Advances in second messenger and phosphoprotein research. 1988; 22:139-173.

61. Kramer R, Fuh G-M, Karachek M. Type IV collagen synthesis by cultured human microvascular endothelial cells and its deposition into the subendothelial basement membrane. Biochemistry 1985; 24:7423-30.

62. Tuder RM, Karasek MA, Bensch KG. Cyclic adenosine monophosphate levels and the function of skin microvascular endothelial cells. J Cell Physiol 1990; 142(2):272-283.

63. Haegerstrand A, Dalsgaard C-J, Jonzon B, Larsson O, Nilsson J. Calcitonin gene-related peptide stimulates proliferation of human endothelial cells. Proc Natl Acad Sci 1990; 87(9):3299-3303.

64. Watkins M, Sharefkin J, Zajtchuk R, Maciag T, D'Amore P, Ryan U, van Wart H, Rich N. Adult human saphenous vein endothelial cells: Assessment of their reproductive capacity for use in endothelial seeding of vascular prostheses. J Surg Res 1985; 36(6):588-596.

65. Hackett SF, Friedman Z, Campochiaro PA. Cyclic 3', 5'-adenosine monophosphate modulates vascular endothelial cell migration in vitro. Cell Biol Int Rep 1987; 11(4):279-287.

66. Klein-Soyer C, Archipoff G, Beretz A, Cazenave JP. Opposing effects of heparin with TGF-beta or afgf during repair of a mechanical wound of human endothelium. Influence of cAMP on cell migration. Biol Cell 1992; 75(2):155-162.

67. Ogawa S, Koga S, Kuwabara K. Hypoxia-induced increased permeability of endothelial monolayers occurs through lowering of cellular cAMP, Am J Physiol 1992; 262(3 Pt 1):C 546-554.

68. Archipoff G, Beretz A, Bartha K, Brisson C, de la Salle D, Froget-Leon C, Klein-Soyer C, Cazenave JP. Role of cyclic AMP in promoting the thromboresistance of human endothelial cells by enhancing thrombomodulin and decreasing tissue factor activities. Br J Pharm 1993; 109:18-28.

69. Graier WF, Groschner K, Schmidt K, Kukovetz WR. Increases in endothelial cAMP levels amplify agonist-induced formation of endothelium derived relaxing factor (EDRF). Biochem J 1992; 288(Pt 2):345-349.

70. Sung C-P, Arleth A, Shikano K, Zabko-Potapovich B, Berkowitz B. Effects of trypsination in cell culture on bradykinin receptors in vascular endothelial cells. Bio Pharm 1989; 38:696-99.

71. Flugelman MY, Virmani R, Leon MB, Bowman RL, Dichek DA. Retroviral vector-mediated gene transfer into endothelial cells. Mol Biol Med 1991; 8(2):257-66.

72. Newman KD, Nguyen N, Dichek DA. Enhancement of the fibrinolytic activity of sheep endothelial cells by retroviral vector-mediated gene transfer. Blood 1991; 77(3):533-41.

73. Lee SW, Kahn ML, Dichek DA. Optimization of retroviral vector-mediated gene transfer into endothelial cells in vitro. Circ Res 1992; 71(6):1508-17.

74. Dichek DA, Nussbaum O, Degen SJ, Anderson WF. Genetically engineered endothelial cells remain adherent and viable after stent deployment and exposure to flow in vitro. Circ Res 1992; 70(2):348-54.

75. Moldovan F, Bennani H, Fiet J, Cussenot O, Dumas J, Darbord C, Soliman HR. Establishment of permanent human endothelial cells achieved by transfection with Large T antigen that retain typical phenotypical and functional characteristics. In vitro Cell Dev Biol Anim 1996; 32(1):16-23.

CHAPTER 15

Risk Factors for Autologous Endothelial Cell Cultures

Johann Meinhart, Manfred Deutsch, Peter Zilla

Introduction

The history of cell culture started over a hundred years ago, when Wilhelm Roux showed in 1885 that embryonic cells can survive outside the animal body. Since then the knowledge of how to culture cells in vitro has steadily increased. Today, cell cultures are a powerful tool to address many fundamental questions in biology and medicine. Recent advances have made it possible to utilize cultured human cells for therapeutic use. Cultured cells have been used to reconstruct skin, bone and many other tissues, including the endothelium. As a consequence, endothelial cells can be used clinically for the physiological masking of synthetic vascular grafts in order to reduce their thrombotic risk. Several studies were performed in past years with different methods[1-7] to achieve endothelialization of otherwise nonhealing grafts. The presence of endothelial cells on synthetic vascular grafts reportedly diminishes the thromboembolic risk[8,9] and it seems to inhibit the formation of anastomotic hyperplasia.[10] Additionally, endothelial cell-covered grafts are probably less prone to graft infection.[11] One method of actively facilitating graft endothelialization is in vitro lining with cultured autologous endothelial cells.[12-14] This technique could prove its effectiveness in long term clinical applications.[15-19] However, despite optimized culture and harvesting procedures, cultures may fail to grow. Since reproducibility of viable autologous cell cultures is a prerequisite for routine clinical use, we have investigated the influence of certain patient-related risk factors on the growth capability of autologous endothelial cells.

Standard Cell Culture Technique for Autologous Endothelial Cell Cultures

Optimal cell harvesting and culture conditions for human vascular endothelial cells have been established and described accurately in previous publications[20-22] and also reviewed in this volume (see chapter 14). For autologous in vitro endothelialization, a short segment of a subdermal vein (mainly jugular and cephalic) is taken under local anesthesia. The vessel is cannulated in situ and filled with collagenase. Primary cells are plated in one T12 culture flask. At a well defined stage of preconfluence (90% surface coverage; p index equal 0.9), primary cultures are passaged to two T162 culture flasks. Culture medium is renewed twice a week by replacing half of the volume with fresh culture medium, consisting of medium 199 with Earls's salts, supplemented with 180 µg/ml preservative-free heparin, 10 ng/ml bFGF, 10 µg/ml and 20% autologous serum. For autologous serum preparation, 250 ml blood is taken from patients and allowed to clot over night at 4°. For both the assessment of 90% confluence in the primary culture and the continual quantification of cells in the two T162 flasks, a microgrid technique is routinely applied.[23] This method provides a partial coverage index ("p" index) of a given cell culture area ranging from 0 (no cells) to 1.0 (confluent cell culture). Thus, the p index semiquantitatively reflects the growth capacity of primary endothelial cells in culture.

Apart from the evaluation of endothelial cell growth, cultures are also morphologically assessed. Vacuolization and cell shape are classified on a scale ranging from 0 (typical polygonal) to 5 (dendritic) for cell shape and from 0 (no vacuoles) to 5 (predominantly vacuoles) for vacuolization. The morphology index ("m") is therefore m=0 for ideal polygonal, nonvacuolized endothelial cells and m=10 for maximally vacuolized, highly dendritic but still viable cells.

Continuous light microscopic assessment of morphological appearance and quantification of cultures provides a good estimation of cell viability and proliferative capacity. Thus, mitigation of cell growth can be detected at an early stage. The most frequent problems with autologous endothelial cell cultures will be described in the following chapters.

Procedure Related Risk Factors

Surgical Vein Harvest

Naturally, autologous human venous endothelial cell cultures need a sufficient vein segment as a cell source. This vein should be easily accessible for surgical excision in order to keep dissection time short and, therefore, mechanical damage low. To further reduce premature mechanical detachment of endothelial cells, a no touch technique for vein harvesting is in use.[23] In brief, after careful touch-free dissection, the vessel is cannulated in situ with two free-flow vessel cannulas with attached 3-way taps. In order to remove remaining blood, the vein is flushed with culture medium in a pulsatile manner and filled with a collagenase solution. The solution is kept under minor pressure within the vein by closing the 3-way taps. After excision, the cannulated and collagenase-filled vein segment is transferred to the laboratory in a thermos container at 37°C for further incubation. If cannulation takes too long, the endothelium might be damaged by air drying. Thus, if cannulation is difficult due to a small vessel diameter or other circumstances, the vein should be flushed intermittently with medium. All manipulations with the vein should be done gently, wearing starch free gloves, since glove powder has been found to be cytotoxic for endothelial cell cultures.[24]

Cell Culture

A 15 minute incubation time with a 0.1% collagenase solution guarantees a maximal yield of endothelial cells. Since all proteolytic enzymes are potentially cytotoxic to cells and commercially available collagenases vary in activity, it might be necessary to test each vial separately. Since the initial goal of in vitro endothelialization was to use only pure endothelial cell cultures for the lining of synthetic vascular prostheses, we tried to avoid the concomitant harvesting of undesirable cells like fibroblasts and smooth muscle cells by fine tuning the enzymatic digestion time and enzymatic activity. These supposedly "contaminating" cells can be detected by immunofluorescence or, in a later stage of cultiva-

tion, by their typical morphological appearance. However, as more information on clinical long term results emerges, smooth muscle cells and fibroblasts appear in a different light, as they play a substantial role in vessel wall formation.[18,25] In future, one will probably tend to have a mixture of vascular cells seeded onto the graft surface, which would de facto mean a convergence of culture and mass harvest procedures.

After successful growth of primary cultures, trypsin is the standard enzyme for the detachment of cells from the surface of culture flasks in order to passage them into larger containers. Trypsinization, especially of primary human endothelial cell cultures, should be performed very carefully. When using 37°C 0.05% trypsin-0.02% EDTA solution, incubation time should not exceed 2 minutes.[23]

For endothelial cell cultures, different media like RPMI, MEM or medium 199 have been used by different authors, with satisfactory results. Medium 199 was originally formulated for the growth of chick fibroblasts, but with Earl's salts is now widely used for endothelial cell culture. Liquid media have a limited shelf life due to the decay of several compounds over time, even at 4°C. This is especially true for L-glutamine. Complete medium should therefore not be kept at 37°C for a prolonged time, since this will result in pH and osmolality change. Moreover, free radical formation might occur, which would result in severe cell damage.

Substitution of the culture medium with growth factors is necessary to reach optimal proliferation, even when serum is supplemented. A multitude of growth factors for endothelial cells, like PDGF, EGF and FGFs have been identified and have been described in numerous publications. For standard endothelial cell culture, bFGF is the most frequently used growth factor. The importance of FGF exceeds mere acceleration of proliferation, as total FGF deprivation in the culture medium also leads to apoptosis of endothelial cells.[26]

Supplementation with antibiotics might be necessary, but they should be used with great care, due to their potential cytotoxicity. Microbial contamination can occur from time to time. Serious infections with yeasts, molds and bacteria are macroscopically visible in cultures. However, chronically infected cultures can be inconspicuous, often only distinguished by decreased cell proliferation. Therefore, microbiological tests should be routinely performed for clinically used cultures. Decreased proliferation capacity without substantial morphological deterioration might also be an indication for an infection with mycroplasms. Several test kits are available for mycoplasm detection. In contrast, the detection of viruses in cell cultures is more difficult than that of bacteria or fungi. Detection methods include coculture systems, transmission electron microscopy and immunofluorescence. Some viruses cause cytological changes like cell rounding, vacuolization or syncytium formation. Since these morphological changes are often similar to other deteriorating influences like cell aging or increased lipid content of serum, the existence of viruses should be kept in mind.[27]

Standard cell culture flasks made of polystyrene are surface treated to promote adhesion and proliferation of attachment dependent cells. Endothelial cells cultured in

20% autologous serum readily adhere to polystyrene with subsequent spreading and growth. This might be facilitated by serum vitronectin and serum fibronectin.[28] The role of fibronectin as a promoter of cell migration and tight anchorage of endothelial cells to many biomaterials has been described extensively.[29-31] Therefore, polystyrene culture dishes are frequently precoated with fibronectin, but other adhesion substances like collagen or gelatin are also used.

The quality of practically all reagents varies from supplier to supplier. Additionally, quality might even be different between batches from the same supplier. These facts should be kept in mind when encountering cell culture problems. Defective machines, like centrifuges, rotation devices and incubators, might also lead to culture problems and should be mentioned briefly here. Above all, incubators should be checked for accurate temperature, humidity and CO_2. Incubators might also be a source of repeated contaminations.

Patient Related Risk Factors

Influences of age or genetic constitution on cell viability and proliferative capacity are well known. In the cardiovascular system, age-associated alterations in vascular cell function lead to vessel wall thickening, increased dilation and aberrant distribution of smooth muscle cells. It is believed that these changes play a fundamental role in the onset of atherosclerosis.[33] Besides these intrinsic factors, acquired factors may alter cellular functions as well. Patients enrolled in our endothelialization of vascular grafts program already had quite a long history of vascular disease before they had to undergo surgical reconstruction for peripheral arterial occlusion. They were treated conservatively and many of them were already operated for other vascular diseases like coronary heart disease or occlusion of the iliac artery. A substantial number had already undergone PTA (percutaneous transluminal angioplasty) before they had to be treated surgically. The majority of patients had one or more risk factors for atherosclerosis. Therefore, these patients formed a quite homogenous group with respect to age, risk factors and clinical stage of disease. Despite this fact, we found differences with regard to the in vitro growth behavior of the endothelial cells of these patients. Thirty-four percent of all cultures showed impaired growth capacity. Cells displayed strong vacuolization and were partially dendritic (Fig. 15.1), a morphological appearance which was previously shown to lead to imminent cell death.[16] When we measured a multitude of serum parameters we found all three main lipid constituents, triglycerides, cholesterol and lipoprotein A, significantly ($p < 0,05$) elevated in sera of patients whose cell cultures initially failed to grow (Table 15.1). Numerous studies have previously shown that hyperlipidemia causes endothelial changes. This includes increased endocytotic activity[34] inhibition of prostacyclin production,[35] increased monocyte-endothelial cell adhesion,[36] disruption of the barrier function,[37] apoptosis[38] and

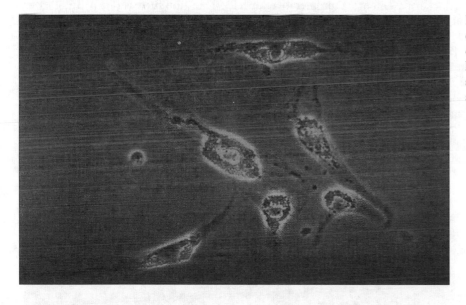

Fig. 15.1. Day 3 culture of a patient's endothelial cells cultured in medium containing 20% autologous serum with high levels of serum lipids. Cells exhibit strong vacuolation and have a dendritic appearance.

Table 15.1. Content of cholesterol, triglycerides, lipoprotein A and glucose in sera of patients with normal growth characteristics of cells compared to sera of patients with initial growth failure of cells and to nonrecovering cell cultures after serum change.

mg/dl ± SD	cholesterol	triglycerides	lipoprotein	glucose
normal growth	220.1±51.1	250.9±202.0	22.2±26.6	139.1±76.3
initial growth failure	262.0±56.8	421.4±298.0	35.9±28.3	108.25±66.25
nonrecovering cultures	222.8±57.5	265.0±166.1	56.25±16.7	205.0±97.1

cytotoxicity.[39] From experimentally induced rabbit atherosclerotic aortas, an increased number of multinucleated giant endothelial cells have been harvested and cultured,[40] a finding quite similar to our own observation. Moreover, lipoprotein A has previously been found to be an independent risk factor for atherosclerosis.[41]

Apart from hyperlipidemia, diabetes is another major risk factor for pathological changes of the vasculature. On the cellular basis it has been shown that endothelial cells cultured in the presence of high glucose levels have a reduced proliferative capacity. Accelerated endothelial cell death[42] is believed to be due to facilitated apoptosis,[43] but may also have osmotic causes. In this context it was interesting that we found higher glucose levels in the serum of patients with normally growing cultures than in sera of patients whose cultures initially failed to grow. Therefore, moderately increased glucose does not seem to affect viability and growth capacity of primary endothelial cell cultures.

The third well established risk factor for the vasculature is smoking tobacco. Its negative influence on endothelial cells has previously been described.[44] Particularly, a lower harvest efficiency and a suppressed reproductive capacity has been reported for autologous endothelial cell cultures from smokers.[45] This is in accordance with our finding that the mean number of harvested cells from smokers was significantly lower in smokers than nonsmokers. However, since the subsequent proliferative behavior of endothelial cells did not significantly differ, our observation supports the previous interpretation that a considerably thicker basement membrane may be responsible for a stronger endothelial cell attachment in smokers.[46]

However, in contrast to other risk factors influencing the successful growth of autologous endothelial cells, the damaging effects of hyperlipidemia can be reversed. When serum is changed from autologous to pooled homologous serum in cultures with morphological signs of growth failure, all cultures, with a few exceptions, regain their proliferative capacity together with a typical morphological appearance (Figs. 15.2 and 15.3). It was also interesting to see that reversibility applied especially to elevated triglyceride and cholesterol levels. The fact that those cultures which irreversibly failed to grow had unproportionally increased levels of lipoprotein A might be an indication that this serum lipid has a particularly damaging effect on endothelial cells.

Summary and Future Aspects

The successful cultivation of autologous endothelial cells is endangered by both procedure dependent and patient dependent risk factors. Reasons for failing cultures due to procedure-related problems are mechanical damage during vein dissection, contaminations and inadequate reagents. However, the most frequent problems with autologous endothelial cell cultures are related to patient factors. Most of the patients who have to undergo bypass surgery have a multitude of major risk factors. Numerous clinical and experimental studies have revealed smoking, diabetes and hyperlipidemia to be major independent risk factors for atherosclerosis. The additive detrimental effect of these risk factors on the vasculature has been further documented.[47-49] Our data seem to reflect these findings in vitro. We found significantly different contents of cholesterol, triglycerides, lipoprotein A and glucose in the sera of patients with initial growth failure as compared to sera of patients with normal primary growth. However, by replacing the patient's own serum as a culture supplement with pooled serum from healthy young donors, the majority of cultures recovered, regaining their normal morphological appearance and full proliferative capacity. Thus, the success rate of autologous endothelial cells cultured for the endothelialization of synthetic vascular grafts was increased from the previous 73-95%. This improvement, together with a further simplification of the seeding process, makes in vitro endothelialization even more clinically practicable. The beneficial long term results in peripheral revascularization and the first promising data for clinically used endothelialized synthetic coronary bypass grafts[50] provide encouraging arguments for a wider application.

Fig. 15.2. Same culture as in Figure 15.1, but 48 h after change from autologous serum to low-lipid pooled homologous serum. The vacuolation has almost completely disappeared.

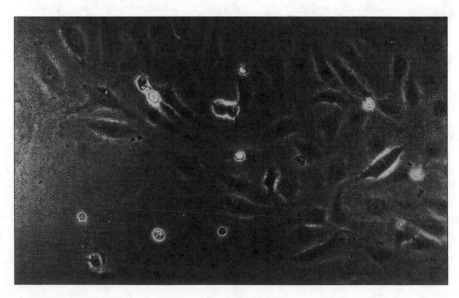

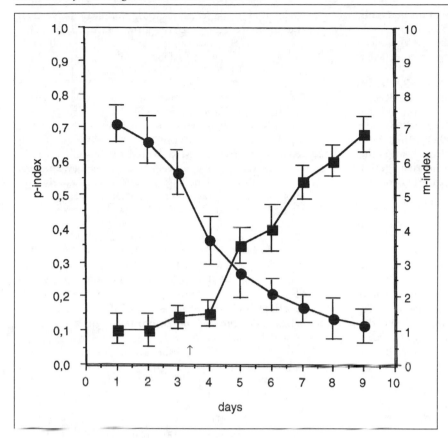

Fig. 15.3. Double y-curve of p indexes (squares) and m indexes (circles) of primary cultures with initial growth failure. Serum change led to an increase in proliferative capacity with a decrease of altered morphological appearance at the same time.

It is quite obvious and desirable that tissue engineering is directing its effort towards fascinating goals like high tech, ready to implant grafts with features of a native artery. However, the fact that a substantial number of patients will have an impaired endothelium, not able to regenerate or fulfill necessary physiological functions, should be considered when discussing these future approaches. Until the successful introduction of a fully engineered vascular prosthesis which emulates native arteries structurally and functionally, in vitro endothelialization will remain a feasible method of improving the performance of synthetic vascular grafts. Centers of excellence could provide endothelialized grafts to a number of neighboring hospitals. This prospect is even more exciting in view of the possibility to genetically modify endothelial cells.[51] Moreover, endothelialization could be used as a generalized hemocompatible drug delivery system which enables the creation of individual delivery schemes for each single patient. Vascular grafts and endothelialization could also be used for the development of various tissue engineered organs. Different cell types, allogenic or xenogenic, could be seeded on the graft surface. These cells would be subsequently covered confluently by autologous endothelial cells, in order to inhibit the immune response. Thus some fascinating prospectives still inhere to endothelialization.

References

1. Herring MB, Gardner AL, Glover JL et al. A single staged technique for seeding vascular grafts with autogenous endothelium. Surgery 1978; 4:498-504.
2. Graham LM, Burkel WE, Ford JW et al. Immediate seeding of enzymatically derived endothelium in dacron vascular grafts. Arch Surg 1980; 115:289-94.
3. Zilla P, Fasol R, Deutsch M et al. Endothelial cell seeding of polytetrafluoroethylene vascular grafts in humans: A preliminary report. J Vasc Surg 1987; 6:535-41.
4. Meerbaum SO, Sharp WV, Schmidt SP. Lower extremity revascularization with polytetrafluoroethylene grafts seeded with microvascular endothelial cells. In Zilla P, Fasol R, Callow A, eds. Applied Cardiovascular biology 1990-1991. Basel: Karger, 1992;107-119.
5. Williams SK, Rose DG, Jarrell BE. Microvascular endothelial cell sodding of ePTFE vascular grafts: Improved patency and stability of the cellular lining. J Biomed Mat Res 1994; 28:203-212.
6. Pasic M, Müller-Glauser W, Odermatt B et al. Seeding with omental cells prevents late intimal hyperplasia in small-diameter Dacron grafts. Circulation 1995; 92:2605-16.
7. Greisler HP, Cziperle DJ, Kim DU et al. Enhanced endothelialization of expanded polytetrafluoroethylene grafts by fibroblast growth factor pretreatment. Surgery 1992; 112:244-54.
8. Örtenwall P, Wadenvik H, Risberg B. Reduced platelet deposition on seeded versus unseeded segments of expanded polytetrafluoroethylene grafts: Clinical observations after a 6-month follow-up. J Vasc Surg 1989; 10:374-380.
9. Örtenwal P, Wadenvik H, Kutti J. Endothelial cell seeding reduces thrombogeneicity of dacron grafts in humans. J Vasc Surg 1990; 11:403-10.
10. Graham LM, Brothers TE, Vincent CK et al. The role of an endothelail cell lining in limiting distal anastomotic

intimal hyperplasia of 4-mm-i.d.dacron grafts in a canine model. J Biomed Mat Res 1991; 25:525-533.

11. Rosenman JE, Kempczinski RF, Berlatzky Y et al. Bacterial adherence to endothelial-seeded polytetrafluoroethylene grafts. Surgery 1985; 98:816-823.

12. Zilla P, Fasol R, Dudeck U, Siedler S, Preiss P, Fischlein T, Müller-Glauser W, Baitella G,Sanan D, Odell J, Reichart B. In situ cannulation, microgrid follow-up and low density plating provide first pasage endothelial cell mass cultures for in vitro lining. J Vasc Surg 1990; 12:180-189.

13. Zilla P, Fasol R, Preiss P, Kadletz M, Deutsch M, Schima H, Tsangaris S, Groscurth P. Use of fibrin glue as a substrate for in vitro endothelialization of PTFE vascular grafts. Surgery 19989; 105:515-522.

14. Zilla P, Preiss P, Groscurth P, Rösemeier F, Deutsch M, Odell J, Heidinger C, Fasol R, von Oppell U. In vitro-lined endothelium: Initial integrity and ultrastructural events. Surgery 1994; 116:524-534.

15. Magometschnigg H, Kadletz M,Vodrazka M et al. Prospective clinical study with in vitro endothelial cell lining of expanded polytetrafluoroethylene grafts in crural repeat reconstruction. J Vasc Surg 1992; 15:527-35.

16. Zilla P, Deutsch M, Meinhart J, Puschmann R, Eberl T, Minar E, Dudczak R, Lugmaier H, Schmidt P, Noscian I, Fischlein T. Clinical in vitro endothelialization of femoropopliteal bypass graft: An actuarial follow-up over three years. J Vasc Surg 1994; 19:540-548.

17. Fischlein T, Zilla P, Meinhart J, Puschmann R, Vesely M, Eberl T, Balon R, Deutsch M. In vitro endothelialization of a mesosystemic shunt: A clinical case report. J Vasc Surg 1994: 19:549-554.

18. Deutsch M, Meinhart J, Vesely M, Groscurth P, Von Oppell U, Zilla P. In vitro endothelialization of ePTFE grafts: A clinical case report after 41 months of implantation. J Vasc Surg 1997; 25:757-763.

19. Meinhart J, Deutsch M, Zilla P Eight years of clinical endothelial cell transplantation. Closing the gap between prosthetic grafts and vein grafts. ASAIO J 1997; 43:M515-M521.

20. Jaffe E, Nachmann R, Becker C et al. Culture of human endothelial cells derived from umbilical veins.Identification by morphological and immunological criteria. J Clin Invest 1973; 52:2757-2764.

21. Haegerstrand A, Gillis C, Bengtsson L et al. Serial cultivation of adult human endothelium from the great saphenous vein. J Vasc Surg 1992; 16:280-285.

22. Gillis C, Jonzon B, Haegerstrand A. Effects of sera, basic fibroblast growth factor, heparin and cyclic AMP-stimulation on proliferation of human vascular endothelial cells. Cell Mol Biol 1995; 41:1131-1138.

23. Zilla P, Fasol R, Dudeck U, Siedler S, Preiss P, Fischlein T, Müller-Glauser W, Baitella G, Sanan D, Odell J, Reichart B. In situ cannulation, microgrid follow-up and low density plating provide first passage endothelial cell mass cultures for in vitro lining. J Vasc Surg 1990; 12:180-189.

24. Sharefkin JB, Fairchild KD, Albus RA et al. The cytotoxic effects of surgical glove powder particles on adult human vascular endothelial cell cultures: Implications for use of tissue culture techniques. J Surg Res 1986; 41:463-72.

25. Baitella-Eberle G, Groscurth P, Zilla P et al. Long term results of tissue development and cell differentiation on Dacron prostheses seeded with microvascular cells in dogs. J Vasc Surg 1993; 18:1019-28.

26. Araki S, Shimada Y, Hayashi H. Apoptosis of vascular endothelial cells by fibroblast growth factor deprivation. Biochem Biophys Res Comm 1990; 168:1194-1200.

27. Cell and Tissue Culture: Laboratory Procedures. In: Doyle A, Griffiths JB, Newell DG, eds. Chichester: John Wiley & Sons Ltd, 1993; 7:7A-7C.

28. Steele JG, Johnson G, Underwood PA. Role of serum vitronectin and fibronectin in adhesion of fibroblasts following seeding onto tissue culture polystyrene. J Biomed Mat Res 1992; 26:861-884.

29. Keseler KA, Herring MB, Arnold MP et al. Enhanced strength of endothelial cell seeding using expanded polytetrafluoroethylene vascular grafts: A comparison of four substrates. J Vasc Surg 1986; 3:58-64.

30. Vohra R, Thomson JL, Carr HMH et al In vitro aherence and kinetics studies of adult human endothelial cell seeded polytetrafluoroethylene and gelatin impregnated Dacron grafts. Eur J Vasc Surg 1991; 5:93-103.

31. Poot A, Beugeling T, Dekker A, Spijkers J et al. Dependence of endothelial cell growth on substrate bound fibronectin. Clinical Materials 1992; 11:151-155.

32. Carr HM, Vohra R, Sharma H et al. Endothelial cell kinetics under chronic flow in prosthetic grafts. Ann Vasc Surg 1996; 10:469-75.

33. Crow MT, Boluyt MO, Lakatta EG. The molecular and cellular biology of aging in the cardiovascular system. In: Holbrook NJ, Martin GR, Lockshin RA, eds. Cellular aging and cell death. Chichester: John Wiley & Sons, 1996:81-107.

34. Holland JA, Pritchard KA, Rogers NJ et al. Atherogenic levels of low density lipoprotein increase endocytotic activity in cultured human endothelial cells. Am J Pathol 1992; 140:551-558.

35. Peng SK, Hu B, Peng A et al. Effect of cholesterol oxides on prostacyclin production and platelet adhesion. Artery 1993; 20:122-134.

36. De Gruijter M, Hoogerbrugge N, van Rijn M et al. Patients with combined hypercholesterolemia-hypertriglyceridemia show an increased monocyte-endothelial cell adhesion in vitro: Triglyceride level as a major determinant. Metabolism 1991; 40:1119-1121.

37. Guretzki HJ, Gerbitz KD, Olgemöller B et al. Atherogenic levels of low density lipoprotein alter the permeability and composition of the endothelial barrier. Atherosclerosis 1994; 107:15-24.

38. Lizard G, Deckert V, Dubrez L et al. Induction of apoptosis in endothelial cells treated with cholesterol oxides. Am J Pathol 1996; 148:1625-1638.

39. Sevanian A, Berliner J, Peterson H. Uptake, metabolism, and cytotoxicity of isomeric cholesterol-5,6-epoxides in rabbit aortic endothelial cells. J Lipid Res 1991; 32:147-155.

40. Tashiro K, Shimokama T, Haraoka S et al. Endothelial cell heterogeneity in experimentally-induced rabbit atherosclerosis. Demonstration of multinucleated giant endothelial cells by scanning electron microscopy and cell culture. Virchows Archiv 1994; 425:521-529.

41. Schreiner PJ, Morrisett JD, Sharrett R et al. Lipoprotein (a) as a risk factor for preclinical atherosclerosis. Arteriosclerosis and Thrombosis 1993; 13:826-833.

42. Cagliero E, Roth T, Taylor AW, Lorenzi M. The effect of high glucose on human endothelial cell growth and gene expression are not mediated by transformtin growth factor-b. Lab Investig 1995; 73:667-673.

43. Baumgartner-Parzer S, Wagner L, Pettermann M et al. High-glucose-triggered apoptosis in cultured endothelial cells. Diabetes 1995; 44:1323-1327.

44. Strohschneider T, Oberhoff M, Hanke H, Hannekum A, Karsch KR. Effect of chronic nicotine delivery on the proliferation rate of endothelial and smooth muscle cells in experimentally induced vascular wall plaques. Clin Investig 1994; 72:908-912.

45. Zilla P, Siedler S, Fasol R et al. Reduced reproductive capacity of freshly harvested endothelial cells in smokers: A possible shortcoming in the success of seeding? J Vasc Surg 1989; 10:143-8.

46. Asmusen I, Kjelsen K. Intima ultrastructure of human umbilical arteries: Observations of arteries from newborn children of smoking and non-smoking mothers. Circ Res 1975; 36:579-589.

47. Bartens W, Rader D, Talley G et al. Decreased plasma levels of lipoprotein (a) in patients with hypertriglycerdemia. Atherosclerosis 1994; 108:149-157.

48. Pech-Ansellem MA, Myara I, Storogenko M et al. Enhanced modification of low-density lipoproteins (LDL) by endothelial cells from smokers: A possible mechanism of smoking-related atherosclerosis. Cariovascular Research 1996; 31:975-983.

49. Blache D, Bouthillier D, Davignon J. Acute influence of smoking on platelet behaviour, endothelium and plasma lipids and normalization by aspirin. Atherosclerosis 1992; 93:179-188.

50. Laube HR, Duwe J, Claus M et al. Autologous endothelial cell seeded PTFE vascular grafts for coronary artery bypass: First clinical results. 15th International Cardiovascular Surgical Symposion. Zürs: Austria, 1997, March 8-15.

51. Dichek DA. Therapeutic potential of genetic engineering: Enhancement of endothelial cell fibrinolysis. In: Zilla P, Fasol R, Callow A, eds. Applied vardiovascular Biology 1990-1991. Basel: Karger, 1992:197-204.

CHAPTER 16

Adhesion Molecule Expression Following In Vitro Lining

Caroline Gillis-Hægerstrand

Introduction

The possibility that human ECs can be seeded on vascular prosthetic grafts to create a "look-alike" to the natural blood vessel is intriguing. The new field of tissue engineering has awakened an interest in many scientists from different disciplines which makes the research area fascinating. Important breakthroughs have greatly enhanced our understanding of the functions of the human endothelial cell. Today it is well accepted that the endothelium is indeed a very active "organ". The endothelium is crucial in maintenance of hemostasis, coagulation and fibrinolysis, as well as in the regulation of vascular tonus, inflammation, immune reactions, angiogenesis and vascular permeability.[1-6]

Long term patency of artificial vascular grafts for hemodialysis access and for bypass or interposition in small caliber arteries is limited due to neointimal hyperplasia and associated graft thrombosis. If these grafts could be seeded with well functioning, adherent ECs which are not activated and expresses adhesion molecules to which leukocytes can adhere, these problems could partly be overcome. The same reasoning is valid for biological heart valves.

In this chapter, I will try to cover aspects of how the endothelium interacts with circulating leukocytes and how an endothelial lining of artificial, cell free materials may effect the adherence of leukocytes.

Vascular Grafts

There are different kinds of grafts to be used for different purposes in vascular surgery.

Autologous Grafts

Autologous vessels are still the preferred vascular substitute. They are superior to all other available alternatives, although it has been demonstrated that surgical preparation partly denudes the vessels and damages the endothelium.[7] A complete re-endothelialization after implantation of these grafts has been shown.[8] The obvious drawback to using autologous vessels is the limited supply. Another problem is intimal hyperplasia, which is thought to be initiated when the endothelium is damaged during the operation. Hyperplasia is a major reason for re-operation or repeated PTCA procedures after open heart surgery and peripheral vascular surgery.

Prosthetic Grafts

One feature that distinctly distinguishes the cardiovascular prosthetic graft from its natural counterpart is its lack of a confluent endothelium. The development of the ideal prosthetic vascular graft has been one of the major goals of vascular surgery since the first

Tissue Engineering of Prosthetic Vascular Grafts, edited by Peter Zilla and Howard P. Greisler.
©1999 R.G. Landes Company.

grafts were used over 40 years ago. The aim has been to achieve a completely endothelialized prosthetic graft where the cells not only remain when the blood flow is restored, but also retain their wide range of functions. Synthetic grafts have acceptable patency rates when used in areas of high blood flow and good run-off to replace vessels of an inner diameter greater than 5-6 mm.[9] When used in low flow areas, the expectations regarding patency are not currently being fulfilled. The two types of synthetic vascular grafts that have gained the widest acceptance are Dacron and ePTFE. Glutaraldehyde-tanned homologous grafts are another alternative but their use is under debate.

Dacron

The manufacturing process allows defined variation of porosity. The pores are larger in Dacron grafts than in ePTFE grafts. After Dacron graft implantation, platelet adhesion and aggregation occurs, followed by fibrin formation. Then there is a gradual ingrowth of fibroblasts and capillaries, and a deposition of matrix proteins. A fibrous tissue is formed on the inner lining of the graft as capillaries grow from the exterior to the interior.

ePTFE

ePTFE grafts are made by controlled expansion of the material by heating. The initial thrombus formation on the inner surface of ePTFE grafts when platelets adhere and aggregate is similar to that in Dacron grafts. However, the porosity is much less than that in Dacron grafts, which prevents ingrowth of fibrous tissue and capillaries. No or little spontaneous ingrowth of ECs from anastomoses occurs in man.[10]

Glutaraldehyde-Tanned Grafts

Glutaraldehyde treatment is implemented to reduce antigenicity, sterilize the graft and stabilize the tissue by crosslinking of collagen.[11] Two of the side effects of this treatment are that calcification of the tissue is promoted and a spontaneous ingrowth of ECs is prohibited.[12,13] The hostile environment to any adhering or ingrowing cell type due to toxic residues of glutaraldehyde may delay an inflammatory/ foreign body reaction to the graft. However, inflammatory cells, macrophages and T cells in the tissue at explantation have been described by several groups.[14]

Heart Valve Prostheses

Mechanical heart valves, or heart valve bioprostheses, similar to the native are frequently used in cardiac surgery. Patients receiving the former, most often containing one or more pyrolytic carbon disks attached to a sewing ring, need life long anticoagulant medication to prevent thromboembolic events, which is associated with a higher risk of bleeding disorders. The degenerative process of a bioprosthetic graft has a multifactorial etiology. Inflammatory,[15] mechanical,[16] and metabolic processes[17,18] as well as the glutaraldehyde per se,[12,13] have been discussed as contributing factors. These bioprostheses are slowly deteriorated due a complex reaction involving stepwise calcification, resulting in poor hemodynamic performance.

Inflammation

Inflammation is the reaction of living tissues to all forms of injury. It involves vascular, neurologic, humoral and cellular responses at the site of injury. The adherence of neutrophils and monocytes to the vascular endothelium is a hallmark of acute inflammation. At sites of inflammation, vascular ECs undergo functional and morphological changes collectively referred to as endothelial activation.[19,20] Cytokines such as IL-1[21] and TNF-α[22] induce functional changes in human ECs in vitro, including increased adhesiveness for leukocytes.[23] In vivo models have also shown that cytokines induce changes corresponding to endothelial activation when introduced to tissues.[24] When stimulated with histamine, thrombin or superoxides the ECs rapidly express P-selectin for approximately 20 min. When activated by cytokines such as IL-1 or TNF-α, the endothelium expresses an array of inducible adhesion molecules, e.g., P-selectin, E-selectin, VCAM-1 and ICAM-1 (Fig. 16.1).

The improvement of cardiovascular prosthetic materials, to reduce thrombus formation and inflammatory/immunological reactions, is a technological as well as a biological challenge. By mediating adhesion and by expressing adhesion molecules to which leukocytes adhere, ECs play a key role in inflammatory reactions. The process of leukocyte adherence, activation and migration involves an interplay between ECs, leukocyte activation and local cytokine activity. An activated leukocyte is likely to adhere to the endothelium even if the endothelium itself is expressing a "normal" range of adhesion-promoting molecules on its surface. A firm adhesion and transmigration into the subendothelial tissue requires an interplay between the leukocyte and the ECs, where activation and structural changes occur in the endothelium. Although the neutrophil is considered more reactive and has been most extensively studied in this respect, the monocyte expresses a similar range of adhesion molecules as do neutrophils and respond to similar stimuli. T lymphocytes are likely to play an important role in the body's reaction to a foreign material. Less is known about T lymphocyte-endothelial interactions.

Endothelial cells express three families of adhesion molecules which interact with leukocytes: selectins, immunoglobulins and integrins.

Selectins

Selectins are cell surface glycoproteins found on the endothelium, leukocytes and platelets. Selectins binds to carbohydrate rich domains on white blood cells. Platelet selectin (P-selectin) is found in granules of the ECs, known as Weibel-palade bodies. Upon stimulation with, e.g., thrombin, P-selectin is rapidly mobilized to the cell surface of ECs as well as platelets.[25] The expression is short lived, declining substantially within a few minutes.

Endothelial cell selectin (E-selectin) expression is largely restricted to activated ECs.[26] Cultured ECs express E-selectin after exposure to interleukin-1 (IL-1), tumor necrosis factor alpha (TNF-α) or lipopolysacharide (LPS).[23,27] Maximal surface expression is observed at 4-6 h, followed by a decline. The basal levels are usually reached 24-48 h after stimulation.

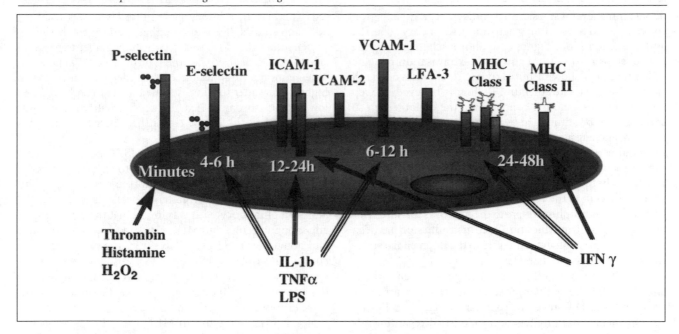

Fig. 16.1. Induction and peak expression of endothelial cell adhesion molecules. H_2O_2 = superoxide, IL = interleukin, TNF = tumor necrosis factor, LPS = lipopolysacchariode (endotoxin), IFN = interferon, ICAM = intercellular adhesion molecule, VCAM = vascular cell adhesion molecule, MHC = major histomcompatibility complex. Please note that ICAM-2 and LFA-3 are constitutively expressed and that MHC class I is both constitutively expressed and inducible.

Ig Superfamily

Unlike E-selectin expression, the elevated expression of the Ig superfamily is not transient but is, rather, sustained over several days. The Ig superfamily binds to integrins on the surface of the white blood cells. Intercellular adhesion molecule-1 (ICAM-1) is expressed on ECs after 8-12 h of stimulation with IL-1 or TNF-α.[28] ICAM-2 expression on ECs does not appear to be regulated by cytokines.[29]

ICAM-3 is a ligand for the leukocyte integrins LFA-1 (Cd11a/cd18) and $\alpha_d\beta_2$.[30,31] ICAM-3 is constitutively expressed at high levels by all resting leukocytes, such as monocytes, lymphocytes and neutrophils, and antigen presenting cells. It shows a pattern clearly distinct from ICAM-1 and ICAM-2. ICAM-3 also seems to be inducible on vascular endothelium in certain disease states, especially lymphomas and myelomas.[32]

Vascular cell adhesion molecule-1 (VCAM-1) is also upregulated by stimulation of IL-1 or TNF-α, with maximal activity reached after 8-12 h.[33] The expression of immunoglobulin superfamily adhesion molecules occurs more slowly and is prolonged in comparison to E-selectin, as stated earlier. The expression of these adhesion molecules on ECs characterizes a later phase of inflammation, usually when leukocytes adhere to the vessel wall. In cardiac transplant rejection the correlation between endothelial expression of VCAM-1 and infiltration of T lymphocytes is strong.[34] Consequently, the ECs play an important role in transplant rejection. In the experimental situation, this function is emphasized by the reduced rate of allograft rejection described when the native endothelium was removed.[35]

CD31 is another member of the immunoglobulin superfamily. It is expressed on the EC surface as well as on the surface of other cells, e.g., neutrophils and monocytes.[36] CD31 binding is homophilic and is thought to participate in the EC-EC interaction.[37] CD31 antibodies have been shown to inhibit granulocyte transmigration, suggesting that neutrophil-EC CD31 binding is important for the inflammatory process.[38]

Integrins

The integrins are heterodimers consisting of noncovalently associated α and β subunits which mediate both cell-substratum and cell-cell adhesion. They are important in cell adhesion, platelet adhesion and cell migration. Integrin ligands, e.g., RGD (arginine-glycine-aspartic acid) sequences on extracellular matrix proteins, are crucial for attachment of ECs to natural or other surfaces.

The ECs may actively participate in specific immune reactions by expressing the ABO antigen system. They express major histocompatibility complex (MHC) antigens.[39,40] MHC class I is expressed constitutively by ECs and class II (HLA-DR) can be induced by interferon-γ.[41] Once ECs express the MHC class II antigen, they can be considered to act as antigen presenting cells.

Furthermore, activated neutrophils often release oxygen free radicals and other short-lived substances that activate the endothelial cells to release platelt activating factor (PAF) and interleukin-8 (IL-8).[42] Platelet selectin (P-selectin) and PAF, coexpressed on the surfaces of activated ECs, presumably perpetuate the neutrophil-EC interaction.

Leukocyte Adhesion Under Flow Conditions

One of the most important aspects of leukocyte extravasation is that it is a multistep process. This process is divided into several steps: initial contact, primary adhesion (often referred to as rolling), activation, secondary adhesion and transmigration. Figure 16.2 shows schematically the several steps involved in neutrophil extravasation in acute inflammation. Following initial contact, leukocytes often roll slowly along the endothelium. Rolling is believed to keep the cells in close enough contact with the endothelium so that they can be stimulated by substances in the local environment and engage additional binding mechanisms.[43] Rolling requires a definite adhesive interaction, as was first demonstrated by the observation that neuotrophils roll much more slowly than predicted for cells tumbling in the fluid stream adjacent to the vessel wall without any adhesion.[44,45] Stimulated neutrophils adhere to the microvasculature. This is referred to as firm adhesion. Once firm adhesion has been established, the leukocytes migrate to the intercellular junctions, where they can diapedese.[46]

There is a great interest in in vitro endothelialization of cardiovascular prosthetic materials to achieve a confluent and flow-resistant vascular lining.[14,47-51] But, to my knowledge, nothing has been published regarding adhesion molecule expression on EC surface when seeded on prosthetic grafts and exposed to shear stress. More has been written about neutrophil-endothelial cell interactions. Quantitative studies of neutrophil adhesion under flow conditions have shown that overall adhesion decreases with increased flow and wall shear stress.[52,44] It has been shown that the leukocyte adherence is optimal in the postcapillary venular wall, where it is about 1-4 dyn per cm^2. It decreases rapidly at higher shear stresses. However, there are some results suggesting that integrin mediated adhesion in the absence of selectins appears to be effective only at wall shear stresses well below 1 dyn cm^2.[53,54]

Endothelialization Reduces Monocyte Adhesion to Xenogeneic Tissue in a Time Dependent Manner

Our group published a paper in 1995 wherein we investigated monocyte adhesion to de-endothelialized and re-endothelialized porcine aorta (PA) before and after cytokine stimulation.[55] In addition, the expression of a selection of adhesion molecules on the EC surface before and after cytokine stimulation after 1, 3 and 7 days were studied. The human monocytic cell line U937 was used for adhesion studies. It was shown that monocyte adhesion to nonendothelialized PA was significantly higher than adhesion to endothelialized specimens on days 3 and 7. The spontaneous monocyte adhesion to EC-seeded porcine aorta was highest 1 day after seeding, declined on day 3 and remained low on the 7th day. When the endothelialized tissue was stimulated with IL-1β, the adhesion of monocytes increased significantly.

Human saphenous vein ECs (HSVECs) seeded on xenogeneic vascular tissue were shown to express E-selectin, ICAM-1, VCAM-1 and MHC class II in a time-dependent manner. This expression pattern correlates well with the adhesion of monocytes. It was found that the expression of adhesion molecules and MHC class II was similar on viable and nonviable tissue, as well as on ECs seeded on gelatin-coated culture plastic. However, it was also shown that nonspecific mouse IgG binding to the HSVECs was higher one day after seeding, although not as high as the adhesion molecule expression. A significant increase in cellular adhesion molecule expression and in MHC class II expression was observed after stimulation with IL-1β or IFN-γ. The nonspecific binding was not affected after cytokine stimulation. Although mechanical de-endothelialization is a relatively imprecise technique, porcine aorta was used as a biological model tissue, mainly because of its availability. Furthermore, the matrix proteins exposed after scraping are reasonably representative of the matrix on a bioprosthetic graft.

The human monocytic cell line U937 is a relatively immature clone derived from a human histiocytoma. However, the U937 cells present leukocyte surface integrins to allow adequate attachment to ECs.[56] To our knowledge, the expression of U937 integrins, and their role in adhesion to subendothelial tissue, is not well characterized. However, it is likely that "normal" integrins are present on U937 and contribute to the increased binding to de-endothelialized collagenous tissue as compared to endothelialized tissue.[57] The time dependent manner in which the adhesion molecule expression declines, which was found in this study, is interesting for several reasons. It indicates that perhaps one should wait 3-7 days before operating an endothelialized graft in a patient. This notion is supported by other findings such as that the maturation of the cytoskeleton may be

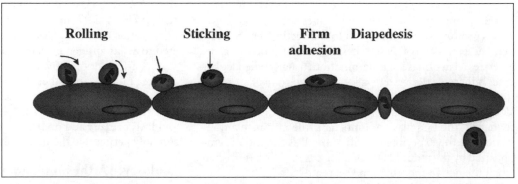

Fig. 16.2. Schematic illustration of adhesion molecule dependent leukocyte interaction with endothelial cells. Initial rolling is a carbohydrate dependent event, whereas sticking and firm adhesion is dependent on Ig-superfamily adhesion molecules on the endothelium binding to integrins on the leukocyte. The diapedesis is at least partly dependent on the homologous binding of the autorecepetor CD31 on both the endothelium and the leukocytes. See text.

Rolling **Sticking** **Firm adhesion** **Diapedesis**

more pronounced after 7-9 days.[58] Furthermore, it has been shown that ECs exposed to chronic shear stress in vitro, applied in a stepwise fashion over several days, are induced to become tightly adherent to the substratum and exhibit more differentiated features.[59] Most likely this assay also gives a better cell retention in seeded grafts after the blood flow has been restored.

There was no difference in the expression of EC adhesion molecules in cells seeded on viable and nonviable tissue specimens. This can be explained by the fact that no immunocompetent cells were present. Apparently, the viable smooth muscle cells, fibroblasts or matrix proteins which were communicating with or exposed to the human ECs, did not influence the ECs' expression of adhesion molecules in this model.

Interestingly, the high levels of monocyte adhesion and nonspecific binding of antibodies on the first day after seeding were also true for ECs seeded on gelatin. This may suggest a nonspecfic activation of ECs by passaging.

In conclusion, there are several findings suggesting that the endothelium is more ready to cope with and survive the conditions in vivo if they are allowed to mature on the graft before transplantation. These findings include the adhesion molecule expression, at least in vitro.

Future Prospect: Antiadhesive Therapy?

Inflammatory response is a crucial consideration in the understanding of many disease processes and in the development of tissue engineering approaches towards therapy. The pharmaceutical industry is developing new anti-inflammatory agents which interfere with leukocyte-endothelial adhesion. In diseases such as rheumatism, this new way of looking at the problem is very promising. One can speculate that such anti-inflammatory agents have a potentially huge market. One approach that can be used is the development of antibodies directed against adhesive molecules on the endothelium, leukocytes and other cell types. However, there will be some difficulties with such a project. The inherent difficulties of this approach include development of serum sickness after injection of foreign protein, diminishing therapeutic effects after prolonged therapy. There will also be a potential for promotion of infections. Other approaches include injection of soluble adhesion molecules which compete with cell-associated adhesion molecules for appropriate counterreceptors.[60] If cultured cells are used, there is a potential of in vitro knock out of specific adhesion molecules to reduce inflammatory responses to a vascular graft. This type of technology would require optimized cell culture and transfection techniques.

Concluding Remarks

Knowledge of the fundamental cellular and molecular mechanisms involved in adhesion and mechanical force modulation of metabolism under conditions that mimic those seen in vivo is essential for real progress to be made in tissue engineering. Bioengineers trained in cell and molecular biology can make unique contributions to this important field. Maybe we are entering a new era of therapeutics: patient-specific therapeutics.[61] This will include tissues, cells

and organs for transplantation and various gene therapy techniques. Because of the integrated systems, and analysis required to understand intracellular functions and intercellular interactions, this development should be done in close cooperation with researchers with training in biology and bioengineers.

The human body is a marvelous feat of engineering. Many vital systems continuously interact with each other in ways that are simultaneously extremely complex yet beautifully simple. Our understanding at the molecular level has made major advances in the last decade. Because these interactions occur dynamically and are subject to various levels of control, much of our increase in knowledge has been possible because of the awareness that real advances require cross-disciplinary teams of bioengineers and biological scientists. This interaction has been and will be extremely beneficial in vascular biology.

Acknowledgments

I wish to thank Associate Professor Anders Hægerstrand for fruitful comments on the manuscript. This study was supported by grants from The Swedish Heart Lung Foundation, The Memorial Foundation of Carl Jeppsson and R & E Lundström.

References

1. Jaffe EA, Nachman RL, Becker CG, Minick CR. Culture of human endothelial cells derived from umbilical veins. Identification by morphologic and immunologic criteria. J Clin Invest 1973; 52:2745-2756.
2. Bloom AL. Physiology of blood coagulation. Haemostasis 1990; 20:14-29.
3. Vane J, Änggård E, Botting R. Regulatory functions of the vascular endothelium. New Engl J Med 1990; 323:27-36.
4. Pober J, Cotran R. The role of endothelial cells in inflammation. Transplantation 1990; 50:537-544.
5. Pober J, Doukas J, Hughs C et al. The potential role of vascular endothelium in immune response. Human Immunology 1990; 28:258-262.
6. Pearson JD. Endothelial cell biology. Radiology 1991; 179:9-14.
7. Risberg B. Fibrinolysis in grafted arteries and veins. Thromb Haemost 1979; 40:512-517.
8. Sottiurai V, Yao J, Flinn W, Batson R. Intimal hyperplasia and neointima: An ultrastructural analysis of thrombosed grafts in humans. Surgery 1983; 93:809-817.
9. Callow A. Current status of vascular grafts. Surg Clin North Am 1982; 62:501-513.
10. Örtenwall P. Endothelial cell seeding-effects on vascular graft thrombogenicity. Thesis 1989.
11. Woodroof A. Use of glutaraldehyde and formaldehyde to process tissue heart valves. J Bioeng 1978; 2:1-9.
12. Gendler E, Gendler S, Nimni ME. Toxic reactions evoked by glutaraldehyde fixed pericardium and cardiac valve tissue bioprosthesis. J Biomed Mater Res 1984; 18:727-736.
13. Eybl E, Griesmachher A, Grimm M, Wolner E. Toxic effects of aldehydes released from fixed pericardium on bovine aortic endothelial cells. J Biomed Res 1989; 23:1355-1365.
14. Bengtsson L. Lining of cardiovascular prosthetic materials with cultured adult human endothelium. Thesis. Karolinska Institute 1992.

15. Grabenwöger M, Grimm M, Eybl E et al. New aspects of the degeneration of bioprosthetic heart valves after long-term implantation. J Thorac Cardiovasc Surg 1992; 104:14-21.

16. Warnes C, Scott M, Silver G et al. Comparison of late degenerative changes in porcine bioprostheses in the mitral and aortic valve position in the same patient. Am J Cardiol 1983; 51:956-68.

17. Sanders S, Levy R, Freed M, Norwood W, Castaneda A. Use of Hancock porcine xenografts in children and adolescents. Am J Cardiol 1980; 46:429-38.

18. Schoen F, Kujovich J, Levy R, St John T, Sutton M. Bioprosthetic valve failure. Cardiovasc Clin 1988; 18:289-316.

19. Cotran R. New roles for the endothelium in inflammation and immunity. Am J Pathol 1987; 129:407-13.

20. Pober JS. Cytokine-mediated activation of vascular endothelium: Physiology and pathology. Am J Pathol 1988; 133:426-433.

21. Bevilacqua M, Pober J, Majeau G, Cotran R, Gimbrone M. Interleukin (IL-1) induces biosynthesis and cell surface expression of procoagulant activity in human vascular endothelial cells. J Exp Med 1984; 160:618-623.

22. Old LJ. Tumour necrosis factor. Nature 1986; 320:584-588.

23. Bevilacqua M, Pober J, Wheeler M, Cotran R, Gimbrone M. Interleukin-1 acts on cultured human vascular endothelium to increase the adhesion of polymorphonuclear leucocytes, monocytes, and related leucocyte cell lines. J Clin Invest 1985; 76:2003-2011.

24. Rosenbaum JT, Howes EL, Rubin RM, Samples JR. Ocular inflammatory effects of intravitreally injected tumor necrosis factor. Am J Pathol 1988; 133:47-53.

25. McEver RP, Beckstead JH, Moore KL, Marshall-Carlson L, Bainton DF. GMP-140, a platelet alpha-granulae membrane protein, is also synthesized by vascular endothelial cells and is localized in Weibel-palade bodies. J Clin Invest 1989; 84:92-99.

26. Gimbrone MAJ, Bevilacqua MP. Vascular endothelim: Functional modulation at the blood interface. In: Simionescu N, Simionescu M, eds. Endothelial cell biology in health and in disease. New York: Plenum Press 1998:255-273.

27. Bevilacqua MP, Stengelin S, Gimbrone MA Jr, Seed B. Endothelial leukocyte molecule-1: An inducible receptor for neutrophils related to complement regulatory proteins and lectins. Science 1989; 243:1160-1165.

28. Pober JS, Gimbrone MA, Lapierre LA et al. Overlapping patterns of activation of human endothelial cells by interleukin-1, tumor necrosis factor and immune interferon. J Immunol 1986; 137:1893-1896.

29. Staunton DE, Dustin ML, Springer TA. Functional cloning of ICAM-2, a cell adhesion ligand for LFA-1 homologous to ICAM-1. Nature 1989; 339:61-64.

30. van der Vieren M, Le Trong H, Wood CL, Moore PF, St John T, Staunton DE, Gallatin WM. A novel leucointegrin, alpha d beta 2, binds preferentially to ICAM-3. Immunity 1995; 3:683-690.

31. Holness CL, Bates, PA, Little AJ, Buckley CD, McDowall A, Bossy D, Hogg N, Simmons DL. Analysis of the binding site on intercellular adhesion molecule 3 for the leukocyte integrin lymphocyte function-associated antigen 1. J Biol Chem 1995; 270:877-884.

32. Doussis-Anagnostopoulou I, Kaklamanis L, Cordell J, Jones M, Turley H, Pulford K, Simmons D, Mason D,

Gatter K. ICAM-3 expression on endothelium in lymphoid malignancy. Am J Path 1993; 143:1040-1043.

33. Rice GE, Munro JM, Bevilacqua MP. Inducible cell adhesion molecule 110 (INCAM-110) is an endothelial receptor for lymphocytes. A CD11/CD18-independent adhesion mechanism. J Exp Med 1990; 171:1369-1374.

34. Briscoe D, Shoen F, Rice G et al. Induced expression of endothelial-leucocyte adhesion molecules in human cardiac allografts. Transplantation 1991; 51:537-539.

35. Galumbeck M, Sanfilippo F, Hagen P-O, Seaver A, Urbaniak J. Inhibition of vessel allograft rejection by endothelial removal. Ann Surg 1987; 206:757-64.

36. Newman PJ, Albelda SM. Cellular and molecular aspects of PECAM-1. Nouv Rev Fr Hematol 1992; 34:S7-S11.

37. Albelda SM, Müller WA, Buck C, Newman PJ. Molecular and cellular properties of PCAM-1 (endo-CAM/CD-31): A novel vascular cell-cell adhesion molecule. J Cell Biol 1991; 114:1059-1068.

38. Vaporciyan AA, DeLisser HM, Yan HC et al. Involvement of platelet-endothelial cell adhesion molecule-1 in neutrophil recruitment in vivo. Science 1993; 262:1580-2.

39. Pober J, Collins T, Gimbrone M, Libby P, Reiss C. Inducible expression of class II major histocompatibility complex antigens and the immunogenicity of vascular endothelium. Transplantation 1986; 41:141-146.

40. Libby P, Hansson GK. Biology of disease. Involvement of the immune system in human atherogenesis: Current knowledge and unanswered questions. Lab Invest 1991; 64:5-15.

41. Basham T, Merigan T. Recombinant interferon-γ increases HLA-DR synthesis and expression. J Immunol 1983; 130:1492-1494.

42. Carlos TM, Harlan JM. Leukocyte-endothelial adhesion molecules. Blood 1994; 84:2068-2101.

43. Jones AD, Smith CW, McIntire VL. Leucocyte adhesion under flow conditions: Principles important in tissue engineering. Biomaterials 1996; 17:337-347.

44. Atherton ABG. Relationship between the velocity of rolling granulocytes and that of the blood flow in venules. J Physiol 1973; 233:157-165.

45. Goldman AJ, Cox RG, Brenner H. Slow viscous motion of a sphere parallel to a plane wall. Chem Engng Sci 1967; 22:637-660.

46. Smith CW. Endothelial adhesion molecules and their role in inflammation. Can J Physiol Pharmacol 1993; 70:76-87.

47. Zilla P, Preiss P, Groscurth P et al. In vitro lined endothelium: Initial integrity and ultrastructural events. Surgery 1994; 116:524-534.

48. Zilla P, Fasol R, Deutsch M et al. Endothelial cell seeding of polytetrafluoroethylene vascular grafts in humans: A preliminary report. J Vasc Surg 1987; 6:535-541.

49. Zilla P, Fasol R, Preiss P et al. Use of fibrin glue as a substrate for in vitro endothelialization of PTFE vascular grafts. Surgery 1989; 105:515-522.

50. Hægerstrand A, Bengtsson L, Gillis C. Serum proteins provide a matrix for cultured endothelial cells on expanded polytetrafluoroethylene vascular grafts. Scand J Thor Cardiovasc Surg 1993; 27:21-26.

51. Bengtsson L, Rådegran K, Hægerstrand A. A new and simple technique to achieve a confluent and flow resistant endothelium on vascular ePTFE-grafts using human serum. Eur J Vasc Surg 1994; 8:182-187.

52. Jones DA, McIntire LV, McEver RP, Smith CW. P-selectin supports neutrophil rolling on histamine-stimulated endothelial cells. Biophys J 1993; 65:1560-1569.

53. Lawerence MB, Smith CW, Eskin SG, McIntire LV. Effect of venous shear stress on CD18-mediated neutrophil adhesion to cultured endothelium. Blood 1990; 75:227-237.

54. Lawrence MB, Springer TA. Leukocytes roll on a selectin at physiologic flow rates: Distinction from and prerequisite for adhesion through integrins. Cell 1991; 65:859-873.

55. Gillis C, Bengtsson L, Hægerstrand A. Reduction of monocyte adhesion to xenogeneic tissue by endothelialization: An adhesion and time-dependent mechanism. J Thorac Cardiovasc Surg 1995; 110:1583-1589.

56. Prieto J, Eklund A, Patarroyo M. Regulated expression of integrins and other adhesion molecules during differentiation of monocytes into macrophages. Cell Immunol 1994; 156:191-211.

57. Patarroyo M. Short analytical review: Leukocyte adhesion in host defence and tissue injury. Clin Immunol Immunopathol 1991; 60:333-348.

58. Schnittler HJ, Franke RP, Fuhrmann R. Influence of various substrates on the actin filament exposed to fluid shear stress. Basel: Karger 183-188.

59. Ballermann BJ, Ott MJ. Adhesion and differentiation of endothelial cells by exposure to chronic shear stress: A vascular graft model. Blood Purification 1995; 13:125-134.

60. Cronstein NB, Weissmann G. The adhesion molecules of inflammation. Arthritis and Rheumatism 1993; 36:147155.

61. McIntire LW. 1992 ALZA Distinguished Lecture: Bioengineering and Vascular Biology. Annals of Biomedical Engineering 1994; 22:2-13.

CHAPTER 17

In Vitro Endothelialization Elicits Tissue Remodeling Emulating Native Artery Structures

Manfred Deutsch, Johann Meinhart, Peter Zilla

In humans, the retrieval of samples from cardiovascular implants is a rare event. Therefore, it is almost impossible to evaluate the long term healing pattern of cardiovascular prostheses. At the same time, animal experiments do not offer a satisfying solution either. The significantly shorter length of the prostheses and an incomparably short implantation time make transanastomotic tissue ingrowth their predominant healing mode. Therefore, there is hardly an opportunity to histologically study blood surfaces of clinical implants which are not affected by transanastomotic ingrowth. This is particularly frustrating in an exciting field such as clinical in vitro endothelialization of arterial grafts, in which the patency results are highly encouraging but the proof for the ongoing existence of functional intimal tissue has only sporadically been provided.

When the techniques for in vitro lining were refined in the mid 1980s, the seeding community was haunted by the fear of so called "contaminating" smooth muscle cells. With the strong emphasis on intimal hyperplasia of those days, the smooth muscle cell was the declared enemy. As a result, much of the research effort went into purification of endothelial cell cultures.[1,2]

Preclinical primate experiments[3] confirmed that a mature and functional endothelium continued to form a confluent cell coverage after weeks of implantation. Moreover, the opportunity to obtain a specimen of a clinically in vitro lined ePTFE graft also showed that a single layer of pure endothelial cells confluently covered the protein precoated ePTFE surface of the graft 5 weeks after implantation.[4] Nevertheless, fears of fibrinolytic degradation of the underlying matrix, with the concomitant detachment of the endothelium, were justified in view of the lack of long term specimens. Furthermore, in native arteries endothelial cells closely interact with their underlying smooth muscle cells in an adaptive attempt to standardize flow and shear stress conditions.[5] Therefore, the presence of a monolayer resting almost directly on the synthetic graft structure seemed more and more unphysiological, and perhaps even unsustainable. However, clinical long term studies increasingly indicated that a functional endothelium continued to cover the graft surface, even after years of implantation. Eventually, we got the chance to morphologically analyze a significant piece of explanted graft 41 months after clinical in vitro lining. Since the healing pattern of a certain prosthetic implant does not principally differ from case to case, the extrapolation of a case report to a principal healing response seems justified, particularly in view of the fact that a representative number of samples cannot be expected in the clinical setup.

Tissue Engineering of Prosthetic Vascular Grafts, edited by Peter Zilla and Howard P. Greisler.

Case Report[6]

A 69 year old man who had undergone a bilateral femoro-popliteal bypass graft procedure with in vitro endothelialized ePTFE grafts was readmitted 41 months later for graft revision. The original indication for an in vitro lined graft was the fact that both saphenous veins had already been taken due to previous coronary artery bypass grafting. The reason for readmission and revision of one graft was the recurrence of severe claudication and a deterioration of the ankle-brachial index from 0.89-0.59. Furthermore, angiography demonstrated a significant stenosis in the midsegment of the affected graft.

The lining procedure with cultured autologous venous endothelial cells has been extensively described elsewhere.[7-10] Endothelial cells were harvested by the in situ no-touch technique previously reported.[1] Routine immunohistochemical screening of the preseeding mass cultures with factor VIII confirmed the purity of endothelial cells. The precoating of the ePTFE structure prior to lining was done with a fibrinolytically inhibited fibrin glue.[3,4,6-10] On light microscopy of freshly lined grafts and of preimplantation controls, a confluent endothelial cell layer rested on a homogenous and evenly covering protein matrix. The postseeding maturation of the confluent endothelium on the fibrin matrix did not result in a diminished thickness of this adhesion matrix (7.3 µm versus 7.0 µm). By scanning electron microscopy, the freshly lined graft surface showed a completely covering, confluent endothelium at the end of the lining procedure. Nine days later, at the time of implantation, the endothelium was still confluent, but the cells were flatter, with better pronounced marginal overlapping.

Forty-one months later at the time of revision, the angiographic appearance of the stenosed area resembled a native arteriosclerotic lesion. A 21 cm long graft segment was subsequently replaced by an equally in vitro endothelialized piece of ePTFE graft. The distance of the affected segment to the anastomoses was approximately 15 cm on both sides. On gross examination of the explant, the inner surface of the entire specimen was smooth and gray-white, showing multiple yellow and white plaques again resembling native atherosclerosis. Histologically, the inner surface was completely covered by a single layer of flattened cells which were strongly positive for factor VIII, CD31 and CD34 (Fig. 17.1). Between this intima and the graft, a continuous tissue layer of 1.21 ± 0.19 mm thickness was demonstrable (Fig. 17.2) showing all histological and immunohistochemical criteria of an arterial tunica media. It contained numerous actin (Fig.17.3) and desmin-positive cells resembling smooth muscle cells. A well developed internal elastic membrane could regularly be found underneath a collagen iv-positive basement membrane of the endothelium (Fig. 17.4). In atheromatous areas the internal elastic membrane was disintegrated to various degrees (Fig. 17.4).

The outside of the graft was surrounded by a rim of histiocytes with multiple multinucleated giant cells. The prosthesis itself did not show any capillary ingrowth. In addition, multiple fatty streaks, fibrous plaques and atheromas (indistinguishable from conventional atherosclerotic

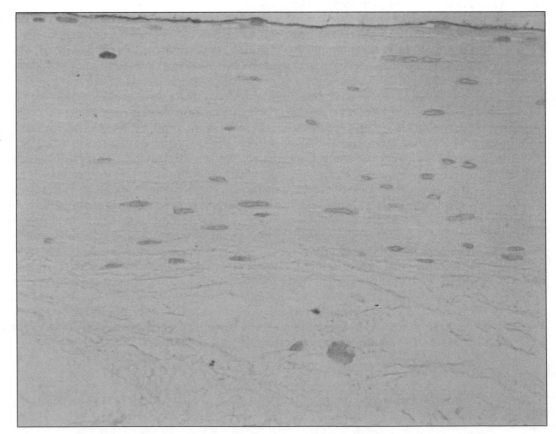

Fig. 17.1. Confluent monolayer of CD34 positive endothelial cells resting on a well developed, concentrically aligned neo-media. The structure of the expanded PTFE graft is clearly visible underneath (APAP technique; x200).

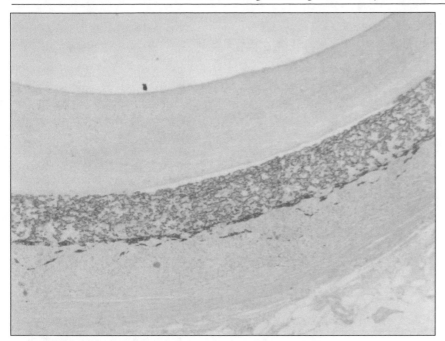

Fig. 17.2. Transverse section of in vitro endothelialized ePTFE graft 41 months after implantation. Typical extraprosthetic foreign body reaction on the outside along the low porosity PTFE wrap of the prosthesis. The inside surface of the graft is covered by cell rich, regularly aligned tissue (H.E.; x40).

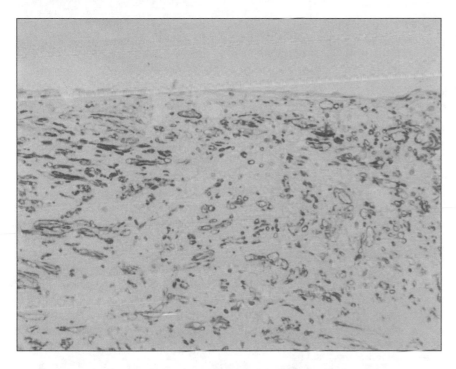

Fig. 17.3. Immunohistochemical proof of the presence of actin in the cells of the neomedia. Negative staining of the cell monolayer at the surface (APAP technique; x200).

lesions) could be seen. Only in these areas, KP-1 and PG-M1 positive foamy macrophages were found (Fig. 17.5). A neovascularization of the intima by small capillaries growing in from the luminal surface of the graft was only found in fibrous plaques, but not in the unaffected parts of the graft.

On scanning electron microscopy, the entire graft segment was covered by a mature and confluent endothelium whose cells were mostly elongated parallel to the bloodstream (Fig. 17.6). These endothelial cells showed numerous microvilli and pronounced marginal overlapping. The entire surface was free of thrombotic adherences, either fibrin or platelets. Areas with macroscopically visible plaques were characterized by surface protrusions of approximately 1 mm in diameter. These protrusions were only partially covered by intact endothelium, whose cells were polygonal rather than aligned with the blood stream (Fig. 17.7). In contrast to the unaffected graft areas, highly polarized leukocytes were adherent. Occasionally, only lamellopodia of these leukocytes were visible, indicating subendothelial leukocyte migration. Between these endothelial remnants the subendothelial matrix was openly exposed (Fig. 17.7).

Ultrastructurally, transmission electron microscopy demonstrated a well differentiated endothelium with numerous Weibel-Pallade bodies in those areas which were not affected by arteriosclerotic changes (Fig. 17.8). Confluence was maintained through complex intercellular contacts. In

Fig. 17.4. Border area between non-diseased part of in vitro lined ePTFE graft and atheromatous lesion. The well defined internal elastic membrane (left) becomes disintegrated (right), together with increasing intimal thickening (Orcein; x200).

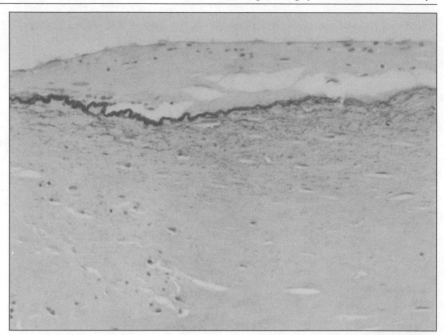

Fig. 17.5. Intimal plaque protruding into the lumen of the in vitro endothelialized prosthesis. CD68 positive foamy macrophages are only found in this area, in the depth of the neo-media close to the ePTFE graft (APAP technique; x200).

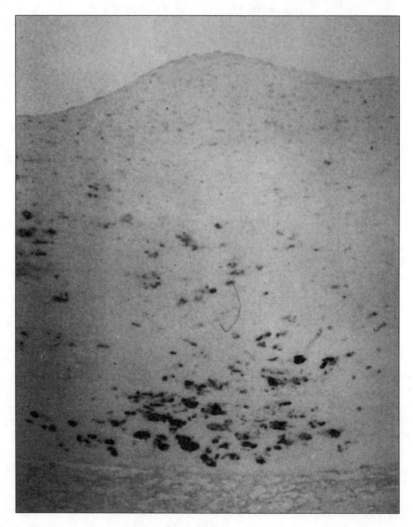

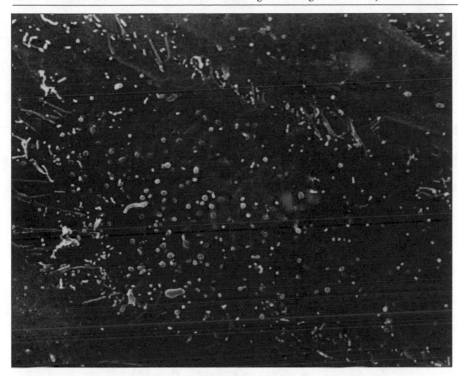

Fig. 17.6. Typical scanning electron microscopic appearance of the mature endothelium which covered the entire 21 cm long graft segment. The elongated endothelial cells show numerous short microvilli and pronounced marginal overlapping (x4,000).

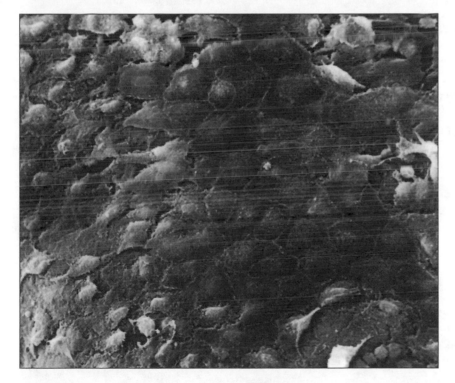

Fig.17.7. Surface morphology of a macroscopically visible atherosclerotic plaque. The endothelium is partly denuded and characterized by polygonal rather than longitudinally aligned cells. Occasionally, adherent blood cells are seen on freely exposed subendothelial matrix (x530).

immediate proximity to the endothelial cells a delicate and noncontinuous basal membrane was found. The endothelium and its basal membrane rested on a dense network of collagen fibrils. The subendothelial matrix was characterized by mature myofibroblasts embedded in densely packed collagen strands (Fig. 17.9). Although these cells had well differentiated peripheral actin filaments they also showed characteristics of secretory cells: a well developed Golgi complex and often a pronounced endoplasmic reticulum. In the proximity of a plaque, these cells contained strikingly large lipid vacuoles (Fig. 17.10).

Conclusions

In vitro endothelialization of small diameter vascular prostheses has significantly improved prosthetic graft patency.[9-12] Due to the difficulty in obtaining specimens from human implants, it could only be assumed that a persistent endothelium was the underlying reason for this better

Fig. 17.8. Transmission electron micrograph of unaffected part of in vitro endothelialized graft. A well differentiated endothelium rests on a collagen-rich sub-endothelial matrix. The cytoplasm shows numerous Weibel-Pallade bodies (⇒) and normal organelles. Complex intercellular contact (→) and incompletely visible basal lamina (Δ) (TEM; x33,000).

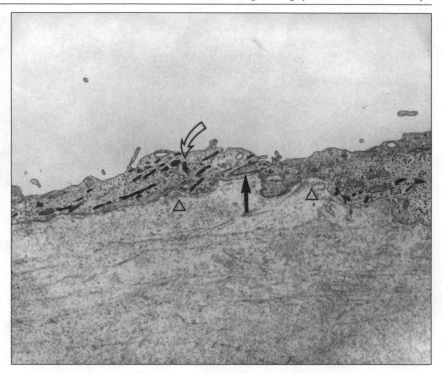

Fig. 17.9. Mature myofibroblasts from the depth of the neo-media with perinuclear organelles. These cells typically contain a well differentiated actin filament system at the periphery and are embedded in a collagen-rich extracellular matrix (TEM; x47,000).

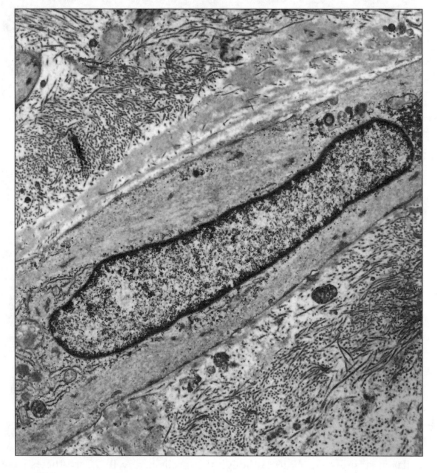

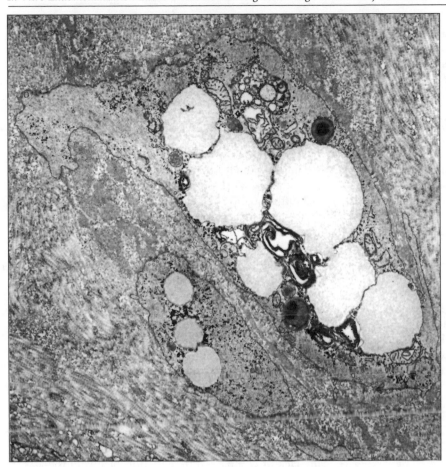

Fig. 17.10. Myofibroblast from the atherosclerotic plaque area with huge lipid vacuoles in the center. Note the peripheral actin filament bundles, as well as the membrane-bound dense bodies which are characteristic of myofibroblasts (TEM; x42,000).

performance. Although the short term integrity of the lined endothelium has previously been proved in a 5 week explant,[4] long term developments remained speculative. With the opportunity to investigate a 41 month implant we were eventually able to substantiate the clinical success with morphological evidence. We could show that in vitro lined grafts maintain an intact endothelial coverage even after 3 1/2 years of implantation. Unexpected, however, was the finding that a neomedia had developed between the prosthesis and the endothelium throughout the entire length of the graft. The cells of this neomedia contained actin filaments and were separated from the intima by a true internal elastic membrane which distinguished them from a neointima. Since untreated ePTFE grafts do not develop a tissue layer on their luminal side, it is evident that this neomedia was enabled or caused by the in vitro lining procedure. Considering the fact that cell ingrowth on conventional grafts is limited to the immediate perianastomotic region,[13] the most eminent question is: How did these neomedia cells get there?

The three principal options are:
1. Through coseeding during the initial endothelialization process;
2. Subendothelial migration from the adjacent artery; or
3. Colonization from the blood.

Coseeding During the Initial Endothelialization

If the progenitor cells of the neo-media were seeded together with the endothelial cells, they must have remained undetectable during cultivation. Even if the assessment of purity of endothelial cell cultures was based on phenotypic characteristics, connective tissue cells can usually be easily detected. Smooth muscle cells and fibroblasts lack the contact inhibition of endothelial cells and therefore tend to overgrow each other in a typical elongated, spindle shape. Since our lining technique only uses first passage mass cultures,[1] endothelial cells do not show signs of phenotypic senescence.[14] This renders them even more the typical cobblestone monolayer in their morphology. Furthermore, first passage mass cultures necessitate prolonged cultivation in one and the same flask,[1] which usually allows connective tissue cells to develop their typical shape. Therefore, only a very insignificant number of connective tissue cells might have been inoculated. To achieve an evenly distributed neomedia with such a low inoculum in a graft of 50-60 cm length, cells would need to migrate over long distances. Thus, even if the neo-media originates from initially coseeded smooth muscle cells, cell migration would remain a significant phenomenon. Alternatively, a higher inoculum might have been achieved by cells which barely differ phenotypically from endothelial cells and were therefore not detected in the initial culture. This would be feasible because the vascular wall intima contains a stem cell population which is epitheloid in culture but still represents a subpopulation of smooth muscle cells. However, such a scenario would mean that two screening methods failed, the immunohistochemical staining because of the small sample size and the phenotypic because of the presence of a rare subpopulation of smooth muscle cells.

Subendothelial Migration from the Adjacent Artery

If the progenitor cells of the neo-media were not seeded but migrated from the anastomotic region, the question is: Why was this possible? For reasons not fully understood yet, connective tissue ingrowth onto synthetic vascular prostheses stops shortly after the anastomosis.[13] One explanation may lie in an inhibitory fibrin layer on the blood surface[16] which gradually builds up. If, however, an endothelial cell population of the surface was possible through apt transmural ingrowth before this change in biological surface environment, smooth muscle cells grow well on the same synthetic surface on which they ceased to proliferate before. Therefore, it seems as if the presence of a PDGF-producing endothelium[17] makes the difference with regard to the presence of a subendothelial smooth muscle cell population. Although quiescent endothelial cells barely produce any PDGF, a significant PDGF production occurs in regenerating endothelium.[18,19] In spite of continual integrity of the lined endothelium we have seen a significant regeneration in the primate model.[3] Others have also found a 8- to 10-fold increase in endothelial replication on ePTFE prostheses[20] accompanied by a significant production of growth factors.[21]

Colonization from the Blood

Finally, as a third option, circulating multipotent stem cells must be considered. All four cell types, fibroblasts, myocytes, endothelial cells and blood borne cells, are embryologically of the same origin. Since they represent various differentiations of one common stem cell, transformation within this cell family appears to be a reasonable option. The differentiation of mononuclear blood cells to fibroblasts, myocytes and endothelial cells has been described.[22-24] Our finding that white blood cells were not only adherent, but also clearly migrated underneath the endothelium, might be explained not only with an inflammatory reaction, but might well fit into the multipotent blood cell theory, which is currently best suited to explain isolated islands of endothelial cells in the center of prosthetic grafts.[25-27]

Whichever theory will eventually explain the formation of a differentiated neo-media on a 55 cm long prosthetic graft, distinct migration and intermesenchymal transformation of cells appear to be pivotal events in this process.

Apart from explaining the origin of this neo-media, another question seems to be of imminent practical importance: Does this neo-media formation represent a pathological process in the sense of a nonself-limiting hyperplastic cell proliferation or rather a self-limiting mechanism of tissue remodeling? To answer this question, mixed microvascular seeding seems to provide an explanatory analogy. When Park et al[28] presented a case report on a seeded human prosthesis, an unusually thick subendothelial cell layer had raised

exactly this concern. In order to clarify this issue we have observed tissue development following mixed microvascular seeding over a long-term period.[29] The major outcome of this study was the concurrence of two events: the maturation of the subendothelial cell matrix from fibroblastoid towards myocytoid and the accomplishment of an equilibrium of cell proliferation. After the long lasting disputes of the 1980s over the method of choice for actively achieving graft endothelialization, it is exciting to see that two methods as diverse as in vitro lining and mixed microvascular seeding eventually lead to an identical result: the healing of a prosthetic graft accompanied by initial tissue proliferation, cell differentiation and endothelialization. This realization further underlines the current redefinition of standpoints in prosthetic graft research. In contrast to previous beliefs, host tissue appears to be capable of physiologically incorporating synthetic grafts, provided it happens prior to a buildup of adverse conditions.[16] Therefore, the manipulation of the chronology of events may well hold the key to ingrowth facilitation. What seems unchallenged is the fact that early endothelialization facilitates the subsequent musculogenesis within the graft wall. All nonbiological aspects like compliance or porosity—as important as they might be—were previously overemphasized[16] although they will need to be an integral part of an entirely engineered arterial graft. Nevertheless, it is quite possible that these nonbiological aspects are the limiting factors of currently available methods of graft endothelialization: Both noncompliance and low porosity might well be responsible for the lack of complete differentiation of myofibroblasts to myocytes and for the early appearance of true arteriosclerotic lesions in endothelialized prosthetic grafts. The most striking observation, however, was that newly formed vessel structures can emulate a native artery even to the extent that they participate in the generalized arteriosclerotic disease of the arterial tree.

References

1. Zilla P, Fasol R, Dudeck U, Kadletz M, Siedler S, Preiss P, Sanan D, Odell J, Reichart B. In situ canulation, microgrid follow-up and low density plating provide first passage endothelial cell mass cultures for in vitro lining. J Vasc Surg 1990; 12:180-9.
2. Haegerstrand A, Gillis C, Bengtsson L. Serial cultivation of adult human endothelium from the great saphenous vein. J Vasc Surg 1992; 16:280-285.
3. Zilla P, Preiss P, Groscurth P, Rösemeier F, Deutsch M, Odell J, Heidinger C, Fasol R, Von Oppell U. In vitro lined endotheliaum: Initial integrity and ultrastructural events. Surgery 1994; 16:524-534.
4. Fischlein T, Zilla P, Meinhart J, Puschmann R, Vesely M, Eberl T, Balon R, Deutsch M. In vitro endotheliaization of a meso-systemic shunt—A clinical case report. J Vasc Surg 1994; 19:549-554.
5. Kaufman BR, De Luca DJ, Folsom DL, Mansell SL, Gorman ML, Fox PL, Graham LM. Elevated platelet-derived growth factor production by aortic grafts implanted on a long-term basis in a canine model. J Vasc Surg 1992; 15:806-816.
6. Deutsch M, Meinhart J, Vesely M, Fischlein T, Groscurth P, Von Oppell U, Zilla P. In vitro endothelialization of

expanded polytetrafluoroethylene grafts: A clinical case report after 41 months of implantation. J Vasc Surg 1997; 25:757-763.

7. Zilla P, Fasol R, Preiss P, Kadletz M, Deutsch M, Schima H, Tsangaris S, Groscurth P. Use of fibrin glue as a substrate for in vitro endothelialization of PTFE vascular grafts. Surgery 1989; 105:515-522.

8. Müller-Glauser W, Zilla P, Lachat M, Bisang B, Rieser F, von Segesser L, Turina M. Immediate shear stress resistance of endothelial cell monolayers lined in vitro on fibrin glue-coated ePTFE prostheses. Europ J Vasc Surg 1994; 7:324-328.

9. Zilla P, Deutsch M, Meinhart J, Puschmann R, Eberl T, Minar E, Dudczak R, Lugmaier H, Schmidt P, Noszian I, Fischlein T. Clinical in vitro endothelialization of femoropopliteal bypass grafts—an actuarial follow-up over 3 years. J Vasc Surg 1994; 19:540-548.

10. Meinhart J, Deutsch M, Zilla P. Eight years of clinical endothelial cell transplantation. Closing the gap between prosthetic grafts and vein grafts. ASAIO Journal 1997; 43:M515-M521.

11. Magometschnig H, Kadletz M, Vodrazka M, Dock W, Grimm M, Grabenwöger M, Minar E, Staudacher M, Fenzel G, Wolner E. Prospective clinical study with in vitro endothelial cell lining of expanded polytetrafluoroethylene grafts in crural repeat reconstruction. J Vasc Surg 1997; 15:527-535.

12. Leseche G, Ohan J, Bouttier S, Palombi S, Bertrand P, Andreassian B. Above-knee femoropopliteal bypass grafting using endothelial cell seeded PTFE grafts: Five year clinical experience. Ann Vasc Surg 1995; 9:S15-S23.

13. Berger K, Sauvage LR, Rao AM, Wood SJ. Healing of arterial prostheses in man: Its incompleteness. Ann Surg 1972; 175:118-127.

14. Watkins MT, Sharefkin JB, Zajtchuk R. Adult human saphenous vein endothelial cells: Assessment of their reproductive capacity for use in endothelial seeding of vascular grafts. J Surg Res 1984; 36:588-596.

15. Schwartz SM, Foy L, Bowen-Pope DF, Ross R. Derivation and properties of platelet derived growth factor-independent rat aortic smooth muscle cells. Am J Path 1990; 136:1417-1428.

16. Davids L. The lack of healing in conventional vascular grafts. In: Zilla P, Greisler H, eds. Tissue Engineering of prosthetic vascular grafts. Georgetown: R.G. Landes Co., 1998.

17. Clowes AW. Platelet-derived growth factor activity and MRNA expression in healing vascular grafts in baboons. J Clin Invest 1991; 87:406-414.

18. Kraiss LW, Raines EW, Wilcox JN, Seifert RA, Barraett BT, Kirkman TR, Hart CE, Bowen-Pope DF, Ross R, Clowes AW. Regional expression of the platelet-derived growth factor and its receptors in a primate graft model of vessel wall assembly. J Clin Invest 1993; 92:338-348.

19. Golden MA, Au YPT, Kirkman TR, Wilcox JN, Raines EW, Ross R, Clowes AW. Platelet-derived growth factor activity and mRNA expression in healing vascular grafts in baboons. J Clin Invest 1991; 87:406-414.

20. Reidy MA, Chao SS, Kirkman TR, Clowes AW. Endothelial regeneration: VI: Chronic non-denuding injury in baboon vascular grafts. Am J Path 1986; 123:432-439.

21. Zacharis RK, Kirkman TR, Kenagy RD, Bowen-Pope DF, Clowes AW. Growth factor production by polytetrafluoroethylene grafts. J Vasc Surg 1988; 7:607-610.

22. Lue HJ, Feigl W, Susani M, Odermatt B. Differentiation of mononuclear blood cels into macrophages, fibroblasts and endothelial cells in thrombus organization. Exp Cell Biol 1988; 56:201-210.

23. Shibuya T, Kambayashi J, Okahara K, Kim DI, Kawasaki T, Shiba E, Mori T. Subendothelial layer of pseudointima of polytetrafluoroethylene grafts is formed by transformation of fibroblasts migrated from extravascular space. Eur J Vasc Surg 1994; 8:276-285.

24. Fujiwara T. Endothelial cells transformed from fibroblasts during angiogenesis. In: Zilla P, Greisler H, eds. Tissue Engineering of prosthetic vascular grafts. Georgetown: R.G. Landes Co., 1998.

25. Shi Q, Hong M, Onuki Y, Ghali R, Huner GC, Johansen KH, Sauvage LR. Endothelium on the flow surface of human aortic dacron vascular grafts. J Vasc Surg 1997; 25:736-742.

26. Hammond W. Surface population with blood-born cells. In: Zilla P, Greisler H, eds. Tissue Engineering of prosthetic vascular grafts. Georgetown: R.G. Landes Co., 1998.

27. Koen W. Entrapment of circulating cells. In: Zilla P, Greisler H, eds. Tissue Engineering of prosthetic vascular grafts. Georgetown: R.G. Landes Co., 1998.

28. Park PK, Jarrell B, Williams SK, Carter TL, Rose DG, Martinez A, Carabasi RA. Thrombus free human endothelial surface in the midregion of a Dacron vascular graft in the splanchnic venous circuit—Observation after nine months of implantation. J Vasc Surg 1990; 11:468-475.

29. Baitella-Eberle G, Groscurth P, Zilla P, Lachmat M, Müller-Glauser W, Schneider J, Neudecker A, Segesser L, Dardel E, Turina M. Long term results of tissue development and cell differentiation on Dacron prostheses seeded with microvascular cels in dogs. J Vasc Surg 1993; 18:1019-1028.

─────────────── CHAPTER 18 ───────────────

In Vitro Endothelialization of Synthetic Vascular Grafts in Long Term Clinical Use

Manfred Deutsch, Teddy Fischlein, Johann Meinhart, Peter Zilla

Introduction

Primary patency of synthetic vascular grafts varies between 30% and 55%, whereas it is between 68% and 85% for autologous reversed saphenous vein grafts after 5 years of implantation.[1-3] Apart from technical errors and anastomotic intimal hyperplasia, surface thrombogenicity appears to be a major reason for the limited performance of synthetic conduits. The tendency of surgical disciplines towards ready to use products led to efforts aiming at improved synthetic materials, delaying the overdue adoption of biological principles. When endothelial seeding was eventually introduced as a first attempt to overcome the problem of graft thrombogenicity with biological tools,[4] an elaborate approach soon surrendered to the clinicians' demand for a single staged procedure. Predictably, the first studies in humans were controversial and mostly disappointing. The most likely reason for the failure of these approaches was an insufficient seeding density which did not allow the formation of a sufficient endothelial coverage. One way to overcome a low cell inoculum is by immediate harvesting of large numbers of cells like microvascular cells from adipose tissue.[5-7] The alternative method of actively facilitating graft endothelialization is in vitro lining with cultured autologous endothelial cells.[8-10] After the preclinical proof of this concept in the non human primate model,[10] our group performed a randomized clinical study involving 49 patients between 1989 and 1991. Based on the encouraging three year results[11] and on the histological proof of an endothelium on a 5 week explant[12] and a central graft segment after 41 months of implantation,[13] we commenced a clinical program of routine implantation of in vitro endothelialized grafts.

Laboratory Procedure

In a step by step approach, reliable culture techniques for autologous endothelial cells,[8] as well as precoating[14] and lining techniques[15] which achieved shear stress resistance of the endothelium,[16] were developed. In brief, in vitro endothelialization is a two staged procedure. It needs a laboratory stage before graft implantation in order to provide a high cell number, sufficient for a complete cellular lining on the luminal graft surface. Therefore, a small segment of a patient's subdermal vein (mostly jugular or cephalic) is used as the cell source and taken out under local anesthesia. After careful, touch-free dissection, the vessel is cannulated in situ with two free-flow vessel cannulas with attached 3-way taps. In order to remove remaining blood, the vein is flushed with culture medium in a pulsatile manner. It is subsequently filled with a 0.1% solution of collagenase. The solution is kept under minor

Tissue Engineering of Prosthetic Vascular Grafts, edited by Peter Zilla and Howard P. Greisler.
©1999 R.G. Landes Company.

pressure within the vein after closing the 3-way taps. Following excision, the cannulated and collagenase-filled vein segment is transferred to the laboratory in a container filled with prewarmed phosphate buffered saline. An enzyme incubation time of 15 minutes with collagenase guarantees a maximal yield of endothelial cells without contaminating fibroblasts or smooth muscle cells. After centrifugation of the cell suspension, the pellet is resuspended in complete culture medium. Complete culture medium consists of Medium 199 supplemented with preservative-free heparin, 10 ng/ml bFGF, 50 μg/ml gentamycin and 20% autologous serum. For autologous serum preparation, 250 ml blood was previously taken from each patient and allowed to clot overnight at 4°C in order to guarantee a maximum release of growth factors into the serum. Cells are subsequently plated in 25 cm² culture flasks. The culture medium is renewed twice weekly by replacing half the culture medium with fresh complete medium. Having reached 90% confluency, primary cultures are passaged to two 162 cm² culture flasks. After having reached the required cell number, the autologuous cells are seeded onto the graft surface by using a rotation device which facilitates an even cell distribution under controlled conditions (Fig. 18.1). However, prior to this, grafts are preclotted with a special dilution of clinically approved and fibrinolytically inhibited fibrin glue in order to provide an adequate matrix for endothelial cells. In our pilot clinical study, we further pretreated grafts with virologically tested fibronectin, to increase adhesion and shear stress resistance of endothelial cells. However, in our second phase of clinical routine application of in vitro endothelialization, no clinically approved fibronectin was commercially available. In order to control the success of the seeding procedure, specimens for scanning electron microscopy were taken immediately after rotation and shortly before implantation (Fig. 18.2). At the time of implantation, the majority of grafts show a confluent endothelial cell lining. Only a few grafts occasionally show a preconfluent endothelium or even small cell-free areas. The whole in vitro procedure from vein excision to graft implantation took 36.9 days in our first clinical study and could be reduced to 30.3 days in the second phase of clinical routine application. Since most procedures are elective, this time span appears to be tolerable for a great number of patients.

Surgical Procedure and Clinical Follow Up

Patients were admitted to the study when their saphenous veins were unavailable, unsuitable or had to be spared for other surgical procedures like aortocoronary bypass grafting. All patients received the same anti-aggregatory treatment, namely oral dipyridamole, 75 mg/day, and oral acetyl salicylic acid, 330 mg/day, beginning two days prior to implantation and continuing throughout the observation period. For endothelialized graft implantation, only minor changes were necessary as compared to standard surgical procedure. Graft implantation was performed as previously described,[18] with the exception that the culture medium was kept inside the graft without clamping the prosthesis. Patients were anesthetized with a continuous epidural block using Bupivacaine-Hydrochloride. Thin-walled reinforced PTFE (6 mm inner diameter) was used as graft material in both phases of implantation.

All patients underwent a tight postoperative follow up. During the first year of our randomized clinical study we assessed the resistance of the endothelium by means of [111]Indium labeling. Patency was determined by clinical evaluation as well as by Duplex sonography. Angiography was routinely performed on an annual basis and in patients with suspected graft thrombosis. This follow up also applied to clinical routine in vitro endothelialization, with the exception of [111]Indium labeling of platelets.

Randomized Clinical Study

Between June 1989 and December 1991, the clinical benefit of graft endothelialization was evaluated in a ran-

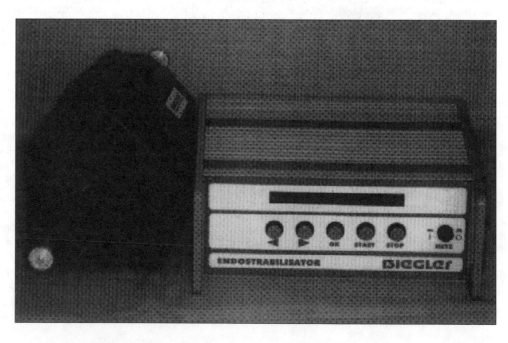

Fig. 18.1. New rotation device for quick in vitro endothelialization of vascular grafts, consisting of a motor unit and a control unit. Grafts are placed in sterile filter protected glass tubes and mounted on the motor unit, which can be easily placed in standard CO₂ incubators. Rotation speed and time can be regulated continuously.

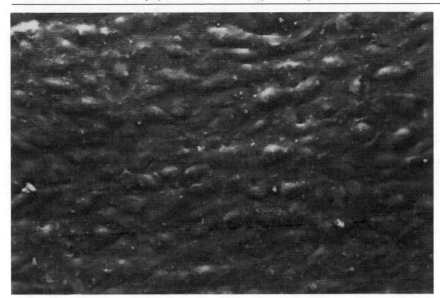

Fig. 18.2. Scanning electron micrograph of an in vitro endothelialized graft surface shortly before implantation. The whole surface is covered confluently with endothelial cells.

domized control study comprising 49 patients. After a 1:2 randomization pattern, 33 patients were assigned to the endothelialized group and 16 to the control group. Growth failure of cell cultures eliminated 9 patients of the endothelialized group. The remaining 24 patients received 27 endothelialized grafts. Patients were monitored for more than 7 years. [111]Indium labeling revealed a significant reduction of surface thrombogenicity of lined grafts. Throughout the first year of phase 1 of our endothelialization program, the difference in platelet activation index (PAI) between the endothelialized group and the control was significant ($p < 0.05$). Although it was most obvious 9 days post implantation, the difference remained significant even after one year. In the endothelialized group the PAI (platelet activation index) was -2.5 ± 9.4 at 9 days, -4.4 ± 13.5 at 3 months -0.7 ± 7.1 at 6 months and 7.0 ± 15.2 at 12 months. In contrast, the control group's values were as high as $37.1 \pm$ at 9 days, 27.8 ± 22.8 at 3 months, 37.2 ± 22.9 at 6 months and 29.0 ± 17.4 at 12 months.

After 3 years a Kaplan-meier analysis showed a primary patency rate of 84.7% for endothelialized grafts and 55.4% for control grafts. After 5 years, it was 73.8% for the endothelialized group and 31.5% for controls.[11] After 7 years, primary patency for control grafts dropped to zero, whereas that for endothelialized grafts remained high, at 73.8%.[18] One patient who underwent bilateral in vitro endothelialized grafting had a unilateral stenosis after 41 months. We decided to remove the stenosed portion of the graft and to implant a newly endothelialized graft. This explant proved the persistence of the transplanted endothelium. Except for the immediate atherosclerotic plaque area, a confluent endothelium covered the entire length of the 21 cm long specimen. Endothelial cells were mostly elongated and orientated parallel to the bloodstream. They were situated on a continuos tissue layer, which showed many morphologic criteria of an arterial tunica media[13] (see also chapter 17).

Clinical Routine Endothelialization

These favorable results encouraged us to transfer in vitro endothelialization to clinical routine in vascular surgery. So far, 93 in vitro lined femoropopliteal bypass grafts have been implanted in 82 patients. The primary patency rate for all endothelialized femoropopliteal reconstructions was 68% after 4 years; this is equivalent to that of reversed saphenous vein grafts. Above-knee procedures were done in 71, and below-knee procedures in 22 cases. Analysis of patency clearly revealed that endothelialization especially exerts its beneficial effect in the below-knee position. Primary patency was 61% in above-knee grafts but was 82% in below-knee grafts (Fig. 18.3). Secondary patency for all femoropopliteal reconstructions was 94% and limb salvage rate was 99%, since only one limb had to be amputated within the entire observation period.

However, although the patency rate for in vitro lined ePTFE grafts was comparable to that of vein grafts during both phases of our clinical endothelialization program, the primary patency rate of phase 2 was lower than that of phase 1. This difference may have several causes:

1. Phase 1—as an initial randomized trial—included considerably fewer patients than phase 2;
2. The follow up time of phase 2 was shorter and implantations were conducted as clinical routine procedures, including substantially more redo operations than phase 1;
3. Grafts of phase 2 had not been precoated with fibronectin, a potent adhesion molecule, due to the unavailability of a clinically approved product. Although the fibrin glue used for precoating contains fibronectin and endothelial cells deposit their own fibronectin-rich extracellular matrix with time, initial cell adherence may well have been diminished with a lower density of binding sites. When HFN-pretreated grafts were compared with untreated ones,

Fig. 18.3. Patency rate of routinely endothelialized femoropopliteal grafts according to the distal anastomoses. Below-knee grafts (n=22; top line) have a significantly higher patency rate than above-knee grafts (n=71; bottom line) after 4 years of implantation.

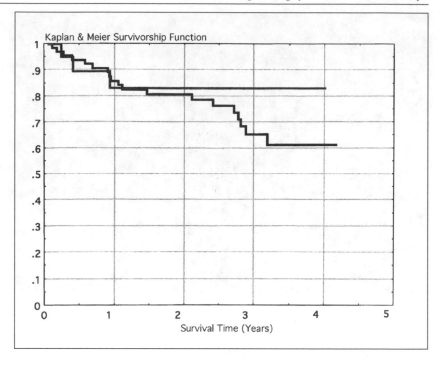

the difference was indistinct (77.8% versus 72.6%; p = 0.3). However, this difference was more pronounced when above-knee grafts were compared (80.0% versus 68.9%, p = 0.17) after 3.5 years of implantation. Although the differences between fibronectin pretreated or nonpretreated grafts were not statistically significant (which might be due to the different number of observed grafts), the curve may suggest that nonfibronectin treated grafts have a higher failure risk within the first year of implantation, a fact probably especially true in the above-knee position with its high flow, high shear stress condition. As a solution, pretreatment of the protein matrix with synthetic or recombinant RGD (arginine-glycine-aspartic acid)-containing molecules could be considered.

Our overall 7 year experience with endothelialized femoropopliteal ePTFE grafts shows a patency of 66.0%. When pretreated with HFN the seven year patency was 72.1%. In the above-knee group the 7 year patency was even as high as 75.8%[20] (Fig. 18.4).

Conclusion

At the end of this century, biological awareness is steadily rising among a new generation of cardiovascular surgeons. Today's research no longer focuses solely on surface endothelialization, but rather on the understanding of complex events that might eventually lead to real graft healing. Nevertheless, biological events facilitating spontaneous graft healing are not yet fully understood and it might take many more years until such a prosthesis is available for clinical implantation. Until then, an active method of graft endothelialization which was shown to significantly improve patency rates could provide us with both an indispensable

clinical tool and the motivation for intensified further attempts searching for an equally effective or even better product from the shelf.

With this goal in mind, we were one of the few groups which did not abandon the idea of surface endothelialization of vascular grafts in the mid-1980s. We decided to rectify procedural weaknesses before declaring endothelial cell transplantation inefficient. Since a low cell inoculum and an immature cytoskeleton seemed to be the main culprits for the failure of single-staged venous seeding, we elected to defy the surgical aversion towards cell culture procedures by confluently in vitro endothelializing prosthetic grafts with autologous mass cultures of endothelial cells.

Eight years of experience with clinical in vitro endothelialization not only provided us with patency data which eventually verified the assumption that surface endothelialization improves the performance of synthetic grafts. It also helped us to diminish three major concerns linked to in vitro lining: infection, failure rate of cultures and the proof of a persisting endothelium after graft implantation. In 120 in vitro endothelialized ePTFE grafts which have been implanted altogether since the start of our in vitro endothelialization program, only one graft showed late infection in a patient with IDDM and lymph fistula. This graft needed to be removed and amputation could be avoided. However, routine microbiological examination of this graft has been performed before implantation and was found to be negative for infections. One lined graft which was diagnosed to be contaminated during the cultivation period was discarded and remained the only occurrence of its kind. The analysis of risk factors for culture conditions enabled us to bring the failure rate for autologous endothelial cell cultures down from 27.3-5% (see chapter 15). Considering the fact that this two staged procedure provides 93% of patients with an

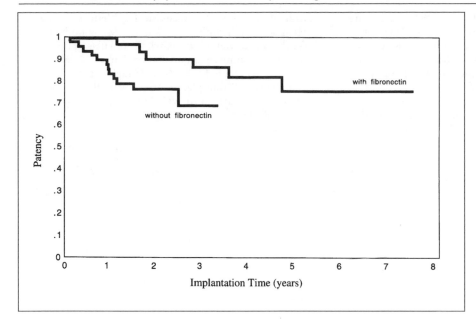

Fig. 18.4. Kaplan-Meier survivorship function for patency rates of all endothelialized above-knee femoro-popliteal grafts grouped according to fibronectin pretreatment. After 7 years, the patency rate was 75.8% for the fibronectin pretreated grafts (n=36).

arterial prosthesis which equals a vein graft, and that the remaining 7% end up with the prosthesis which they would have had without this procedure, one can accept the low probability of growth failure without ethical concerns. Finally, the proof of the existence of a confluently covering endothelium 5 weeks and 41 months after in vitro lining dissipated concerns regarding the continual presence of an endothelium after implantation. In summary, eight years of clinical in vitro endothelialization were able to prove two main hypotheses: Autologous endothelial cell lining significantly improves the patency of prosthetic small diameter vascular grafts, and a cell culture-dependent procedure can be carried over into clinical routine.

References

1. Veith FJ, Gupta SK, Ascer E et al. Six year prospective multicenter randomized comparison of autologous saphenous vein and expanded polytetrafluoroethylene grafts in infrainguinal arterial reconstructions. J Vasc Surg 1986; 3:104-14.
2. Cacciatore R, Inderbitzi R, Stirnemann P. Five years experience with infra-inguinal arterial reconstructions: A comparison of venous with PTFE bypass. VASA 1992; 21:171-176.
3. Quiñones-Baldrich WJ, Prego AA, Ucelay-Gomez R, Freischlag JA, Ahn SS, Baker JD, Machleder HI, Moor WS. Long-term results of infrainguinal revascularization with polytetrafluorethylene: A ten-year experience. J Vasc Surg 1992; 16:209-217.
4. Herring M, Gardner A, Glover J. A single-staged technique for seeding vascular grafts with autogenous endothelium. Surgery 1978; 84:498-504.
5. Vici M, Pasquinelli G, Preda P, Martinelli G, Gibellini D, Freyrie A, Curti T, D'Addato M. Electron microscopic and immunocytochemical profiles of human sucutaneous fat tissue microvascular endothelial cells. Ann Vasc Surg 1993; 7:541-548.
6. Jarrell B, Williams S, Stokes G, Hubbard A, Carabasi A, Koolpe E, Greener D, Pratt K, Moritz M, Radomski J, Speicher L. Use of freshly isolated capillary endothelial cells for the immediate establishment of a monolayer on a vascular graft at surgery. Surgery 1986; 100:392-399.
7. Baitell-Eberle G, Groscurth P, Zilla P, Lachat M, Müller-Glauser W, Schneider J, Neudecker A, von Segesser L, Dardel E, Turina M. Long term results of tissue development and cell differentiation on dacron prostheses seeded with microvascular cells in dogs. 1993; 18:1019-1028.
8. Zilla P, Fasol R, Dudeck U, Siedler S, Preiss P, Fischlein T, Müller-Glauser W, Baitella G, Sanan D, Odell J, Reichart B. In situ cannulation, microgrid follow-up and low density plating provide first passage endothelial cell mass cultures for in vitro lining. Vasc Surg 1990; 12:180-189.
9. Zilla P, Fasol R, Preiss P, Kadletz M, Deutsch M, Schima H, Tsangaris S, Groscurth P. Use of fibrin glue as a substrate for in vitro endothelialization of PTFE vascular grafts. Surgery 1989; 105:515-522.
10. Zilla P, Preiss P, Groscurth P, Rösemeier F, Deutsch M, Odell J, Heidinger C, Fasol R, von Oppell U. In vitro-lined endothelium: Initial integrity and ultrastructural events. Surgery 1994; 116:524-534.
11. Zilla P, Deutsch M, Meinhart J, Puschmann R, Eberl T, Minar E, Dudczak R, Lugmaier H, Schmidt P, Noscian I, Fischlein T. Clinical in vitro endothelialization of femoropopliteal bypass graft: An actuarial follow-up over three years. Vasc Surg 1994; 19:540-548.
12. Fischlein T, Zilla P, Meinhart J, Puschmann R, Vesely M, Eberl T, Balon R, Deutsch M. In vitro endothelialization of a mesosystemic shunt: A clinical case report. Vasc Surg 1994; 19:549-554.
13. Deutsch M, Meinhart J, Vesely M, Groscurth P, Von Oppell U, Zilla P. In vitro endothelialization of ePTFE grafts: A clinical case report after 41 months of implantation. Vasc Surg 1997; 25:757-763.
14. Kaehler J, Zilla P, Fasol R, Deutsch M, Kadletz M. Precoating substrate and surface configuration determine

adherence and spreading of seeded endothelial cells on polytetrafluoroethylene grafts. J Vasc Surg 1989; 9:535-541.

15. Zilla P, Fasol R, Preiss P, Kadletz M, Deutsch M, Schima H, Tsangaris S, Groscurth P. Use of fibrin glue as a substrate for in vitro endothelialization of PTFE vascular grafts. Surgery 1989; 105:515-522.

16. Franke RP, Graefe M, Schnittler H, Seiffge D, Mittermayer C. Induction of human vascular endothelial stress fibres by fluid shear stress. Nature 1984; 307:648-649.

17. Zilla P, Fasol R, Deutsch M, Fischlein T, Minar E, Hammerle A, Krupicka O, Kadletz M. Endothelial cell seeding of polytetrafluoroethylene vascular grafts in humans: A preliminary report. J Vasc Surg 1987; 6:535-541.

18. Meinhart J, Deutsch M, Zilla P. Eight years of clinical endothelial cell transplantation. Closing the gap between prosthetic grafts and vein grafts. ASAIO J 1997; 43:M515-M521.

Part III

Biointeractive Prostheses: Complete Healing

Biological Components

Taming of Adverse Responses

Prevention of the Inflammatory Reaction

─────────────── CHAPTER 19 ───────────────

Inflammatory Reaction: The Nemesis of Implants

James M. Anderson

Introduction

Nemesis is the Greek goddess of retributive justice or vengeance. Thus, the term "nemesis" has been used to identify one that inflicts retribution or vengeance. Alternatively, nemesis has been defined as a source of harm or destruction. Following the implantation of a medical device, biomaterial or prosthesis, the inflammatory reaction is the first host defense system which interacts with the medical device, biomaterial or prosthesis, and may be the source of harm or destruction to the implant or may result in untoward inflammatory and healing responses which lead to failure of the device in its intended function. In considering the inflammatory response to prosthetic vascular grafts, the inflammatory response is a complex series of cellular and humoral interactions which are time-dependent and lead to the healing response. Given these perspectives, the purpose of this chapter is to review the inflammatory response to prosthetic vascular grafts and provide a current state of the art perspective on the inflammatory response to prosthetic vascular grafts and the potential for inflammatory response interactions with tissue-engineered prosthetic vascular grafts.

Inflammation and the Healing Response

Inflammation is generally defined as the reaction of vascularized living tissue to local injury.[1-3] With porous vascular grafts, i.e., Dacron or ePTFE, a dual perspective of the injury which initiates the inflammatory and wound healing responses must be considered. The surgical procedure itself causes local injury to vascularized living tissue, and inflammation is initiated by injury to soft tissue or muscle. This form of injury produces a response to the outer or periadventitial surface of the vascular graft. The second response which initiates injury is the blood-material interaction which follows implantation and re-establishment of blood flow of the vascular graft. Blood-material interactions and the inflammatory response are intimately linked and, in fact, early responses to injury involve mainly blood and the vasculature. The interaction of blood and its components with the luminal surface of vascular grafts must also be considered as an initiator of the inflammatory response. Some types of porous vascular grafts with relatively high porosity must be rendered impermeable prior to implantation by a process called preclotting. Preclotting of vascular grafts with blood and its humoral and cellular components can be expected to initiate the inflammatory response to the prosthesis immediately prior to surgical implantation of the prosthesis.

Following the implantation of a vascular graft, a series of local events occur. These local events (Table 19.1) are described as the tissue response continuum or, more commonly, the inflammatory and healing responses. In the 1950s and '60s, woven, knitted and velour types of fabrics of various polymers were evaluated or utilized as vascular grafts. Initially, vascular grafts were conceptually considered to be scaffolds over which the vasculature would

Tissue Engineering of Prosthetic Vascular Grafts, edited by Peter Zilla and Howard P. Greisler.
©1999 R.G. Landes Company.

recapitulate itself, with the formation of intimal, medial and adventitial components of the vessel wall and the reestablishment of an endothelial lining which separated blood from vascular wall components with their attendant adverse blood-tissue interactions.[4,5] This concept has not been realized in humans to date, although use of highly porous ePTFE vascular grafts have produced endothelial linings in baboons. In lower species, i.e., rabbits, pigs, dogs and others, the re-endothelialization process does occur on an inner capsule (pseudointima) and thus constitutes a neointima in these species.

Immediately following injury, changes occur in vascular flow, caliber and permeability. Fluid, proteins and blood cells escape from the vascular system into the injured tissue in a process called exudation. Following changes in the vascular system, which also include changes induced in blood and its components, cellular events occur and characterize the inflammatory response. Although injury initiates the inflammatory response, chemicals and agents released from plasma, cells and injured tissue, as well as blood, mediate the response to vascular grafts.

Figure 19.1 illustrates the temporal variation in the tissue response continuum, i.e., the acute inflammatory response, chronic inflammatory response, granulation tissue development and foreign body reaction to implanted vascular grafts. The intensity and time variables are dependent upon the extent of injury created in the implantation and the size, shape and topography, and chemical and physical properties of the biomaterial as well as the porosity of the vascular graft.

Table 19.1. Sequence of local events following implantation

Injury
Acute inflammation
Chronic inflammation
Granulation tissue
Foreign body reaction
Fibrosis

While little is known regarding the acute and chronic inflammatory responses to the luminal surfaces of vascular grafts, some understanding of the series of events following injury in the inflammatory and wound healing responses to the porous periadventitial surface of vascular grafts is appreciated. Acute inflammation is of relatively short duration, lasting from minutes to days, and is characterized by the exudation fluid and plasma proteins and the immigration of leukocytes, predominantly neutrophils. Neutrophils are short lived and disintegrate and disappear after 24-48 h, depending on the form and topography of the vascular graft. Highly porous prostheses may have a longer lived neutrophil response, as these cells migrate into the porous body of the vascular graft. This is especially true with loosely knitted and velour Dacron vascular grafts and has not been a prominent observation with ePTFE grafts.

The accumulation of leukocytes, in particular neutrophils and monocytes, is the most important feature of the inflammatory reaction. Leukocytes accumulate through a series of processes including margination, adhesion, integration, phagocytosis, and extracellular release of leukocyte products. Leukocyte immigration is controlled in part by chemotaxis, which is the unidirectional migration of cells along the chemical gradient. A wide variety of exogenous and endogenous substances have been identified as chemotactic agents. Important to the immigration is movement of leukocytes, as is the presence of specific receptors for chemotactic agents on the cell membranes of leukocytes. These and other receptors may also play a role in the activation of leukocytes.

Blood protein adsorption to the luminal, periadventitial and interstitial surfaces of porous vascular graft biomaterials is a significant early response which is poorly understood. The protein adsorption phenomenon occurs prior to any cellular interaction. Prior to the immigration of leukocytes to and within the vascular graft, blood protein has coated the surfaces of the graft material and thus presents a protein-modified surface to cellular interactions. The physical and chemical characteristics of the vascular graft material itself may play little role in subsequent cellular and humoral responses. Obviously, preclotting of the

Fig. 19.1. The temporal variation in the tissue response continuum.

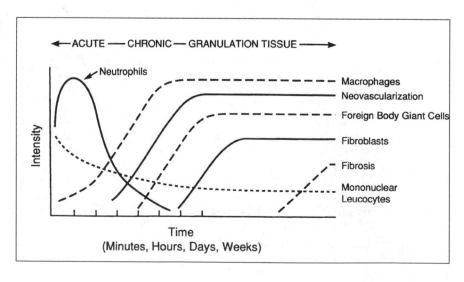

vascular graft accomplishes the protein precoating in an excessive fashion.[6]

To better understand the early blood protein adsorption onto vascular graft materials, we have utilized a surface radioimmunoassay technique and an immunogold labeling technique with scanning electron microscopy to characterize human blood protein adsorption onto Dacron and ePTFE vascular grafts in an in vitro human blood recirculation system.[7-10] The detection of the various proteins deposited on the surfaces of the Dacron, ePTFE and control materials fell into two groups: Fibrinogen, IgG and albumin were found in the highest amounts; Hageman factor (factor XII), factor VIII/vWF, fibronectin and hemoglobin were found in moderate amounts. Of the proteins assayed, IgG showed the greatest degree of adsorption and affinity to all of the materials tested and particularly to Dacron and ePTFE. After exposure of the tested materials for five minutes, IgG accounted for approximately 25% of the radioactivity bound to Dacron and to ePTFE. In the recirculation system, significant protein adsorption had occurred within 5 minutes of blood contact and did not significantly increase out to 180 minutes. Fibrinogen adsorption to Dacron and ePTFE decreased as the time of exposure to blood increased. Hageman factor (factor XII) significantly decreased on Dacron as the time of exposure increased, but its adsorption to other materials, i.e., ePTFE and silica-free PDMS, remained constant over the 180 minute time period. Adsorption of IgG to Dacron decreased with time, but IgG adsorption to ePTFE and PDMS did not change over 180 minutes.

These studies demonstrate that early adsorption of blood proteins which are adhesion receptor ligands (fibronectin, fibrinogen), opsonins which can facilitate complement activation (IgG), and significant coagulation cascade proteins (Hageman factor) adsorb quickly and readily to the luminal surfaces, where they may participate in subsequent inflammatory, coagulation and thrombotic processes.

Our human blood recirculation system has been also utilized to investigate vascular graft-associated complement activation and leukocyte adhesion.[11] Materials tested were ePTFE, crimped Dacron Bionit (C.R. Bard) and preclotted Dacron Bionit. A decrease in the total blood leukocyte concentration with perfusion time was seen for all materials tested, and increasing leukocyte adhesion to the graft surface was observed by scanning electron microscopy. The most dramatic decrease in leukocyte concentration was observed for the interaction of heparinized whole blood with Dacron. This was due to the selective decrease in neutrophils and monocytes, and was correlated with an increase in both leukocyte adhesiveness and complement activation, as measured by C5a elevation. Minimal complement activation or leukocyte adhesion was observed for ePTFE and the silicone rubber control. Interestingly, Dacron Bionit exhibited the highest C5a levels when compared to Dacron Bionit which had been preclotted in whole blood. Dacron Bionit preclotted in platelet-poor plasma gave C5a levels which were slightly greater than ePTFE which was comparable to the silicone rubber control. These studies demonstrated the significance of utilizing an appropriate anticoagulant in in vitro studies with human blood and vascular grafts. Heparin was used as the anticoagulant for these studies; this anticoagulant permits complement activation with subsequent leukocyte activation. The utilization of citrate, EDTA or EGTA will deplete or bind calcium ions significantly, thus inhibiting complement activation by the calcium-dependent pathway.

With highly porous grafts, i.e., knits and velours, acute and chronic inflammatory cell infiltration into the interstices of the vascular grafts occurs. The time dependent nature of these responses and the extent of their duration within the interstices of the vascular grafts are dependent upon the porosity and structure of the vascular grafts. As described earlier, preclotting of Dacron vascular grafts provides a barrier to this response and little is known regarding inflammatory cell infiltration into preclotted vascular grafts.

In the early 1980s, Meadox Medicals provided a collagen coated Dacron vascular graft, Hemashield with Microvel, in which a thin layer of collagen was present on the luminal and adventitial surfaces as well as within the interstices of the vascular graft. This simple concept, originally considered to replace preclotting of the Dacron vascular grafts, also had a significant inhibition of the inflammatory cell infiltrate in the early response. The collagen coating converted a highly porous material into a nonporous material which developed its porosity in vivo by the biodegradation of the collagen coating. The biodegradation of the collagen coating occurs within 4-12 weeks, and thus porosity develops after the inflammatory responses and during the granulation tissue and fibrosis phases of the healing response. As the porosity develops, macrophages and fibroblasts present at the graft/tissue interface migrate into the vascular graft to produce the foreign body reaction and fibrosis without having to contend with the detritus of the inflammatory reaction.[12] The collagen coated Dacron grafts are an early example of vascular graft tissue engineering.

Foreign Body Reaction

The foreign body reaction consisting of macrophages and foreign body giant cells develops at the periadventitial tissue-material interface coincidentally with the development of granulation tissue, with its attendant fibroblast proliferation and neovascularization, i.e., capillary formation. At the same time, smooth muscle cells and fibroblasts from the wall of the native artery migrate and proliferate along the surface of the vascular graft to produce a pseudointima. Endothelial cells also migrate and proliferate from the native artery at the anastomosis, but in humans their migration into the vascular graft is limited in extent as compared to animal models where endothelialization is extensive. This lack of endothelialization of the pseudointimal surface of the vascular graft in humans has remained a challenge and a profound problem with human vascular grafts. Of special note is the apparent lack of inflammatory cell interaction at the luminal surface of human vascular grafts.[13] Given the potential for complement activation and leukocyte adhesion, one might have expected early monocyte adhesion and differentiation into macrophages which can fuse into foreign body giant cells at the luminal surfaces of vascular graft materials. Studies of retrieved human vascular grafts, however, suggest that this sequence of events does not occur, as foreign body giant cells are not identified at the material-blood, material-blood protein or material-pseudointimal interface on the luminal surface of ePTFE vascular grafts. With Dacron, FBGCs at the luminal surface of the graft material are seen following the healing response and neovascularization within the graft interstices. Studies in our laboratory have suggested that leukocyte adhesion is dependent on both complement C3 and fibronectin deposition, as well as being sensitive to the levels of shear stress in flowing blood.[14] High levels of shear stress and/or turbulence, as well as low levels of complement C3 and fibronectin deposition, may result in minimal to no leukocyte adhesion, and thus macrophage development and foreign body giant cell formation at the luminal surfaces is limited.

The histological evaluation of retrieved human vascular grafts shows the presence of macrophages and foreign body giant cells interacting with the prosthetic material within the graft interstices and at the periadventitial surface. The foreign body reaction with macrophages and foreign body giant cells has been demonstrated as early as several weeks following implantation. In vascular grafts which have been implanted for over two decades, these cells are still present at the tissue-material interface. As the foreign body reaction appears to be virtually an all-inclusive interaction at soft tissue-material interfaces, we have focused our attention on the potential roles played by macrophages and foreign body giant cells not only in modulating the wound healing response but also their potential participation in failure mechanisms of human vascular grafts, i.e., anastomotic hyperplasia and stenosing pseudointimal hyperplasia.

In 1984, we began to address the hypothesis that adherent macrophages which were activated released chemical mediators, in particular cytokines, which in an autocrine, paracrine and endocrine fashion modulated the formation of the foreign body reaction at the tissue-material interface and the development of the fibrous capsule.[3,15,16] Figure 19.2 illustrates this early concept, in which activated macrophages on protein-coated biomedical polymer surfaces produce and secrete various cytokines and growth factors which can modulate platelet activity, fibroblast proliferation and se-

cretion of extracellular matrix materials, and endothelial cell proliferation, which can affect the hemostatic, thrombotic balance, and smooth muscle cell proliferation which may participate in anastomotic or pseudointimal hyperplasia. This hypothesis developed from two aspects of our research. First, the consistent and all-inclusive finding that macrophages and foreign body giant cells were present at the interface of clinically retrieved human vascular grafts regardless of implant time pointed toward the importance of the macrophage and foreign body giant cells in tissue-material interactions. Secondly, our in vivo cage implant studies with a wide variety of vascular graft materials, including polyether polyurethanes, demonstrated the early—as soon as three days—adhesion of monocytes/macrophages on the surfaces of the materials.

The second area of research was the first demonstration that adherent activated macrophages and foreign body giant cells on polyether polyurethane surfaces were responsible for the biodegradation of these materials.[17,18] This finding explained the earlier clinical studies of polyurethane degradation in cardiac pacemaker leads, and also explains the biodegradation of polyether polyurethanes when they are utilized as vascular graft materials. Numerous academic and industrial scientists have attempted to utilize polyether polyurethanes as porous and nonporous vascular grafts, but long term implant studies indicate biodegradation with attendant dilatation of the vascular graft or loss of integrity of the wall of the polyether polyurethane vascular graft. These studies, in part, have led to the development of more stable polyurethanes by the incorporation of more efficient antioxidants, substitution of the degradable polyether soft segments by more stable soft segment prepolymers such as polydimethylsiloxane or polycarbonates, and the chemical modification of polyether polyurethanes by so-called "end-capping," where more stable moieties are bonded to the chain ends to produce polymers which are inherently less biodegradable.[19]

These new materials are in the early stages of development and testing for application as vascular graft materials, and it is anticipated that the desirable elastomeric

Fig. 19.2. The tissue/implant interface with protein adsorption, macrophage adhesion and activation, cytokine and growth factor production, and cellular synthesis and proliferation.

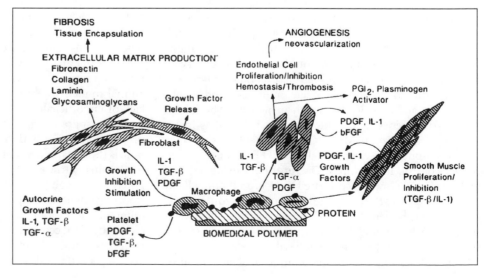

and biocompatible properties of the polyurethanes will prove to be efficacious and not undergo inflammatory cell-mediated biodegradation when utilized in various vascular applications.

Macrophage Motility, Adhesion and Activation

The accumulation of macrophages in vascular graft implant sites is achieved through selective cellular and humoral mechanisms that both attract and immobilize macrophages and macrophage precursors where their functional activity can be directed at resolution and/or repair of tissue. Monocytes contact stimulatory factors within blood vessels around the vascular graft and adhere to endothelial cells lining the vessels. These monocytes then pass through the vessel wall and into the tissue undergoing transformation in response to the stimuli and differentiate into macrophages. Monocyte and macrophage movement within the tissue toward the site of injury is controlled and directed by chemotaxis or chemokinesis. Chemokinesis is the accelerated random locomotion in response to, and the speed of turning of the cells toward, chemical stimuli, whereas chemotaxis is the highly directed movement of cells along a chemical gradient. Table 19.2 shows important agents which mediate chemotaxis and are integral features of the inflammatory process. These agents can both sustain and control the severity of the inflammatory response. In addition to dead or dying cells, chemotactic stimuli include fragments derived from the activation of complement protein, mediators of the kinin, clotting and fibrinolytic systems, and products produced by leukocytes themselves.

Our early studies on human monocyte/macrophage activation and interleukin-1 generation by biomedical polymers were carried out in in vitro cell culture systems where the interleukin-1 production was assayed by a biological thymocyte proliferation biological assay.[20-26] In the mid to late 1980s, a paucity of reagents was available to study specific cytokines and growth factors produced by macrophages and foreign body giant cells in contact with vascular graft materials. Later, when radioimmunoassays and ELISAs became available for interleukin-1 quantitation, these were incorporated into our studies. It is noteworthy that biomedical polymers have a very low potential for activating macrophages with the release of interleukin-1. In our studies, we utilized lipopolysaccharide to additionally stimulate the adherent monocytes/macrophages, as we believe that this is

more indicative of the inflammatory reaction at the tissue/material interface. Studies under these conditions demonstrated that Dacron and polyethylene exhibited a high reactivity as measured by IL-1 release, ePTFE was intermediate and Biomer and polydimethylsiloxane were low in their abilities to activate macrophages and release interleukin-1.[24] To examine the paracrine effect of interleukin-1 on fibroblast proliferation, we studied the effect of supernatants produced by the in vitro interaction of monocytes/macrophages on various biomedical polymers including Dacron and ePTFE and subsequently measured the fibroblast-stimulating potential for these supernatants. For Dacron and ePTFE, the fibroblast stimulatory potential was equivalent, but the interleukin-1 activity for Dacron was much higher than that exhibited for ePTFE. Neutralization experiments utilizing specific antibodies to interleukin-1 in our experiments demonstrated the potential production and paracrine effects of other cytokines and growth factors which may also be produced in the macrophage activation and secretory process.

Table 19.3 illustrates some monocyte/macrophage molecules important in modulation of inflammation and wound healing with vascular graft materials. The potential role for the molecules is shown; these molecules may be either secreted to produce an autocrine, paracrine or endocrine effect or may be cell membrane associated, such as important adhesion molecules and receptors which may participate in the adhesion of monocytes/macrophages to protein-coated vascular graft materials or in cell-cell interactions important in the inflammatory and wound healing processes. Table 19.4 provides a partial list of chemoattractants and growth modulators produced by macrophages. This table is limited to only those agents thought to be important in the tissue-material interaction in the inflammatory response to vascular graft materials. It is noteworthy that interleukin-1 and tissue growth factor-β (TGF-β) may function as growth agonists or growth antagonists. The schizophrenic nature of cytokines and growth factors must be considered when attempting to explain the autocrine, paracrine or endocrine activity of cytokines and growth factors.

Greisler and colleagues have utilized monocyte/macrophage molecules released during the inflammatory and wound healing processes to modulate cellular proliferation in the wound healing and neointimal response to vascular graft materials.[27] In in vitro studies, fibroblast growth factor type I (FGF-I) and heparin placed into suspensions of fibrinogen polymerized by addition of thrombin (fibrin glue) promoted endothelial cell proliferation while suppressing smooth muscle cell proliferation. These studies demonstrated the potential for controlled release systems coupled with vascular graft materials which could cellularly engineer the wound healing response with vascular grafts. Preliminary in vivo experiments utilizing growth factor release from vascular grafts in canines demonstrated this concept and identified the potential for the direct control of inflammatory and healing responses directly by cytokines and growth factors.[28] From a tissue engineering perspective, this is a promising avenue of exploration which requires additional effort.

Table 19.2. Major mediators of macrophage chemotaxis

Complement Components
Lymphokines
Fibronectin Fragments
Leukotriene B$_4$
Interleukins (IL-1, IL-8)
Endothelial Cell Products
Monocyte Chemotactic Peptide 1 (MCP-1)
Thrombin
Fibrinopeptides

Table 19.3. Monocyte/macrophage molecules important in the modulation of inflammation and wound healing

Molecule	Expression	Role
Interleukin-1 (IL-1) Receptor	Secreted	Increased Adhesion Molecule Expression, Smooth Muscle Cell Migration and Proliferation, Inhibit Endothelial Cell Proliferation
Interleukin-1 Receptor Antagonist (IL-1Ra)	Secreted	Decreases Interleukin-1 Response
Interleukin-6 (IL-6)	Secreted	Activation of Coagulation, Smooth Muscle Cell Secondary Gene Induction
Interleukin-8 (IL-8)	Secreted	Recruitment of Lymphocytes and Endothelial Cells
Monocyte Chemoattractant Protein-1 (MCP-1)	Secreted	Monocyte Chemoattractant, Activation of β_2 Integrin Receptors
Monocyte Colony-Stimulating Factor (M-CSF)	Secreted	Monocyte Chemoattraction, Proliferation, and Survival
Granulocyte/Monocyte Colony Stimulating Factor (GM-CSF)	Secreted	Chemoattractant for Monocytes
Tumor Necrosis Factor-α (TNF-α)	Secreted	Increase Endothelial Cell Adhesion Molecule Expression, Monocyte Chemoattractant, Smooth Muscle Cell Proliferation, Inhibits Endothelial Cell Proliferation
Transforming Growth Factor-β (TGF-β)	Secreted	Monocyte Chemoattractant, Increases Smooth Muscle Cell Proliferation Inhibits Endothelial Cell Proliferation
Interferon-γ (INF-γ)	Secreted	Inhibits Endothelial Cell and Smooth Muscle Cell Proliferation
Osteopontin	Secreted	Cell Adhesion and Migration, Neovessel Formation, and Calcification
SPARC, Osteonectin	Secreted	Cell Migration, Proliferation, and Neovessel Formation
Thrombospondin	Secreted	Cell Migration, Neovessel Formation
Oxidized Low Density	Secreted	Increases Monocyte Chemotaxis and Macrophage Secretion of IL-1 and TNF-α
Lipoprotein (oxLDL)		Increases VCAM-1 Expression on Endothelium
basic Fibroblast Growth Factor (bFGF)	Secreted	Endothelial Cell Chemoattractant, Increases Endothelial Cell and Smooth Muscle Cell Proliferation
Vascular Endothelium Growth Factor (VEGF)	Secreted	Increases Endothelial Cell Proliferation
Insulin-like Growth Factor (IGF-1)	Secreted	Smooth Muscle Cell Chemoattractant, Increases Smooth Muscle Cell Proliferation
acidic Fibroblast Growth Factor (aFGF)	Secreted	Endothelial Cell Chemoattraction and Proliferation
Heparin-Binding Epidermal Growth Factor (HB-EGF)	Secreted	Smooth Muscle Cell Chemoattraction and Proliferation
Platelet-Derived Growth Factor (PDGF)	Secreted	Smooth Muscle Cell Chemoattraction and Proliferation
Vascular Adhesion Molecule-1 (VCAM-1)	Cell-Associated	Monocyte/Macrophage Activation and Retention
Intercellular Cell Adhesion Molecule (ICAM-1)	Cell-Associated	Monocyte/Macrophage Activation and Retention
Complement C3bi Receptor	Cell-Associated	Thrombosis and Macrophage Adhesion
Thrombin Receptor	Cell-Associated	Monocyte/Macrophage Activation

To complement our in vitro human monocyte/macrophage activation and cytokine secretion studies, we have continued to evaluate retrieved human vascular grafts and our latest effort involves cytokine and growth factor analysis utilizing immunohistochemistry and steady state mRNA analysis with in situ hybridization techniques. Cytokines and growth factors/inhibitors studied included interleukin-1α (IL-1α), interleukin-1β (IL-1β), tumor necrosis factor-α (TNF-α), transforming growth factor-β1 (TGF-β1), and platelet derived growth factor A and B (PDGF-A and -B). For analysis, five contiguous zones or areas on or within retrieved vascular grafts were evaluated: luminal surface, pseudointima (inner capsule), pseudointima-graft interface (including the luminal portion of the graft), periadventitia-graft interface (including the outer portion of the graft), and periadventitia (outer capsule).

The luminal surface of the vascular graft specimens showed no to some endothelium at the blood-pseudointima interface. The pseudointima (inner capsule) was predominantly acellular but isolated areas of fibroblasts and smooth muscle cells were identified. In situ hybridization studies identified IL-1α, IL-1β, TNF-α, TGF-β, and PDGF-A and -B in the pseudointima. The pseudointima-graft interface showed the presence of macrophages and foreign body giant cells adjacent to the ePTFE graft nodes and fibrils and Dacron fibers and fiber bundles. These components of the foreign body reaction were localized at the synthetic graft fiber interface but not in areas distant from the luminal surface of the graft. The interstitial network of the synthetic vascular grafts contained isolated fibroblasts. In situ hybridization and immunohistochemistry analysis identified the presence of IL-1α, IL-1β, TNF-α, TGF-β, and PDGF-A and

Table 19.4. Chemoattractants and growth modulators produced by macrophages

Chemoattractants	Growth Agonists	Growth Antagonists
Granulocyte/Monocyte-Colony Stimulating Factor (GM-CSF)	Granulocyte/Monocyte-Colony Stimulating Factor (GM-CSF)	Interferon-γ (IFN-γ)
Monocyte-Colony Stimulating Factor (M-CSF)	Monocyte-Colony Stimulating Factor (M-CSF)	Interleukin-1 (IL-1)
Basic Fibroblast Growth Factor (bFGF)	Heparin-Binding Epidermal Growth Factor (HB-EGF)	Transforming Growth Factor-β (TGF-β)
Monocyte Chemotactic Protein-1 (MCP-1)	Insulin-like Growth Factor (IGF-1)	
Tissue Growth Factor-β (TGF-β)	Vascular Endothelial Growth Factor (VEGF)	
Platelet Derived Growth Factor (PDGF)	Basic Fibroblast Growth Factor (bFGF)	
Vascular Endothelial Growth Factor (VEGF)	Interleukin-1 (IL-1)	
Oxidized Low Density Lipoprotein (oxLDL)	Tumor Necrosis Factor-α (TNF-α)	
	Transforming Growth Factor-α (TGF-α)	
	Transforming Growth Factor-β (TGF-β)	
	Platelet Derived Growth Factor (PDGF)	

-B in the pseudointima-graft interface. The graft-periadventitial tissue interface exhibited a foreign body reaction with the presence of macrophages and foreign body giant cells localized at the synthetic graft surface. This interface also exhibited the same cytokines and growth factors identified at the pseudointima-graft interface by immunohistochemical and in situ hybridization techniques. The periadventitial fibrous capsule (outer capsule) showed a well-healed fibrous capsule with fibroblasts and capillaries within a type I collagen matrix. These histopathologic features were similar for all types of retrieved human vascular grafts. In situ hybridization and immunohistochemical analysis showed the presence of IL-1α, IL-1β, TNF-α, TGF-β, and PDGF-A and -B within the outer capsule.

Overall, for IL-1α, high levels of expression of steady state IL-1α mRNA were identified by in situ hybridization, and protein expression as determined by immunohistochemistry was also high. Higher levels of steady state IL-1α mRNA were present in the periadventitial fibrous (outer) capsule relative to the pseudointima, the pseudointima-graft interface and the periadventitia-graft interface. Fibroblast-like cells were the predominant cell type in the outer capsule and expressed higher levels of IL-1α mRNA, as compared to other cell types including smooth muscle cells and endothelial cells in the capillaries. In the pseudointima, fibroblast-like cells expressed high levels of IL-1α mRNA, whereas smooth muscle cells did not appear to express IL-1α mRNA. In contrast to the pseudointima and the periadventitial fibrous capsule, macrophages and foreign body giant cells in the pseudointima-graft and periadventitia-graft interfaces were predominant cell types that expressed IL-1α mRNA and protein. Relative levels of IL-1β mRNA and protein detected in Dacron and ePTFE vascular graft sections were similar to that of the IL-1α mRNA detected. Overall, the periadventitial fibrous (outer) capsule expressed higher levels of steady state IL-1β mRNA relative to the other areas. However, with the ePTFE vascular grafts, very low levels of IL-1β mRNA were found in all of the areas studied. IL-1β mRNA was predominantly ex-

pressed by macrophages and foreign body giant cells. Steady state TNF-α mRNA expression was variable, with moderate amounts of mRNA and protein being associated with macrophages and foreign body giant cells.

TGF-β1 mRNA expression was low compared to IL-1α and IL-1β mRNA. Likewise, protein levels of TGF-β as determined by immunohistochemistry were also lower than IL-1α and IL-1β. Fibroblast-like cells in the pseudointima and periadventitial fibrous (outer) capsule, and macrophages and foreign body giant cells at the graft-tissue interfaces, were the predominant cells that expressed TGF-β1 mRNA. The expression of steady state PDGF-A and -B mRNAs was examined, and the relative levels were similar. Relatively low levels were identified, and immunohistochemical analysis indicated no or little protein.

Our preliminary study focused on the utilization of mRNA for transcriptional analysis and cell localization in combination with protein expression by immunohistochemistry as an indicator of translational events. Detection of IL-1α and -β mRNAs and protein suggests that IL-1 may act as a regulatory protein in the induction of intimal/anastomotic hyperplasia. In addition, the presence of IL-1α mRNA in fibroblast-like cells and myofibroblast-like cells suggests that it may function as a paracrine messenger, stimulating fibroblasts and myofibroblasts to proliferate and differentiate. Activated fibroblasts also produce a number of soluble mediators including bFGF, PDGF and IL-1 which can activate other inflammatory cells in addition to smooth muscle cells. Although not as strong as IL-1α mRNA, steady state IL-1β mRNA was identified and may stimulate smooth muscle cell proliferation in a paracrine fashion.

Transformtin growth factor-β1 (TGF-β1) was identified at low levels of steady state mRNA expression in macrophages and foreign body giant cells. TGF-β1 is an important regulator of the duration of the inflammatory response and also is a potent inhibitor of cell proliferation, as well as a stimulator of connective tissue formation by cells. The enhanced activity of macrophages and foreign body giant cells was exhibited by the detection of steady state TNF-α mRNA.

TNF-α is known to enhance the phagocytic activity of macrophages and foreign body giant cells. Our in situ hybridization study found low levels of steady state mRNAs for PDGF-A and -B in macrophages and foreign body giant cells, and very little to no protein was detected by immunohistochemistry.

The detection of various cytokine mRNAs and protein implicates cytokine-mediated interactions of cellular components in the ePTFE and Dacron vascular grafts. The paracrine interaction mediated by IL-1 in macrophages/foreign body giant cells and fibroblasts/myofibroblasts with vascular smooth muscle cells is strongly suggested by these findings.

Foreign Body Giant Cell Formation

As part of our ongoing investigation into the role of the monocyte/macrophage in biocompatibility, a major goal has been to identify the adhesion and fusion mechanisms that initiate and promote the observed in vivo morphologic progression of monocyte to macrophage to foreign body giant cell on biomaterials and vascular graft materials. Adherent monocyte-derived macrophages and foreign body giant cells (FBGCs), formed by macrophage fusion, are prominent and persistent cell types on implanted vascular grafts and, through their numerous secretory capacities, are believed to exert multiple and complex influences on the inflammatory response at the implant site and on the biocompatibility of vascular grafts. Although monocyte adhesion to implanted vascular grafts is critical to biocompatibility outcome, as it initiates macrophage development and FBGC formation, it is unknown how monocytes recognize biomaterials and how surface properties might influence this event.

Material surface property-dependent blood protein adsorption occurs immediately upon surgical implantation of a vascular graft, and it is the protein-modified biomaterial that inflammatory cells subsequently encounter. Monocytes express receptors for various blood components, but they recognize naturally occurring foreign surfaces by receptors for opsonins such as fragments of complement component C3. Because complement activation by biomaterials has been well documented, we investigated monocyte interactions with foreign surfaces. Exposure to blood during vascular graft implantation may permit extensive opsonization with the labile fragment C3b and the rapid conversion of C3b to its hemolytically inactive but nevertheless opsonic and more stable form, C3bi. C3b is bound by the Cd35 receptor, but C3bi is recognized by distinct receptors, Cd11b/cd18 and Cd11c/cd18. Fibrinogen, a major plasma protein that adsorbs to vascular grafts, is another described ligand for these molecules, which together with Cd11a/cd18 constitutes a subfamily of integrins that is restricted to leukocytes. Studies with monoclonal antibodies to their common β$_2$ subunit (CD18) and distinct α chains (Cd11a,b,c) have implicated Cd11a/cd18 in cell-cell adhesive interactions and Cd11b/cd18 and Cd11c/cd18 in multiple phagocytic cell responses. Other potential adhesion-mediating proteins that adsorb to biomaterials include IgG, which may interact with monocytes via receptors to its Fc constant region, and fibronectin, for which monocytes also express multiple types of receptors.

Because of experimental complexities in dealing with the three dimensional structures of Dacron and ePTFE, we initiated our studies utilizing chemically-modified polystyrene surfaces to explore the role of surface chemistry in monocyte adhesion, macrophage phenotypic expression and foreign body giant cell formation.[29] Human monocyte in vitro adhesion with fluorinated, siliconized, nitrogenated and oxygenated surfaces were reduced by 50-100% when complement component C3-depleted serum was used for adsorption. The fluorinated surfaces exhibited the greatest inhibition of monocyte adhesion with C3-depleted serum. Monocyte adhesion was restored on all surfaces when C3-depleted serum was replenished with purified C3. Monocyte adhesion to serum-adsorbed surfaces was inhibited by monoclonal antibodies to the leukocyte integrin beta subunit, CD18, and partially inhibited by a monoclonal antibody to the alpha subunit Cd11b. These findings suggest adhesive interactions between adsorbed C3bi, the hemolytically inactive form of the C3b fragment, and the leukocyte integrin Cd11b/cd18. Additional studies demonstrated that adsorbed fibrinogen reduced the effectiveness of these inhibiting monoclonal antibodies, indicating that alternative adhesion mechanisms may operate, depending on the critical adhesion-mediating components adsorbed onto the different surfaces.

Recent studies in our laboratory have implicated IL-4 and IL-13 cytokines in the in vitro formation of foreign body giant cells derived from human monocytes/macrophages.[30-33] These studies have resulted in the development of an in vitro culture system that may now be utilized for testing various materials for their ability to participate in foreign body giant cell formation. When IL-4 or IL-13 are added to human monocyte cultures at day 3, foreign body giant cells containing as many as 100 nuclei and measuring 1.0 mm^2 in surface area are formed on various modified surfaces. Critical to these experiments was the addition of the cytokine at day 3 of the culture and not at day 0 of the culture. Simultaneous addition of the cytokine and the cells at the beginning of the culture does not lead to foreign body giant cell formation and may result in the lack of monocyte/macrophage adhesion to the substrate. This sequential addition of the cytokine points out the importance of temporal variations which may occur in addressing cytokine/cell interactions.

IL-4 and IL-13 are lymphokines secreted predominantly by Th2 lymphocytes in humans. Thus, lymphocytes present transiently in the early chronic inflammatory phase of the inflammatory response may participate in the foreign body reaction through facilitation of the formation of foreign body giant cells. IL-4 and IL-13 downregulate the secretion of proinflammatory cytokines such as IL-1, IL-6 and TNF-α; growth factors such as granulocyte-macrophage CSF and granulocyte CSF; and chemokines such as IL-8 and macrophage inflammatory protein-1α. FcγR expression, reactive oxygen intermediate secretion and cytotoxic activities are also inhibited by these cytokines. Conversely, IL-4 and IL-13 upregulate monocyte/macrophage production of

IL-1R antagonist, antigen-presenting capacity and cell surface expression of several adhesion molecules including Cd11b/cd18 and Cd11c/cd18. Although IL-4 and IL-13 negatively regulate several cytotoxic and inflammatory functions of monocytes/macrophages, they are not generally viewed as downregulators of monocyte/macrophage activity.

The role for IL-4 in foreign body giant cell formation in vivo has been demonstrated in a rat cage implant system with polyurethane.[31] Utilization of both recombinant IL-4 and anti-IL-4 injected into the cage demonstrates the enhancement and inhibition of foreign body giant cell formation on the polyurethane surface, respectively. The in vivo studies also point out the lack of effect by IL-4 in facilitating macrophage adhesion to the polyurethane surface. Thus, the IL-4 appears to facilitate foreign body giant cell formation through mechanisms not related to the surface density of adherent macrophages.

Complementary experiments with IL-4-induced macrophage fusion in foreign body giant cell development has shown the prevention of macrophage fusion and the formation of foreign body giant cells by the use of inhibitors of mannose receptor activity. α-Mannan and synthetic neoglycoprotein conjugates inhibit the fusion of macrophages to form foreign body giant cells. Inhibition of macrophage activity in the formation of foreign body giant cells may be facilitated by blocking inhibitors which participate in the macrophage fusion process. This offers a pathway by which the foreign body reaction may be controlled.

Future Perspectives on Inflammatory Responses to Tissue Engineered Prosthetic Vascular Grafts

The future development of tissue engineered prosthetic vascular grafts requires new knowledge and information on normal and directed healing mechanisms, biological signals and signal mechanisms, and delivery and phenotypic expression of cells in and on tissue-engineered prosthetic vascular grafts. Research efforts in the tissue engineering area must be directed towards developing new information, i.e., biologically-based design criteria, and an expansion of our current knowledge base regarding these processes and mechanisms. There is no doubt that we are exceptionally limited in our knowledge base as it applies to the research and development of tissue-engineered prosthetic vascular grafts. In considering the early responses to implanted tissue engineered prosthetic vascular grafts, emphasis must be placed on developing an understanding of the inflammatory response interactions with the tissue-engineered prosthetic vascular graft with its unique characteristics. As such, the evaluation must take into consideration the unique function and application of the tissue-engineered prosthetic vascular graft. A major hurdle to this effort is the apparent species differences which exist with prosthetic vascular grafts and in particular the process of endothelialization which occurs in primates and other mammals, but not in human prosthetic vascular grafts. Coupled with this problem is the lack of knowledge regarding the phenotypic expression of cellular components in the inflammatory response in different species.

The second major barrier that must be confronted is the highly complex and time-dependent nature of the cellular and humoral components of the inflammatory responses. Our approach has been to utilize human material whenever possible, but this limits one to in vitro experiments. As humans cannot ethically be used in preliminary experiments to test the safety of devices, animal models must be utilized. The question resulting from the use of animal models is the equivalency of, and similarity and differences between, the animal model and the response in humans. Not only must the various components of the inflammatory response be considered, but also the extent and duration of the components of the inflammatory response and the time-dependent nature, i.e., kinetics, of the inflammatory responses and their components. These factors may or may not vary when comparing animal model responses to human responses.

These barriers and lack of knowledge of inflammatory responses offer new challenges that must be met in the research and development of tissue-engineered prosthetic vascular grafts. New paradigms must be developed with new perspectives based on new information, and older paradigms, while comfortable to some investigators, may not adequately and appropriately address the significant scientific issues that are necessary in the development of tissue-engineered prosthetic vascular grafts.

A third major barrier facing us in the development of tissue-engineered prosthetic vascular grafts is the adequate and appropriate evaluation of new concepts or products from a safety and efficacy perspective. Unique devices will require unique testing and evaluation protocols. Appropriate rationale and justification must be provided for the inclusion or omission of test methods, which will be based on the unique characteristics of the tissue-engineered prosthetic vascular graft under consideration. New materials and devices designed for deliberate and specific interactions with blood and tissue components must be based on those deliberate and specific interactions, which are a component of the design of the tissue engineered prosthetic vascular graft. In the development of tests for tissue-engineered prosthetic vascular grafts, it is important that we emphasize the complex and interactive milieu of the cellular and humoral components that interact or are anticipated to interact with the tissue-engineered prosthetic vascular graft. We must appreciate the interactive environment provided by the numerous humoral enzyme systems (kinin, fibrinolytic, coagulation and complement), formed elements (platelets), and cells (polymorphonuclear leukocytes, monocytes, lymphocytes and eosinophils) which provide for positive (activating) and negative (inhibiting) interactions. Failure to appreciate these types of interactions and feedback control mechanisms may lead to false interpretations of results from single or isolated test methods. Furthermore, emphasis must be placed on the quantitative determination of parameters in the biological response evaluation. As our knowledge base for the research and development of new tissue-engineered prosthetic vascular grafts increases, enhanced integration of disciplines affecting not only the basic research but also the development of test methods will be necessary.

It is our perspective that the inflammatory response to prosthetic vascular grafts and tissue-engineered prosthetic vascular grafts is not necessarily a nemesis. In the past, we have tended to label the inflammatory response as a nemesis, i.e., source of harm or destruction, based upon our incomplete knowledge of the inflammatory and wound healing responses. With the expansion of our knowledge base of inflammatory cell interactions with prosthetic vascular grafts and tissue-engineered prosthetic vascular grafts, we can anticipate that the new and expanded knowledge base of inflammatory responses and interactions will be utilized to modify inflammatory cell responses to these new devices, and possibly convert a foe into a friend or ally.

References

1. Anderson JM. Mechanisms of inflammation and infection with implanted devices. Cardiovasc Pathol 1993; 2:199S-208S.
2. Anderson JM. Inflammation and the foreign body response. Problems in General Surgery 1994; 11:147-160.
3. Anderson JM. Inflammatory response to implants. ASAIO J 1988; 11:101-107.
4. Wesolowski SA. Evaluation of Tissue and Prosthetic Vascular Grafts. Springfield:Charles C. Thomas, 1962.
5. Wesolowski SA and Dennis C, eds. Fundamentals of Vascular Grafting. New York:McGraw-Hill Book Company, Inc., 1963.
6. Yates SG, Barros AAB, Berger K et al. The preclotting of porous arterial prostheses. Ann Surg 1978; 188:611-622.
7. Ziats NP, Pankowsky DA, Tierney BP et al. Adsorption of Hageman factor (factor XII) and other human plasma proteins to biomedical polymers. J Lab Clin Med 1990; 116:687-696.
8. Pankowsky DA, Ziats NP, Topham NS et al. Morphological characteristics of adsorbed human plasma proteins on vascular grafts and biomaterials. J Vasc Surg 1990; 11:599-606.
9. Anderson JM, Bonfield TL, Ziats NP. Protein adsorption and cellular adhesion and activation on biomedical polymers. Int J Artif Org 1990; 13:375-382.
10. Ziats NP, Topham NS, Pankowsky DA, Anderson JM. Analysis of protein adsorption on retrieved human vascular grafts using immunogold labelling with silver enhancement. Cells & Materials 1991; 1:73-82.
11. Kottke-Marchant K, Anderson JM, Miller KM et al. Vascular graft associated complement activation and leukocyte adhesion in an artificial circulation. J Biomed Mater Res 1987; 21:379-397.
12. Anderson JM. Microvel with Hemashield vascular grafts. A preliminary report of the healing response in humans. Angio Archiv 1985; 9:73-77.
13. Anderson JM, Abbuhl MF, Hering T, Johnston KH. Immunohistochemical identification of components in the healing response of human vascular grafts. ASAIO J 1985; 8:79-85.
14. Kao WJ, Sapatnekar S, Hiltner A, Anderson JM. Complement-mediated leukocyte adhesion on poly(etherurethane ureas) under shear stress in vitro. J Biomed Mater Res 1996; 32:99-109.
15. Hering TM, Marchant RE and Anderson JM. Type V collagen during granulation tissue development. Experimental and Molecular Pathology 1983; 39:219-229.
16. Marchant RE, Miller KM, Hiltner A, Anderson JM. Selected aspects of cell and molecular biology of in vivo biocompatibility. In: Shalaby S, Hoffman A, Horbett T and Ratner B, eds. Polymers as Biomaterials. New York:Plenum Press, 1984:209-223.
17. Zhao Q, Agger MP, Fitzpatrick M et al. Cellular interactions with biomaterials: in vivo cracking of prestressed Pellethane 2363-80A. J Biomed Mater Res 1990; 24:621-637.
18. Zhao Q, Topham N, Anderson JM et al. Foreign-body giant cells and polyurethane biostability: in vivo correlation of cell adhesion and surface cracking. J Biomed Mater Res 1991; 25:177-183.
19. Mathur AB, Collier TO, Kao WJ et al. In vivo biocompatibility and biostability of modified polyurethanes. J Biomed Mater Res 1997; 36:246-257.
20. Miller KM, Anderson JM. Human monocyte/macrophage activation and interleukin 1 generation by biomedical polymers. J Biomed Mater Res 1988; 22:713-731.
21. Miller KM, Huskey RA, Bigby LF, Anderson JM. Characterization of biomedical polymer-adherent macrophages: Interleukin 1 generation and scanning electron microscopy studies. Biomaterials 1989; 10:187-196.
22. Bonfield TL, Colton E, Anderson JM. Plasma protein adsorbed biomedical polymers: Activation of human monocytes and induction of interleukin 1. J Biomed Mater Res 1989; 23:535-548.
23. Miller KM, Anderson JM. In vitro stimulation of fibroblast activity by factors generated from human monocytes activated by biomedical polymers. J Biomed Mater Res 1989; 23:911-930.
24. Miller KM, Rose-Caprara V, Anderson JM. Generation of IL1-like activity in response to biomedical polymer implants: A comparison of in vitro and in vivo models. J Biomed Mater Res 1989; 23:1007-1026.
25. Bonfield TL, Colton E, Marchant RE, Anderson JM. Cytokine and growth factor production by monocytes/macrophages on protein preadsorbed polymers. J Biomed Mater Res 1992; 26:837-850.
26. Bonfield TL, Anderson JM. Functional versus quantitative comparison of IL-1β from monocytes/macrophages on biomedical polymers. J Biomed Mater Res 1993; 27:1195-1199.
27. Greisler HP. Growth factor release from vascular grafts. J Contr Rel 1996; 39:267-280.
28. Kang SS, Gosselin C, Ren D, Greisler HP. Selective stimulation of endothelial cell proliferation with inhibition of smooth muscle cell proliferation by FGF-1 plus heparin delivered from fibrin glue suspensions. Surgery 1995; 118:280-287.
29. McNally AK, Anderson JM. Complement C3 participation in monocyte adhesion to different surfaces. Proc Natl Acad Sci USA 1994; 91:10119-10123.
30. McNally AK, Anderson JM. Interleukin-4 induces foreign body giant cells from human monocytes/macrophages. Differential lymphokine regulation of macrophage fusion leads to morphological variants of multinucleated giant cells. Amer J Pathol 1995; 147:1487-1499.
31. Kao WJ, McNally AK, Hiltner A, Anderson JM. Role for interleukin-4 in foreign-body giant cell formation on a poly(etherurethane urea) in vivo. J Biomed Mater Res 1995; 29:1267-1276.
32. McNally AK, DeFife KM, Anderson JM. Interleukin-4-induced macrophage fusion is prevented by inhibitors of mannose receptor activity. Am J Pathol 1996; 149:975-985.
33. DeFife KM, McNally AK, Colton E, Anderson JM. Interleukin-13 induces human monocyte/macrophage fusion and macrophage mannose receptor expression. J Immunol 1997; 158:3385-3390.

Taming of Adverse Responses

Prevention of the Inflammatory Reaction

--------------------------------- CHAPTER 20 ---------------------------------

Molecular Determinants of
Acute Inflammatory Responses to Biomaterials

Liping Tang, John W. Eaton

Introduction

Despite the fact that most biomaterials are inert, nontoxic and nonimmunogenic, biomaterial implants often cause adverse reactions. Typically, shortly after implantation, biomaterial surfaces attract a layer of phagocytic cells (especially, macrophages/monocytes and neutrophils)[1-4] and fibroblast-like cells.[5] This very much resembles the acute inflammatory response seen with many other types of foreign bodies and, to an extent, with focal bacterial infections. The acute inflammatory responses to tissue contact biomaterials are very often followed by chronic inflammation[6-8] and the appearance of fibrotic tissue surrounding many types of implants.[7,9-18] Chronic inflammation and fibrosis are also associated with the degradation and failure of many types of implants, including pacemaker leads,[19-21] mammary prostheses,[22,23] temporomandibular[24,25] and other joint implants.[26]

At first glance, these inflammatory responses to inert, nonimmunogenic and nontoxic materials are difficult to understand. Why should such unreactive and so-called "biocompatible" materials cause recruitment and evident activation of phagocytes? The following represents a brief summary of our present understanding of the inflammatory responses to implanted biomaterials.

Surface-Protein Interactions

Because biomaterial surfaces spontaneously and rapidly acquire a layer of host proteins upon contact with blood or proteinaceous body fluids, it is generally believed that these absorbed proteins likely influence, or absolutely dictate, the ensuing adverse responses.[27-30] Because this protein adsorption occurs much faster than the arrival of cells on the foreign surface, host cells almost certainly interact with surface-adsorbed proteins, rather than with the material itself.[29-31] Therefore, the types and states of adsorbed proteins are probably critical determinants of biocompatibility.[30,32-35]

The composition of adsorbed proteins varies with different biomaterials.[29,36] Unfortunately, due in part to the bewildering variety of model materials and protein types which have been used to investigate protein adsorption by biomaterials, the general principles governing surface-protein interactions under real life conditions are by no means clear. Generally speaking, albumin, fibrinogen and immunoglobulin G (IgG) predominate on many types of blood-contact biomaterials, including Dacron® (a woven form of polyester terephthalate; hereafter, 'PET'), expanded polytetrafluoroethylene, polydimethylsiloxane ('silastic'), polyurethanes and polyethylene.[29,36,37] Especially on hydrophobic surfaces such as these

Tissue Engineering of Prosthetic Vascular Grafts, edited by Peter Zilla and Howard P. Greisler
©1999 R.G. Landes Company.

(which are typical of the majority of implanted biomaterials), the adsorbed proteins may undergo conformational changes over a period of hours, becoming tightly adherent.[38-41] These conformational changes of adsorbed proteins have been detected using many different techniques, including sodium dodecyl sulfate (SDS) elution,[42,43] scanning angle reflectometry,[44] scanning force microscopy,[45] attenuated total reflectance Fourier transform infrared spectroscopy[39] and differential scanning calorimetry.[46] It has been assumed that, upon binding to hydrophobic surfaces, many proteins tend to unfold[47] and, within a short period, undergo surface "denaturation" (perhaps via loss of the normal sphere of hydration encouraged by contact with the hydrophobic surface).[48] The resulting conformational changes of adsorbed protein may expose hidden epitope(s) which, in turn, help initiate adverse reactions such as coagulation and inflammation.[49-52] However, a direct link between protein conformational changes and these adverse responses has not been established.

Which Adsorbed Host Protein(s) Might Be Important in Mediating Inflammatory Responses to Biomaterial Implants?

In order to investigate the mechanisms of biomaterial-mediated inflammatory responses, we developed a simple animal implantation model. Biomaterial films are cut into 1.2 cm diameter disks. After repetitive washes with ethanol, the disks are precoated with various types of proteins and then implanted in the mouse peritoneal cavity for 16-18 h (in this model, the time of maximal phagocyte accumulation).[53] The surface associated activities of myeloperoxidase (MPO) and nonspecific esterase (NSE) are measured to estimate the numbers of adherent neutrophils and macrophages/monocytes, respectively.[53,54] Although a number of other investigators have used subcutaneous implants or cage implants (e.g., refs. 2,3,19,20), these experimental systems have some shortcomings compared to intraperitoneal implants.[7] The peritoneal cavity provides a good site for studying inflammatory responses because reactions elicited by the polymer are clearly defined with minimal participation of the coagulation system.[7,53-57] Furthermore, it appears that at least the majority of phagocytic cells found adherent to explants are, indeed, recruited de novo and by the implant itself. Thus, mice subjected to sham surgery show only a small increment in numbers of phagocytes in peritoneal lavage fluids compared to implant-bearing animals.

As indicated above, albumin, IgG, fibrinogen and (to a lesser extent) complement are the most abundant proteins in plasma and are found to predominate on many blood-contact and tissue-contact biomaterials, including polyethylene terephthalate, expanded polytetrafluoroethylene, polydimethylsiloxane, polyurethanes and polyethylene.[29,36,37,53,54] Especially on hydrophobic surfaces, these adsorbed proteins tend to assume an altered conformation and become tightly adherent.[38-41,53,54] Taking advantage of this property, we were able to determine the possible role of various plasma proteins—precoated on implant surfaces—in initiating biomaterial-mediated inflammatory responses. In agreement with many previous reports, we find that albumin, the most abun-

dant protein on biomaterial surfaces, can "passivate" biomaterials, blunting both inflammatory and thrombogenic responses.[1,33,53,58] We therefore initially hypothesized that IgG, which is also adsorbed on biomaterial surfaces in large amounts,[29,31,36,53] might be the crucial mediator of phagocyte responses to biomaterial implants.

Adsorbed IGg Is Not Required for Phagocyte Accumulation on Biomaterial Implants

The possible involvement of adsorbed IgG in acute inflammatory responses to biomaterial implants was supported by several observations. First, immunoglobulins are important in the opsonization of foreign particles, which makes them more readily ingested by phagocytes.[59] Second, both surface-bound and heat-denatured IgG and IgA are potent activators of human neutrophils, causing the release of lysosomal enzymes (lysozyme, β-glucuronidase and myeloperoxidase) and stimulation of phagocyte oxidative metabolism.[60-62] Finally, in our experimental animal implantation model we found that IgG-coated surfaces accumulated as many inflammatory cells (both neutrophils and macrophages/monocytes) as did uncoated or plasma-coated surfaces.[53]

However, further experimental evidence indicates that adsorbed immunoglobulins are not essential to acute inflammatory responses to implants. We placed implants in mice with severe combined immunodeficiency (SCID) which have extremely low plasma IgG levels (< 1 μg/ml vs. 4 mg/ml in normal, otherwise syngeneic, animals). In SCID mice, the inflammatory response to uncoated PET disks as evidenced by the recruitment of both neutrophils (Fig. 20.1) and macrophages (not shown) is almost as great as in immunocompetent animals. The modest decrement in neutrophils and macrophage recruitment in SCID vs. normal mice probably reflects a general defect in phagocyte mobilization, because this difference is apparent on both uncoated and IgG-coated surfaces.

Complement Activation Is Not Required for Phagocyte Accumulation on Biomaterial Implants

A few blood-contact biomaterials may trigger complement activation and (during, e.g., hemodialysis or leukapheresis) transient neutropenia, suggesting that complement activation might contribute to the inflammatory effects of blood-contact biomaterials (e.g., see refs. 32, 63-67). This hypothesis is well supported by the known effects of activated complement components. For example, surface-induced complement activation will generate C3a and C5a fragments,[68,69] which are known to mediate granulocyte aggregation,[67] chemotaxis,[70] and adhesiveness to endothelial cells.[71] In addition, complement activation by some polymeric materials has been shown in vitro to cause phagocyte adhesion.[65,72] By extrapolation, one might anticipate that similar events might be involved in acute inflammatory responses to tissue contact biomaterials. However, complement depleted mice (pretreated with cobra venom factor) exhibit normal recruitment of inflammatory cells to implant surfaces.[53] Consequently, it appears that although activated complement components may powerfully

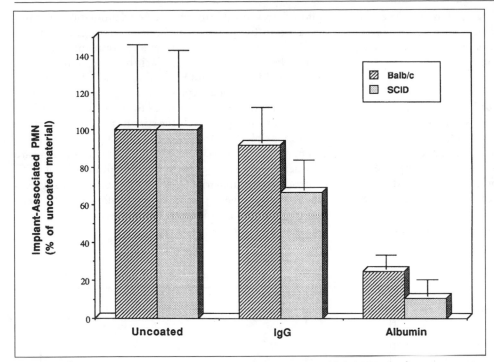

Fig. 20.1. Numbers of surface-associated neutrophils (PMN) on clean PET implants and PET implants precoated with either immunoglobulin G (IgG) or human albumin. The implants were placed either in control Balb/c mice or congeneic animals with severe combined immunodeficiency (SCID) and extremely low levels of circulating IgG. Following 16 h implantation, the material was removed and numbers of PMN estimated by analyses of surface-associated myeloperoxidase. Calculated numbers of PMN from explants in Balb/c mice: $166,000 \pm 74,000/cm^2$ on uncoated implants (numbers similar to those recovered from plasma-coated implants), $153,000 \pm 31,000/cm^2$ on IgG-coated implants and $41,000 \pm 11,000/cm^2$ on albumin-coated implants. In SCID mice: $225,000 \pm 94,000/cm^2$ on uncoated implants (similar values obtained for plasma-coated implants), $150,000 \pm 36,000/cm^2$ on IgG-coated implants and $24,000 \pm 19,000/cm^2$ on albumin-coated implants. Vertical lines denote $\pm$ 1 SD (n = 4 in all cases). In both control and SCID animals, values for albumin-coated material differ significantly from both IgG-precoated implants and uncoated implants at p<0.05 (Student's 't' test, two tailed). (Data from ref. 53.)

stimulate phagocytes, complement activation is not important in acute inflammatory responses to biomaterial implants (or, at least to implants of hydrophobic polymers such as polyethylene terephthalate, polyvinyl chloride or polyether urethane).

Fibrin(ogen) Is Necessary for Phagocyte Accumulation on Biomaterial Implants

The foregoing results indicate that, insofar as our experimental murine model is analogous to the human circumstance, neither complement activation nor adsorbed IgG is a *necessary* mediator of acute inflammatory reactions to implanted materials such as Dacron (PET). Together, albumin, IgG and fibrinogen may comprise > 80% of adsorbed surface proteins, at least on certain polymers.[29,36,73,74] Consequently, it seemed that fibrinogen—also present in large amounts on implant surfaces[36]—might be the host protein most important in triggering inflammatory reactions.

This hypothesis was supported by a surprising observation: Serum coated surfaces, like albumin coated surfaces, fail to prompt inflammatory responses.[54] The major difference between plasma and serum is that plasma, but not serum, contains fibrinogen. We therefore reconstituted serum by adding a physiological concentration of fibrinogen and used this to coat experimental implants. Disks precoated with fibrinogen-repleted serum attract as many phagocytes as do disks coated with fresh, minimally heparinized plasma. In addition, fibrinogen alone is sufficient to trigger inflammatory responses; PET disks preincubated with purified human (or murine) fibrinogen also attract large numbers of

both neutrophils and macrophages. In order to exclude the possible involvement of activated coagulation factors, similar studies were done using afibrinogenemic plasma in which fibrinogen was undetectable. PET coated with afibrinogenemic plasma attracted very few phagocytes (roughly equal to the numbers which accumulate on albumin-coated material). However, when physiologic levels (3 mg/ml) of purified fibrinogen were restored to this afibrinogenemic plasma, PET disks incubated in this mixture prompted normal recruitment of phagocytes.[54]

Most importantly, the requirement for fibrinogen adsorption to the surface of PET implants would appear to hold in vivo as well. Mice having undetectable plasma fibrinogen were produced by repetitive injections of ancrod.[75-80] Ancrod infusion causes severe hypofibrinogenemia and hypoplasminogenemia, but does not disturb the number or turnover of platelets or the levels of other coagulation factors and plasma proteins (including fibronectin).[76,78,81,82] Ancrod-treated mice (having undetectable fibrinogen at the time of implantation) show almost no neutrophil accumulation on untreated disks, but do so if the disks are precoated with purified murine fibrinogen (Fig. 20.2).[54] The same dependence on adsorbed fibrin(ogen) was also observed in similar experiments employing subcutaneous, rather than intraperitoneal, implants. Finally, we should note that although some studies have shown that fibronectin can serve as a bridge for phagocyte-surface fibrin(ogen) interactions,[83,84] our preliminary experiments have revealed no difference in in vitro phagocyte adherence to materials coated with normal plasma vs.

fibronectin-depleted plasma (Tang et al, unpublished observations). This may, however, reflect the absence of exposure of these phagocytes to factors which, e.g., upregulate cell adherence molecules (vide infra).

Which Portion of Fibrinogen Is Critical in Mediating Phagocyte Adhesion?

The foregoing results provide strong support for the proposition that the spontaneous adsorption of host fibrinogen to the surfaces of implanted PET is a necessary precedent to the subsequent inflammatory and fibrotic processes. We reasoned that the adsorbed fibrinogen probably displayed one or more epitopes normally occult in the soluble protein but exposed by surface-mediated "denaturation" of the protein. In order to determine the location of the hypothetical

epitope(s) responsible for phagocyte accumulation, plasmin degradation fragments of fibrinogen were generated and used to coat implant surfaces (Fig. 20.3). Implants precoated with the plasmin degradation fragment D100 (MW = 105 kDa), but not E50 (MW = 50 kDa), accumulate large numbers of phagocytes (both neutrophils and macrophages/monocytes), as many as fibrinogen-coated disks. To determine more precisely the specific portion of fibrinogen responsible, D100 was digested to D80 (MW = 80 kDa) and further to D30 (MW = 30 kDa). Both D80 and D30 are fully active in fostering the in vivo accumulation of both neutrophils and macrophages/monocytes.[85] This suggests that at least one necessary motif for phagocyte accumulation is within the fibrinogen D30 fragment.

Fig. 20.2. Numbers of surface-associated phagocytes on clean ('uncoated') PET implants and PET implants precoated with either fibrinogen or human albumin. The implants were placed either in (A) control Balb/c mice or (B) mice pretreated with ancrod to produce a state of hypo- or afibrinogenemia at the time of implant placement. Following 16 h implantation, the material was removed and the numbers of PMN estimated by analyses of surface-associated myeloperoxidase while the numbers of monocytes/macrophages were assessed by assay of nonspecific esterase. Calculated numbers of PMN from explants in control mice: 84,000 ± 32,000/cm² on uncoated implants, 46,000 ± 25,000/cm² on fibrinogen-coated implants and 100 ± 500/cm² on albumin-coated implants. In ancrod-treated mice: 12,000 ± 6,000/cm² on uncoated implants, 49,000 ± 25,000/cm² on fibrinogen-coated implants and 2,000 ± 2,000/cm² on albumin-coated implants. Vertical lines denote ± 1 SD (n = 6 in all cases). In both control and ancrod-treated animals, values for albumin-coated material differ significantly from both fibrinogen-precoated implants and uncoated implants at p < 0.01, and values for uncoated materials in control vs. ancrod-treated mice differ significantly at p < 0.01 (Student's 't' test, two tailed). (Data from ref. 54.)

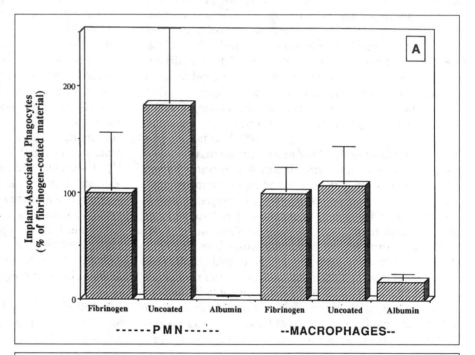

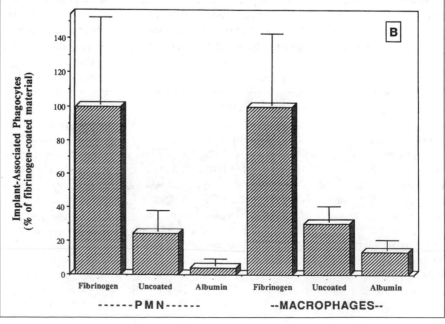

Altieri and colleagues[87] had earlier found that one segment of D30, γ190-202 (hereafter abbreviated as 'P1'), is critically important in mediating phagocyte-fibrinogen interactions. Thus, we thought that this particular short sequence might be a crucial determinant of phagocyte interactions with adsorbed fibrinogen on implant surfaces. To test this, P1 and a P1-based scrambled peptide were synthesized and covalently linked to human albumin (which has been used widely as a carrier to enhance cellular responses to peptides[88-90]). Indeed, implant surfaces precoated with P1 peptide, but not with the scrambled peptide, induce substantial phagocyte accumulation, roughly equivalent to that caused by fibrinogen-coated surfaces (Fig. 20.4).

How Does Adsorbed Fibrinogen Become Pro-Inflammatory?

The preceding results indicate that fibrinogen γ190-202 is the most important factor in mediating the accumulation of phagocytes on fibrinogen-bearing implant surfaces. However, it remains unclear how the simple adsorption of fibrinogen to implant surfaces might modify the protein, converting it into a pro-inflammatory signal. It is very likely that the pro-inflammatory nature of adsorbed fibrinogen reflects the occurrence of a conformational change, probably also reflected by the progressive resistance of adsorbed fibrinogen to elution by detergents.[38] For

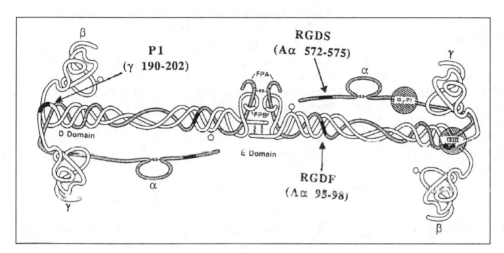

Fig. 20.3. Schematic drawing of the various domains of a single fibrinogen molecule showing the three (α, β and γ) chain types, two major plasmin cleavage domains (D and E) and the site of the evidently important 13 amino acid epitope P1 at γ190-202. Redrawn from ref. 86, with permission from the author and publishers.

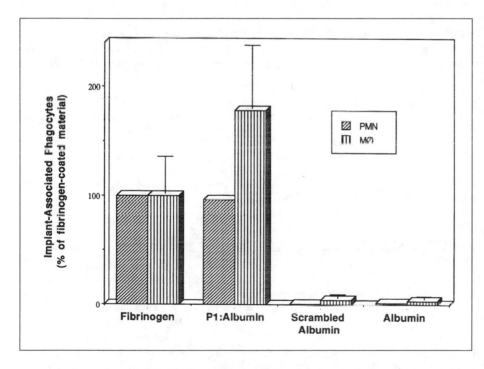

Fig. 20.4. Phagocyte accumulation on the surfaces of PET disks precoated with human fibrinogen, a covalent adduct between a synthesized version of γ190-202 (P1) ('P1:albumin'), a covalent adduct between a synthetic 13 amino acid peptide containing the same amino acids in random sequence ('scrambled albumin') or unmodified albumin. Values shown represent the numbers of neutrophils (PMN; cross-hatched bars) and monocytes/macrophages (MØ; vertical striped bars) on the surfaces of explants following 16 h implantation in Balb/c mice. Vertical lines denote ± 1 SD (n = 6 in all cases). Estimated numbers of PMN: 120,000 ± 51,000/cm² on fibrinogen-coated disks, 115,000 ± 64,000/cm² on 'P1:albumin'-coated disks, 400 ± 900/cm² on 'scrambled: albumin'-coated disks and 2,100 ± 2,500/cm² on albumin-coated disks. Calculated numbers of monocytes/macrophages: 221,900 ± 76,000/cm² on fibrinogen-coated disks, 393,000 ± 128,000/cm² on 'P1:albumin'-coated disks, 9,100 ± 7,300/cm² on 'scrambled: albumin'-coated disks and 7,300 ± 5,500/cm² on albumin-coated disks. Values obtained for fibrinogen vs. P1:albumin-coated surfaces do not differ, whereas both of these differ at p < 0.001 when compared to either albumin or 'scrambled albumin'-coated surfaces. (Data from ref. 85.)

example, after PET film has been incubated with purified fibrinogen for 4 h, more than 60% of adsorbed protein is resistant to elution by sodium dodecyl sulfate.[53] The conformational changes of adsorbed fibrinogen also have been recently probed by differential scanning calorimetry (DSC),[46] based on the assumption that denaturation of adsorbed protein will prevent some or all further thermal transitions. The DSC thermograms of native bovine fibrinogen have two transition peaks at 55°C and 96°C, reflecting denaturation of the D and E domains of fibrinogen, respectively. After prolonged interaction with low temperature isotropic carbon (which has a highly hydrophobic surface), the transition peaks for both domains are diminished, but the peak for the fibrinogen D domain is reduced more than that of the E domain. This suggests that the D domain may be more susceptible to surface induced denaturation than the E domain. Because the P1 epitope is within the D domain and the D domain is very susceptible to conformational changes, we now believe that the interaction between fibrinogen and surfaces mediates the conformational changes of the D fragment causing the exposure of P1. As a result, otherwise inert and unreactive surfaces displaying this epitope are recognized by phagocytes. The exposure of normally hidden epitopes as a result of adsorption to polymeric surfaces has some precedent; upon adsorption to plastic tissue culture surfaces (which, having been plasma discharge treated, are not precisely analogous to most hydrophobic implant surfaces), fibrinogen changes conformation and exposes multiple receptor-induced binding sites (RIBS) γ112-119 and Aα95-98.[91]

Thus, we now believe that surface fibrin(ogen) undergoes changes in conformation, becoming fibrin-like and that this anomalous fibrin(ogen) is critical in the attraction and adherence of phagocytic cells to implant surfaces. The ensuing responses of phagocytic cells to this product may also occur naturally in the normal course of hemostasis and wound resolution. The presence of fibrin has long been recognized as coeval with inflammatory and fibrotic responses, and fibrin deposition is typical of both acute and chronic inflammatory processes.[92-95] Furthermore, patients who are hypo- or afibrinogenemic are known to have abnormal inflammatory and wound healing responses. Therefore, it may be that the body interprets the presence of fibrin as an indication that vascular barriers have been breached and that invasion by microorganisms might have occurred. In this light, the attraction of phagocytic cells—important in both host defense and in the ultimate dissolution of the coagulum—makes perfect biological sense.

The Mechanism of Biomaterial-Mediated Inflammatory Responses

Although the above may represent some small progress in understanding the importance of surface protein adsorption in the response to biomaterial implants, there remain many mysteries concerning the mechanisms involved in the overall inflammatory response. The evolution of biomaterial-mediated inflammatory responses may be somewhat arbitrarily divided into three consecutive events (Fig. 20.5):

1. Phagocyte transmigration through the endothelial barrier;
2. Chemotaxis toward the implants; and, finally,
3. Adherence to the biomaterial.

A fuller understanding of these processes—discussed below in reverse order of occurrence—may help in the development of strategies to moderate biomaterial-mediated inflammatory responses and associated tissue responses.

Phagocyte Adherence to Biomaterial Implants

In order to interact with implant surfaces, receptors on cell surfaces must interact with adsorbed fibrinogen. We

Fig. 20.5. Hypothetical (and simplified) sequence of events important in acute inflammatory responses to implanted biomaterials.

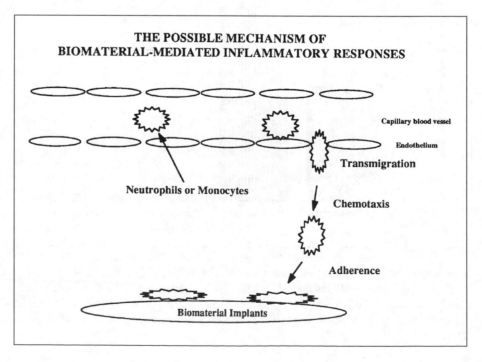

presently think that the phagocyte integrin Mac-1 (Cd11b/cd18) is required for this interaction. This is partly because earlier investigators had shown that the critical fibrin(ogen) epitope, P1, is recognized by Mac-1.[87] As a partial test of this hypothesis, we employed recombinant neutrophil inhibitory factor (hereafter, 'NIF'), which blocks Cd11b-dependent binding of Mac-1 to fibrinogen (which presumably occurs through the P1 epitope) without affecting other Mac-1 integrin functions such as binding to coagulation factor X.[96,97] Indeed, when mice were given repetitive injections of NIF before and during implantation, phagocytes failed to accumulate on fibrinogen-coated surfaces. Further support for the importance of Mac-1 in these phagocyte-implant interactions derives from recent experiments in animals lacking this integrin. In Cd11b knockout (KO) and CD18 KO mice, the 'normal' accumulation of phagocytes on implant surfaces fails to occur. Interestingly, this impairment of phagocyte accumulation is not caused by decreased phagocyte recruitment; the numbers of macrophages and neutrophils in peritoneal lavage fluids following implantation in both types of KO animals are roughly equivalent to those in wild type controls.[98]

Thus, the Mac-1 integrin appears to be crucial in the adhesion of inflammatory cells to implant surfaces. However, unstimulated phagocytes normally express only low levels of surface Mac-1 and most of this is in the 'low-affinity' state. This raises the question of what factors might prompt the apparent upregulation of this phagocyte integrin. Earlier studies indicated that TNF-α is a potent stimulator of the expression of Mac-1 on cell surfaces.[99-101] Furthermore, by ELISA assays, we have found that TNF-α is present in peritoneal lavage fluids from implant-bearing mice within four hours after implantation (unpublished results). This suggested the possibility that TNF-α might be critical in upregulating Mac-1 integrin expression on incoming phagocytes. In at least partial support of this possibility, we find that administration of neutralizing anti-TNF-α antibodies to implant-bearing mice blocks phagocyte accumulation on implant surfaces. Furthermore, as was the case with the Mac-1 KO mice described above, we find that neutralizing antibodies against TNF-α do not affect the extent of phagocyte recruitment to the site of the implant because the numbers of recruited cells are roughly equivalent in treated and control animals.[98]

Therefore, the adhesion of inflammatory cells to implant surfaces appears to depend on three separable events:
1. Precedent adherence of fibrin(ogen) accompanied by exposure of the P1 epitope;
2. The release of TNF-α in response to implantation; and
3. Consequent TNF-α-mediated upregulation of Mac-1 on incoming phagocytes.

Phagocyte Chemotaxis Toward Implant Surfaces

The accumulation of phagocytes on implant surfaces is clearly not a random event. In the peritoneum of an animal implanted ~16 h previously, ~20% of total neutrophils and ~50% of total macrophages are found on the implant surface (as opposed to being recovered in peritoneal lavage). Inasmuch as the implant represents only ~2% of the total

intraperitoneal surface phagocytic cells are obviously preferentially accumulated on the implant. We have assumed that certain chemokines might participate in attracting the incoming phagocytic cells toward implant surfaces. A number of chemokines have been reported to foster the recruitment of inflammatory cells in a variety of inflammatory diseases.[102-105] In searching for possible candidates among many potential chemokines we employed reverse transcript polymerase chain reaction to estimate levels of chemokine mRNA produced by implant adherent cells. We observed high levels of mRNA production for two particular chemokines: macrophage inflammatory protein-1α (MIP-1α) and monocyte chemoattractant protein-1 (MCP-1), both of which appear to be involved in phagocyte-implant interactions.

Neutralizing antibodies to both MIP-1α and MCP-1, but not to MIP-1β and MIP-2, block 70-90% of the accumulation of both macrophages and neutrophils on implant surfaces. However, the numbers of recruited phagocytes do not differ amongst control and treated groups.[106] Therefore, it is likely that the reduction in numbers of adherent phagocytes is caused by impairment of directed phagocyte chemotaxis (although other interpretations are possible at the moment). Indeed, these results are in accord with prior studies indicating that MIP-1α and MCP-1 contribute to inflammatory and immune tissue responses via promotion of chemotaxis and activation of both phagocytes and T lymphocytes.[107-112] Because many different types of cells are able to generate either MIP-1α and MCP-1,[109,113,114] it is still not clear which cell type is responsible for the production of MIP-1α and MCP-1 in the course of biomaterial-mediated inflammatory responses.

Thus, in interim summary, we are gaining some idea of the mechanisms involved in implant surface-protein interactions and in phagocyte chemotaxis towards, and adherence to, tissue contact biomaterials. However, the processes involved in the critical initial step—phagocyte transmigration through the endothelial barrier—remain undefined.

Phagocyte Transmigration Through the Endothelial Barrier

For a number of reasons, we hypothesized that the release of histamine might be important for the recruitment of inflammatory cells to implantation sites. The most direct evidence favoring this idea was the observation made by us and others[115] that the tissue surrounding biomaterial implants is often hyperemic and edematous, features of a classical histaminic response. In order to test the possible involvement of histamine, we administered the histamine receptor antagonists pyrilamine (an H1 receptor antagonist) and famotidine (an H2 receptor antagonist) to animals receiving implants. When given separately, neither receptor antagonist significantly diminishes the accumulation of inflammatory cells on implant surfaces. However, combined treatment of implant recipients with both H1 and H2 receptor antagonists significantly reduces the numbers of phagocytes on implant surfaces and the numbers of macrophages and neutrophils recruited de novo to the peritoneal cavity (down to values of 50% and 40% of untreated controls, respectively).[116] We tentatively conclude that histamine enhances the transmigration of phagocytes through the endothelial barrier via both H1 and H2 receptors.

Mast cells are the most likely source of the histamine which may be involved (although macrophages also are reported to produce and release histamine).[117-119] Indeed, the peritoneal space contains relatively large numbers of mast cells (2-5% of total lavage cells)[8,120] and mast cells have the largest amounts of stored histamine, which can be released in a short period of time. The importance of mast cells in the pathogenesis of other types of inflammatory responses has been investigated by others using mast cell deficient mice (WBB6F1-Wv/W).[121-123] In part, the results indicate that mast cell degranulation is important in neutrophil recruitment,[121] macrophage activation,[124] IL-1 production by monocytes and macrophages,[125] fibroblast proliferation and collagen accumulation,[126] fibrin deposition,[123] and, not surprisingly, the Arthus reaction.[123] In fact, several years ago, Christenson and coworkers[8] made the prescient suggestion that mast cells might play a key role in the inflammatory responses to intraperitoneal implants.

We therefore tested the possible importance of mast cells in phagocyte recruitment using mast cell deficient mice.[116] After intraperitoneal implantation for 16 h, far fewer PMN (< 50% of normal) and macrophages/monocytes (< 30% of normal) accumulated on implant surfaces in mast cell deficient mice than in their congenic controls. Furthermore, as was the case with normal animals treated with combined histamine receptor antagonists, the reduction of the numbers of adherent phagocytes is accompanied by greatly decreased recruitment of phagocytes to the peritoneum. Therefore, the results obtained with two different models in which histamine-dependent signaling events are disrupted—histamine receptor antagonist administration and mast cell deficient animals—are in complete agreement.

However, once again mysteries remain. It is anything but clear how implant surfaces may cause the activation of mast cells and, indeed, whether other released products of mast cells (such as TNF-α) might be important in the overall inflammatory response. Nonetheless, we can tentatively conclude that biomaterial implants do trigger the activation of mast cells, which release histamine. The subsequent histaminic responses—obvious as localized hyperemia and edema—facilitate the arrest and diapedesis of phagocytic cells at sites of biomaterial implantation.

Conclusions

Although typically inert, nontoxic and non-immunogenic, tissue-contact biomaterials often prompt a variety of unwanted host responses. Our present ignorance of the mechanisms involved in these implant-mediated host responses hinders the rational development of more biocompatible materials. Despite the efforts of a large number of excellent investigators, there remain many more questions than answers.

What little we do know can be very briefly summarized:

1. Implants (and blood-contact devices) made of hydrophobic polymers almost instantly acquire a layer of spontaneously adsorbed host protein;
2. The adsorbed protein gradually 'denatures';
3. The presence of the implant is sensed by the host either through mechanical properties of the material itself or through the presence of these 'denatured' surface proteins;
4. Guardian cells—especially mast cells—are activated, releasing histamine and, perhaps, other pro-inflammatory products;
5. The resultant histaminic response promotes the diapedesis of phagocytic cells across the endothelial barrier;
6. Acting on the instructions of particular cytokines (especially MIP-1α, MCP-1 and TNF-α) the incoming phagocytes migrate towards the implant whilst simultaneously upregulating surface adherence molecules such as Mac-1;
7. Upon encountering the surface of the implant, the phagocytic cells bind to the proteinaceous coat of the implant, a binding facilitated by interactions between Mac-1 and a small 13 amino acid epitope displayed by adsorbed fibrinogen.

And then? Clearly, a great deal more work will be required to unravel the intricacies involved in the above steps and, as importantly, the nature of subsequent responses which may eventuate in chronic inflammation and fibrosis. Nonetheless, this knowledge, once won, should eventually enable the purposeful engineering of materials with vastly improved biocompatibility.

References

1. Kottke-Marchant K, Anderson JM, Umemura Y, Marchant RE. Effect of albumin coating on the in vitro blood compatibility of Dacron arterial prostheses. Biomaterials 1989; 10:147-155.
2. Marchant RE, Phua K, Hiltner A, Anderson JM. In vivo biocompatibility studies: II. Biomer: Preliminary cell adhesion and surface characterization studies. J Biomed Mater Res 1984; 18:309-315.
3. Marchant RE, Miller KM, Anderson, JM. In vivo biocompatibility studies: V. In vivo leukocyte interactions with biomer. J Biomed Mater Res 1984; 18:1169-1190.
4. Marchant RE, Anderson JM, Dillingham EO. In vivo biocompatibility studies: VII. Inflammatory responses to polyethylene and to a cytotoxic polyvinylchloride. J Biomed Mater Res 1986; 20:37-50.
5. Tang L, Eaton JW. Mechanism of acute inflammatory response to biomaterials. Cells Mater 1994; 4:429-436.
6. Desai NP, Hubbell JA. Tissue response to intraperitoneal implants of polyethylene oxide-modified polyethylene terephthalate. Biomaterials 1992; 13:505-510.
7. Christenson L, Aebischer P, McMillan P, Galletti PM. Tissue reaction to intraperitoneal polymer implants: Species difference and effects of corticoids and doxorubicin. J Biomed Mater Res 1989; 23:705-718.
8. Christenson L, Wahlberg L, Aebischer P. Mast cells and tissue reaction to intraperitoneally implanted polymer capsules. J Biomed Mater Res 1991; 25:1119-1131.

9. Stark GB, Gobel M, Jaeger K. Intraluminal cyclosporine A reduces capsular thickness around silicon implants in rats. Ann Plast Surg 1990; 24:156-161.

10. Behling CA, Spector M. Quantitative characterization of cells at the interface of long-term implants of selected polymers. J Biomed Mater Res 1986; 20:653-666.

11. Gordon M, Bullough PG. Synovial and osseous inflammation in failed silicone rubber prostheses. A report of six cases. J Bone Joint Surg 1982; 64:574-580.

12. Kossovsky N, Millett D, Juma S et al. In vivo characterization of the inflammatory properties of poly(tetrafluoroethylene) particulates. J Biomed Mater Res 1991; 25:1287-1301.

13. Nelson GD. Complications from the treatment of fibrous capsular contracture of the breast. Plast Reconstr Surg 1981; 68:969-980.

14. Smahel J. Foreign material in the capsules around breast prostheses and the cellular reaction to it. Br J Plast Surg 1979; 32:35-42.

15. Vistness LM, Ksander GA, Kosek J. Study of encapsulation of silicon rubber implants in animals. A foreign reaction. Plast Reconstr Surg 1978; 62:580-588.

16. Domanskis EJ, Owsley JQ Jr. Histological investigation of the etiology of capsule contracture following augmentation mammaplasty. Plast Reconstr Surg 1976; 58:689-693.

17. Yates SG II, Nakagawa Y, Berger K, Sauvage LR. Surface thrombogenicity of arterial prostheses. Surg Gynec Obstet 1973; 136:12-16.

18. Berger K, Sauvage LR, Rao AM, Wood SJ. Healing of arterial prostheses in man. Its incompleteness. Ann Surg 1972; 175:118-127.

19. Zhao Q, Agger MP, Fitzpatrick M et al. Cellular interactions with biomaterials: in vivo cracking of prestressed pellethane 2363-80A. J Biomed Mater Res 1990; 24:621-637.

20. Zhao Q, Topham N, Anderson JM et al. Foreign-body giant cells and polyurethane biostability: In vivo correlation of cell adhesion and surface cracking. J Biomed Mater Res 1991; 25:177-183.

21. Sutherland K, Mahoney JR II, Coury AJ, Eaton JW. Degradation of biomaterials by phagocyte-derived oxidants. J Clin Invest 1993; 92:2360-2367.

22. Chan SC, Birdsell DC, Gradeen CY. Detection of toluenediamines in the urine of a patient with polyurethane-covered breast implants. Clin Chem 1991; 37:756-758.

23. Picha GJ, Goldstein JA, Stohr E. Natural-Y Meme polyurethane versus smooth silicone: Analysis of the soft-tissue interaction from 3 days to 1 year in the rat animal model. Plast Reconstr Surg 1990; 85:903-916.

24. Trumpy I, Lyberg T. In vivo deterioration of proplast-teflon temporomandibular joint interpositional implants: A scanning electron microscopic and energy-dispersive X-ray analysis. J Oral Maxillofac Surg 1993; 51:624-629.

25. Henry CH, Wolford LM. Treatment outcomes for temporomandibular joint reconstruction after Proplast-Teflon implant failure. J Oral Maxillofac Surg 1993; 51:352-358.

26. Kozinn SC, Johanson NA, Bullough PG. The biologic interface between bone and cementless femoral endoprostheses. J Arthroplasty 1986; 1:249-259.

27. Lindsay R. Blood surface interactions. Trans Am Soc Artif Internal Org 1980; 26:603-610.

28. Leininger RI, Hutson TB, Jakobsen RJ. Spectroscopic approaches to the investigation of interactions between artificial surfaces and proteins. Ann NY Acad Sci 1987; 516:173-183.

29. Anderson JM, Bonfield TL, Ziats NP. Protein adsorption and cellular adhesion and activation on biomedical polymers. Int J Artif Org 1990; 13:375-382.

30. Bohnert JL, Horbett TA. Changes in adsorbed fibrinogen and albumin interactions with polymers indicated by decreases in detergent elutability. J Colloid Interface Sci 1986; 111:363-377.

31. Pitt WG, Park K, Cooper SL. Sequential protein adsorption and thrombus deposition on polymeric biomaterials. J Colloid Interface Sci 1986; 111:343-362.

32. Kuwahara T, Markert M, Wauters JP. Protein adsorption on dialyzer membranes influences their biocompatibility properties. Contrib Nephrol (Basel, Karger) 1989; 74:52-57.

33. Sevastianov VI. Role of protein adsorption in blood biocompatibility of polymers. CRC Crit Rev Biocompat 1988; 4:109-154.

34. Horbett TA. Adsorption of proteins from plasma to a series of hydrophilic-hydrophobic copolymers. II. Compositional analysis with the prelabeled protein technique. J Biomed Mater Res 1981; 15:673-695.

35. Shinoda BA, Mason RG. Reaction of blood with artificial surfaces of hemodialyzers. Studies of human blood with platelet defects or coagulation factor deficiencies. Biomat Med Dev Art Org 1978; 6:305-329.

36. Pankowsky DA, Ziats NP, Topham NS et al. Morphologic characteristics of adsorbed human plasma proteins on vascular grafts and biomaterials. J Vasc Surg 1990; 11:599-606.

37. Andrade J, Hlady V. Plasma protein adsorption: The big twelve. Ann NY Acad Sci 1987; 516:158-172.

38. Lenk TJ, Horbett TA, Ratner BD, Chittur KK. Infrared spectroscopic studies of time-dependent changes in fibrinogen adsorbed to polyurethanes. Langmuir 1991; 7:1755-1764.

39. Lu DR, Park K. Effect of surface hydrophobicity on the conformational changes of adsorbed fibrinogen. J Colloid Interfac Sci 1991; 144:271-281.

40. Slack SM, Horbett TA. Changes in the strength of fibrinogen attachment to solid surfaces: An explanation of the influence of surface chemistry on the Vroman effect. J Colloid Interfac Sci. 1989; 133:148-165.

41. Vroman L, Adams AL, Klings M et al. Reactions of formed elements of blood with plasma proteins at interfaces. Ann NY Acad Sci 1977; 283:65-75.

42. Chinn JA, Posso SE, Horbett TA, Ratner BD. Postadsorption transition in fibrinogen adsorbed to polyurethanes: Changes in antibody binding and sodium dodecyl sulfate elutability. J Biomed Mater Res 1992; 16:757-778.

43. Rapoza RJ, Horbett TA. Changes in the SDS elutability of fibrinogen adsorbed from plasma to polymers. J Biomater Sci Polym Ed 1989; 1:99-110.

44. Schaaf P, Dejardin P. Structural changes within an adsorbed fibrinogen layer during the adsorption process: A study by scanning angle reflectometry. Colloids Surfaces 1988; 31:89-100.

45. Wigren R, Elwing H, Erlandsson R et al. Structure of adsorbed fibrinogen obtained by scanning force microscopy. FEBS Letts 1991; 280:225-258.

46. Feng L, Andrade JD. Protein adsorption on low-temperature isotropic carbon: I. Protein conformation change

probed by differential scanning calorimetry. J Biomed Mater Res 1994; 28:735-743.

47. MacRichie F. The adsorption of proteins at the solid/liquid interface. J Colloid Interfac Sci 1972; 38:484-490.

48. Lee R. Adsorption of proteins onto hydrophobic polymer surfaces: Adsorption isotherms and kinetics. J Biomed Mater Res 1974; 8:251-259.

49. Andrade JD, Hlady VL, Van Wagenen RA. Effects of plasma protein adsorption on protein conformation and activity. Pure Appl Chem 1984; 56:1345-1350.

50. Absolom DR, Zingg W, Policova Z, Neumann AW. Determination of the surface tension of protein coated materials by means of the advancing solidification front technique. Trans Am Soc Intern Artif Organs 1983; 29:146-151.

51. Morrissey BW, Han CC. The conformation of γ-globulin adsorbed on polystyrene lattices determined by quasielastic light scattering. J Colloid Interfac Sci 1978; 65:423-431.

52. Morrissey BW, Fenstermaker CA. Conformation of adsorbed γ-globulin and β-lactoglobulin. Effect of surface concentration. Trans Am Soc Artif Intern Org 1976; 22:278-284.

53. Tang L, Lucas AH, Eaton JW. Inflammatory responses to Dacron: Role of surface adsorbed IgG. J Lab Clin Med 1993; 122:292-300.

54. Tang L, Eaton JW. Fibrin(ogen) mediates acute inflammatory responses to biomaterials. J Exp Med 1993; 178:2147-2156.

55. Freyria AM, Chignier E, Guidollet J, Louisot P. Peritoneal macrophage response: An in vivo model for the study of synthetic materials. Biomaterials 1991; 12:111-118.

56. Merhi Y, Roy R, Guidoin R et al. Cellular reactions to polyester arterial prosthesis impregnated with cross-linked albumin: in vivo studies in mice. Biomaterials 1989; 10:56-58.

57. Uenoyama K, Kanagawa R, Tamura M et al. Experimental intraocular lens implantation in the rabbit eye and in the mouse peritoneal space. Part 1. Cellular components observed on the implanted lens surface. J Cat Refract Surg 1988; 14:187-191.

58. Guidoin R, Snyder R, Martin L et al. Albumin coating of a knitted polyester arterial prosthesis: An alternative to preclotting. Ann Thorac Surg 1984; 37:457-465.

59. Stossel TP. Medical progress—phagocytosis (first of three parts). New Engl J Med 1974; 290:717-723.

60. Henson PM, Oades ZG. Stimulation of human neutrophils by soluble and insoluble immunoglobulin aggregates. Secretion of granule constituents and increased oxidation of glucose. J Clin Invest 1975; 56:1053-1061.

61. Henson PM, Johnson HB, Spiegelberg HL. The release of granule enzymes from human neutrophils stimulated by aggregated immunoglobulins of different classes and subclasses. J Immunol 1972; 109:1182-1192.

62. Chuang HYK, Mohammad SF, Mason RG. Prostacyclin (PGI2) inhibits the enhancement of granulocyte adhesion to cuprophane induced by immunoglobulin G. Thromb Res 1980; 19:1-9.

63. Cappelli G, Lucchi L, Bonucchi D et al. Polymorphonuclear oxygen free radical production and complement activation induced by dialysis membranes as assayed in an experimental model. Blood Purif 1989; 7:293-300.

64. Shepard AD, Gelfand JA, Gallow AD, O'Donnell TF Jr. Complement activation by synthetic vascular prostheses. J Vasc Surg 1984; 1:829-838.

65. Herzlinger GA, Cumming RD. Role of complement activation in cell adhesion to polymer blood contact surface. Trans Am Soc Artif Intern Org 1980; 26:165-171.

66. Nusbacher J, Rosefeld SI, MacPherson JL et al. Nylon fiber leukapheresis: Associated complement component changes and granulocytopenia. Blood 1978; 51:359-365.

67. Craddock PR, Fehr J, Dalmasso AP et al. Hemodialysis leukopenia. Pulmonary vascular leukostasis resulting from complement activation by dialyzer cellophane membrane. J Clin Invest 1977; 59:879-888.

68. Janatova J. C3, C5 and C3a, C4a, and C5a fragments of the complement system. Meth Enzymol 1988; 162:579-625.

69. Janatova J, Cheung AK, Parker CJ. Biomedical polymers differ in their capacity to activate complement. Complement Inflamm 1991; 8:61-69.

70. Dahlgren C, Hed J, Stendahl O. Chemotaxis of polymorphonuclear leukocytes in response to surface-bound complement-derived chemoattractants generated in situ. Inflammation 1984; 8:201-208.

71. O'Flaherty JT, Rossi AG, Redman JR, Jacobson DP. Tumor necrosis factor regulates expression of receptors for formyl-methionyl-leucyl-phenylalanine, leukotriene B4 and platlet activating factor. Dissociation from priming in human polymorphonuclear neutrophils. J Immunol 1991; 147:3842-3847.

72. Cumming RD. Important factors affecting initial blood-material interactions. Trans Am Soc Artif Intern Org 1980; 26:304-308.

73. Miale JB. Laboratory Medicine Hematology. Sixth edn. C. V. Mosby Co., p. 1084, 1982.

74. Dittmer DS (edited), Altman PL (analysis and compilation). Blood and other body fluids. Biology Handbook. Federation of American Societies for Experimental Biology, Washington, DC, p. 540, 1961.

75. McRitchie DI, Girotti MJ, Glynn MFX et al. Effect of systemic fibrinogen depletion on intraabdominal abscess formation. J Lab Clin Med 1991; 118:48-55.

76. Cole EH, Glynn FX, Laskin CA et al. Ancrod improves survival in murine systemic lupus erythematosus. Kidney Internat 1990; 37:29-35.

77. Pollak VE, Glueck HI, Weiss MA et al. Defibrination with ancrod in glomerulonephritis: Effects on clinical and histologic findings and on blood coagulation. Am J Nephr 1982; 2:195-207.

78. Bell WR, Shapiro SS, Martinez J, Nossel HL. The effects of Ancrod, the coagulation enzyme from the venom of Malayan pit viper (A. rhodostoma) on prothrombin and fibrinogen metabolism and fibrinopeptide A release in man. J Lab Clin Med 1978; 91:592-604.

79. Silberman S, Bernik MB, Potter EV, Kwuan HC. Effects of ancrod (Arvin) in mice: Studies of plasma fibrinogen and fibrinolytic activity. Br J Hæmat 1973; 24:101-113.

80. Reid HA, Chen KE, Thean PC. Prolonged coagulation defect (defibrination syndrome) in malayan viper bite. Lancet 1963; i:621-626.

81. Barcelli U, Rademacher PR, Ooi BS, Pollak VE. Defibrination with Ancrod: Effect of reticuloendothelial clearance of circulating immune complexes. Nephron 1982; 30:314-317.

82. Esnouf MP, Tunnah GW. The isolation and properties of the thrombin-like activity from Ancistrodon rhodostoma venom. Br J Hæmat 1967; 13:581-590.

83. Blystone S, Weston L, Kaplan JE. Fibronectin dependent macrophage fibrin binding. Blood 1991; 78:2900-2907.

84. Kaplan JE, Cardarelli PM, Rourke FJ et al. Fibronectin augments binding of fibrin to macrophages. J Lab Clin Med 1989; 113:168-176.

85. Tang L, Ugarova TP, Plow EF, Eaton JW. Molecular determinants of acute inflammatory responses to biomaterials. J Clin Invest 1996; 97:1329-1334.

86. Mossesson MW. Fibrin polymerization and its regulatory role in hemostasis. J Lab Clin Med 1990; 116:8-17.

87. Altieri DC, Plescia J, Plow EF. The structural motif glycine190-valine202 of the fibrinogen γ chain interacts with Cd11b/cd18 integrin ($\alpha_M\beta_2$, Mac-1) and promotes leukocyte adhesion. J Biol Chem 1993; 268:1847-1853.

88. Humphries M, Komoriya A, Akiyama K et al. Identification of two distinct regions of the type IIIcs connecting segment of human plasma fibronectin that promote cell type-specific adhesion. J Biol Chem 1987; 262:6886-6892.

89. McCarthy JB, Skubitz APN, Zhao Q, Yi X-Y et al. RGD-independent cell adhesion to the carboxy-terminal heparin-binding fragments of fibronectin involves heparin dependent and independent activities. J Cell Biol 1990; 110:777-787.

90. Haugen PKJ, McCarthy JB, Skubitz APN et al. Recognition of the A chain carboxyl-terminal heparin binding region of fibronectin involves multiple sites: Two contiguous sequences act independently to promote neural cell adhesion. J Cell Biol 1990; 111:2733-2745.

91. Ugarova TP, Budzynski AZ, Shattil SJ et al. Conformational changes in fibrinogen elicited by its interaction with platelet membrane glycoprotein GPIIb-IIIa. J Biol Chem 1993; 268:21080-21087.

92. Cooper JA, Lo SK, Malik AB. Fibrin is a determinant of neutrophil sequestration in the lung. Circ Res 1988; 63:735-741.

93. Behrens BL, Clark RA, Presley DM et al. Comparison of the evolving histopathology of early and late cutaneous and asthmatic responses in rabbits after a single antigen challenge. Lab Invest 1987; 56: 101-113.

94. Rowland TN, Donovan M, Gillies C et al. Fibrin mediator of in vivo and in vitro injury and inflammation. Curr Eye Res 1985; 4:537-553.

95. Colvin RB, Johnson RA, Mihm MC Jr, Dvorak HF. Role of the clotting system in cell-mediated hypersensitivity. 1. Fibrin deposition in delayed skin reaction in man. J Exp Med 1973; 138:686-698.

96. Muchowski PG, Zhang L, Chang ER et al. Functional interaction between the integrin antagonist neutrophil inhibitory factor and the I domain of the Cd11b/cd18. J Biol Chem 1994; 269:26419-26423.

97. Moyle M, Foster DL, McGrath DE et al. A hookworm glycoprotein that inhibits neutrophil function is a ligand of the integrin Cd11b/cd18. J Biol Chem 1994; 269:10008-10015.

98. Tang L, Welty S, Smith CW, Eaton JW. The participation of adhesion molecules in inflammatory responses to biomaterials. Trans Soc Biomat 1997a; 20:261.

99. Lo SK, Detmers PA, Levin SM, Wright SD. Transient adhesion of neutrophils to endothelium. J Exp Med 1989; 169:1779-1794.

100. Witthaut R, Farhood A, Smith C, Jaeschke H. Complement and TNFα contribute to Mac-1 (Cd11b/cd18) upregulation and systemic neutrophil activation during endotoxemia in vivo. J Leuk Biol 1994; 55:105-111.

101. Nathan C, Sporn M. Cytokines in context. J Cell Biol 1991; 113:981-986.

102. Oppenheim JJ, Zachariae CO, Mukaida N, Matsushima K. Properties of the novel proinflammatory supergene "intercrine" cytokine family. Ann Rev Immunol 1991; 9:617-648.

103. Harrison LC, Campbell IL. Cytokines: An expanding network of immuno-inflammatory hormones. Molec Endocrin 1988; 2:1151-1156.

104. Ward PA. Cytokines, inflammation, and autoimmune diseases. Hosp Practice 1995; 30:35-41.

105. Arai K-I, Lee F, Miyajima A et al. Cytokines: Coordinators of immune and inflammatory responses. Ann Rev Biochem 1990; 59:783-836.

106. Tang L, Chesney J, Sherry B, Eaton JW. The pivotal role of cytokines in the recruitment and adhesion of inflammatory cells to implanted biomaterials. Trans Soc Biomat 1997b; 20:127.

107. Standiford TJ, Kunkel SL, Lukacs NW et al. Macrophage inflammatory protein-1 alpha mediates lung leukocyte recruitment, lung injury, and early mortality in murine endotoxemia. J Immunol 1995; 155:1515-1524.

108. Kristensen MS, Deleuran BW, Larsen GG et al. Expression of monocyte chemotactic and activating factor (MCAF) in skin related cells: a comparative study. Cytokines 1995; 5:520-524.

109. Smith RE, Streiter RM, Zhange K et al. A role of C-C chemokines in fibrotic lung diseases. J Leukoc Biol 1995; 57:782-787.

110. Alam R, Kumar D, Anderson-Walters D, Forsythe PA. Macrophage Inflammatory protein-1 alpha and monocyte chemoattractant peptide-1 elicit immediate and late cutaneous reactions and activate murine mast cells in vivo. J Immunol 1994; 152:1298-1303.

111. Koch AE, Kunkeln SL, Harlow LA et al. Macrophage inflammatory protein-1 alpha—A novel chemotactic cytokine for macrophages in rheumatoid arthritis. J Clin Invest 1994; 93:921-928.

112. Strieter RM, Koch AE, Antoney VB et al. The immunopathology of chemotactic cytokines: The role of interleukin-8 and monocyte chemoattractant protein-1. J Lab Clin Med 1994; 123:183-197.

113. Wolpe SD, Cerami A. Macrophage inflammatory proteins 1 and 2: members of a novel superfamily of cytokines. FASEB J 1989; 3:2565-2573.

114. Kasama T, Strieter RM, Standiford TJ et al. Expression and regulation of human neutrophil-derived macrophage inflammatory protein-1 alpha (MIP-1 alpha). J Exp Med 1994; 178:63-72.

115. Guo W, Willen R, Andersson R et al. Morphological response of the peritoneum and spleen to intraperitoneal biomaterials. Internat J Artif Organs 1993; 16:276-284.

116. Tang L, Jennings TA, Eaton JW. Mast cells mediate acute inflammatory responses to implanted biomaterials. Proc Natl Acad Sci 1998; 95:8841-8846.

117. Riley JF, West GB. The presence of histamine in tissue mast cells. J Physiol 1953; 129:528-537.

118. Okamoto H, Nakano K. Regulation of interleukin-1 synthesis by histamine produced by mouse peritoneal macrophages per se. Immunology 1990; 69:162-165.

119. Zwadlo-Klarwasser G, Braam U, Muhl-Zurbes P, Schmutzler W. Macrophages and lymphocytes: Alternative sources of histamine. Agents Actions 1994; 41:C99-C100.

120. Franzen L. Further studies on the relationship between drug-induced mast cell secretion and local cell proliferation. Acta Path Microbiol Scand 1981; 89:57-62.

121. Zhang Y, Ramos BF, Jakschik BA. Neutrophil recruitment by tumor necrosis factor from mast cells in immune complex peritonitis. Science 1992; 258:1957-1959.

122. Ramos BF, Zhang Y, Qureshi R, Jakschik BA. Mast cells are critical for the production of leukotrienes responsible for neutrophil recruitment in immune complex-induced peritonitis in mice. J Immunol 1991; 147:1636-1641.

123. Ramos BF, Zhang Y, Angkachatchai V, Jakschik BA. Mast cell mediators regulate vascular permeability changes in Arthus reaction. J Pharmacol Exp Therap 1992; 262:559-565.

124. Norrby K, Enestrom S. Cellular and extracellular changes following mast-cell secretion in avascular rat mesentery. Cell Tissue Res 1984; 235:339-345.

125. Yoffe JR, Taylor DJ, Woolley DE. Mast-cell products and heparin stimulate the production of mononuclear-cell factor by cultured human monocyte/macrophages. Biochem J 1985; 230:83-88.

126. Watanabe S, Watanabe K, Ohnishi T et al. Mast cells in the rat alveolar septa undergoing fibrosis after ionizing irradiation. Lab Invest 1974; 31:555-567.

Taming of Adverse Responses

Prevention of Fibrosis

--- CHAPTER 21 ---

The Accumulation of Inflammatory Mediators: A Target for the Prevention of Fibrosis

John Zagorski, Sharon M. Wahl

Introduction

The primary purpose of the mammalian immune response is to eliminate foreign objects from the body. Most typically, immune surveillance is directed against pathogenic microorganisms that have entered the body via the respiratory or gastrointestinal tracts or through inadvertent ruptures in epithelial tissues. Circulating leukocytes are rapidly recruited from the circulation in response to infection and accumulate at the afflicted site. There, leukocytes release a variety of microbicidal compounds including reactive oxygen intermediates (ROIs) such as superoxide anion, hydroxyl radicals and hydrogen peroxide which are toxic to bacteria.[1-5] These cells also play an important early role in the resolution of the trauma that usually accompanies infection. Wounds or ruptures in epidermal or epithelial tissue must be repaired to restore the integrity of the tissue. However, prior to repair, the debris associated with the wound must be sequestered and cleared. Leukocytes are highly secretory cells and, when activated, release a variety of strong proteolytic enzymes including elastase,[6 8] collagenase[9-10] and members of the cathepsin family.[11-13] Digestion of the tissue debris during wound clearance is essential for remodeling of the wound site and its subsequent re-epithelialization and repair.

Killing of bacteria by neutrophils via chemical secretion and by phagocytosis constitutes an early phase of the host inflammatory response. Subsequent migration of monocytes and lymphocytes adds to the host response. Monocytes not only produce microbicidal molecules and proteases, but are also prodigious producers of pro-inflammatory cytokines and growth factors including interleukin-1 (IL-1) and tumor necrosis factor (TNF), transformtin growth factor-b (TGF-β), members of the fibroblast growth factor (FGF) family and numerous chemotactic factors including members of the chemokine superfamily.[14-16] Indeed, the pivotal role of monocytes in wound repair is emphasized by the observations that wound repair proceeds when other cell types are eliminated from experimental animals, but is retarded when monocytes are selectively removed.[17-21] Monocytes thus play a dual role in wound resolution by secreting inflammatory mediators that act directly at the wound site to promote repair and regrowth of the surrounding tissue, but also are the key cell type in orchestrating recruitment of additional cells, both myeloid and stromal. It is therefore not surprising that dysregulation of the repair process, the subject of this review, is in large part a consequence of impaired monocyte function.

Expansion of the inflammatory response can be a dangerous process. While extensive recruitment of immune cells to a site of inflammation is intended to promote elimination of microorganisms or antigen removal and subsequent tissue healing, a prolonged response invariably begins to damage the inflamed tissue.[22] Thus, chronic inflammation is almost always deleterious, and may in fact be viewed as a pathology distinct from the transient and generally beneficial acute inflammatory response.[23] Expansion of the immune response is mediated in large part by cytokine networks which have evolved to regulate inflammation, with numerous pro-inflammatory proteins functioning to promote, and equally numerous immune-suppressive proteins acting to attenuate, the inflammatory response. So long as a proper balance of pro- and anti-inflammatory mediators is maintained within traumatized tissue, normal clearance of pathogens and tissue repair proceed. Dysregulation of the cytokine balance, by various mechanisms, is at the core of persistent, chronic inflammation, leading to the seemingly contradictory results of tissue destruction and hyperproliferation (fibrosis).[24-26]

The grafting of an artificial prosthesis within normal tissue, the deliberate placement of a foreign object within a body, may be considered as several distinct and deliberate pathological insults. First, the surgery involved is a controlled wound which must be managed in such a way as to maximize normal wound healing. Second, some degree of infection often accompanies the grafting procedure and an acute inflammatory response is then inevitable. Lastly, and most importantly, the emplacement of a prosthetic device into a host may be interpreted by the host immune system as an immense "pathogen", and may initiate chronic rejection attempts by effector cells of the innate and/or adaptive immune system. Ideally, the process of grafting should not interfere with the normal acute inflammatory response, but also should not evoke such a prolonged and unresolvable stimulus that a chronic response spins out of control. As such, it is critical that the prosthesis be constructed in such a manner that it evokes as little recognition by the immune system as possible. In particular, the biomaterials used in the construction of the prosthesis should be inert in the sense that they do not promote activation of immune cells.[27-28] In this review we will attempt to review the mechanisms by which inflammatory responses become prolonged and attempt to identify pro-inflammatory mediators which may be attractive targets for mitigating some of the side effects of prostheses and preventing fibrosis.

Inflammation

Emigration of circulating cells from the vasculature to the tissues is a hallmark feature of inflammation. The mechanism of this emigration has been proposed to occur via a three step model (Fig. 21.1).[29] In the initial step, circulating leukocytes adhere transiently to activated endothelial cells in the proximity of the emerging inflammatory site. When this process is observed by intravital microscopy, leukocytes are seen to adhere to endothelial surfaces, roll along the surface, detach and then re-attach, sometimes within a single microscope field.[30-32] Rolling is mediated by complementary adhesion molecules expressed on the leukocytes and the activated endothelial cells, including members of the selectin family.[33-36] L-selectin is expressed on the surface of rolling leukocytes and binds carbohydrate ligands on acti-

vated endothelial cells while E- and P-selectins, expressed on the surfaces of activated endothelial cells, bind similar ligands on circulating leukocytes[37-39] (Fig. 21.1). Leukocyte rolling on activated endothelia most likely allows the leukocytes time to survey the local environment for additional pro-inflammatory stimuli without requiring firm adhesive interactions that might commit the leukocyte to remaining at that site. These additional stimuli may in large part be contributed by locally expressed chemoattractants, primarily members of the chemokine superfamily.[40-43] Exposure of rolling leukocytes to sufficiently high concentrations of chemoattractants causes a marked alteration in the adhesive interactions between leukocytes and endothelial cells. Selectin-mediated adhesion is dramatically reduced, in part, by proteolytic shedding of L-selectin from the leukocyte surface.[44] However, prolonged expression of endothelial P-selectin has been observed.[45]

Concurrent with loss of selectin-mediated adhesion, leukocytes begin the second step in vascular emigration, adherence to endothelium via tight integrin-mediated interactions.[46-49] The three leukocyte integrins, LFA-1, Mac-1 and p150,95, are heterodimeric proteins containing a shared β_2 subunit (CD18) and one of three different α subunits, α_L, (Cd11a), α_m (Cd11b) or α_x (CD11c). Among the multiple other integrins present on leukocytes, β_1 integrins can interact with both endothelial cells and extracellular matrix molecules.[46] For example, $\alpha_4\beta_1$ (VLA-4) receptors bind to regions of fibronectin, but also recognize VCAM, the corresponding ligand on endothelial cells. Integrin-mediated leukocyte-endothelial adhesion is, at least in part, directly increased by the actions of chemoattractants on leukocytes.[48,49] This helps to insure that as leukocytes lose selectin-mediated adhesive interactions in the intimate proximity of endothelial cells, a second type of adhesion is rapidly initiated. Endothelial ligands for the leukocyte integrins include the ICAM family of immunoglobulin-like adhesion molecules and VCAM.[50-51] These molecules are differentially regulated on the endothelial cell surface and are upregulated by such pro-inflammatory mediators as IL-1, TNF-α and IFN-γ. Integrin-ICAM and -VCAM adhesive interactions serve to secure the leukocytes at the inflammatory site and also transduce signals which are necessary for migration through the endothelial monolayer and underlying basement membrane, the final step in emigration (diapedesis)[52,53] (Fig. 21.1).

Regulation of Leukocyte Recruitment

The long established paradigm that neutrophils are recruited early in inflammation while mononuclear lymphocytes and monocytes are recruited later strongly suggests that chemotactic signals unique for each cell type are generated near the inflammatory site in a temporally restricted manner.[54] However, until relatively recently, cell type specific chemotactic factors had not been identified. The classic chemoattractants, complement fragments, leukotrienes and bacterial N-formyl peptides, as well as TGF-β, are chemotactic for a wide variety of leukocytes and are not selective chemoattractants for promoting the accumulation of specific cell populations at any stage of inflammation.[55,56] Rather, it is more likely that these factors serve as pleiotropic distress signals, initiating the recruitment of a spectrum

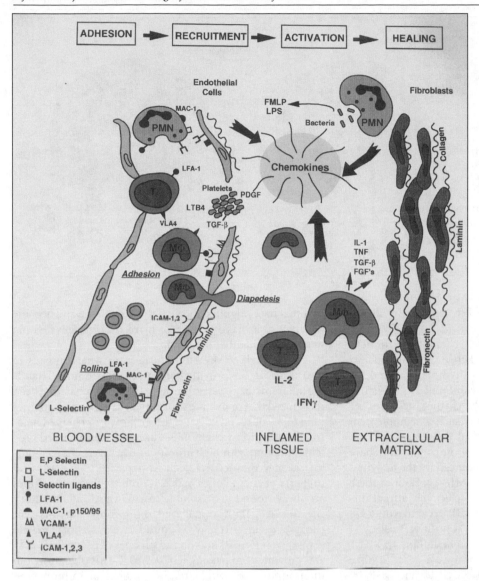

Fig. 21.1. Sequential events in recruitment and activation of circulating leukocytes at sites of inflammation. In response to inflammatory signals, leukocytes in the blood vessel adhere and roll through selectin-mediated attachment, and then via a firmer integrin-ligand interaction commence diapedesis from the vessel into the tissue. Within the inflammatory site, the neutrophils (PMN), monocytes (Mφ) and T lymphocytes (T) are activated to generate additional chemoattractants and cytokines to augment the immune response. In turn, cytokines and growth factors promote fibroblast recruitment, proliferation and extracellular matrix generation essential for wound healing. Excess cellular infiltration and production of these molecules eventuates in tissue fibrosis and pathogenesis. Adapted from Zagorski and Wahl, Encyclopedia of Immunology, 1998.[113]

of immune cells from the vasculature. It is clear, however, that mechanisms do exist for the recruitment of specific cell populations, since this has been observed histologically in many pathological conditions.[57-59]

Within the past decade, a new group of related polypeptides, the chemokines, has emerged as a major source of chemotactic activity responsible for promoting immune cell recruitment in numerous inflammatory pathologies.[40-43] Chemokines are a large superfamily of related proteins characterized by their close similarities in size and protein tertiary structure. This superfamily draws its name from the most important characteristic of the individual proteins, namely, that they are *chemo*tactic cyto*kines*. An additional hallmark of the chemokine superfamily is the presence in each protein of four positionally conserved cysteine residues. The organization of the cysteines allows a convenient and functionally significant subdivision of the proteins into two major chemokine families (Fig. 21.2). In the β-chemokines, these first two cysteines are adjacent ("CC") while in the α-chemokines the first two cysteines are separated by a single apparently nonconserved amino acid ("CXC"). The genes for CC and CXC chemokines are arranged in clusters and in

humans, the CC gene cluster is located on chromosome 17, while the CXC cluster is located on human chromosome 4.[43] It seems likely that the various members of each family arose through recombination-mediated gene duplication of single ancestral CC and CXC progenitors, a hypothesis with interesting implications concerning the evolution of the mammalian inflammatory response.

Members of the CXC chemokine family include IL-8, MIG, NAP-2, IP-10, ENA-78, and the three GRO/MIP-2 proteins (GROα, β, and γ). The CC chemokines are a somewhat more diverse family and include MCP-1, -2, -3, -4 and -5, Rantes, I-309, Eotaxin-1 and -2, and MIP-1α, β and γ (Fig. 21.2). The advent of high throughput DNA sequencing continues to add putative chemokines to the databases far faster than they can be characterized for function, and the list above is only partial. While most of the current repertoire of chemokines were first isolated as cDNAs, either from specific or subtracted library screens or from random sequencing, many of the chemokine proteins were first purified by traditional biochemical methods based on their activities.[60-63] For two very recent, but rapidly outdated, compilations of chemokines and chemokine ESTs (expressed

Fig. 21.2. Chemokine receptors and their ligands. Selective expression of chemokine receptors on polymorphonuclear neutrophils (PMN) and mononuclear cells (MNL) and the chemokines which specifically interact with these receptors. Adapted from Zagorski and Wahl, Encyclopedia of Immunology, 1998.[113]

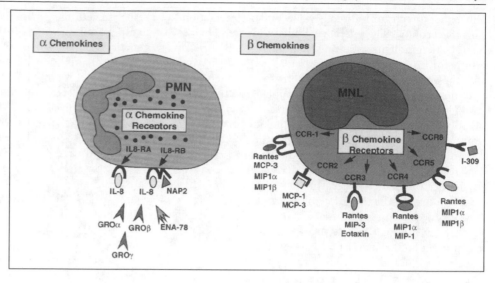

sequence tags) the reader is referred to Wells and Peitsch[42] and Baggiolini et al.[43]

In general, CXC chemokines are chemotactic for neutrophils while CC chemokines are active on mononuclear cells, predominantly monocytes and T lymphocytes and, for some chemokines, basophils and eosinophils.[64-69] It is this cell type selectivity that separates the chemokines from the more "traditional" chemoattractants such as complement fragments, leukotrienes and bacterial fMLP and that has stimulated research on them. In fact, some chemokines have exquisite cell type specificity as evidenced by the activities of the CC chemokines, MIP-1α and MIP-1β. Both of these proteins attract monocytes but also selectively attract different populations of T cells, with MIP-1α active on CD8 positive cells but MIP-1β active on CD4 positive T cells.[70,71] In contrast, the recently reported CC chemokine DC-CK1 is chemotactic for naive, CD45RA positive T cells,[72] unlike other T cell active chemokines like MIP-1α and MIP-1β, which only recruit activated T lymphocytes. The specificities exhibited by chemokines in in vitro assays support the numerous observations demonstrating cell type specific recruitment in vivo, and offer them as strong candidates for mediators in the associated pathologies. It is possible that the unique combination of specificity and redundancy within the chemokine superfamily may allow therapeutic inhibition of single chemokines to be efficacious in treating human inflammatory disease without simultaneously suppressing immune surveillance.

Chemotactic activities are usually measured in in vitro assays. While many devices are currently used, most are derivations of the Boyden chamber.[73,74] However, the physical nature of chemotactic gradients in vitro and in vivo may be very different, leading to some profound physiological consequences. In Boyden chamber type assays, leukocytes in an upper chamber are separated from the putative chemoattractant in a lower chamber by a polycarbonate membrane containing 3 μm-8 μm diameter pores. The membrane mimics an endothelial cell layer, separating the leukocytes from the source of chemoattractant and minimizing random cell migration. Cells that migrate in response to the chemoattractant are usually quantitated by staining and counting

cells that have migrated through the membrane and become adherent to its basal surface, or by recovering cells floating in the basal chamber medium.[75]

Although an oversimplification of what happens in vivo, this assay has provided the foundation for understanding inflammatory cell recruitment. However, it has long been recognized that one of the properties shared by chemokines (and many other proteins) is their affinity for charged macromolecules. Most chemokines are positively charged proteins and bind with high affinity to negatively charged biological macromolecules such as heparin.[43] This physical property of chemokines makes it unlikely that chemokines are always found in a "soluble" form at pro-inflammatory sites in vivo. Rather, it is becoming more obvious that chemokines in vivo may be bound by extracellular matrix (ECM) components and on the surfaces of cells, where they are "presented" to passing leukocytes.[76] This phenomenon, the migration of cells along a gradient of immobilized chemoattractants, is commonly referred to as haptotaxis. The soluble phase chemotaxis induced by chemokines in vitro may only be an approximation of the haptotaxis that is actually generated by solid phase gradients in vivo.

The likely physiological significance of chemokine adherence on tissue ECM has important implications for prostheses. A priori, polymers used for the construction of prosthetic devices dictate the electrostatic charge of the prosthesis in vivo.[27] Studies have demonstrated that charged polymers are differentially coated with plasma proteins when implanted into animals and that the kinetics of protein deposition do not necessarily reflect the relative plasma abundance of the adhering proteins.[27,77] Thus, implanted polymers are not necessarily preferentially coated with the most abundant serum proteins, namely, albumin and immunoglobulins.

Circulating or locally expressed proteins with high affinity for a synthetic matrix may preferentially deposit on the matrix even if they are present at relatively low concentrations. Simplistically, since many biopolymers are negatively charged, and most chemokines are positively charged, it is reasonable to speculate that an implanted polymer may become coated with significant amounts of chemokine protein, either directly or indirectly via secondary interactions. This effect could easily generate very high and persistent local haptotactic gradients, resulting in sustained leukocyte recruitment from adjacent microvascular endothelia. Worse still, the very high densities of adherent chemotactic proteins that may decorate implanted biopolymers are likely to strongly activate freshly recruited cells (see below). Since the biopolymer "matrix" to which the chemokines may become immobilized is not likely to turn over, implanted biopolymers may become "sinks" for concentrating chemotactic factors, resulting in indefinite leukocyte recruitment. It is this persistence of leukocyte recruitment and activation which results in overproduction of cytokines and growth factors, leading to chronic inflammatory diseases and fibrosis (Fig. 21.1). Although these growth factors are essential for recruitment of fibroblasts, fibroblast proliferation, and matrix synthesis in the induction of tissue repair, excess quantities of such factors in the microenvironment of a chronic inflammatory lesion are causative in pathologic fibrotic sequelae.

Mitigation of Recruitment

Termination of the inflammatory response is as important as its initiation, and the persistence of chronic inflammatory states may best be considered as a failure to modulate the immune response rather than its uncontrolled initiation. It is notable in this respect that most chemoattractants have inherent self-limiting properties. In general, the chemotactic dose-response curve for most chemoattractants is bell shaped, and as protein concentration increases beyond a maximum effective concentration, chemotactic activity decreases. However, at these higher concentrations, chemoattractants tend to activate their target cells, inducing in neutrophils, for example, degranulation, oxidative burst and increased adhesiveness. Chemotactic dose dependence may automatically trigger cells responding to a local chemotactic gradient to cease migration near the inflammatory site and commence their effector functions (Fig. 21.1). Combining chemotactic and activating functions into single molecules may ensure a smooth transition from one phenotype to another as leukocytes migrate up the chemokine gradient to their intended destination. This potential adaptive advantage is, however, offset by the consequence that local conditions supporting leukocyte recruitment and activation may become self-sustaining.

There exists in the current pharmacopia of medicine a wide variety of drugs used for the control of inflammation. The most commonly used and effective anti-inflammatories can probably be assigned to one of two categories, glucocorticosteroids and nonsteroidal anti-inflammatory drugs (NSAIDs).[78] Steroids, such as prednisolone and dexamethasone, are very powerful anti-inflammatory agents that exert their effects through regulation of gene expression. Many pro-inflammatory cytokine genes contain glucocorticoid responsive elements within their promoters which contribute to the regulation of their expression.[79] Exogenous administration of high levels of steroids as therapeutics suppresses gene expression of these cytokines, with the obvious result of limiting accumulation of the proteins themselves. Glucocorticoids can also promote a Th2 cytokine

response with the generation of IL-4 and IL-10, which can dampen immune functions.[80] Thus, glucocorticoids act as genetic switches, turning off or on entire sets of genes which control inflammation[81,82] and cellular proliferation.[83] Unfortunately, chronic use of glucocorticoids is associated with severe side effects,[84] including antifibrotic effects which may impair wound healing.

The other major category of drugs, the NSAIDs, inhibit the cyclo-oxygenase pathway to reduce biosynthesis of prostaglandins, with resulting anti-inflammatory, and analgesic, consequences.[85,86] Though useful for the treatment of minor inflammatory disease or as part of a combination therapy, NSAIDs such as aspirin, indomethacin, acetaminophen, and ibuprofen, are relatively weak, and when used at high doses can have toxic gastrointestinal and renal side effects.[87]

There is no doubt that powerful new anti-inflammatory agents are needed which combine the potency of glucocorticoids without the negative side effects. Some such products are now emerging as a consequence of the successes of molecular biology and biotechnology over the past two decades. The systematic dissection of the mammalian immune system has led to the identification of many pro- and anti-inflammatory cytokines with clinical potential. In addition, the numerous adhesion molecules that are a prerequisite for both normal and aberrant migration of leukocytes between lymphoid and systemic circulatory pathways and between the circulation and tissues make attractive targets for synthetic inhibitors.

An obvious approach for suppressing inflammation is by inhibiting leukocyte recruitment to the inflammatory site. The "three step" model leading to leukocyte diapedesis discussed earlier offers several options for intervention. It might be possible to inhibit the rolling of cells along activated endothelia, thus preventing any possibility of subsequent adhesion and chemotaxis. Synthetic analogs of the carbohydrate ligand for L-selectin have shown promise in preclinical models of acute inflammation.[88-90] However, selectins are crucial for normal recirculation of leukocytes between the lymphoid and systemic circulations, and anti-selectin drugs may adversely perturb this process. Integrins are also excellent candidates as targets for inhibitors. Reducing the strong adhesion between leukocytes and endothelial cells necessary for diapedesis should limit cellular recruitment into inflamed tissue, and many studies have supported this concept in vivo.[46,91,92] In this regard, synthetic peptides derived from the A chain of fibronectin have been shown to not only block integrin-dependent adhesion,[91,92] but also to interfere with matrix augmented cytokine signal transduction and cellular activation.[93] These promising anti-inflammatory peptides have proven beneficial in animal models of arthritis, autoimmunity[91,92,94,95] and liver fibrosis (Wahl SM, unpublished data).

Another possibility for suppressing cellular recruitment might be to target chemotactic factors themselves, in particular by identifying chemoattractant receptor antagonists. If a specific chemokine can be identified as the major chemoattractant associated with a given disease, antagonists of that chemokine might demonstrate efficacy without significant adverse effects or immune suppression. The latter hypothesis derives from the obvious redundancy among members of the chemokine superfamily, and assumes that any systemic immune defect caused by specific inhibition of one chemokine will be obscured by the remaining, overlapping activities of other chemokines.

The specificity of chemokines for their respective target cells is determined by the relative distribution of chemokine receptors expressed by the various populations of myeloid cells. Not surprisingly, there exist separate receptors for the two families of chemokines, CXC receptors and CC receptors.[96-98] Interestingly, the chemokine receptors display a wide range of specificities for the chemokines themselves, with some receptors binding a single ligand and others binding many ligands within a chemokine family. When all the data are combined, they reveal the existence of networks of redundant ligands and receptors for all types of myeloid cells, suggesting that recruitment of specific cell types in inflammation is dependent on temporal and spatial sequestration of chemokine expression.

Two neutrophil receptors have been identified for CXC chemokines which have very different properties (Fig. 21.2). Both receptors were originally characterized as receptors for IL-8 and were thus named type A and type B IL-8 receptors. However, the type B receptor binds several other CXC chemokines besides IL-8, including GROα, β and γ, NAP-2 and ENA-78. In contrast to the type B receptor, the type A IL-8 receptor is selective for IL-8 and binds other CXC-chemokines with approximately 100-fold lower affinity. Binding of CXC-chemokines to both IL-8 receptors is mediated largely, but not entirely, by the important sequence motif "ELR" which is located immediately upstream of the signature CXC domain of these chemokines. Significantly, the three CXC chemokines that do not bind the type B receptor, IP-10, MIG and PF4, all lack the ELR domain.

The family of CC chemokine receptors is far more complicated than that for the two IL-8 receptors. At least eight receptors for CC chemokines have been identified on various mononuclear leukocytes and are designated CCR1 through CCR8.[96-102] Each of the receptors is expressed on the surfaces of specific mononuclear cells and binds a specific subset of the CC chemokines, as shown in Figure 21.2, although the receptors CCR6 and CCR7 and their ligands are very poorly characterized. Alone among the well characterized CC chemokine receptors, CCR8 is apparently unique in having only one well defined ligand, the T lymphocyte chemoattractant I-309.[102]

The development of chemokine receptor antagonists (ra) is at the earliest research stage. Structure-function analysis of CXC and CC chemokines has revealed that the N-termini of both families of chemokines are crucial for both receptor binding and signal transduction.[43] Interestingly, chemokine mutants containing N-terminal truncations have been described which have the desired properties of high affinity receptor binding but negligible receptor activation.[103-106] These chemokine receptor antagonists generally retain the receptor type specificities of their normal counterparts, suggesting that they might selectively block a limited number of chemokines in vivo. The potential efficacy of chemokine receptor antagonists in treating human disease has yet to be demonstrated, but such proteins have shown promise in animal studies. An MCP-1ra has been used to successfully ameliorate experimental arthritis in mice,[107] and a CINCra (cytokine-induced neutrophil chemoattractant, a rat CXC chemokine) reduced peritoneal inflammation induced by injection of zymosan.[106] The specificity that chemokine receptor antagonists predictably inherit from their normal counterparts might initiate a new paradigm for anti-inflammatory selectivity, which is desirable for any new generation of drugs. The need for specificity is exemplified by observations that similar CXC chemokines such as IL-8 (ELR-containing) and IP-10 (non-ELR) exert opposing influences in idiopathic pulmonary fibrosis, with IL-8 promoting, and IP-10 suppressing, angiogenic activity.[108]

A simpler, but perhaps less obvious approach toward antagonizing chemoattractants derives from the spatial restrictions necessary for generating gradients. In vivo, endothelial layers and basement membranes serve a barrier function between leukocyte and chemoattractant to generate a chemotactic gradient. With leukocytes circulating in the vasculature and chemoattractants originating in the tissues, the gradient flows inward towards the blood. It follows that by intentionally increasing the concentration of chemoattractant in the blood, local gradients associated with inflammatory sites should collapse. Simply put, administering chemokines or other factors intravenously should have a paradoxically anti-inflammatory effect. Some data support this concept. Systemic administration of the potent chemoattractant TGF-β has been shown to reduce arthritis in rats, whereas direct tissue injection of the cytokine into joints aggravated the disease.[109,110] Similarly, systemic administration of the CC chemokine MCP-1 protected mice from lethal endotoxemia, although the mechanism of action was clearly complex, since the treatment notably altered plasma TNF-α, IL-10 and IL-12 levels as well.[111] Thus, by blocking the recruitment of leukocytes from the circulation to tissue sites of persistent infection, injury and/or implantation, it may be possible to attenuate the cascade of events responsible for chronic inflammation, tissue damage and fibrotic repair. Once fibropathogenesis has developed, it becomes more difficult to effectively intervene.

Summary and Perspectives

Technology often outstrips our ability to understand and adequately control it. Medical technology, and in particular surgery, is no exception. For instance, the techniques of whole organ transplant were successfully developed during the 1950s and 1960s, and are now common. However, the barrier to successful transplantation was not the physical act of moving the organ from donor to recipient, but convincing the recipient's immune system to accept, or more precisely ignore, the foreign tissue. It was the advent of immunosuppressive anti-rejection drugs like cyclosporin A that finally allowed the full potential of surgical transplants to be realized.[112] Yet, though we can sometimes fool the immune system into accepting our interventions, our level of control remains incomplete.

The discovery and characterization of an ever increasing number of cytokines and their receptors offers the possibility that new drugs will be developed that can exercise more selective control over inflammation than is currently possible. Such selectivity almost certainly offers the additional possibility that future therapeutics will have more limited adverse effects to complement their efficacy. While it is unlikely that we will be able to completely discount drug toxicity in humans, the increasing selectivity of anti-inflammatory drugs engendered by a better understanding and control of the immune response will undoubtedly provide improved therapeutic opportunities.

References

1. Hircsch JG. Antimicrobial factors in tissues and phagocytic cells. Bacteriol Rev 1960; 21:133-147.
2. Klebanoff SJ. Phagocytic cells: Products of oxygen metabolism. In: Gallin JI, Goldstein IM, Snyderman R, eds. Inflammation: basic principles and clinical correlates. New York: Raven Press, 1988:391-444.
3. Babior GL, Rosin RE, McMurrich BJ et al. Arrangement of the respiratory burst oxidase in the plasma membrane of the neutrophil. J Clin Invest 1981; 67:1724-1728.
4. Elsbach P, Weiss J. A re-evaluation of the roles of the O_2-dependent and O_2-independent microbicidal systems of phagocytes. Rev Infect Dis 1983; 5:843-853.
5. Elsbach P, Weiss J. Oxygen-dependent and oxygen-independent mechanisms of microbicidal activity of neutrophils. Immunol Lett 1985; 11:159-163.
6. Janoff A, Scherer J. Mediators of inflammation in leukocyte lysosomes. IX. Elastinolytic activity in granules of human polymorphonuclear leukocytes. J Exp Med 1968; 128:1137-1155.
7. Rabinovitch MC. Elastase and cell matrix interactions in the pathobiology of vascular disease. Acta Paediatr Jpn 1995; 37:657-666.
8. Doring G. The role of neutrophil elastase in chronic inflammation. Am J Resp Crit Care Med 1994; 150:S114-117.
9. Lazarus GS, Brown RS, Daniels JR et al. Human granulocyte collagenase. Science 1968; 159:1483-1485.
10. Shingleton WD, Hodges DJ, Brick P et al. Collagenase: A key enzyme in collagen turnover. Biochem Cell Biol 1996; 74:759-775.
11. Yamamoto K. Cathepsin E and cathepsin D: Biosynthesis, processing and subcellular location. Adv Exp Med Biol 1995; 362:223-229.
12. Peterson MW, Walter ME, Nygaard SD et al. Effect of neutrophil mediators on epithelial permeability. Am J Resp Cell Mol Biol 1995; 13:719-727.
13. Chapman HA, Biese RJ, Shi GP. Emerging roles for cysteine proteases in human biology. Ann Rev Physiol 1997; 59:63-88.
14. Durum SK, Oppenheim JJ. Macrophage derived mediators: Interleukin 1, tumor necrosis factor, interleukin 6, and related cytokines. In: Gallin JI, Goldstein IM, Snyderman R, eds. Inflammation: Basic Principles and Clinical Correlates. New York: Raven Press, 1988:639-662.
15. Wahl SM. Acute and chronic inflammation. In: Asherson GL, Zembala M, eds. Human monocytes. New York: Academic Press, 1989:361-371.
16. Nathan C. Mechanisms and modulation of macrophage activation. Behring Inst Mitt 1991; 88:200-207.
17. Stein JM, Levinson SM. Effect of the inflammatory reaction on subsequent wound healing. Surg Forum 1966; 17:484-485.
18. Hugo NE, Thompson LW, Zook EG et al. Effect of chronic anemia on the tensile strength of healing wounds. Surgery 1969; 66:741-745.
19. Simpson DM, Ross R. The neutrophilic leukocyte in wound repair. A study with antineutrophil serum. J Clin Invest 1972; 51:2009-2023.
20. Wahl SM, Arend WP, Ross R. The effect of complement depletion on wound healing. Am J Pathol 1974; 74:73-83.
21. Leibovich SJ, Ross R. The role of the macrophage in wound repair: A study with hydrocortisone and antimacrophage serum. Am J Pathol 1975; 78:71-91.
22. Border WA, Ruoslahti E. Transformtin growth factor-beta in disease, the dark side of tissue repair. J Clin Invest 1992; 90:1-7.
23. Fassbender, HG. The disease picture in rheumatoid arthritis as a result of different pathomechanisms. Z Rheumatol 1985; 44:33-46.
24. Wahl SM. Fibrosis: Bacterial-cell-wall-induced hepatic granulomas. In: Gallin JI, Goldstein IM, Snyderman R, eds. Inflammation: Basic principles and clinical correlates. New York: Raven Press, 1988: 841-859.
25. Friedman SL. Molecular mechanisms of hepatic fibrosis and principles of therapy. J Gastroenterol 1997; 32:424-430.
26. Morris W, Knauer CM. Cardiopulmonary manifestations of shistosomiasis. Semin Respir Infect 1997; 12:159-170.
27. Marchant RE, Wang IW. Physical and chemical aspects of biomaterials used in humans. In: Greco RS, ed. Implantation Biology: The Host Response to Biomedical Devices. Boca Raton: CRC Press, 1994:13-38.
28. Choi ET, Callow AD. The effect of biomaterials on the host. In: Greco RS, ed. Implantation Biology: The Host Response to Biomedical Devices. Boca Raton: CRC Press, 1994:39-54.
29. Butcher EC. Leukocyte-endothelial cell recognition: Three (or more) steps to specificity and diversity. Cell 1991; 67:1033-1036.
30. Arfors KE, Lundberg C, Lindhorm I et al. A monoclonal antibody to the membrane glycoprotein complex CD18 inhibits polymorphonuclear leukocyte accumulation and plasma leakage in vivo. Blood 1987; 69:338-340.
31. Ley K, Lundgren E, Berge E et al. Shear dependent inhibition of granulocyte adhesion to cultured endothelium by dextran sulfate. Blood 1989; 73:1324-1330.
32. Argenbright LW, Letts LG, Rothlein R. Monoclonal antibodies to the leukocyte membrane CD18 glycoprotein complex and to intracellular adhesion molecule-1 inhibit leukocyte-endothelial adhesion in rabbits. J Leuk Biol 1991; 49:253-257.
33. Springer TA. Traffic signals on endothelium for lymphocyte recirculation and leukocyte emigration. Ann Rev Physiol 1995; 57:827-872.
34. McEver RP, Moore KL, Cummings RD. Leukocyte trafficking mediated by selectin-carbohydrate interactions. J Biol Chem 1995; 270:11025-11028.
35. Rossitter II, Alon R, Kupper TS. Selectins, T-cell rolling and inflammation. Mol Med Today 1997; 3:214-222.
36. Lasky LA. Selectin-carbohydrate interactions and the initiation of the inflammatory response. Ann Rev Biochem 1995; 64:113-139
37. Varki A. Selectin ligands. Proc Natl Acad Sci USA 1994; 91:7390-7397.
38. Kansas GS. Selectins and their ligands: Current concepts and controversies. Blood 1996; 88:3259-3287.

39. Varki A. Selectin ligands: Will the real ones please stand up? J Clin Invest 1997; 99:158-162.

40. Oppenheim JJ, Zachariae COC, Mukaida N et al. Properties of the novel proinflammatory supergene "intercrine" family. Ann Rev Immunol 1991; 9:617-648.

41. Kelvin DJ, Michiel DF, Johnston JA et al. Chemokines and serpentines: the molecular biology of chemokine receptors. J Leuk Biol 1993; 54:604-612.

42. Wells TNC, Peitsch MC. The chemokine information source: Identification and characterization of novel chemokines using the worldwideweb and expressed sequence tag databases. J Leuk Biol 1997; 61:545-550.

43. Baggiolini M, Dewald B, Moser B. Human chemokines: An update. Ann Rev Immunol 1997; 15:675-705.

44. Kahn J, Ingraham RH, Shirley F et al. Membrane proximal cleavage of L-selectin; identification of the cleavage site and a 6kD transmembrane peptide fragment of L-selectin. J Cell Biol 1994; 125:461-470.

45. Gober JS, Bowen BL, Ebling H et al. Monocyte-endothelial adhesion in chronic rheumatoid arthritis: In situ detection of selectin and integrin-dependant interactions. J Clin Invest 1993; 91:2609-2619.

46. Wahl SM, Feldman GM, McCarthy JB. Regulation of leukocyte adhesion and signaling in inflammation and disease. J Leuk Biol 1996; 59:789-796.

47. Loftus JC, Liddington RC. Cell adhesion in vascular biology. New insights into integrin-ligand interaction. J Clin Invest 1997; 99:2302-2306.

48. Carr MW, Alon R, Springer TA. The C-C chemokine MCP-1 differentially modulates the avidity of β1 and β2 integrins on T lymphocytes. Immunity 1996; 4:179-187.

49. Burns AR, Simon SI, Kukielka GL et al. Chemotactic factors stimulate CD18-dependent canine neutrophil adherence and motility on lung fibroblasts. J Immunol 1996; 156:3389-3401.

50. Madri JA, Graesser D, Haas T. The roles of adhesion molecules and proteinases in lymphocyte transendothelial migration. Biochem Cell Biol 1996; 74:749-757.

51. Lefkowith, JB. Leukocyte migration in immune complex glomerulonephritis: Role of adhesion receptors. Kidney Int 1997; 51:1469-1475.

52. Newton RA, Thiel M, Hogg N. Signaling mechanisms and the activation of leukocyte integrins. J Leuk Biol 1997; 61:422-426.

53. Ruoslahti E. Integrins as signaling molecules and targets for tumor therapy. Kidney Int 1997; 51:1413-1417.

54. Ryan GB. The origin and sequence of the cells found in the acute inflammatory response. Aust J Exp Biol Med Sci 1967; 45:149-162.

55. Wahl SM. Transforming growth factor beta in inflammation. A cause and a cure. J Clin Immunol 1992; 12:61-74.

56. Frank MM, Fries LF. Complement. In: Gallin JI, Goldstein IM, Snyderman R, eds. Inflammation: Basic principles and clinical correlates. New York: Raven Press, 1988: 679-702.

57. Standiford TJ, Kunkel SL, Greenberger MJ et al. Expression and regulation of chemokines in bacterial pneumonia. J Leuk Biol 1996; 59:24-28.

58. Schroder JM, Noso N, Sticherling M et al. Role of eosinophil-chemotactic C-C chemokines in cutaneous inflammation. J Leuk Biol 1996; 59:1-5.

59. Baggiolini M, Dahinden CA. CC chemokines in allergic inflammation. Immunol Today 1994; 15:127-133.

60. Yoshimura TK, Matsushima K, Tanaka S et al. Purification of a human monocyte-derived neutrophil chemotactic factor that shares sequence homology with other host defense cytokines. Proc Natl Acad Sci USA 1987; 84:9233-9236.

61. Matsushima K, Larsen CG, DuBois GC et al. Purification and characterization of a novel monocyte chemotactic and activating factor produced by a human myelomonocytic cell line. J Exp Med 1989; 169:1485-1490.

62. Sherry B, Tekamp-Olson P, Gallegos C et al. Resolution of the two components of macrophage inflammatory protein 1, and cloning and characterization of one of those components, macrophage inflammatory protein 1β. J Exp Med 1988; 168:2251-2259.

63. Nakagawa H, Komorita N, Shibata F et al. Identfication of cytokine-induced neutrophil chemoattractants (CINC), rat GRO/CINC-2α and CINC-2β, produced by granulation tissue in culture: Purification, complete amino acid sequences and characterization. Biochem J 1994; 301:545-551.

64. Geiser T, Dewald B, Ehrengruber MU et al. The interleukin-8-related chemotactic cytokines GROα, GROβ, and GROγ activate human neutrophil and basophil leukocytes. J Biol Chem 1993; 268:15419-15424.

65. Weber M, Uguccioni M, Ochensberger B et al. Monocyte chemotactic protein MCP-2 activates human basophil and eosinophil leukocytes similar to MCP-3. J Immunol 1995; 154:4166-4172.

66. Forssmann U, Uguccioni M, Loetscher P et al. Eotaxin-2, a novel CC chemokine that is selective for the chemokine receptor CCR3, and acts like eotaxin on human eosinophil and basophil leukocytes. J Exp Med 1997; 185:2171-2176.

67. Proost P, Wuyts A, Van Damme J. Human monocyte chemotactic proteins-2 and -3: Structural and functional comparison with MCP-1. J Leuk Biol 1996; 59:67-74.

68. Garcia-Zepeda EA, Rothenberg ME, Ownbey RT et al. Human eotaxin is a specific chemoattractant for eosinophil cells and provides a new mechanism to explain tissue eosinophilia. Nature Med 1996; 2:449-456.

69. Kita H, Gleich GJ. Chemokines active on eosinophils. Potential roles in allergic inflammation. J Exp Med 1996; 183:2421-2426.

70. Schall TJ, Bacon K, Camp RDR et al. Human macrophage inflammatory protein 1α (MIP-1α) and MIP-1β chemokines attract distinct populations of lymphocytes. J Exp Med 1993; 177:1821-1830.

71. Taub D, Conlon K, Lloyd AR et al. Preferential migration of activated CD4+ and CD8+ T cells in response to MIP-1α and MIP-1β. Science 1993; 260:355-358.

72. Adema GJ, Hartgers F, Verstraten R et al. A dendritic-cell-derived C-C chemokine that preferentially attracts naive T cells. Nature 1997; 387:713-717.

73. Snyderman R, Altman LC, Hausman MS et al. Human mononuclear leukocyte chemotaxis: A quantitative assay for mediators of humoral and cellular chemotactic factors. J Immunol 1972; 109:857-860.

74. Altman LC, Snyderman R, Oppenheim JJ et al. A human mononuclear leukocyte chemotactic factor: Characterization, specificity and kinetics of production by homologous leukocytes. J Immunol 1973; 110:801-810.

75. Zagorski J, DeLarco JE. Expression of active human GROβ and GROγ neutrophil chemotactic proteins in E. coli. Prot Exp Purif 1994; 5:337-345.

76. Tanaka Y, Adams DH, Hubscher S et al. T-cell adhesion induced by proteoglycan-immobilized cytokine MIP-1β. Nature 1993; 361:79-82.

77. Andrade JD, Hlady V. Plasma protein adsorption; the big twelve. Ann NY Acad Sci 1987; 516:158-172.

78. Brooks PM, Day RO. Nonsteroidal antiinflammatory drugs-differences and similarities. N Engl J Med 1991; 324:1716-1721

79. Saatcioglu F, Claret FX, Karin M. Negative transcriptional regulation by nuclear receptors. Seminars Cancer Biol 1994; 5:347-359.

80. Ramierz F, Fowell DJ, Puklavec M, Simmonds S, Mason D. Glucocorticoids promote a TH2 cytokine response by CD4+ T cells in vitro. J Immunol 1996;156:2406-2412.

81. Brattsand R, Linden M. Cytokine modulation by glucocorticoids: Mechanisms and actions in cellular studies. Aliment Pharmacol Ther 1996; 10:81-90.

82. Barnes PJ, Karin M. Nuclear factor-kappaβ: A pivotal transcription factor in chronic inflammatory disease. N Engl J Med 1997; 336:1066-1071.

83. Armelin MC, Oliveira ML, Mercado JM et al. Molecular genetic approach to cell proliferation control and neoplasia. Braz J Med Biol Res 1996; 29:911-919.

84. Harris ED. The role of glucocorticoids. In: Rheumatoid arthritis. Philadelphia: WB Saunders, 1997:350-363.

85. Lewis RA, Austen KF. Leukotrienes. In: Gallin JI, Goldstein IM, Snyderman R, eds. Inflammation: Basic Principles and Clinical Correlates. New York: Raven Press, 1988:121-128.

86. Vane JR, Botting RM. Mechanism of action of aspirin-like drugs. Semin Arthritis Rhem 1997; 26:2-10.

87. Clements PJ, Paulnott R. Nonsteroidal anti-rheumatic drugs. In: Kelly WN, Harris ED, Ruddy S et al., eds. Textbook of Rhematology, 5th edition. Philadelphia: WB Saunders, 1996:707-740.

88. Kubes P, Jutila M, Payne D. Therapeutic potential of inhibiting leukocyte rolling in ischemia/reperfusion. J Clin Invest 1995; 95:2510-2519.

89. Turunen JP, Majuri ML, Seppo A et al. De novo expression of endothelial sialyl Lewis(a) and sialyl Lewis(x) during cardiac transplant rejection: Superior capacity of a tetravalent sialyl Lewis(x) oligosaccharide in inhibiting L-selectin-dependent lymphocyte adhesion. J Exp Med 1995; 182:1133-1141.

90. Seppo A, Turunen JP, Penttila I. et al. Synthesis of a tetravalent Lewis x glycan, a high affinity inhibitor of L-selectin-mediated lymphocyte binding to endothelium. Glycobiology 1996; 6:65-71.

91. Hines KL, Kulkarni AB, McCarthy JB et al. Synthetic fibronectin peptides interrupt inflammatory cell infiltration in TGF-β1 knockout mice. Proc Natl Acad Sci USA 1994; 91:5187-5191.

92. Wahl SM, Allen JB, Hines KL et al. Synthetic fibronectin peptides suppress arthritis in rats by interrupting leukocyte adhesion and recruitment. J Clin Invest 1994; 94:655-662.

93. McCarthy JB, Vachhani BV, Wahl SM, Finbloom DS, Feldman MF. Human monocyte binding to fibronectin enhances IFN-γ-induced early signaling events. J Immunol 1997; 159:2424-2430.

94. McCartney-Francis N, Mizel D, Frazier-Jessen M, Kulkarni A, McCarthy J, Wahl SM. Lacrimal gland inflammation is responsible for ocular pathology in TGF-β1-null mice. Am J Pathol 1997; in press.

95. McCartney-Francis N, Mizel D, Redman R et al. Autoimmune Sjogren's-like lesions develop in salivary glands of TGF-β1 deficient mice and can be inhibited by adhesion-blocking peptides. J Immunol 1996; 157:1306-1312.

96. Murphy PM. The molecular biology of leukocyte chemoattractant receptors. Annu Rev Immunol 1994; 12:593-633.

97. Raport CJ, Schweickart VL, Chantry D et al. New members of the chemokine receptor gene family. J Leuk Biol 1996; 59:18-23.

98. Wells TNC, Power CA, Lusti-Narasimhan M et al. Selectivity and antagonism of chemokine receptors. J Leuk Biol 1996; 59:53-60.

99. Baba M, Imai T, Nishimura M et al. Identification of CCR6, the specific receptor for a novel lymphocyte-directed CC chemokine LARC. J Biol Chem 1997; 272:14893-14898.

100. Yoshida R, Imai T, Hieshima K et al. Molecular cloning of a novel human CC chemokine EBI1-ligand chemokine that is a specific functional ligand for EBI1, CCR7. J Biol Chem 1997; 272:13803-13809.

101. Tiffany HL, Lautens LL, Gao JL et al. Identification of CCR8: A human monocyte and thymus receptor for the CC chemokine I-309. J Exp Med 1997; 186:165-170.

102. Roos RS, Loetscher M, Legler DF et al. Identification of CCR8, the receptor for the human CC chemokine I-309. J Biol Chem 1997; 272:17251-17254.

103. Moser B, Dewald B, Barella L et al. Interleukin-8 antagonists generated by N-terminal modification. J Biol Chem 1993; 268:7125-7128.

104. Gong JH, Clark-Lewis I. Antagonists of monocyte chemoattractant protein 1 identified by modification of functionally critical NH2-terminal residues. J Exp Med 1995; 181:631-640.

105. Gong JH, Uguccioni M, Dewald B et al. Rantes and MCP-3 antagonists bind multiple chemokine receptors. J Biol Chem 1996; 271:10521-10527.

106. Zagorski J, Wahl SM. Inhibition of acute peritoneal inflammation in rats by a cytokine-induced neutrophil chemoattractant receptor antagonist. J Immunol 1997; 159:1059-1062.

107. Gong JH, Ratkay LG, Waterfield JD et al. An antagonist of monocyte chemoattractant protein 1 (MCP-1) inhibits arthritis in the MRL-lpr mouse model. J Exp Med 1997; 186:131-137.

108. Keane MP, Arenberg DA, Lynch JP et al. The CXC chemokines, IL-8 and IP-10, regulate angiogenic activity in idiopathic pulmonary fibrosis. J Immunol 1997; 159:1437-1443.

109. Allen JB, Manthey CL, Hand AR et al. Rapid onset synovial inflammation and hyperplasia induced by transforming growth factor β. J Exp Med 1990; 171:231-247.

110. Brandes ME, Allen JB, Ogawa Y et al. Transforming growth factor β1 suppresses acute and chronic arthritis in experimental animals. J Clin Invest 1991; 87:1108-1113.

111. Zisman DA, Kunkel SL, Strieter RM et al. MCP-1 protects mice from lethal endotoxemia. J Clin Invest 1997; 99:2832-2836.

112. Rao A, Luo C, Hogan PG. Transcription factors of the NFAT family: Regulation and function. Annu Rev Immunol 1997; 15:707-747.

113. Zagorski J, Wahl SM. Recruitment. In: Roitt IM, Delves PJ, eds. Encyclopedia of Immunology, Second Edition. London: Academic Press, 1998; in press.

Taming of Adverse Responses

Prevention of a Hyperplastic Intimal Response

―――――――――――――――― CHAPTER 22 ――――――――――――――――

Pathobiology of Hyperplastic Intimal Responses

Erik L. Owens, Alexander W. Clowes

Introduction

Understanding the pathologic response of blood vessels to injury remains a primary research focus of the vascular surgeon and vascular biologist. In addition to learning more about the primary atherosclerotic lesion, the ultimate goal of this effort is to favorably influence the healing process after intervention, thus allowing the re-establishment of a widely patent lumen not narrowed by thrombus, intimal hyperplasia, or vasoconstriction.

This hyperplastic healing response has been established as a cause for angioplasty and vascular graft failure.[1-3] Although the available interventional modalities (stents, endovascular grafts, etc.) and the anatomic locations in which they are used (cerebral angioplasty, coronary stenting, etc.) continue to grow rapidly, no clinically proven method exists for preventing the late failure of these treatments by intimal hyperplasia.

In the peripheral vascular surgery literature, restenosis is a clinical term commonly used to describe the loss of more than 50% of luminal diameter in a vessel or graft after intervention.[4] It was previously thought that intimal hyperplasia was the principal cause of restenosis. We now believe that it is just one of several contributory components. Other mechanisms responsible for restenosis include vasoconstriction and accumulation of mural thrombus. Understanding the relationship between intimal hyperplasia and restenosis is crucial to properly interpreting results from pertinent clinical trials and animal models.

Clinical Relevance

Percutaneous transluminal coronary angioplasty (PTCA) has an excellent primary success rate (about 90-95%). However, approximately 30% of dilated coronary arteries develop marked restenosis by 6 months.[5,6] Coronary vein grafts have a 10 year patency of 50%.[7,8] Infra-inguinal saphenous vein grafts have a 24% failure rate at 4 years.[9] Polytetrafluoroethylene (PTFE) grafts in the same position have a 46% failure rate at 4 years.[9] Renal artery stenting appears to have a restenosis rate of about 44% at 1 year.[10] These observations are just a sampling of the known clinical data related to restenosis and graft failure after therapeutic intervention. The failure of a vascular graft placed during reconstruction or the development of restenosis in an artery that has previously undergone angioplasty (or stenting) exposes the patient to the risk of significant morbidity and mortality. Repeat intervention or vascular reconstruction is often the only remedy for the situation, further increasing the risk for the patient. From an economic viewpoint, considerable costs are incurred as a result of repeat vascular intervention. If one considers the frequency with which vascular procedures are currently performed and the incidence of graft failure or arterial restenosis after intervention, it becomes clear why such intense interest exists in understanding intimal hyperplasia.

Tissue Engineering of Prosthetic Vascular Grafts, edited by Peter Zilla and Howard P. Greisler.
©1999 R.G. Landes Company.

The development of methods to successfully control intimal hyperplasia promises both improved patient outcomes and overall cost effectiveness of our vascular interventions.

Mechanisms of Restenosis in Human Vessels

A clearer picture of the mechanisms of stenosis and restenosis in humans is emerging. Restenosis is most likely related to several factors, including the type of intervention performed and the relevant risk factors for each patient. Until recently, our knowledge about restenosis in humans was largely based on the examination of pathologic specimens at the time of reoperation. New technology that generates morphologic images in a non- or minimally-invasive manner has allowed serial observations of restenotic lesions in vessels, grafts, and stents.

After carotid endarterectomy, hemodynamically significant restenosis detected by duplex ultrasound occurs in about 20% of patients, although only a small percentage of these patients require reoperation.[11] The endarterectomy specimens removed during reoperations within the first two years of the primary procedure have the histologic appearance of intimal hyperplasia.[12] Lesions removed after two years resemble atherosclerotic plaque, not intimal hyperplasia.[13] Evidence exists that some lesions regress with time.[11]

Autogenous saphenous vein grafts placed during lower extremity revascularization have been extensively studied. Early failure of these grafts (within 0-30 days of operation) is commonly related to either technical defects or inadequate runoff. Hemodynamically significant stenoses requiring intervention occur in 30% of these grafts within two years and are caused by intimal hyperplasia.[2] Lesions in grafts failing later than two years after placement, designated as long term failures, appear to result from a combination of other factors, including intimal hyperplasia, progression of the patient's underlying disease, and atherosclerosis.[14]

Intraluminal, tubular, slotted stents placed in the coronary circulation inhibit the acute recoil and chronic remodeling of the vessel wall. Theoretically, restenosis in this setting should result primarily from tissue proliferation. Studies using intravascular ultrasound (IVUS) have confirmed that in-stent stenosis is solely a result of intimal hyperplasia.[15,16] While the clinical applications for vascular stents are still being investigated, it appears that stent restenosis serves as a pure model for investigating strategies to inhibit intimal hyperplasia.

When atheroma form, arteries can dilate to preserve arterial lumen size, a phenomenon called remodeling. Evidence of remodeling was first reported in monkeys[17] and then in human coronary and carotid arteries.[18] Remodeling has been demonstrated in a hypercholesterolemic rabbit model,[19] and may occur after angioplasty in human vessels. The ability of an artery or graft to remodel in response to intimal thickening may determine whether graft stenosis or restenosis after angioplasty in humans will occur.

Other processes may play significant roles in human restenosis but are not easily studied in animal models. Such processes include vasospasm, dissection, plaque instability or rupture, and thrombosis.

Models of Intimal Hyperplasia

Most of what we know about intimal hyperplasia is derived from animal studies. The majority of this information has been obtained from models in which the hyperplastic healing response is observed after injuring normal vessels, usually with balloon dilation. The injury response depends on the type of vessel injured (artery (normal or diseased, elastic or muscular) or vein graft (new or old)) and the severity of the injury (vessel dilation, valvulotomy, arterial angioplasty, stenting, atherectomy, or endarterectomy). It is unlikely that each of these maneuvers invokes the same degree, or even type, of injury response.

Intimal hyperplasia in grafts may be a very distinct form of healing. Vein grafts start with a normal cellular architecture which we know then undergoes adaptive changes upon exposure to the arterial circulation. Prosthetic grafts, however, have only an acellular, fibrous scaffolding on which a neointima forms.

Several studies performed in animals have suggested that certain drugs prevent intimal hyperplasia. However, when similar studies have been performed in human clinical trials, no reduction in restenosis was observed. This may be a result of the previously mentioned inability to equate intimal hyperplasia with restenosis. However, species-specific responses also appear to exist and offer one more potential limitation of the current animal model data.[20,21,22]

It is clear that intimal hyperplasia is a complex process that occurs in many different clinical settings and is influenced by a myriad of factors. Animal models have, however, identified common threads in the basic pathophysiologic responses to vascular injury. In vitro studies performed in numerous vascular biology laboratories have also contributed greatly to our current understanding. Successful application of this knowledge to the human clinical setting remains the daunting challenge.

Arteries

Intimal hyperplasia develops after many types of injury, including the removal of adventitia (which causes ischemia in the media due to loss of blood supply from adventitial capillaries), electrical injury, external clamping, blunt trauma, chemical or endotoxin infusion, as well as luminal damage by passage of a dilated balloon catheter.[23] Most of these forms of injury have limited clinical relevance.

The severity of injury is important in determining the ultimate pathophysiologic response.[24-27] A classification system based upon the immediate histologic effect of the injury might be considered.[4]

Type I injuries result in no significant loss of the vessel's basic cellular architecture. There may be a slight change of the endothelial architecture and associated cellular adhesion. The fatty streak, an early atherosclerotic lesion, can be thought of as a type I injury. Hemodynamic factors and flow disturbances represent type I injuries because they produce, at most, only a modification of the established cellular architecture.

Type II injuries involve loss of the endothelial layer. The internal elastic lamina (IEL) remains intact, and there is little or no damage to the media. These injuries occur during simple arterial catheterization, endovascular procedures, or vein graft preparation. A rat model of a type II injury uses gentle filament endothelial denudation of the carotid artery.[24] In areas of endothelial loss, platelets may adhere and begin to form a thrombus.

Type III injuries are inflicted upon countless human vessels each day in the form of balloon angioplasty, endarterectomy, atherectomy, and other forms of surgical repair or reconstruction. A type III injury results in transmural damage. The endothelium is removed. The IEL is often disrupted, and a significant portion of the medial cells are killed.[24,28] An inflammatory response is initiated within the vessel wall. Upon loss of the endothelium, platelets deposit and thrombus forms.

Molecular Mechanisms of Intimal Hyperplasia after Injury

Much has been learned about the basic pathophysiology of intimal hyperplasia from the response of a rat carotid artery to a type III injury. The model is a modification of a method described by Baumgartner.[28] A small Fogarty embolectomy catheter is passed into the common carotid artery via the external carotid artery. The balloon is inflated and pulled through the common carotid artery, denuding the endothelium and damaging the underlying tissue. Progressive luminal thrombosis does not typically occur. Intimal thickening occurs within 2 weeks and reaches a maximum at about 3 months. Luminal area declines transiently, partly because of intimal thickening and partly because the injured vessel contracts. The histologic and molecular changes that have been documented after injury in this rat

model form the basis for the proposed three phase paradigm for the development of intimal hyperplasia.

Table 22.1 summarizes many of the putative regulatory factors and their proposed role in intimal lesion formation or inhibition.

First Phase: Proliferation

The first cellular event after injury is the proliferation of a proportion of medial smooth muscle cells (SMCs). Medial SMCs in a normal artery proliferate at a very low level (0.06% per day). As soon as 24 hours after injury, 10-30% of the medial SMCs are induced to enter the growth cycle.[29,30] The proportion of proliferating cells remains high for several days but by 4 weeks returns to baseline levels. Early observations of the events surrounding vascular injury resulted in the "reaction to injury" hypothesis which implicated platelets in the development of intimal hyperplasia.[31,32] This theory was based upon three key observations:

1. Platelets appear on the luminal surface of injured vessels immediately;
2. Platelets deposit α–granules which contain numerous growth factors for cultured SMCs including platelet derived growth factor (PDGF), transforming growth factor (TGF)-β, and epidermal growth factor; and
3. Thrombocytopenic animals experience less intimal thickening after balloon injury.[33-35]

While overall intimal thickening is reduced in thrombocytopenic animals, the first wave of SMC proliferation is unaltered.[35] Additionally, balloon-injured vessels (a type III

Table 22.1. Molecular mechanisms of intimal hyperplasia after arterial injury

Potential Stimulatory Factors	Proposed Role in Lesion Formation
Basic fibroblast growth factor (bFGF)	Medial SMC proliferation
Platelet-derived growth factor (PDGF)	SMC migration/ECM formation
Angiotensin II (AII)	Medial and intimal SMC proliferation/SMC migration
Transforming growth factor (TGF)-β	Intimal SMC proliferation/matrix formation
urokinase-like plasminogen activator (uPA)	SMC migration
tissue-type plasminogen activator (tPA)	SMC migration
Metalloproteinases (MMP)-2 and -9	SMC migration
Integrins	SMC migration
Thrombin	Promotes platelet aggregation/medial SMC proliferation
Endothelin	Medial SMC proliferation/produces vasoconstriction
Insulin-like growth factor (IGF)-β	Medial SMC proliferation
Catecholamines	Intimal and medial SMC proliferation
Cytokines	Intimal SMC proliferation
Potential Inhibitory Factors	**Proposed Role in Lesion Inhibition**
Nitric oxide (NO)	Blocks platelet aggregation/SMC proliferation and migration/produces vasorelaxation
Prostacyclin (PGI2)	Blocks platelet aggregation/produces vasorelaxation
Heparin-like molecules	Limits thrombosis/intimal SMC proliferation/SMC migration
Tissue inhibitor of metalloproteinases (TIMP)-1	SMC migration
Plasminogen activator inhibitor (PAI)-1	SMC migration

injury) develop more medial SMC proliferation and intimal thickening than filament-injured vessels (a type II injury).[35] In both of these models, the endothelial layer is removed and platelets adhere to the exposed subendothelium, releasing their cytoplasmic granules. Thus, platelet-related effects in the two models should be similar. The fact that more injury is inflicted upon the medial layer in the balloon injury model suggests that the specific stimulus for proliferation is related to the degree of injury in this area. The most logical conclusion is that a nonplatelet derived factor released by injury is primarily responsible for the initial wave of medial SMC proliferation and that the platelet factors must affect a portion of the process other than proliferation.

Lindner and Reidy demonstrated that the initial stimulus for proliferation is most likely basic fibroblast growth factor (bFGF).[36-38] In vitro, bFGF is a strong mitogen and is released from disrupted cultured SMCs.[39,40] Endothelial cells, SMCs, and extracellular matrix all store various amounts of bFGF.[39] In the extracellular matrix (ECM), bFGF is stored bound to heparan sulfate proteoglycans. Treatment with heparin infusion has been shown to blunt the proliferative response, presumably by displacing the bFGF from the matrix.[41] Proliferating SMCs express the relevant receptor to bFGF.[38] SMC proliferation is significantly enhanced by the administration of bFGF and antibodies to bFGF reduce SMC proliferation by approximately 80%.[36,37,42,43]

The renin-angiotensin system may also play a role in the early injury response.[44] In vitro, angiotensin ii is a mitogen for SMCs.[45] Additionally, AII induces the expression of other known mitogens.[46-48] In vivo, AII receptor antagonists and angiotensin converting enzyme (ACE) inhibitors delivered after injury each reduce SMC proliferation and inhibit intimal thickening.[49] SMC proliferation and intimal thickening are enhanced by infusion of AII.[50,51]

Other growth factors might have roles in this early proliferative stage of lesion development including PDGF,[52] thrombin,[53] endothelin,[54-56] insulin-like growth factor-1 (IGF-1),[57] and catecholamines.[58] The evidence for their involvement is, however, not as strong as that for bFGF or AII.

Second Phase: Migration

As early as 4 days after injury, SMCs begin to appear in the intima.[59] This results from migration of cells across the IEL, since normal rat intima contains no SMCs. This process continues for up to one month. Only about 50% of migrating cells continue to proliferate.[28, 30]

Two distinct events must take place for cells to traverse the IEL and enter the forming intima. First, there must be a chemoattractant or some form of signal for the SMCs to initiate the journey. Secondly, the cells must be freed from their surrounding matrix. Multiple factors are certainly involved in the migratory process. Some may have dual roles as both chemoattractants and as initiators of matrix detachment.

As previously mentioned, platelet factors might play a role in intimal thickening, perhaps by influencing SMC migration. Platelet α-granules are known to contain PDGF. Most of the evidence now seems to point to one of the isoforms of PDGF, PDGF-BB, and stimulation of the PDGF-β receptor as the major migratory signal. While PDGF was initially isolated from platelets, all vascular wall cells including endothelial cells, SMCs, and macrophages can express this factor. PDGF is a strong mitogen in vitro, but its main effect in vivo appears to be on migration. (For a review on PDGF, see ref. 60.)

In vitro work in our lab has demonstrated a strong migratory response of baboon SMCs to PDGF-BB but not to PDGF-AA.[61] Of the three possible isoforms, AA, BB, and AB, PDGF-BB is the predominant isoform in platelet α-granules in rat, pig, and baboon. Human platelets contain all three isoforms in equal amounts.[62] Since PDGF-BB is able to bind to both the α and the β form of the PDGF receptor and PDGF-AA is only able to bind to the α receptor,[60] this strongly suggests that activation of the β receptor plays a leading role in SMC migration.

When a polyclonal antibody to human PDGF is administered to rats undergoing balloon injury, intimal thickening is inhibited by 40%.[63] Smooth muscle proliferation is not affected. When the recombinant form of PDGF-BB is administered intravenously or intraarterially, SMC migration is markedly stimulated and intimal thickening is increased.[64] SMC proliferation in the media is only slightly increased. In our lab, an antibody to the PDGF receptor-β (PDGFR-β) administered to baboons subjected to balloon injury of the saphenous artery or PTFE graft bypass significantly reduces intimal hyperplasia (unpublished results). Similar results have been obtained using specific antibodies to the PDGFR-β in baboons and in rats.[62] Sirois et al have recently shown using immunohistochemical analysis that both PDGF receptors (PDGFR-α and -β) are present in the normal artery wall and are markedly upregulated after injury.[65] Treatment with antisense oligonucleotides to PDGFR-β significantly decreases PDGFR-β expression and inhibits intimal thickening.

The roles of PDGF-A chain and the PDGFR–α are not yet clear. Animal studies using neutralizing antibodies to PDGF-A have shown no observable effect during injury.[62] In a Boyden chamber used to measure migration, activation of the PDGFR-α by either PDGF-AA or -BB generates an inhibitory signal for baboon SMC migration.[61] Analysis of human fetal, normal adult, and atherosclerotic aortas suggests a maintenance role for PDGFR-α, since levels of PDGF-A message ribonucleic acid (mRNA) by reverse transcription-polymerase chain reaction (RT-PCR) were 100 times higher in normal vessels than either developing (fetal) or diseased (atherosclerotic) vessels.[66] The idea that PDGF-A is a "survival factor" has also been proposed.[67-69]

In order for the SMCs to break their attachments with the extracellular matrix, proteases are required. The act of detachment itself may serve to further activate the migratory process.[35] Plasmin is the main fibrinolytic enzyme in the body and is also able to degrade most matrix components. It is derived from plasminogen through the action of urokinase-like plasminogen activator (uPA) and tissue-type plasminogen activator (tPA).[70] Urokinase-like plasminogen activator (uPA) is activated within 2-3 hours after injury.[71,72] Tissue-type plasminogen activator (tPA) appears several days later, around the same time as SMCs are seen entering the intima.[73] Tranexamic acid, a plasmin inhibitor, inhibits SMC migration after injury.[74] Knockout mice studies reveal that deletion of uPA reduces intimal thickening after injury. Deletion of tPA has no effect and deletion of the naturally occurring plasminogen activator inhibitor (PAI)-1 increases thickening.[75] We have observed that overexpression of PAI-1 in the rat carotid inhibits intimal hyperplasia (unpublished results).

A second class of enzymes also linked to SMC migration is the matrix metalloproteinases (MMP). The MMPs are a group of proteases found in the ECM. They digest collagen, elastin, fibronectin, laminin, and proteoglycans.[76] Plasmin activates MMPs.[77] These proteinases have been observed in stimulated SMCs in culture and in SMCs from injured arteries and atherosclerotic plaques. Hours after injury, MMP-9 (gelatinase b) appears and remains elevated for approximately one week. Several days later, at about the same time as tPA appears, MMP-2 (gelatinase a), which is present in normal artery walls, increases.[72] Conditioned media containing tissue inhibitor of metalloproteinases (TIMP)-1 (a natural inhibitor of MMP) completely inhibits the PDGF-BB induced migration of SMCs in vitro, a process that can be overcome by treatment with an antibody to TIMP-1. Local overexpression of TIMP-1 suppresses intimal thickening in the injured rat carotid model.[78] In an explant model using baboon tissue developed by Kenagy, antibodies to urokinase, tPA, and MMP-2 and -9 each inhibit migration, while addition of plasminogen increases migration.[22]

Detachment of the SMCs from their extracellular matrix might be further regulated by integrins, a family of transmembrane proteins that link the cytoskeleton to the ECM and to adhesion molecules on other cells. Integrins are heterodimers made up of two noncovalently linked subunits, designated α and β. Blockade of the integrin receptor $\alpha_v\beta_3$ reduces PDGF-induced SMC migration in vitro and inhibits intimal hyperplasia in a rabbit carotid injury model.[79] Blockade of another receptor, $\alpha_{IIb}\beta_3$, appears to prevent platelet aggregation after injury.[80] Human clinical trials using a monoclonal antibody fragment (c7E3 Fab) that blocks both the $\alpha_v\beta_3$ and the $\alpha_{IIb}\beta_3$ receptors as a result of their common β_3 component decreases the frequency of ischemic events after PTCA and reduces restenosis by 26%.[81] Whether this is the result of the inhibitory effect on platelet aggregation or SMC migration or a combination of the two is unknown.

New proteins or proteins that are normally present in only small quantities begin to appear in abundance in the matrix of the newly formed intima of the injured rat carotid. It is thought that many of these proteins, including osteopontin,[82] versican,[83] tenascin,[84] thrombospondin,[85] and splice products of fibronectin, may play a role in the adhesion of cells in the injured vascular wall. Peptides with the amino acid sequence arginine-glycine-aspartic acid (RGD) interfere with integrin binding.[86] RGD peptides inhibit migration of SMCs in vitro and reduce intima formation in the rat.[79] Integrins that bind these peptides have been demonstrated in the injured rat carotid and are also abundant in normal human and atherosclerotic human arteries.[87]

The role of SMC migration in the injured atherosclerotic lesion is unclear, since SMCs are already present in diseased human arteries. It does appear, however, from analysis of atherectomy specimens, that migration might be the predominant mode of intimal formation in human lesions.[88]

Third Phase: Intimal Expansion

The lesion continues to expand by SMC migration and intimal proliferation. These cells also synthesize and secrete matrix proteins. The largest contribution to lesion formation is made by the deposition of these matrix proteins including elastin, collagen, and proteoglycan.[89] It would seem logical that some of the factors present in early lesion development might play a role in intimal expansion. Some of the aforementioned factors, especially TGF-β and PDGF, are known to stimulate ECM production.[90] Unlike the earlier stages, where a single factor appears to control activity, control of the later expansion phase appears multifactorial in nature. No one stimulatory factor has yet been shown to predominate.

Regarding lesion expansion, studies seem to indicate that bFGF is unlikely to be involved in regulating intimal SMC proliferation. Antibodies to bFGF do not affect SMC proliferation when administered 5 days after balloon injury of the rat carotid.[91] Furthermore, no convincing evidence exists that PDGF plays a role. PDGF-BB infusion weeks after injury does produce a modest but measurable increase in intimal SMC proliferation.[63] However, PDGF-B has not been detected to any measurable extent in the forming intima, only in the endothelium near the wound edge.[92] Rather, PDGF-A ligand and PDGFR-β predominate in the intima during this time period.[52] Since PDGF-A ligand can only bind to PDGFR-α, it appears unlikely that PDGF plays a significant role in this phase.

As discussed previously, evidence does indicate that the angiotensin system may play a role in SMC proliferation after injury. A possible role in SMC migration[49] and intimal expansion has been demonstrated as well.[23] Angiotensin ii may influence intimal growth indirectly through either its interactions with other growth factors (AII stimulates PDGF-A and TGF-β production) or its stimulation of the sympathetic nervous system.[50] Catecholamines have been shown to be SMC mitogens in vitro. Angiotensin ii administration produces a vigorous increase in intimal SMC proliferation and lesion area, even when infused at a time when the rat carotid lesion is already well developed.[23] Infusion of ACE inhibitors and angiotensin receptor blockers inhibit intimal thickening after balloon injury in the rat independent of blood pressure effects.[36-38] Cilazapril, an ACE inhibitor, as well as other ACE inhibitors, and Dup 753, a specific angiotensin ii receptor antagonist, block intimal thickening in rats after balloon injury.[93] A human clinical trial using Cilazipril during coronary angioplasty, however, has shown no effect on either restenosis or angiographic outcome.[94,95]

Messenger RNAs for insulin-like growth factor (IGF)-1 and TGF-β have been detected in the newly formed intima and could play a role in regulating cell proliferation or extracellular matrix production.[96,97]

After about 3 months, intimal thickening stops. The final composition of the intima, once it achieves a resting state, is generally 80% ECM by volume.[98] What determines the endpoint at which growth ceases? Most probably, the lesion reaches the point at which either the stimulatory signals subside or the inhibitory signals develop strongly enough to counter the stimulatory signals, or both.

Evidence exists that endothelial cells play a role in this aspect of lesion growth. In the rat carotid injury model, an endothelial surface is formed by the ingrowth of cells from uninjured areas proximal and distal to the zone of denudation. The central portion remains uncovered indefinitely, and the growing edge appears to stop 1 cm to 1.2 cm from the untraumatized zone.[99,100] Smooth muscle cell proliferation stops sooner (approximately 2 weeks) in areas covered by a new endothelial layer. After about 4 weeks, SMC growth returns to baseline even in areas left devoid of endothelium.[89] SMC proliferation may slow as a result of growth inhibitor release by the endothelial cells.

Cultured endothelial cells are known to secrete heparin-like heparan sulfates.[101] The growth inhibitory properties of this family of molecules are well known.[102,103] Heparin has also been shown to alter the composition of the ECM.[104] Nitric oxide (NO) is another inhibitory factor produced by endothelial cells. Nitric oxide here is produced via constitutive nitric oxide synthase or cNOS, the form of NOS unique to endothelial cells.[105] In vitro data suggest that NO is a potent inhibitor of cell proliferation and migration.[106,107] In vivo, NO may control lesion development through both its vasoactive properties and its inhibitory effects on other growth factor pathways. Since endothelial cells serve as the major source of NO, loss of endothelium during injury results in the loss of an important SMC growth inhibitor. Once endothelial regeneration occurs, the pace of intimal hyperplasia and SMC proliferation may slow simply by restoring the inhibitory NO signal. In both a rat and rabbit balloon injury model, L-arginine added to the drinking water increases NO production and reduces intimal hyperplasia.[108,109] In vivo gene transfer with a plasmid containing a cDNA encoding for cNOS or an adenovirus containing iNOS after rat carotid artery injury restores NO to levels seen in normal, untreated vessels and inhibits intimal formation by 70%.[110,111] Rats kept in an atmosphere of 80 ppm NO after balloon injury also develop significantly less intimal hyperplasia at both 1 and 2 weeks after injury.[112] A single, locally delivered treatment of bovine serum albumin modified to carry multiple NO groups inhibits intimal hyperplasia after balloon injury in a rabbit model in a dose dependent manner.[113] Administration of this molecule decreases platelet adhesion and SMC migration in association with elevations in platelet and vascular guanosine 3',5'-cyclic monophosphate (cGMP) content, the result of guanylate cyclase activation by NO. Aside from its inhibition of SMC proliferation and migration, NO also affects vascular smooth muscle relaxation,[114] platelet inhibition,[63] leukocyte adhesion,[115] and vascular permeability.[116] It is apparent that NO inhibits lesion formation after arterial injury. Whether this is a result of one specific effect or a combination of several is not yet known.

In areas that remain devoid of endothelium, the luminal SMCs may assume some endothelial functions, including the production of inhibitory factors. For example, NO is generated via the inducible form of nitric oxide synthase (iNOS) and prostacyclin (PGI$_2$) via cyclooxygenase (COX).[117,118] Smooth muscle cell iNOS is upregulated in areas of injury.[117] The administration of a NO synthase inhibitor (N-omega-nitro-L-arginine methylester (L-NAME)) accelerates intimal formation after balloon injury, most likely by inhibiting NO production by iNOS since very little cNOS is present once the endothelium is removed.[119]

Hemodynamic factors also influence lesion formation. Increases in blood flow after balloon injury appear to have a protective effect. In a rat carotid injury model, intimal hyperplasia is reduced in rats that undergo contralateral common carotid artery ligation (high flow) when compared to rats that undergo ipsilateral internal carotid artery ligation (low flow).[120] Since SMC proliferation is not different between the two groups of animals, this implies an alteration in SMC migration as the possible mechanism.

Could the ultimate control mechanism in lesion development be related to flow (shear stress)? Endothelial cells serve as the primary sensor for flow related phenomena through shear stress receptors.[121] Activation of these pathways may cause changes in the secretion of growth or inhibitory factors. It has been well documented that increasing shear stress increases NO production by endothelial cells in vitro[122] and in vivo.[123] In areas of endothelial denudation, SMCs have been shown to undergo phenotypic changes to render themselves more endothelial-like.[124] As the lesion size increases, luminal area decreases, resulting in increased shear stress (assuming constant blood flow and no significant change in vessel contraction or dilation). There is some evidence that the vessel itself dilates in an attempt to compensate for the loss of luminal area.[18] This response is, however, probably limited. During the early period of luminal dilation (relatively low shear stress) and loss of endothelium, NO production is low. Lack of a strong inhibitory signal allows continued SMC growth. However, as the luminal area decreases, the shear stress begins to increase. As the shear stress approaches some critical level and endothelial cells begin to repopulate the area, NO production occurs, inhibiting further growth of the lesion. The artery wall's stimulatory and inhibitory factors once again become balanced and the system returns to an equilibrium that more closely resembles the quiescent artery wall.

As we know, this is not the end of the story. Many lesions continue to grow, ultimately causing significant compromise of the lumen. Most probably, these advanced lesions result from a persistent imbalance of the growth and inhibitory factors in favor of continued lesion growth. As an example, endothelial regrowth in an injured area might not be complete, resulting in the absence of inhibitory signals. It should be noted, however, that endothelial cells also have the ability to produce stimulatory growth factors. This suggests that their role in lesion formation is variable depending upon their local environment. Additionally, the lesion may create focal turbulence in the flowstream, resulting in persistent growth factor stimulation via the previously mentioned mechanoreceptors. In humans, atherogenic risk factors also contribute to altered healing after injury.

As has been noted before, there is an inflammatory response after injury. The role of leukocytes in lesion formation is not entirely clear. It is known, however, that T lymphocytes are a major component of human atherosclerotic plaque.[125] T lymphocytes are seen in the rat carotid artery injury model. The most significant evidence that they play a role here is the fact that they express γ–interferon, a known inhibitor of SMC growth. Most of the nondividing SMCs seen in the rat intima express the class II major histocompatibility antigen Ia, which is known to be induced only by γ–interferon.[126] This raises the possibility that other cytokines, including interleukin-1, might be active in the wall.

Atherosclerotic Artery Injury

The arteries of cholesterol-fed rabbits and larger species develop atherosclerosis. To accelerate the atherosclerotic process and generate lesions that resemble advanced human disease, investigators have combined cholesterol feeding with balloon injury. In the rabbit, these lesions cause stenosis and become restenotic after a second injury (Gruntzig angioplasty). Unfortunately, these lesions are distinct from human lesions, typically consisting of a concentric foam cell infiltration of the intima and media.

Lesions produced in nonhuman primate models more closely resemble those of humans.[127,128] These animals first develop a fatty streak with infiltrates of lipid-filled macrophages and later proceed to develop intermediate and advanced lesions similar to those seen in humans. Balloon injury of diseased, but not stenotic, iliac arteries in hypercholesterolemic monkeys demonstrate a repair response involving intimal hyperplasia, recoil, and remodelling.[129] These three mechanisms are felt to form the basis of the restenotic pathway in humans. While this model is not characterized by a high degree of stenosis or restenosis, the basic mechanisms resemble the known human mechanisms more closely than those seen in other animal models.[12] This model has been used especially to characterize remodeling, the process by which the arterial lumen size is preserved by vessel dilation during atheroma formation.

Grafts

Vein

Autologous vein is the most widely used conduit in both coronary and peripheral bypass surgery. Vein grafts develop intimal hyperplasia upon exposure to the arterial circulation.[130] During reconstruction, vigorous distention of a vein graft already in spasm or passage of a valvulotome damages the endothelium and the graft wall. However, these defects are relatively minor and are repaired within a few days.[131] Restenosis due to intimal hyperplasia occurs in about 10% of peripheral vein grafts and usually during the time period 6-24 months after reconstruction. Intimal thickening is most pronounced at anastomoses, valve cusps, and clamp injury sites.[132] It is also known to occur in vein grafts placed using the in situ technique, despite the fact that this technique is thought to be less traumatic to the vessel.[133]

Preexisting venous disease might account for some degree of lesion formation at nontraumatized sites.[134,135] At later times, vein grafts fail due to the development of frank atherosclerotic lesions. This is particularly prevalent in the aortocoronary bypass grafts.[136] It is noteworthy that when the internal mammary artery, a conduit which requires no adaptation to the arterial circulation, is used for coronary grafting, a much lower failure rate occurs.[7] Renewed interest also exists in using the radial artery as a coronary artery bypass conduit in hopes of achieving similar results. Previously, its propensity to spasm and the increased likelihood of subclinical atheroma discouraged its use. Recent studies seem to indicate that if appropriate intraoperative steps are taken to inhibit radial artery vasoreactivity, long term patency is excellent.[137] The improved success achieved with arterial conduits suggests that the adaptive process that occurs in vein grafts might make them more susceptible to lesion formation.

Regardless of the actual technique employed (in situ or reversed), vein graft injury undoubtedly occurs during reconstruction, even in the best of hands. The immediate, histologic effects of this injury do not differ significantly from that of arterial injury. Several differences have, however, been observed despite this similar starting point. Re-endothelialization is fast and complete in injured veins.[138] Additionally, SMC proliferation appears to take place even after endothelial coverage is restored. This is in contrast to the artery, where endothelial coverage appears to inhibit intimal SMC proliferation.[28] The time course of wall thickening differs as well. Maximal arterial wall intima formation occurs at 2 weeks. Vein graft thickening continues for up to 12 weeks.[138] What is responsible for these differences?

One apparent difference is that vein graft endothelium appears to possess altered physiologic properties from that of the arterial endothelium. Vein graft endothelium has impaired vasomotor properties[139] and increased permeability.[140] In addition, the arterial circulation exposes the thin venous wall to a continuous type I hemodynamic injury. While not as dramatic as arterial balloon dilation, this injury provides a persistent stimulus for wall thickening. When the vein dilates immediately upon exposure to the high pressure arterial circulation, two phenomena occur. First, the wall of the vein is exposed to a dramatically higher shear stress. Shear stress responsive elements present on the endothelial surface are thought to play a role in the activation of certain stimulatory pathways. The ultimate result is SMC proliferation and migration toward the lumen, possibly through some of the same mechanisms that have been characterized in the rat injury model. Second, the increased luminal blood pressure has been shown to invoke medial thickening, primarily through a response to increased wall stress.[141,142] It is not yet clear which of these mechanisms is primarily responsible for wall thickening in vein grafts. What is clear, however, is that hemodynamic factors play an important role in vein graft patency.[14]

Prosthetic

The prosthetic graft is a man-made, acellular, fibrous scaffolding upon which the body constructs a modified vessel wall. The anastomoses appear to be the areas of maximal intimal hyperplasia as a result of surgical trauma and the presence of flow disturbance. It is thought that human prosthetic grafts heal via two main mechanisms, capillary ingrowth through the graft wall, depending upon the characteristics of the graft, and growth along the luminal surface from each anastomosis.[143] New evidence in a canine model supports fallout endothelialization from the blood stream as another possible mode of graft healing.[144] No current evidence exists that prosthetic grafts inserted into the human circulation are able to develop an endothelialized intima along the entire flow surface. Rather, endothelial cells manage to populate the lumen in just the few centimeters near the anastomoses.[145] The remainder of the graft is lined by thrombus containing fibrin, platelets, and leukocytes.

In our experience with prosthetic PTFE grafts placed in baboons, the development of an endothelial layer is dependent upon porosity.[146] In low porosity grafts (10 and 30 μm internodal distance), luminal endothelial coverage is limited to small areas near the anastomoses. In high porosity grafts, (60 and 90 μm), luminal endothelial coverage is complete. The 90 μm grafts, for unknown reasons, develop areas of endothelial loss. The 60 μm grafts perform optimally regarding endothelial coverage and intimal layer stability. Similar results have been obtained in dogs.[147]

Once an endothelial layer is present, intimal thickening forms. It is perplexing that in the rat carotid injury model, the endothelial layer serves to inhibit intimal thickening, while in the prosthetic grafts, intimal thickening occurs only once endothelium is present. This observation appears to confirm the variable role of endothelial cells in the development of intimal hyperplasia.

Our laboratory has extensively characterized the healing of prosthetic grafts in baboons. Since there is no significant thrombotic response, it is unlikely that the growth factors responsible for intimal formation are derived from platelets. Endothelial cells, however, can produce growth factors, among them, PDGF. Golden observed that healing aortoiliac PTFE grafts removed after 2, 8, and 12 weeks and perfused ex vivo released more mitogenic factors than control arteries.[148] This activity was blocked by an antibody to PDGF. Furthermore, PDGF-A mRNA and protein levels were detectable in the graft intima by both Northern analysis and in situ hybridization. SMC proliferation was seen by thymidine labeling in the same region (inner third of the intima) as PDGF mRNA expression. PDGF-B was nearly undetectable.[149]

As discussed earlier, flow-related effects are seen in vein graft healing. Studies have also demonstrated flow-dependent formation of intima in PTFE grafts in baboons.[150] Grafts placed in the aorto-iliac position under high flow conditions created by placement of a distal fistula form smaller intimal layers than those that heal under normal flow. If normal flow is returned to the graft previously allowed to heal during high flow, the intima undergoes a vigorous thickening. This "flow switch" model has been used in an attempt to identify the stimuli responsible for intimal thickening in the PTFE graft in primates.

Four days after flow switch, PDGF-A mRNA and protein levels are significantly increased.[149] Levels of PDGF-B ligand do not appear to change, while mRNA levels for both

the α and β receptor are increased, but not to a significant level. We have recently completed a study using monoclonal human/mouse chimeric antibodies to both the PDGFR-α and -β receptor in this model. The α receptor antibody had no effect, possibly because circulating serum concentrations did not achieve desirable levels. Adequate levels of the β receptor antibody were achieved and the intimal thickening normally observed after "flow switch" was significantly inhibited in this group of animals (unpublished results). This lends further credence to the theory that PDGF-BB and the β receptor play a significant role in intimal development. It is unclear, however, why the PDGF-B ligand has not been detectable at higher levels in the developing intimal lesion. One possible explanation is that it is being produced primarily by the endothelial cells in small but sufficient quantities and serves mainly as a powerful chemoattractant to attract SMCs towards the lumen. While other factors may participate in the development of intimal hyperplasia in PTFE grafts, we feel that the flow-related effects and the resultant production of PDGF and NO play significant roles. Further studies are needed to better characterize this relationship.

Summary

Vascular injury can induce intimal hyperplasia. The ultimate response depends upon the severity of the injury and the change in the overall balance of stimulatory and inhibitory factors at the site of injury. Based upon animal models, the essential components of this exuberant healing response are SMC proliferation, SMC migration, and extracellular matrix deposition. SMC proliferation after injury is predominantly stimulated by bFGF released mostly from damaged cells but also from the vessel wall matrix. PDGF-BB, deposited at the site of injury by platelets and released by cells in the vessel wall, serves as the primary stimulus for SMC migration. Release of SMCs from their surrounding matrix is accomplished by plasmin and MMPs. Cellular adhesion receptors or integrins are also involved in this process. Control of matrix production is not yet as well defined. In addition to causing the release and production of stimulatory factors, vascular injury also transiently reduces the availability of important inhibitory factors such as NO. Intimal hyperplasia occurring in atherosclerotic arteries, vein grafts, and prosthetic grafts is not as well understood as in the rat carotid artery injury model, although similarities in the basic pathophysiology most likely exist. The challenge for the future is to further define the human response in a systematic manner and to successfully apply this knowledge towards improving the effectiveness of our vascular interventions.

References
  1. Topol EJ, Leya F, Pinkerton CA et al. A comparison of directional atherectomy with coronary angioplasty in patients with coronary artery disease. New Engl J Med 1993; 329:221-27.
  2. Mills JL, Fujitani RM, Taylor SM. The characteristics and anatomic distribution of lesions that cause reversed vein graft failure: A five year prospective study. J Vasc Surg 1993; 17:195-204.

3. Lytle BW, Loop FD, Cosgrove DM et al. Long-term (5 to 12 years) serial studies of internal mammary artery and saphenous vein coronary bypass grafts. J Thorac Cardiovasc Surg 1985; 89:248-258.

4. Kraiss LW, Clowes AW. Response of the arterial wall to injury and intimal hyperplasia. In: Sidawy AN, Sumpio BE, DePalma RG, eds. The Basic Science of Vascular Disease. Armonk, NY: Futura Publishing Company, Inc.;1997:289-317.

5. Holmes DR, Vliestra RE, Smith HC et al. Restenosis after percutaneous transluminal coronary angioplasty (PTCA): A report from the PTCA Registry of the National Heart, Lung, and Blood Institute. Am J Cardiol 1984; 53:77C.

6. Fanelli C, Aronoff R. Restenosis following coronary angioplasty. Am Heart J 1990; 119:357-68.

7. Grondin CM, Campeau L, Lesperance J et al. Comparison of late changes in internal mammary artery and saphenous vein grafts in two consecutive series of patients 10 years after operation. Circulation 1984; 70:1208-12.

8. Campeau L, Enjalbert M, Lesperance J et al. The relation of risk factors to the development of atherosclerosis in saphenous-vein bypass grafts and the progression of disease in the native circulation. N Engl J Med 1984; 311:1329-32.

9. Veith FJ, Gupta SK, Ascer E et al. Six-year prospective multicenter randomized comparison of autologous saphenous vein and expanded polytetrafluoroethylene grafts in infrainguinal arterial reconstructions. J Vasc Surg 1986; 3:104-114.

10. Tullis MJ, Zierler RE, Glickerman DJ et al. Results of percutaneous transluminal angioplasty for atherosclerotic renal artery stenosis: A follow-up study with duplex ultrasonography. J Vasc Surg 1977; 25:46-54.

11. Healy DA, Clowes AW, Zierler RE et al. Immediate and long-term results of carotid endarterectomy. Stroke 1989; 20:1138-1142.

12. Clagett GP. Morphogenesis and clinicopathologic characteristics of recurrent carotid disease. J Vasc Surg 1986; 3:10-23.

13. Das MB, Hertzer NR, Ratliff NB et al. Recurrent carotid stenosis: A five-year series of 65 reoperations. Ann Surg 1985; 202:28-35.

14. Davies MG, Hagen P-O. Pathophysiology of vein graft failure: A review. Eur J Vasc Endovasc Surg 1995; 9:7-18.

15. Becker GJ. Intravascular stents. General principles and status of lower-extremity arterial applications. Circulation 1991; 83:I122-36.

16. Mintz GS, Popma JJ, Hong MK et al. Intravascular ultrasound to discern device-specific effects and mechanisms of restenosis. Am J Cardiol 1996; 78:18-22.

17. Bond MG, Adams MR, Bullock BC. Complicating factors in evaluating coronary artery atherosclerotic coronary arteries. Artery 1981; 9:21-29.

18. Glagov S, Weisenberg E, Zarins CK et al. Compensatory enlargement of human atherosclerotic coronary arteries. N Engl J Med 1987; 316:1371-75.

19. Kakuta T, Currier JW, Haudenschild CC et al. Differences in compensatory vessel enlargement, not intimal formation, account for restenosis after angioplasty in the hypercholesterolemic rabbit model. Circulation 1994; 89:2809-15.

20. Popma JJ, Califf RM, Topol EJ. Clinical trials of restenosis after coronary angioplasty. Circulation 1991; 84:1426-36.

21. MARCATOR Study Group. Does the new angiotensin converting enzyme inhibitor cilazapril prevent restenosis after percutaneous transluminal coronary angioplasty? Results of the MARCATOR study: A multicenter, randomized, double-blind placebo-controlled trial. Circulation 1992; 86:100-10.

22. Kenagy RD, Vergel S, Mattsson E et al. The role of plasminogen, plasminogen activators, and matrix metalloproteinases in primate arterial smooth muscle cell migration. Arterioscler Thromb Vasc Biol 1996; 16:1373-82.

23. Schwartz SM, deBlois D, O'Brien ERM. The intima: Soil for atherosclerosis and restenosis. Circ Res 1995; 77:445-465.

24. Fingerle J, Au YPT, Clowes et al. Author: Please provide initials for author Clowes. Intimal lesion formation in rat carotid arteries after endothelial denudation in absence of medial injury. Arteriosclerosis 1990; 1082-87.

25. Sarembock IJ, LaVeau PJ, Sigal SL et al. Influence of inflation pressure and balloon size on the development of intimal hyperplasia after balloon angioplasty: A study in the atherosclerotic rabbit. Circulation 1989; 80:1029-40.

26. Schwartz RS, Huber KC, Murphy JG et al. Restenosis and the proportional neointimal response to coronary artery injury: Results in a porcine model. J Am Coll Cardiol 1992; 19:267-74.

27. Clowes AW, Clowes MM, Fingerle J et al. Regulation of smooth muscle cell growth in injured artery. J Cardiovasc Pharmacol 1989; 14:S12-15.

28. Clowes AW, Reidy MA, Clowes MM. Kinetics of cellular proliferation after arterial injury. I. Smooth muscle growth in the absence of endothelium. Lab Invest 1983; 49:327-33.

29. Majesky MW, Schwartz SM, Clowes AW et al. Heparin regulates smooth muscle S phase entry in the injured rat carotid artery. Circ Res 1987; 61:296-300.

30. Clowes AW, Schwartz SM. Significance of quiescent smooth muscle migration in the injured rat carotid artery. Circ Res 1985; 56:139-145.

31. Ross R, Glomset JA. The pathogenesis of atherosclerosis. N Engl J Med 1976; 295:369-77.

32. Ross R, Glomset JA. The pathogenesis of atherosclerosis. N Engl J Med 1976; 295:420-25.

33. Friedman RJ, Stemerman MB, Wenz B et al. The effect of thrombocytopenia on experimental atherosclerotic lesion formation in rabbits. Smooth muscle cell proliferation and re-endothelialization. J Clin Invest 1977; 60:1191-201.

34. Ross R, Glomset J, Kariya B et al. A platelet-dependent serum factor that stimulates the proliferation of arterial smooth muscle cells in vitro. Proc Natl Acad Sci USA 1974; 71:1207-10.

35. Fingerle J, Johnson R, Clowes AW et al. Role of platelets in smooth muscle cell migration and proliferation after vascular injury in rat carotid artery. Proc Natl Acad Sci USA 1989; 86:8412-16.

36. Lindner V, Lappi DA, Baird A et al. Role of basic fibroblast growth factor in vascular lesion formation. Circ Res 1991; 68:106-13.

37. Lindner V, Reidy MA. Proliferation of smooth muscle cells after vascular injury is inhibited by an antibody against basic fibroblast growth factor. Proc Natl Acad Sci USA 1991; 88:3739-43.

38. Lindner V, Reidy MA. Expression of basic fibroblast growth factor and its receptor by smooth muscle cells and endothelium in injured rat arteries: An en face study. Circ Res 1993; 73:589-95.

39. D'Amore PA. Modes of FGF release in vivo and in vitro. Canc Metastasis Rev 1990; 9:227-38.

40. Mignatti P, Morimoto T, Rifkin DB. Basic fibroblast growth factor, a protein devoid of secretory signal sequence, is released by cells via a pathway independent of the endoplasmic reticulum-Golgi complex. J Cell Physiol 1992; 151:81-93.

41. Thompson RW, Whalen GF, Saunders KB et al. Heparin-mediated release of fibroblast growth factor-like activity into the circulation of rabbits. Growth Factors 1990; 3:221-29.

42. Lindner V, Olson NE, Clowes AW et al. Inhibition of smooth muscle cell proliferation in injured rat arteries. Interaction of heparin with basic fibroblast growth factor. J Clin Invest 1992; 90:2044-49.

43. Lindner V, Majack RA, Reidy MA. Basic fibroblast growth factor stimulates endothelial regrowth and proliferation in denuded arteries. J Clin Invest 1990; 85; 2004-8.

44. Campbell DJ. Circulating and tissue angiotensin systems. J Clin Invest 1987; 79:1-6.

45. Campbell-Boswell M, Robertson AL Jr. Effects of angiotensin ii and vasopressin on human smooth muscle cells in vitro. Exp Mol Pathol 1981; 35:265-76.

46. Battegay EJ, Raines EW, Seifert RA et al. TGF-β induces bimodal proliferation of connective tissue cells via complex control of an autocrine PDGF loop. Cell 1990; 63:515-24.

47. Naftilan AJ, Pratt RE, Dzau VJ. Induction of platelet-derived growth factor A-chain and c-myc gene expression by angiotensin ii in cultured rat vascular smooth muscle cells. J Clin Invest 1989; 83:1419-24.

48. Naftilan AJ, Pratt RE, Eldridge CS et al. Angiotensin ii induces c-fos expression in smooth muscle via transcriptional control. Hypertension 1989; 13:706-11.

49. Prescott MF, Webb RL, Reidy MA. Angiotensin-converting enzyme inhibitor versus angiotensin ii, AT1 receptor antagonist: Effects on smooth muscle cell migration and proliferation after balloon catheter injury. Am J Pathol 1991; 139:1291-96.

50. Daemen MJ, Lombardi DM, Bosman FT et al. Angiotensin ii induces smooth muscle cell proliferation in the normal and injured rat arterial wall. Circ Res 1991; 68:450-56.

51. Laporte S, Escher E. Neointima formation after vascular injury is angiotensin ii mediated. Biochem Biophys Res Comm 1992; 187:1510-16.

52. Majesky MW, Reidy MA, Bowen-Pope DF et al. PDGF ligand and receptor gene expression during repair of arterial injury. J Cell Biol 1990; 111:2149-58.

53. Sarembock IJ, Gertz SD, Gimple LW et al. Effectiveness of recombinant desulphatohirudin in reducing restenosis after balloon angioplasty of atherosclerotic femoral arteries in rabbits. Circulation 1991; 84:232-43.

54. Douglas SA, Louden C, Vickery-Clark LM et al. A role for endogenous endothelin-1 in neointimal formation after rat carotid artery balloon angioplasty. Protective effects of the novel nonpeptide endothelin receptor antagonist SB 209670. Circ Res 1994; 75:190-97.

55. Trachtenberg JD, Sun S, Choi ET et al. Effect of endothelin-1 infusion on the development of intimal hyperplasia after balloon catheter injury. J Cardiovasc Pharmacol 1993; 22:S355-39.

56. Takuwa Y, Yanagisawa M, Takuwa N et al. Endothelin, its diverse biological activities and mechanisms of action. Prog Growth Factor Res 1989; 1:195-206.

57. Bornfeldt KE, Arnqvist HJ, Capron L. In vivo proliferation of rat vascular smooth muscle in relation to diabetes mellitus insulin-like growth factor I and insulin. Diabetologia 1992; 35:104-8.

58. Jackson CL, Schwartz SM. Pharmacology of smooth muscle cell replication. Hypertension 1992; 20:713-36.

59. Thyberg J, Blomgren K, Hedin U et al. Phenotypic modulation of smooth muscle cells during the formation of neointimal thickenings in the rat carotid artery after balloon injury: An electronic-microscopic and stereological study. Cell Tissue Res 1995; 281:421-428.

60. Raines EW, Bowen-Pope DF, Ross R. Platelet-derived growth factor. In: Sporn MB, Roberts AB, eds. Handbook of Experimental Pharmacology: Peptide Growth Factors. New York: Springer-Verlag, Inc; 1990:173-189.

61. Koyama N, Hart CE, Clowes AW. Different functions of the platelet-derived growth factor-α and -β receptors for the migration and proliferation of cultured baboon smooth muscle cells. Circ Res 1994; 75:682-91.

62. Hart CE, Clowes AW. Platelet-derived growth factor and arterial response to injury. Circulation 1997; 95:555-56.

63. Ferns GAA, Raines EW, Sprugel KH. Inhibition of neointimal smooth muscle accumulation after angioplasty by an antibody to PDGF. Science 1991; 253:1129-1132.

64. Jawien A, Bowen-Pope DF, Lindner V et al. Platelet-derived growth factor promotes smooth muscle migration and intimal thickening in a rat model of balloon angioplasty. J Clin Invest 1992; 89:507-11.

65. Sirois MG, Simons M, Edelman ER. Antisense oligonucleotide inhibition of PDGF-β receptor subunit expression directs suppression of intimal thickening. Circulation 1997; 95:669-676.

66. Murry CE, Bartosek T, Giachelli CM et al. Platelet-derived growth factor-A mRNA expression in fetal, normal adult, and atherosclerotic human aortas. Circulation 1996; 93:1095-1106.

67. Barres BA, Hart IK, Coles HSR. Cell death in the oligodendrocyte lineage. J Neurobiol 1992; 23:1221-1230.

68. Bennett MR, Evan GI, Schwartz SM. Apoptosis of human vascular smooth muscle cells derived from normal vessels and coronary atherosclerotic plaques. J Clin Invest 1995; 95:2266-74.

69. Harrington EA, Bennett MR, Fanidi A. c-myc-induced apoptosis in fibroblasts is inhibited by specific cytokines. EMBO J 1994; 13:3286-95.

70. Wakefield TW. Coagulation and disorders of hemostasis. In: Sidawy AN, Sumpio BE, DePalma RG, eds. The Basic Science of Vascular Disease. Armonk, NY Futura Publishing Company, Inc.;1997:289-317.

71. Clowes AW, Clowes MM, Au YPT et al. Smooth muscle cells express urokinase during mitogenesis and tissue-type plasminogen activator during migration in injured rat carotid artery. Circ Res 1990; 67:61-7.

72. Zempo N, Kenagy RD, Au YPT et al. Matrix metalloproteinases of vascular wall cells are increased in balloon-injured rat carotid artery. J Vasc Surg 1994; 20:209-17.

73. Reidy MA, Irvin C, Lindner V. Migration of arterial wall cells. Expression of plasminogen activators and inhibitors in injured rat arteries. Circ Res 1996; 78:405-14.

74. Bendeck MP, Zempo N, Clowes AW et al. Smooth muscle cell migration and matrix metalloproteinase expression after arterial injury in the rat. Circ Res 1994; 75:539-45.

75. Carmeliet P, Stassen JM, De Mol M et al. Arterial neointima formation after trauma in mice with inactivation of the tPA, uPA, or PAI-1 genes. Fibrinolysis 1994; 8:280a.

76. Matrisian LM. Metalloproteinases and their inhibitor in matrix remodeling. Trends in Genet 1990; 6(4):121-25.

77. HE CS, Wilhelm SM, Pentland AP. Tissue cooperation in a proteolytic cascade activating human interstitial collagenase. Proc Natl Acad Sci USA 1989; 86:2632-36.

78. Forough R, Koyama N, Hasentstab D et al. Overexpression of tissue inhibitor of matrix metalloproteinase-1 inhibits vascular smooth muscle cell functions in vitro and in vivo. Circ Res 1996; 79:812-20.

79. Choi ET, Engel L, Callow AD et al. Inhibition of neointimal hyperplasia by blocking $\alpha_v\beta_3$ integrin with a small peptide antagonist GpenGRGDSPCA. J Vasc Surg 1994; 19:125-34.

80. Matsuno H, Hoylaerts MF, Vermylen J et al. Inhibition of integrin function prevents restenosis following vascular injury. Nippon Yakurigaku Zasshi 1995; 106:143-55.

81. The EPIC Investigation. Use of a monoclonal antibody directed against the platelet glycoprotein IIb/IIIa receptor in high-risk coronary angioplasty. New Engl J Med 1994; 330:956-61.

82. Giachelli CM, Liaw L, Murry CE et al. Osteopontin expression in cardiovascular diseases. Ann N Y Acad Sci 1995; 760:109-26.

83. Wolf YG, Rasmussen LM, Ruoslahti E. Antibodies against transformtin growth factor-β-1 suppress intimal hyperplasia in a rat model. J Clin Invest 1994; 93:1172-78.

84. Hedin U, Holm J, Hansson GK. Induction of tenascin in rat arterial injury; relationship to altered smooth muscle cell phenotype. Am J Pathol 1991; 139:649-56.

85. Majesky MW. Neointima formation after acute vascular injury. Role of counteradhesive extracellular matrix proteins, Texas Heart Inst J 1994, 21:78-85.

86. Hynes RO. Integrins: Versatility, modulation, and signaling in cell adhesion. Cell 1992; 69:11-25.

87. Hoshiga M, Alpers CE, Smith LL et al. $\alpha_v\beta_3$ integrin expression in normal and atherosclerotic artery. Circ Res 1995; 77:1129-35.

88. Garratt KN, Edwards WD, Kaufmann UP et al. Differential histopathology of primary atherosclerotic and restenotic lesions in coronary arteries and saphenous vein bypass grafts: Analysis of tissue obtained from 73 patients by directional atherectomy. J Am Coll Cardiol 1991; 17:442-48.

89. Clowes AW. Pathologic intimal hyperplasia as a response to vascular injury and reconstruction. In: Rutherford RB, ed. Vascular Surgery. 4th Edition. Philadelphia: W.B. Saunders, 1995:285-95.

90. Raines EW, Dower SK, Ross R. Interleukin-1 mitogenic activity for fibroblasts and smooth muscle cells is due to PDGF-AA. Science 1989; 243:393-96.

91. Olson NE, Chao S, Lindner V et al. Intimal smooth muscle cell proliferation after balloon catheter injury: The role of basic fibroblast growth factor. Am J Pathol 1992; 140:1017-23.

92. Lindner V, Reidy MA. Platelet-derived growth factor ligand and receptor expression by large vessel endothelium in vivo. Am J Pathol 1995; 146:1488-97.

93. Powell, JS, Clozel JP, Muller RKM et al. Inhibitors of angiotensin-converting enzyme prevent myointimal proliferation after vascular injury. Science 1989; 245:186-88.

94. Faxon DP. Effect of high dose angiotensin-converting enzyme inhibition on restenosis: Final results of the MARCATOR Study, a multicenter, double-blind, placebo-controlled trial of cilazapril. The Multicenter American Research Trial With Cilazapril After Angioplasty to Prevent Transluminal Coronary Obstruction and Restenosis (MARCATOR) Study Group. J Am Coll Cardiol 1995; 25:362-69.

95. Heyndricks GR, MARCATOR. Angiotensin-converting enzyme inhibitor in a human model of restenosis. Basic Res Cardiol 1993; 88:169-82.

96. Cercek B, Fishbein MC, Forrester JS et al. Induction of insulin-like growth factor-β messenger RNA in rat aorta after balloon denudation. Circ Res 1990; 66:1755-60.

97. Majesky MW, Lindner V, Twardzik DR et al. Angiotensin ii induces smooth muscle cell proliferation in the normal and injured rat arterial wall. Circ Res 1991; 88:904-10.

98. Clowes AW, Reidy MA, Clowes MM. Mechanisms of stenosis after arterial injury. Lab Invest 1983; 49:208-15.

99. Reidy MA. A reassessment of endothelial injury and arterial lesion formation. Lab Invest 1985; 53:513-20.

100. Schwartz SM, Haudenschild CC, Eddy EM. Endothelial regeneration. I. Quantitative analysis of endothelial regeneration in rat aortic intima. Lab Invest 1978; 38:568-80.

101. Castellot JJ Jr, Addonizio ML, Rosenberg R et al. Cultured endothelial cells produce a heparin-like inhibitor of smooth muscle cell growth. J Cell Biol 1981; 90:372-79.

102. Clowes AW, Karnovsky NJ. Suppression by heparin of smooth muscle cell proliferation in injured arteries. Nature 1977; 265:625-26.

103. Clowes AW, Clowes MM. Kinetics of cellular proliferation after arterial injury. IV. Heparin inhibits rat smooth muscle mitogenesis and migration. Circ Res 1986; 58:839-45.

104 Au YP, Montgomery KF, Clowes AW. Heparin inhibits collagenase gene expression mediated by phorbol ester-responsive element in primate arterial smooth muscle cells. Circ Res 1992; 70:1062-69.

105. Lloyd-Jones DM, Bloch KD. The vascular biology of nitric oxide and its role in atherogenesis. Annu Rev Med 1996; 47:365-75.

106. Garg UC, Hassid A. Nitric oxide-generating vasodilators and 8-bromo-cyclic guanosine monophosphate inhibit mitogenesis and proliferation of cultured rat vascular smooth muscle cells. J Clin Invest;38:1774-77.

107. Sarkar R, Meinberg EG, Stanley JC et al. Nitric oxide inhibits the migration of cultured vascular smooth muscle cells. Circ Res 1996; 78:225-30.

108. McNamara DB, Bedi B, Aurora H et al. L-arginine inhibits balloon catheter-induced intimal hyperplasia. Biochem Biophys Res Commun 1993; 193:291-96.

109. Taguchi J, Junichi A, Takuwa Y et al. L-arginine inhibits neointimal formation following balloon injury. Life Sci 1993; 53:387-92.

110. von der Leyen HE, Gibbons GH, Morishita R et al. Gene therapy inhibiting neointimal vascular lesion: In vivo transfer of endothelial cell nitric oxide synthase gene. Proc Natl Acad Sci USA 1995; 92:1137-1141.

111. Tzeng E, Shears LL II, Robbins PD et al. Vascular gene transfer of the human inducible nitric oxide synthase: Characterization of activity and effects on myointimal hyperplasia. Mol Med 1996; 2:211-25.

112. Lee JS, Adrie C, Jacob HJ et al. Chronic inhalation of nitric oxide inhibits neointimal formation after balloon-induced arterial injury. Circ Res 1996; 78:337-342.

113. Marks DS, Vita JA, Folts JD et al. Inhibition of neointimal proliferation in rabbits after vascular injury by a single treatment with a protein adduct of nitric oxide. J Clin Invest 1995; 96:2630-38.

114. Myers PR, Minor Jr RL, Guerra R et al. Vasorelaxant properties of the endothelium-derived relaxing factor more closely resembles S-nitrosocysteine than nitric oxide. Nature 1990; 345:161-163.

115. Kubes P, Suzuki M, Granger DN. Nitric oxide: and endogenous modulator of leukocyte adhesion. Proc Natl Acad Sci USA 1991; 88:4651-4655.

116. Kubes P, Granger DN. Nitric oxide modulates microvascular permeability. Am J Physiol 1993; 262:H611-H615.

117. Hansson GK, Geng Y, Holm J. Arterial smooth muscle cells express nitric oxide synthase in response to endothelial injury. J Exp Med 1994; 180:733-38.

117. Pritchard KA Jr, O'Banion MK, Miano JM et al. Induction of cyclooxygenase-2 in rat vascular smooth muscle cells in vitro and in vivo. J Biol Chem 1994; 269:8504-9.

118. Cayatte AJ, Palocino JJ, Horten K et al. Chronic inhibition of nitric oxide production accelerates neointimal formation and impairs endothelial-type function in hypercholesterolemic rabbits. Arterioscler Thromb 1994; 14:753-59.

119. Kohler TR, Jawien A. Flow affects development of intimal hyperplasia after arterial injury in rats. Arterioscler Thromb 1992; 12:963-71.

120. Berk BC, Corson MA, Peterson TE et al. Protein kinases as mediators of fluid shear stress stimulated signal transduction in endothelial cells: A hypothesis for calcium-dependent and calcium-independent events activated by flow. J Biomechanics 1995; 28:1439-50.

121. Corson MA, James NL, Latta SE et al. Phosphorylation of endothelial nitric oxide synthase in response to fluid shear stress. Circ Res 1996; 79:984-91.

122. Nadaud S, Philippe M, Arnal JF et al. Sustained increase in aortic endothelial nitric oxide synthase expression in vivo in a model of chronic high blood flow. Circ Res 1996; 79:857-63.

123. Davies PF, Remuzzi A, Gordon EJ et al. Turbulent fluid shear stress induces vascular endothelial turnover in vitro. Proc Natl Acad Sci USA 1986; 83:2114-17.

124. Libby P, Hansson GK. Involvement of the immune system in human atherogenesis: Current knowledge and unanswered questions. Lab Invest 1991; 64:5-15.

125. Hansson GK, Jonasson L, Holm J et al. Gamma interferon regulates vascular smooth muscle proliferation and Ia expression in vitro and in vivo. Circ Res 1988 63; 712-19.

126. Clarkson TB, Bond MG, Bullock BC et al. A study of atherosclerosis regression in Macaca mulatta, V:
Changes in abdominal aorta and carotid and coronary arteries from animals with atherosclerosis induced for 38 months and then regressed for 24 or 48 months at plasma cholesterol concentrations of 300 or 200 mg/dl. Exp Mol Pathol 1984; 41:96-118.

127. Faggiotto A, Ross R, Harker L. Studies of hypercholesterolemia in the nonhuman primate. I. Changes that lead to fatty streak formation.   Arteriosclerosis 1984; 4:323-340.

128. Geary RL, Williams JK, Golden D et al. Time course of cellular proliferation, intimal hyperplasia, and remodeling following angioplasty in monkeys with established atherosclerosis. A nonhuman primate model of restenosis. Arterioscl Thromb Vasc Biol 1996; 16:34-43.

129. Zwolak RM, Adams MC, Clowes AW. Kinetics of vein graft hyperplasia: Association with tangential stress. J Vasc Surg 1987; 5:126-36.

130. LoGerfo FW, Quist WC, Cantelmo NL et al. Integrity of vein grafts as a function of initial intimal and medial preservation. Circulation 1983; 68:II117-24.

131. Fuchs JC, Mitchener JS III, Hagen P-O. Postoperative changes in autologous vein grafts. Ann Surg 1978; 188:1-15.

132. Bandyk DF, Kaebnick HW, Stewart GW et al. Durability of the in situ saphenous vein arterial bypass. A comparison of primary and secondary patency. J Vasc Surg 1987; 5:256-68.

133. Panetta TF, Marin ML, Veith FJ et al. Unsuspected preexisting saphenous vein disease: An unrecognized cause of vein bypass failure. J Vasc Surg 1992; 15:102-12.

134. Varty K, Allen KE, Bell PRF et al. Infrainguinal vein graft stenosis. Br J Surg 1993; 80:825-33.

135. Spray TL, Roberts WC. Changes in saphenous used as aorto-coronary bypass grafts. Am Heart J; 1977; 94:500-16.

136. Buxton B, Fuller J, Gaer J et al. Curr Opin Cardiol 1996; 11:591-98.

137. Kohler TR, Kirkman TR, Clowes AW. Effect of heparin on adaptation of vein grafts to arterial circulation. Arteriosclerosis 1989; 9:523-28.

138. Luscher TF. Vascular biology of coronary bypass grafts. Coronary Artery Disease 1992; 3:157-65.

139. Cox JL, Chaisson DA, Gotlieb AI. Stranger in a strange land: The pathogenesis of saphenous vein graft stenosis with emphasis on structural and functional differences between veins and arteries. Prog Cardiovasc Dis 1991; 34:45-68.

140. Dobrin PB, Littooy FN, Golan J et al. Mechanical and histologic changes in canine vein grafts. J Surg Res 1988; 14:259-60.

141. Dobrin PB, Litooy FN, Endean ED. Mechanical factors predisposing to intimal hyperplasia and medial thickening in autogenous vein grafts. Surgery 1989; 105:393-400.

142. Clowes AW, Kirkman TR, Reidy MA. Mechanisms of arterial graft healing. Rapid transmural capillary ingrowth provides a source of intimal endothelium and smooth muscle in porous PTFE prostheses. Am J Pathol 1986; 123:220-30.

143. Shi Q, Wu MH, Hayashida N et al. Proof of fallout endothelialization of impervious Dacron grafts in the aorta and inferior vena cava of the dog. J Vasc Surg 1994; 20:546-56.

144. Clowes AW, Kohler T. Graft endothelialization: The role of angiogenic mechanisms. J Vasc Surg 1991; 13:734-36.

145. Golden MA, Hanson SR, Kirkman TR et al. Healing of polytetrafluoroethylene arterial grafts is influenced by graft porosity. J Vasc Surg 1990; 11:838-45.

146. Tsuchida H, Kashyap A, Cameron BL et al. In vivo study of a high-porosity polytetrafluoroethylene graft: Endothelialization, fluid leakage, and the effect of fibrin glue sealing. J Invest Surg 1993; 6:509-18.

147. Golden MA, Au YPT, Kenagy RD et al. Growth factor gene expression by intimal cells in healing polytetrafluoroethylene grafts. J Vasc Surg 1990; 11:580-85.

148. Kraiss LW, Geary RL, Mattsson EJR et al. Acute reductions in blood flow and shear stress induce platelet-derived growth factor-A expression in baboon prosthetic grafts. Circ Res 1996; 79:45-53.

149. Kohler TR, Kirkman TR, Kraiss LW et al. Increased blood flow inhibits neointimal hyperplasia in endothelialized vascular grafts. Circ Res 1991; 69:1557-65.

Taming of Adverse Responses

Prevention of a Hyperplastic Intimal Response

─────────────── CHAPTER 23 ───────────────

Cell Cycle Interruption to Inhibit Intimal Hyperplasia

Michael J. Mann, Ruediger C. Braun-Dullaeus, Victor J. Dzau

Neointimal hyperplasia is the hallmark of occlusive vascular graft disease. It is largely responsible for the primary failures of up to 30% of infrainguinal grafts within two years, and it is believed to form the substrate for the accelerated atherosclerosis that is linked to the failures of 30-50% of coronary bypass grafts.[1-3] Migration and proliferation of medial vascular smooth muscle cells (VSMC) provide the bulk of the neointimal cell mass, and antiproliferative regimens have therefore been sought as a means to curb this process.[4-7] Targeting the molecular machinery that regulates cell cycle progression has proven to be among the most potent of such antiproliferative strategies in experimental models of neointimal disease, as this network of kinases and transcription factors offers a final common pathway to the myriad signaling cascades known to trigger the activation and proliferation of vascular cells.

Recent studies suggest that the cell's ability to enter and progress through the cell cycle at a critical point during the onset of vascular remodeling is an essential element in the pathogenesis of vascular graft disease.[8,9] Data suggest that the activation of quiescent vascular cells results not only in cell division, but also in the abnormal expression of adhesion molecules and cytokines that facilitate cell migration, enhance the inflammatory response and perpetuate a cycle of vascular cell dysfunction. The results of these investigations further indicate that manipulation of cell cycle regulatory events can induce alternative pathways of vessel wall adaptation to the traumatic and hemodynamic stresses associated with bypass grafting. For example, cell cycle arrest has been shown to tip the balance away from neointima formation and toward other, more salutary, pathways of graft remodeling that result in a vessel wall architecture, hemodynamic stability and resistance to accelerated atherosclerosis reminiscent of the native artery.

The process of cell cycle regulation has been dissected in recent years through in vitro studies in numerous cell types. These studies have revealed an intricate system of checks and balances that is initiated upon stimulation of quiescent cells to enter the proliferative cycle of DNA replication and cell division. This system involves the regulation of specialized cell cycle proteins on many levels: the initiation of new mRNA transcription, the translation and accumulation of proteins at or above threshold levels, and the activation or inactivation of these proteins through phosphorylation, dephosphorylation and protein-protein complex formation. Proliferative diseases have been linked to alteration in these patterns of genetic and biochemical regulation of cell biology. The elucidation of these pathways may therefore yield the sophisticated tools necessary for clinicians to overcome pathobiological processes that have until now proven elusive to traditional therapeutic approaches.

The role of cell cycle regulation in neointima formation has been most extensively explored in models of arterial balloon injury. Recently, studies in our laboratory and others have documented analogous events in the development of neointimal hyperplasia in

Tissue Engineering of Prosthetic Vascular Grafts, edited by Peter Zilla and Howard P. Greisler.
©1999 R.G. Landes Company.

autologous vein grafts.[8,10-12] We have therefore developed strategies designed to alter patterns of vascular cell gene expression associated with the onset of this abnormal accumulation of intimal cells. We initially hypothesized that vein graft failures linked to neointima formation and/or accelerated atherosclerosis were the downstream result of phenotypic changes in vascular cells. We subsequently observed that genetic blockade of cell cycle progression during a critical phase of vein graft response to the surgical, hemodynamic and inflammatory insults of grafting results in a shift of graft biology toward a more adaptive remodeling process characterized by medial hypertrophy and stabilization of endothelial function.

The Molecular and Cellular Biology of Neointimal Vascular Graft Disease

Despite progress in the development of artificial vascular prostheses, autologous vein grafts continue to have higher long term patency rates of approximately 70% and 50% at three and five years, respectively.[1,2] Vein graft occlusions, however, have been linked to neointimal hyperplasia, and "activated" VSMC are known to express an array of proteins that can contribute to a pro-atherogenic environment in the graft wall. These upregulated molecules include cytokines such as interleukins -1, -2 and -6, and tumor necrosis factor (TNF), adhesion molecules such as intercellular adhesion molecule-1 (ICAM-1) and chemoattractants such as monocyte chemoattractant protein-1 (MCP-1).[12-15] In addition to midgraft thrombosis, anastomotic stenosis contributes significantly to the failures of artificial graft conduits, and this anastomotic disease is similarly characterized by a neointimal proliferative response stemming from the adjacent artery.[16] Inhibition of neointimal hyperplasia has therefore become a focal point for research aimed at improving the long term success of surgical revascularization (Fig. 23.1).

The molecular and cellular biology of neointimal hyperplasia have been best characterized in animal models of arterial injury that mimic the vessel's response to balloon angioplasty.[17] A primary process of neointimal hyperplasia is the activation of medial VSMC, and their subsequent proliferation and migration across the internal elastic lamina. Numerous factors have been found to stimulate VSMC pro-

liferation in vitro, including basic fibroblast growth factor (bFGF) and platelet derived growth factor (PDGF),[18,19] and these factors have been identified in the vessel wall in vivo in arterial and venous models of neointimal hyperplasia, as well.[20,21] Increased platelet adherence and degranulation and release from injured vascular cells were initially thought to be the primary sources of PDGF and bFGF, respectively, although it is now recognized that vascular cells themselves initiate the autocrine and paracrine production of these factors after arterial injury and vein grafting.[18,19]

Proliferation among medial VSMC has been documented within 24-48 hours after balloon injury, and migration of VSMC across the internal elastic lamina is established by days 3 and 4.[17,22] Early neointimal cells have demonstrated rates of bromo-deoxyuridine incorporation, indicative of DNA synthesis, as high as 50%, and this rapid proliferation establishes approximately 90% of the neointimal cell mass within two weeks of injury.[22] Cell cycle progression and cell division subsequently slows, while further increases in neointimal thickness result primarily from continued extracellular matrix production.[23] In addition to PDGF and bFGF, other factors, such as transformtin growth factor-β (TGF-β), angiotensin II and insulin-like growth factor-1 (IGF-1), are also expressed in the vessel wall after injury, and may play important roles in determining the extent of lesion formation.[24-26]

A dramatic increase in VSMC DNA synthesis has also been documented during the first week after operation in experimental vein grafts.[8,10] In a study of rabbit jugular to carotid interposition grafts, this proliferative rate returned to a low level by postoperative weeks 2-4, by which time a thick, highly cellular neointimal layer had been formed. Zwolack and colleagues further demonstrated that neointimal thickening proceeded over the subsequent 4-8 weeks, primarily via increased extracellular matrix production, and that the neointimal layer then remained morphometrically stable up to 12 months, establishing a pattern of cellular kinetics parallel to those observed after rat carotid balloon injury. Francis et al[27] succeeded in demonstrating the release of PDGF in porcine vein grafts at 1 and 4 weeks after surgery, while Hoch et al[12] established the time course of both TGF-β1 and PDGF-A expression by rat vein graft cells and the relationship of this growth factor expression to

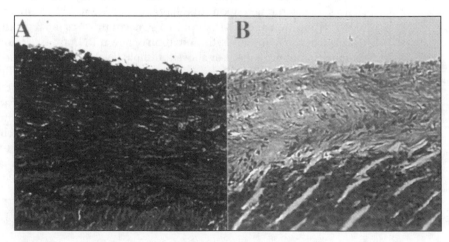

Fig. 23.1. Vascular graft neointimal hyperplasia. Proliferation and migration of medial vascular smooth muscle cells (VSMC) leads to development of a thick layer of abnormal cells on the lumenal aspect of the internal elastic lamina of an experimental vein graft (A), and migration of cells from the adjacent artery leads to a similar VSMC layer on the lumenal aspect of a PTFE graft placed in the rabbit aorta (B).

the development of graft neointimal hyperplasia. Further studies have since documented the elaboration of cytokines such as IL-1β, TNF and MCP-1 in the vein graft wall during the first 1-4 weeks after operation;[14,28] these proteins may play roles in the further "activation" of vascular cells, and may enhance the infiltration of the vessel wall by pro-inflammatory cells.

Neointimal growth also occurs in vascular prostheses made of artificial materials. Ingrowth of endothelial and VSMC from the anastomotic ends of experimental grafts comprised of either Dacron or polytetrafluoroethylene (PTFE) progresses along the length of the graft to varying degrees, depending upon the species and material.[29] Neointimal thickness, however, is always greatest near the anastomosis, and this heightened perianastomotic thickening correlates to the clinical phenomenon of anastomotic stenosis in artificial grafts.[30] Increased porosity of the graft material also allows direct ingrowth of capillaries through the graft wall in animal models, with subsequent acceleration of neointima formation in the grafts' midportions,[31] As in the injured artery and the healing vein graft, prosthetic vascular graft neointima formation tends to reach a point of stable equilibrium, after which cellular proliferation ceases to contribute to neointimal thickness.[30] Several animal models, including dog and baboon, exhibit complete coverage of Dacron and high porosity PTFE grafts with neointimal and endothelial linings, although neointima formation in human grafts is generally limited to the perianastomotic region.[29] Clowes and associates have documented the production of both PDGF and TGF-β in the walls of prosthetic vascular grafts, by both inflammatory and proliferating vascular cells.[32]

A wide array of growth factors, such as PDGF, bFGF and IGF, have all been shown to stimulate the VSMC proliferation that is a necessary part of neointimal hyperplasia. Strategies to inhibit this proliferative process via blockade of any one or two of these redundant molecular targets are therefore likely to be unsuccessful. There is a final common pathway, however, onto which these various proliferative stimuli and their secondary messengers converge: the molecular and genetic machinery controlling entry into and progression through the cell cycle (Fig. 23.2). Scientists now have a growing understanding of the complex regulation of the movement of cells from quiescence (G_0-phase) into the phases of:

1. Preparation for chromosomal duplication (G_1-phase);
2. DNA synthesis (S-phase);
3. Preparation for cell division (G_2-phase); and finally
4. Mitosis (M-phase), and opportunities for targeted intervention in these processes have therefore become available.

Cell Cycle Progression: A Careful Orchestration

The precision with which cellular growth and proliferation are governed during normal development and healing has necessitated the development of an elaborate system of checkpoints and regulatory events in the molecular control of cell cycle progression (Fig. 23.3). Although a number of details have been found to vary slightly in different cell types and in different species, a remarkably conserved pattern of gene upregulation and enzymatic activity has been observed during the movement of cells through the various stages of new DNA synthesis and cellular division. In this context, several classes of molecules have been described as playing well defined roles in the management of cell cycle progression, and studies have confirmed many of these roles in VSMC in vitro.

One of the first responses of cells to stimulation by growth factors or other mitogens is the upregulated expression of a series of protooncogenes, also known as immediate early genes. Among these genes, *c-fos* and *c-myc* are known to be important not only for entry of cells into the

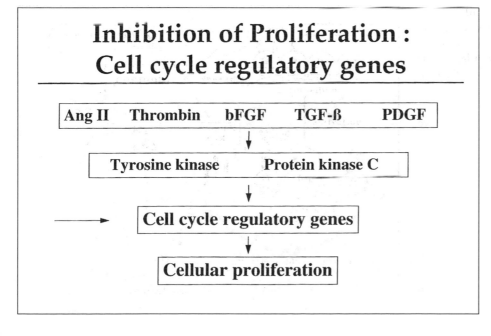

Fig. 23.2. Multiple growth factors and hormones are known to stimulate VSMC proliferation both in vitro and in vivo. Their multiple secondary messenger systems, however, converge on a final common pathway: the cell cycle regulatory machinery and the coordinated upregulation of cell cycle regulatory genes.

cell cycle, but for successful progression through all four stages as well.[33,34] The protein products of these genes act as transcription factors that increase the expression of other molecules (in particular the cyclin-dependent kinases described below) whose activities are required to trigger cell cycle switches. The product of another protooncogene, *c-myb*, acts similarly to upregulate cell cycle proteins, whereas the *ras* gene encodes a membrane-bound, guanine nucleotide-binding protein that couples signals from surface tyrosine kinase growth factor receptors to cytoplasmic secondary messenger systems.[35]

The cyclin-dependent kinases (Cdks) form another class of molecules that directly regulate the progression of cells through the cell cycle. Other proteins, termed cyclins, act as cofactors for the Cdks, and the binding of specific cyclins to specific Cdks leads to formation of active holoenzymes. Both cyclins and Cdks are expressed only at low levels in quiescent cells, and are upregulated at various intervals after stimulation of the cell into cell cycle progression. Once upregulated, Cdk expression remains high as long as the cell continues to progress through rounds of the cell cycle, whereas cyclin protein levels fluctuate at different points through cell cycle progression. Early in the G_1-phase, cyclin D and Cdk4 are upregulated and form a complex together with another cell cycle regulatory protein, proliferating cell nuclear antigen (PCNA). Cdk4 further requires phosphorylation by a Cdk activating kinase (CAK) to complete its activation. Cdk2, which forms a holoenzyme with cyclin E, is the other primary G_1-phase Cdk, and it is responsible, along with cyclin D/Cdk4, for hyperphosphorylation of the retinoblastoma gene product Rb.[36-38]

In quiescent cells, Rb exists in its hypophosphorylated form, pRb, and resides in a complex with cyclin A, Cdk2 and the transcription factor E2F. Hyperphosphorylation to the ppRb state results in a release of E2F from this complex.[39] E2F then transactivates a number of other genes whose products are essential for progression through the S-, G_2- and M-phases of the cell cycle.[40] These genes include

protooncogenes such as *c-myc*, genes encoding enzymes such as dihydrofolate reductase, and those for cell cycle regulatory proteins such as Cdk2 and cyclin E. Hyperphosphorylation of Rb and activation of E2F comprises the restriction point R in the cell cycle, beyond which the cell is committed to DNA synthesis and after which the cell cycle can be completed without further stimulation from external growth factors.[39]

After DNA replication has taken place in S-phase, another cyclin-Cdk complex, that of cyclin B and Cdk1 (also known as cell division cycle 2 kinase or cdc2 kinase) is responsible for final progression of the cell through the G_2/M transition. This complex, the mitosis promoting factor (MPF), requires phosphorylation by CAK and dephosphorylation by cdc25 phosphatase for activation.[41,42] An example of the coordination of cell cycle events is reflected in the fact that c-myc protein not only contributes to the upregulation of Cdk1 protein levels, but also to induction of cdc25 phosphatase and thereby to Cdk1 activation.[43] Activated MPF initiates mitosis, and also triggers a proteosomal pathway involving ubiquination that not only facilitates anaphase, but also leads to destruction of cyclin B itself in a negative feedback loop.[44]

In addition to cell cycle promoting factors, a number of natural inhibitors of cell cycle progression are known to play important roles in the management of cell cycle progression. One group of these molecules is the cyclin-dependent kinase inhibitors (CKIs). These inhibitors bind to cyclin/Cdk complexes and block their enzymatic activation. In several cell types, including VSMC, the CKI p27^{Kip1} is expressed at high levels during G_0-phase, and a drop in this protein level is seen during entry into G_1-phase.[45] This drop is believed to be necessary for effective phosphorylation of pRb at the R point. Interestingly, another CKI, p21^{Cip1}, is expressed only after cell cycle entry has been initiated, and it is believed to play a role in controlling cell cycle progression.[45] The tumor suppressor p53 acts as a transcription factor to inhibit cell cycle progression under certain conditions.[46] Beta

Fig. 23.3. The cell cycle. The upregulated expression and coordinated activation of cyclin-dependent kinases (Cdks) is required at various points during cell cycle progression. These enzymes are regulated by inhibitory proteins such as p27 and p21. At the R point, the hypophosphorylated retinoblastoma gene product (pRb) is hyperphosphorylated by G_1 Cdks, releasing the transcription factor E2F, which in turn transactivates up to a dozen genes that encode proteins required for completion of the cell cycle. (See text.)

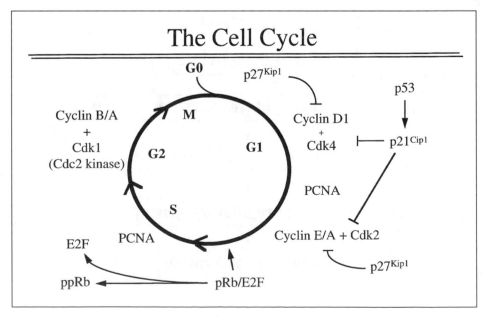

particle and ultraviolet light irradiation, for example, lead to a p53-mediated upregulation of p21^{Cip1} expression, thereby preventing progression to S-phase and DNA replication in the context of radiation-induced DNA damage.[47] In the presence of free E2F protein, p53 has also been linked to induction of programmed cell death, or apoptosis, providing a mechanism for prevention of propagation of damaged DNA in cells that have passed the R point of the cell cycle.[48] The homeobox proteins, such as GAX, are another class of natural cell cycle inhibitors, and are believed to help maintain differentiated cells in a quiescent state.[49]

Cell Cycle Arrest and Neointimal Hyperplasia

The molecular and genetic basis of cell cycle regulation has also been explored in the context of the intact vessel wall during the proliferative response to vascular injury. Increases in mRNA levels of the protooncogenes *c-myc, c-fos,* and *c-jun* have been documented within hours after arterial balloon injury, whereas protein levels of the cell cycle inhibitors GAX and p27^{Kip1} are rapidly downregulated.[50-52] Expression of the "immediate early" genes *c-fos* and *c-jun* has also been demonstrated in human saphenous vein segments within hours after harvest, even without re-implantation as bypass grafts.[53] Expression of *c-myc* peaks a second time 7 days after arterial injury, when VSMC proliferative activity has been shown to reach its highest levels.[50] The upregulation of immediate early genes is followed in turn by increases in both the mRNA and protein levels of cyclins and Cdks in the arterial wall, within 1-4 days after injury.[54,55] Cell cycle gene activation has further been documented in medial and neointimal VSMC via the immunohistochemical staining of increased levels of PCNA in this time period after injury, and increased PCNA and Cdk1 protein levels have similarly been measured in autologous rabbit vein grafts at 4 days after surgery.[8]

Understanding the control of cell cycle progression at the level of cell cycle regulatory gene expression has led to a number of gene-based approaches at inhibiting VSMC proliferation after vascular injury. Genetic manipulation can involve either the blockade of target genes using oligonucleotide transfection, or the introduction of genes using lipids or viral vectors. Antisense oligodeoxynucleotides (ODN) are short chains of single stranded DNA that bear an antisense, or Watson-Crick complementary, sequence to that of a region of the target gene mRNA. After delivery to a target cell, the ODN bind to this mRNA and prevent its translation into protein. Several mechanisms of antisense activity have been proposed; the most commonly accepted, however, involves the destruction of DNA-RNA hybrids via RNAse H. An alternative gene blockade strategy utilizes double-stranded "decoy" ODN that bear a consensus binding site for a target transcription factor protein (Fig. 23.4). The factor becomes bound by the excess of decoy ODN, and is prevented from interacting with its binding site in the promoter region of a gene under its control. Upregulation of target gene transcription is therefore inhibited. Ribozymes, chains of RNA that catalyze cleavage of mRNA in a sequence-specific manner, offer another alternative for gene blockade.

The first report of in vivo intervention in vascular cell cycle gene expression was made by Simons et al,[56] and involved antisense ODN inhibition of *c-myb* expression after rat carotid balloon injury. A porcine arterial balloon injury model was subsequently used to demonstrate a similar reduction in neointimal lesion size after treatment of the vessel wall with antisense ODN against *c-myc*.[57] Whereas single antisense ODN targeting PCNA, Cdk1 or Cdk2 have also been shown to reduce neointimal hyperplasia after balloon injury, the simultaneous inhibition of a combination of cell cycle genes, such as Cdk1 and cyclin B or Cdk1 and PCNA, was found to have a more profound, nearly complete inhibition of neointima formation in a rat carotid injury model that lasted up to 8 weeks after injury.[54,58] Blockade of the latter combination of genes using ribozymes has also successfully inhibited neointimal hyperplasia in a similar arterial injury model.[59]

The synergy observed with inhibition of multiple cell cycle regulatory genes led to studies of in vivo inhibition of the transcription factor E2F using decoy ODN transfection after carotid injury.[60] Fusigenic liposomes comprised of coat proteins from inactivated hemagglutinating virus of Japan (HVJ) particles and neutral lipids were used to enhance delivery of the decoy ODN. Free E2F is responsible for the transactivation of up to a dozen cell cycle regulatory proteins, including c-myc, Cdk1 and PCNA, and its blockade with the single decoy ODN proved as effective as combinations of antisense ODN directed against multiple cell cycle gene targets.

The transfer of genes encoding several bioengineered or naturally occurring cell cycle inhibitory proteins has also succeeded in reducing neointimal hyperplasia after arterial balloon injury. Overexpression of either p21^{Cip1} or GAX, for example, has been shown to reduce neointimal hyperplasia in injured porcine and rabbit arteries, respectively, and neointima formation has similarly been reduced via transduction of porcine femoral arteries with a nonphosphorylatable mutant of Rb and of rat carotid arteries with a dominant negative mutant of Ras.[61-64] Cell cycle interruption via gene transfer, however, is likely to require a very high transduction efficiency to achieve a clinically significant effect on VSMC proliferation and neointimal growth, since cell cycle progression will be blocked only in transduced cells. The studies described all used replication-deficient, recombinant adenoviral vectors to achieve transgene delivery to the target vessels. Although these recombinant adenoviruses are the most widely studied and efficient vectors yet described in vascular tissue, transgene expression is generally limited to approximately 30-50% of cells in an arterial wall, and only after some form of vessel wall injury.[63,65] Furthermore, infection with these vectors is associated with a prominent inflammatory reaction, transient gene expression and the hazard of possible viral mutation. Nonviral means of manipulating cell cycle gene expression may therefore provide a more practical opportunity at the present time for influencing vascular proliferative disease in both human arteries and vein grafts.

Fig. 23.4. The transcription factor "decoy" approach. The transcription factor E2F is bound to a regulatory complex and is inactive in quiescent cells (A). Upon activation, E2F is released and is free to interact with the consensus binding site in promoters of target genes (B). "Decoy" ODN bearing the consensus binding site compete for transcription factor binding and prevent gene transactivation (C).

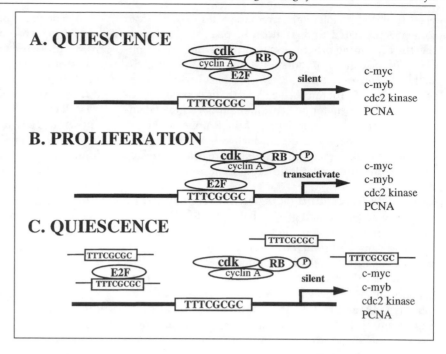

Genetic Engineering of Vein Graft Resistance to Atherosclerosis via Cell Cycle Gene Blockade

Neointimal hyperplasia plays a particularly important role in the pathogenesis of autologous vein graft failure, not only through direct encroachment upon the vessel lumen, but also because it acts as a substrate for accelerated graft atherosclerosis. Neointima formation is a well characterized response to multiple forms of vascular injury, ranging from gentle denudation to desiccation to balloon distention. The ischemic, mechanical and inflammatory injuries associated with vein graft harvest and implantation are therefore likely to provide a strong stimulus for neointima formation. The authors have hypothesized that blockade of gene expression necessary for cell cycle progression can prevent the initiation of neointimal hyperplasia as a response to these multiple factors and stimuli. Furthermore, once graft healing has progressed and the stimulation from these injuries has subsided, the graft can respond to the hemodynamic impetus for wall thickening via vascular hypertrophy and medial thickening. Stabilization of vascular cell phenotype and function during the postoperative period of graft healing may therefore allow vein graft adaptation to the hemodynamic stresses of the arterial circulation without incurring increased susceptibility to graft disease and failure associated with neointimal hyperplasia.

This hypothesis was tested in a series of experiments utilizing the delivery of ODN to cells of rabbit jugular veins at the time of grafting into the carotid artery. A combination of antisense ODN against both Cdk1 and PCNA inhibited neointimal hyperplasia by 90%, and this inhibition persisted for up to 10 weeks after grafting.[8] By week 6, however, adaptive graft wall thickening approached levels seen in untreated grafts largely through hypertrophy of the medial layer. This thickening translated into an effective reduction in tangential wall stress. Most importantly, in the absence of

significant neointimal hyperplasia, these genetically engineered grafts resisted the accelerated, diet-induced deposition of foam cells and generation of atherosclerotic plaque observed in control grafts (Fig. 23.5).

Vein graft susceptibility to accelerated atherosclerosis is associated with endothelial dysfunction similar to that seen in early arterial atherosclerosis.[66] In addition to blockade of VSMC proliferation during the immediate postoperative period, inhibition of cell cycle regulatory gene expression had a long term stabilizing effect on vein graft endothelial function.[9] This phenotypic alteration was documented via enhanced endothelial cell nitric oxide synthase activity and maintenance of normal jugular vasoreactivity, as well as through reduced superoxide anion generation, adhesion molecule expression and monocyte binding to graft endothelium. This preservation of endothelial function may represent either a direct effect of cell cycle gene blockade in endothelial cells, or it may reflect a change in the influence normally exerted by underlying abnormal neointimal VSMC.

Transfection of the vein graft wall with the single agent E2F decoy ODN has subsequently been shown to similarly influence vein graft biology and prevent both neointimal disease and atherosclerosis.[67] This observation has been extended to six months after operation, at which time E2F decoy ODN-treated grafts remain free of significant neointima formation and resist diet-induced atherosclerosis. Studies have also documented that ODN can be delivered efficiently to human saphenous vein segments ex vivo, and in an organ culture system these ODN have inhibited target gene function in a sequence specific manner. These findings have served as the basis for initiation of a large scale human clinical trial to test the efficacy of intraoperative vein graft engineering via E2F decoy ODN transfection in preventing infrainguinal bypass graft failures.[68] This study rep-

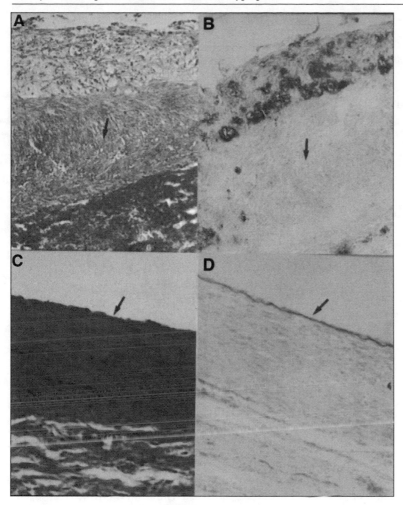

Fig. 23.5. Inhibition of neointimal hyperplasia and resistance to accelerated atherosclerosis in vein grafts transfected intraoperatively with ODN that block cell cycle regulatory gene upregulation (C,D). Plaque in a control graft is comprised largely of foam cells (A) and demonstrated positive immunohistochemical staining for macrophages (B). From Mann et al. Proc Natl Acad Sci USA 1995; 92:4502-4506.

resents the first attempt at integrating a gene therapy strategy into a routine cardiovascular surgical procedure, and the first large scale testing of our ability to influence cell cycle biology and its role in human vascular pathogenesis.

Summary

Vascular cell proliferation is clearly a requisite component of the neointimal hyperplasia that is known to compromise the long term success of autologous and prosthetic vascular reconstruction. Cell cycle regulation that is at the heart of this proliferation is regulated by a complex and well orchestrated series of molecular and genetic events. Interruption of these events at critical points of cell cycle progression has been shown to influence neointimal hyperplasia in models of arterial injury. Although a powerful tool to block cellular proliferation, inhibition of cell cycle progression, and blockade of cell cycle regulatory gene expression in particular, may have even more profound effects on the development of vascular graft disease through its stabilizing influence on vascular cell phenotype and tissue behavior.

Current studies are probing the molecular links between cell cycle entry and other aspects of cellular activation, such as adhesion molecule expression and cytokine secretion. Even as our understanding of vascular cell cycle biology continues to grow, clinical studies are already underway that may establish the practical, long term benefits that a one time intervention in cell cycle regulation may have for vascular graft compatibility and adaptation. The results of these basic science and clinical studies will likely yield vascular biologists, bioengineers and clinicians new tools to aid in the design of vascular prostheses with enhanced durability and performance.

References

1. Campeau LM, Enjalbert J, Lesperance MC, Bourassa P, Kwiterowich S, Wacholder A. Sniderman A. The relation of risk factors to the development of atherosclerosis in saphenous vein bypass grafts and the progresion of disease in the native circulation: A study 10 years after aortocoronary bypass surgery. N Engl J Med 1984; 311:1329-1334.
2. Grondin CM, Campeau L, Thornton JC, Engle JC, Cross FS, Schreiber H. Coronary artery bypass grafting with saphenous vein. Circ 1989; 79:I-24-I-29.
3. Cox JL, Chaisson DA, Gotleib AI. Stranger in a strange land: The pathogenesis of saphenous vein graft stenosis. Prog Cardiovasc Dis 1991; 34:45-68.
4. Clowes AW, Reidy MA. Prevention of stenosis after vascular reconstruction: Pharmocologic control of intimal hyperplasia—A review. J Vasc Surg 1991; 13:885-91.

5. Hirsch GM, Karnovsky MJ. Inhibition of vein graft intimal proliferative lesions in the rat by heparin. Am J Path 1991; 139:581-7.

6. Chen C, Mattar SG, Hughes JD, Pierce GF, Cook JE, Ku DN, Hanson SR, Lumsden AB. Recombinant mitotoxin basic fibroblast growth factor-saporin reduces venous anastomotic intimal hyperplasia in the arteriovenous graft. Circ 1996; 94:1989-95.

7. Davies MG, Dalen H, Kim JH, Barber L, Svendsen E, Hagen PO. Control of accelerated vein graft atheroma with the nitric oxide precursor: L-arginine. J Surg Res 1995; 59:35-42.

8. Mann MJ, Gibbons GH, Kernoff RS, Diet FP, Tsao P, CookeJP, Kaneda Y, Dzau VJ. Genetic engineering of vein grafts resistant to atherosclerosis. Proc Natl Acad Sci USA. 1995; 92:4502-4506.

9. Mann MJ, Gibbons GH, Tsao PS, von der Leyen HE. Buitrago R, Kernoff R, Cooke JP, Dzau VJ. Cell cycle inhibition preserves endothelial function in genetically engineered vein grafts. J Clin Invest 1997; 99:1295-1301.

10. Zwolak RM, Adams MC, Clowes AW. Kinetics of vein graft hyperplasia: Association with tangential stress. J Vasc Surg 1987; 5:126-136.

11. Moggio RA, Ding JZ, Smith CJ, Tota RR, Stemerman MB, Reed GE Immediate-early gene expression in human saphenous veins harvested during coronary artery bypass graft operations. J Thorac Cardiovasc Surg 1995; 110:209-13.

12. Hoch JR, Stark VK, Turnipseed WD. The temporal relationship between the development of vein graft intimal hyperplasia and growth factor gene expression. J Vasc Surg 1995; 22:51-58.

13. Tanaka H, Sukhova GK, Swanson SJ, Clinton, SK, Ganz P, Cybulsky MI, Libby P. Sustained activation of vascular cells and leukocytes in the rabbit aorta after balloon injury. Circ 1993; 88:1788-1803.

14. Faries PL, Marin ML, Veith FJ, Ramirez JA, Suggs WD, Parsons RE, Sanchez LA, Lyon RT. Immunolocalization and temporal distribution of cytokine expression during the development of vein graft intimal hyperplasia in an experimental model. J Vasc Surg 1996; 24:463-71.

15. Yu X, Dluz S, Graves DT, Zhang L, Antoniades HN, Hollander W, Prusty S, Valente AJ, Schwartz CJ, Sonenshein GE. Elevated expression of monocyte chemoattractant protein 1 by vascularsmooth muscle cells in hypercholesterolemic primates. Proc Natl Acad Sci USA 1992; 89:6953-7.

16. Hamdan AD, Misare B, Contreras M, LoGerfo FW, Quist WC. Evaluation of anastomotic hyperplasia progression using the cyclin specific antibody MIB-1. Am J Surg 1996; 172:168-70.

17. Clowes AW, Reidy MA, Clowes MM. Kinetics of cellular proliferation after arterial injury. I. Smooth muscle growth in the absence of endothelium. Lab Invest 1983; 49:327-333.

18. Gospodarowics D, Ferrara N, Haaparanta T, Neufeld G. Basic fibroblast growth factor: Expression in cultured bovine vascular smooth muscle cells. Eur J Cell Biol 1988; 46:144-151.

19. Walker LN, Bowen-Pope DF, Ross R, Reidy MA. Production of platelet-derived growth factor-like molecules by cultured arterial smooth muscle cells accompanies proliferation after arterial injury. Proc Natl Acad Sci USA 1986; 83:7311-7315.

20. Reidy MA, Fingerle J, Lindner V. Factors controlling the development of arterial lesions after injury. Circulation 1992; 86:III43-46.

21. Sterpetti AV, Cucina A, Randone B, Palumbo R, Stipa F, Proietti P, Saragosa MT, Santoro-D'Angelo L, Cavallaro A. Growth factor production by arterial and vein grafts: relevance to coronary artery bypass grafting. Surgery 1996; 120:460-7.

22. Clowes AW, Schwartz SM. Significance of quiescent smooth muscle migration in the injured rat carotid artery. Circ Res 1985; 56:139-145.

23. Clowes AW, Reidy MA, Clowes MM. Mechanisms of stenosis after arterial injury. Lab Invest 1983; 49:208-215.

24. Majeski MW, Lindner V, Twardzik DR, Reidy MA. Production of transforming growth factor beta-1 during repair of arterial injury. J Clin Invest 1991; 88:904-910.

25. Grant MB, Wargovich TJ, Ellis EA, Caballero S, Mansour M, Pepine CJ. Localization of insulin-like growth factor I and inhibition of coronary smooth muscle cell growth by somatostatin analogues in human coronary smooth muscle cells. A potential treatment for restenosis? Circ 1994; 89:1511-1517.

26. Rakugi H, Wang DS, Dzau VJ, Pratt RE. Potential importance of tissue angiotensin-converting enzyme inhibition in preventing neointima formation. Circ 1994; 90:449-455.

27. Francis SE, Hunter S, Holt CM, Gadsdon PA, Rogers S, Duff GW, Newby AC, Angelini GD. Release of platelet-drived growth factor activity from pig venous arterial grafts. J Thor Cardiovasc Surg 1994; 108:540-548.

28. Stark VK, Hoch JR, Warner TF, Hullett DA. Monocyte chemotactic protein-1 expression is associated with the development of vein graft intimal hyperplasia. Arterioscler Thromb Vasc Biol 1997; 17:1614-21.

29. Zacharias RK, Kirkman TR, Clowes AW. Mechanisms of healing in synthetic grafts. J Vasc Surg 1987; 6:429-36.

30. Clowes AW, Kirkman TR, Clowes MM. Mechanisms of arterial graft failure. II. Chronic endothelial and smooth muscle cell proliferation in healing polytetrafluoroethylene prostheses. J Vasc Surg 1986; 3:877-84.

31. Golden MA, Hanson SR, Kirkman TR, Schneider PA, Clowes AW. Healing of polytetrafluoroethylene arterial grafts is influenced by graft porosity. J Vasc Surg 1990; 11:838-44.

32. Zacharias RK, Kirkman TR, Kenagy RD, Bowen-Pope DF, Clowes AW. Growth factor production by polytetrafluoroethylene vascular grafts. J Vasc Surg 1988; 7(4):606-10.

33. Karn J, Watson JV, Lowre AD, Green SM, Vedeckis W: Regulation of cell cycle duration by c-myc levels. Oncogene 1989; 4:773-787.

34. Pai SR, Bird RC. c-fos expression is required during all phases of the cell cycle during exponential cell proliferation. Anticancer Res 1994; 14:985-994.

35. Avruch J, Zhang XF, Kyriakis JM. Raf meets Ras: Completing the framework of a signal transduction pathway. Trends Biochem Sci 1994; 19:279-283.

36. Pardee AB. G1 events and regulation of cell proliferation. Science 1989; 246:603-608.

37. Morgan DO. Principles of CDK regulation. Nature 1995; 374:131-134.

38. Sherr CJ. Mammalian G1 cyclins. Cell 1993; 73:1059-1065.

39. Weinberg RA. The retinoblastoma protein and cell cycle control. Cell 1995; 81:323-330.

40. DeGregori J, Kowalik T, Nevins JR. Cellular targets for activation by the E2F1 transcription factor include DNA synthesis- and G1/S-regulatory genes. Mol Cell Biol 1995; 15:4215-4224.

41. King RW, Jackson PK, Kirschner MW. Mitosis in transition. Cell 1994; 79:563-571.

42. Coleman TR, Dunphy WG. cdc2 regulatory factors. Curr Opin Cell Biol 1994; 6:877-882.

43. Galaktionov K, Chen X, Beach D. cdc25 cell-cycle phosphatase as a target of c-myc. Nature 1996; 382:511-517.

44. King RW, Deshaies RJ, Peters JM, Kirschner MW. How proteolysis drives the cell cycle. Science 1996; 274:1652-1658.

45. Sherr CJ, Roberts JM. Inhibitors of mamalian G1 cyclin-dependent kinases. Gen Dev 1995; 9:1149-1163.

46. Levine AJ. p53, the cellular gatekeeper for growth and division. Cell 1997; 88:323-331.

47. el-Deiry WS, Tokino T, Velculescu VE, Levy DB, Parsons R, Trent JM, Lin D, Mercer WE, Kinzler KW, Vogelstein B. WAF1, a potential mediator of p53 tumor suppression. Cell 1993; 75:817-825.

48. Kastan MB, Onyekwere O, Sidransky D, Vogelstein B, Craig RW. Participation of p53 protein in the cellular response to DNA damage. Cancer Res 1991; 51:6304-6311.

49. Gorski DH, Patel CV, Walsh K. Homeobox transcription factor regulation in the cardiovascular system. Trends Cardiovasc Med 1993; 3:184-190.

50. Miano JM, Vlasic N, Tota RR, Stemerman MB. Smooth muscle cell immediate-early gene and growth factor activation follows vascular injury. A putative in vivo mechanism for autocrine growth. Arterioscler Thromb 1993; 13:211-219.

51. Weir L, Chen D, Pastore C, Isner JM, Walsh K. Expression of gax, a growth arrest homeobox gene, is rapidly down-regulated in the rat carotid artery during the proliferative response to balloon injury. J Biol Chem 1995; 270:5457-5461.

52. Braun-Dullaeus RC, von der Leyen HE, Mann MJ, Zhang L, Morris RE, Dzau VJ. Loss of p27Kip1 and induction of Cdk1 in the rat carotid artery following balloon catheter injury. In vivo and in vitro influence of rapamycin (abstract). FASEB J 1997; 11:A153.

53. Sterpetti AV, Cucina A, Randone B, Palumbo R, Stipa F, Proietti P, Saragosa MT, Santoro-D'Angelo, Cavallaro A. Growth factor production by arterial and vein grafts: Relevance to coronary artery bypass grafting. Surgery 1996; 120:460-7.

54. Kaneda Y, Ogihara T, Dzau VJ. Intimal hyperplasia after vascular injury is inhibited by antisense cdk 2 kinase oligonucleotides. J Clin Invest 1994; 93:1458-1464.

55. Abe J, Zhou W, Taguchi J, Takuwa N, Miki K, Okazaki H, Kurokawa K, Kumada M, Takuwa Y. Suppression of neointimal smooth muscle cell accumulation in vivo by antisense cdc2 and cdk2 oligonucleotides in rat carotid artery. Biochem Biophys Res Commun 1994; 198:16-24.

56. Simons M, Edelman ER, DeKeyser JL, Langer R, Rosenberg RD. Antisense c-myb oligonucleotides inhibit intimal arterial smooth muscle cell accumulation in vivo. Nature 1992; 359:67-70.

57. Shi Y, Fard A, Galeo A, Hutchinson HG, Vermani P, Dodge GR, Hall DJ, Shaheen F, Zalewski A. Transcatheter delivery of c-myc antisense oligomers reduce neointimal formation in a porcine model of coronary artery balloon injury. Circ. 1994; 90:944-951.

58. Morishita R, Gibbons GH, Kaneda Y et al. Pharmacokinetics of antisense oligodeoxynucleotides (cyclin B1 and cdc2 kinase) in the vessel wall in vivo: Enhanced therapeutic utility for restenosis by HVJ-liposome delivery. Gene 1994; 149:13-9.

59. Dev V, Parikh A, Ren M, Goldenberg T, Fishbein MC, Eigler N, Rossi J, Litvack F. Ribozymes to cell division cycle (CDC-2) kinase and proliferating cell nuclear antigen (PCNA) prevent intimal hyperplasia in rat carotide artery (abstract). Circulation (suppl I) 1995; 92:I-634.

60. Morishita R, Gibbons GH, Horiuchi M et al. A novel molecular strategy using cis element "decoy" of E2F binding site inhibits smooth muscle proliferation in vivo. Proc Natl Acad Sci USA 1995; 92:5855-9.

61. Chang MW, Barr E, Lu MM, Barton K, Leiden JM. Adenovirus-mediated over-expression of the cyclin/cyclin-dependent kinase inhibitor, p21 inhibits vascular smooth muscle cell proliferation and neointima formation in the rat carotid artery model of balloon angioplasty. J Clin Invest 1995; 96:2260-2268.

62. Maillard L, Belle EV, Perlman H, Branellec D, Barry J, Steg C, Walsh K. GAX adenovirus percutaneous gene transfer inhibits neointima formation in a rabbit model of balloon angioplasty (abstract). Circulation (suppl I) 1996; 94:I-637.

63. Chang MW, Barr E, Seltzer J, Jiang YQ, Nabel GJ, Nabel EG, Parmacek MS, Leiden JM. Cytostatic gene therapy for vascular proliferative disorders with a constitutively active form of the retinoblastoma gene product. Science 1995; 267:518-522.

64. Indolfi C, Avvedimento EV, Rapacciuolo A, Di Lorenzo E, Esposito G, Stabile E, Feliciello A, Mele E, Giuliano P, Condorelli G et al. Inhibition of cellular ras prevents smooth muscle cell proliferation after vascular injury in vivo. Nat Med 1995; 1:541-545.

65. Schulick AH Dong G Newman KD Virmani R Dichek DA. Endothelium-specific in vivo gene transfer. Circ Res 1995; 77:475-85.

66. Ku DD, Caulfield JB, Kirklin JK. Endothelium-dependent responses in long-term human coronary artery bypass grafts. Circ 1991; 83:402-411.

67. Mann MJ, Kernoff R, Dzau VJ. Intraoperative transfection with E2F decoy oligonucleotide yields long term resistance to vein graft atherosclerosis. Journal of Investigative Medicine, 1997; 45:224A.

68. Mann MJ, Whittemore AD, Donaldson MC, Belkin MA, Orav EJ, Polak J, Dzau VJ. Preliminary clinical experience with genetic engineering of human vein grafts: Evidence for target gene inhibition. Circ. 1997; 96:I4.

Facilitation of Healing

Chemotaxis

---------- CHAPTER 24 ----------

Signaling Mechanisms for Vascular Cell Migration

Ian Zachary

Introduction

It is increasingly recognized that migration of vascular smooth muscle cells (VSMC) from the media is a key event in progressive intimal thickening leading to atherosclerosis and other occlusive vasculoproliferative complications.[1,2] Transendothelial migration into the tunica intima of other cell types, particularly monocytes and T lymphocytes, is thought to be central both to the formation of the mature atherosclerotic lesion and to the pathogenesis of the disease.[1,2] Arterial bypass graft surgery is one of the commonest treatments for atherosclerotic cardiovascular disease, and a major cause of failure of bypass graft surgery is stenosis of the graft, which occurs predominantly at, or contiguous to, the sites of anastomosis.[3-6] Stenosis of the grafted vessel is primarily due to the proliferation and migration of VSMC.[7] The use of prosthetic grafts in place of autogenous vessels has been an important development in vascular surgery, but prosthetic materials have lower patency rates compared to veins. The lower patency of prosthetic grafts is widely attributed to their inability to form an endothelial lining, thus contributing to enhanced thrombogenicity and VSMC proliferation/migration. Animal studies indicate that seeding prosthetic grafts with endothelial cells (EC) prior to implantation can significantly reduce neointimal hyperplasia and thrombogenicity.[8,9] As these brief introductory remarks suggest, vascular cell migration may be relevant for cardiovascular disease from more than one perspective. Thus, while VSMC and monocyte migration contribute to progression of the primary disease and—in the case of VSMC—complications consequent upon treatment, the *promotion* of EC migration and proliferation may be of equal importance in clinical situations, either where prosthetic grafts are used or where the endothelium is damaged (e.g., angioplasty).

The aim of this chapter is to provide an overview of the extracellular factors and intracellular mechanisms implicated in the regulation of vascular cell migration. Emphasis will be placed on the migration of VSMC and EC, though the role of the migration of other cell types in the arterial wall and the atherosclerotic microenvironment (e.g., monocytes) will also be considered. Emphasis will be placed on recent developments in our understanding of the molecular basis of cell migration, such as the role of focal adhesion kinase (FAK) and Rho proteins. Inevitably, many of the findings that will be discussed have come from studies in other nonvascular cell types, but it is anticipated that these findings will have relevance for the migration of vascular cells. The first section of the chapter (Migration Factors) will describe the major factors known to modulate vascular cell locomotion in cell culture. The second section (Chemotactic Signal Transduction) will go on to discuss intracellular mechanisms implicated in cell migration and linked cellular processes.

Tissue Engineering of Prosthetic Vascular Grafts, edited by Peter Zilla and Howard P. Greisler
©1999 R.G. Landes Company.

Migration Factors

Chemotaxis is the directed movement of cells along a gradient of a chemoattractant and should be distinguished from the random movement or chemokinesis of cells in the absence of a gradient. In what follows, migration will generally be understood as synonymous with chemotaxis, i.e., the directed movement of cells in response to a specific factor. A diverse array of molecules have been shown to influence the movement of vascular cells in vitro and are therefore potential regulators of vascular cell migration in vivo. The most important known chemoattractants and migration factors, together with their cellular and noncellular sources and principal target cells are summarized in Table 24.1.

PDGF and Other Growth Factors

Platelet-derived growth factor-BB (PDGF-BB) is the most potent known chemoattractant for cultured VSMC derived from a variety of species.[1,2] The mRNA for PDGF ligand and receptors are upregulated both in human atherosclerotic plaques[10] and in rat and baboon neointimal tissue induced by injury or vascular grafting.[11,12] It has been reported that PDGF-stimulated neointima formation in the rat model of balloon angioplasty predominantly involves migration of VSMC from the media. Thus, intimal thickening following infusion of PDGF-BB into rats subjected to injury of the carotid artery was primarily the result of migration and was accompanied by only a small increase in VSMC proliferation.[13] Furthermore, neointimal VSMC accumulation in the rat carotid can be inhibited by an antibody to PDGF.[14] These findings suggest that PDGF-induced chemotaxis of medial VSMC may play a major role in the formation of a neointima both in atherosclerosis and in restenosis following angioplasty.

PDGF in atherosclerotic lesions and following vascular injury may be derived from several sources. PDGF exists as disulfide-linked dimers of two homologous isoforms, the A- and B chains, which give rise to three dimeric bioactive isoforms, AA, AB and BB. The BB form is the major species in porcine platelets[15], while PDGF-AB is the predominant form in human platelets.[16,17] Expression of PDGF-A and -B chains is induced in EC by interleukin-1 (IL-1), tumor necrosis factor-α and by transformtin growth factor-β (TGF-β).[18-21] Adult rat VSMC apparently produce only A chains[22,23] and PDGF-AA expression is upregulated in these cells by TGF-β and IL-1.[24-27] Macrophages also produce PDGF-B and are an additional source of this factor in the atherosclerotic plaque.[1,28,29]

Two isotypes of the PDGF receptor have been identified, the α and β receptors, which exhibit different affinities for PDGF ligand isoforms. The α receptor (PDGFRα) recognizes all three possible isoforms of PDGF ligand while the β receptor (PDGFRβ) exhibits high-affinity binding only of the PDGF-B chain.[30-33] Evidence is accumulating that the different isoforms of PDGF ligand and receptor may mediate distinct cellular functions in VSMC.[34-36] The BB homodimer is chemotactic for a variety of cell types including every species of VSMC so far tested.[34-38] The AB heterodimer is also chemotactic where it has been examined.[35,36] In contrast, the chemotactic response to PDGF-AA is highly cell type dependent. Thus, PDGF-AA promotes the migration of granulocytes but not of monocytes.[35] Furthermore, in VSMC of several species and in monocytes and fibroblasts this isoform has no chemotactic effects[34-38] and has been shown to antagonize migratory responses to PDGF-BB.[34-36] Our recent findings show that rabbit VSMC do not respond chemotactically to PDGF-AA and lack func-

Table 24.1. Factors regulating vascular cell migration

Factor	Sources	Target Cell(s)	Biological Activities
PDGF-BB	Platelets EC Macrophages	VSMC	Stimulates chemotaxis and proliferation
PDGF-AA	VSMC/EC	VSMC	Stimulates proliferation and inhibits chemotaxis
IGF-1	Circulation EC/VSMC Platelets	VSMC	Stimulates chemotaxis and and is a co-mitogen
HB-EGF	Macrophages EC/VSMC	VSMC	Stimulates chemotaxis and proliferation
VEGF	VSMC macrophages	EC Monocytes	Stimulates EC proliferation and EC and monocyte chemotaxis
bFGF	VSMC/EC	VSMC/EC	VSMC mitogen, mitogen and chemoattractant for EC
MCP-1	VSMC/EC	Monocytes	Specific monocyte chemoattractant
IL-1	Macrophages EC/VSMC	VSMC	Possible chemotactic factor and mitogen; induces PDGF expression in EC and VSMC
CSFs	T-lymphocytes EC/VSMC	Monocytes	Chemoattractant
TGF-beta	Platelets EC/T-lymphocytes	VSMC/EC	Indues expression of ECM, beta 3 integrins and PDGF-A in VSMC; induces PDGF in EC. Bimodal effects on VSMC proliferation. Possible direct bimodal effects on VSMC and EC migration.

This table lists polypeptide ligands for receptor PTKs and cytokines. For the effects of ECM components, the reader is referred to the text. Abbreveiations: EC, endothelial cells. Other abbreviations are explained in the text.

tional α receptors.[38] Low α receptor expression cannot entirely account for the lack of chemotactic responsiveness to PDGF-AA, however. For example, though human foreskin fibroblasts express 20,000-30,000 PDGF-AA binding sites per cell, and rat and baboon VSMC possess PDGF α receptors albeit at relatively low levels, the AA isoform failed to stimulate migration of all these cells and inhibited their migratory response to the BB isoform.[34-36] In addition, TGF-β1 decreased migration of rat VSMC as a consequence of PDGF-AA secretion.[36] Koyama et al[34] showed that the PDGF-AA inhibition of baboon VSMC migration stimulated either by PDGF-BB or by fibronectin was abolished by specific antibodies to the α receptor and is therefore mediated through this specific receptor isotype. These findings suggest that the stimulation of directed migration of VSMC is mediated by the β receptor, while the α receptor may play a specific role in the negative regulation of chemotaxis. It is at present unclear, however, whether these conclusions can be extended either to human VSMC or to VSMC migration in vivo. Human VSMC express α receptors[37,38] and respond mitogenically to PDGF-AA.[39] Relatively few studies of the effects of PDGF-AA on the migration of these cells have been published, but it was reported that PDGF-AA stimulates chemotaxis in human VSMC and that this response correlated with the ability of human VSMC to respond mitogenically to the AA isoform.[39] It is unknown whether the α receptor has an inhibitory effect on migration of human VSMC.

Of the other polypeptide ligands for receptor protein tyrosine kinases (PTKs), heparin-binding epidermal growth factor-like growth factor (HB-EGF) has been reported to stimulate migration of bovine aortic smooth muscle cells in a heparin-dependent manner.[40] Insulin-like growth factor-I (IGF-1) is present at high levels in platelet α-granules, is secreted by cultured VSMC and EC[41,42] and has increased expression in rat aorta following balloon injury.[43] IGF-1 has been reported to be a migration factor for human VSMC,[37] and results from our laboratory show that IGF-1 promotes chemotaxis in rabbit aortic VSMC (Abedi H, Zachary I, unpublished observations). In both cell types, IGF-1 produces a weaker migratory response compared to PDGF-BB.

Basic fibroblast growth factor (bFGF) is a mitogen for VSMC[1,42] but there is little evidence that this factor has stimulatory effects on VSMC migration in vitro. This factor may play a role in VSMC migration in vivo, however. Administration of bFGF and neutralizing antibodies to bFGF respectively stimulated and inhibited VSMC migration following balloon injury of the rat carotid artery.[44] There is much stronger evidence that bFGF is a potent migration factor for EC. Both basic and acidic FGF stimulate movement of EC in vitro[45-47] and have been reported to promote re-endothelialization following balloon injury.[48,49] It is likely that the repertory of polypeptide migration factors for VSMC will be extended in the future. For example, a 58 kDa autocrine migration factor which appears to be different from PDGF was recently purified from the conditioned medium of rat aortic VSMC.[50]

The secreted polypeptide vascular endothelial growth factor (VEGF) (also known as vascular permeability factor) is a distant relative of PDGF and is a member of a new family of growth factors, which also includes VEGF-B, VEGF-C and placenta growth factor (PlGF).[51-55] VEGF expression is upregulated by hypoxia and by cytokines and growth factors in several cell types, including arterial VSMC[56-58] and EC.[59,60] It has been established that VEGF plays a central role in angiogenesis in a variety of biological processes and disease states, including embryogenesis, wound healing, tumor growth, and collateral blood vessel formation in myocardial ischemia.[61,62]

Most of the biological effects of VEGF are attributed to its ability to stimulate EC mitogenesis and recently this has focused interest on the role of VEGF in accelerating re-endothelialization following balloon angioplasty. Initial studies in animal models of balloon injury have proved promising, and administration of VEGF protein and VEGF gene transfer have been shown to inhibit intimal thickening following balloon angioplasty and improve blood flow in ischemic limbs, effects mediated through stimulation of EC regrowth and angiogenesis respectively.[63-66]

In addition to its mitogenic effects in EC, VEGF also promotes the migration of EC and it is increasingly recognized that EC migration plays an essential role in angiogenesis and vascular modelling.[61,62,67,68] VEGF also has a number of biological activities which may contribute to vessel wall pathology. VEGF is a permeability-increasing factor,[51,69] and also stimulates monocyte chemotaxis and tissue factor production.[70,71] It has also been proposed that VEGF may play a role in neovascularization of the advanced atherosclerotic plaque.[57,72-74] Induction of VEGF expression in the arterial wall may therefore be pro-atherogenic both through its effects on the permeability of the endothelium, thereby facilitating the infiltration of monocytes, platelets and T cells, and by a direct effect on monocyte migration. At later stages of atherogenesis, neo-vascularization induced by hypoxia and mediated by VEGF may also contribute to disease progression.

Angiotensin II

The vasoconstrictor angiotensin II is implicated in the regulation of VSMC proliferation, but it is unclear whether it contributes significantly to migration of these cells. Data from in vitro studies are conflicting. Thus, it was reported that angiotensin II stimulates migration of bovine aortic VSMC,[75] while MII and co-workers found no effect of angiotensin II on migration of human VSMC.[76] It is possible, however, that angiotensin II may play a role in migration of VSMC in vivo. Consistent with this notion, infusion of angiotensin II enhanced neointima formation following balloon injury of the rat carotid artery[77] and, using the same model, it was shown that both inhibitors of angiotensin-converting enzyme and antagonists of the angiotensin type 1 (AT$_1$) receptor inhibited the accumulation of intimal VSMC.[78] It is unclear from these studies, however, whether the effects of angiotensin II are direct or indirectly mediated through increased expression of another migration factor(s) and/or receptor(s).

Cytokines

A variety of cytokines are released from macrophages, T lymphocytes, platelets and VSMC in the atherosclerotic microenvironment and stimulate monocyte chemotaxis and endothelial transmigration.[1,27] They include interleukins, colony-stimulating factors, monocyte chemotactic protein-1 (MCP-1), oxidized low-density lipoprotein (ox LDL) and TGF-β (Table 24.1). TGF-β is produced by activated macrophages,[79] VSMC[80] and the α-granules of platelets[81] and has been reported to have bimodal effects on VSMC migration.[82] Interleukin-1 has also been shown to stimulate migration of VSMC.[83] The specific monocyte chemoattractant MCP-1 is secreted by arterial VSMC in hypercholesterolemic primates.[84]

TGF-β regulation of vascular cell migration is as complex as its effects on VSMC proliferation, which can be both positive and negative.[25,85] TGF-β is a potent inducer of the production of ECM components and also upregulates expression of integrins in VSMC,[85] so it is unclear whether the modulation of VSMC chemotaxis by TGF-β is direct or indirectly mediated. In theory, TGF-β could also either stimulate or inhibit VSMC migration indirectly through its respective abilities, mentioned above, to induce PDGF-B chain expression in EC and PDGF-A expression in VSMC. TGF-β may also regulate EC migration. In cocultures of bovine EC and smooth muscle cells, TGF-β is secreted in a latent form which is activated by plasmin and subsequently inhibits EC movement.[86]

Extracellular Matrix

Dynamic adhesive interactions between cell surface integrins and components of the ECM play a central role in cell migration by providing cell-substrate traction for the generation of intracellular mechanical stresses.[87,88] The ECM-integrin network can regulate cell motility in at least three ways:

1. Through specific ECM-integrin interactions;
2. By changes in the concentration of particular ECM substrates; and
3. As a result of varying cell surface integrin density.

The last of these possibilities will be considered in the next section.

Deposition of matrix is a major feature of the fibrous atherosclerotic lesion.[1,2] Several ECM components, including fibronectin[34,89] and vitronectin,[90] promote migration of VSMC. The RGD-motif ECM molecule osteopontin is upregulated in proliferating rat VSMC, during rat neointima formation and in human atherosclerotic lesions.[91,92] It was recently reported that osteopontin promotes adhesion, spreading and chemotaxis of rat VSMC.[93,94] TGF-β1 induces expression of collagen types I, III and V and of fibronectin in VSMC.[95-97] Other ECM components such as laminin, collagen and the glycosaminoglycan heparin may have inhibitory effects on migration in vivo.[1] However, VSMC do migrate on collagen substrates in vitro.[37,38,98] It was recently reported that maximal migration of human VSMC occurs on fibronectin and collagen IV substrates at intermediate attachment strengths.[98] Since ECM concentration is one of the key parameters determining the 'stickiness' of cell-substrate interactions, this finding may suggest that, at least in

the case of these ECM components, it is the strength of attachment as much as adhesion to the matrix itself that is one of the critical variables regulating cell motility.

Recently, attention has focused on the role of matrix-degrading metalloproteinases (MMPs) in VSMC migration. MMP expression and secretion are upregulated in proliferating VSMC cultures and during neointimal thickening induced by balloon injury of rat and pig carotid arteries.[99-101] Components of the plasminogen activator system, and in particular the urokinase-type plasminogen activator have also been implicated in the regulation of VSMC migration.[101-104] Receptors for the urokinase-type plasminogen activator are upregulated in atherosclerotic lesions. The identification of endogenous tissue inhibitors of mmps (TIMPs) has generated considerable interest in targeting MMPs for the treatment of restenosis and stenosis. Overexpression of TIMP-1 inhibited VSMC migration in vitro and attenuated neointimal hyperplasia in the balloon-injured rat carotid artery.[105]

The findings discussed above indicate that VSMC migration in the arterial wall is modulated by a delicate balance between degradation and deposition of matrix components as well as by the differential effects of distinct matrix components. It is now increasingly recognized that integrin-matrix interactions do not simply play a structural and biomechanical role in the regulation of cell movement. As discussed below, it has become well established that integrins transduce signals into cells which may be important in the regulation of cell adhesion and motility.[106]

Chemotactic Signal Transduction

The Role of the Actin Cytoskeleton and Focal Adhesions

Three distinct processes occur during the movement of animal cells: protrusion, in which lamellipodia and microspikes (or filopodia) extend from the leading edge of the cell; attachment, in which focal adhesion plaques form adhesive interactions with the substratum; and traction, through which the intracellular mechanical forces generated by the locomotive cell machinery moves the cell body forward. All of these processes are crucially dependent on the actin cytoskeleton and associated ultrastructural elements such as the focal adhesion.

Migration is a highly dynamic process involving the rapid, organized and coordinated polymerization and depoylmerization of actin filaments, crosslinking between actin filaments, cell adhesion and detachment at focal contacts, and the assembly and disassembly of macromolecular complexes associated with both actin stress fibers and focal adhesions. Furthermore, directed cell movement implies that these dynamic changes in the configuration and organization of components of the actin cytoskeleton is highly organized in cells both spatially and temporally. While actin polymerization is essential for the rapid formation and protrusion of lammellipodia at the leading edge of a migrating cell, depolymerization of actin elsewhere is vital both to provide a source of monomeric actin for localized and rapid stress fiber formation and to release or weaken adhesions and thus allow cell movement. Similar considerations apply to focal adhesions, whose rate of turnover and/or detachment/attachment to the cellular substrate is also a crucial parameter determining the rate and direction of cell locomotion. In addition to dynamic adhesive interactions between the cell and its substrate, eukaryotic cell locomotion requires the generation of force by the cytoskeleton and associated components.[87,88]

Actin filaments organized in stress fibers and their sites of attachment at focal adhesions are both thought to play a critical role in the regulation of cell adhesion and locomotion.[107,108] Focal adhesions are specialized juxtamembrane regions which form at the termini of stress fibers and at sites of attachment of cells to the ECM. Integrins, the adhesive receptors for ECM components, aggregate at focal contacts and many nonstructural cytoskeletal-associated components are localized to these subcellular structures (Table 24.2).

Interactions between integrins and the cytoskeleton are themselves very dynamic.[109,110] For example, in nonmotile cells, β_1 integrins are localized in focal adhesions at the ends of stress fibers while in motile cells, integrins are found in organized, but dynamic substructures termed macroaggregates that are in less intimate association with focal contacts.[109]

The formation of stress fibers and the assembly of focal contacts is stimulated in adherent cells including VSMC and EC by a variety of extracellular factors including PDGF, VEGF, bombesin, angiotensin II, the serum component lysophosphatidic acid (LPA) and the ceramide sphingosine.[68,111-115] In serum-starved Swiss 3T3 cells and at relatively low concentrations, PDGF has been reported to induce a slow increase in focal adhesion assembly and stress fiber formation as well as intense membrane ruffling.[115] The function of membrane ruffling is unclear but it appears to be closely associated with pinocytosis.[115-117] In Swiss 3T3 fibroblasts, PDGF appears to have bimodal effects on actin cytoskeleton organization and, at higher concentrations, induces a marked disruption of the actin cytoskeleton.[118] The relevance of findings in Swiss 3T3 cells for the potent chemotactic effects of PDGF-BB in VSMC are unclear, however. PDGF-BB causes no disruption of the actin cytoskeleton in cultured human and rabbit VSMC.[38] There are no reports as yet showing unambiguous PDGF-BB stimulation of stress fiber or focal contact formation in vascular cells, suggesting that regulation of actin cytoskeleton organization is complex.

Given their pivotal cellular location at a point of close juxtaposition between the ECM and the actin cytoskeleton, attention has naturally focused on the role of components associated with actin and with focal adhesions in regulating signal transmission between the matrix and the actin cytoskeleton.

Actin-Binding Proteins

A large number of actin-binding proteins have been identified, some of which are thought to play an important role in regulating the dynamics of actin polymerization. The scope of this review precludes a comprehensive discussion, and brief consideration will be directed to some of the findings most directly relevant to chemotactic signaling (see ref. 108 for a recent review).

Profilin is a 12-17 kDa protein which is associated with actin filaments in dynamic areas of the cell such as the leading lamellae and at the termini of newly-formed stress fibers.[108,119] In vitro profilin binds to actin, and phosphatidylinositol 4,5-bisphosphate (PIP_2). Earlier findings suggested that profilin had a strong inhibitory effect on actin polymerization, but it is now believed that the effect of this protein on actin polymerization may be considerably more complex. Profilin binds and sequesters G-actin, thus reducing the concentration of free actin monomers and lowering the rate of polymerization. On the other hand, profilin also stimulates ATP/ADP exchange on G-actin, thereby promoting actin polymerization.[120] Gelsolins are a large family of proteins, the most dominant form of which is 80 kDa and contains multiple actin binding sites.[108,121] Gelsolins are associated with focal adhesions and can both sever actin filaments and also cap the barbed (fast growing) ends of actin filaments.[121] Like profilin, gelsolin binds to PIP_2, and a role for this protein in modulating agonist-induced actin filament organization through PIP_2 hydrolysis has been proposed (see below).

Table 24.2. Cellular components implicated in cytoskeletal reorganization and cell migration

Focal Adhesion Components		Small GTP-binding proteins	SH2/SH3 Domain Proteins
β_1, β_3 Integrins	90-110 kDa	p21 rho	p85-a/PI3 kinase
Vinculin	116 kDa		pp60[src]
Tensin	215 kDa	p25 rac	p130[Cas]
Talin	220 kDa		GRB-2
Zyxin	82 kDa	Cdc42Hs	PLC-γ
α-actinin	90 kDa		Csk
FAK	125 kDa		Crk
FRNK	41-43 kDa		
Paxillin	68 kDa		

Components implicated in the signaling mechanisms underlying cytoskeletal reorganization and cell migration. Alpha-actinin is a cross-linking protein which binds to the cytoplasmic domain of beta-integrins, and to vinculin and zyxin. Talin binds to vinculin and beta-integrins in vitro. Tensin is tyrosine phosphorylated in reponse to integrin activation and in cells over-expressing p125[FAK]. Other components listed are discussed in the text. All non-standard terms and abbreviations are defined in the text.

Several lines of evidence suggest that the level of expression of actin-binding proteins may influence vascular cell motility. Gelsolin has been implicated in EGF-stimulated cell motility and in histamine-induced changes in actin filament organization in HUVEC.[122] Overexpression of both gelsolin and CapG did not have significant effects on actin filament content or organization, but did increase the rates of wound healing and chemotaxis. On the other hand, in rat aortic VSMC, it was reported that gelsolin protein and mRNA are reduced during intimal thickening induced by endothelial injury of rat aortas.[123]

Integrins

VSMC express β_1 and β_3 integrins as well as a variety of α subunits including α_v and α_1.[94,124-129] The β_1 integrin is constitutively expressed in most cells in the body[106] and this also appears to be true for VSMC.[127,128] In contrast, expression of β_3 is upregulated in VSMC by TGF-β and by PDGF-BB, and TGF-β was also reported to induce expression of α_1 subunits.[127,128] Recent results suggest that β_1 and β_3 integrins may have different functions in VSMC adhesion and migration. Thus, antibodies to β_1 inhibit attachment and spreading of rabbit arterial VSMC on collagen and fibronectin substrates[126] while osteopontin-stimulated migration of VSMC was inhibited by antibodies to β_3 but not anti-β_1 antibody.[94] Interestingly, it has been reported that in the early stages of VSMC migration β_1 integrins are organized into focal adhesions which gradually cover the basal surface of the cells, while β_3 integrins remain at the leading edges of cells.[129] These findings suggest that β_1 integrins are both necessary and probably sufficient for cell adhesion, while β_3 integrins may play a more specific role during chemotaxis or migration.

Most integrins have small cytoplasmic domains which lack any intrinsic enzymatic activity, and this suggests that the mechanisms involved in integrin-mediated signaling are fundamentally distinct from those of receptor PTKs or G-protein linked receptors. In the past few years it has become clear that integrin-mediated cell adhesion stimulates several signaling pathways.[106,130] In particular, it is now well established that activation of β_1 integrins in adherent cells induces tyrosine phosphorylation of focal adhesion kinase (FAK) and the focal adhesion-associated protein paxillin.[107,131-133] Attachment of fibroblasts, EC and lymphocytes to fibronectin also causes an increase in intracellular pH,[106] and this response is implicated in cell proliferation.[130] Attachment of Swiss 3T3 fibroblasts to fibronectin and laminin has also been reported to activate mitogen-activated protein (MAP) kinases,[134-6] but, as will be discussed below, the role of this pathway in cell migration is a matter of debate. Recent findings suggest that integrins may act synergistically with receptors for extracellular growth factors.[130] In particular, attachment of some cells to fibronectin and antibody-induced aggregation of the $\alpha_5\beta_1$ integrin enhances the increase in cytoplasmic pH stimulated by PDGF.[137] Such cooperative interactions may underlie the well known but poorly understood phenomenon of adhesion-dependent proliferation.

Focal Adhesion Kinase

FAK is a member of a growing family of protein tyrosine kinases (PTKs) which also includes the recently identified FAKB and PYK-2.[131-133,138,139] FAK was originally identified as one of a group of proteins that are highly tyrosine phosphorylated in chicken embryo fibroblasts transformed with the *v-src* oncogene.[140] The cDNA for FAK encodes a protein with a predicted molecular weight of 119-121 kDa depending on the species, though on the basis of its migration in gels it is often designated p125[FAK]. FAK is widely expressed in tissues, and is present in fibroblasts, VSMC, EC, platelets, lymphocytes, monocytes and neuronal cells. A 41-43 kDa protein corresponding to the noncatalytic carboxyl-terminal FAK domain, termed FRNK (FAK-related nonkinase) is autonomously expressed in some cells.[139] A salient feature of FAK is its subcellular localization to focal adhesions and this has stimulated intense interest in the role of this kinase in the regulation of cell adhesion, cytoskeletal organization and cell locomotion.[131-133]

The structure of FAK is unique, comprising a central catalytic region flanked by two large noncatalytic domains with no homologies to other PTKs (Fig. 24.1). Tyrosine phosphorylation of FAK is stimulated through the signal transduction pathways initiated by *v-src* transformation,[140,141] activation of β_1 integrins in fibroblasts[142-144] and α_{IIb}/β_3 integrins in platelets,[145,146] by aggregation of high-affinity IgE receptors in mast cells,[147] and in Swiss 3T3 fibroblasts by regulatory peptides including bombesin and endothelin[148,149] and by LPA[111] and sphingosine.[112] It was recently reported that tyrosine phosphorylation of FAK is also induced by hepatocyte growth factor in oral squamous cell carcinoma cells.[150] The integrity of the actin cytoskeleton is essential for FAK tyrosine phosphorylation.[68,111,112,118,149]

Much evidence suggests that the noncatalytic amino- and carboxyl-terminal domains mediate associations with integrins, other focal adhesion components, and signaling molecules.[132,133] Little is known about the function of the amino-terminal domain of FAK, but as mentioned above it may associate directly with the cytoplasmic domains of integrins.[151] The COOH-terminal noncatalytic domain is sufficient for targeting of FAK to focal adhesions[152] and is also implicated in the association of FAK with paxillin, a 68 kDa protein which colocalizes to focal contacts.[153] Bombesin, PDGF-BB, VEGF and cell adhesion to fibronectin all induce paxillin tyrosine phosphorylation in fibroblasts concomitantly with FAK phosphorylation[38,68,143,154] and paxillin is a putative substrate for FAK.[155,156] Paxillin has recently been molecularly cloned and its sequence reveals a number of interesting features, including a proline-rich region which is a potential binding site for SH3 domains, a putative binding region for the focal adhesion proteins talin and vinculin and several consensus binding sites for v-Crk.[157] Another component called p130[Cas] (Cas stands for Crk-associated substrate) is also tyrosine phosphorylated in response to bombesin concomitantly with FAK in Swiss 3T3 cells.[148] P130[Cas] contains an SH3 domain and multiple binding sites for v-Crk,[158] and has been shown to associate with FAK.[159,160]

Several factors which potently stimulate stress fiber and focal adhesion formation, including LPA, sphingosine

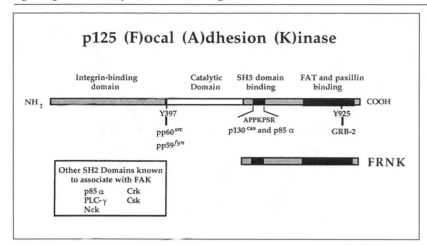

Fig. 24.1. The structure of FAK and its associations with other cellular components. The functions of the catalytic region and the noncatalytic amino and carboxy-terminal domains are indicated above the schematic. Paxillin is known to interact with the carboxy-terminal domain of FAK. Specific binding sites for pp60[Src], GRB-2 and p85α are indicated. A proline-rich sequence has been shown to interact with the SH3 domain of p85α. Other SH2 domain proteins reported to associate with FAK but for which the site of association is unknown are boxed.

and bombesin, also increase tyrosine phosphorylation of FAK. Recent findings have implicated FAK in the migration of other cell types.[150,161] In oral squamous cell carcinoma cells the protein tyrosine kinase inhibitor herbimycin blocked the stimulation of FAK tyrosine phosphorylation and cell migration by hepatocyte growth factor.[150] Intriguingly, the ECM glycosaminoglycan hyaluronan has been shown to promote both the rapid assembly and disassembly of focal adhesions and a rapid phosphorylation-dephosphorylation of FAK in a *c-H-ras*-transformed fibroblast cell line.[161] In VSMC and in EC, effects of several factors on FAK tyrosine phosphorylation correlate with a chemotactic response.[38,68] Results from our laboratory show that LPA induces FAK tyrosine phosphorylation and directed migration in rabbit aortic VSMC (Abedi H, Zachary I, unpublished observations). Angiotensin II stimulates FAK and paxillin tyrosine phosphorylation in rabbit VSMC (Abedi H, Zachary I, unpublished observations),[89] but as already indicated it is unclear whether this factor can induce a direct migratory response in VSMC. PDGF-BB stimulates FAK and paxillin tyrosine phosphorylation in VSMC through the β receptor[38,118] and VEGF stimulates FAK and paxillin tyrosine phosphorylation in human EC.[68] IGF-1 has been reported to stimulate FAK and paxillin tyrosine phosphorylation concomitantly with lammellipodial advance in neuroblastoma cells,[162] and our recent findings show that in VSMC, IGF-1 promotes tyrosine phosphorylation of FAK, directed migration and an increase in immunolocalization of FAK to focal adhesions (Abedi H, Lobo M, Zachary I, unpublished observations). Taken together, these findings suggest that tyrosine phosphorylation of FAK might represent a convergent point in the signaling pathways stimulated by several migration factors for vascular cells and other cell types. The role of FAK as a common target in the action of diverse factors and cell surface receptors is highlighted in Figure 24.2. FAK tyrosine phosphorylation may not be a common pathway for all migration factors, however. There are, for example, no reports to date that bFGF, a potent chemoattractant for EC, can regulate this pathway.

The signal transduction pathways which mediate tyrosine phosphorylation and presumably increased activity of FAK are unclear. LPA appears to act through a membrane

receptor coupled to two G-protein pathways, one pertussis-toxin sensitive which is implicated in activation of p21[Ras],[163] the other pertussis toxin-insensitive leading to activation of phospholipase C and tyrosine phosphorylation of FAK.[164,165] Consistent with the involvement of this second PLC-mediated pathway, LPA-induced stress fiber formation was pertussis toxin-insensitive.[113] Though FAK lacks both src homology-2 (SH2) and SH3 domains,[166] several recent reports indicate that FAK can associate with SH2 domain proteins. FAK was originally identified as a prominently tyrosine phosphorylated protein in *v-src*-transformed fibroblasts,[140] and it has subsequently been shown that FAK associates with pp60[c-src] and pp59[c-Fyn] via an interaction between the SH2 domain of Src-family PTKs and the major autophosphorylation site of FAK, Y397.[167] Several other SH2 domains (listed in Table 24.2) including those of the PDGF receptor substrates p85α,[168] GRB-2, NCK and phospholipase C-γ[169] have also been found to associate with FAK. Moreover, in the case of the GRB-2 SH2 domain, association appears to result from the tyrosine phosphorylation of FAK at a specific residue, Y925, induced by cell attachment to fibronectin.[170] Two other SH2 domain-containing proteins have recently been implicated in the regulation of focal adhesion-associated components. The adapter protein p47Crk associates with paxillin[171] and the carboxy-terminal src kinase (Csk), which phosphorylates and negatively regulates pp60[Src], has been shown to bind to both paxillin and FAK.[169,172] FAK also associates with SH3 domain-containing proteins. In platelets, FAK associates with the SH3 rather than the SH2 domain of the p85α subunit of phosphatidylinositol 3' kinase (PI3 kinase) via a proline-rich sequence (residues 706-711) in the noncatalytic carboxy-terminal domain of FAK_{128}.[170] The same FAK motif also mediates association with p130[Cas], and FAK-p130[Cas] complexes are enriched in cytoskeleton-associated fractions in an adhesion-dependent manner.[159,160] The associations of FAK with other cellular components are summarized in Figure 24.1.

Rho-Related GTP-binding Proteins

One of the most exciting developments in chemotactic signal transduction has been the discovery that

Fig. 24.2. FAK as a convergent point in signaling pathways for β_1 and β_3 integrins, receptor PTKs and seven transmembrane domain, G-protein coupled receptors. The diagram illustrates current evidence concerning the signal transduction mechanisms distal to FAK activation and downstream of FAK. Small GTP-binding proteins of the Rho/Rac family are implicated in mediating regulation of FAK tyrosine phosphorylation through G-protein coupled receptors and less certainly through the PDGF receptor. Integrin-dependent activation of FAK is thought to involve direct associations, possibly with the amino-terminal domain of FAK. The substrates of FAK which are important in vivo are still unknown, but FAK has been shown to associate in vivo and in vitro with several components in the focal adhesion (paxillin, talin) and with proteins containing either SH2 and/or SH3 domains (p130[Cas], Src, PI3 kinase). How signals are relayed from FAK through FAK-associated proteins to the focal adhesion remains unknown. Key: RPTK, receptor PTK; PI3K, PI3 kinase. Other nonstandard terms and abbreviations are defined in the text.

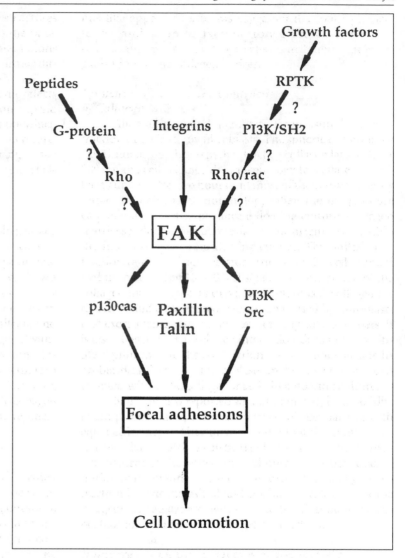

Ras-related small GTP-binding proteins of the Rho and Rac family are implicated in regulation of cytoskeletal organization.[115,117,173] The first evidence for the role of Rho proteins in actin filament organization came from studies of the exoenzyme C3 transferase, which is produced by the bacterium *Clostridium botulinum* and which ADP-ribosylates Rho at residue Asn 41 and thereby inactivates it. Introduction of C3 transferase into cells causes a loss of actin stress fibers.[173] Microinjection into fibroblasts of either wild type recombinant Rho proteins[174] or constitutively activated Rho proteins with a valine residue instead of glycine at residue 14[115] causes a rapid formation of stress fibers and an increase in the localization of the focal adhesion associated proteins vinculin and talin to focal adhesions. Importantly, introduction of either C3 transferase or of ADP-ribosylated and inactivated rhoA into cells blocked the stimulation of stress fiber formation and focal adhesion assembly caused by bombesin, LPA or serum.[115] Recent evidence suggests that Rho-related proteins perform specialized roles in the regulation of actin filament organization. While Rho appears to be important for stress fiber and focal adhesion formation, Rac promotes membrane ruffling and lammellipodia for-

mation and cdc42 induces peripheral actin microspikes and filipodia.[175,176]

Despite the interest in Rho and other members of the Rho/Rac family in regulating actin cytoskeleton organization, there are few studies of these proteins in vascular cells, and consequently their role in the migration (or other functions) of vascular cells remains poorly understood. A few studies have, however, implicated Rho in some biological responses in smooth muscle, including contractility and myosin light chain phosphorylation.[107]

Recent findings have implicated Rho in mediating phosphorylation of FAK (Fig. 24.2). C3 transferase inhibits FAK tyrosine phosphorylation induced either by LPA, bombesin or by the nonhydrolyzable GTP analog GTPγS.[165,177,178] Introduction of Rho into cells has also been shown to stimulate tyrosine phosphorylation of FAK, paxillin and p130[Cas].[179] These findings argue strongly that Rho is involved in the activation of FAK through some G-protein-coupled seven transmembrane domain receptors. Interestingly, it was reported that the SH2/SH3 domain protein crk, which as mentioned above binds to paxillin, associates via its SH3 domains with the guanine nucleotide exchange factor C3G.[180] Since C3G may regulate the activity of Ras proteins, this finding suggests that other small GTP-binding proteins may participate in the regulation of FAK and associated proteins in the focal adhesion complex.

Very little is known about the role of Rho family proteins in the activation of the FAK pathway through receptor tyrosine kinases. The recent finding that PDGF-BB stimulates an increase in the GTP-bound form of Rac, and that Rac activation is inhibited by the PI3 kinase inhibitor wortmannin,[181] suggests that this small GTP-binding protein may play a role in mediating PDGF stimulation of the FAK pathway (Fig. 24.2). Regardless of the precise sequence of interactions involved, it is likely that versatile proteins containing SH2 and SH3 modules will provide the crucial mediating links between the PDGF receptor, GTP-binding proteins of the Rho family and FAK.

How Rho is itself activated by these (or indeed any other) receptors is unclear, but recent progress has been made towards the identification of candidate downstream effectors which mediate the actions of Rho. Two serine/threonine protein kinases have been identified which associate with Rho, called Rho-kinase and PKN.[107] Rho-kinase has been reported to phosphorylate MLC in vitro.[182] The primary phosphorylation site for Rho-kinase, Ser19, is identical to the major phosphorylation site utilized by MLC kinase,[183] and phosphorylation of this residue is required to enable actin activation of the myosin ATPase.[184] Evidence supporting a direct role for Rho-kinase in stress fiber and focal adhesion formation has come from microinjection studies.[185] Rho has also been reported to stimulate phosphatidylinositol 4-phosphate 5-kinase (PI4P5K) which catalyzes formation of PIP_2 and promotes actin polymerization (see below). The central role of Rho in signaling pathways regulating actin cytoskeletal organization is illustrated in Figure 24.3.

Receptor Protein Tyrosine Kinase Signaling

Given the importance of ligands for receptor PTKs in the regulation of cell migration, it will be helpful to give a brief general discussion of some of the principal themes which have emerged in studies of receptor PTK activation and signal transmission. The PDGF receptor will serve as a

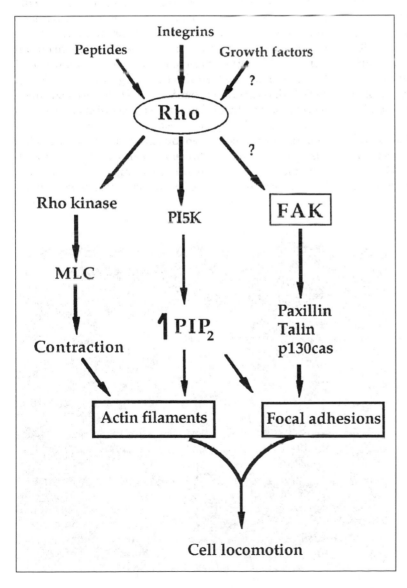

Fig. 24.3. The central role of Rho proteins in the regulation of actin cytoskeleton. Regulation of Rho activity is still poorly understood, partly because it has been difficult to directly measure Rho-bound GTP/GDP ratios. Studies with C3 exoenzyme and dominant negative Rho mutants suggest that Rho lies downstream of integrins and G-protein coupled receptors. Little evidence is available for receptor PTKs, though Rac may be activated by PDGF. Effectors for Rho include phosphatidylinositol 4-phosphate 5-kinase (PI5K) and Rho kinase. FAK activation may also be mediated by Rho, though the mechanism is unclear. Both PI5K and Rho-kinase have been shown to stimulate actin filament and focal adhesion formation. Effects of Rho-kinase may in part be mediated through phosphorylation of myosin. Key: MLC, myosin light chain. Other abbreviations are explained in the text.

paradigm. The receptor(s) for PDGF consists of an extracellular ligand-binding domain, a single membrane-spanning region and a cytoplasmic domain with intrinsic PTK activity. Binding of PDGF in the form of homo- or heterodimers of A and B chains induces dimerization of the receptor and subsequent receptor autophosphorylation. Autophosphorylation is thought to occur mainly by transphosphorylation of each dimerized receptor molecule by its partner. Homodimers of α and β receptors as well as α/β heterodimers have all been identified, but as indicated above the relative abundance of a given receptor dimer is highly dependent on cell-type and species. Dimerization and receptor autophosphorylation are essential for the activation of the receptor.[186] Subsequently, the receptor associates with and tyrosine phosphorylates its intracellular targets via SH2 domain interactions with specific tyrosine phosphorylated residues in the cytoplasmic domain of the receptor.[186,187]

Though an increasing number of the cellular components which are phosphorylated by the PDGF β receptor have been identified,[186,187] it remains unclear which components or intracellular signaling pathways specifically mediate the effects of PDGF-BB on cell migration and locomotion. In addition, most studies of PDGF Receptor signal transduction have been performed on the β receptor, which as discussed above is able to transduce mitogenic and chemotactic signals in a wide variety of cells. In contrast, α receptor signaling has not been intensively examined. As a result, little is known concerning either cell type-specific or receptor isotype-specific differences in PDGF signal transduction.[187]

The main features of the activation mechanism that have been identified for the PDGF receptor have also been demonstrated for other receptor PTKs. In some cases, however, the signal transduction mechanisms are not yet particularly well understood.[188-190] The VEGF receptor will serve as an example. The diverse biological effects of VEGF are mediated through two specific PTK receptors, KDR/Flk-1 and Flt-1. Both receptor isotypes are expressed in ECs[67] and Flt-1 is expressed in monocytes.[71] Expression of VEGF receptors has to date only been reported in these two cell types. KDR/Flk-1 is thought to be the receptor largely responsible for the angiogenic effects of VEGF and its mitogenic effects in EC.[191,192] The signal transduction pathways which mediate the diverse biological effects of VEGF either in EC or in monocytes remain unclear. Studies of VEGF signal transduction have so far produced varying results.[67,68,193,194] In porcine aortic EC which have been transfected either with KDR or Flt-1, VEGF stimulated migration and proliferation but had little effect on tyrosine phosphorylation of phospholipase C-γ (PLC-γ), p120 GTPase-activating protein (GAP) or on phosphatidylinositol 3 kinase (PI3 kinase) activity.[67] In contrast, VEGF has been reported to stimulate tyrosine phosphorylation of p120[GAP], PLC-γ and p85α subunit of PI3 kinase in bovine aortic EC and NIH 3T3.[193,194] Our recent findings show, however, that in HUVEC, VEGF activates MAP kinase and stimulates tyrosine phosphorylation of PLC-γ, FAK and paxillin.[68]

Phosphatidylinositol Lipids and Calcium

Many chemoattractants for vascular cells, including PDGF, IGF-1, bFGF and VEGF, stimulate hydrolysis of PIP$_2$ through the tyrosine phosphorylation and activation of PLC-γ. PIP$_2$ binds to the actin-binding proteins profilin and gelsolin. and it has been proposed that PIP$_2$ can modulate actin filament formation through the sequestration of actin-binding proteins like profilin and gelsolin. Anti-sense oligonucleotides to gelsolin and expression of a peptide which competes for the PIP$_2$-binding site on gelsolin both reduced epidermal growth factor-induced cell movement in NR6 cells.[195] In platelets, gelsolin-derived PIP$_2$-binding peptides also inhibited uncapping of F-actin induced by thrombin receptor activation.[196]

PIP$_2$ has also been reported to bind to vinculin and unmask its talin and actin binding sites, thereby promoting focal adhesion and stress fiber formation.[197] Profilin binding to PIP$_2$, the substrate of PLC-γ, inhibits PLC-γ activity and this inhibition is overcome by tyrosine phosphorylation. By effectively lowering the concentration of PIP$_2$, activation of PLC-γ can potentially promote actin filament disassembly both by raising the level of free profilin and gelsolin and by reducing its vinculin unmasking activity (Fig. 24.4). As indicated above, however, the role of profilin may be more complex. Another consequence of PIP$_2$ hydrolysis is the formation of inositol 1,4,5 trisphosphate, which in turn leads to the mobilization of intracellular Ca^{2+}. Ca^{2+} also affects the equilibrium between actin polymerization and depolymerization and also activates calcium-dependent enzymes such as Ca^{2+}/calmodulin-dependent protein kinase II and the Ca^{2+}/calmodulin-activated protein phosphatase calcineurin, both of which have been implicated in the regulation of VSMC migration (see Fig. 24.4).[198,199]

PIP$_2$ levels can be increased in cells through the activation of phosphatidylinositol 4-phosphate 5-kinase (PI4P5K). Overexpression of PI4P5K in COS-7 cells causes a striking increase in actin polymerization.[200] This kinase has been shown to be regulated by Rho,[201] thus providing a link with the pathway thought to be responsible for activation of FAK by bombesin and LPA and potentially of other factors which act through seven transmembrane domain, G-protein coupled receptors. It is not known which extracellular factors are responsible for activating PI4P5K, but it may be speculated that activation of this kinase and the consequent increase in cellular levels of PIP$_2$ may contribute to the striking increase in actin filament and focal adhesion formation caused by bombesin, LPA and other factors which activate FAK through a Rho-dependent pathway. Integrin engagement has also been reported to activate PI4P5K.[202]

PI3 Kinase

Activation of PI3 kinase is an early event in the action of several receptor PTK ligands, including PDGF-BB and IGF-1. Recent findings have implicated PI3 kinase in PDGF-induced chemotaxis.[203-205] PDGF-BB failed to stimulate migration in Chinese hamster ovary cells expressing mutant forms of the PDGFRβ which are unable to associate with the p85α subunit of PI3 kinase.[203] In addition, p85α/PI3 kinase has also been implicated in membrane ruffling induced by PDGF[204] and IGF-1.[205] PI3 kinase has also been implicated in mediating PDGF-stimulated FAK tyrosine phosphorylation. In Swiss 3T3 cells, inhibitors of PI3 kinase blocked PDGF-induced FAK and paxillin tyrosine phospho-

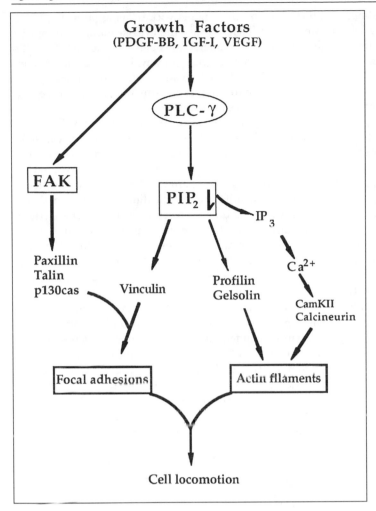

Growth Factors
(PDGF-BB, IGF-I, VEGF)

PLC-γ

FAK

PIP$_2$

IP$_3$

Paxillin
Talin
p130cas — Vinculin

Profilin
Gelsolin

Ca^{2+}

CamKII
Calcineurin

Focal adhesions

Actin filaments

Cell locomotion

Fig. 24.4. The role of phosphoinositide metabolism in the regulation of actin cytoskeleton organization. Many migration factors, particularly ligands for receptor PTKs, activate PLC-γ, leading to hydrolysis of PIP$_2$, and the generation of inositol 1,4,5-trisphosphate (IP$_3$). Hydrolysis of PIP$_2$ may release actin-binding proteins (profilin and gelsolin) which can promote depolymerization of actin. Similarly, since PIP$_2$ has been reported to allow vinculin to bind to talin and actin, thereby promoting focal adhesion formation, hydrolysis of PIP$_2$ may also reduce focal adhesion assembly. As explained in the text, at least in the case of profilin, the role of PIP$_2$-binding actin-associated proteins may be more complex than suggested by this model. Ca^{2+} mobilized from intracellular stores by IP$_3$ may also promote cell migration through its effects on Ca^{2+}/calmodulin-dependent protein kinase (CamKII) and calcineurin.

rylation without affecting stimulation by bombesin. The significance of these findings for cell migration are unclear, especially since PDGF causes a profound inhibition of FAK tyrosine phosphorylation, migration and actin cytoskeleton organization at concentrations higher than 10 ng/ml in the same cells. Our own studies in rabbit aortic VSMC indicate that the PI3 kinase inhibitors wortmannin and LY294002 at concentrations which inhibit PDGF-BB-stimulation of PI3 kinase activity do not impair either the migratory response to PDGF-BB or PDGF-BB-induced FAK tyrosine phosphorylation (Abedi H, Cospedal R, Zachary I, manuscript submitted).

Arachidonic Acid Metabolism

Studies in several cell types implicate arachidonic acid and products of its metabolism in chemotactic signaling. The best evidence so far is for a role of the products of the lipoxygenase pathway in the migration of monocytes and eosinophils. 5-oxo-15-HETE is a potent chemoattractant for eosinophils,[206,207] and other lipoxygenase products, lipoxin A4 and lipoxin B4, have been shown to stimulate chemotaxis of human monocytes.[208] Other studies have implicated the cytosolic phospholipase A$_2$, thought to catalyze the agonist-driven release of arachidonic acid, in migration of monocytes in response to the chemokines RANTES and MCP-1,[209] and in migration of EC stimulated by bFGF.[210]

The mechanisms by which products of arachidonic acid metabolism stimulate chemotaxis in vascular cells are at present not well understood.

Nitric Oxide

Recent evidence suggests that NO may play a role in angiogenesis and in the migration of both epithelial cells and EC.[211-213] In particular, NO production has been shown to be permissive for endothelin-induced migration of HUVECs.[213] These findings indicate that NO production is at least permissive for EC migration in response to factors such as endothelin, but the mechanism through which the NO pathway could act is unknown. Other EC migration factors may also act through the NO pathway. Our recent findings show that VEGF is able to induce NO production in EC (Zachary I, unpublished findings).

The MAP Kinase Pathway

Recent findings have established that the engagement of integrins can activate the MAP kinase pathway.[134-136] The role of integrin-mediated stimulation of this pathway in cytoskeletal changes is unclear, however. Thus, Clark and Hynes showed that while adhesion-dependent activation of Erk-2 is dependent upon Ras, inhibition of Ras signaling by expression of a dominant negative Ras mutant (N17Ras) blocked Erk-2 activation but had no effect either on FAK tyrosine phosphorylation or on cell adhesion, spreading, focal adhesion formation or stress fiber assembly.[136] Other investigators have provided evidence that integrin activation of Erks is mediated through Rho rather than Ras.[202] Integrins failed to activate Erk-1/2 in the absence of Rho/Rac activity, and integrin-dependent MAP kinase activity was blocked by C3 exoenzyme and was enhanced by expression of a constitutively active Rho mutant (RhoQ63L).[214] Though some chemoattractants for VSMC and EC, including PDGF-BB, activate the MAP kinase cascade, other factors such as IGF-1 stimulate chemotaxis of human VSMC without activation of MAP kinase.[37] These findings suggest that the MAP kinase pathway is at least not obligatory for VSMC migration, and it has been proposed that mitogenic and chemotactic signaling pathways can be fairly sharply dissociated.[37,215] A degree of functional segregation of signal transduction mechanisms underlying these processes is attractive, especially since the same factor (e.g., PDGF-BB) is often able to stimulate both mitogenesis and migration. It is possible, however, that MAP kinases may cooperate with other signaling pathways to augment a migratory response. Unpublished results from our laboratory show that a selective inhibitor, PD98059, of MAP kinase kinase, the enzyme which specifically phosphorylates and activates Erk 1 and 2, caused partial inhibition of PDGF-BB-stimulated migration without reducing FAK tyrosine phosphorylation. Stimulation of rat VSMC migration by PDGF-BB has also been shown to be partially inhibitable by PD98059.[216] Since IGF-1 is a less potent chemoattractant for VSMC than PDGF-BB, it might be speculated that activation of MAP kinase by the latter factor could help to explain this difference. This possibility remains to be tested.

Future Perspectives

Elucidation of the signal transduction mechanisms underlying the movement of cells remains a major unresolved problem in molecular cell biology. In the past few years, however, our understanding of these mechanisms has been transformed by the identification of a variety of components which are implicated in key cellular processes linked to cell locomotion, including assembly of focal adhesions and the formation of stress fibers. Neither the precise role played by these components in the molecular and cellular sequelae leading to cell migration nor the relationships and interactions between them have been defined as yet. Future effort will also need to address the relevance of putative chemotactic signaling pathways both for the action of specific migration factors and for the migration of vascular cells such as VSMC and EC.

This chapter has highlighted recent work suggesting that FAK and other focal adhesion-associated molecules may play a role in vascular cell migration in response to growth factor ligands for receptor PTKs. The latter notion is especially attractive in the light of recent findings that FAK has the ability to associate both with components of focal adhesions and with certain SH2 domain-containing substrates of the PDGF receptor. The role of small GTP-binding proteins of the Rho family has also been emphasized, as has the possibility that FAK and Rho proteins may be constituents

of a common signaling network relaying information between the cell surface and the cytoskeleton. More precise delineation of the interactions between the FAK and Rho pathways and of both with pathways involving proteins containing SH2 and SH3 domains, is likely to yield important new insights into the mechanisms underlying the regulation of vascular cell migration.

In the case of the most potent known VSMC migration factor, PDGF-BB, the migratory response appears to be determined by a complex interplay between surface expression of receptor isotypes, the bioavailability of ligand isoforms and other as yet unidentified cell type specific determinants. Identification of the differences in signaling in different cells via α and β receptor is likely to be a crucial prerequisite for understanding the mechanisms underlying the PDGF chemotactic response. It is plausible that alterations in the VSMC signaling pathways induced by PDGF and associated changes in biological responsiveness, mediated in part by changes either in autocrine/paracrine ligand production and/or receptor isotype expression, could also have important implications for our understanding of the mechanisms underlying the long term pathogenesis of atherosclerosis and other vascular pathologies. Whether a similar complexity underlies the chemotactic effects of other factors such as bFGF, IGF-1 and VEGF awaits further study.

A further challenge, with particular relevance to the vessel wall, is posed by the diversity of extracellular factors which may regulate vascular cell migration. It is probable that this diversity will grow and that the repertory of VSMC migration factors will be extended in the future both by the discovery of novel regulatory molecules and by identifying new functions for existing components of the hemostatic system. The dependence of VSMC migration on the complex interplay between diverse environmental factors has important ramifications for chemotactic signal transduction. The finding that FAK is a point of convergence in signaling mediated both by integrins and by several receptor PTKs raises the possibility that, in part at least, chemotactic signaling mechanisms through distinct receptors may share common features. It is equally likely that important differences also exist creating scope for complementary, crosstalk and synergistic interactions between different receptor-mediated pathways. Establishing the relationships between the pathways regulated by integrins, receptor PTKs, and other receptor types will be crucial for understanding the molecular basis of the migratory response in the vessel wall. The roles of metalloproteinases and the plasminogen activator system are likely to prove of particular importance for vascular cell migration in vivo.

Paracrine interactions between VSMC, EC, monocytes and other cells in the atherosclerotic microenvironment adds a further layer of complexity to the regulation of migration of vascular cells. The production of PDGF by EC in response to monocyte-, platelet- and T lymphocyte-derived cytokines, and the induction in VSMC of VEGF, an angiogenic factor whose target cells are monocytes and EC, are two striking examples of such interactions. The production of VEGF by VSMC and the role of this factor in promoting re-endothelialization may have a special relevance for tissue engineering of prosthetic grafts. The use of VEGF gene transfer for accelerating endothelial regrowth following balloon injury raises the possibility of using a similar approach to promote endothelial growth over prosthetic grafts.

Studies of the mechanisms regulating vascular cell migration have considerable implications for the clinical treatment of cardiovascular disease. One potentially important inference to be drawn from the experience of bypass graft surgery and the use of prosthetic grafts is that combinatorial therapeutic strategies aimed at either suppressing the migration of VSMC leading to stenosis, and/or at enhancing the migration of EC and thus promoting more effective re-endothelialization, may both constitute rational approaches for the treatment of the vasculoproliferative complications of arterial bypass grafting. Elucidation of the molecular mechanisms underlying vascular cell migration and the identification of cell type-specific migration factors will be of crucial importance in effectively targeting such therapies. The rapidly growing knowledge of signaling networks, together with the ability to isolate specific components and model component-specific agents, make the targeting of specific signal transduction components or pathways for the treatment of human disease increasingly an attainable goal. Understanding the mechanisms involved in vascular cell migration will therefore be of considerable value both in identifying novel targets for the design of new useful drugs, and for opening up novel perspectives for treatment of vasculoproliferative disorders.

Acknowledgments

The work on the regulation of FAK tyrosine phosphorylation in VSMC is supported by the British Heart Foundation. Dr. Ian Zachary is a BHF (Basic Science) Lecturer.

References

1. Ross R. The pathogenesis of atherosclerosis: A perspective for the 1990's. Nature 1993; 362:801-809.
2. Ross R. Cell biology of atherosclerosis. Annu Rev Physiol 1995; 57:791-804.
3. Wells N. Coronary heart Disease: The need for action. London: Office of Health Economics, 1987.
4. Wolfe JHN, Harris PL, Vaughan Ruckley C. Trust Hospitals and vascular Services. Br Med J 1994; 309:414-419.
5. Hillegass WB, Ohman EM, Califf RM. Restenosis: The clinical issues. In: Topol EJ, ed. Textbook of Interventional Cardiology. Philadelphia USA: W.B. Saunders Co., 1994:415-435.
6. Hertzer NR, Bevan EG, Young JR et al. Coronary disease in vascular patients. A Classification of 1000 coronary angiograms and the results of surgical management. Ann Surg 1984; 199:223-233.
7. Schwartz SM, Campbell GR, Campbell JH. Replication of Smooth Muscle Cells in Vascular Disease. Circ Res 1986; 58:427-444.
8. Pasic M, Muller-Glauser W, Odermatt B et al. Seeding with omental cells prevents late neointimal hyperplasia in small-diameter Dacron grafts. Circulation 1995; 92:2605-2616.
9. Zilla P, Preiss P, Groscurth P et al. In vitro-lined endothelium: Initial integrity and ultrastructural events. Surgery 1994; 116:524-534.
10. Wilcox JN, Smith KM, Williams LT et al. Platelet derived growth factor mRNA detection in human atherosclerotic plaques by in situ hybridisation. J Clin Invest 1988; 82:1134-1143.
11. Majesky MW, Reidy MA, Bowen-Pope DF et al. Role of PDGF-A expression in the control of vascular smooth muscle cell growth by TGF-β. J Cell Biol 1990; 111:2149-2158.
12. Golden MA, Au YPT, Kirkman TR et al. Platelet derived growth factor activity and mRNA expression in healing vascular grafts in baboons. J Clin Invest 1991; 87:406-414.
13. Jawien A, Bowen-Pope DF, Lindner V et al. Platelet derived growth factor promotes smooth muscle migration and intimal thickening in a rat model of balloon angioplasty. J Clin Invest 1992; 89:507-511.
14. Ferns GAA, Raines EW, Sprugel KH et al. Inhibition of neointimal smooth muscle accumulation after angioplasty by an antibody to PDGF. Science 1991; 253:1129-1132.
15. Stroobant P, Waterfield MD. Purification and properties of platelet-derived growth factor. EMBO J 1984; 3:2963-2967.
16. Hart CE, Bailey M, Curtis DA et al. Purification of PDGF-AB and PDGF-BB from human platelet extracts and identification of all three platelet derived growth factor dimers in human platelets. Biochemistry 1990; 29:166-172.
17. Hammacher A, Hellman U, Johnsson A et al. A major part of the platelet derived growth factor purified from human platelets is one A and one B chain. J Biol Chem 1988; 263:16493-16498.
18. Kavanaugh WM, Harsh GR, Starksen NF et al. Transcriptiocgulation of the A and B chain genes of platelet-derived growth factor in microvascular endothelial cells. J Biol Chem 1988; 263:8470-8472.
19. Daniel TO, Gibbs VC, Milfay DF et al. Agents that increase cAMP accumulation block endothelial c-sis induction by thrombin and transformtin growth factor-β. J Biol Chem 1987; 262:11893-11896
20. Starksen NF, Harsh GR, Gibbs VC et al. Regulated expression of the PDGF A chain gene in microvascular endothelial cells. J Biol Chem 1987; 262:14381-14384.
21. Newby AC, Henderson AH. Stimulus secretion coupling in vascular endothelial cells. Annu Rev Physiol 1990; 52:661-674.
22. Sejersen T, Betsholtz C, Sjolund M et al. Rat skeletal myoblasts and arterial smooth muscle cells express the gene for the A chain but not the gene for the B chain (c-sis) of platelet-derived growth factor (PDGF) and produce a PDGF-like protein. Proc Natl Acad Sci USA 1986; 83:6844-6848.
23. Majesky MW, Benditt EP, Schwartz SM. Expression and developmental control of PDGF-A chain and B chain/sis genes in rat aortic smooth muscle cells. Proc Natl Acad Sci USA 1988; 85:1524-1528.
24. Majack RA, Majesky MW, Goodman LV. Role of PDGF-A expression in the control of vascular smooth muscle cell growth by TGF-β. J Cell Biol 1990; 111:239-247.
25. Battegay EJ, Raines EW, Seifert RA et al. TGF-β induces bimodal proliferation of connective tissue cells via complex control of an autocrine PDGF loop. Cell 1990; 63:515-524.
26. Raines E, Dower S, Ross R. Interleukin-1 mitogenic activity for fibroblasts and smooth muscle cells is due to PDGF-AA. Science 1989; 243:393-396.
27. Nilsson J. Cytokines and smooth muscle cells in atherosclerosis. Cardiovasc Res 1993; 27:1184-1190.

28. Ross R, Masuda J, Raines EW et al. Localization of PDGF-B protein in macrophages in all phases of atherogenesis. Science 1990; 248:1009-1012.

29. Shimokado K, Raines EW, Madtes DK et al Significant part of macrophage-derived growth factor consists of at least two forms of PDGF. Cell 1985; 43:277-286.

30. Bowen-Pope DF, Hart CE, Seifert RA. Sera and conditioned media contain different isoforms of platelet-derived growth factor which bind to different classes of PDGF receptor. J Biol Chem 1989; 264:2502-2508.

31. Hart CE, Forstrom JW, Kelly JD et al. Two classes of PDGF receptor recognize different isoforms of platelet derived growth factor. Science 1988; 240:1529-1531.

32. Gronwald RGK, Grant FJ, Haldeman BA et al. Cloning and expression of a cDNA coding for the human platelet-derived growth factor receptor. Evidence for more than one receptor class. Proc Natl Acad Sci USA 1988; 85:3435-3439.

33. Seifert RA, Hart CE, Phillips PE et al. Two different subunits associate to create isoform-specific PDGF receptors. J Biol Chem 1989; 264:8771-8778.

34. Koyama N, Hart CE, Clowes, AW. Different functions of the PDGF α and β receptors for the migration and proliferation of cultured baboon smooth muscle cells. Circ Res 1994; 75:682-691.

35. Siegbahn A, Hammacher A, Westermark B et al. Differential effects of the various isoforms of PDGF in chemotaxis of fibroblasts, monocytes and granulocytes. J Clin Invest 1990; 85:916-920.

36. Koyama N, Morisaki N, Saito Y et al. Regulatory effects of PDGF-AA homodimer on migration of vascular smooth muscle cells. J Biol Chem 1992; 267:22806-22812.

37. Bornfeldt KE, Raines EW, Nakano T et al. Insulin-like growth factor-I and platelet-derived growth factor-BB induce directed dirceted migration of human arterial smooth muscle cells via signalling pathways that are distinct from those of proliferation. J Clin Invest 1994; 93:1266-1274.

38. Abedi H Dawes KE, Zachary I. Differential effects of platelet-derived growth factor BB on p125 focal adhesion kinase and paxillin tyrosine phosphorylation and on cell migration in rabbit aortic vascular smooth muscle cells and Swiss 3T3 fibroblasts. J Biol Chem 1995; 270:11367-11376.

39. Ferns GA, Sprugel KH, Seifert RA et al. Relative platelet-derived growth factor receptor subunit expression determines migration to different dimeric forms of PDGF growth factors. 1990; 3:315-324.

40. Higashiyama S, Abraham JA, Klagsbrun M. Heparin-binding EGF-like growth factor stimulation of smooth muscle cell migration: Dependence on interactions with cell surface heparan sulfate. J Cell Biol 1993; 122:933-940.

41. Delafontaine P, Bernstein KE, Alexander RW. Insulin-like growth factor I gene expression in vascular cells. Hypertension 1991; 17:693-699.

42. Newby AC, George SJ. Proposed roles for growth factors in mediating smooth muscle proliferation in vascular pathologies. Cardiovasc Res 1993; 27:1173-1183.

43. Cercek B, Fishbein MC, Forrester JS et al. Induction of insulin-like growth factor I messenger RNA in rat aorta after balloon denudation. Circ Res 1990; 66:1755-1760.

44. Jackson CL, Reidy MA. Basic fibroblast growth factor: Its role in the control of smooth muscle cell migration. Amer J Pathol 1993; 143:1024-1031.

45. Terranova VP, DiFloria R, Lyall R et al. Human EC are chemotactic to EC growth factor and heparin. J Cell Biol 1985; 101:2330-2334.

46. Sato Y, Rifkin DB. Inhibition of EC movement by pericytes and smooth muscle cells: Activation of a latent transformtin growth factor-β-like molecule by plasmin during coculture. J Cell Biol 1988; 107:1199-1205.

47. Tsuboi R, Sato Y, Rifkin DB. Correlation of cell migration, cell invasion, receptor number, proteinase production, and basic fibroblast growth factor levels in EC. J Cell Biol 1990; 110:511-517.

48. Lindner V, Majack RA, Reidy MA. Basic fibroblast growth factor stimulates endothelial regrowth and proliferation in denuded arteries. J Clin Invest 1990; 85:2004-2008.

49. Bjornsson TD, Dryjski M, Tluczek J et al. Acidic fibroblast growth factor promotes vascular repair. Proc Natl Acad Sci USA 1991; 88:8651-8655.

50. Koyama N, Harada K, Yamamoto A et al. Purification and characterisation of an autocrine migration factor for vascular smooth muscle cells (SMC), SMC-derived migration factor. J Biol Chem 1993; 268:13301-13308.

51. Ferrara N, Houck KA, Jakeman LB et al. Molecular and biological properties of the vascular endothelial growth factor family of proteins. Endocrine Rev 1992; 13:18-32.

52. Plate KH, Breier G, Weich HA et al. Vascular endothelial growth factor is a potential tumor angiogenesis factor in human gliomas in vivo. Nature 1992; 359:845-848.

53. Park JE, Chen HH, Winer J et al. Placenta growth factor: Potentiation of vascular endothelial growth factor bioactivity, in vitro and in vivo, and high-affinity binding to Flt-1 but not to Flk-1/KDR. J Biol Chem 1994; 269:25646-25654.

54. Olofsson B, Pajusola K, Kaipainen A et al. Vascular endothelial growth factor B, a novel growth factor for EC. Proc Natl Acad Sci USA 1996; 93:2576-2581.

55. Joukov V, Pajusola K, Kaipainen A et al. A novel vascular endothelial growth factor, VEGF-C, is a ligand for the Flt-4 (VEGFR-3) and KDR (VEGFR-2) receptor tyr kinases. EMBO J 1996; 15:290-298.

56. Stavri G, Zachary I, Baskerville P et al. Basic fibroblast growth factor upregulates the expression of vascular endothelial growth factor in vascular smooth muscle cells. Circulation 1995; 91:5-8.

57. Stavri G, Hong Y, Zachary I et al. Hypoxia and platelet-derived growth factor-BB synergistically upregulate the expression of vascular endothelial growth factor in vascular smooth muscle cells. FEBS Lett 1995; 358:311-315.

58. Brogi E, Wu T, Namiki A et al. Indirect angiogenic cytokines upregulate VEGF and bFGF gene expression in vascular smooth muscle cells, whereas hypoxia upregulates VEGF expression only. Circulation 1994; 90:649-652.

59. Liu Y, Cox SR, Morita T et al. Hypoxia regulates vascular endothelial growth factor gene expression in EC. Identification of a 5' enhancer. Circ Res 1995; 77:638-643.

60. Kourembanas S, Bernfield M. Hypoxia and endothelial-smooth muscle cell interactions in the lung. Am J Respir Cell Mol Biol 1994; 11:373-374.

61. Folkman J. Angiogenesis in cancer, vascular, rheumatoid and other disease. Nature Med 1995; 1:27-31.

62. Risau W. Mechanisms of angiogenesis. Nature 1997; 386:671-674.

63. Asahara T, Bauters C, Pastore C. et al. Local delivery of vascular endothelial growth factor accelerates reendothelialization and attenuates intimal hyperplasia in

balloon-injured rat carotid artery. Circulation 1995; 91:2793-2801.

64. Bauters C, Asahara T, Zheng LP et al. Recovery of disturbed endothelium-dependent flow in the collateral-perfused rabbit ischemic hindlimb after administration of vascular endothelial growth factor. Circulation 1995; 91:2802-2809.

65. Isner JM, Pieczek A, Schainfeld R, Blair R, Haley L, Asahara T, Rosenfield K, Razvi S, Walsh K, Symes JF. Clinical evidence of angiogenesis after arterial gene transfer of phVEGF$_{165}$ in patient with ischemic limb. Lancet 1996; 348:370-374.

66. Asahara T, Chen D, Tsurum, Y et al. Accelerated restitution of endothelial integrity and endothelial-dependent function after phVEGF$_{165}$ gene transfer. Circulation 1996; 94:3291-3302.

67. Waltenberger J, Claesson-Welsh L, Siegbahn A et al. Different signal transduction properties of KDR and Flt1, two receptors for vascular endothelial growth factor. J Biol Chem 1994; 269:26988-26995.

68. Abedi H, Zachary I. Vascular endothelial growth factor stimulates tyrosine phosphorylation and recruitment to new focal adhesions of focal adhesion kinase and paxillin in EC. J Biol Chem 1997; 272:15442-15451.

69. Connolly DT, Olander JV, Heuvelman D et al. Human vascular permeability factor. Isolation from U937 cells. J Biol Chem 1989; 264:20017-20024.

70. Clauss M, Gerlach H, Brett J et al. Vascular permeability factor: A tumor derived poypeptide that induces endothelial cell and monocyte procoagulant activity and monocyte migration. J Exp Med 1990; 172:1535-1545.

71. Clauss M, Weich H, Breier G et al. The vascular endothelial growth factor receptor Flt-1 mediates biological activities. J Biol Chem 1996; 271:17629-17634.

72. Barger AC, Beeuwkes R, Lainey LL et al. Hypothesis: Vasa vasorum and neo-vascularisation of human coronary arteries. Possible role in the pathophysiology of atherosclerosis. N Eng J Med 1984; 310:175-178.

73. Geiringer E. Intimal vascularisation and atherosclerosis. J Path Bacteriol 1951; 63:201-211.

74. O'Brien ER, Garvin MR, Dev R et al. Angiogenesis in human coronary atherosclerotic plaques. Amer J Pathol 1994; 145:883-894.

75. Bell L, Madri, JA. Influence of the angiotensin system on endothelial and smooth muscle cell migration. Amer J Pathol 1990; 137:7-12.

76. Mii S, Ware JA, Mallette SA et al. Effect of angiotensin II on human vascular smooth muscle cell growth. J Surg Res 1994; 57:174-178.

77. Daemen MJAP, Lombardi DM, Bosman FT et al. Angiotensin II induces smooth muscle cell proliferation in the normal and injured rat arterial wall. Circ Res.1991; 68:450-456.

78. Prescott MF, Webb RL, Reidy MA. Angiotensin-converting enzyme inhibitor versus angiotensin II, AT$_1$ receptor antagonist: Effects on smooth muscle cell migration and proliferation after balloon catheter injury. Amer Pathol 1991; 139:1291-1296.

79. Assoian RK, Fleurdelys BE, Stevenson HC et al. Expression and secretion of type beta transforming growth factor by activated human macrophages. Proc Natl Acad Sci USA 1987; 84:6020-6024.

80. Majesky MW, Lindner V, Twardzik DR et al. Production of transforming growth factor beta 1 during repair of arterial injury. J Clin Invest 1991; 88:904-910.

81. Assoian RK, Sporn MB. Type beta transforming growth factor in human platelets: release during platelet degranulation and action on vascular smooth muscle cells. J Cell Biol 1986; 102:1217-1223.

82. Koyama N, Koshikawa T, Morisaki N et al. Bifunctional effects of transformtin growth factor-β on migration of cultured rat aortic smooth muscle cells. Biochem Biophys Res Commun 1990; 169:725-729.

83. Nomoto A, Mutoh S, Hagihara H et al. Smooth muscle cell-migration induced by inflammatory cell products and its inhibition by a potent calcium antagonist, Nilvadipine. Atherosclerosis 1988; 72:213-219.

84. Yu X, Dluz S, Graves DT, Zhang L, Antoniades HN, Hollander W, Prusty S, Valente AJ, Schwartz CJ, Sonenshein GE. Elevated expression of monocyte chemoattractant protein 1 by vascular smooth muscle cells in hypercholesterolemic primates. Proc Natl Acad Sci USA 1992; 89:6953-6957.

85. Massague J. The transformtin growth factor-β family. Annu Rev Cell Biol 1990; 6:597-641.

86. Sato Y, Rifkin DB. Inhibition of endothelial cell movement by pericytes and smooth muscle cells: Activation of a latent transformtin growth factor-β1-like molecule by plasmin during coculture. J Cell Biol 1989; 109:309-315.

87. Singer SJ, Kupfer A. The directed migration of eukaryotic cells. Annu Rev Cell Biol 1986; 2:337-365.

88. Devroetes PN, Zigmund SH. Chemotaxis in eukaryotic cells: A focus on leukocytes and Dictyostelium. Annu Rev Cell Biol 1988; 4:649-686.

89. Koyama N, Koshikawa T, Morisaki N et al. Secretion of a potent new migration factor for smooth muscle cells (SMC) by cultured SMC. Atherosclerosis 1991; 86:219-226.

90. Naito M, Hayasi T, Funaki C et al. Vitronectin-induced haptotaxis of vascular smooth muscle cells in vitro. Exp Cell Res 1991; 194:154-156.

91. Giachelli CM, Bae N, Almeida M et al. Osteopontin is elevated during neointima formation in rat arteries and is a novel component of human atherosclerotic plaques. J Clin Invest 1993; 92:1686-1696.

92. Shanahan CM, Weissberg PL, Metcalfe JC. Isolation of gene markers of differentiated and proliferating vascular smooth muscle cells. Circ Res 1991; 73:193-204.

93. Liaw L, Almeida M, Hart CE et al. Osteopontin promotes vascular cell adhesion and spreading and is chemotactic for smooth muscle cells in vitro. Circ Res 1994; 74:214-224.

94. Yue TL, Mckenna RJ, Ohlstein EH et al. Osteopontin-stimulated vascular smooth muscle cell migration is mediated by β$_3$ integrin. Exp Cell Res 1994; 214:459-464.

95. Liau G, Chan LM. Regulation of extracellular matrix RNA levels in cultured smooth muscle cells. Relationship to cellular quiescence. J Biol Chem 1989; 264:10315-10320.

96. Nugent MA, Lane EA, Keski-Oja J et al. Growth stimulation, altered regulation of epidermal growth factor receptors and autocrine transformation of spontaneously transformed normal rat kidney cells by transformtin growth factor-beta. Cancer Res 1989; 49:3884-3890.

97. Lawrence R, Hartmann DJ, Sonenshein GE. Transforming growth factor β$_1$ stimulates type V collagen expression in bovine vascular smooth muscle cells. J Biol Chem 1994; 269:9603-9609.

98. DiMilla PA, Stone JA, Quinn JA et al. Maximal migration of human smooth muscle cells on fibronectin and

type IV collagen occurs at an intermediate attachment strength. J Cell Biol 1993; 122:729-737.

99. Southgate KM, Davies M, Booth RFG et al. Involvement of extracellular-matrix-degrading metalloproteinases in rabbit aortic smooth muscle cell proliferation. Biochem J 1992; 288:93-99.

100. Southgate KM, Fisher M, Banning AP et al. Upregulation of basement membrane-degrading metalloproteinase secretion after balloon injury of pig carotid arteries. Circ Res 1996; 79:1177-1187.

101. Kenagy RD, Vergel S, Mattsson E et al The role of plasminogen, plasminogen activators, and matrix metalloproteinases in primate arterial smooth muscle cell migration. Arterioscler Thromb Vasc Biol 1996; 16:1373-1382.

102. Okada SS, Grobmyer SR, Barnathan ES. Contrasting effects of plasminogen activators, urokinase receptor, and LDL receptor-related protein on smooth muscle cell migration and invasion. Arterioscler Thromb Vasc Biol 1996; 16:1269-1276.

103. Wang W, Chen HJ, Giedd KN et al. T-cell lymphokines, interleukin-4 and gamma-interferon modulate the induction of vascular smooth muscle cell tissue plasminogen activator and migration by serum and platelet-derived growth factor. Circ Res 1995; 77:1095-1106.

104. Noda-Heiny H, Sobel BE. Vascular smooth muscle cells migration mediated by thrombin and urokinase receptor. Am J Physiol 1995; 268: C1195-C1201.

105. Forough R, Koyama N, Hasenstab D et al. Overexpression of tissue inhibitor of matrix metalloproteinase-1 inhibits vascular smooth muscle cell functions in vitro and in vivo Circ Res 1996; 79:812-820.

106. Hynes RO. Integrins: Versatility, modulation and signalling in cell adhesion. Cell 1992; 69:11-25.

107. Burridge K, Chrzanowska-Wodnicka M. Focal adhesions, contractility, and signalling. Annu Rev Cell Dev Biol 1996; 12:463-519.

108. Jockusch BM, Bubeck P, Giehl K et al. The molecular architecture of focal adhesions. Annu Rev Cell Dev Biol 1995; 11:379-416.

109. Regan CM, Horvitz AF. Dynamics of β_1 integrin-mediated adhesive contacts in motile fibroblasts. J Cell Biol 1992; 117:1347-1359.

110. Schmidt CE, Horwitz AF, Lauffenburger DA et al. Integrin-cytoskeletal interactions in migrating fibroblasts are dynamic, asymmetric and regulated. J Cell Biol 1993; 123:977-991.

111. Seufferlein T, Rozengurt E. Lysophosphatidic acid stimulates tyrosine phosphorylation of focal adhesion kinase, paxillin and p130. Signalling pathways and crosstalk with platelet-derived growth factor. J Biol Chem 1994; 269:9345-9351.

112. Seufferlein T, Rozengurt E. Sphingosine induces focal adhesion kinase (FAK), and paxillin tyrosine phosphorylation, actin stress fiber formation and focal contact assembly in Swiss 3T3 cells. J Biol Chem 1994; 269:27610-27617.

113. Chrzanowska-Wodnicka M, Burridge K. Tyrosine phosphorylation is involved in reorganization of the actin cytoskeleton in response to serum or LPA stimulation. J Cell Sci 1994; 107:3643-3654.

114. Turner CE, Pietras KM, Taylor DS et al. Angiotensin II stimulation of rapid paxillin tyrosine phosphorylation correlates with the formation of focal adhesions in rat aortic smooth muscle cells. J Cell Sci 1995; 108:333-342.

115. Ridley. A, Hall A. The small GTP-binding protein rho regulates the assembly of focal adhesions and actin stress fibers. Cell 1992; 70:389-399.

116. Bar-Sagi D, Feramisco JR. Induction of membrane ruffling and fluid-phase pinocytosis in quiescent fibroblasts by ras proteins. Science 1986; 233:1061-1068.

117. Ridley A, Paterson HF, Johnston C L et al. The small GTP-binding protein rac regulates growth factor-induced membrane ruffling. Cell 1992; 70:401-410.

118. Rankin S, Rozengurt E. Platelet-derived growth factor modulation of focal adhesion kinase (FAK) and paxillin tyrosine phosphorylation in Swiss 3T3 cells. Bell shaped dose response and crosstalk with bombesin. J Biol Chem 1994; 269:704-710.

119. Haarer BK, Brown SS. Structure and function of profilin. Cell Motil Cytoskelet 1990; 17:71-74.

120. Theriot JA, Mitchieson TJ. The three faces of profilin. Cell 1993; 75:835-838.

121. Yin HL. Gelsolin: Calcium- and polyphosphoinositide-regulated actin-modulating protein. Bioessays 1987; 7:176-179.

122. Carson MR, Shasby SS, Lind SE, Shasby DM. Histamine, actin-gelsolin binding, and polyphosphoinositides in human umbilical vein EC. Am J Physiol 1992; 263: L664-L669.

123. Chaponnier C, Kocher O, Gabbiani G. Modulation of gelsolin content in rat aortic smooth muscle cells during development, experimental intimal thickening and culture. Eur J Biochem 1990; 190:559-565.

124. Clyman RI, McDonald KA, Kramer RH. Integrin receptors on aortic smooth muscle cells mediate adhesion to fibronectin, laminin and collagen. Circ Res 1990; 67:175-186.

125. Clyman RI, Turner DC, Kramer RH. An α_1/β_1-like integrin receptor on rat aortic smooth muscle cells mediates adhesion to laminin and collagen types I and IV. Arteriosclerosis 1990; 10:402-9.

126. Yamamoto K, Yamamoto M. Cell Adhesion receptors for native and denatured type I collagens and fibronectin in rabbit arterial smooth muscle cells in culture. Exp Cell Res 1994; 214:258-263.

127. Janat MF, Argraves WS, Liau G. Regulation of vascular smooth muscle cell integrin expression by transformtin growth factor-β and platelet-derived growth factor-BB. J Cell Physiol 1992; 151:588-595.

128. Basson CT, Kocher O, Basson MD et al. Differential modulation of vasuclar cell integrin and extracellular matrix expression in vitro by transformtin growth factor-b1 correlates with reciprocal effects on cell migration. J Cell Physiol 1992; 153:118-128.

129. Clyman RI, Mauray F, Kramer RH. β_1 and β_3 integrins have different roles in the adhesion and migration of vascular smooth muscle cells on extracellular matrix. Exp Cell Res 1992; 200:272-284.

130. Damsky CH, Werb Z. Signal transduction by integrin receptors for extracellular matrix: Cooperative processing of extracellular information. Curr Opin Cell Biol 1992; 4:772-781.

131. Zachary I, Rozengurt E. Focal adhesion kinase (FAK): A point of convergence in the action of neuropeptide, integrins and oncogenes. Cell 1992; 71:891-894.

132. Schaller MD, Parsons JT. Focal adhesion kinase and associated proteins. Curr Opin Cell Biol 1994; 6:705-710.

133. Abedi H, Zachary I. Signalling mechanisms in the regulation of vascular cell migration. Cardiovasc Res 1995; 30:544-556.

134. Chen Q, Kinch MS, Lin TH et al. Integrin-mediated cell adhesion activates mitogen-activated protein kinases. J Biol Chem 1994; 269:26602-26605.

135. Morino N, Mimura T, Hamasaki K et al. Matrix-integrin interaction activates the mitogen-activated protein kinase, pp44erk-1 and pp42erk-2. J Biol Chem 1995; 270:269-273.

136. Clark EA, Hynes RO. Ras activation is necessary for integrin-mediated activation of extracellular signal-regulated kinase 2 and cytosolic phospholipase A_2 but not for cytoskeletal organization. J Biol Chem 1996; 271:14814-14818.

137. Schwartz MA, Lechene C. Adhesion is required for protein kinase c-dependent activation of the Na^+/H^+ antiporter by PDGF. Proc Natl Acad Sci USA 1992; 89:6138-6141.

138. Lev S, Moreno H, Martinez R et al. Protein tyrosine kinase PYK-2 is involved in Ca^{2+}-induced regulation of ion channel function and MAP kinase functions. Nature 1995; 376:737-745.

139. Richardson A, Parsons JT. A mechanism for regulation of the adhesion-associated tyrosine kinase p125 focal adhesion kinase. Nature 1996; 380:538-540.

140. Kanner SB, Reynolds AB, Vines RR et al. Monoclonal antibodies to individual tyrosine phosphorylated protein subtrates of oncogene encoded tyrosine kinases. Proc Natl Acad Sci USA 1990; 87:3328-3332.

141. Guan J-L, Shalloway D. Regulation of focal adhesion associated protein tyrosine kinase by both cellular adhesion and oncogenic transformation. Nature 1992; 358:690-692.

142. Hanks SK, Calalb MB, Harper MC et al. Focal adhesion protein tyrosine kinase phosphorylated in response to cell attachment to fibronectin. Proc Natl Acad Sci USA 1992; 89:8487-8491.

143. Burridge K, Turner CE, Romer LH. Tyrosine phosphorylation of paxillin and p125 focal adhesion kinase accompanies cell adhesion to extracellular matrix: A role in cytoskeletal assembly. J Cell Biol 1992; 119:893-903.

144. Kornberg L, Earp HS, Parsons JT et al. Cell adhesion or integrin clustering increases phosphorylation of a focal adhesion associated tyrosine kinase. J Biol Chem 1992; 267:23439-23442.

145. Lipfert L, Haimovich B, Schaller MD et al. Integrin-dependent phosphorylation and activation of the protein tyrosine kinase p125 focal adhesion kinase (FAK) in platelets. J Cell Biol 1992; 119:905-912.

146. Huang M-M, Lipfert L, Cunningham M et al. Adhesive ligand binding to integrin alpha (IIb) beta 3 stimulates tyrosine phosphorylation of novel protein substrates before phosphorylation of p125 focal adhesion kinase (FAK). J Cell Biol 1993; 122:473-483.

147. Hamawy MM, Mergenhagen SE, Siraganian RP. Tyrosine phosphorylation of p125 focal adhesion kinase (FAK) by the aggregation of high affinity immunoglobin E receptors requires cell adherence. J Biol Chem 1993; 268:6851-6854.

148. Zachary I, Sinnett-Smith J, Rozengurt E. Bombesin, vasopressin and endothelin stimulation of tyrosine phosphorylation in Swiss 3T3 cells. Identification of a novel tyrosine kinase as a major substrate. J Biol Chem 1992; 267:19031-19034.

149. Sinnett-Smith J, Zachary I, Valverde A et al. Bombesin stimulation of FAK focal adhesion kinase tyrosine phos-

phorylation. Role of Protein kinase c, Ca^{2+} mobilisation, and the actin cytoskeleton. J Biol Chem 1993; 268:14261-14268.

150. Matsumoto K, Matsumoto K, Nakamura T et al. Hepatocyte growth factor/ scatter factor induces tyosine phosphorylation of focal adhesion kinase (FAK) and promotes migration and invasion by oral squamous cell carcinoma cells. J Biol Chem 1994; 269:31807-31813.

151. Schaller MD, Otey CA, Hildebrand JD et al. Focal adhesion kinase and paxillin binds to peptides mimicking β integrin cytoplasmic domains J Cell Biol 1995; 130:1181-1187.

152. Hildebrand JD, Schaller MD, Parsons JT. Identification of sequences required for the efficient localization of the focal adhesion kinase, p125 focal adhesion kinase (FAK), to cellular focal adhesions. J Cell Biol 1993; 123:993-1005.

153. Turner CE, Glenny JR Jr, Burridge K. Paxillin: A new vinculin binding protein present in focal adhesions. J Cell Biol 1990; 111:1059-1068.

154. Zachary I, Sinnett-Smith J, Turner C et al. Bombesin, vasopressin and endothelin stimulate tyrosine phosphorylation of the focal adhesion-associated protein paxillin in Swiss 3T3 cells. J Biol Chem 1993; 268:22060-22065.

155. Turner CE, Schaller MD, Parsons JT. Tyrosine phosphorylation of the focal adhesion kinase p125 focal adhesion kinase (FAK) during development: Relation to paxillin. J Cell Sci 1993; 105:637-645.

156. Tachibana K, Sato T, D'Avirro N et al. Direct association of pp125^{FAK} with paxillin, the focal adhesion-targetting mechanism of pp125^{FAK}. J Exp Med 1995; 182:1089-1100.

157. Salgia R, Li J-L, Lo SH et al. Molecular cloning of human paxillin, a focal adhesion protein phosphorylated by p210$^{BCR/ABL}$. J Biol Chem 1995; 270:5039-5047.

158. Sakai R, Iwamatsu A, Hirano N et al. A novel signalling molecule, p130, forms stable complexes in vivo with v-Crk and v-Src in a tyrosine phosphorylation-dependent manner. EMBO J 1994; 13:3748-3756.

159. Polte TR, Hanks SK. Interaction between focal adhesion kinase and Crk-associated tyrosine kinase substrate p130^{Cas}. Proc Natl Acad Sci USA 1995; 92:10678-10682.

160. Polte TR, Hanks SK. Complexes of focal adhesion kinase (FAK) and Crk-associated substrate (p130^{Cas}) are elevated in cytoskeleton-associated fractions following adhesion and src transformation J Biol Chem 1997; 272:5501-5509.

161. Hall CL, Wang C, Lange LA et al. Hyaluronan and the hyaluronan receptor RHAMM promote focal adhesion kinase turnover and transient tyrosine kinase activity J Cell Biol 1994; 126:575-588.

162. Leventhal PS, Shelden EA, Kim B et al. Tyrosine phosphorylation of paxillin and focal adhesion kinase during insulin-like growth factor-I-stimulated lamellipodial advance J Biol Chem 1997; 272:5214-5218.

163. van Corven EJ, Hordijk PL, Medema RH et al. Pertussis toxin-sensitive activation of p21^{ras} by G protein-coupled receptor agonists in fibroblasts. Proc Natl Acad Sci USA 1993; 86:1259-1261.

164. Hordijk RJ, Verlaan L, van Corven PL et al. Protein tyrosine phosphorylation induced by lysophosphatidic acid in Rat-1 fibroblasts. Evidence that phosphorylation of MAP kinase is mediated by the Gi-p21^{ras} pathway. J Biol Chem 1994; 269:645-651.

165. Kumagai N, Morii N, Fujisawa K et al. ADP-ribosylation of Rho p21 inhibits lysophosphatidic acid -induced protein tyrosine phosphorylation and phosphatidylinositol

3-kinase activation in cultured Swiss 3T3 cells. J Biol Chem 1993; 268:24535-24538.

166. Schaller MD, Borgman CA, Cobb BS et al. P125 focal adhesion kinase, a structurally distinctive protein-tyrosine kinase associated with focal adhesions. Proc Natl Acad Sci USA 1992; 89:5192-5196.

167. Cobb BS, Schaller MD, Leu T-H et al. Stable association of pp60^{Src} and pp59^{fyn} with the focal adhesion-associated protein tyrosine kinase, p125 focal adhesion kinase. Mol Cell Biol 1994; 14:147-155.

168. Chen H-C, Guan J-L. Association of focal adhesion kinase with its potential substrate phosphatidylinositol 3-kinase. Proc Natl Acad Sci USA 1994; 91:10148-10152.

169. Schlaepfer DD, Hanks SK, Hunter T et al. Integrin-mediated signal transduction linked to Ras pathway by GRB2 binding to focal adhesion kinase. Nature 1994; 372:786-791.

170. Guinebault C, Payrastre B, Racaud-Sultan C et al. Integrin-dependent translocation of phosphoinositide 3-kinase to the cytoskeleton of thrombin-activated platelets involves specific interactions of p85α with actin filaments and focal adhesion kinase. J Cell Biol 1995; 129:831-842.

171. Birge RB, Fajardo JE, Reichman C et al. Identification and characterisation of a high-affinity interaction between v-Crk and tyrosine-phosphorylated paxillin in CT 10-transformed fibroblasts. Mol Cell Biol 1993; 13:4648-4656.

172. Sabe H, Hata A, Okada M et al. Analysis of the binding of the Src homology 2 domain of Csk to tyrosine-phosphorylated proteins in the suppression and mitotic activation of C-src. Proc Natl Acad Sci USA 1994; 91:3984-3988.

173. Ridley A. Rho-related proteins: Actin cytoskeleton and cell cycle. Curr opin Gen and Develop 1995; 5:24-30.

174. Paterson HF, Self AJ, Garrett MD et al. Microinjection of recombinant p21rho induces rapid changes in cell morphology. J Cell Biol 1990; 111:1001-1007.

175. Kozma R, Ahmed S, Best A, Lim L. The ras-related protein cdc42Hs and bradykinin promote formation of peripheral actin microspikes and filipodia in Swiss 3T3 fibroblasts. Mol Cell Biol 1995; 15:1942-1952.

176. Nobes CD, Hall A. Rho, rac and cdc42 GTPases regulate the assembly of multimolecular focal complexes associated with actin stress fibers, lamellipodia and filopodia. Cell 1995; 81:53-62.

177. Rankin S, Morii N, Narumiya S et al. Botulinum C3 exoenzyme blocks the tyrosine phosphorylation of FAK and paxillin induced by bombesin and endothelin. FEBS Letts 1994; 354:315-319.

178. Seckl M, Morii N, Narumiya S et al. Guanine 5'-3-O-(thio)triphosphate stimulates tyrosine phosphorylation of FAK and paxillin in permeabilized Swiss 3T3 cells. J Biol Chem 1995; 270:6984-6990.

179. Flinn HM, Ridley AJ. Rho stimulates tyrosine phosphorylation of focal adhesion kinase, p130 and paxillin. J Cell sci 1996; 109:1133-1141.

180. Tanaka S, Morishita T, Hashimoto Y et al. C3G, a guanine nucleotide-releasing protein expressed ubiquitously, binds to the Src homology 3 domains of CRK and GRB2/ASH. Proc Natl Acad Sci USA 1994; 91:3443-3447.

181. Hawkins PT, Eguinoa A, Qui R-G et al. PDGF stimulates an increase in GTP-Rac via activation of phosphoinositide 3-kinase. Curr Biol 1995; 5:393-403.

182. Amano M, Ito M, Kimura K et al. Phosphorylation and activation of myosin by Rho-associated kinase (Rho-kinase) J Biol Chem 1996; 271:20246-20249.

183. Ikebe M, Hartshorne DJ. Effects of Ca2+ on the conformation and enzymatic activation of smooth muscle myosin. J Biol Chem 1985; 260:10027-10031.

184. Kamisoyama H, Araki Y, Ikebe M. Mutagenesis of the phosphorylation site (serine 19) of smooth muscle myosin regulatory light chain and its effects on the properties of myosin. Biochemistry 1994; 33:840-847.

185. Amano M, Chihara K, Kimura K et al. Formation of actin stress fibers and focal adhesions enhanced by rho-kinase. Science 1997; 275:1308-1311.

186. Cantley LC, Auger KR, Carpenter C et al. Oncogenes and signal transduction. Cell 1991; 64:281-302.

187. Claesson-Welsh L. Platelet-derived growth factor receptor signals. J Biol Chem 1994; 269:32023-32026.

188. de Vries C, Escobedo JA, Ueno H, Houck K, Ferrara N, Williams LT. The fms-like tyrosine kinase, a receptor for vascular endothelial growth factor. Science 1992; 255:989-991.

189. Matthews W, Jordan CT, Gavin M, Jenkins NA, Copeland NG, Lemischka IR. A receptor tyrosine kinase cDNA isolated from a population of enriched primitive hematopoietic cells and exhibiting close genetic linkage to c-kit. Proc Natl Acad Sci USA 1991; 88:9026-9030.

190. Quinn TP, Peters KG, De Vries C, Ferrara N, Williams LT. Fetal liver kinase-1 is a receptor for vascular endothelial growth factor and is selectively expressed in vascular endothelium. Proc. Natl. Acad. Sci. USA 1993; 90:7533-7537.

191. Millauer B, Wizigmann-Voos S, Schnuch H, Martinez R, Moller NPH, Risau W, Ullrich A. High affinity VEGF binding and developmental expression suggest Flk-1 as a major regulator of vasculogenesis and angiogenesis. Cell 1993; 72:835-846.

192. Shweiki D, Itin A, Neufeld G, Gitay-Goren H, Keshet E. Patterns of expression of vascular endothelial growth factor (VEGF) and VEGF receptors in mice suggest a role in hormonally regulated angiogenesis. J. Clin. Invest. 1993; 91:2235-2243.

193. Guo D, Jia Q, Song H-Y, Warren RS, Donner DB. Vascular endothelial cell growth factor promotes tyrosine phosphorylation of mediators of signal transduction that contain SH2 domains. J Biol Chem 1995; 270:6729-6733.

194. Seetharam L, Gotoh N, Maru Y, Neufeld G, Yamaguchi S, Shibuya M. A unique signal transduction from Flt tyrosine kinase, a receptor for vascular endothelial growth factor VEGF. Oncogene 1995; 10:135-147.

195. Chen P, Murphy-Ullrich JE, Wells A. A role for gelsolin in actuating epidermal growth factor receptor-mediated cell motility. J Cell Biol 1996; 134:689-698.

196. Hartwig JH, Bokoch GM, Carpenter CL et al. Thrombin receptor ligation and activated Rac uncap actin filament barbed ends through phosphoinositide synthesis in permeabilized human platelets. Cell 1995; 82:643-653.

197. Gilmore AP, Burridge K. Regulation of vinculin binding to talin and actin by phosphatidylinositol-4-5-bisphosphate. Nature 1996; 381:531-535.

198. Pauly RR, Bilato C, Sollott SJ et al. Role of calcium/calmodulin dependent protein kinase II in the regulation of vascular smooth muscle cell migration. Circulation 1995; 91:1107-1115.

199. Lawson MA, Maxfield FR. Ca2+-and calcineurin-dependent recycling of an integrin to the front of migrating neutrophils. Nature 1995; 377:75-79.

200. Shibasaki Y, Ishihara H, Kizuki N et al. Massive actin polymerization induced by phosphatidylinositol-4-phosphate 5-kinase in vivo J. Biol Chem 1997; 272:7578-7581.

201. Chong LD, Traynor-Kaplan A, Bokoch GM et al. The small GTP-binding protein Rho regulates a phosphatidylinositol 4-phosphate 5-kinase in mammalian cells. Cell 1994; 79:507-513.

202. Renshaw MW, Toksoz D, Schwartz MA. Involvement of the small GTPase Rho in integrin-mediated activation of mitogen-activated protein kinase. J Biol Chem 1996; 271:21691-21694.

203. Kundra V, Escobedo JA, Kazlauskas A et al. Regulation of chemotaxis by the platelet-derived growth factor receptor-beta. Nature 1994; 367:474-476.

204. Wennstrom S, Siegbahn A, Yokote K et al. Membrane ruffling and chemotaxis transduced by the PDGF beta receptor require the binding site for phosphatidylinositol 3' kinase. Oncogene 1994; 9:651-660.

205. Kotani K, Yonezawa K, Hara K et al. Involvement of phosphoinositide 3-kinase in insulin- or IGF-1-induced membrane ruffling. EMBO J 1994; 13:2313-2321.

206. Powell WS, Chung D, Gravel S. 5-oxo-6,8,11,14-eicosatetraenoic acid is a potent stimulator of human eosinophil migration. J Immunol 1995; 154:4123-4132.

207. Schwenk U, Schroder JM. 5-oxo-eicosanoids are potent eosinophil chemotactic factors. J Biol Chem 1995; 270:15029-15036.

208. Maddox JE, Serhan CN. Lipoxin A4 and B4 are potent stimuli for human monocyte migration and adhesion: Selective inactivation by dehydrogenation and reduction. J Exp Med 1996; 183:137-146.

209. Locati M, Lamorte G, Luini W, Introna M, Bernasconi S, Mantovani A, Sozzani S. Inhibition of monocyte chemotaxis to C-C chemokines by antisense oilgonucleotide for cytosolic phospholipase A$_2$. J Biol Chem 1996; 271:6010-6016.

210. Sa G, Fox PL. Basic fibroblast growth factor-stimulated EC movement is mediated by a pertussis toxin-sensitive pathway regulating phospholipase A$_2$ activity. J Biol Chem 1994; 269:3219-3225.

211. Leibovich SJ, Polverini PJ, Fong TW et al. Production of angiogenic activity by human monocytes requires an L-arginine/nitric oxide-synthase-dependent effector mechanism. Proc Natl Acad Sci USA 1994; 91:4190-4194.

212. Noiri E, Peresleni T, Srivastava N et al. Nirtric oxide is necessary for a switch from stationary to locomoting phenotype in epithelial cells. Am J Physiol 1996; 270:C794-C802.

213. Noiri E, Hu Y, Bahou WF et al. Permissive role of nitric oxide in endothelin-induced migration of endothelial cells. J Biol Chem 1997; 272:in press.

214. Hotchin NA, Hall A. The assembly of inyegrin adhesion complexes requires both extracellular matrix and intracellular rho/rac GTPases. J Cell Biol 1995; 131:1857-1865.

215. Bornfeldt KE. Intracellular signalling in arterial smooth muscle: Migration versus proliferation. Trends Cardiovasc Med 1996; 6:143-151.

216. Graf K, Xi XP, Yang D et al. Mitogen-activated protein kinasde activation is involved in platelet-derived growth factor-directed migration by vascular smooth muscle cells. Hypertension 1997; 29:334-339.

Facilitation of Healing

Chemotaxis

CHAPTER 25

Adhesion Molecules: Potent Inducers of Endothelial Cell Chemotaxis

Zoltan Szekanecz, Alisa E. Koch

Introduction

Angiogenesis, the formation of new blood vessels, plays an important role in a number of physiological processes including development and tissue repair. Thus, it may also be involved in the integration of newly implanted vascular grafts. Neovascularization is also essential in a number of pathological situations, such as atherosclerosis, diabetic angiopathy, rheumatoid arthritis, psoriasis and tumor growth.[1-3]

During angiogenesis, endothelial cells produce proteolytic enzymes, which leads to the degradation of the basement membrane, followed by the emigration of endothelial cells. Although there is another chapter on angiogenesis in this volume, here we will discuss the role of cellular adhesion molecules and adhesive mechanisms in the induction of endothelial cell migration and chemotaxis, which are essential steps in capillary formation. There is evidence that certain adhesion molecules and extracellular matrix molecules may be chemotactic for endothelial cells and thus may stimulate the migration of these cells into sites of angiogenesis. It is possible that the induction of endothelial cell migration and neovascularization around the vascular graft may facilitate its healing.

In this chapter, we will summarize our current understanding of the role of adhesion factors in endothelial cell migration and chemotaxis. We will discuss the involvement of extracellular matrix components and cellular adhesion molecules in these processes, also highlighting our recently published data on recombinant, soluble adhesion molecule-induced endothelial cell chemotaxis and neovascularization. We will also discuss the interactions of other soluble mediators, such as growth factors and cytokines, with extracellular matrix molecules and cellular adhesion molecules during endothelial cell migration and angiogenesis. With regard to vascular surgery, we will present information on the role of cellular adhesion molecules in the formation of human abdominal atherosclerotic aortic aneurysms, as well as in wound healing. These data may support our theory that, after vascular graft implantation, extracellular matrix macromolecules and cellular adhesion molecules are involved in attracting endothelial cells and in the formation of new capillaries. Thus, the induction of adhesion molecule expression may stimulate the revascularization of the surrounding extracellular matrix, enhance blood supply and enable the survival of the graft.

Tissue Engineering of Prosthetic Vascular Grafts, edited by Peter Zilla and Howard P. Greisler
©1999 R.G. Landes Company.

The Role of Extracellular Matrix Macromolecules in Endothelial Cell Motility During Vessel Formation

The extracellular matrix surrounding the emigrating endothelial cells consists of two major compartments: the basement membrane and the interstitial extracellular matrix. The basement membrane contains various extracellular matrix macromolecules synthesized by the endothelium, including mainly type IV collagen and laminin, but also other types of collagen, fibronectin, proteoglycans, entactin and thrombospondin.[1,4-6] Many of these extracellular matrix components play a role in the direction of endothelial cells during capillary formation.[4-6] The interstitial, extravascular extracellular matrix contains mainly type I collagen, as well as other extracellular matrix components including fibronectin, fibrinogen, vitronectin, tenascin and thrombospondin.[4-6]

It has been postulated that endothelial cell migration and chemotaxis are stimulated by type I, and, to a lesser extent types II, III, IV and V collagen.[1,7-9] In the in vitro collagen gel assay, capillary endothelial cells adhere to type I collagen, acquire elongated morphology, begin to produce extracellular matrix components, and form tubular structures when placed within, but not when layered onto, the gel.[6,10] These data suggest that collagen types in the interstitial extracellular matrix stimulate endothelial cell chemotaxis. Fibronectin is also chemotactic for endothelial cells, promotes the elongation of microvessels in explant cultures in vitro and wound healing in vivo.[1,8,11,12] Laminin is secreted during endothelial cell proliferation[1] and is chemotactic for human endothelial cells.[8] Matrigel, a laminin-rich basement membrane-like substrate, induces endothelial cell migration and the formation of new vascular structures.[9,13] Tenascin is also an important stimulator of endothelial sprouting.[14] Fibrinogen also promotes endothelial cell motility.[15] Heparin and heparan sulfate proteoglycans are essential for neovascularization, as a number of angiogenic growth factors bind to these proteoglycans in the extracellular matrix.[1-3] Heparin itself is chemotactic for human endothelial cells and potentiates the chemotactic effect of growth factors.[8]

In contrast to other extracellular matrix components described above, thrombospondin-1, which interacts with a number of other extracellular matrix components such as heparin, fibronectin, fibrinogen and collagen, inhibits endothelial cell chemotaxis to basic fibroblast growth factor as reported by most investigators.[16,17] The downregulation of the thrombospondin-1 gene expression by antisense oligonucleotides resulted in increased bovine aortic endothelial cell chemotaxis to basic fibroblast growth factor on collagen gels.[17] Others, however, reported that soluble thrombospondin-1 itself was chemotactic for bovine aortic and murine lung capillary endothelial cells. This chemotactic effect was highly β_3 integrin-dependent, as determined by blocking studies using monoclonal antibody to this integrin.[18] It is likely that, while recombinant thrombospondin-1 promotes endothelial cell migration, it suppresses the chemotactic effect of angiogenic mediators, such as basic fibroblast growth factor.

The endothelial cell cytoskeleton is reorganized during endothelial cell migration and capillary formation on Matrigel. These processes can be blocked in vitro by colchicine, cytochalasin D and cycloheximide, indicating the involvement of microfilaments, microtubules and active protein synthesis, respectively.[19]

Adhesion Molecules in Endothelial Cell Migration and Angiogenesis

Cellular adhesion molecules play an important role in endothelial cell adhesion to and migration into the extracellular matrix (Table 25.1). Endothelial cells also utilize a number of cellular adhesion molecules for their adhesion to each other, as well as to other cell types. Endothelial cell-extracellular matrix interactions are mostly mediated by integrins, while intercellular adhesion molecules include the $\alpha_4\beta_1$ integrin, all β_2 (leukocyte) integrins, members of the immunoglobulin superfamily of cellular adhesion molecules, selectins, cadherins and other cellular adhesion molecules.[20-24]

Among integrins, the $\alpha_1\beta_1$ and $\alpha_2\beta_1$ heterodimers mediate endothelial cell adhesion to types I and IV collagen, as well as to laminin.[20-22,24-26] The main endothelial cell laminin

---

Table 25.1. Endothelial cellular adhesion molecules involved in endothelial cell migration and neovascularization.

Cellular adhesion molecule superfamily	Adhesion molecule receptor*	Reference(s)
1. Integrins	β_1 integrins (most)	10, 18, 24, 25, 29-31
	β_3 integrins ($\alpha_v\beta_3$)	
2. Immunoglobulin superfamily	Vascular cell adhesion molecule-1	23, 27, 35
	CD31	
3. Selectins	E-selectin	24, 27, 35
4. Cadherins	VE-cadherin	23
5. Others	Sialyl Lewis-X	23, 24, 32-34
	CD34	
	Endoglin	

* See text for cellular adhesion molecule ligands and more information.

receptor, however, is $\alpha_6\beta_1$. There are two important receptors for fibronectin, the RGD (arginine-glycine-aspartic acid)-dependent $\alpha_5\beta_1$, as well as the RGD-independent $\alpha_4\beta_1$.[20-22,24,25] The former is present on most endothelial cells,[25] while we and others have confirmed that $\alpha_4\beta_1$ is also expressed by some endothelial cells.[27,28] Another fibronectin, laminin and collagen receptor, $\alpha_3\beta_1$, is also present on endothelial cells.[25,26] Integrins containing the β_3 subunit are involved in endothelial cell adhesion to fibronectin, vitronectin, thrombospondin, von willebrand factor and fibrinogen. The α_v integrin subunit can be associated with several β chains (β_1, β_3, β_5, β_6, β_8), and mediates endothelial cell adhesion to a variety of extracellular matrix components, depending on the β subunit.[20-22,25,26]

Extracellular matrix binding integrins can be classified into subgroups of "basement membrane" (collagen-laminin)-binding integrins ($\alpha_1\beta_1$, $\alpha_2\beta_1$, $\alpha_3\beta_1$ and $\alpha_6\beta_1$) and "inflammatory matrix" integrins (fibronectin-fibrinogen receptors: $\alpha_4\beta_1$, $\alpha_5\beta_1$, α_v and β_3). While microvessels express the former, but not the latter type of integrins in situ, cellular adhesion molecules belonging to both subgroups are present on capillary endothelial cells in vitro. These data suggest that endothelial cells have a potential to alter their cellular adhesion molecule profile during vascular morphogenesis.[25] Additional studies have shown that the $\alpha_2\beta_1$ molecule is involved in type I collagen-induced endothelial cell migration and neovascularization.[10,24] The $\alpha_v\beta_3$ molecule was found to be involved in endothelial cell migration on vitronectin.[24] $\alpha_v\beta_3$ is necessary for capillary formation in tumors and wound granulation tissue and promotes endothelial cell cord formation in vitro.[29,30] It has recently been shown that the $\alpha_v\beta_3$ integrin is required for the survival and maturation of new blood vessels.[30] As described above, β_3 integrins may also be important in thrombospondin-1-mediated endothelial cell chemotaxis.[18] The $\alpha_6\beta_1$ integrin stimulates angiogenesis on Matrigel.[31]

Adhesion molecules mediating endothelial cell adhesion to other cells include vascular cell adhesion molecule-1, intercellular adhesion molecules-1 and -2, CD31, E- and P-selectin, CD34 and other carbohydrate ligands for L-selectin, and the transformtin growth factor-β1 receptor endoglin.[20-23,32,33] Antibodies to E-selectin, as well as to its ligands sialyl Lewis-X and sialyl Lewis-A, inhibit the migration and tube formation of capillary endothelial cells.[24,34] CD31 has been implicated in tumor-associated neovascularization.[35] The L-selectin ligand CD34 shows high endothelial cell expression in developing tissues and healing wounds.[32]

Endothelial adherens junctions, which contain clustered cellular adhesion molecules and other membrane proteins, were also implicated in endothelial cell migration, adhesion and angiogenesis. VE-cadherin, a major constituent of these junctions, mediates homophilic binding between endothelial cells. Many other adhesive proteins, such as CD31, CD34, endoglin, occludin and connexins show colocalization with VE-cadherin.[23] As endothelial cells bind to each other through these cellular adhesion molecules, these cells can migrate in organized clusters during capillary formation.

We have recently shown the role of certain soluble, recombinant endothelial cellular adhesion molecules in endothelial cell chemotaxis, as well as in vivo neovascularization. Soluble vascular cell adhesion molecule-1 and soluble E-selectin have been tested in endothelial cell chemotaxis assays in vitro and the rat corneal neovascularization model in vivo.[27] Recombinant E-selectin and vascular cell adhesion molecule-1 as chemotactic factors dose-dependently increased the chemotaxis of human umbilical vein endothelial cells and dermal microvascular endothelial cells above the basal level. The chemotactic action of these soluble cellular adhesion molecules was comparable to that of basic fibroblast growth factor, a "classical" angiogenic mediator. We have also shown in checkerboard analyses that both soluble E-selectin and soluble vascular cell adhesion molecule-1 were chemotactic rather than chemokinetic for endothelial cells. These soluble cellular adhesion molecules seem to be mediating a direct effect, as they did not stimulate umbilical endothelial cells to produce the angiogenic basic fibroblast growth factor, tumor necrosis factor-α or interleukin-8 in vitro.[27]

In addition, monoclonal antibodies to the E-selectin ligand sialyl Lewis-X and to the vascular cell adhesion molecule-1 counterreceptor $\alpha_4\beta_1$ integrin on endothelial cells, significantly reduced soluble cellular adhesion molecule-mediated human umbilical vein endothelial cell chemotaxis. We and others have detected both sialyl Lewis-X and $\alpha_4\beta_1$ on umbilical vein endothelial cells by immunohistochemistry.[27,30] Although sialyl Lewis-X has been implicated in bovine capillary morphogenesis in vitro,[34] our novel results suggest a link between the soluble E-selectin-sialyl Lewis-X, as well as soluble vascular cell adhesion molecule-1-$\alpha_4\beta_1$, adhesion pathways, which mediate leukocyte-endothelial cell interactions, endothelial cell recruitment and angiogenesis.[27] These data are supported by those of other investigators showing that sugars, which are also major constituents of selectins and sialyl Lewis-X, are chemotactic for bovine corneal endothelial cells.[36] In the rat corneal neovascularization assay both soluble cellular adhesion molecules induced in vivo capillary formation at low concentrations in most experiments. We have also shown in neutralization studies that soluble E-selectin and soluble vascular cell adhesion molecule-1 account for a portion of rheumatoid arthritic synovial fluid-mediated chemotactic activity for human umbilical vein endothelial cells.[27]

In summary, we have shown that soluble E-selectin and soluble vascular cell adhesion molecule-1 may act as proangiogenic factors. They may directly trigger the migration and chemotaxis of endothelial cells by binding to their respective endothelial cell ligands.[27]

Interactions of Soluble Mediators with Cellular Adhesion Molecules and Extracellular Matrix Components During Endothelial Cell Recruitment and Neovascularization

Cellular adhesion molecules and extracellular matrix macromolecules may interact with other soluble mediators during endothelial cell migration and neovascularization. In fact, basic fibroblast growth factor treatment of endothelial cells in vitro resulted in an increased expression of the integrin subunits α_2, α_3, α_5, α_6, β_1, β_3, β_4 and β_5, as well as in better adherence to type I collagen, fibronectin, laminin and vitronectin compared to untreated cells.[37,38] Interactions between basic fibroblast growth factor, thrombospondin and cellular adhesion molecules have also been demonstrated. Thrombospondin inhibits angiogenesis by blocking the effects of basic fibroblast growth factor on endothelial cell chemotaxis.[16,17,39] In addition, thrombospondin receptors, such as β_3 integrins, have been implicated in endothelial cell migration and neovascularization.[18,26,30]

Transformtin growth factor-β and basic fibroblast growth factor differentially modulate the integrin profile on human microvascular endothelial cells, as transformtin growth factor-β downregulates integrin expression on human dermal microvascular endothelial cells, both at the mRNA and protein level.[38,40] This growth factor also inhibits fibronectin-mediated endothelial cell chemotaxis.[40] One receptor for transformtin growth factor-$\beta1$, endoglin, contains an RGD motif and thus serves as a cellular adhesion molecule for endothelial cells.[23,33] We found increased, well correlated expression of endoglin and transformtin growth factor-$\beta1$ in the highly vascularized synovium of rheumatoid arthritis patients.[33]

Treatment of endothelial cells with tumor necrosis factor-α stimulates $\alpha_1\beta_1$ expression and adhesion to laminin, while the combination of tumor necrosis factor-α and interferon-g downregulates $\alpha v \beta 3$ expression on these cells, suggesting the modulating effect of angiogenic and angiostatic mediators in endothelium-extracellular matrix interactions.[26] Tumor necrosis factor-α can also induce the expression of intercellular adhesion molecule-1, vascular cell adhesion molecule-1, E-selectin and some integrins on synovial and other types of endothelial cells.[3,20,21,25,26] The increasing production of endothelial cellular adhesion molecules may result in the perpetuated shedding of these cellular adhesion molecules from the cell surface. The serum and synovial fluid concentrations of soluble E-selectin and soluble vascular cell adhesion molecule-1 are high in rheumatoid arthritis, a well-known "angiogenic disease".[41,42] As described above, these soluble cellular adhesion molecules, in turn, may stimulate endothelial cell chemotaxis and angiogenesis.[27]

Chemokines, which are chemotactic for endothelial cells, as well as for leukocytes, may also be involved in this regulatory network. Some C-X-C chemokines containing the ELR motif, such as interleukin-8, have high angiogenic activity and they promote endothelial cell chemotaxis. In contrast, C-X-C chemokines lacking the ELR sequence, such as interferon-inducible protein-10 and platelet factor IV, inhibit endothelial cell migration and angiogenesis.[43] Although very little is known about the effects of C-X-C chemokines on cellular adhesion molecules, interleukin-8 stimulates β_2 integrin expression on neutrophils,[44] while interferon-inducible protein-10 induces integrin-dependent T cell adhesion to fibronectin, laminin and collagen, as well as to recombinant human intercellular adhesion molecule-1 and vascular cell adhesion molecule-1.[45] There are a number of data available showing that C-C chemokines such as RANTES, macrophage inflammatory protein-1α and monocyte chemoattractant protein-1 stimulate the expression and avidity of both β_1 and β_2 integrins on T cells and monocytes.[45,46] These chemokines also promote the adhesion of mononuclear cells to extracellular matrix components, as well as recombinant human intercellular adhesion molecule-1 and vascular cell adhesion molecule-1.[45,46] However, most of these data are available on leukocytes, and not on endothelial cells. Therefore, the possibility that either C-X-C or C-C chemokines may also influence endothelial cell migration and chemotaxis via the modulation of endothelial cell adhesion molecule expression needs to be elucidated.

The Relevance of Angiogenesis Studies in Vascular Surgery: Aortic Aneurysms and Wound Healing

We have performed a number of studies on the possible role of angiogenic mediators and adhesion molecules in the pathogenesis of human abdominal aortic aneurysms. In this disease, atherosclerotic and inflammatory mechanisms occurring in the aneurysm wall are accompanied by the escalation of neovascularization. Small vessels of the vasa vasorum in the adventitial layer proliferate and the migration of endothelial cells into the aortic wall plays an important role in the formation of new vessels and the growth of aneurysm.[47-50]

Our immunohistochemical analysis carried out on aortic aneurysm explants revealed that there was an increased expression of intercellular adhesion molecule-1 on endothelial cells found in aortic aneurysm tissues compared to normal control aortas.[50] Moreover, aortic aneurysm explants released significantly more soluble intercellular adhesion molecule-1 into their culture supernatants than did normal aortic tissues.[47] We have used human aortic endothelial cell culture as an in vitro model for studying the interactions of angiogenic cytokines and cellular adhesion molecules. The angiogenic cytokine tumor necrosis factor-α stimulated intercellular adhesion molecule-1 expression of, and soluble intercellular adhesion molecule-1 production by, these endothelial cells compared to control, unstimulated aortic endothelial cells.[47] We have also determined that aortic aneurysm explants produce more tumor necrosis factor-α, interleukin-6 and interleukin-8 into their conditioned media, than do normal aortic tissues.[48,49,51,52] These cytokines induced neovascularization in both in vitro and in vivo models for angiogenesis.[2,3,53-55] Moreover, we have shown, that tumor necrosis factor-α and interleukin-8 account for a portion of aortic aneurysm-associated endothelial cell chemotaxis.[48]

Thus, soluble angiogenic and chemotactic mediators and certain cellular adhesion molecules, at least intercellular adhesion molecule-1, can be detected in aortic aneurysm tissues. The increased production of these mediators results in increased endothelial intercellular adhesion molecule-1 expression. In conclusion, the interactions of angiogenic and chemotactic cytokines with cellular adhesion molecules may be important in the perpetuation of endothelial cell recruitment and capillary formation underlying the growth of aortic aneurysms.

Regarding wound healing, in the normal skin cellular adhesion molecule expression is restricted to the basal layer of the epidermis. These cellular adhesion molecules mediate the adhesion of the basal cells to the basement membrane.[56,57] During injury and wound healing, cellular adhesion molecules, mostly β_1 and β_3 integrins, appear in the suprabasal layers of the skin, accompanied by the influx of fibroblasts and endothelial cells, their adhesion to fibronectin, vitronectin and fibrinogen, as well as angiogenesis and scarring.[56,58] Similarly, we have found strong vascular cell adhesion molecule-1, P-selectin and CD44 expression in the injured, desquamating skin of scleroderma patients.[57]

A Regulatory Network in Sites of Endothelial Cell Migration: Potential Target Promoting Graft Healing

In conclusion, in "angiogenic states", such as rheumatoid arthritis, aortic aneurysms, wound healing or vascular graft implantation, cellular adhesion molecules such as β_1 and β_3 integrins, vascular cell adhesion molecule-1, E-selectin, sialyl Lewis-X and others, as well as extracellular matrix molecules including collagen, fibronectin, laminin, tenascin, fibrinogen and heparin may be involved in endothelial cell chemotaxis, migration and adhesion to extracellular matrix components. A number of soluble mediators secreted mainly by macrophages and endothelial cells in the extracellular matrix may interact with these cellular adhesion molecules and extracellular matrix components. Some of these factors, such as basic fibroblast growth factor, tumor necrosis factor-α, and possibly chemokines may induce cellular adhesion molecule expression on and shedding from the endothelial cell surface. Increased cellular adhesion molecule expression may result in stronger endothelial cell adhesion to extracellular matrix components. As we and others have suggested, soluble, and possibly surface-bound endothelial cellular adhesion molecules can act as direct mediators of endothelial cell migration and angiogenesis. In addition, as one of the possible ligands for E-selectin is closely related to basic fibroblast growth factor, these cellular adhesion molecules may also participate in neovascularization-associated signaling triggered by other mediators. Thus, the complex interactions between endothelial cells, extracellular matrix macromolecules, cellular adhesion molecules and other angiogenic factors may lead to the perpetuation of angiogenesis. There are antagonistic factors, such as transformtin growth factor-b and thrombospondin-1, which inhibit endothelial cell chemotaxis, as well as neovascularization. The net balance of these factors result in the perpetuation or downregulation of endothelial cell migration in the sites of angiogenesis. The detection of these factors, as well as functional studies using in vitro chemotaxis assays or in vivo animal models, can lead us to the better understanding of the role of adhesive mechanisms around the healing vascular graft (Fig. 25.1).

In addition, targeting cellular adhesion molecules, extracellular matrix components or other angiogenic mediators by local injections of any mediators described above may result in the local enhancement of endothelial cell chemotaxis and neovascularization, and thus may be useful for the healing and the prolonged survival of implanted vascular grafts. Recently, putative progenitor endothelial cells for angiogenesis were isolated from human peripheral blood. These originally hematopoietic stem cells carry the CD34 antigen, as well as Flk-1, a receptor for the angiogenic vascular endothelial growth factor. While mononuclear cells lose these two antigens during in vivo differentiation, progenitor cells plated onto fibronectin attach and become spindle-shaped within days, and continue expressing CD34 and Flk-1, as well as endothelial cell marker cellular adhesion molecules, such as E-selectin and CD31. In in vivo animal models of hindlimb ischemia, where one femoral artery is excised, the progenitor endothelial cells isolated by magnetic bead separation using anti-CD34 or anti-Flk-1 monoclonal

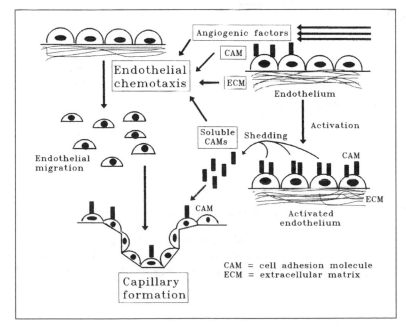

Fig. 25.1. Interactions between cellular adhesion molecules, extracellular matrix components and angiogenic mediators in the regulation of endothelial migration and angiogenesis. See text for details.

antibodies migrated into sites of ischemia and angiogenesis. Preliminary data suggest that these endothelial cells, possibly with the administration of angiogenic cytokines that enhance endothelial cell migration, could be used in autologous endothelial cell transplantation in order to promote neovascularization.[59] Similar techniques may be applied in vascular surgery as well.

Acknowledgments

This work was supported by NIH grants AR30692 and AR41492 (A.E.K.), funds from the Veterans' Administration Research Service (A.E.K.), Hungarian Scientific Foundation grant No. T013239 (Z.S.) and Hungarian Medical Research Council grant No. 156/93 (Z.S.).

References

1. Colville-Nash PR, Scott DL. Angiogenesis in rheumatoid arthritis: Pathogenic and therapeutic implications. Ann Rheum Dis 1992; 51:919-925.
2. Folkman J, Shing Y. Angiogenesis. J Biol Chem 1992; 267:10931-10934.
3. Klagsbrun M, D'Amore PA. Regulators of angiogenesis. Annu Rev Physiol 1991; 53:217-239.
4. Diaz-Flores L, Gutierrez R, Varela H. Angiogenesis: An update. Histol Histopathol 1994; 9:807-843.
5. Sage EH, Vernon, RB. Regulation of angiogenesis by extracellular matrix: The growth and the glue. J Hypertens 1994; 12(Suppl 10):S145-S152.
6. Montesano R, Pepper MS, Vassalli J-D et al. Modulation of angiogenesis in vitro. EXS 1991; 59:129-136.
7. Madri JA, Williams KS. Capillary endothelial cell cultures: Phenotypic modulation by matrix components. J Cell Biol 1983; 97:153-165.
8. Terranova VP, DiFlorio R, Lyall RM et al. Human endothelial cells are chemotactic to endothelial cell growth factor and heparin. J Cell Biol 1985; 101:2330-2334.
9. Garrido T, Riese HH, Aracil M et al. Endothelial cell differentiation into capillary-like structures in response to tumour cell conditioned medium: A modified chemotaxis chamber assay. Br J Cancer 1995; 71:770-775.
10. Jackson CJ, Jenkins K, Schrieber L. Possible mechanisms of type I collagen-induced vascular tube formation. EXS 1991; 59:198-204.
11. Nicosia RF, Bonanno E, Smith M. Fibronectin promotes the elongation of microvessels during angiogenesis in vitro. J Cell Physiol 1993; 154:654-661.
12. Clark RA. Potential roles of fibronectin in cutaneous wound repair. Arch Dermatol 1988; 124:201-206.
13. Schnaper HW, Kleinman HK, Grant DS. Role of laminin in endothelial cell recognition and differentiation. Kidney Int 1993; 43:20-25.
14. Canfield AE, Schor AM. Evidence that tenascin and thrombospondin-1 modulate sprouting of endothelial cells. J Cell Sci 1995; 108:797-809.
15. Dejana E, Languino LR, Polentarutti N et al. Interaction between fibrinogen and cultured endothelial cells. Induction of migration and specific binding. J Clin Invest 1985; 75:11-18.
16. Vogel T, Guo NH, Krutzsch HC et al. Modulation of endothelial cell proliferation, adhesion, and motility by recombinant heparin-binding domain and synthetic peptides from the type I repeats of thrombospondin. J Cell Biochem 1993; 53:74-84.
17. DiPietro LA, Nebgen DR, Polverini PJ. Downregulation of endothelial cell thrombospondin 1 enhances in vitro angiogenesis. J Vasc Res 1994; 31:178-185.
18. Taraboletti G, Roberts D, Liotta LA et al. Platelet thrombospondin modulates endothelial cell adhesion, motility, and growth: A potential angiogenesis regulatory factor. J Cell Biol 1990; 111:765-772.
19. Grant DS, Lelkes PI, Fukuda K. et al. Intracellular mechanisms involved in basement membrane induced blood vessel differentiation in vitro. In Vitro Cell Dev Biol 1991; 27A: 327-336.
20. Albelda SM, Buck CA. Integrins and other cell adhesion molecules. FASEB J 1990; 4:2868-2880.
21. Springer TA. Adhesion receptors of the immune system. Nature 1990; 346:425-433.
22. Szekanecz Z, Szegedi G. Cell surface adhesion molecules: Structure, function, clinical importance. Orv Hetil 1992; 133:135-142.
23. Dejana E. Endothelial adherens junctions: Implications in the control of vascular permeability and angiogenesis. J Clin Invest 1996; 98:1949-1953.
24. Bischoff J. Approaches to studying cell adhesion molecules in angiogenesis. Trends Cell Biol 1995; 5:69-74.
25. Albelda SM. Differential expression of integrin cell-substratum adhesion receptors on endothelium. EXS 1991; 59:188-192.
26. Defilippi P, Bozzo C, Geuna M et al. Modulation of extracellular matrix receptors (integrins) on human endothelial cells by cytokines. EXS 1991; 59:193-197.
27. Koch AE, Halloran MM, Haskell CJ et al. Angiogenesis mediated by soluble forms of E-selectin and vascular cell adhesion molecule-1. Nature 1995; 376:517-519.
28. Massia SP, Hubbell JA. Vascular endothelial cell adhesion and spreading promoted by the peptide REDV of the IIICS region of plasma fibronectin is mediated by integrin alpha 4 beta 1. J. Biol Chem. 1992; 267:14019-14026.
29. Brooks PC, Clark RA, Cheresh DA. Requirement of vascular integrin alpha v beta 3 for angiogenesis. Science 1994; 264:569-571.
30. Brooks PC, Montgomery AM, Rosenfeld M et al. Integrin alpha v beta 3 antagonists promote tumor regression by inducing apoptosis of angiogenic blood vessels. Cell 1994; 79:1157-1164.
31. Bauer J, Margolis M, Schreiner C et al. In vitro model of angiogenesis using a human endothelium-derived permanent cell line: Contributions of induced gene expression, G-proteins, and integrins. J Cell Physiol 1992; 153:437-449.
32. Ito A, Nomura S, Hirota S et al. Enhanced expression of CD34 messenger RNA by developing endothelial cells of mice. Lab Invest 1995; 72:532-538.
33. Szekanecz Z, Haines GK, Harlow LA et al. Increased synovial expression of transforming growth factor (TGF)-β receptor endoglin and TGF-β1 in rheumatoid arthritis: Possible interactions in the pathogenesis of the disease. Clin Immunol Immunopathol 1995; 76:187-194.
34. Nguyen M, Strubel NA, Bischoff J. A role for sialyl Lewis-X/A glycoconjugates in capillary morphogenesis. Nature 1993; 365:267-269.
35. Horak ER, Leek R, Klenk N et al. Angiogenesis, assessed by platelet/endothelial cell adhesion molecule antibodies, as indicator of node metastases and survival in breast cancer. Lancet 1992; 340:1120-1124.

36. Vogel T, Blake DA, Whikehart DR et al. Specific simple sugars promote chemotaxis and chemokinesis of corneal endothelial cells. J Cell Physiol 1993; 157:359-366.

37. Klein S, Giancotti FG, Presta M et al. Basic fibroblast growth factor modulates integrin expression in microvascular endothelial cells. Mol Biol Cell 1993; 4:973-982.

38. Enenstein J, Walehm NS, Kramer RH. Basic FGF and TGF-beta differentially modulate integrin expression of human microvascular endothelial cells. Exp Cell Res 1992; 203:499-503.

39. Taraboletti G, Belotti D, Giavazzi R. Thrombospondin modulates basic fibroblast growth factor activities on endothelial cells. EXS 1991; 59:210-213.

40. Frank R, Adelmann-Grill BC, Herrmann K et al. Transformtin growth factor-beta controls cell-matrix interaction of microvascular dermal endothelial cells by downregulation of integrin expression. J Invest Dermatol 1996; 106:36-41.

41. Mason JC, Kapahi P, Haskard DO. Detection of increased levels of circulating intercellular adhesion molecule 1 in some patients with rheumatoid arthritis but not in patients with systemic lupus erythematosus. Lack of correlation with levels of circulating vascular cell adhesion molecule 1. Arthritis Rheum 1993; 36:519-527.

42. Koch AE, Turkiewicz W, Harlow LA et al. Soluble E-selectin in arthritis. Clin Immunol Immunopathol 1993; 69:29-35.

43. Strieter RM, Polverini PJ, Kunkel SL et al. The functional role of the ELR motif in CXC chemokine-mediated angiogenesis. J Biol Chem 1995; 270:27348-27357.

44. Strieter RM, Kunkel SL. Acute lung injury: The role of cytokines in the elicitation of neutrophils. J Investig Med 1994; 42:640-651.

45. Lloyd AR, Oppenheim JJ, Kelvin DJ et al. Chemokines regulate T cell adherence to recombinant adhesion molecules and extracellular matrix proteins. J Immunol 1996; 156:932-938.

46. Weber C, Alon R, Moser B et al. Sequential regulation of alpha 4 beta 1 and alpha 5 beta 1 integrin avidity by CC chemokines in monocytes: implications for transendothelial chemotaxis. J Cell Biol 1996; 134:1063-1073.

47. Szekanecz Z, Shah MR, Pearce WH et al. Intercellular adhesion molecule-1 (ICAM-1) expression and soluble ICAM-1 (sIcellular adhesion molecule-1) production by cytokine-activated human aortic endothelial cells: A possible role for ICAM-1 and sICAM-1 in atherosclerotic aortic aneurysms. Clin Exp Immunol 1994; 98:337-343.

48. Szekanecz Z, Shah MR, Harlow LA et al. Interleukin-8 and tumor necrosis factor-alpha are involved in human aortic endothelial cell migration. Pathobiology 1994; 62:134-139.

49. Szekanecz Z, Shah MR, Pearce WH et al. Human atherosclerotic abdominal aortic aneurysms produce interleukin (IL)-6 and interferon-gamma but not IL-2 and IL-4. Agents Actions 1994; 42:159-162.

50. Davis CA III, Pearce WH, Haines GK et al. Increased ICAM-1 expression in aortic disease. J Vasc Surg 1993; 18:875-880.

51. Pearce WH, Sweis I, Yao JST et al. Interleukin-1β and tumor necrosis factor-α release in normal and diseased human infrarenal aortas. J Vasc Surg 1992; 16:784-789.

52. Koch AE, Kunkel SL, Pearce WH et al. Enhanced production of the chemotactic cytokines interleukin-8 and monocyte chemoattractant protein-1 in human abdominal aortic aneurysms. Am J Pathol 1993; 142:1423-1428.

53. Leibovich SJ, Polverini PJ, Shepard HM et al. Macrophage-induced angiogenesis is mediated by tumour necrosis factor-α. Nature 1987; 329:630-632.

54. Koch AE, Polverini PJ, Kunkel SL et al. Interleukin-8 as a macrophage-derived mediator of angiogenesis. Science 1992; 258:1798-1801.

55. Rosen EM, Liu D, Setter E et al. Interleukin-6 stimulates motility of vascular endothelium. EXS 1991; 59:194-205.

56. Van Waes C. Cell adhesion and regulatory molecules involved in tumor formation, hemostasis, and wound healing. Head Neck 1995; 17:140-147.

57. Koch AE, Kronfeld-Harrington LB, Szekanecz Z et al. In situ expression of cytokines and cellular adhesion molecules in the skin of patients with systemic sclerosis. Pathobiology 1993; 61:239-246.

58. Gailit J, Clark RA. Studies in vitro on the role of alpha v and beta 1 integrins in the adhesion of human dermal fibroblasts to provisional matrix proteins fibronectin, vitronectin, and fibrinogen. J Invest Dermatol 1996; 106:102-108.

59. Asahara T, Murohara T, Sullivan A et al. Isolation of putative progenitor endothelial cells for angiogenesis. Science 1997; 275:964-967.

Facilitation of Healing

Angiogenesis

—————————————————— CHAPTER 26 ——————————————————

Angiogenesis in Tissues and Vascular Grafts

Paula K. Shireman, Howard P. Greisler

Overview of Angiogenesis

Angiogenesis is a cellular process that starts during embryogenesis and continues throughout the life of the organism. It is defined as the formation of new blood vessels by a process of sprouting from preexisting vessels, while vasculogenesis is the differentiation of endothelial cells from mesodermal precursors and their subsequent organization into a primary capillary plexus. Unlike angiogenesis, vasculogenesis is limited to the embryonic period of life.[1]

Angiogenesis is a highly regulated process that is predominantly inhibited except for brief periods of time in which the normally quiescent vasculature is stimulated to form new blood vessels. Many disease states such as arthritis, ocular neovascularization, and tumor growth and metastasis, occur due to unregulated angiogenesis.[2] Although the factors that induce angiogenesis are poorly understood, hypoxia is thought to be a potent stimulus. Hypoxia induces various cell lines to secrete angiogenic molecules. It is not understood how cells sense hypoxia or how this triggers secretion of angiogenic molecules.[3]

Stimulating factors for angiogenesis are often categorized as direct or indirect. This often leads to confusing, and sometimes conflicting, data in the literature due to the various systems in which the molecules are tested. Target cell specificity for an angiogenic molecule is usually determined using in vitro methods such as endothelial cell proliferation and migration assays. Angiogenic activity, however, is analyzed in vivo using bioassays such as the chicken chorioallantoic membrane assay. When the two methods correlate, the angiogenic factor is classified as being "direct" because it stimulates endothelial cell proliferation or migration directly. When the angiogenic factor fails to stimulate activity in vitro, it is classified as "indirect" because it is assumed that the endothelial cell activity observed in vivo must be induced by some other factor or cell type that the indirect angiogenic molecule elicits.[2]

The formation of new vessels occurs by activation of endothelial cells from pre-existing capillaries or venules. Pericytes are cells that closely resemble smooth muscle cells. Pericytes closely envelop endothelial cells in quiescent capillaries, and they become sparse or absent in growing vessels. They reappear in mature, nongrowing capillaries where they downregulate endothelial cell proliferation.[3]

Angiogenesis is thought to occur in four basic steps. Endothelial cells of a capillary become activated by a variety of factors including hypoxia, acidosis and cytokines. This is followed by local vasodilation and increased vascular permeability, both of which are caused, at least in part, by vascular endothelial growth factor (VEGF). The initial step of angiogenesis involves degradation of the basement membrane of the parent vessel. This allows the

Tissue Engineering of Prosthetic Vascular Grafts, edited by Peter Zilla and Howard P. Greisler.
©1999 R.G. Landes Company.

endothelial cells to migrate toward the angiogenic stimulus, which is the second step of angiogenesis. Migrating endothelial cells elongate and align with one another to form a capillary sprout. Thirdly, endothelial cells proliferate, which occurs proximal to the migrating tip, further increasing the length of the sprout. The solid sprout gradually develops a lumen proximal to the region of proliferation. Contiguous sprouts anastomose at their tips to form a functional capillary loop in which blood flow can be established. The fourth step is vessel maturation, which is accomplished by reconstitution of the basement membrane and the reappearance of surrounding pericytes (see Fig. 26.1).[1,4]

New capillaries, as well as blood vessels that are stimulated by VEGF, tend to be "leaky" and thus have an increased vascular permeability. This leads to the accumulation of extravascular fibrin, which acts as a provisional matrix that is progressively removed and replaced by other matrix components.[1] Fibrin itself is chemotactic for inflammatory cells and has been shown to regulate endothelial cell and fibroblast migration.[5]

Degradation of the extracellular matrix is a highly regulated process that occurs secondary to the interplay of proteolytic enzymes, their inhibitors, and angiogenic molecules that induce the formation of these enzymes. Endothelial cells produce both plasminogen activators, tissue-type plasminogen activator (tPA) and urokinase-type plasminogen activator (uPA), as well as the plasminogen activator inhibitor (PAI-1).[6] The plasminogen activators cleave the inactive plasminogen to form plasmin, a proteolytic enzyme with broad specificity for fibrin, laminin, gelatin, and other extracellular components. Plasmin also activates the matrix metalloproteinases, a family of proteolytic enzymes that also degrade extracellular matrix components.[7] Fibroblast growth factor-2 (FGF-2), also known as basic FGF, is another important angiogenic molecule that enhances endothelial growth, proliferation, and migration. It also enhances endothelial cell expression of uPA and collagenase. In contrast, transformtin growth factor-β (TGF-β) dramatically increases PAI-1 synthesis in endothelial cells. The interplay

of FGF-2 and TGF-β allow extracellular matrix degradation to occur in a controlled fashion, thereby allowing endothelial cell migration for angiogenesis. A feedback mechanism has been described for these two angiogenic molecules. Increased plasminogen activation by FGF-2 results in high pericellular plasmin activity. Plasmin activates TGF-β by releasing it from its latent complex. Activated TGF-β decreases the overall proteolytic capacity by increasing synthesis of PAI-1 and decreasing synthesis of uPA. The resulting decrease in plasmin activity blocks the activation of further TGF-β. When active TGF-β is no longer present, the effects of FGF-2 again prevail, thereby increasing plasmin and uPA levels. Plasmin also releases FGF-2 that is bound to the extracellular matrix by heparan sulfate proteoglycans. The cleavage of the proteoglycan core releases FGF-2 in an active form that is protected from proteolytic degradation and can diffuse to affect target cells.[8]

Degradation of the extracellular matrix and the release of the growth factors stored there are also enhanced by macrophages. Macrophages contribute to angiogenesis in several ways. Macrophages release proteolytic enzymes, including plasminogen activators and matrix metalloproteinases, that assist in extracellular matrix breakdown. Macrophages also degrade heparan sulfate, which binds many growth factors to the extracellular matrix, thus releasing active cytokines to affect endothelial cells. Finally, macrophages themselves secrete many angiogenic factors such as FGF-2, TGF-β, VEGF, and angiotropin as well as factors that inhibit angiogenesis. Macrophages are important regulators of inflammation and tissue healing, and angiogenesis is an integral part of both of these processes.[9]

Many different cytokines and growth factors have been implicated in either promoting or inhibiting angiogenesis, and in some cases the same factor may have both stimulating and inhibitory properties depending upon local conditions. We will review the functions of several of these major cytokines: FGF, VEGF, TGF-β, and angiostatin.

The FGF family of growth factors plays an important role in angiogenesis. FGF-2 stimulates endothelial cell pro-

Fig. 26.1. Four steps in angiogenesis. Parent mature vessel is on the left. (1) Basement membrane and ECM degradation. (2) Endothelial migration. (3) Endothelial proliferation (mitoses). (4) Organization and maturation. (Used with permission from ref. 4).

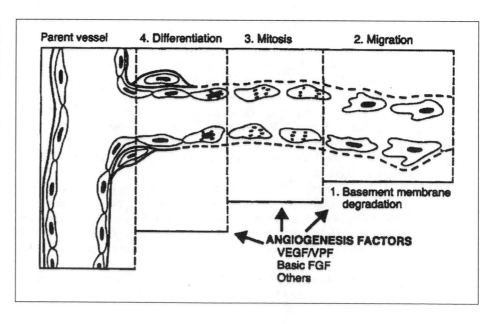

liferation, migration, and promotes formation of differentiated capillary tubes in vitro.[9] Endothelial cell production of FGF-2 leads to its sequestration in the extracellular matrix where it can be released to participate in angiogenesis during the degradation of the extracellular matrix. FGF-2 also induces the formation of plasminogen activators and collagenase, thereby promoting extracellular degradation and its own activation.[10] Both FGF-1, also known as acidic FGF, and FGF-2 are synthesized by a broad range of cell types including endothelial cells, fibroblasts, macrophages, and smooth muscle cells. Both forms of FGF lack a signal sequence for secretion, and it is not entirely clear how FGF release is regulated. As previously discussed, FGF binds to heparan sulfate and can be released from the extracellular matrix. Furthermore, FGF is released from damaged and dying cells and may therefore be important in inducing angiogenesis in ischemic and injured tissues.[3] For a more detailed review of the functions of the FGF family of growth factors in angiogenesis, see chapter 28.

VEGF, also known as vascular permeability factor, is another important angiogenic molecule that is expressed in many different cell types including macrophages, fibroblasts, smooth muscle cells and endothelial cells. Hypoxia may, in part, control the expression of VEGF.[11] Unlike FGF, VEGF has a peptide leader sequence which probably controls cellular secretion of VEGF.[10] Endothelial cells exhibit VEGF receptors, which explains the exquisite specificity of VEGF for endothelial cells. Unlike FGF and other cytokines that induce endothelial proliferation as well as proliferation of other cell lines, VEGF is generally considered to be a specific endothelial cell mitogen. Binding of VEGF to its receptor induces a sequence of protein phosphorylation. VEGF increases intracellular calcium levels and induces the release of von Willebrand factor from endothelial cells.

VEGF was originally discovered because of its ability to increase the permeability of blood vessels, primarily postcapillary venules and small veins. This increased permeability occurs rapidly and is transient and reversible, persisting for less than 30 minutes; it is not associated with any detectable cell damage.[12] This increased permeability leads to the accumulation of extravascular fibrin, which acts as a provisional matrix for migrating endothelial cells during angiogenesis.

VEGF induces endothelial cells to invade collagen gels in vitro and also incites endothelial cell sprouting. Synergism between VEGF and FGF-2 was shown in a microvascular endothelial cell assay which demonstrated endothelial invasion of a three dimensional collagen gel with formation of capillary-like tubules. Both FGF-2 and VEGF were angiogenic in this model, with VEGF being about half as potent as FGF-2 in equimolar concentrations. However, when both cytokines were added simultaneously, the angiogenic response was far greater than the additive effect of each cytokine separately and occurred at a more rapid rate.[13] VEGF also promotes expression of tPA and matrix metalloproteinases in endothelial cells, which as already discussed, induces degradation of the extracellular matrix as well as the provisional fibrin matrix, releasing angiogenic factors. PAI-1 is also increased by VEGF and may provide a negative feedback mechanism to balance the proteolytic process.[8,14]

There are 4 major isoforms of VEGF and the relative affinity to heparin binding may affect the bioavailability of the various isoforms. VEGF-121 fails to bind heparin and is therefore a freely diffusible protein that is secreted from cells. VEGF-165, the major isoform, has an intermediate affinity for heparin and is secreted from cells, although a significant portion remains bound to the cell surface and the extracellular matrix. Both VEGF-189 and VEGF-206 have a high affinity for heparin and these isoforms are almost completely sequestered in the extracellular matrix (see Fig. 26.2.).[15,16]

The important role that VEGF plays in angiogenesis and vasculogenesis in embryo development is demonstrated by mouse VEGF knockout models. A heterozygous VEGF

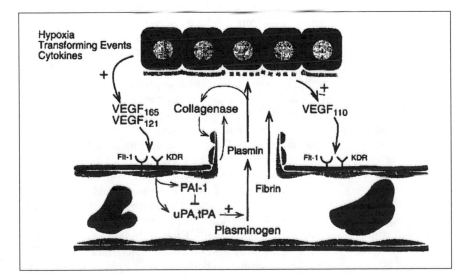

Fig. 26.2. Schematic representation of the actions of VEGF isoforms on the vascular endothelium. Several stimuli may result in the release of the diffusible alternatively spliced VEGF isoforms (VEGF-165 and VEGF-121) from a variety of cell types. These proteins may induce a complex series of effects on the vascular endothelium, including cell sprouting, induction of interstitial collagenase, plasminogen activators (PA), and plasminogen activator inhibitor-1 (PAI-1), as well as extravasation of plasma proteins. Plasminogen activation results in generation of plasmin, which may cleave extracellular matrix-bound VEGF (VEGF-189 or VEGF-206) to release a diffusible proteolytic fragment (VEGF-110). Plasmin may also activate procollagenase. Activation of PAI-1 may constitute a negative regulatory step, by inhibiting the action of PA. (Used with permission from ref. 15).

knockout resulted in embryonic lethality between days 11 and 12. Homozygous knockouts of the VEGF receptor results in embryonic lethality.

Another growth factor that exhibits both angiogenic and antiangiogenic properties is TGF-β. TGF-β is angiogenic in vivo but inhibits macrovascular proliferation of endothelial cells and the proliferation of endothelial cells not engaged in angiogenesis in vitro. TGF-β promotes proliferation of endothelial cells engaged in angiogenesis in vitro and induces the formation of capillary-like tubes of microvascular endothelial cells. TGF-β potentiates FGF-2 and VEGF induced angiogenesis in vitro at low, but not high, doses.[3] As previously discussed, TGF-β modulates extracellular degradation by inducing PAI-1 synthesis and thus downregulates plasmin-mediated proteolysis. In view of its capacity to directly inhibit endothelial cell proliferation and migration, reduce extracellular proteolysis, and promote matrix deposition in vitro, TGF-β has been proposed to be a potential mediator of the resolution phase of angiogenesis.[1]

Although many factors promote angiogenesis, uncontrolled angiogenesis is associated with many disease states, including tumor formation and metastasis. It is therefore the delicate balance of angiogenic and antiangiogenic molecules that leads to controlled, appropriate angiogenesis. Folkman and associates[17] have recently isolated angiostatin, an antiangiogenic molecule that inhibits the formation of tumor metastases in the Lewis mouse lung model. Angiostatin is a 38 kDa fragment of plasminogen that inhibits endothelial cell proliferation in vitro. The primary tumor secretes angiostatin, which inhibits the growth of metastases. Removing the primary tumor decreases angiostatin levels and this allows the metastases to reestablish their blood supply and grow.

Angiogenesis in Vascular Grafts

Synthetic, small diameter vascular grafts fail primarily because of interactions at the blood-material and tissue-material interfaces.[18] Currently available prostheses elicit inflammatory and regenerative reactions, yielding graft thrombosis and intimal hyperplasia.[19] In humans, clinically utilized grafts of Dacron and 30 μm internodal distance expanded polytetrafluorethylene (ePTFE) do not allow capillary infiltration despite the small wall thickness. Many researchers have attempted to improve synthetic grafts by using various techniques such as endothelial seeding[20,21] and bioresorbable grafts.[19] Clowes and associates studied the effect of porosity on ePTFE grafts and demonstrated that these grafts could be lined by endothelial cells that were derived from graft transmural capillaries. This induction of "graft angiogenesis" occurred in ePTFE grafts with 60 μm internodal distance. Previous studies had shown that ePTFE grafts with a 30 μm internodal distance were covered by an ingrowth of endothelium from the adjacent artery as a continuous sheet across the anastomosis and along the graft.[22] This process was relatively slow with only 60% of grafts 6-9 cm in length exhibiting complete coverage by 12 months in an aortoiliac baboon model.[23] In contrast, when 60 μm internodal grafts were used, endothelial cells began to appear on the graft surface at 1-2 weeks after surgery and be-

came confluent at 4 weeks. Transmural capillaries were observed to connect the graft lumen to extravascular granulation tissue. At 2 weeks, multiple small orifices 100-500 μm apart were located between the ridges of the graft. At 4 and 12 weeks, the entire graft surface was covered with endothelial cells and the number of small vessel orifices had diminished. Smooth muscle cells were seen underneath the endothelial cells in the network of microvessels within the graft as early as 2 weeks. A progressive thickening of the intima, which was the greatest at 12 weeks, was seen throughout the graft. Smooth muscle cells, which were thought to be derived from pericytes, accompanied the capillary endothelial cells into the graft lumen. In contrast, intimal thickening occurred only at the anastomotic ends in the 30 μm internodal grafts (see Fig. 26.3.). These results indicate that capillary endothelium and smooth muscle cells can function in the same manner as their large vessel counterparts and could provide coverage of synthetic graft surfaces in contact with the arterial circulation.[24]

The 60 μm internodal graft appeared to provide the "optimal" porosity in the baboon model. In low porosity grafts, 10 and 30 μm internodal distance, endothelial coverage was incomplete and was limited to the graft surface near the anastomoses. In contrast, high porosity grafts, 60 and 90 μm internodal distance, revealed complete endothelial coverage with a uniformly distributed intimal thickening throughout the graft. However, the 90 μm graft developed areas of focal endothelial loss at 3 months, suggesting that the larger pore size resulted in intimal instability and endothelial cell loss in the ePTFE.[25]

Dacron, another porous graft material, was compared to the 60 μm internodal ePTFE grafts in the baboon model. The Dacron grafts showed incomplete endothelialization at 12 weeks while all the ePTFE grafts revealed a confluent endothelial layer. Although both types of grafts healed by proliferation of cells derived from invading capillaries, the authors hypothesized that the Dacron material itself may somehow inhibit graft endothelialization.[26]

Dacron may induce various cell types to secrete factors that could inhibit angiogenesis and graft endothelialization. Evidence supporting this hypothesis is provided by Greisler et al.[27] Rabbit peritoneal macrophages, grown in the presence of Dacron particles in vitro, released more TGF-β than control macrophages. The effects of TGF-β on angiogenesis and endothelial proliferation are complex. In vitro, TGF-β inhibits endothelial cell proliferation.[28] TGF-β instillation into newborn mice[29] and into the chorioallantoic membrane assay[30] induces angiogenesis, while higher doses of TGF-β resulted in inhibition of angiogenesis in these models.[31] The higher levels of TGF-β released by macrophages in the presence of Dacron may contribute to the inhibition of endothelialization seen in Dacron grafts.

In an attempt to apply the above research to the clinical setting, 10 above-knee femoropopliteal composite grafts were placed into 8 patients. Each of these grafts consisted of equal lengths of 30 and 60 μm internodal distance ePTFE with the 60 μm portion being randomly placed in either the proximal or distal position. In contrast to the baboon experiments which used unwrapped ePTFE, these grafts were reinforced with a thin, nonexpanded wrap for human use. Noninvasive assessment of endothelialization was performed using [111]Indium-labeled platelet imaging at 1 week and 3 months after surgery. There was no difference in indium uptake between the 60 and 30 μm segments at either time point. Histologic sections were available from 60 μm segments from 2 patients who underwent operations for graft thrombosis. Capillary ingrowth into the graft was observed, but it rarely extended more than half the distance from the outside of the graft to the lumen. Smooth muscle cells were not seen on the luminal surface, indicating that a neointima had not formed. The finding that capillary ingrowth can occur in the 60 μm internodal graft, but does not lead to an endothelial lining in humans, could possibly be attributed to an inadequacy of angiogenesis in adult humans or retardation of capillary ingrowth by the reinforcing wrap.[32]

Other attempts at inducing graft angiogenesis by coating the luminal surface of synthetic grafts with FGF-1 incorporated into a fibrin glue have been made by Greisler and associates. FGF-1 is a potent endothelial cell mitogen and the greater adhesivity of the FG surface for seeded endothelial cells plus the slow release of the suspended FGF-1 suggest the tissue engineering applicability of this substrate[33,34] For a more thorough review of this work, see chapter 28.

Therapeutic Angiogenesis in Ischemic Tissues

Unregulated angiogenesis can be seen in many cancers and is a biologically undesirable situation that often leads to the death of the host. On the other hand, tissue ischemia caused by occlusive arteriosclerosis represents a relative deficiency of angiogenesis. Various cytokines have been used to induce angiogenesis in animal models of tissue ischemia. Perhaps one of the most commonly used is the rabbit hindlimb ischemia model. The hindlimb is made ischemic by tying off the external iliac artery and removing the common femoral and superficial femoral arteries. Growth factors, such as FGF (reviewed in chapter 28) and VEGF, are then introduced into the ischemic limb and their angiogenic effect is measured by counting the new vessels seen on angiography. VEGF has been extensively studied by Isner's group using this model. They found that a single bolus injection of VEGF via the ipsilateral internal iliac artery caused an increase in flow at rest, in maximum flow velocity, and in maximum blood flow at 30 days as compared to saline controls.[35] VEGF treated rabbits also re-established an increased endothelium-dependent blood flow in response to serotonin and acetylcholine injection as compared to saline treated animals which did not respond to the serotonin or acetylcholine injections, suggesting that VEGF facilitated endothelial recovery after ischemic injury.[36] VEGF also increased endothelial cell proliferation 2.8-fold at day 5, followed by a decrease to baseline by day 7 as compared to controls, while smooth muscle cell proliferation increased by 2.7-fold.[37] Endogenous VEGF production in the ischemic hindlimb model was found to be decreased in older (4-5 years) as compared to younger (6-8 months) rabbits and the angiogenic response was also decreased in the older rabbits. Exogenous

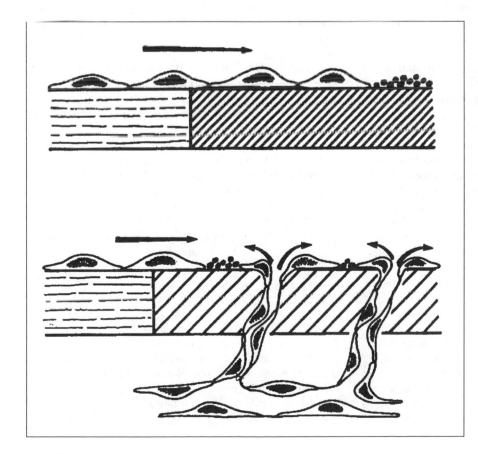

Fig. 26.3. Diagrammatic representation of healing by endothelial and smooth muscle cells of low-porosity (top) and high-porosity (bottom) ePTFE grafts. In low-porosity grafts endothelium is derived from the cut edges of adjacent artery and grows as a continuous monolayer toward the center of the graft. In high-porosity grafts, capillaries derived from surrounding granulation tissue penetrate the graft matrix and provide multiple sources of endothelium at the luminal surface. (Used with permission from ref. 24).

administration of VEGF induced a similar angiogenic response in both older and younger rabbits, suggesting that a relative VEGF deficiency may occur with aging and that replacement of VEGF may overcome this defect.[38] This relative VEGF deficiency in response to ischemia was also seen in diabetic mice. The diabetic mice exhibited less angiogenesis and produced less VEGF than their normal mice counterparts.[39] Another model used by this group involved balloon injury to the rat carotid artery with a 30 minute inoculation with either saline or VEGF. The VEGF treated animals re-endothelialized more quickly and exhibited less neointimal thickening.[40]

After establishing the angiogenic effect of the VEGF protein in ischemia, Isner's group then proceeded to study the effect of naked plasmid DNA encoding for human VEGF-$_{165}$ (phVEGF-$_{165}$). Using the rabbit ischemic hindlimb model, they injected the phVEGF-$_{165}$ intramuscularly; 30 days later, there were increased collateral vessels and histologically identifiable capillaries were also seen. In addition, there was a superior calf blood pressure ratio in the phVEGF-$_{165}$ treated group. They felt that ischemic skeletal muscle was a good target for gene therapy and that VEGF was a good gene to use.[41] Hypoxia upregulates VEGF receptor gene expression making ischemic tissues more likely to respond to VEGF than normal tissues. VEGF also promotes physiological maturation of newly formed collateral channels and restores appropriate endothelium-derived relaxing factor as well as the nitric oxide-dependent vasorelaxation response initiated by the endothelium, thereby increasing the blood flow through the expanding vascular bed.[42]

An alternate method to deliver the phVEGF-$_{165}$ involved transfecting endothelial cells by balloon catheter angioplasty in the rabbit femoral artery. The phVEGF-$_{165}$ treated animals showed enhanced endothelialization in the transfected side as well as the nontransfected, control side, decreased intimal thickening, decreased thrombotic occlusion, and accelerated recovery of endothelial-dependent vasomotor reactivity as compared to transfection with the LacZ gene in control animals.[43]

Recently, this work with the phVEGF-$_{165}$ has been performed in humans. A patient with nonreconstructable occlusive disease received an angioplasty in a normal-appearing section of her distal popliteal artery to transfect the surrounding endothelial cells with phVEGF-$_{165}$. A normal section of artery was chosen to enhance cellular transfection and to avoid the confounding factor of increased blood flow that may result from treating a stenotic segment of artery. The patient exhibited increased collaterals at 4 and 12 weeks as demonstrated by angiography and increased resting and maximal blood flows. Three sporadic angiomas developed on the foot and ankle of the treated leg. One of the angiomas was excised, revealing a proliferative endothelium and the other 2 regressed spontaneously. The patient also developed leg edema 1 week after gene transfer which resolved in 4 weeks, corresponding to the time course of VEGF production observed in animal models after transfection. The treatment, however, was ultimately unsuccessful and the patient required a below-knee amputation 5 months after the transfection.[44]

Another human trial with transfection of phVEGF-$_{165}$ by intramuscular injection or intraarterially revealed increased serum levels of VEGF. Furthermore, 63% of the patients had edema and the response seemed to correlate with disease severity, with no edema occurring in patients with claudication, variable amounts of edema occurring in patients with rest pain, and profound edema occurring in patients with ischemic tissue loss.[45] Isner's group also reported on a trial of 10 limbs in 9 patients with ulcers and rest pain that received IM gene transfer two times at 4 week intervals. The clinical status was improved in 8, unchanged in 1, and worse in 1 limb after a 3.7 month follow up. The patients overall demonstrated an increased ankle-brachial index, improved blood flow by magnetic resonance angiography, and angiographic evidence of new collaterals in 6/10 limbs.[46] Further clinical trials are currently being performed using this gene transfer technique.

Yet another route for delivering VEGF to promote graft angiogenesis was used by Weatherford and associates.[47] They incorporated VEGF and heparin into fibrin glue and found that human aortic endothelial cell proliferation on this glue was increased as compared to fibrin glue alone. The addition of heparin to the VEGF increased endothelial cell proliferation while inhibiting smooth muscle cell proliferation. The application of VEGF and heparin in fibrin glue to a prosthetic vascular graft may be used in the future to promote graft patency and endothelialization.

Future Directions

Research into the mechanisms of angiogenesis is a relatively new scientific endeavor and much progress has been made in a relatively short period of time. Control of angiogenesis could provide enormous clinical benefits. Inhibition of angiogenesis could result in new treatment strategies for cancer, while promoting angiogenesis could relieve myocardial and peripheral ischemia from atherosclerotic occlusive disease. Other emerging technologies will probably utilize our increasing knowledge of angiogenesis regulation to induce new vessel formation in ischemic tissues, perhaps someday making bypass grafting for chronic arterial occlusive disease obsolete.

References

1. Pepper MS. Manipulating angiogenesis, from basic science to the bedside. Arteriosclerosis Thromb Vasc Biol 1997; 17:605-619.
2. Folkman J, Shing Y. Angiogenesis. J Biol Chem 1992; 267:10931-10934.
3. Battegay EJ. Angiogenesis: Mechanistic insights, neovascular diseases, and therapeutic prospects. J Mol Med 1995; 73:333-346.
4. Cotran RS. Inflammation and repair. In: Cotran RS, Robbins SL, Kumar V, eds. Robbins Pathologic Basis of Disease, 5th Edition. Philadelphia: WB Saunders Co., 1994:51-92.
5. Brown LF, Dvorak AM, Dvorak HF. Leaky vessels, fibrin deposition, and fibrosis: A sequence of events common to solid tumors and to many other types of diseases. Am Rev Respir Dis 1989; 140:1104-1107.

6. Loskutoff DJ, Curriden SA. The fibrinolytic system of the vessel wall and its role in the control of thrombosis. Ann NY Acad Sci 1990; 598:238-247.

7. Murphy G, Atkinson S, Ward R, Gavrilovic J, Reynolds JJ. The role of plasminogen activators in the regulation of connective tissue metalloproteinases. Ann of NY Acad Sci 1992; 667:1-12.

8. Pintucci G, Bikfalvi A, Klein S, Rifkin DB. Angiogenesis and the fibrinolytic system. Seminars in Thrombosis and Hemostasis. 1996; 22:517-524.

9. Sunderkotter C, Steinbrink K, Goebeler M, Bhardwaj R, Sorg C. Macrophages and angiogenesis. J Leukoc Biol 1994; 55:410-422.

10. Schott RJ, Morrow LA. Growth factors and angiogenesis. Cardio Res 1993; 27:1155-1161.

11. Namiki A, Brogi E, Kearney M, Kim EA, Wu T, Couffinhal T, Varticovski L, Isner JM. Hypoxia induces vascular endothelial growth factor in cultured human endothelial cells. J Biol Chem 1995; 52:31189-31195.

12. Brown LF, Detmar M, Claffey K, Nagy JA, Feng D, Dvorak AM, Dvorak HF. Vascular permeability factor/vascular endothelial growth factor: A multifunctional angiogenic cytokine. EXS 1997; 79:233-269.

13. Pepper MS, Ferrara N, Orci L, Montesano R. Potent synergism between vascular endothelial growth factor and basic fibroblast growth factor in the induction of angiogenesis in vitro. Biochem and Biophys Res Comm 1992; 189:824-831.

14. Pepper MS, Ferrara N, Orci L, Montesano R. Vascular endothelial growth factor (VEGF) induces plasminogen activators and plasminogen activator inhibitor-1 in microvascular endothelial cells. Biochem and Biophys Res Comm 1991; 181:902-906.

15. Ferrara N, Davis-Smyth T. The biology of vascular endothelial growth factor. Endocrine Rev 1997; 18:4-23.

16. Park JE, Keller G A, Ferrara N. The vascular endothelial growth factor (VEGF) isoforms: Differential deposition into the subepithelial extracellular matrix and bioactivity of extracellular matrix-bound VEGF. Mol Biol Cell 1993; 4:1317-1326.

17. O'Reilly MS, Holmgren L, Shing Y, Chen C, Rosenthal RA, Moses M, Lane WS, Cao Y, Sage EH, Folkman J. Angiostatin: A novel angiogenesis inhibitor that mediates the suppression of metastases by a Lewis lung carcinoma. Cell 1994; 79:315-328.

18. Greisler HP, Ellinger J, Henderson SC, Shaheen AM, Burgess WH, Kim DU, Lam TM. The effects of an atherogenic diet on macrophage/biomaterial interactions. J Vasc Surg 1991; 14:10-23.

19. Greisler HP, Schwarcz TH, Ellinger J, Kim DU. Dacron inhibition of arterial regenerative activities. J Vasc Surg 1986; 3:747-756.

20. Zilla P, Deutsch M, Meinhart J, Puschmann R, Eberl T, Minar E, Dudczak R, Lugmaier H, Schmidt P, Noszian I, Fischlein T. Clinical in vitro endothelialization of femoropopliteal bypass grafts: An actuarial follow-up over three years. J Vasc Sug. 1994; 19:540-548.

21. Zilla P, Preiss P, Groscurth P, Rosemeier F, Deutsch M, Odell J, Heidinger C, Fasol R, von Oppell U. In vitro-lined endothelium: Initial integrity and ultrastructural events. Surgery 1994; 116:524-534.

22. Clowes AW, Gown AM, Hanson ST, Reidy MA. Mechanisms of graft failure. I. Role of cellular proliferation in early healing of PTFE prosthesis. Am J Pathol 1985; 118:43-54.

23. Clowes AW, Kirkman TR, Clowes MM. Mechanism of arterial graft failure. II. Chronic endothelial and smooth muscle cell proliferation in healing poytetrafluoroethylene prostheses. J Vasc Surg 1986; 3:877-884.

24. Clowes AW, Kirkman TR, Reidy MA. Mechanisms of arterial graft healing, rapid transmural capillary ingrowth provides a source of intimal endothelium and smooth muscle in porous PTFE prostheses. Am J Pathol 1986; 123:220-230.

25. Golden MA, Hanson SR, Kirkman TR, Schneider PA, Clowes AW. Healing of polytetrafluoroethylene arterial grafts is influenced by graft porosity. J Vasc Surg 1990; 11:838-845.

26. Zacharias RK, Kirkman TR, Clowes AW. Mechanisms of healing in synthetic grafts. J Vasc Surg 1987; 6:429-436.

27. Greisler HP, Petsikas D, Cziperle DJ, Murchan PM, Henderson SC, Lam TM. Dacron stimulation of macrophage transformtin growth factor-β release. Cardiovasc Surg 1996; 4:169-173.

28. Frater-Schroeder M, Risau W, Hallmann R et al. Tumor necrosis factor type α, a potent inhibitor of endothelial cell growth in vitro, is angiogenic in vivo. Proc Natl Acad Sci USA. 1987; 84:5277-5281.

29. Roberts AB, Sporn MB, Assoian RK et al. Transforming growth factor type β: Rapid induction of fibrosis and angiogenesis in vivo and stimulation of collagen formation in vitro. Proc Natl Acad Sci USA. 1986; 83:4167-4171.

30. Yang EY, Moses HL. Transforming growth factor beta 1-induced changes in cell migration, proliferation, and angiogenesis in the chicken chorioallantoic membrane. J Cell Biol 1990; 111:731-741.

31. Moses HL, Yang EY, Pietenpol JA. TGF-β stimulation and inhibition of cell proliferation: New mechanistic insights. Cell 1990; 63:245-247.

32. Kohler TR, Stratton JR, Kirkman TR, Johansen KH, Zierler BK, Clowes AW. Conventional versus high-porosity polytetrafluoroethylene grafts: Clinical evaluation. Surgery 1992; 112:901-907.

33. Greisler HP, Cziperle DJ, Petsikas D, Murchan PM, Appelgren EO, Drohan W, Burgess WH, Kim DU. Enhanced endothelialization of expanded PTFE grafts by heparin binding growth factor-type 1 (HBGF-1) pretreatment. Surgery 1992; 112:244-255.

34. Zarge JI, Huang P, Husak V, Kim DU, Haudenschild CC, Nord RM, Greisler HP. Fibrin glue containing fibroblast growth factor type 1 and heparin with autologous endothelial cells reduces intimal hyperplasia in a canine carotid artery balloon injury model. J Vasc Surg 1997; 25:840-849.

35. Bauters C, Asahara T, Zheng LP, Takeshita S, Bunting S, Ferrara N, Symes JF, Isner JM. Physiological assessment of augmented vascularity induced by VEGF in ischemic rabbit hindlimb. AM J Physiol. 1994; 267 (Heart Circ Physiol. 36): H1263-H1271.

36. Bauters C, Asahara T, Zheng LP, Takeshita S, Bunting S, Ferrara N, Symes JF, Isner JM. Recovery of disturbed endothelium-dependent flow in the collateral-perfused rabbit ischemic hindlimb after administration of vascular endothelial growth factor. Circulation 1995; 91:2802-2809.

37. Takeshita S, Rossow ST, Kearney M, Zheng LP, Bauters C, Bunting S, Ferrara N, Symes JF, Isner JM. Time course of increased cellular proliferation in collateral arteries after administration of vascular endothelial growth factor in a rabbit model of lower limb vascular insufficiency. Am J Pathol 1995; 147:1649-1660.

38. Rivard A, Fabre J-E, Silver M, Murohara T, Chen D, Asahara T, Isner JM. Age-dependent impairment of angiogenesis. Circulation (Suppl) 1997; 96:I-18.

39. Rivard A, Silver M, Fabre J-E, Magner M, Kearney M, Isner JM. Diabetes impairs angiogenesis in limb ischemia. Circulation (Suppl) 1997; 96:I-175.

40. Asahara T, Bauters C, Pastore C, Kearney M, Rossow S, Bunting S, Ferrara N, Symes JF, Isner JM. Local delivery of vascular endothelial growth factor accelerates reendothelialization and attenuates intimal hyperplasia in balloon-injured rat carotid artery. Circulation 1995; 91:2793-2801.

41. Tsurumi Y, Takeshita S, Chen D, Kearney M, Rossow ST, Passeri J, Horowitz JR, Symes JF, Isner JM. Direct intramuscular gene transfer of naked DNA encoding vascular endothelial growth factor augments collateral development and tissue perfusion. Circulation 1996; 94:3281-3290.

42. Majesky MW. A little VEGF goes a long way, therapeutic angiogenesis by direct injection of vascular endothelial growth factor-encoding plasmid DNA. Circulation 1996; 94:3062-3064.

43. Asahara T, Chen D, Tsurumi Y, Kearney M, Rossow S, Passeri J, Symes JF, Isner JM. Accelerated restitution of endothelial integrity and endothelium-dependent function after phVEGF$_{165}$ gene transfer. Circulation 1996; 94:3291-3302.

44. Isner JM, Pieczek A, Schainfeld R, Blair R, Haley L, Asahara T, Rosenfield K, Razvi S, Walsh K, Symes JF. Clinical evidence of angiogenesis after arterial gene transfer of phVEGF-165 in patient with ischaemic limb. Lancet 1996; 348:370-374.

45. Baumgartner I, Pieczek AM, Blair R, Manor O, Walsh K, Isner JM. Evidence of therapeutic angiogenesis in patients with critical limb ischemia after intramuscular phVEGF-$_{165}$ gene transfer. Circulation (Suppl) 1997; 96:I-32.

46. Baumgartner I, Magner M, Pieczek AM, Isner JM. Clinical evidence that vascular endothelial growth factor enhances vascular permeability. Circulation (Suppl) 1997;-96:I-4.

47. Weatherford DA, Sackman JE, Reddick TT, Freeman MB, Stevens SL, Goldman MH. Vascular endothelial growth factor and heparin in a biologic glue promotes human aortic endothelial cell proliferation with aortic smooth muscle cell inhibition. Surgery 1996; 120:433-439.

Facilitation of Healing

Angiogenesis

――――――――――――――――――― CHAPTER 27 ―――――――――――――――――――

Polypeptide Growth Factors with a Collagen Binding Domain: Their Potential for Tissue Repair and Organ Regeneration

Bo Han, Lynn L.H. Huang, David Cheung, Fabiola Cordoba, Marcel Nimni

Introduction

Tissue engineering is an emerging interdisciplinary field that applies the principles of engineering to the life sciences, with the aim of developing biological substitutes that restore, maintain or improve tissue function. In this process, extracellular matrix, cells and regulatory signals are important in guiding, modulating and facilitating regenerative events.

Cellular activities are regulated by a large number of polypeptides which behave as growth modulating factors. Such growth factors can either stimulate or inhibit cell division, differentiation, migration or expression. The effects of such factors are cell type dependent and can vary with the frequency and way of administration. As we increase our understanding of growth factor functions and their clinical applications, the need for useful pharmaceutical forms becomes more apparent. Growth factor targeting to responsive cells and maintenance of adequate tissue levels becomes essential, particularly in view of their sometimes opposite effects on various cells and the dose dependence of their response.

The extracellular matrix provides a scaffold for cell growth and differentiation, and may eventually help to regenerate tissues. Since collagen is a major constituent of extracellular matrices and connective tissues, its use in designing a synthetic matrix becomes of special interest. When growth factors contain collagen-binding domains, they can be targeted to collagen matrices, their activities localized, and together with the collagen matrix, synergistically affect the biological activities of cells. Therefore, collagen matrices impregnated with growth factors become potentially useful for tissue repair and organ regeneration, stimulating cell growth and extracellular restoration as well as remodeling.

In this chapter, currently developed collagen derived matrices, their interactions with cells and related growth factors for tissue regeneration are reviewed. In addition, we will discuss means of modulating growth factor release, including the use of recombinant protein strategies for targeting their delivery.

Development of the potential for addition of growth factors to bioprostheses in the design of synthetic matrices is anticipated.

The Collagen Derived Matrix

The advantages of using collagen derived matrices as scaffoldings for tissue regeneration include its excellent biocompatibility, its ability to resorb and to be obtained in a pure form. In addition, collagen can be processed to generate minimal immune response and crosslinked for attaining optimal degradation rates.[1]

Tissue Engineering of Prosthetic Vascular Grafts, edited by Peter Zilla and Howard P. Greisler
©1999 R.G. Landes Company.

Many investigators and manufacturers have established the use of various collagen-derived matrices in dermatology, cardiovascular surgery, neurosurgery, periodontal and oral surgery, ophthalmology, orthopedic surgery, drug delivery systems and other applications. Hyaluronan, chondroitin sulfate, and other polysaccharides, as well as growth factors and pharmacologically active compounds, are frequently added to such collagen-derived matrices. These matrices may be processed to attain different forms such as sponges, films, sheets, tubes, membranes, felts, gels, etc. Chemical modifications which include crosslinking with glutaraldehyde, epoxy, or other chemicals may be carried out to prolong the duration of such matrices.

Collagen Fibrillar Matrices / Hyaluronan Composites

In our laboratories, we have developed numerous collagen derived matrices and the biological response to these matrices has been studied.[2-5] Various concentrations of bovine skin type I collagen solutions were reconstituted to fibrillar matrices under physiological conditions. The contractility of these matrices by fibroblasts, a potentially undesirable side effect, has been investigated. To facilitate the process of wound healing, hyaluronan has been added to collagen fibrillar matrices. Through a contraction model with a floating collagen fibrillar matrix, it has demonstrated that high concentrations (> 1 mg/ml) of hyaluronan can significantly reduce matrix contraction by fibroblasts and the specificity documented. In addition, hyaluronan stimulates cell outgrowth and migration.[4]

In order to prolong the beneficial effects of hyaluronan, CNBr-activated hyaluronan was covalently linked to the collagen fibrillar matrix to stabilize the interactions of hyaluronan and collagen. It is found that covalently linked hyaluronan not only strengthens the collagen fibrils, but also blocks the direct communication between fibroblasts and collagen fibrils.[5] Contractility of such developed hyaluronan-collagen fibrillar matrix by fibroblasts is therefore abolished.[3,4]

In implantation studies, full-thickness wounds in the dorsal skin of guinea pigs were filled with such noncontractible hyaluronan-collagen fibrillar matrix, or collagen fibrillar matrix, or hyaluronan, or nothing as a control. The wounds filled with hyaluronan-collagen fibrillar matrices healed faster than the open control group. In addition, they manifest superior healing. The structure of the neomatrix can be hardly distinguished from the normal counterpart evaluated by pathological examination and scanning electron micrographs.[6] The results indicate that the hyaluronan-collagen fibrillar matrix could provide ideal tissue templates for big areas of wounds and may be very useful for the development of bioprostheses and implants (Fig. 27.1).

Collagen / Glycosaminoglycan Networks

Yannas et al[7-10] proposed a two stage artificial skin model for severe burn related healing. Clinical data show that stage 1 grafts are able to form a neodermis, but that the epidermis layer has to be replaced by an autograft in the second stage. The membrane in stage 1 is a wound closure

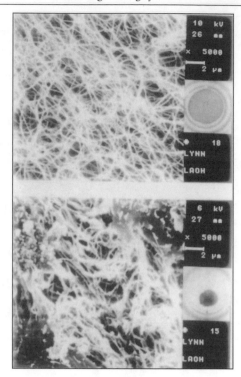

Fig. 27.1. (A) Network of reconstituted type I collagen coating tissue culture well. (B) Same as (A). but after seeding with human skin fibroblasts. Note contraction of the collagen network.

designed for emergency treatment to prevent infection or excessive fluid loss. The bilayer membrane consists of a polydimethylsiloxane (silicone) top layer and a porous biodegradable collagen-glycosaminoglycan network bottom layer. The glycosaminoglycan used in the network was mainly chondroitin sulfate. Physicochemical and mechanical properties such as moisture/air permeability, surface energy, flexural rigidity, and tear strength of the membrane are carefully controlled. About 14 days after covering the wounds with stage 1 membrane, the silicone layer must be removed and the stage 2 membrane transplanted. The stage 2 membrane with basal cells seeded into the collagen-glycosaminoglycan layer can help the formation of neoepidermis. Silicone still covers the top of the membrane. The confluency between new dermis and new epidermis is achieved about 15 days later. The result, after the silicone layer is peeled off at zero strength, is a reconstructed skin.

The choice of collagen-glycosaminoglycan network was claimed to be an important feature of their design (Fig. 27.2). The advantages of this crosslinked network are as follows:

1. Both collagen and glycosaminoglycan are biodegradable and relatively nonantigenic;
2. Coprecipitation of collagen with one of several glycosaminoglycans (including chondroitin 6-sulfate, chondroitin 4-sulfate, dermatan sulfate, heparin and heparan sulfate) can control the biodegradation rate, which is evaluated by collagenase susceptibility;

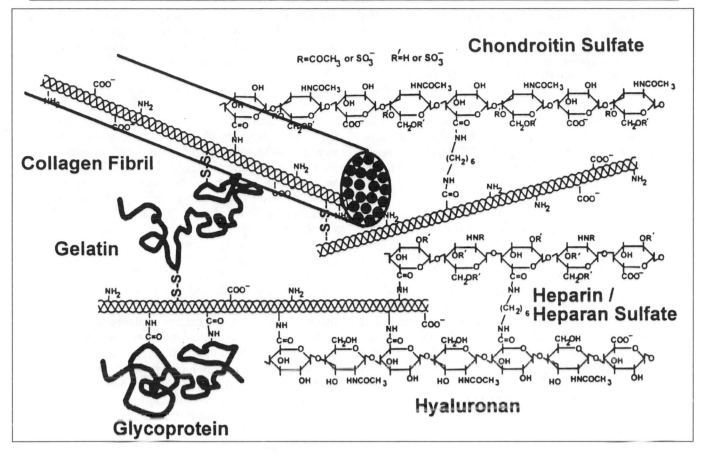

Fig. 27.2. Modified reconstituted or engineered biosynthetic extracellular matrices containing various portions of native components and thiolated gelatin.

3. Glycosaminoglycan are also used to control the mechanical behavior, e.g., as a modulator of the elasticity.

It has been reported that certain collagen-glycosaminoglycan polymers have delayed or arrested the contraction of full-thickness skin wounds. At least three conditions must be met to prevent wound contraction:

1. The enzymatic degradation rate of the implant must be below a certain threshold value;
2. The average pore size must within the range of 20-500 μm in order to allow proper distribution of mesenchymal cells;
3. Epidermal (basal) cells must be seeded into the porous implant before grafting.

Interactions of Biosynthetic Matrices with Cells

Cell Migration on Biosynthetic Matrices

Cell migration requires a solid support such as an extracellular matrix or a basement membrane. In the process of wound healing, certain cells migrate extensively in a highly organized manner.[11] Evidence for the mechanisms of organized cell movement are:

1. Cells are bound to the extracellular matrix through a variety of large glycoproteins;[11-13]

2. Fibronectin molecules can assemble into fibrils as 'cables and connectors' for linking cells to collagen and fibrin;[11]
3. Through binding to cell surface receptors, fibronectin can transduce signals internally to modulate cellular function.[14]

Yaffe and Shoshan[15] studied the behavior of gingival epithelial cells cultured in dishes with gingival epithelial extracellular matrix. It was found that the movement of epithelial cells stops at the contact point with extracellular matrix, and that this results in the piling of cells into several layers. This suggested that the movement of epithelial cells may be influenced by collagen fibers in vivo. This also implies a role for collagen in preventing epithelial cells from penetrating into the lower layer.

The studies of Donaldson et al[16] failed to demonstrate collagen type specificity for supporting the migration of epidermal cells. Denatured collagen and glutaraldehyde crosslinked collagen gels are also able to support the migration of epidermal cells. It is found that the tertiary structure of the collagen molecule is unimportant for the binding of epidermal cells. It is also reported that the α1 chain of type I collagen has at least three, and most likely more, epidermal binding sites.

Epidermal growth factor (EGF) and transformtin growth factor-β (TGF-β) have been shown to play a role in stimulating the growth of epithelial cells.[17,18] The structures of EGF and TGF-β are similar and both bind to the same cell surface receptor, tyrosine kinase.[19] The interactions between the receptor and growth factors lead to intracellular changes in preparing cells for DNA synthesis and proliferation. Barrandon and Green[18] found that the effects of EGF and TGF-β in promoting cell proliferation depend on their abilities to increase the rate of cell migration, which is essential in the process of wound healing. Therefore, appropriate application of EGF or TGF-β during tissue regeneration should be able to promote the re-epithelialization process.

Cell Infiltration into Biosynthetic Matrices

When cells are cultured on a hydrated collagen gel, the shape and motility of cells are very similar to cells in vivo.[13] In addition to the biological effects of hyaluronan demonstrated by Huang et al[5,6] Doillon et al[20] have shown that the presence of either fibronectin or hyaluronic acid or both in a collagen sponge can enhance wound healing in vivo. It has been found that fibroblasts can infiltrate and proliferate through the entire sponge, and subsequently increase collagen biosynthesis. The effect of hyaluronic acid is to promote cellular infiltration and that of fibronectin is to mediate cell attachment to the collagen fibrils. Therefore, incorporation of hyaluronic acid or fibronectin into collagen sponges appears to improve the properties of the regenerated tissue.[21]

Influence of Cells on Matrix Reorganization

Denefle et al[22,23] used unstriated fibrils of purified type I collagen gels to study the anchoring process of keratinocytes and their influences on collagen organization. Two types of collagen striated fiber assemblies seem to appear when isolated epithelium is superimposed on a collagen gel. Numerous extended filopodia of cells arise at the contact sides with one type of collagen fiber assembling around and along them. In the inner side of the gel matrix, collagen fibers assume different shapes and widths depending on the concentration of acid soluble collagen.[22] To further distinguish the effect of preexisting fibronectin from that of keratinocytes on the reorganization of collagen gels, frog skin fragments opposed to collagen coatings were studied either in the presence or absence of fetal calf serum. The results indicate that keratinocytes in the absence of serum appear to influence fibril organization of purified type I collagen gel. Pre-existing fibronectin appears to enhance the capability of keratinocytes to modify collagen fibers, since the presence of serum causes the collagen morphology to closely resemble that of the native wound healing process.[23]

Grinnell and Lamke[24] studied the reorganization of hydrated collagen lattices by human skin fibroblasts. They found collagen reorganization to be similar whether the cells were cultured on the top or at the bottom of the lattices. Initially, proximal collagen fibrils were aligned along the plane of cell spreading. Subsequently, the collagen fibrils distal to the cells underwent reorganization. If the collagen lattice is detached from the underlying substratum, the collagen fibrils roll up into a compact form which has a der-

mis-like appearance. It was suggested that both physical forces and secreted factors from fibroblasts such as fibronectin or other proteoglycans contribute to the reorganization of the collagen lattices.

Influence of Cells on the Contraction of Collagen Matrices

Allen and Schor[25] quantitatively measured the contraction of collagen by fibroblasts. The spherical fibroblasts were initially incubated in the attached collagen lattice. Over 90% of the cells change the morphology to stellate cells after incubation for two hours, but most of them subsequently retract to a spherical morphology when the matrices are carefully detached to produce a floating culture. Collagen matrices reduce to about one half of the original size within the first two hours in a floating culture. This initial contraction rate of collagen is proportional to the cell number within the range of 10^5-10^6 cells/gel. The contraction of the collagen matrix appears to be the result of cell-collagen interaction and collagen reorganization caused by fibroblasts that exert a tension upon the surrounding collagen fibers. It is also suggested that cell-cell interaction does not contribute significantly to the contraction process, since stellate fibroblasts and spherical fibroblasts are homogeneously distributed within the collagen matrix in a floating culture.

Bell et al also reported that human fibroblasts of different proliferative potential contract collagen lattices with equal efficiency.[26] They further found that the contraction rate of collagen lattices can be regulated by varying the protein content of the lattice, the cell number, or the concentration of inhibitors such as colcemid. Inhibition of gel contraction by cytochalasin B and colchicine indicate that the integrity of the cytoskeletons inside the fibroblasts is important for the mechanism of gel contraction.

Influence of Collagen Derived Matrices on Cells

To improve the hematocompatibility of cardiovascular materials, Lee et al[27,28] chemically crosslinked collagen to polyurethane and investigated the growth of endothelial cells on the surface. A flossy-like collagen formed on the polyurethane surface when the crosslinking reaction was carried out with (N-ethyl-N'-3-dimethyl aminopropyl)carbodiimide at pH 5. A fibrillated collagen network was further reconstituted on the polyurethane surface under physiological conditions, using either the flossy-like collagen as a nucleus or an epoxy crosslinking reaction. When cultured with endothelial cells, the collagen fibrillar networks better supported the cell growth. The amounts as well as the density and diameter of collagen fibrils grafted on the polyurethane surfaces correlated with the proliferation of endothelial cells.

Endothelial cells in Tissue Engineering

The main function of endothelial cells is to maintain surface integrity, such as in the lining of heart, blood vessels and lymphatic vessels. They reduce the friction at the fluid to lumen interface, as well as control the flow of blood and passage of cells in the circulation out of the vascular system into the surrounding tissues.[29] Resting endothelium expresses low levels of adhesion molecules that prevent the binding of leukocytes and inhibit coagulation. Infection or injury stimulates the endothelium to express cell surface molecules and adhesion proteins that promote cell interactions.[30] There has been a tremendous resurgence of interest concerning the modulation of endothelial cell function by factors, especially cytokines, and by the composition of the extracellular matrix; this has encouraged the development of endothelial cell culture techniques.[31,32] Endothelial cells cultured from the umbilical vein can be induced to switch to a capillary-like morphology on interaction with basement.[33-35] This morphogenesis results in formation of cellular cords containing a central lumen surrounded by one to three endothelial cells, and is thought to parallel capillary formation in later stages of angiogenesis in vivo.[33-35] Since endothelial cells in vivo are organized in monolayers covering the basement membrane of the vessels, much work has been done using in vitro models with endothelial cells seeded on basement membrane equivalents such as Matrigel, reconstituted from solubilized basement membrane components such as type IV collagen, laminin and fibronectin extracted from Engelbreth-Holm-Swam mouse sarcoma.[36-39] However, endothelial cells can also be successfully cultivated on gelatin or poly-L-lysine-coated surfaces. The cultivation of microvascular endothelial cells in Matrigel can result in the formation of vessel-like cell assembly.[40] Ingber and Folkman studied the effects of coating density of fibronectin, type IV collagen or gelatin on culture dishes (adhesiveness) on the behavior of FGF-stimulated endothelial cells.[41] They observed extensive cell spreading and growth in dishes coated with a high density of fibronectin or type IV collagen, while cell rounding, detachment and loss of viability occurred in dishes with low density coating. Intermediate coating density promoted cell extension and partial retraction of multicellular aggregates; cessation of growth and formation of branching tubular networks occurred. Based on these results they proposed that FGF-stimulated endothelial cells may be "switched" between growth and differentiation as a response to the mechanical integrity of their extracellular matrices. The influence of the extracellular matrix on endothelial behavior is likely to be mediated through integrins, a family of heterodimeric cell surface receptors which transmit signals from the extracellular matrix by organizing the cytoskeleton, thus regulating cell shape, internal cellular architecture and other cell functions.[42] While Matrigel supports the attachment, proliferation and differentiation of endothelial cells, type I collagen containing alpha-elastin was found to inhibit the proliferation and migration of vascular endothelial cells. While others found that type I collagen inhibits the growth of endothelial cells, Lee et al found that endothelial cell growth is supported by large reconstituted type I collagen fibrils formed from collagen dialyzed in phosphate buffered saline.[28] Chen et al studied human and bovine capillary cells grown on surfaces coated with micropatterned extracellular matrix substrates.[43] As the extracellular matrix-coated adhesive islands decreased in size, cell extension became more restricted and the endothelial cells began to switch from growth to apoptosis. Spacing between different adhesive islands also affected cell spreading. Changes in the size and spacing of the micropattern of the adhesive islands caused alteration in cell shape, which governed whether individual cells grow or die. The effect of the extracellular adhesiveness on cell growth and viability was independent of the type of matrix protein used to mediate adhesion in the islands (Fig. 27.3).

Modified Growth Factors: TGF-β with a Collagen Binding Domain

TGF-β appears to be an important regulator of the cardiovascular system. The TGF-β proteins are highly

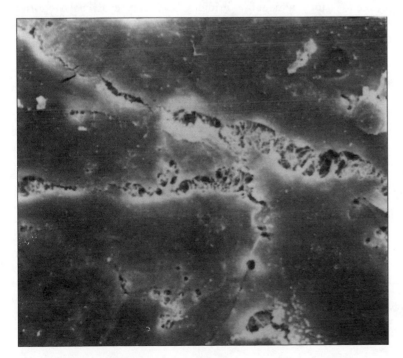

Fig. 27.3. Endothelial cells grown on collagen matrix.

expressed during embryonic development of the heart, and can be elevated after hemodynamic stress. Hence, they possess the potential to significantly influence the progression of a number of vascular disorders, in particular those involving vessel remodeling and repair, such as hypertension following percutaneous balloon catheter angioplasty, atherosclerosis and under some circumstances, angiogenesis. These and many other effects of TGF-β proteins in cardiovascular development, physiology and pathophysiology are dependent upon processes that regulate their expression and release from latent complexes, the receptor types available for binding and the interactions between receptor-mediated intracellular signaling events, which ultimately lead to tissue responses.[44]

Major problems that hamper the use of growth factors in tissue engineering are:

1. The activity is quickly lost due to the protease digestion;
2. They are not retained at the application site;
3. They are carried away by the circulation.

Therefore, targeting growth factors to the application site and controlling their release and activity becomes crucial when applying growth factors as regulatory signals for tissue engineering. In addition to approaches that rely on adsorption of ionically bound, physically entrapped or covalently bound growth factors to resorbable matrices, a novel approach developed in our laboratory relies on the construction of fusion proteins which include a matrix or cell binding domain for targeted delivery of such growth factors[45] (Fig. 27.4).

Transformtin growth factor-β (TGF-β) was used as an example for studying a ECM targeted growth factor. TGF-β is a secreted multifunctional protein that regulates many aspects of cellular functions, including cell proliferation, differentiation, and extracellular matrix metabolism.[46] Based on the different physiological effects of TGF-β, a variety of potential clinical applications for this growth factor have been suggested.[47,48] Since TGF-β is a pleotropic agent which can stimulate, inhibit, and modulate cellular events in a time and concentration dependent manner, it is important to control the biological activity of this growth factor during its use as regulatory signal for tissue engineering.

A collagen targeted TGF-β recombinant fusion protein has been designed, expressed, and renatured into active forms.[45,49] In these fusion proteins, a collagen targeting decapeptide derived from von willebrand factor[50] was modified[49] and fused at the N-terminus of the active TGF-β fragment by molecular manipulation. A protease sensitive site was also inserted in the sequence between the collagen binding domain and the active TGF-β fragment, in order to release the growth factor at appropriate times and sites. Bacterial expression systems provided a good source for this recombinant protein and appear to guarantee sufficient amounts for tissue engineering applications. BL21 (DE3) *E. coli* strain was transformed with a pET 28b expression vector which carried recombinant DNA. Under IPTG induction, this fusion protein can be induced to express at high yield. The induced fusion proteins were found in insoluble inclusion bodies. After being solubilized by a denaturant and purified by Ni-chelating column, the purified TGF-β monomer was refolded in an in vitro optimized system, in which reduced and oxidized forms of glutathione assist TGF-β inter- and intradisulfide bond exchange.[45]

Binding Characteristics

Active TGF-β, a highly hydrophobic basic protein, is rapidly lost from the medium or extracellular fluid by protease digestion. Many extracellular matrix components bind to TGF-β in a reversible manner and may serve as a reservoir for the growth factors.[51,52] TGF-β binding proteins could sequester TGF-β to the extracellular matrix and act as a buffer for its activities.[53,54] Since collagen is a major component of the extracellular matrix, and the structural protein of most tissues, it was chosen as functional carrier of soluble growth factors in this study. In the fusion of TGF-β proteins, a collagen binding domain derived from von willebrand factor was incorporated at the N-terminal of the active growth factor fragment by a bridging Gly. Takagi et al[50] have reported that the primary structure of the von willebrand factor contains a high-affinity collagen binding domain. They further

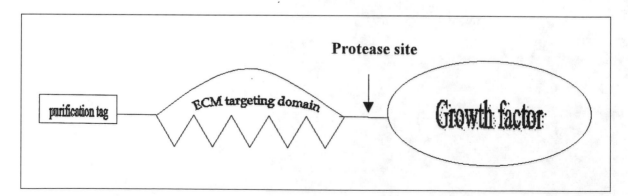

Fig. 27.4. A schematic representation of the genetically engineered growth factor(s). The constructs contain: a collagen binding sequence derived from von willebrand factor; a purification tag (e.g., (His)₆ or GST); and a protease-sensitive site for control release.

delimited the collagen binding site to a decapeptide with the amino acid sequence WREPSFCALS. The collagen targeting characteristics were assayed as described below.

Collagen targeted TGF-β fusion proteins from bacterial inclusion bodies were isolated, dehydrated in DMF, and labeled by [³H]NaBH₄ (100 mCi, Amersham) DMF solution.[55] Labeled recombinant proteins were purified and renatured as described and the bioactivity was also checked. Different doses of labeled TGF-β1-F1 or -F2 fusion proteins were then added to the collagen precoated wells. After incubation and extensive washes in PBS, the labeled TGF-β remaining bound to the collagen was counted after collagenase digestion. The results are shown in Figure 27.5. TGF-β1-F2, which has a collagen binding domain, binds to collagen in a dose dependent manner. TGF-β1-F1, which lacks the collagen binding domain, binds to collagen with less affinity through nonspecific interactions. The only difference in F1 and F2 constructs is the auxiliary collagen binding decapeptide; this suggests that with a collagen binding domain, TGF-β can be specifically targeted to collagen matrices.

To determine the affinity of such binding, F2 fusion protein was first immobilized on a Ni-NTA column and then exposed to biosynthetically labeled [³H]collagen, which was subsequently loaded onto the column. Under these conditions a large portion of the radioactivity was found to bind to the column. Washing the column with a linear gradient of NaCl from 0.15 to 2.0 did not release the [³H]collagen. However, application of a urea gradient (0-5.0 M) was able to quantitatively elute all bound radioactivity (Fig. 27.6). By contrast, when the F1 fusion protein containing only a (His)₆ tag and the TGF-β1 active fragment was applied to the Ni-NTA column under the same conditions, most [³H]collagen was eluted in the void volume, suggesting that the auxiliary

collagen binding domain in F2 afforded this high affinity interaction with collagen.

Biological Activity

Released Collagen Targeted TGF-β Retains Biological Activity

TGF-β activity was assessed by transfected mink lung cell with PAI-1 promoter/luciferase reporter genes.[45] The specificity and sensitivity are the result of using a truncated PAI-1 promoter which retains the two regions responsible for maximal response to TGF-β (56). Collagen bound TGF-β1-F1/F2 fusion proteins were released from the collagen gels with collagenase. The released solubilized TGF-β1-F1 and TGF-β1-F2 proteins were assayed for their biological activity. It was found that collagen bound TGF-β1-F2 was still active when released with collagenase. These experiments demonstrate that the collagen binding domain enables TGF-β1-F2 to be sequestered by the collagen matrix and that it can be released by collagenase digestion to display its biological activity.

Collagen Bound TGF-β1 Activity

Even though we had proven that collagen-targeted TGF-β can bind selectively to the collagen matrix, the biological activity of bound TGF-β2-F2 was unclear. When we precoated culture wells with type I collagen, and then added TGF-β2-F1 and TGF-β2-F2 on the collagen gels, then washed extensively with PBS, only bound TGF-β2-F1/F2 remained on the gel. Subsequently, osteoblastic osteosarcoma cells were plated on top of the collagen gel. After 72 hrs, alkaline phosphatase activity was tested in the cell layer. Results (Fig. 27.7) showed that when TGF-β2-F1/F2 was added to the medium, the cellular responses to these two factors were similar; for

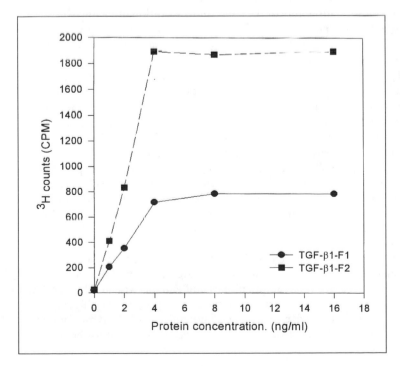

Fig. 27.5. Binding curve of renatured TGF-β2-F2 for collagen matrices. [³H]labeled fusion proteins bind to collagen in a dose-dependent manner. Radio-labeled TGF-β1-F1 or -F2 was incubated with collagen gel. After extensive washing, the collagenase digest solution was counted for radioactivity.

Fig. 27.6. Binding of TGF-β1-F1 and -F2 proteins with collagen. The tripartite fusion proteins F1 (dashed line) and F2 (solid line) were first bound to the Ni-NTA column (3 ml). [³H]collagen was then applied to the column and bound protein was eluted with a gradient of 0-5 M urea in 0.05 M phosphate buffer at pH 7.0 (3 ml/ fraction).

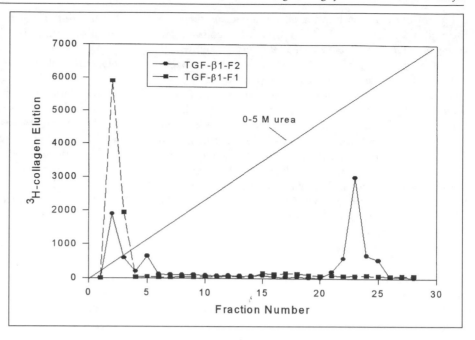

the collagen-bound TGF-β2, cells could still 'recognize' bound TGF-β2 and display increased alkaline phosphatase activity. On the other hand, TGF-β2-F1, washed away by PBS from the collagen gel because it lacks a collagen binding domain, exhibited no effect on induction of alkaline phosphatase activity above control. These results not only confirmed that TGF-β2-F2 could specifically target collagen, but also demonstrated that extracellular matrix-associated TGF-β still performed its biological function.

Other Growth Factors Which May Individually or Synergistically Contribute to Organogenesis

Growth factor targeting to responsive cells and maintenance of adequate pharmacological levels becomes essential, particularly in view of their different effects on various cells and the dose dependence of their response. Using the same recombinant strategy, other growth factors besides TGF-β have also been engineered with an ECM targeting domain. These growth factors include basic fibroblast growth factor (bFGF), epidermal growth factor (EGF), vascular endothelial growth factor (VEGF), α-ECGF and bone morphogenic protein-3 (BMP-3). The targeting sites of growth factors are not limited to the collagen matrix, since fibronectin and heparin targeting domains can also be incorporated into the growth factor molecules. The tissue distribution and cellular effects of platelet-derived growth factor (PDGF), basic fibroblast growth factor (bFGF), transformtin growth factor-b1 (TGF-β1) and insulin-like growth factor 1 (IGF-1) suggest a potential role for these factors in cardiovascular matrix regeneration. Fibroblast replication is stimulated by PDGF and by bFGF. IGF-1 and TGF-β1 have no effect on fibroblast replication. Collagen production is stimulated by all of the growth factors tested: in order of potency, TGF-β1. PDGF, IGF, bFGF. None of the growth factors affected the proportion of rapidly degraded newly synthesized collagen.[57] The sensitivity of cardiac fibroblasts to these factors is con-

sistent with their playing a role during the rapid changes seen in cardiovascular tissues in during development and induced anomalies.

bFGF

bFGF is present in many tissues, intracellularly or bound to heparin-like molecules of the extracellular matrix. It is thought to exert its physiological functions in tissue repair and neovascularizatoion after being released from the extracellular matrix.[58,59] bFGF causes mesenchyme formation and stimulates skin wound healing by increasing cell recruitment, mitosis, and extracellular protein production. Though very potent, bFGF is rapidly degraded when injected or ingested and applications of bFGF are hampered by the instability of the compound. Additionally, a bFGF dose-response curve on bone growth study exhibits biphasic effects, reflected by an exaggerated inhibited cell ingrowth.[60] Controlling bFGF activity therefore becomes meaningful for proper use and clinical application of this growth factor. Preservation and stabilization of bFGF was previously accomplished by binding the factor to heparin-Sepharose beads. This permitted its prolonged storage, repeated handing and encapsulation within a microspherical controlled-released device.[61] Recently our laboratory has engineered collagen targeting bFGF recombinant fusion proteins to enable this fusion protein to be targeted to collagen matrices. Its in vitro activities have been evaluated and their application is under investigation.

VEGF

Recent studies show that exogenously administered angiogenic factors can induce the formation of new blood vessels in adult animals and enhance collateral blood flow to ischemic tissues. It has been suggested that this approach may have a therapeutic potential.[62] VEGF (vascular endothelial growth factor) is a specific mitogen for endothelial

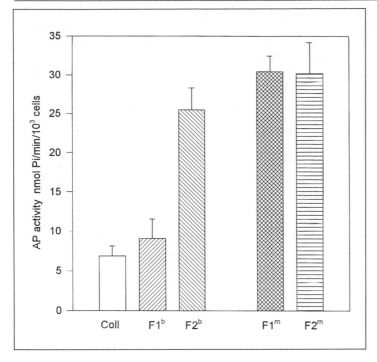

Fig. 27.7. Collagen bound TGF-β2-F2 increases alkaline phosphatase activity of MG-63 cells. F1^m and F2^m: 1 ng TGF-β2-F1 or -F2 fusion protein in the medium. F1^b and F2^b: 5 ng TGF-β2-F1 or -F2 incubated with precoated collagen gel for 1 hour at 37°C followed by three extensive washes with PBS. Cells were then plated on top of gel. Alkaline phosphatase activity was evaluated after a 72 hour incubation.

cells in general and for vascular endothelial cells in particular. It has been shown to promote angiogensis, accelerate endothelial repaving, and to attenuate intimal hyperplasia after arterial injury. The active forms of VEGF are disulfide-linked, dimeric glycoproteins. The presence of two tyrosine kinase receptors for VEGF have been identified in vascular endothelial cells.

EGF and ECGF

Epidermal growth factor (EGF), a 53 amino acid mitogenic polypeptide present in many mammalian species, is one of a number of growth factors being investigated for their potential to expedite the healing process. EGF has been shown to stimulate keratinocyte division in vitro and epidermal regeneration in vivo. It had been shown to have an effect on mesenchymal cells by producing marked proliferation of the dermis in partial thickness wounds and by increasing the tensile strength of surgical incisions. In experimental animals a modified fibrin glue containing 1 μg of α-endothelial cell growth factor (ECGF) was implanted between the aorta and the myocardium of the left ventricle.[63] After 9 weeks of implantation, angiography and histologic investigation showed a newly grown vascular structure between the aorta and the myocardium in all experimental animals, but none in the controls. These studies proved the feasibility of initiating site-directed formation of new blood vessel structures to the heart by a modified fibrin glue implant containing angiogenic growth factor α-ECGF.

BMP-3

One of the few tissues that can regenerate in mammals is bone. To a great extent this is due to the activity of specific growth factors which stimulate its formation. Bone morphogenetic protein-3 (BMP-3, osteogenin) is one of the

several BMP family members which belongs to the transformtin growth factor-beta superfamily. BMP-3 has been characterized by its ability to stimulate osteoblastic differentiation and bone formation.[64,65] It was first identified and then purified from bovine bone by Reddi and colleagues.[65] Although in vivo tests support the role of BMP-3 in bone formation, its mechanism of action is poorly understood. In our laboratory, we bioengineered human recombinant BMP-3 fusion proteins from *E. coli* and renatured them into their native dimer conformation. The large quantities of BMP-3 obtained enabled us to do extensive studies on this growth factor in animal models. When combined with collagen sponge matrices or porous hydroxyapatite ceramics, it appears to generate a potential bone substitute for fracture repair and regeneration.[66]

Applications of the Growth Factor Matrix Technology to the Design of Bioprostheses

One of the significant advances in medicine in this century is associated with the ability of the surgeon to replace defective heart valves, veins and arteries with bioprosthetic devices. Nevertheless, these implants have associated disadvantages since they may require anticoagulation, periodic monitoring for possible failure and in some cases have a limited durability or only be usable in selected cases or locations. It is obvious that if we can provide a scaffolding which after being implanted would allow a tissue or organ to regenerate, that we would be achieving a very meritorious objective. Our current understanding of cell biology, that is, how cells differentiate from stem cells into differentiated cells, how cells interact with the extracellular matrix and the consequences of controlled cell-cell interactions, should be able to lead to the ordered repair of tissues and even organ regeneration in the near future.

Collagen is an ideal biomatrix, as it is the major component of the extracellular matrix. It can be rendered relatively nonantigenic, even if obtained from another species, after removal of the nonhelical antigenic determinants and may soon be available in a recombinant form from human DNA. Reconstituting soluble collagen into fibrous matrices, alone or in combination with the other major component of the extracellular space, namely the proteoglycans, is a relatively simple procedure. Specific collagen types, including those which give rise to basement membranes, are also becoming available in the design of biomatrices.

Growth factors are part of a large number of polypeptides that transmit signals affecting cellular activities. Cells may communicate with each other through direct molecular interactions involving their cell membranes, as a result of the movement of molecules such as peptides or steroids, that can act locally or systematically to modulate cell functions. Growth factors are included in the latter group.[1]

Growth factors can either stimulate or inhibit cell division, differentiation, migration or gene expression, depending on the cells involved. Depending on the concentration present in the cellular environment, growth factors can act in an opposing manner and up or downregulate the synthesis of receptors. In general, both growth factors and mRNAs that code for them turn over very rapidly. They usually exist as inactive or partially active precursors that require proteolytic activation, and may need to bind to matrix molecules for activity or stabilization. They may perform differ-

Fig. 27.8. Collagen-derived matrices combined with collagen-targeted growth factor as tissue substitutes. (A) Modified, reconstituted or engineered biosynthetic extracellular matrices containing various proportions of native components, rearranged and crosslinked to each other, provide sui carriers for the local delivery of such factors. (B) Recombinant collagen-targeted growth factors are specifically targeted to collagen matrices and therefore their effects become localized. Growth factor release can be controlled by proteases due to the insertion of protease sensitive sites between the collagen targeting domain and the active growth factor fragment or by the action of collagenase, which slowly degrades the matrix. (C) Growth factor and collagen composite materials serve as scaffold for cell growth, migration, and differentiation. Under growth factor modulation, cells reorganize and synthesize new extracellular matrix and tissue can be regenerated.

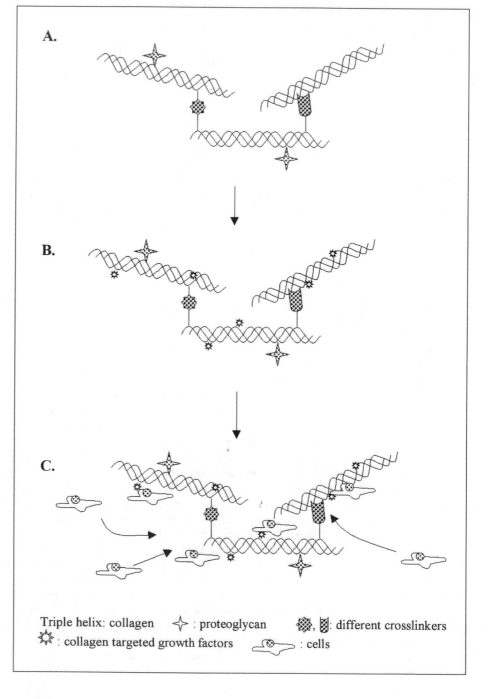

A.

B.

C.

Triple helix: collagen   ✛ : proteoglycan   ▦, ▨ : different crosslinkers

✵ : collagen targeted growth factors   ⊶ : cells

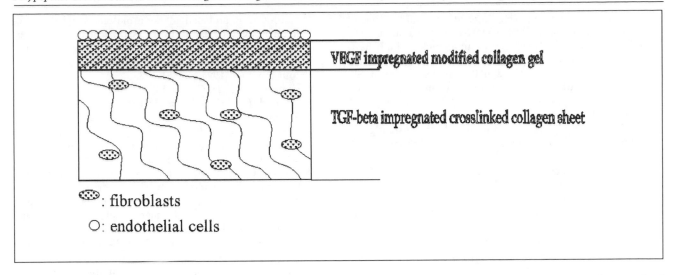

Fig. 27.9. Schematic diagram of vascular graft substitute. A TGF-β impregnated crosslinked collagen sheet supports the growth of fibroblast. VEGF impregnated modified collagen gel supports the growth of vascular endothelial cell growth.

ent functions on different cell types: For instance, TGF-β is stimulatory for fibroblasts and inhibitory for keratinocytes.

With the increasing availability of growth factors derived from cultured human cells and their expansion through recombinant technologies, coupled with an increasing understanding of their functions and clinical applications, the need for useful pharmaceutical forms is becoming more and more apparent. Growth factor targeting to responsive cells and maintenance of adequate pharmacological levels becomes essential, particularly in view of their different effects on various cells and the dose dependence of their response.

An important issue is the short biological half life of growth factors. For example, platelet-derived growth factor (PDGF), an important growth factor first isolated from platelets, cannot be detected in the circulation, and when injected intravenously its half life is less than 2 min.[67]

Our ability to target growth factors to the extracellular matrix components and to couple their release to native ability or inducible enzymatic activity, and our understanding of stem cell biology, as well as our ability to cause such cells to differentiate under the influence of specific growth factors, should allow us to generate functional tissues as replacement for damaged ones. In Figures 27.8 and 27.9 we have provided models for the design of such a matrix, with an emphasis on the construction of a vascular graft. Further experimental work along these lines is very likely to generate functional tissues which, starting with vascular grafts, will continue to increase in complexity until we eventually are able to generate more complex functional organs.

Summary and Conclusion

The design of artificial vascular prostheses and reconstruction with collagen scaffoldings of damaged vessels represents a very important field of endeavor. Vascular grafts should be soft, pliable, flexible, puncturable, and compatible with the surrounding tissue and should be able to anastomose readily to the existing viable tissue.

Our increased understanding of the extracellular matrix, and of the role of agents such as cytokines and growth factors in the various aspects of cellular activity associated with tissue repair and remodeling, can now provide us with sufficient insight into the design of tissue compatible scaffoldings. These scaffoldings can be populated with cells and via processes of cell-matrix and cell-cell interactions modulated to acquire shapes and functions compatible with their endothelial and mesenchymal cells. There should have a decreased tendency to attract platelets and be able to retain growth modulating polypeptides which encourage systematic repopulation by selected cells and yield functional vascular prostheses. We hope that the data present as well as the suggestions made during the course of this review continue to assist and encourage others to move in this direction.

References

1. Nimni ME. Polypeptide growth factors: Targeted delivery systems. Biomaterials 1997; 18:1201-1225.
2. Huang-Lee LLH, Nimni ME. Preparation of type I collagen fibrillar matrices and the effects of collagen concentration on fibroblast contraction. Biomed Eng Appl Basis Comm 1993; 5:664-675.
3. Huang-Lee LLH, Nimni ME. Fibroblast contraction of collagen matrices with and without covalently bound hyaluronan. J Biomater Sci Polymer Edn 1993; 5:99-109.
4. Huang-Lee LLH, Nimni ME. Crosslinked CNBr-activated hyaluronan-collagen matrices: Effects on fibroblast contraction. Matrix Biology, 1994; 14:147-157.
5. Huang-Lee LLH, Wu JH, Nimni ME. Effects of hyaluronan on collagen fibrillar matrix contraction by fibroblasts. J Biomed Mater Res, 1994; 28:123-132.

6. Huang LLH, Chung CH. Superior wound healing of hyaluronan-collagen fibrillar matrix. In Preparation. 1997.

7. Yannas IV, Burke JF. Design of an artificial skin. I. Basic design principles. J Biomed Mater Res 1980; 14:65-81.

8. Yannas IV, Burke JF, Gordon PL, Huang C, Rubenstein RH. Design of an artificial skin. II. Control of chemical composition. J Biomed Mater Res 1980; 14:107-131.

9. Yannas IV. What criteria should be used for designing artificial skin replacements and how do the current grafting materials meet these criteria? J.Trauma 1984; 24(9):s29-s39.

10. Yannas IV. Regeneration of skin and nerve by use of collagen templates. In: Nimni ME, ed. Collagen Biotechnology, Vol. 3. CRC Press, Inc. 1988:87-115.

11. Hynes RO. Fibronectins. Scientific American. 1986; 256(6):42-51.

12. Kleinman HK, Klebe RJ, Martin GR. Role of collagenous matrices in the adhesion and growth of cells. J Cell Biol 1981; 88:473-485.

13. Grinnell F. Cell-collagen interactions: Overview. Meth Enzym 1982; 82:499-503.

14. Bretscher MS. How animal cells move. 1987; 257(6):72-90.

15. Yaffe A, Shoshan S. Cessation of epithelial cell movement at native type I collagen-epithelial interface in vitro. Collagen Res Rel 1985; 5:533-540.

16. Donaldson DJ, Smith GN, Kang AH. Epidermal cell migration on collagen and collagen-derived peptides. J Cell Sci 1982; 57:15-23.

17. Brunt JV, Klausner A. Growth factors speed wound healing. Biotechnology 1988; 6(1): 25-30.

18. Barrandon Y, Green H. Cell migration is essential for sustained growth of keratinocyte colonies: The roles of transformtin growth factor-b and epidermal growth factor. Cell 1987; 50:1131-1137.

19. Berridge MJ. The molecular basis of communication within the cell. Scientific American 1985; 253(4):142-152.

20. Doillon CJ, Silver FH. Collagen wound dressing: Effect of hyaluronic acid and fibronectin. Biomaterials 1986; 7:3-8.

21. Doillon CJ, Silver FH. Fibroblast growth on a porous collagen spone containing hyaluronic acid and fibronectin. Biomaterials 1987; 8:195-200.

22. Denefle JP, Lechaire JP, Miskulin M. Frog skin epithelium interactions with a bovine purified type I collagen gel in culture. J Submicrosc Cytol 1985; 17(1):41-47.

23. Denefle JP, Lechaire JP, Zhu QL. Cultured epidermis influences the fibril organization of purified type I collagen gels. Tissue & Cell 1987; 19(4):469-478.

24. Grinnell F, Lamke CR. Reorganization of hydrated collagen lattices by human skin fibroblasts. J Cell Sci 1984; 66:51-63.

25. Allen TD, Schor SL. The contraction of collagen matrices by dermal fibroblasts. J Ultrastructure Res 1983; 83:205-219.

26. Bell E, Ivarsson B, Merrill C. Production of a tissue-like structure by contraction of collagen lattices by human fibroblasts of different proliferative potential in vitro. Proc Natl Acad Sci USA 1979; 76(3):1274-1278.

27. Lee PC, Chen LW, Huang LLH. Comparison of carbodiimide and epoxy reactions to graft collagen on polyurethane. Biomed Eng Appl Basis Comm 1996; 8:22-29.

28. Lee PC, Huang LL, Chjen LW, Hsieh KH, Tsai CL. Effect of forms of collagen linked to polyurethane on endothelial cell growth. J Biomed Mater Res 1996; 32:645-653.

29. Smith CW Endothelial adhesion molecules and their role in inflammation. Can J Physiol Pharmacol 1993; 71:76-86.

30. Bevilacqua MP, Nelson RM, Mannori G, Cecconi O. Endothelial-leukocyte adhesion molecules in human disease. Ann Rev Med 1994; 45:361-378.

31. Gimbrone MA Jr, Cotran RS, Folkman J. Human vascular endothelial cells in culture. J Cell Biol 1974; 60:675-684.

32. Moyer CF, Dennis PA, Majno G, Joris I. Vascular endothelium in vitro, isolation and characterization. In vitro Cell Dev Biol 1988; 24:359-368.

33. Bauer J, Margolis M, Schreiner C, Edgell CJ, Azizkhan J, Lazarowski E, Juliano RL. In vivo model of angiogenesis using a human endothelium-derived permanent cell line: Contributions of induced gene expression, G-protein, and integrins. J Cell Physiol 1992; 153:427-449.

34. Grant DS, Tashiro KI, Segui-Real B, Yamada Y, Martin HK. Intracellular mechanisms involved in basement membrane induced blood vessel differentiation in vitro. In Vitro cell Dev Biol 1991; 27A:327-336.

35. Kubota Y, Kleinmam HK, Martin GR, Lawley TJ. Role of laminin and basement membrane in the morphological differentiation of human endothelial cells into capillary-like structures. J Cell Biol 1988; 107:1589-1598.

36. Schiffrin EL. The endothelium and control of blood vessel function in health and disease. Clin Invest Med 1994; 17:602-620.

37. Yao J, Bone RC, Sawnhey RS. Different effects of tumor necrosis factor-alpha on the expression of fibronectin and collagen genes in cultured bovine endothelial cells. Cell Mol Biol Res 1995; 41:17-28.

38. Fournier N, Doillon CJ. In vitro angiogenesis in fibrin matrices containing fibronectin or hyaluronic acid. Cell Biol Int Rep 1992; 16:1251-1263.

39. Schnaper HW, Kleinman HK, Grant DS. Role of laminin in endothelial cell recognition and differentiation. Kidney Int. 1993; 43:20-25.

40. Passaniti A, Taylor RM, Pili R, Guo Y, Long PV, Haney JA, Pauly RR, Grant DS, Martin GR. Methods in laboratory investigation. A simple, quantitative method for assessing angiogenesis and antiangiogenic agents using reconstituted basement membrane, heparin, and fibroblast growth factor. Lab Invest 1992; 67:519-528.

41. Ingber DE, Folkman J. Mechanochemical switching between Growth and differentiation during fibroblast growth factor-stimulated angiogenesis in vitro: Role of extracellular matrix. J Cell Biol 1989; 109:317-330.

42. Jullano RL, Haskill S. Signal transduction from the extracellular matrix. J Cell Biol 1993; 120:577-585.

43. Chen CC, Mrksich M, Huang S, Whitesides GM, Ingber DE. Geometric control of cell life and death. Science 1997; 276:1425-1428.

44. Saltis J, Agrotis A, Bobik A. Regulation and interactions of transformtin growth factor-β with cardiovascular cells: Implications for development and disease. Clin Exp Pharm Phys 1996; 23:193-200.

45. Han B, Hall FL, Nimni ME. Purification of a recombinant collagen-targeted TGF-β2 fusion protein expressed in E. coli. Protein Expression and Purification. 1997; 11:169-1778.

46. Massague J. The transformtin growth factor-beta family. Annu Rev Cell Biol 1997; 6:597-641.

47. Miyazono K, Heldin CH. Latent forms of TGF-β: Molecular structure and mechanisms of activation. In: Clini-

cal Applications of TGF-β. CIBA Foundation Symposium 157. Chichester: John Wiley and Sons, 1991:81-90.

48. Roberts AB, Sporn MB. Physiological actions and clinical applications of transformtin growth factor-β (TGF-β). Growth Factor 1993; 8:1-9.

49. Tuan T, Cheung DT, Wu L, Yee A, Gabriel S, Han B, Nimni EM, Hall F. Engineering, expression and renaturation of targeted TGF-β fusion protein. Connect Tissue Res 1996; 34:1-9.

50. Takagi J, Asai H, Satio Y. A collagen/gelatin binding decapeptide derived from bovine peopolypeptide of von willebrand factor. Biochemistry 1992; 31:8530-4.

51. Mooradian DL, Lucas RC, Weatherbee JA, Furcht LT. Transformtin growth factor-beta 1 binds to immobilized fibronectin. J Cell Biochem 1989; 41:189-200.

52. Butzow R, Fukushima D, Twardzik DR, Ruoslahti E. A 60 kD protein mediates the binding of transformtin growth factor-β to cell surface and extracellular matrix proteoglycans. J Cell Biol 1993; 256:5575-727.

53. Omitted in proof.

54. Massague J. Betaglycan can act as a dual modulator of TGF-β access to signaling receptor: Mapping of ligand bonding and GAG attachment sites. J Cell Biol 1994; 124:557-68.

55. Cheung DT, Benya PD, Gorn A, Nimni ME. An efficient method for in vitro labeling proteins to high specific radioactivity using [³H]-NaBH₄ in dimethylformamide. Anal Biochem 1981; 116:69-74.

56. Abe M, Harpel JG, Metz CN, Nunes I, Loskutoff DJ, Rifkin DB. An assay for transformtin growth factor-β using cells transfected with a plasminogen activator inhibitor-1 promoter-luciferase construct. Analy Biol 1994; 216:276-284.

57. Butt RP, Laurent GJ, Bishop JE. Collagen production and replication by cardiacfibroblasts is enhanced in response to diverse classes of growth factors. Eurp J Cell Biol 1995; 68:330-335.

58. Baird A, Klagsbrun M. Annals of the New York Academy of Science: the fibroblast growth factor family, Volume 638. New York Academy of Science. 1991.

59. Voldavsky I, Fuks Z, Ishai-Michaeli R, Bashkin P, Korner G, Bar-Shavit R, Klagsbrun M. Extracellular matrix-resident basic fibroblast growth factor: Implication for the control of angiogenesis. J. Cell Biochem 1991; 45:167-76.

60. Wang JS, Aspenberg P. Basic fibroblast growth factor increases allograft incorporation. Acta Orthop Scand 1994; 65:27-31.

61. Edelman ER Mathiowitz E, Langer R, Klagsbrun. Controlled and modulated release of basic fibroblast growth factor. Biomaterial 1991; 12:619-626.

62. Safi J Jr, Gloe TR, Riccioni TR, Riccioni T, Kovesdi I, Capogrossi MC. Gene therapy with angiogenic factors: A new potential approach to the treatment of ischemic diseases. J Mol Cell Cardiol 1997; 29:2311-2325.

64. Sampath TK, Reddi AH. Dissociative extraction and reconstitution of extracellular matrix components involved in local bone differentiation. Proc Natl Acad Sci USA 1981; 78:7599-603.

65. Luyten FP, Cunnungham NS, Ma S, Muthukumaran N, Hammonds RG, Nevin WB, Wood WI, Reddi AH. Purification and partial amino acid sequence of osteogenin, a protein initiating bone differentiation. J Biol Chem 1989; 264:13377-13380.

66. Han B, Perelman N, Hall F, Shors E, Nimni M. Bone induction by a recombinant collagen targeted BMP-3 fusion protein composite, (in prepration).

67. Bowen-Pope DF, Malpass TW, Foster DM, Rodd R. Platelet-derived growth fctor in vivo: Levels, activity, and rate of clearance. Blood 1984; 64:458-469.

Facilitation of Healing

Angiogenesis

--------- CHAPTER 28 ---------

Fibroblast Growth Factors in Angiogenesis and Tissue Engineering

Karin A. Blumofe, Timothy J. Heilizer, Paula K. Shireman, Howard P. Greisler

Introduction

The main treatment for arterial occlusive disease has become reconstruction. This involves utilizing a graft, either in the form of a vein or synthetic material. These treatments have been found to be limited in their long term therapeutic value due to stenosis formation, a process in which there is luminal narrowing of the vessel due to smooth muscle cell proliferation and connective tissue deposition in the intima of the vessel wall or at the vessel-synthetic graft interface. The smooth muscle cells can continue to proliferate for up to one year after the initial injury. This response is in part modulated by a variety of growth factors such as fibroblast growth factor (FGF), platelet derived growth factor, angiotensin ii, insulin-like growth factor I, and so forth. This course of events results in intimal hyperplasia, ultimately leading to a decrease in blood flow, thrombosis and failure of the interventional reconstruction.

A major focus of vascular research has been to investigate ways in which to decrease the smooth muscle cell migration and proliferation, ultimately decreasing the intimal hyperplasia response. Fibroblast growth factor, as mentioned above, is one of the growth factors that stimulates smooth muscle cell migration and proliferation. Additionally, it serves as a potent stimulator of endothelial cells, inducing angiogenesis, the formation of new blood vessels. The process of neovascularization has also been studied extensively as a therapeutic treatment for ischemic disease. With this in mind, the goal of this chapter is to discuss properties of FGF and its role in tissue engineering.

History

In the mid-1900s the brain was found to be a rich source of growth factors that stimulated fibroblast proliferation. However, it was not until the 1970s that partially purified pituitary extracts were shown to contain potent mitogens, particularly for 3T3 fibroblasts.[1] In 1974 a mitogenic polypeptide from the pituitary was identified[2-4] which was named fibroblast growth factor. Attempts to further characterize the growth factor were hampered by high levels of contaminating fragments of myelin basic protein.[5] Thomas in 1980 used isoelectric points to isolate acidic FGF.[6] The acidic form did not interact with antibodies against myelin basic protein. It was also found that the acidic form possessed mitogenic activity for endothelial cells.[7] Bovine brain contained another type of FGF which had different properties from the acidic FGF, as it was a basic mitogen. Thus, FGF was separated into two forms: FGF-1 and FGF-2. The structural characterization of acidic FGF[8] and basic FGF[9]

Tissue Engineering of Prosthetic Vascular Grafts, edited by Peter Zilla and Howard P. Greisler.
©1999 R.G. Landes Company.

demonstrated that these growth factors are related polypeptides and established the basis for a larger family of polypeptide growth factors. Over the next 13 years eight more isoforms of FGF would be identified, most recently FGF-9 in 1993.[10]

Angiogenesis

Angiogenesis is the formation of new blood vessels from the microcirculation, by a process of cellular outgrowth. In contrast, the development of new vessels from stem cells, as found in an embryo, is termed vasculogenesis. Angiogenesis plays a major role in a variety of natural and disease processes significant in the adult life, such as reproduction (placenta, corpus luteum formation, etc.), wound healing, bone repair, inflammation, neoplasia and collateralization in response to ischemia (heart disease and peripheral vascular disease).

The phenomenon of angiogenesis begins with vascular sprouts that originate from the walls of preexisting capillaries and small venules.[11] It is possible that endothelial cells are recruited from venular segments, because these cells are less constrained by a well formed basal lamina. More recently, larger vessels have been shown to play a role in the formation of new blood vessels. For example, it has been demonstrated that the rat femoral vein, with a discontinuous layer of internal elastic lamina and smooth muscle cells, can contribute to angiogenesis. When the vein is treated with prostaglandins E1 and E2, vascular sprouts arise from the endothelial cells in the intima layer of the vessel.[12] Angiogenesis does not seem to originate from the arterial side of the circulation.[13]

Scanning electron microscopy has been used to study the early changes in vasculature and sprouts appear rapidly, as early as 27 hours after exposure to angiogenic stimuli.[14] From three to five days these sprouts continue to flourish, ultimately forming a rich anastomosing plexus.

On a cellular level, there are multiple processes involved in angiogenesis. Early on there is an increase in the vascular permeability. There is an association of inflammatory cells with intravascular accumulation of platelets and polymorphonuclear leukocytes. The new vessels arise following the margination and diapedesis of the leukocytes.[13] Then the endothelial cells become activated. They display a number of morphological changes, including hypertrophy with bulging into the vascular lumen, nuclear enlargement, increase in the number of organelles and formation of projections from their surfaces.[13] The fragmentation and disintegration of the basal lamina is a necessary step for the migration of endothelial cells to occur.[15] This degradation is due to proteolytic enzymes synthesized and secreted by the activated endothelial cells.[16]

Angiogenesis then proceeds with the migration of endothelial cells, moving into the interstitial space. Two different types of endothelial cell migration have been described:

1. Bicellular or telescoping formation; and
2. Linear formation.

In the bicellular type of migration, two or more endothelial cells move from the wall of the parent vessel towards the perivascular space, forming parallel processes. With linear movement, a single endothelial cell projection or pseudopod migrates from the parent capillary to the surrounding connective tissue.[11,17]

The next phase in this process is that of endothelial cell proliferation. Mature endothelial cells normally have a slow turnover rate of approximately 2 months. However, when necessary, as in response to angiogenic stimuli, the endothelial cell can quickly convert to a proliferative state. The induction of endothelial cell proliferation is associated with disruption of cell-cell contacts[18] and alterations in the cytoskeletal organization, such as microtubule destabilization.[19] Development of the new vessel lumen involves the endothelial cell forming tubular channels. It is thought that the capillary lumen is generated by adjacent endothelial processes, causing intercellular canalization of adjacent endothelial cells.[20] A new basal lamina is generated consisting of fibronectin, laminin and type IV collagen.[13]

Another important cell in the angiogenic process is the pericyte. Initially the pericytes undergo intense proliferation. During the stages of capillary sprouting, the exact role of the pericytes is unclear. These cells appear to bridge the gaps between opposing endothelial sprouts by utilizing the pericytic processes. Capillary sprouts are then able to fuse, forming capillary loops and eventually a plexus network. The pericytes also play a role in the regulation of angiogenesis. There is an absence of pericytes at the tips of migrating endothelial cells while, in contrast, their presence in the older regions of capillaries may inhibit endothelial cell proliferation and migration, leading to vessel maturation.[21]

Many cells, including pericytes, macrophages, mast cells, lymphocytes, connective tissue cells, endothelial cells and tumor cells influence the formation of new vessels by secreting soluble angiogenic molecules. The balance of positive and negative regulators of angiogenesis control when a vessel will proceed to neovascularization. A multitude of molecules have been characterized as influencing this process. Initial studies were done with the chorioallantoic membrane of the chick embryo (CAM) and the corneal pocket of the rabbit. In the CAM system, a quantity of an angiogenic substance was placed on exposed chick chorioallantoic membrane. Similarly with the rabbit experiments, angiogenic substances were introduced into intracorneal pockets. These two models were useful in examining the angiogenic potential of a substance. However, it was not until the development of cultured endothelial cells and biological assays that it became possible to directly examine the mechanisms which regulate cell behavior in angiogenesis. The first purified angiogenic factor was FGF-2. This was followed by numerous other molecules such as vascular endothelial growth factor (VEGF), transformtin growth factor-beta, tumor necrosis factor, interleukin-8, platelet derived endothelial cell growth factor (PD-ECGF), angiogenin and angiotropin, to name a few.

FGF serves as a chemotactic stimulator for endothelial cells. If a monolayer of cultured endothelial cells is damaged, FGF stimulates cellular migration into the denuded area.[22] FGF-2 has been shown to increase the secretion of plasminogen activator and collagenase from bovine aortic endothelial cells. These substances are thought to digest the basement membrane preceding migration of endothelial cells. Antibodies directed against FGF-2 cause impairment of endothelial cell migration and inhibit the release of plasminogen activator.[22] Additional experiments have demonstrated that FGF-2 treatments can induce capillary endothelial cells to invade a collagen matrix. These cells then organize themselves to form characteristic tubules that resemble blood capillaries.[23] In animal studies, when FGF is applied to the rabbit or mouse cornea, directed ingrowth of new vessels is stimulated.[24,25] Increased levels of FGF has not only been implicated in vessel growth but becomes limited when neovascularization ceases.[23]

FGF Characterization

Isoforms

Currently the FGF gene family comprises nine members (FGF-1 through FGF-9) in mammals. All are structurally related, with a homology from 35-55% and generally encode proteins with a molecular mass of 20-30 kDa. Over the course of time and as research has developed, so has the nomenclature and characterization of FGF (Table 28.1).

In 1980, FGF-1 was discovered by detecting the presence of a polypeptide with a distinct acidic isoelectric point from extracts of bovine brain.[6] FGF-2 was purified by Abraham in 1986 by using cDNA clones from kidney, heart, liver, placenta and breast carcinoma.[26] FGF-3 was identified as the site of insertion of the mouse mammary tumor virus. Insertion of viral DNA within genomic *int-2* led to gene activation and transformation of infected cells.[27] FGF-4 and FGF-5 were identified by screening neoplastic cells for the presence of genes capable of transforming 3T3 fibroblasts.[28,29] Delli Bovi transfected DNA from Kaposi's sarcoma into fibroblasts and two new mRNAs were produced. The protein product of one was termed FGF-4. It was 206 amino acids in length had significant homology to both FGF-1 and FGF-2. Subsequently, Zahn discovered FGF-5 after transfecting fibroblasts with human tumor DNA. Using a human *hst* specific probe to screen a mouse cosmid library, Marics found FGF-6. Tanaka showed that a mouse mammary carcinoma cell line was stimulated by a growth factor which was FGF-7.[30] FGF-7 is a keratinocyte cell mitogen[31] which possesses a DNA sequence complementary

to the FGF family, with 30-40% homology. FGF-9, the most recently discovered, was purified from a human glial cell line.[10]

Of these nine FGF genes that have been identified, different isoforms can be created through a variety of methods. For instance, varying isoforms are generated by using alternative initiation codons for translation.[32,33] Novel FGF isoforms can also be generated by alternative splicing such as with FGF-2[34] and FGF-8.[30] Finally, posttranslational modification techniques provide additional isoforms.

Structure

The gene for FGF-1 is located on chromosome 5 between bands 5q31.3 and 5q33.2, while the FGF-2 gene is on chromosome 4.[35] These two genes are similar in their organization, as they both have three exons separated by two large introns. The major difference in these two genes is the location of the amino-terminus of the two proteins. Nucleotide sequence analysis of FGF-1 reveals that the open reading frame is flanked by termination codons. The primary sequence of FGF-2, however, has revealed an amino-terminal sequence that extends 5' to a proposed initiator, methionine.[36] FGFs also possess a distinct structural feature known as a nuclear localization sequence, located near the NH_2 end of the protein. This sequence in FGF-1 plays a role in moving extracellular FGF towards the nucleus in a receptor-dependent manner. FGF-2 has similar features but has been found to be more complicated. FGF-2 mRNA contains multiple translational start sites and the resulting proteins are transferred to either a cytosolic or nuclear locale.[37]

FGF-1 and FGF-2 are single chain polypeptides which share 55% sequence homology. The complete structure of bovine FGF-1 was first described in 1985.[38] The final structure is the result of multiple proteolytic cleavages of a more primitive form. Sequence analysis of human FGF-1 demonstrates similar amino-terminal truncations, with a 92% sequence identity with the bovine protein.[39] FGF-1 is an anionic mitogen with a molecular weight ranging from 15,000-17,000 kDa. The X-ray crystal structure of human FGF-1 has been identified.[40] It has been shown to contain four independent molecules arranged in an asymmetric unit. Each molecule contains a sulfate ion which stabilizes the other molecules through a hydrogen bond interaction, a potential heparin binding site.

FGF-2 is a cationic mitogen with an isoelectric point of 9.6. Its molecular weight is 18,000 kDa. FGF-2 has been found to contain 146 amino acids. Within this structure are two sequences similar to known heparin binding sites.[9]

FGF Secretion

The FGF prototypes regulate biological activities as an extracellular protein; therefore it is important to examine how these proteins are released (or secreted) from cells. FGF-1, FGF-2 and FGF-9 have been found to lack a "traditional" leader sequence (similar to the interleukin family) and consequently secretion via the endoplasmic reticulum does not occur. When the endoplasmic reticulum-Golgi apparatus path is disrupted by chemical agents, the release of FGF-1 is not inhibited.[41] It is thought that FGF is released in

---

Table 28.1. Nomenclature of the FGF family

	Historical Name (23)
FGF-1	acidic FGF, HBGF-1, ECGF
FGF-2	basic FGF, HBGF-2
FGF-3	Int-3
FGF-4	Kaposi's FGF, KS3, Hst-1
FGF-5	
FGF-6	Hst-2
FGF-7	Keratinocyte growth factor (KGF)
FGF-8	Androgen inducible growth factor
FGF-9	

the form of a dimer which is then separated by a reducing agent. The monomer form of FGF is able to interact with the FGF receptors[37,42] (Fig. 28.1). Various methods of FGF release have been proposed. For example, it has been demonstrated that the release of FGF-1 is regulated by temperature. NIH 3T3 cells secrete FGF-1 in response to heat shock,[43] and terminate release following treatment with either actinomycin D or cyclohexamide. Recent studies of the kinetics of FGF-1 release suggest that the FGF-1 secretion pathway may be limited to newly translated FGF-1.[22] Inflammation has also been proposed to serve as the initial stressor releasing FGF. FGF-2 has also been found to be secreted by an independent pathway.[44] FGF-9 also lacks a typical N-terminal signal sequence, but has been found to be secreted following transfection into COS cells.[45]

In contrast, the remaining members of the FGF family possess a functional signal sequence. Some of the FGF genes have been identified as oncogenes, reflecting an ability to function in an autocrine manner. For example, FGF-4 (*hst-1*) is a frequently identified oncogene in transformation assays of NIH 3T3 cells.

Storage of FGF has been localized to the extracellular matrix and basement membranes of medium and large blood vessels, as well as the anastomosis site of branching capillaries. Heaprin sulfate, which is known to prevent proteolytic degradation of FGF, is also found in high concentrations in these areas. FGF is released from the extracellular matrix in a biologically active form.[46]

Interaction with Heparin

In 1983 it was discovered that crude extracts of heparin bind to FGF.[47] This was also demonstrated with pure forms of FGF-1[48] and FGF-2.[49] The use of heparin affinity purification of FGFs allowed for a clearer understanding of its biological activities. These initial studies showed that the binding of FGF-1 and FGF-2 to heparin were different, allowing a means to differentiate between the two. Heparin

potentiates the biological activity of FGF-1 but does not have a profound effect on the mitogenic activity of FGF-2. Both forms of FGF are protected from degradation when associated with heparin. It is suggested that this is due to the stabilization of FGF's tertiary structure and prevention of proteolytic modification. Heparin has additionally been found to protect FGF from heat[50,51] and acid[51] inactivation. FGF-1 is further protected from trypsin, plasmin[50] and thrombin.[52] As previously mentioned, FGF is found in association with heparin in the extracellular matrix and basement membranes of blood vessels. FGF is ultimately released from its interactions with heparin by an enzyme called heparinase, which is expressed by platelets, neutrophils and lymphoma cells.[46]

Biological Activity

Tissue Expression

High levels of FGF-1 are found in neural tissue.[54] The structural characterization of pituitary FGF was described in 1985. In 1987 it was demonstrated that FGF is located in the subendothelial extracellular matrix[53] and basement membrane, particularly in arterial and capillary walls. FGF-1 is not as widely distributed as FGF-2, which is located in brain, kidney, adrenal, corpus luteum and the macrophage cell lines.[23] Using radiolabeled immunoassays, circulating FGF was established in bovine, rat and human serum. Since FGF is involved in cell growth, it stands to reason that its distribution would be widespread.

In Vitro

FGF has been found to affect a variety of cell types in vitro, including endothelial cells (as previously discussed), fibroblasts, smooth muscle cells, and neuroendocrine cells.

Fibroblasts

During tissue repair fibroblasts function as a source of collagen and matrix that participate in the formation of

Fig. 28.1. Mechanism of FGF-1 secretion. In response to a variety of stresses, FGF-1 is released as a homodimer. Reducing agents (RSH) such as glutathione are able to reduce the FGF-1 dimer, enabling it to interact with the heparan sulfate proteoglycan (HSPG). Once associated with HSPG at the cell surface, FGF-1 is able to signal a biological response through the FGF receptor (FGFR-1). (Reproduced with permission from ref. 37)

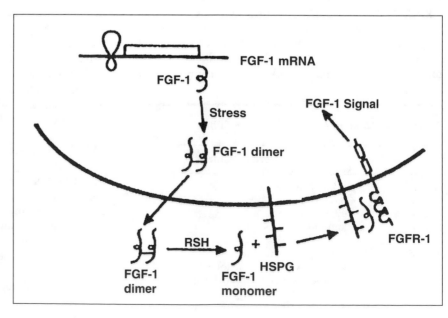

granulation tissue. FGF is chemotactic for fibroblasts. It also acts as a negative regulator of collagen metabolism as demonstrated by a decrease in collagen production in cultured fibroblasts.

Smooth Muscle Cells

FGF-2 has been found to stimulate vascular smooth muscle cell proliferation. Amplification of DNA synthesis occurs within the smooth muscle cell due to autocrine effects of the FGF.[55] Smooth muscle cell proliferation is also stimulated by FGF-1, but only in the presence of heparin (at physiologically relevant concentrations of FGF-1).

Neuroendocrine Cells

Both FGF-1 and FGF-2 are widely distributed throughout the central nervous system. It has been found that FGF has an effect on glial cells, playing a role in the modulation of cell proliferation.[56]

In Vivo

The biological effects of FGF in vivo have been studied in both natural and pathological processes such as angiogenesis (as previously described), intimal hyperplasia, neoplasia, and wound healing.

Intimal Hyperplasia

FGF has been found to be a smooth muscle cell mitogen and may contribute to the initial smooth muscle cell proliferation, playing a critical role in the development of intimal hyperplasia. When rat arteries are injured to induce intimal hyperplasia, the response is limited when antibodies to FGF-2 are applied, causing a significant reduction in the smooth muscle cell response.[57] By encoding porcine arterial endothelial cells with a FGF-1 gene, increased intimal thickening was demonstrated after 3 weeks as compared to a control group.[58] Finding ways to inhibit the smooth muscle cell response to FGF while concomitantly stimulating endothelial cell progression has been a major area of vascular research and tissue engineering.

Neoplasia

Tumor angiogenesis has properties somewhat different from normal angiogenesis. The fast growth of tumor cells requires that angiogenesis takes place at a high rate in order to keep up with the needs of an expanding tumor. FGF-1 and FGF-2 are found to be associated with the majority of adult tumors (for instance, breast, lung, prostate cancer, renal cell and bladder carcinoma, brain tumors, hepatocellular carcinoma, melanoma, Kaposi's sarcoma and others). A study of FGF localization in gastrointestinal tumors found FGF-2 in the extracellular matrix. Cellular staining also revealed FGF to be present in fibroblasts and endothelial cells of the host.[59] There is a reported correlation between blood vessel density versus metastatic lesions in breast, lung, prostate, and head and neck cancers.[60] This correlation was tested by injecting mice with anti-FGF antibodies, and a decrease in tumor blood vessel density was observed. FGF is even detectable at significant levels in the serum and urine of cancer patients.[61]

Since angiogenesis plays such an important role in tumor biology, it has been postulated that the inhibition of angiogenic growth factors may ultimately affect tumor growth and overall outcome. A number of different techniques have been utilized to inhibit the effects of FGF. One particular model uses a monoclonal antibody against FGF-2 and successfully suppressed solid tumor growth.[62] A different approach to inhibit FGF is based on molecular targeting of the gene transcripts. For instance, the use of antisense oligodeoxynucleotides will inhibit translation and reduce the stability of targeted RNA. For FGF-2 this method has been shown to inhibit primary melanoma proliferation in tissue culture.[63]

Wound Healing

Wound healing consists of a series of complex processes comprising inflammation, neovascularization, granulation tissue formation and matrix remodeling, which proceed in an overlapping manner. Exogenously applied FGF-2 has been known to induce potent angiogenesis and granulation tissue formation, and to result in stimulation of wound healing in animal models. Localized immunostaining with antibodies shows increased FGF-2 levels in burn wounds.[64] Using a variety of "healing-impaired" mice (such as obese, diabetic, steroid treated, malnourished, etc.) the effects of FGF were observed. Each mouse sustained an injury (such as a burn wound, decubitus ulcer, excisional wound, and so forth) and each wound was covered with an occlusive dressing, some with the application of FGF-2. The wound healing rate was monitored. It was found that the FGF-2 treatment resulted in an acceleration of wound healing in every condition.[65] FGF has been found to have two major contributions to wound healing: It facilitates neovascularization and causes a decrease in collagen production, ultimately resulting in tissue with a reduced tensile strength.[66]

Receptors

Early studies suggested that FGF-1 and FGF-2 were bound by the same receptor.[67] But later experiments revealed that both high and low affinity binding sites exist.

High Affinity Receptors

The high affinity receptors for FGF-1 and FGF-2 have been located on a wide range of cell types such as endothelial cells, hepatoma cells, smooth muscle cells, fibroblasts, smooth muscle cells, retinal cells, chondrocytes, hepatocytes, myoblasts, and various tumor cells.[68] The number of sites per cell varies from 2,000 to over 100,000 and the molecular weight ranges from 105-165 kDa, depending on the type of cell studied. The majority of FGF receptors are utilized by both FGF-1 and FGF-2. However, there is some heterogeneity among receptors, dependent on varying degrees of glycosylation.

The varying FGF receptor isoforms are produced by the same gene. Since 1989 there have been four FGF receptor genes identified. The nomenclature is varied: FGFR1 (flg, bFGR, Cek1, N-bFGFR, h2, h3, h4, h5), FGFR2 (bek, Cek3, K-sam, TK 14, TK 25, KGFR), FGFR3 (Cek2), and FGFR4. The FGF receptor genes share a large sequence homology with each other. The gene structure reveals two mechanisms for the formation of the receptor isoforms: alternative mRNA splicing, resulting in deletions or alternate exon usage; and internal polyadenylation, resulting in truncated products.[23] Thus the FGF receptor system is redundantly specific. That is, one receptor may bind with several different FGFs or, alternatively, one FGF may interact with a number of varying receptors.

The structure of the high affinity receptor, a transmembrane glycoprotein, is divided into an extracelluar and intracellular component. The extracellular portion contains three Ig-like domains which vary in expression by alternative splicing; this area of the receptor is the least conserved region. The first Ig domain is not essential for the high affinity binding of FGF-1 or FGF-2. There is also a signal peptide and acid box region in the extracellular portion of the receptor. The intracellular component has two tyrosine kinase domains which are the most highly conserved regions (Fig. 28.2).

Low Affinity Receptors

The low affinity receptors have been located on fibroblasts, endothelial cells, epithelial cells, neurons, tumor cells and in the basement membrane of a variety of tissues. These binding sites range from 0.5×10^6 to several million in number.

The low affinity receptor present on the cell surface shows many similarities to heparin. In fact, when cells are incubated with heparin, the interaction of FGF-2 and this receptor is inhibited.[69] Cloning of this receptor demonstrated a cell-surface heparan proteoglycan. Heparan sulfates are N-sulfated polysaccharide components of proteoglycans. It is synthesized by most vertebrate cells, as compared to heparin which is an exclusive product of connective tissue mast cells. Heparan sulfate and heparin synthesis occur within the Golgi complex, beginning with the nonsulfated precursor heparan. This precursor is transformed to heparan sulfate or heparin by a series of polymer modifications. This results in heparin containing a significant higher concentration of sulfate groups as compared to heparan sulfate. Heparan sulfates are mainly present on cell surfaces and in the extracellular matrix as proteoglycans. It is well established that the heparan sulfates bind to a wide variety of cytokines and specifically to FGF-1 and FGF-2.[70]

The low affinity receptor is now known to be syndecan. Syndecan is a proteoglycan initially cloned from mouse. It is a polymorphic molecule with heparan and chondoitin sulfate chains associated with a 31 kDa transmembrane polypeptide. It is mainly found on the surface of epithelial cells from mature tissues such as skin, liver, and breast.[68] Syndecan is a family of proteoglycans (syndecan 1, 2, 3 or 4) based on four specific core proteins. They can interact with

Fig. 28.2. Structure of an FGF receptor (Reproduced with permission from ref. 42)

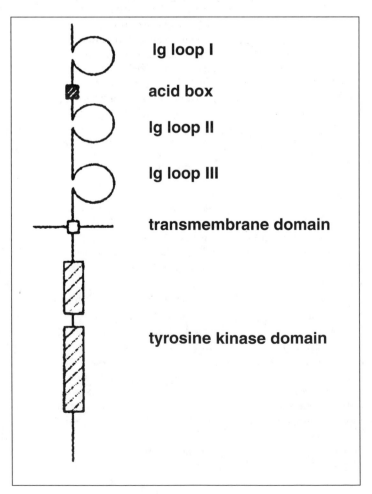

Ig loop I

acid box

Ig loop II

Ig loop III

transmembrane domain

tyrosine kinase domain

varying components of the matrix like fibronectin and collagen as well as FGF-2.[72]

The amino acid sequence of the core protein contains a transmembrane domain with an extracellular region containing six potential attachment sites for glycosaminoglycan side chains.[71] The receptor has been characterized to two major components: a proteoglycan of 250 kDa which appears in the plasma membrane and an 800 kDa which is located in the extracellular matrix. It is the extracellular component that can vary, allowing for diversity.[72]

It is suggested that the low affinity receptor is an accessory molecule required for the binding of FGF to the high affinity receptor. Using cells deficient in heparan sulfates, it was found that FGF-2 could not bind to its high affinity receptor.[73] Similarly, treatment of skeletal muscle or adrenal cells with heparinase demonstrated FGF's inability to interact with its high affinity receptor, with a decrease in cell proliferation.[74,75] All of this data implicates the low affinity FGF receptor as an accessory molecule, required for the complexing of FGF in a biologically active form to its high affinity receptor.

Signal Transduction

FGF signaling immediately follows the binding of FGF to its receptor. Heparin is required for this interaction to occur. Although the exact mechanism is unclear, it is thought that heparin helps stabilize the FGF-FGF receptor complex. The binding leads to FGF receptor dimerization, autophosphorylation and an increase in the tyrosine kinase activity. This initiates a responding cascade of events with activation of a variety of signaling molecules, ultimately resulting in transcription of genes necessary for the FGF response[76] (Fig. 28.3).

FGF and Vascular Grafts

The major cause of failure of vascular grafts is 2-fold: Early on it is due to thrombosis and later the primary cause is myointimal hyperplasia. The interface between the blood and graft wall is where these pathological processes occur.

In 1978 Herring developed the concept that endothelial cells transplanted onto a graft surface could prolong the graft's survival.[77] The presence of a confluent monolayer of endothelial cells could theoretically improve graft thrombo-

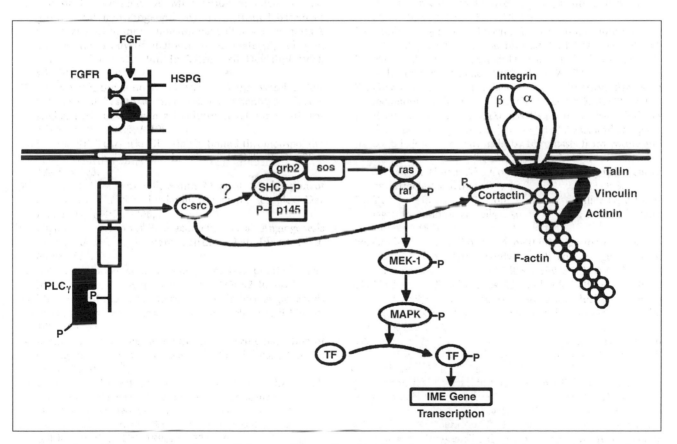

Fig. 28.3. Schematic presentation of intracellular signaling mediated by the FGF receptor (FGFR). The FGFR is activated upon binding FGF and associated heparan sulfate proteoglycan (HSPG). The FGFR undergoes autophosphorylation on tyrosine residues. A signal transduction cascade results in the activation of various proteins, including the F-actin-binding protein cortactin. Further propagation of the signaling cascade induces the activity of MAP kinase (MAPK), which phosphorylates transcription factors (TF), activating the genes necessary for the FGF response. (Reproduced with permission from ref. 37)

resistance and prevent the development of intimal hyperplasia. Three sources of endothelial cells seen on a prosthetic vascular lumen have been observed. Endothelial cells may infiltrate from a native artery over the anastomosis, are observed as ingrowth through the interstices originating from host perigraft tissue, and may occasionally be circulating. In humans it is rare to see complete endothelialization on a prosthetic graft, even after it has been well incorporated into the host tissue. Direct seeding of endothelial cells onto prosthetic grafts has been extensively investigated, but in clinical trials the benefits have been modest.[78-81] One of the difficulties with this technique is the relatively low cell density initially applied to the graft and inadequate cell attachment. The use of specific endothelial cell chemoattractants and mitogens, such as FGF, can theoretically stimulate transinterstitial capillary ingrowth, resulting in enhanced endothelialization of the graft surface.

Work by Greisler's group has evaluated the application of FGF to synthetic surfaces as a means to either enhance spontaneous endothelialization of that surface or to stimulate the proliferation of seeded endothelial cells. In early studies, FGF-1 was applied to both Dacron and polydioxanone (PDS) grafts by means of sequential application of fibronectin, heparin, FGF-1 and a second layer of heparin. Using [^{125}I]FGF-1, the retention of the growth factor in vivo was quantitated. One week after the application, the retention was 44% in the Dacron grafts and 23% in the PDS grafts.[82,83] After the graft was explanted, the FGF-1 was eluted and shown to have retained its mitogenic activity on quiescent lung endothelial cells.[83] A study by Tomizawa used minced canine adipose tissue that was applied to vascular grafts. These were implanted into the abdominal aorta of dogs. When the grafts were removed, endothelial-like cells extending onto luminal thrombus was observed. These cells were immunohistologically positive for FGF-2.[84]

Further studies have utilized fibrin glue (FG), a composite of thrombin and fibrinogen, as a controlled local delivery system for FGF-1 and heparin. Three dimensional analysis of the FGF distribution has revealed that it was even throughout the graft.[85] Studies comparing the fibronectin treatment to the FG illustrated greater endothelial cell retention with the latter.[86] Expanded polytetrafluoroethylene (ePTFE—60 micron internodal distance) grafts were treated with the FG-FGF-1-heparin combination and implanted in dogs as 5 cm aortoiliac grafts and 30 cm thoracoabdominal aortic grafts. When compared to control groups, the pretreated grafts resulted in a significant increase in endothelial cell proliferation as assayed by en face autoradiography. There was also extensive transinterstitial capillary ingrowth observed throughout the graft wall.[87,88] Cross-sectional autoradiography showed a similar increase in subendothelial myofibroblast proliferation in the pretreated grafts at one month. Analysis at 140 days revealed the FG-FGF-1-heparin grafts had developed a significantly thicker inner capsule (139 microns versus <95 microns in the control groups) consisting of myofibroblasts and collagen.[88]

Although heparin and FGF-1 act synergistically to stimulate smooth muscle cell and fibroblast proliferation, in the absence of FGF-1, heparin alone has been shown to inhibit smooth muscle cells.[89,90] Additional in vitro studies have shown that at an optimized FGF-1 to heparin ratio, using a high dose of heparin, endothelial cell proliferation could selectively be stimulated while smooth muscle cells are inhibited.[91]

Others have studied the release of FGF from prosthetic grafts. For instance, Yamamura applied FGF-2 to 0.75 mm disks made of ePTFE. Biodegradable hydroxypropylchitosan acetate (HPCHA) was applied to control the rate of release of FGF from these disks. The disks were implanted into rabbit skin pockets and harvested over 24 hours. The disks treated with HPCHA and FGF released only 60% of the FGF-2, while disks treated with FGF-2 alone released all of the cytokine in a 24 hour period. It was concluded that HPCHA allowed the slow, reliable release of FGF from prosthetic material.[92] In another experiment, bone marrow cells were applied to ePTFE vascular grafts and implanted into the abdominal aorta of dogs. At six months time the grafts were still immunohistochemically reactive to FGF-2.[93]

The following experiments examined the FGF retention within injured vessels. Using a balloon injury model, [^{125}I]FGF-1 in FG was applied to the carotid arteries of dogs. The result revealed a 41% and 37% retention of FGF-1 after 10 and 60 minutes of circulation respectively.[94,95] In a similar fashion, the retention of ^{111}Indium-labelled platelets was quantitated in FG versus untreated identically injured carotids. Platelet deposition was a significant 45% less in the FG group.[95] These studies seem to indicate that the application of FG to arterial surfaces following injury has potential clinical utility. The incorporation of FGF-1 plus heparin within FG onto synthetic grafts may promote neovascularization and prevent pseudointimal hyperplasia, but this is still under investigation.

One technique that is now being utilized is the use of "mutant" forms of FGF-1. In other words, by making specific mutations in the structure of FGF, perhaps a growth factor with a more specific function can be developed. For example, an extensive characterization of FGF-1 mutants of lysine 132 to a glutamic acid or a glycine residue has been completed.[96,97] This altered form of FGF-1 in bone assays has been shown to induce angiogenesis with a decease in fibroblast proliferation. These functional characteristics, selective stimulation of endothelial cells and inhibiting fibroblasts, are qualities that are likely to be beneficial when applied to models of vascular healing.

To determine the relative percent coverage of seeded versus spontaneously ingrowing endothelial cells on FG treated surfaces, a method of fluorescent labeling with PKH-26 has been developed. Proliferation assays in vitro documented virtually identical growth rates for labeled versus unlabeled canine jugular vein endothelial cells. There is nearly a linear relationship between the concentration of applied PKH-26 (from 0-10 μM of PKH-26) and the mean intensity of fluorescence of labeled endothelial cells. Additionally, no PKH-26 induced toxicity or alterations in growth kinetics were observed using concentrations of PKH-26 up to 10 μM (although cellular toxicity was detected at 20 μM concentrations). Labeled endothelial cells are visualized on both Dacron and ePTFE surfaces under fluorescent illumination.[98] This cell labeling technique is now being applied to study the effects on balloon injured carotid arteries treated with FG plus FGF-1 and heparin and PKH-26 labeled autologous endothelial cells.

FGF and Ischemia

Compromised vascular circulation is an important component in many disease processes such as coronary ischemia, congestive heart failure, and peripheral vascular insufficiency. In these conditions there is insufficient capillary flow, which contributes to the extent of the damage to the tissue. It is thought that increasing the number of capillaries, and ultimately the oxygen supply, in these underperfused tissue beds may provide a palliative effect, thus limiting necrosis or loss of function. Angiogenesis has been investigated in terms of its relation to the development of collateral blood flow. Studies examining canine and swine coronary circulations have established that cellular proliferation is a feature of collateral vessel development that occurs as a result of arterial occlusion.[99,100] By using angiogenic growth factors, such as FGF, collateral artery development has been augmented.

Since cardiac disease is a major cause of morbidity and mortality, the effects of FGF on myocardial neovascularization have been studied extensively. When rabbits with chronic myocardial ischemia were subjected to pericardial injections of FGF-2, there was a significant increase in the growth of small vessels.[101] To study the effect of FGF on acute myocardial damage, dog right ventricles were injected with FGF and heparin after an induced myocardial event. Examination after one month revealed less area of infarction in the treated cardiac tissue as compared to the right ventricle.[102] Sellke studied chronic myocardial ischemia, showing that chronic perfusion through collateral vessels in the heart impairs endothelium dependent relaxation and promotes vasoconstriction in the microcirculation.[103] In the pig model Selke administered FGF to coronary arteries and preserved endothelial relaxation in newly formed collaterals.[104] By using endothelial cells cultured from human heart transplant patients, FGF-2 was applied to cells from tissue with either coronary artery disease or idiopathic myopathy (noncoronary artery disease). The number of capillary-like microtubules, a reflection of angiogenesis, was increased in the cells from the coronary artery disease group. This demonstrated that diseased vessels, i.e., coronary artery disease, respond better to FGF with neovascularization.[105] It has been reported that FGF-2 is a circulating peptide and gene expression is increased after myocardial ischemia. Using a FGF-2 enzyme-linked immunoassay, FGF-2 levels in the blood were determined in patients experiencing an acute myocardial infarction. It was found that there was an increased serum level of FGF-2 10 days after the ischemic event, suggesting that FGF-2 at this time mediates the development of collateral coronary circulation.[106]

The development of collateral vessel development in the setting of lower extremity ischemia has also been investigated. Lower limb ischemia is generated by surgically excising the femoral artery in rabbits. FGF-2 is applied through intramuscular injections; after 14 days capillary density and collateral vessels were found to be augmented.[107] In a similar fashion, FGF-1 was administered after the ischemia was allowed to subside for 10 days. Even after 30 days there was evidence of angiogenesis and increased collateral blood flow in the rabbit hindlimb.[108] This method of investigation has been applied to other angiogenic growth factors such as VEGF[109] (see chapter 26 for a full review).

The interest in FGF and ischemic disease has broadened, and research is now being done on brain infarcts (strokes)[110,111] and trauma injuries.[112]

The therapeutic potential of angiogenic cytokines remains to be fully defined, but clearly FGF plays an important role in the development of collateral neovascularization in ischemic disease states.

Conclusions

Over the past 15 years our knowledge and understanding of angiogenic cytokines, FGF in particular, has made great strides. Current vascular research is focused on more bio-interactive grafts that optimize the microenvironment of the tissue-graft-blood interfaces. The application of endothelial cells and growth factors to synthetic grafts to induce angiogenesis and limit the smooth muscle cell response are some of the most promising areas of research.

References

1. Armelin, HA. Pituitary extracts and steroid hormones in the control of 3T3 cell growth. Proc Natl Acad Sci USA 1973; 70:2702-6.
2. Gospodarowicz D, Jones KL, Sato G. Purification of a growth factor for ovarian cells from bovine pituitary glands. Proc Natl Acad Sci USA 1974; 71:2295-99.
3. Gospodarowicz D. Localisation of a fibroblast growth factor and its effect alone and with hydrocortisone on T cell growth. Nature 1974; 249:123-7.
4. Gospodarowicz D. Purification of a fibroblast growth factor from bovine pituitary. J Biol Chem 1975; 250:2519-19.
5. Westfall FC, Lenon VA, Gospodarowicz D. Brain derived fibroblast growth factor: Identity with a fragment of the basic protein myelin. Proc Natl Acad Sci USA 1978; 75:4675-78.
6. Thomas KA, Riley MC, Lemmon SK, Baglan NC, Bradshaw RAS. Brain derived fibroblast growth factor: Non identity with myelin basic protein. J Biol Chem 1980; 255:5517-20.
7. Lemmon SK, Riley MC, Thomas KA, Hoover GA, Maciag T, Bradshaw RA. Bovine fibroblast growth factor: Comparison of brain and piuitary preparations. J Cell Biol 1982; 95:162-9.
8. Gimenez-Gallego G, Rodkey J, Bennett C, Rios-Candelore M, DiSalvo J, Thomas KA. Brain-derived acidic fibroblast growth factr: Complete amino acid sequence and homologies. Science 1985; 230:1385-1388.
9. Baird A, Esch F, Mormede P, Ueno N, Ling N et al. Molecular characterization of FGF: Distribution and biological activities in various tissues. Recent Prog Horm Res 1986; 42:143-205.
10. Miyamoto M, Naruo KI, Seko C, Matsumoto S, Kondo T, Kurokawa T. Molecular cloning of a novel cytokine cDNA encoding the ninth member of the fibroblast growth factor family which has a unique secretion property. Mol Cell Biol 1993; 13:4251-59.

11. Sholley MM, Ferguson GP, Seibel HR, Montuor JL., Wilson JD. Mechanisms of neovascularization. Vascular sprouting can occur without proliferation of endothelial cells. Lab Invest 1984; 51:624-34.

12. Diaz-Flores L, Guiterrez R, Valladares F, Varela H, Perez M. Intense vascular sprouting from rat femoral vein induced by prostaglandins E1 and E2. Anat Rec 1994; 238:68-76.

13. Diaz-Flores L, Gutierrez R, Varela H. Angiogenesis: An update Histol Histopath 1994; 9:807-843.

14. Burger PC, Chandler DB, Klintworth GK. Corneal neovascularization as studied by scanning electron microscopy of vascular casts. Lab Invest 1983; 48:169-80.

15. Ausprunk DH, Folkman J Migration and proliferation of endothelial cells in preformed and newly formed blood vessels during tumor angiogenesis. Microvasc Res 1977; 14:53-65.

16. Rifkin DE, Gross JL, Moscatelli D, Jaffe EA. Proteases and angiogenesis: Production of plasminogen activation and collagenase by endothelial cells. In: Nossel HL, Vogel ID, eds. Pathobiology of the endothelial cell. New York: Academic Press Inc., 1982:191-197.

17. Folkman J. How is blood vessel growth regulated in normal and neoplastic tissue? Cancer Res 1986; 46:467-73.

18. Bavisotto LM, Schwartz SM, Heimark RL. Modulation of Ca-dependent intercellular adhesion in bovine aortic and human umbilical vein endothelial cells by heparin-binding growth factors. J Cell Physiol 1990; 143:39-51.

19. Liaw L, Schwatrz SM. Microtubule disruption stimulates DNA synthesis in bovine endothelial cells and potentiates cellular response to basic fibroblast growth factor. Am J Pathol 1990; 143:937-48.

20. Wakui S. Two and three dimensional ultrastructural observation of two cell type angiogenesis in human granulation tissue. Virchows Arch (B) 1988; 56:127-39.

21. Orlidge A, D'Amore PA. Inhibition of capillary endothelial cell growth by pericytes and smooth muscle cells. J Cell Biol 1987; 105:1455-62.

22. Sato Y, Rifkin DB. Autocrine activities of basic fibroblast growth factor: regulation of endothelial cell movement, plasminogen activator synthesis, and DNA synthesis. J Cell Biol 1988; 107:1199-205.

23. Slavin J. Fibroblast growth factor. At the heart of angiogenesis. Cell Biol International 1995; 19:431-44.

24. Folkman J. Angiogenesis factors. Science 1987; 235:442-7.

25. Kenyon BM, Voest E, Chen C, Flynn E, Folkman J, D'Amato R. A model of angiogenesis in the mouse cornea. Invest Opth. & Visual Science 1996; 37(8):1625-32.

26. Abraham JA, Whang JL, Tumolo A, Mergia A, Friedman J, Gospodarowicz D, Fiddes JC. Human basic fibroblast growth factor: Nucleotide sequence and genomic organization. EMBO J 1986; 5:2523-8.

27. Dickson C, Peters G. Potential oncogene product related to growth factors. Nature 1987; 326:830-33.

28. Deli Bovi P, Curatola AM, Kern FG, Greco A, Ittman M, Bascilico C. An oncogene isolated by transfection of Kaposi's sarcoma DNA encodes a growth factor that is a member of the FGF family. Cell 1987; 50:729-37.

29. Zahn X, Bates B, Hu X, Goldfarb M. The human FGF-5 gene encodes a novel protein related to fibroblast growth factors. Mol Cell Biol 1988; 8:3487-97.

30. Tanaka A, Miyamoto K, Minamino M, Takeda M, Sato B, Matsuo H, Matsumoto K. Cloning and characterisation of an androgen-induced growth factor essential for the androgen-dependent growth of mouse mammary carcinoma cells. Proc Natl Acad Sci USA 1992; 89:8928-32.

31. Finch P, Rubin JS, Miki T, Ron D, Aaronson SA. Human KGF is FGF related with properties of a paracrine effector of epithelial cell growth. Science. 1989; 245:752-55.

32. Acland P, Dixon M, Peters G, Dickson C. Subcellular fate of the Int-2 oncoprotein is determined by choice of intiation codon. Nature 1990; 343:662-65.

33. Powell PP, Klagsbrun M. Three forms of rat basic fibroblast growth factor are made from a single mRNA and localise to the nucleus. J Cell Physiol. 1991; 148:202-10.

34. Zuniga AZM, Meijers C, Zeller R. Expression of alternatively spliced bFGF first coding exons and antisense RNAs during chicken embryogenesis. Dev Biol 1992; 157:110-8.

35. Mergia A, Eddy R, Abraham JA, Fiddes JC, Showes TB. The genes for basic and acidic fibroblast growth factor are on different chromosomes. BioChem Biophys. Res Commun 1986; 136:644-51.

36. Jaye M, Howk R, Burgess WH, Ricca G, Chiu IM, Ravera MW, O'Brien SJ, Modi WS, Maciag T, Drohan WN. Human endothelial cell growth factor: Cloning, nucleotide sequence, and chromosome localization. Science 1986; 233:543-45.

37. Freisel R, Maciag T. Molecular mechanisms of angiogenesis: FGF signal transduction. FASEB J 1995; 920 (9):919-925.

38. Gimenez-Gallego G, Rodkey J, Bennett C, Rios-Candelore M, DiSalvo J, Thomas KA. Brain-derived acidic fibroblast growth factor: Complete amino acid sequence and homolgies. Science. 1985; 230:1385-88.

39. Burgess WH, Maciag T. The heparin-binding (fibroblast) growth factor family of proteins. Annu. Rev BioChem 1989; 58:575-606.

40. Blaber M, DiSalvo J, Thomas K. X-ray crystal structure of human acidic fibroblast growth factor. BioChem 1996; 35:2086-2094.

41. Jackson A, Tarantini F, Gamble S, Friedman S, Maciag T. Release of fibroblast growth factor-1 from NIH 3T3 cells in response to temperature involves the function of cysteine residues. J Biol Chem 1995; 270:33-6.

42. Mason I. The ins and outs of fibroblast growth factors. Cell; 1994; 78:547-552.

43. Jackson A, Freidman S, Zhan X, Engleka KA, Forough R, Maciag T. Heat shock induces the release of fibroblast growth factor-1 from NIH-3T3 cells. Proc Natl Acad Sci USA 1992; 89:10691-5.

44. Mignatti P, Morimoto T, Rifkin DB. Basic fibroblast growth factor, a protein devoid of secretory signal sequence, is released by cells via a pathway independent of the endoplasmic reticulum-Golgi complex. J Cell Physiol 1992; 151:81-93.

45. Miyamoto M, Naruo K, Seko C, Matsumoto S, Kondo T, Kurokawa T. Molecular cloning of a novel cytokine cDNA encoding the ninth member of the fibroblast growth factor family which has a unique secretory property. Mol Cell Biol 1993; 13:4251-4259.

46. Vlodavsky I, Bashkin P, Ishai-Michaeli R, Chajek-Shaul T, Bar-Shavit R, Haimovitz-Friedman A, Klagsburn M, Fuks Z. Sequestration and release of basic FGF. Annals NY Acad Sci 1991; 638:207-220.

47. Thornton SC, Mueller SN, Levine EM. Human endothelial cells: Use of heparin in cloning and long term serial cultivation. Science 1983; 222:623-5.

48. Maciag T, Mehlman T, Freisel R, Schriber AB. Heparin binds endothelial cell growth factor, the principal endo-

thelial cell mitogen in bovine brain. Science 1984; 225:932-35.

49. Shing Y, Folkman J, Sullivan R, Butterfield C, Murray J, Klagsburg M. Heparin affinity: Purification of a tumor derived capillary endothelial cell growth factor. Science 1984; 223:1296-99.

50. Rosengart TK, Johnson W, Friesel R, Clark R, Maciag T. Heparin protects heparin-binding-growth-factor-I from proteolytic inactivation in vitro. BioChem Biophys. Res Commun. 1988; 152:432-40.

51. Gospodarowicz D, Cheng J. Heparin protects basic and acidic FGF from inactivation. J Cell Physiol 1986; 128:475-84.

52. Lobb R. Thrombin inactivates acidic fibroblast growth factor but not basic fibroblast growth factor. BioChem 1988; 27:2572-78.

53. Vlodavsky I, Folkman J, Sullivan R, Fridman R, Ishai-Michaeli R, Sasse J, Klagsbrun M. Endothelial cell-derived basic fibroblast growth factor: Synthesis and deposition into subendothelial extracellular matrix. Proc Natl Acad Sci USA 1987; 84: 2292-6.

54. Lobb R, Sasse J, Sullivan R, Shing Y, D'Amore P, Jacobs J, Klagsbrun M. Purification and characterization of heparin-binding endothelial cell growth factors. J Biol Chem 1986; 261:1924-8.

55. Davis MG, Zhou M, Ali S, Coffin JD, Doetschman T, Dorn GW. Intracrine and autocrine effects of basic fibroblast growth factor in vascular smooth muscle cells. J Mol Cell Cardiol 1997; 29(4):1061-72.

56. Engele J, Bohn MC. Effects of acidic and basic fibroblast growth factors on glial precursor cell proliferation: Age dependency and brain region specificity. Dev Biol 1992; 152:363-72.

57. Reidy M. Factors contolling the development of arterial lesions after injury. Circ Supl 1992; 86(6):43-6.

58. Nabel E. Recombinant FGF-1 promotes intimal hyperplasia and angiogenesis in arteries in vivo. Nature 1993; 363:844-6.

59. Ohtani II, Nakamura S, Watanabe Y, Mizoi T, Saku T, Nagura H. Immunocytochemical localization of basic fibroblast growth factor in carcinomas and inflammatory lesions of the human digestive tract. Lab Invest 1993; 68:520-7.

60. Wellstein A. Inhibition of FGFs. Breast Ca Res and Trmt 1996; 38; 09-19

61. Nguyen M, Watanabe H, Budson AE, Richie JP, Hayes DF, Folkman J. Elevated levels of an angiogenic peptide, basic fibroblast growth factor, in the urine of patients with a wide spectrum of cancers. J Natl Cancer Inst 1994; 86:356-61.

62. Hori A, Sasada R, Matsutani E, Naito K, Sakura Y, Fujita T, Kozai Y. Suppression of solid tumor growth by immunoneutralizing monoclonal antibody against basic fibroblast growth factor. Cancer Res 1991; 51:6180-84.

63. Becker D, Meier CB, Herlyn M. Proliferation of human malignant melanomas is inhibited by antisense oligodeoxynucleotides targeted against basic fibroblast growth factor. EMBO J 1989; 8:3685-91.

64. Girban N. Basic FGF in the early human burn wound. J Surg Res 1994; 56:226-34.

65. Okamura M. Effect of bFGF on wound healing in healing-impaired animal models. Drug Res 1996; 46(1):547-551.

66. Slavin J, Hunt JA, Nash JR, Williams DF, Kingsnorth AN. Recombinant basic fibroblast growth factor in red blood cell ghosts accelerates incisional wound healing. Br J Surg 1992; 79:918-21.

67. Neufeld G, Gospodarowicz D. Basic and acidic growth factors interact with the same cell surface receptors. J Biol Chem 1986; 261:5631-7.

68. Ledoux D, Gannoun-Zaki L, Barritault D. Interactions of FGFs with target cells. Progress in Growth Factor Res 1992; 4:107-20.

69. Moscatelli D. High and low affinity binding sites for basic fibroblast growth factor on cultured cells: Absence of a role for low affinity binding in the stimulation of plasminogen activator production by bovine capillary endothelial cells. J Cell Physiol. 1987; 131:123-30.

70. Gallagher JT, Turnbull JE. Heparan sulfate in the binding and activation of basic fibroblast growth factor. Glycobiology 1992; 2(6):523-8.

71. Kiefer MC, Stephans JC, Crawford K, Okino K, Barr PJ. Ligand-affinity cloning and structure of a cell surface heparan sulfate proteoglycan that binds basic fibrfoblast growth factor. Proc Natl Acad Sci USA 1990; 87:6985-9.

72. Bernfield M, Sanderson RD. Syndecan, a developmentally regulated cell surface proteoglycan that binds extracellular matrix and growth factors. Phil Trans R Soc Lond 1990; 327:171-86.

73. Yayon A, Klagsburn M, Esko JD, Leder P, Ornitz DM. Cell surface, heparin-like molecules are required for binding of basic fibroblast growth factor to its high affinity receptor. Cell. 1991; 64:841-8.

74. Rapraeger AC, Krufka A, Olwin BB. Requirement of heparan sulfate for bFGF-mediated fibroblast growth factor and myoblast differentiation. Science 1991; 252:1705-8.

75. Savona C, Chambaz EM, Feige JJ. Proteoheparan sulfates contribute to the binding of basic FGF to its high affinity receptors on bovine adrenocortical cells. Growth Factors. 1991; 5:273-82.

76. Friesel R, Maciag T. Molecular mechanisms of angiogenesis: Fibroblast growth factor signal transduction. FASEB 1995; 9:919-25.

77. Herring MB, Gardner AL, Glover J. A single staged technique for the seeding of vascular grafts with autogenous endothelium. Surgery 1978; 84:498.

78. Ortenwall P, Wadenvik H, Risberg B. Reduced platelet deposition on seeded versus unseeded segments of expanded polytetrafluoroethylene grafts: Clinical observations after a 6-month follow-up. J Vasc Surg 1989; 10:374-80.

79. Ortenwall P, Wadenvik H, Kutti J, Risberg B. Endothelial seeding reduces thrombogenicity of Dacron grafts in humans. J Vasc Surg 1990; 11:403-10.

80. Park PK, Jarrell BE, Williams SK, Carter TL, Rose DG, Martinez-Hernandez A, Carabasi RA. Thrombus-free, human endothelial surface in the midregion of a Dacron vascular graft in the splanchnic venous circuit- Observations after nine months of implantation. J Vasc Surg 1990; 11:468-75.

81. Baitella-Eberle G, Grosscurth P, Zilla P, Lachat M, Muller-Glauser W, Schneider J, Neudecker A, von Segesser LK, Dardel EE, Turina M. Long-term results of tissue development and cell differentiation on Dacron prostheses seeded with microvascular cells in dogs. J Vasc Surg 1993; 18:1019-28.

82. Greisler HP, Klosak JJ, Dennis JW, Ellinger J et al. Endothelial cell growth factor attachment to biomaterials. Trans ASAIO 1986; 32:346-9.

83. Greisler HP, Klosak JJ, Dennis JW, Karesh SM et al. Biomaterials pretreatment with ECGF to augment endothelial cell proliferation. J Vasc Surg 1987; 5:393-402.

84. Tomizaw Y, Noishiki Y, Okoshi T, Nishida H, Endo M, Koyanagi H. Endogenous basic fibroblast growth factor for endothelialization due to angiogenesis in fabric vascular prostheses. ASAIO J 1996; 42(5):M698-702.

85. Greisler HP. Dacron inhibition of arterial regenerative activity. J Vasc Surg 1986; 3:747-56.

86. Gosselin C, Vorp DA, Warty V, Severyn DA, Dick EK, Borovetz HS, Greisler HP. ePTFE coating with FG, FGF-1, and heparin: Effect on retention of seeded endothelial cells. J Surg Res 1996; 60:327-32.

87. Greisler HP, Cziperle DJ, Kim DU et al. Enhanced endothelialization of expanded polytetrafluoroethylene grafts by fibroblast growth factor type 1 pretreatment. Surgery 1992; 112:244-55.

88. Gray JL, Kang SS, Zenni GC et al. FGF-1 affixation stimulates ePTFE endothelialization without intimal hyperplasia. J Surg Res 1994; 57:596-612.

89. Reilly CF, Kindy MS, Brown KE et al. Heparin prevents vascular smooth muscle cell progression through the G1 phase of the cell cycle. J Biol Chem 1989; 264:6990-6995.

90. Au TYP, Kenagy RD, Clowes MM, Clowes AW. Mechanisms of inhibition by heparin of vascular smooth muscle cell proliferation and migration. Haemostasis 1993; 23:177-82.

91. Kang SS, Gosselin C, Ren D, Greisler HP. Selective stimulation of endothelial cell proliferation with inhibition of smooth muscle cell proliferation by fibroblast growth factor-1 plus heparin delivered from fibrin glue suspensions. Surgery 1995; 118:280-287.

92. Yamamura K, Sakuraj T, Yano K, Nabeshima T, Yotsuyanagi T. Sustained release of bFGF from synthetic vascular prosthesis using hydroxypropylchitosan acetate. J BioChem Mat. Res 1995; 29:203-6.

93. Noishiki Y, Tomizawa Y, Yamane Y, Matsumoto A. Autocrine angiogenic vascular prosthesis with bone marrow transplantation. Nature Medicine. 1996; 2(1):90-3.

94. Zarge J, Huang P, Husak V, Kim D, Haudenschild C, Nord RM, Greisler HP. Fibrin glue containing fibroblast growth factor type 1 and heparin with autologous endothelial cells reduces intimal hyperplasia in a canine carotid artery balloon injury model. J Vasc Surg 1997; 25(5):840-8.

95. Greisler HP, Kang SS, Lin P, Hirko MK. In vivo and in vitro release kinetics of FGF-1 when impregnated into ePTFE grafts using fibrin glue suspensions. Society for Biomaterials Transactions 1995; 18:104.

96. Burgess WH, Shaheen AM, Ravera M, Jaye M, Donohue PJ, Winkles JA. Possible dissociation of the heparin-binding and mitogenic activities of heparin-binding (acidic fibroblast) growth factor-1 from its receptor-binding activities by site directed mutagenesis of a single lysine residue. J Cell Biol 1990; 111:2129-38.

97. Burgess WH, Shaheen AM, Hampton B, Donohue PJ, Winkles JA. Structure-function studies of heparin-binding (acidic fibroblast) growth factor-1 using site-directed mutagenesis. J Cell. BioChem 1991; 45:131-38.

98. Fox D, Kouris G, Blumofe K, Heilizer T, Husak V, Greisler HP. Optimizing fluorescent labeling of endothelial cells for tracking during long term studies of autologous transplantation. Chicago: Presented at the 21st Annual Meeting of the Midwestern Vascular Surgical Society. 1997:Sept 12-13.

99. Cowan DF, Hollenberg NK, Connelly CM, Williams DH, Abrams HL. Increased collateral arterial and venous endothelial cell turnover after renal artery stenosis in the dog. Invest Radiol 1978; 13:143-9.

100. White FC, Carroll SM, Magnet A, Bloor CM. Coronary collateral development in swine after coronary artery occlusion. Circ Res 1992; 71:1490-1500.

101. Landau C, Jacobs AK, Haudenschild CC. Intrapericardial FGF2 induces myocardial angiogenesis in a rabbit model of chronic ischemia. Am Heart J 1995; 129(5):924-31.

102. Uchida Y, Yanagjsawa-Miwa A, Nakamura F, Yamada K, Tomaru T, Kimura K, Morita T. Angiogenic therapy of acute myocardial infarction by intrapericardial injection of basic fibroblast growth factor and heaprin sulfate: An experimental study. Am Heart J 1995; 130(6):1182-8.

103. Sellke FW, Quillen JE, Brooks LA, Harrison DG. Endothelial modulation of the coronary vasculature in vessels perfused via mature collaterals. Circulation 1990; 81:1938-47.

104. Selke F. Basic FGF preserves the endothelial function in the microcirculation perfused by collaterals. Abstracts of the Scientific Conference on the Molecular Cellular Biology of the Vascular Wall. Boston; Vol. 49; 1993:Oct 15-17.

105. Chen CH, Nguyen HH, Weilbaecher D, Luo S, Gotto AM Jr, Henry PD. FGF-2 reverses the atherosclerotic impairment of human coronary angiogenesis-like responses in vitro. Atherosclerosis 1995; 116: 261-8.

106. Cuevas P, Barrios V, Gimenez-Gallego G, Martinez-Coso V, Cuevas B, Benavides J, Garcia-Segovia J, Asin-Cardiel E. Serum levels of basic fibroblast growth factor in acute myocardial infarction. Eur J Med Res 1997; 2(7):282-4.

107. Baffour R, Berman J, Garb JL, Rhee SW, Kaufman J, Friedmann P. Enhanced angiogenesis and growth of collaterals by in vivo administration of recombinant FGF-2 in a rabbit model of acute lower limb ischemia: Dose-response effect of FGF-2. J Vasc Surg 1992; 16:181-91.

108. Pu L, Sniderman AD, Brassard R, Lachapelle KJ, Graham AM, Lisbona R, Symes JF. Enhanced revascularization of the ischemic limb by means of angiogenic therapy. Circulation 1993; 88:208-15.

109. Takeshita S, Rossow S, Kearney M, Zheng L, Bauters C, Bunting S, Ferrara N, Symes J, Isner J. Time course of increased cellular proliferation in collateral arteries after administration of vascular endothelilial growth factor in a rabbit model of lower limb vascular insufficiency. Am J Path. 1995; 147(6):1649-60.

110. Chen HH, Chien CH, Liu HM. Correlation between angiogenesis and basic fibroblast growth factor expression in experimental brain infarct. Stroke 1994; 25:1651-7.

111. Ren JM, Finklestein SP. Time window of infarct reduction by intravenous basic fibroblast growth factor in focal cerebral ischemia. Eur J Pharmacol 1997; 327(1):11-16.

112. Fu X, Sheng Z, Wang Y, Ye Y, Xu M, Sun T, Zhou B. Basic fibroblast growth factor reduces the gut and liver morphologic and functional injuries after ischemia and reperfusion. J Trauma 1997; 42(6):1080-5.

Facilitation of Healing

Matrix Degradation

---------- CHAPTER 29 ----------

Role of Urokinase-Type Plasminogen Activator (uPA) in In Vitro Angiogenesis in Fibrin Matrices

Pieter Koolwijk, Victor W.M. van Hinsbergh

Summary

Tissue repair-associated angiogenesis, the formation of new blood vessels from existing ones, usually involves cell invasion into a fibrin structure and the presence of inflammatory cells. In this chapter the role of plasminogen activators and their receptors in the invasion of endothelial cells into a fibrin matrix is described. At the basolateral side of the endothelial cell, the urokinase-type plasminogen activator (uPA) bound to a specific cellular receptor (uPA receptor) is involved in the proteolytic modulation of matrix proteins and cell-matrix interaction. Interference in the activity of uPA and the binding of uPA to the uPA receptor inhibits the in vitro invasion of human microvascular endothelial cells (HMVEC) and the formation of capillary-like tubular structures of HMVEC in three dimensional fibrin matrices, induced by a combination of the cytokine tumor necrosis factor-α (TNF-α) and the angiogenic factors basic fibroblast growth factor (bFGF) and vascular endothelial growth factor (VEGF).

Introduction

Angiogenesis, the outgrowth of new blood vessels from existing ones, is an essential process during development, but normally stops when the body becomes adult. In the absence of injury, overt angiogenesis in adults is limited to the reproductive system of females (formation of corpus luteum and placenta).[1] However, the formation of new blood vessels is an essential factor in tissue repair (formation and regression of granulation tissue) which is necessary to restore healthy tissue after wounding and/or inflammation. Furthermore, angiogenesis is associated with many pathological conditions, such as chronic inflammation including rheumatoid arthritis,[2] malignancies,[3] and retinopathy caused by metabolic dysregulation in particular diabetes.[4] Common in these conditions is that angiogenesis is accompanied by vascular leakage,[5] the occurrence of inflammatory cells,[6] and the presence of fibrin.[7,8] These latter factors are absent in angiogenesis during embryonic development. Therefore, the possibility exists that "developmental angiogenesis" and adult "repair-associated or pathologic angiogenesis" are two processes with many identical features, but with different properties with respect to their regulation.

Fibrin, a Temporary Repair Matrix

Fibrin is a temporary matrix which is formed after wounding of a blood vessel and when plasma leaks from blood vessels forming a fibrous exudate. The fibrin matrix not only

---

acts as a barrier preventing further blood loss, but also provides a structure in which new microvessels can infiltrate during wound healing. Proper timing of the outgrowth of microvessels as well as the subsequent (partial) disappearance of these vessels is essential to ensure adequate wound healing and to prevent the formation of scar tissue. An important role in the invasion of a fibrin matrix by endothelial cells is played by the plasminogen activator/plasmin system, which lyses fibrin at the basolateral side of the cell. However, the endothelium must respond differently to fibrin depending on whether the fibrin is present at its luminal or abluminal side. If fibrin is generated at the luminal side, the vessel may be occluded, which will cause serious damage of the distal tissues. To prevent this the endothelium is able to instantaneously increase the fibrinolytic activity in the blood compartment. If, however, this would lead to strong systemic fibrinolytic activity, recurrent bleeding might occur. Therefore, fibrinolysis must be restricted to a limited distance of the endothelium. To fulfill the roles of fibrinolysis in both the prevention of local intravascular fibrin accumulation, and a differently timed contribution in neovascularization and tissue repair, endothelial cells are equipped with a complex regulatory system which involves inhibitors, cell polarity and cellular receptors. After discussing the components of the plasminogen activator/plasmin system, we will focus on the contribution of the urokinase-type plasminogen activator (uPA) in pericellular proteolytic events associated with cell migration and the invasion of capillary-like tubular structures into fibrin matrices.

Components of the Plasmin/Plasminogen Activator System

Proteases

Plasmin is formed from its zymogen plasminogen by proteolytic activation by plasminogen activators (PAs) (Fig. 29.1). Two types of mammalian PAs are presently known: tissue-type plasminogen activator (tPA) and urokinase-type plasminogen activator (uPA).[9,10] The three serine proteases, plasminogen, tPA and uPA, are synthesized as single polypeptide chains, and each of them is converted by specific proteolytic cleavage to a molecule with two polypeptide chains connected by a disulphide bond. The C-terminal part of the molecule (the so-called B chain) contains the proteolytically active site, whereas the amino-terminal part of the molecule (the A-chain) is built up of domains that determine the interaction of the proteases with matrix proteins and cellular receptors. The proteolytic cleavage of plasminogen and single chain uPA to their respective two chain forms is necessary to disclose the proteolytically active site and to activate the molecule. The interaction of plasminogen with fibrin or the cell surface occurs predominantly via binding sites in the kringle structures, which recognize lysine residues of proteins, in particular C-terminal lysines. Because B-type carboxypeptidases remove C-terminal lysine residues from potential binding sites for plasminogen in fibrin or on the cell surface, they can act as negative regulators of the fibrinolytic system.[11]

Inhibitors

The activities of the proteases of the fibrinolytic system are controlled by potent inhibitors which are members of the serine protease inhibitor (serpin) superfamily. Plasmin, if not bound to fibrin, is instantaneously inhibited by α_2-antiplasmin.[12] Because this interaction is facilitated by the lysine binding domain of plasmin, it is attenuated when plasmin is bound to fibrin. The predominant regulators of tPA and uPA activities are PAI-1 and PAI-2.[13,14] PAI-1 is a 50 kDa glycoprotein present in blood platelets and synthesized by endothelial cells, smooth muscle cells and many other cell types in culture.[15,16] PAI activity in human plasma is normally exclusively PAI-1. PAI-1 binds to vitronectin, which stabilizes its inhibitory activity. PAI-1 is the main if not the sole inhibitor of PAs synthesized by endothelial cells, vascular smooth muscle cells and hepatocytes, whereas PAI-2 is produced by monocytes/macrophages, placental trophoblasts and certain tumor cell lines.[14] It can be found as a glycosylated secreted molecule and as an nonglycosylated molecule intracellularly.[17]

Receptors

Regulation of fibrinolytic activity also occurs by cellular receptors. These receptors direct the action of PAs and plasmin to focal areas on the cell surface, or are involved in the clearance of the PAs. High affinity binding sites for plasminogen,[18-21] tPA[21,22] and uPA[23-25] are found on various types of cells, including endothelial cells.

Endothelial cells in vitro bind plasminogen with a moderate affinity (120-340 nM depending on whether the Lys or Glu form of plasminogen is used), but with a high capacity (3.9-14 x 10^5 molecules per cell).[19,26] This binding, which is also observed with many other cell types, is mediated by the lysine binding sites of kringles 1-3 of the plasmin(ogen) molecule. Because these lysine binding sites are also involved in the interaction of plasmin with α_2-antiplasmin, occuPAtion of lysine binding sites protects plasmin from instantaneous inhibition by α_2-antiplasmin not only when plasmin is bound to fibrin (see above), but also when it is bound to the cellular receptors. The nature of the plasminogen receptors is not fully resolved. In addition to gangliosides, which directly or indirectly contribute to the plasminogen binding,[27] at least eight proteins have been reported to be involved in plasminogen binding. Among them are members of the low density lipoprotein receptor family, such as gp330 and LRP; annexin II; a not yet identified 45 kDa protein; GbIIb/IIIa and α-enolase (see ref. 21 for review). In neural cells plasminogen binding to amphoterin was found. Lipoprotein LpA, which has strong structural homology with a large part of the plasminogen molecule, can compete for plasminogen binding to endothelial cells.[20,28] This competition also involves lysine binding sites.

Specific binding of tPA to human endothelial cells has been reported.[29-31] tPA binds via its growth factor domain with high affinity to annexin II on human endothelial cells in culture.[32] Different epitopes of the annexin II molecule are involved in plasminogen and tPA binding. It is conceivable that annexin II, like fibrin, forms a ternary complex

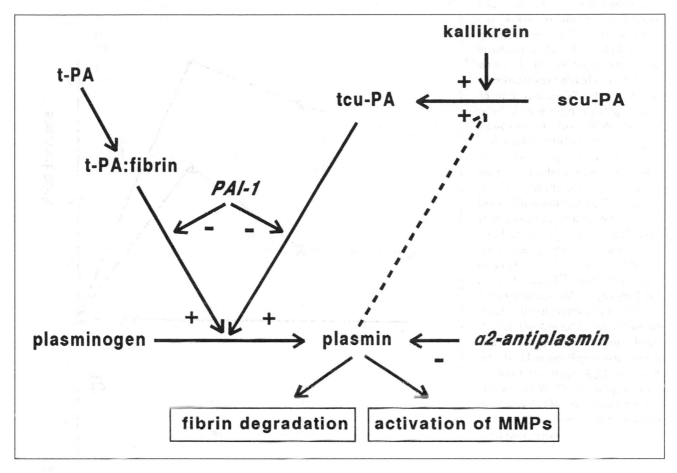

Fig. 29.1. Scheme of the plasminogen activation system. +: activation; -: inhibition. Inhibitors are indicated in italics. PA: plasminogen activator; tPA: tissue-type PA; tcuPA: two chain urokinase-type PA; scuPA: single chain urokinase-type PA; PAI: PA inhibitor.

with tPA and plasminogen on the endothelial cell surface.[21] In addition, tPA interacts with matrix-bound PAI-1.[31]

Binding of uPA with the cell surface limits plasminogen activation to focal areas such as the focal attachment sites and cellular protrusions involved in cell migration and invasion. Furthermore, uPA interaction with the cell evokes signal transduction and phosphorylation of several proteins.[33,34] A specific uPA receptor has been identified and cloned. It is present on many cell types, including endothelial cells.[35] It is a glycosyl phosphatidyl inositol (GPI)-anchored glycoprotein,[25] which binds both single chain uPA and two chain uPA via their growth factor domains.[36] The uPA receptor is heavily glycosylated and belongs to the cysteine-rich cell surface proteins. After synthesis it is proteolytically processed at its carboxyl-terminus and subsequently anchored in the plasma membrane by a GPI group.[37] It comprises three domains, which are structurally homologous to snake venom α-toxins.[25] The uPA receptor has been found in focal attachment sites, where integrin-matrix interactions occur, and in cell-cell contact areas.[38,39] Human endothelial cells in vitro contain about 140,000 uPA receptors per cell.[40]

The uPA receptor both acts as a site for focal pericellular proteolysis by uPA and is involved in the clearance of the uPA-PAI-1 complex. Upon secretion, single chain uPA binds to the uPA receptor and is subsequently converted to the proteolytically active two chain uPA. Since the endothelial cell also contains plasmin(ogen) receptors, an interplay between receptor-bound uPA and receptor-bound plasmin(ogen) and plasmin formation is likely to happen. The generated plasmin can degrade a number of matrix proteins. In addition, a direct plasmin-independent proteolytic action of uPA on matrix proteins may also occur.[41] Like free uPA activity, receptor-bound two chain uPA is subject to inhibition by PAI-1. As a consequence, uPA is only active over a short period of time. In contrast to receptor-bound single chain or noninhibited two chain uPA, the uPA-PAI-1 complex is rapidly internalized together with the uPA receptor,[42] followed by the degradation of the uPA-PAI-1 complex and the return of the empty uPA receptor to the plasma membrane. Internalization of the GPI-linked uPA receptor probably occurs after interaction with another receptor, such as the α_2-macroglobulin/low density lipoprotein receptor-related protein (LRP)[43] or the VLDL receptor.[44] VLDL receptors were demonstrated on capillary and arteriolar endothelial cells in vivo.[45] Recently it has been found that the uPA receptor may have an additional role. The uPA receptor occupied by uPA interacts avidly with vitronectin.[46] Hence, cell adhesion may represent an additional function of the uPA receptor.

The LRP and LRP-like proteins on liver hepatocytes are involved in the clearance of plasmin-α_2-antiplasmin, PA-PAI-1 complexes[47-49] and probably free PAs from the circulation. In addition, tPA can also be cleared by mannose receptors present on macrophages and liver endothelial cells[50] and by α-fucose receptors on hepatocytes.[32]

The Regulation of Plasminogen Activation and Pericellular Proteolysis by Inflammatory and Angiogenic Mediators

Regulation of Proteases And Inhibitors

The primary cytokines interleukin-1 (IL-1) and tumor necrosis factor-α (TNF-α) exert many effects on the vascular endothelium. Their most prominent feature is the induction or increase of the transcription of many genes, such as the leukocyte adhesion molecules E-selectin, VCAM-1 and ICAM-1, cyclooxygenase-2, and a number of proteases and protease inhibitors. The inflammatory mediators TNF-α, IL-1 and the bacterial lipopolysaccharide (LPS) induce the synthesis of uPA in human endothelial cells in vitro.[51] Whereas uPA is normally not found in endothelial cells in vivo, association of uPA with the endothelium was observed in acute appendicitis[52] and in rheumatoid arthritis.[2] Induction of endothelial uPA by TNF-α in vitro is associated by an increased degradation of matrix proteins.[53] The enhanced secretion of uPA occurs entirely towards the basolateral side of the cell, whereas the secretion of tPA and PAI-1 proceeds equally to the luminal and basolateral sides of the cell.[51] The polar secretion of uPA suggests that uPA may be involved in local remodeling of the basal membrane of the cell. uPA activity is controlled in space by interaction of uPA with its cellular receptor and by the inhibitor PAI-1.

TNF-α and IL-1, as well as LPS, also elicit another effect on the regulation of plasminogen activator production in endothelial cells. Simultaneous with the increase in uPA, these inflammatory mediators markedly increase the production of PAI-1 in endothelial cells in vitro.[54-57] This induction was also demonstrated at the transcriptional level, and was largely inhibited by the isoflavone compound genistein.[58] In vivo, administration of TNF-α, IL-1 or LPS causes an increase in PAI-1 concentration in the circulation. After infusion of LPS in animals, PAI-1 mRNA increased in vascularized tissues and PAI-1 mRNA was elevated in the endothelium of various organs.[59,60] The increase of PAI-1 induced by inflammatory mediators may represent a protective mechanism of the cell against uncontrolled uPA activity.

The effect of the angiogenic growth factors basic and acidic fibroblast growth factor (bFGF, aFGF) and vascular endothelial growth factor (VEGF) on the production of uPA by endothelial cells is species dependent. Whereas bFGF and VEGF are potent inducers of both uPA in bovine cells,[61,62,63] bFGF and VEGF do not enhance uPA production in human endothelial cells.[64,65] PAI-1 production by human endothelial cells is slightly decreased by the addition of bFGF or VEGF.[65]

Regulation of the uPA Receptor

The expression of the uPA receptor is enhanced by angiogenic growth factors including basic and acidic fibroblast growth factor (bFGF, aFGF) and vascular endothelial growth factor (VEGF).[65-67] The number of uPA receptors on human and bovine endothelial cells is also enhanced by the activation of protein kinase c and by the elevation of the cellular cAMP concentration.[68,69] Preliminary experiments in our laboratory have demonstrated that the induction of uPA receptor by VEGF in human endothelial cells is inhibited by protein kinase c inhibition. The effects of bFGF and VEGF on the induction of uPA receptor in human endothelial cells are regulated independently of their effects on cell proliferation. Similarly, Presta et al[70] have shown that the induction of uPA by bFGF in bovine endothelial cells proceeds independently from the stimulation of mitogenesis by this growth factor.

In addition to FGFs and VEGF, which induce mitogenesis, TNF-α also can induce angiogenesis, but this occurs without stimulation of cell proliferation.[71,72] TNF-α increases uPA receptor levels in human microvascular endothelial cells[65] and in monocytes,[73] but not in endothelial cells from human umbilical vein or aorta.[65] However, simultaneous exposure of the latter cells to TNF-α (which induces uPA synthesis) to bFGF and VEGF (which enhance the expression of uPA receptors) potently increases cell-bound uPA activity.

Interaction Between the uPA/Plasmin System and Matrix-Degrading Metalloproteases

The observation that TNF-α also increases the production of matrix-degrading metalloproteinases (MMPs) by endothelial cells is consistent with a putative role for TNF-α and IL-1 in inflammation-induced local pericellular proteolysis. In human microvascular and vein endothelial cells, TNF-α increases the mRNA levels and the synthesis of interstitial collagenase (MMP-1), stromelysin-1 (MMP-3) and—if protein kinase c is also activated—gelatinase-B (MMP-9), whereas the mRNAs levels and synthesis of their physiological inhibitors TIMP-1 and TIMP-2 are not changed.[74,75] Furthermore, activation of gelatinase a (MMP-2) was observed after exposure of the cells to TNF-α.[74] Recently, it has been shown that activation of gelatinase a depends on the activity of membrane-type MMP (MT-MMP),[76,77] and that MMP-2 interacts with $\alpha_v\beta_3$ integrin.[78] Interestingly, secretion of gelatinases by bovine endothelial cells occurs predominantly towards the basolateral side of the cells,[79] similarly to the TNF-α-induced production of uPA.[51] A role of MMPs in endothelial cell-matrix remodeling has indeed been shown in a three dimensional collagen matrix in vitro.[80] Furthermore, MMPs have been detected in vivo in proliferating endothelial cells during development,[81] and in endothelial cells present in atherosclerotic plaques and growing tumors.[82-84]

The plasmin-plasminogen activator system and the matrix metalloproteinases cooperate in the degradation of extracellular matrix proteins.[85] Figure 29.2 depicts the interaction between the two systems. It should be noted, however, that this schematic picture is based on in vitro data, and that it is still uncertain whether all the depicted steps also act in vivo. Nevertheless, uPA and MMP expression frequently coincide in time and location in pathological tissues. If these data are taken together, it will be clear that activation of endothelial cells by TNF-α affects multiple sites in the proteolytic cascades involved in the degradation of matrix proteins to such an extent that it markedly enhances the breakdown and remodeling of the endothelial cell basal membrane.

Involvement of uPA and uPA Receptor in Cell Migration and Realignment of Endothelial Cells

Concentration of uPA activity at the cellular protrusions of migrating or invading cells has been frequently observed.[86,87] Blasi[88] suggested that a continuous activation and removal of uPA bound to the receptor could contribute to the formation and detachment of focal attachment sites and hence to locomotion of the cell. Indeed, migrating and invading cells, such as monocytes and tumor cells, express uPA activity bound to uPA receptors on their cellular protrusions[87] and on focal attachment sites.[38,89] Receptor-bound uPA activity is also thought to be involved in smooth muscle and endothelial cell migration and in the formation of new blood vessels (angiogenesis). Inhibition of plasminogen activation interferes with smooth muscle cell migration in vitro[90,91] and affects smooth muscle migration and proliferation in vivo.[92] In mice lacking uPA, intimal hyperplasia of injured arteries is less pronounced than in wild type or tPA-deficient mice.[93] Moreover, PAI-1-deficient mice show an exacerbated intimal proliferation.[93] Animals made deficient for plasminogen show comparable pathological features to those with a combined deficiency of uPA and tPA.[94,95] These data suggest that uPA and plasminogen have a role in cell recruitment.

An involvement of uPA and the uPA receptor in the migration of bovine endothelial cells has been demonstrated by several investigators.[63,96,97] After the wounding of a monolayer of these endothelial cells, the cells that migrate into the wounded area express uPA activity[96] bound to the uPA receptor.[63] The migration and expression of uPA depends on the release of bFGF from the wounded area.[97] bFGF is a potent inducer of plasminogen activator activity, in particular uPA, in bovine endothelial cells,[61,98] but not in human endothelial cells.[65] In both species bFGF increases the number of uPA receptors on endothelial cells.[63,65,66]

Receptor-bound uPA was demonstrated in focal adhesion sites of fibroblasts[89] and endothelial cells.[39] It may act proteolytically on these structures and hence influence cell-matrix interactions and cell migration. After exposure of endothelial cells to shear forces induced by fluid flow, the cells realign according to the direction of flow.[99] This process is paralleled by a movement of the cellular focal contact sites of endothelial cells.[100] Ponfoort et al[101] observed that the production of uPA by human iliac vein endothelial cells was elevated several fold after exposure of the cells to fluid flow. Interestingly, the realignment of iliac vein endothelial cells according to the direction of flow appeared to be related to cell-bound uPA activity. Anti-uPA antibodies, which inhibited uPA activity, reduced the cellular realignment induced by fluid shear forces.[101]

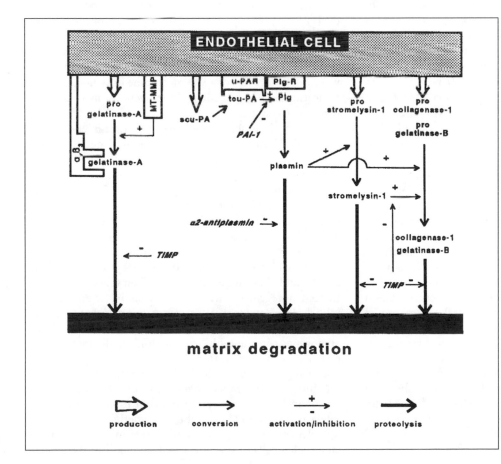

Fig. 29.2. Schematic representation of the interaction between the uPA/plasmin system and the presumed activation of matrix degrading metalloproteinases (MMPs). Abbreviations: PA: plasminogen activator; uPA: urokinase-type PA; sc-uPA: single chain uPA; tc-uPA: two chain uPA; uPAR: uPA receptor; Plg: plasminogen; Plg-R: Plg receptor; PAI-1: PA inhibitor-1; MT-MMP: membrane-bound MMP; TIMP: tissue inhibitor of MMP. +: stimulation; -: inhibition.

Role of the Plasmin/Plasminogen Activator System in the Formation of Endothelial Tubes in a Fibrin Matrix

The outgrowth of new blood vessels from existing ones, angiogenesis, is an essential process during development, but normally stops when the body becomes adult. The half life of endothelial cells in the adult body varies between 100-10,000 days in normal tissues, whereas it is reduced to several days in placenta and tumors.[102] With the exception of the female reproductive system, angiogenesis in the adult is associated with tissue repair after injury by wounding or inflammation. Repair-associated angiogenesis in the adult is usually accompanied by the presence of fibrin and inflammatory cells or mediators, in contrast to developmental angiogenesis in the embryo. Fibrin is a temporary matrix, which is formed after the wounding of a blood vessel and when plasma leaks from blood vessels forming a fibrous exudate, often seen in areas of inflammation and in tumors.[7,103] The fibrin matrix acts as a barrier preventing further blood loss, and provides a structure in which new microvessels can infiltrate during wound healing. A proper timing of the outgrowth of microvessels as well as the subsequent (partial) disappearance of these vessels is essential to ensure adequate wound healing and to prevent the formation of scar tissue. Although essential for the formation of granulation tissue and tissue repair, angiogenesis, once under the control of pathological stimuli, can contribute to a number of pathological conditions, such as tumor neovascularization, pannus formation in rheumatoid arthritis, and diabetic retinopathy. Understanding the mechanisms involved in angiogenesis may provide clues to preventing pathological angiogenesis without seriously impairing tissue repair. A number of studies and reviews have focused on angiogenic factors and the formation of capillary-like structures.[4,5,108-109] Among them, Dvorak[7] and Colvin[8] have pointed to the importance of fibrin in angiogenesis. Furthermore, the work of Polverini and colleagues have demonstrated the involvement of monocytes and their products in the induction of angiogenesis.[6,71,72,110] Because of the specific roles of fibrin and inflammatory cells and mediators in pathological angiogenesis in the adult, we have focused our studies on the invasion of human endothelial cells into three dimensional fibrin matrices and the role of endothelial plasminogen activators in this process. This model resembles recanalization of a fibrin clot by invading endothelial cells. This invasion is usually preceded by the infiltration of inflammatory cells, which interact with the vascular structures from which endothelial cells subsequently migrate into the fibrin clot.[111]

A three dimensional fibrin matrix model was used by Pepper and Montesano to demonstrate a direct correlation between the expression of PA activity and the formation of capillary sprouts by bovine microvascular endothelial cells in vitro.[106,112] The outgrowth of tubular structures was increased by bFGF, which increases both uPA activity and uPA receptor in bovine endothelial cells. Interestingly, the extent of tube formation and the diameter of the formed tubes were reduced by the simultaneous presence of TGF-β.[112] The latter is a growth factor which, amongst others, exerts a strong enhancement of PAI-1 synthesis in cultured endothelial cells, and thus inhibits PA activity.[61] In addition to bFGF, VEGF can also stimulate bovine endothelial cells to form tubular structures. It acts cooperatively with bFGF in this induction.[113]

Studies in human endothelial cells showed that no tubular structures are formed when a quiescent monolayer of human microvascular endothelial cells grown on a fibrin matrix is exposed to bFGF or VEGF. However, when bFGF or VEGF are added simultaneously with TNF-α, a large number of capillary-like tubular structures are formed (Fig. 29.3).[65] The outgrowth of tubular structures requires uPA activity and is completely reduced by anti-uPA immunoglobulins but not by anti-tPA antibodies (Fig. 29.4). It is also reduced by inhibiting the interaction of uPA with its receptor. Furthermore, proteolytic activation of plasminogen appears to be involved, because the plasmin inhibitor aprotinin largely inhibits the formation of tubular structures.[65] Recent immunohistochemical studies performed on cross sections of these invading capillary-like tubular structures showed an enhanced expression of both uPA and the uPAR antigen by invading endothelial cells compared with noninvading endothelial cells (Kroon et al; manuscript submitted for publication). These data agree with the data on bovine endothelial cells, except that in human endothelial cells a second mediator is required to induce uPA synthesis. In animals bFGF and aFGF have been shown to induce neovascularization.[114,115] Because it is difficult to rule out the involvement of a limited number of leukocytes in these experiments in vivo, it remains to be elucidated whether these growth factors act in vivo in conjunction with inflammatory mediators or independently of the latter mediators. Min et al[116] have recently shown that prevention of the binding of uPA to the uPAR by a fusion product of the epidermal growth factor-like domain of murine uPA and the Fc portion of human IgG reduced bFGF-induced angiogenesis in vivo, and the growth of a B16 melanoma in syngeneic mice, indicating that uPA-mediated angiogenesis also occurs in these in vivo systems.

Proteolysis of the basement membrane of endothelial cells and invasion of endothelial cells into the underlying matrix are prerequisites for angiogenesis.[117] However, not only proteolysis, but also the formation of new cell attachment sites, is important for the formation of tubular structures. It should be noted that fibrin contains cell binding domains for endothelial cells: a RGD sequence in its α-chains which binds to the vitronectin receptor, i.e., the $\alpha_v\beta_3$ integrin;[118,119] and another site in the β-chain (residues 5-42),[120] which binds to an 130 kDa receptor.[121] Brooks et al[122,123] and Hammes et al[124] have shown that inhibition of the $\alpha_v\beta_3$ integrin reduces angiogenesis in several in vivo models. Friedlander et al[125] recently reported that both $\alpha_v\beta_3$ and $\alpha_v\beta_5$ integrin are involved in growth factor-stimulated angiogenesis in the rabbit cornea, but via distinct mechanisms. It is of interest to note that bFGF- and TNF-α-induced angiogenesis is inhibited by an antibody against the $\alpha_v\beta_3$ integrin, whereas angiogenesis induced by VEGF or by a protein kinase c activating phorbol ester required $\alpha_v\beta_5$ integrin. It remains to be established whether both $\alpha_v\beta_3$- and $\alpha_v\beta_5$-dependent mechanisms are active in the invasion of endothelial cells into a fibrin matrix. The involvement of

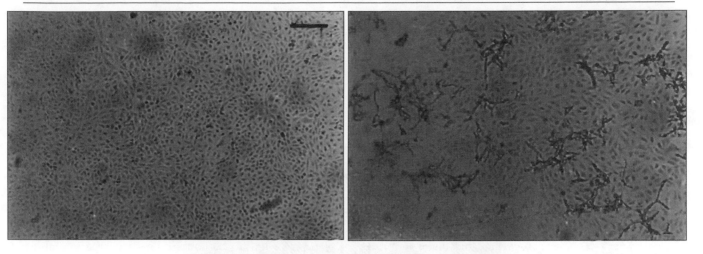

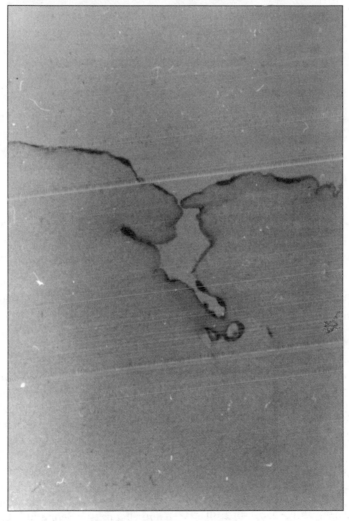

Fig. 29.3. Formation of capillary-like tubular structures in a three dimensional fibrin matrix by human endothelial cells. (A) Phase contrast microscopy of human microvascular endothelial cells grown under control conditions on top of a three-dimensional fibrin matrix. The bar represents 300 μm. (B) Formation of tubular structures is induced by the simultaneous addition of the growth factor bFGF (20 ng/mL) and the cytokine TNF-a (20 ng/mL). (C) Light microscopy of haemotoxylin/ploxin-stained cross-secion perpendicular to the fibrin matrix surface of a capillary-like tubular structure of microvascular endothelial cells.

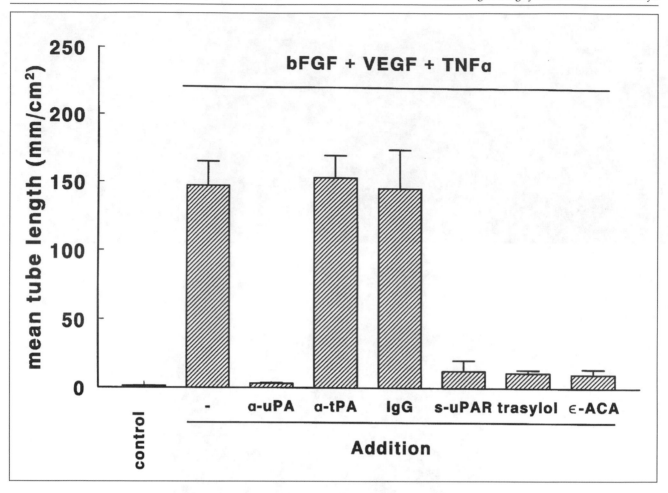

Fig. 29.4. Effect of various inhibitors of the uPA/plasmin system on the bFGF/VEGF/TNF-α-induced formation of tubular structures of human microvascular endothelial cells in a three dimensional fibrin matrix in vitro.

$\alpha_v\beta_3$ integrin interaction with the fibrin matrix is likely,[126] while the role of $\alpha_v\beta_5$ integrin, which more selectively interacts with vitronectin, has to be evaluated. Irrespective of the exact role of fibrin in stimulating angiogenesis, the fibrin structure has important consequences for wound healing, and proteolytic modification of fibrin, e.g., by leukocyte elastase, or interaction of fibrin with other matrix proteins, such as vitronectin and fibronectin, may affect cell invasion and angiogenesis and the success of wound healing. Furthermore, the recent observation that MMP-2 (gelatinase-A) binds to $\alpha_v\beta_3$[78] further points to the complexity of interactions that the $\alpha_v\beta_3$ integrin may have in fibrinous exudates, in which the matrix consists of a mixture of fibrin, collagens and other extracellular matrix components.

Perspective

Delineation of the various cellular pathways that are involved in angiogenesis is essential to selective interference with unwanted angiogenesis, such as in rheumatoid arthritis and tumors, and to stimulation of neovascularization at sites where it is needed, such as in normal wound healing and collateral formation.

The structure of fibrin clot, determined not only by the concentration of fibrinogen and thrombin present in the tissues but also by the presence of matrix molecules such as fibronectin, vitronectin, hyaluronic acid and thrombospondin, and by the environmental conditions like the pH and the ionic strength, determines whether new capillaries are formed or not. The invasion of endothelial cells into a fibrin matrix and the formation of capillary-like structures in the fibrin matrix in vitro is an attractive model to study this essence of the angiogenesis process associated with tissue repair. A recent paper of Nehls and Herrmann[128] points to the importance of the fibrin structure in endothelial cell migration and the formation of tubular structures. These authors show that the rigidity of the fibrin gel has a strong impact on tube formation by bovine endothelial cells in response to bFGF and VEGF. In addition, we have found that this was also the case when human microvascular endothelial cells were used (Collen et al, manuscript submitted for publication). It remains to be determined whether this effect of the fibrin structure reflects a mechanical barrier to movement of cells by a dense fibrin network, or is due to an inadequate spacing of cell-binding epitopes in the fibrin network.

Nevertheless, these data obtained using in vitro experiments may be of great value when fibrin gels are used in vivo as "temporary" matrix with regard to the initiation of site-directed formation of new blood vessel structures or collaterals, as shown by Dvorak et al[129] and Fasol et al.[130]

References

1. Bacharach E, Itin A, Keshet E. In vivo patterns of expression of urokinase and its inhibitor PAI-1 suggest a concerted role in regulating physiological angiogenesis. Proc Natl Acad Sci USA 1992; 89:10686-10690.
2. Weinberg JB, Pippen AMM, Greenberg CS. Extravascular fibrin formation and dissolution in synovial tissue of patients with osteoarthitis and rheumatoid arthritis. Arthitis Rheum 1991; 34:996-1005.
3. Folkman J, Shing Y. Angiogenesis. J Biol Chem 1992; 267:10931-10934.
4. Aiello LP, Avery RL, Arrigg PG, Keyt BA, Jampel HD, Shah ST, Pasquale LR et al. Vascular endothelial cell growth factor in ocular fluid of patients with diabetic retinopathy and other retinal disorders. N Engl J Med 1994; 331:1480-1487.
5. Dvorak HF, Brown LF, Detmar M, Dvorak AM. Vascular permeability factor/vascular endothelial growth factor, microvascular hyperpermeability, and angiogenesis. American J Pathol 1995. 146:1029-1039.
6. Polverini P. Macrophage-induced angiogenesis—A review. Macrophage-Derived Cell Regulatory Factors 1989; 1:54-73.
7. Dvorak HF. Tumors: Wounds that do not heal: similarities between tumor stroma generation and wound healing. N Engl J Med 1986; 315:1650-1659.
8. Colvin RB. Wound healing processes in hemostasis and thrombosis. In: Gimbrone MA Jr, ed. Vascular Endothelium in Hemostasis and Thrombosis. Edinburgh: Churchill Livingstone, 1986:220-241.
9. Bachmann F. Fibrinolysis. In: Verstraete M, Vermylen J, Lijnen R, Arnout J, eds. Thrombosis and Haemostasis. Leuven: Leuven University Press, 1987:227-265.
10. Wallén P. Structure and function of tissue plasminogen activator and urokinase. In: Castellino PJ, Gaffney PJ, Samama MM, Takada A, eds. Fundamental and Clinical Fibrinolysis. Amsterdam: Elsevier, 1987:1-18.
11. Redlitz A, Tan AK, Eaton DL, Plow EF. Plasma carboxypeptidases as regulators of plasminogen system. J Clin Invest 1995; 96:2534-2538.
12. Holmes WF, Nelles L, Lijnen HR, Collen D. Primary structure of human α_2-antiplasmin, a serine protease inhibitor (serpin). J Biol Chem 1987; 262:1659-1664.
13. Fearns C, Samad F, Loskutoff DJ. Synthesis and localization of PAI-1 in the vessel wall. In: van Hinsbergh VWM, ed. Vascular Control of Hemostasis. Amsterdam: Harwood Acad Pub, 1996:207-226.
14. Bachmann F. The enigma PAI-2. Gene expression, evolutionary and functional aspects. Thromb Haemostas 1995; 74:172-179.
15. Sprengers ED, Kluft C. Plasminogen activator inhibitors. Blood 1987; 69:381-387.
16. Loskutoff DJ. Regulation of PAI-1 gene expression. Fibrinolysis 1991; 5:197-206.
17. Wohlwend A, Belin D, Vassalli J-D. Plasminogen activator-specific inhibitors produced by human monocytes/macrophages. J Exp Med 1987; 165:320-339.
18. Miles LA, Plow EF. Plasminogen receptors: Ubiquitous sites for cellular regulation of fibrinolysis. Fibrinolysis 1988; 2:61-71.
19. Plow EF, Felez J, Miles LA. Cellular regulation of fibrinolysis. Thromb Haemostas 1991; 66:32-36.
20. Nachman RL. Thrombosis and atherogenesis: Molecular connections. Blood 1992; 79:1897-1906.
21. Hajjar KA. Cellular receptors in the regulation of plasmin generation. Thromb Haemostas 1995; 74:294-301.
22. Hajjar KA. The endothelial cell tissue plasminogen activator receptor. Specific interaction with plasminogen. J Biol Chem 1991; 266:21962-21970.
23. Vassalli J-D. The urokinase receptor. Fibrinolysis 1994; 8:172-181.
24. Blasi F, Conese M, Møller LB, Pedersen N, Cavallaro U, Cubellis M, Fazioli F, Hernandez-Marrero L, Limongi P, Munoz-Canoves P, Resnati M, Riittinen L, Sidenius N, Soravia E, Soria M, Stoppelli M, Talarico D, Teesalu T, Valcamonica S. The urokinase receptor: Structure, regulation and inhibitor-mediated internalization. Fibrinolysis 1994; 8:182-188.
25. Danø K, Behrendt N, Brünner N, Ellis V, Ploug M, Pyke C. The urokinase receptor protein structure and role in plasminogen activation and cancer invasion. Fibrinolysis 1994; 8:189-203.
26. Hajjar KA, Nachman RL. Endothelial cell-mediated conversion of Glu-plasminogen to Lys-plasminogen. Further evidence for assembly of the fibrinolytic system on the endothelial cell surface. J Clin Invest 1988; 82:1769-1778.
27. Miles LA, Dahlberg CM, Levin EG, Plow EF. Gangliosides interact directly with plasminogen and urokinase and may mediate binding of these fibrinolytic components to cells. Biochem 1989; 28:9337-9343.
28. Miles LA, Fless GM, Levin EG, Scanu AM, Plow EF. A potential basis for the thrombotic risks associated with lipoprotein(a). Nature 1989; 399:301-303.
29. Hajjar KA, Hamel NM, Harpel PC, Nachman RL. Binding of tissue plasminogen activator to cultured human endothelial cells. J Clin Invest 1987; 80:1712-1719.
30. Beebe DP. Binding of tissue plasminogen activators to human umbilical vein endothelial cells. Thromb Res 1987; 46:241-254.
31. Barnathan ES, Kuo A, Van der Keyl H, McCrae KR, Larsen GR, Cines DB. Tissue-type plasminogen activator binding to human endothelial cells. Evidence for two distinct sites. J Biol Chem 1988; 263:7792-7799.
32. Hajjar KA, Reynolds C. α-Fucose-mediated binding and degradation of tissue-type plasminogen activator by HepG2 cells. J Clin Invest 1994; 93:703-710.
33. Dumler I, Petri T, Schleuning W-D. Interaction of urokinase-type plasminogen activator (uPA) with its cellular receptor (uPAR) induces phosphorylation on tyrosine of a 38 kDa protein. FEBS Letters 1993; 322:37-40.
34. Rao NK, Shi G-P, Chapman HA. Urokinase receptor is a multifunctional protein: Influence of receptor occupancy on macrophage gene expression. J Clin Invest 1995; 96:465-474.
35. Barnathan ES. Characterization and regulation of the urokinase receptor of human endothelial cells. Fibrinolysis 1992; 6:1-9.
36. Appella E, Robinson EA, Ullrich SJ, Stoppelli MP, Corti A, Cassani G, Blasi F. The receptor-binding sequence of urokinase A biological function for the growth-factor module of proteases. J Biol Chem 1987; 262:4437-4440.
37. Ploug M, Behrendt N, Lober D, Danø K. Protein structure and membrane anchorage of the cellular receptor for urokinase-type plasminogen activator. Seminars in Thromb Haemostas 1991; 17:183-193.
38. Pöllänen J, Hedman K, Nielsen LS, Danø K, Vaheri A. Ultrastructural localization of plasma membrane-associated urokinase-type plasminogen activator at focal contacts. J Cell Biol 1988; 106:87-95.

39. Conforti G, Dominguez-Jimenez C, Rønne E, Høyer-Hansen G, Dejana E. Cell-surface plasminogen activation causes a retraction of in vitro cultured human umbilical vein endothelial cell monolayer. Blood 1994; 83:994-1005.

40. Haddock RC, Spell ML, Baker CD III, Grammer JR, Parks JM, Speidel M, Booyse FM. Urokinase binding and receptor identification in cultured endothelial cells. J Biol Chem 1991; 266:21466-21473.

41. Quigley JP, Gold LI, Schwimmer R, Sullivan LM. Limited cleavage of cellular fibronectin by plasmin activator purified from transformed cells. Proc Natl Acad Sci USA 1987; 84:2776-2780.

42. Olson D, Pöllänen J, Høyer-Hansen G, Rønne E, Sakaguchi K, Wun T-C, Appella E, Danø K, Blasi F. Internalization of the urokinase-plasminogen activator inhibitor type-1 complex is mediated by the urokinase receptor. J Biol Chem 1992; 267:9129-9133.

43. Nykjœr A, Petersen CM, Møller B, Jensen PH, Moestrup SK, Holtet TL, Etzerodt M, Thogersen HC, Munch M, Andreasen PA, Gliemann J. Purified α_2-macroglobulin receptor/LDL receptor-related protein binds urokinase activator inhibitor type-1 complex—Evidence that the α_2-macroglobulin receptor mediates cellular degradation of urokinase receptor-bound complexes. J Biol Chem 1992; 267:14543-14546.

44. Heegaard CW, Wiborg Simonsen AC, Oka K, Kjøller L, Christensen A, Madsen B, Ellgaard L, Chan L, Andreasen PA. Very low density lipoprotein receptor binds and mediates endocytosis of urokinase-type plasminogen activator-type-1 plasminogen activator inhibitor complex. J Biol Chem 1995; 270:20855-20861.

45. Wyne KL, Pathak RK, Seabra MC, Hobbs HH. Expression of the VLDL receptor in endothelial cells. Arterioscl Thromb Vasc Biol 1996; 16:407-415.

46. Wei Y, Waltz D, Rao N, Drummond R, Rosenberg S, Chapman H. Identification of the urokinase receptor as cell adhesion receptor for vitronectin. J Biol Chem 1994; 269:32380-32388.

47. Orth K, Madison EL, Gething M-J, Sambrook JF, Herz J. Complexes of tissue-type plasminogen activator and its serpin inhibitor plasminogen-activator inhibitor type-1 are internalized by means of the low density lipoprotein receptor-related protein/α_2-macroglobulin receptor. Proc Natl Acad Sci USA 1992; 89:7422-7426.

48. Bu G, Williams S, Strickland DK, Schwartz AL. Low density lipoprotein receptor-related protein/α_2-macroglobulin receptor is an hepatic receptor for tissue-type plasminogen activator. Proc Natl Acad Sci USA 1992; 89:7427-7431.

49. Bu G, Warshawsky I, Schwartz AL. Cellular receptors for the plasminogen activators. Blood 1994; 83:3427-3436.

50. Otter M, Barrett-Bergshoef MM, Rijken DC. Binding of tissue-type plasminogen activator by the mannose receptor. J Biol Chem 1991; 266:13931-13935.

51. Van Hinsbergh VWM, van den Berg EA, Fiers W, Dooijewaard G. Tumor necrosis factor induces the production of urokinase-type plasminogen activator by human endothelial cells. Blood 1990; 75:1991-1998.

52. Grøndahl-Hansen J, Kirkeby L, Ralfkiœr E, Kristensen P, Lund LR, Danø K. Urokinase-type plasminogen activator in endothelial cells during acute inflammtion of the appendix. Am J Pathol 1989; 135:631-636.

53. Niedbala MJ, Stein-Picarella M. Tumor necrosis factor induction of endothelial cell urokinase-type plasminogen activator mediated proteolysis of extracellular matrix and its antagonism by γ-interferon. Blood 1992; 79:678-687.

54. Colucci M, Paramo JA, Collen D. Generation in plasma of a fast-acting inhibitor of plasminogen activator in response to endotoxin stimulation. J Clin Invest 1985; 75:818-824.

55. Emeis JJ, Kooistra T. Interleukin-1 and lipopolysaccharide induce a fast-acting inhibitor of tissue-type plasminogen activator in vivo and in cultured endothelial cells. J Exp Med 1986; 163:1260-1266.

56. Schleef RR, Bevilacqua MJ, Sawdey M, Gimbrone MA, Loskutoff DJ. Cytokine activation of vascular endothelium. Effect on tissue-type plasminogen activator and type 1 plasminogen activator inhibitor. J Biol Chem 1988; 263:5797-5803.

57. Van Hinsbergh VWM, Kooistra T, Van den Berg EA, Princen HMG, Fiers W, Emeis JJ. Tumor necrosis factor increases the production of plasminogen activator inhibitor in human endothelial cells in vitro and in rats in vivo. Blood 1988; 72:1467-1473.

58. Van Hinsbergh VWM, Vermeer M, Koolwijk P, Grimbergen J, Kooistra T. Genistein reduces tumor necrosis factor α-induced plasminogen activator inhibitor-1 transcription but not urokinase expression in human endothelial cells. Blood 1994; 84:2984-2991.

59. Quax PHA, Van den Hoogen CR, Verheijen JH, Padro T, Zeheb R, Gelehrter TD, van Berkel TJC, Kuiper J, Emeis JJ. Endotoxin induction of plasminogen activator and plasminogen activator inhibitor type 1 mRNA in rat tissues in vivo. J Biol Chem 1990; 265:15560-15563.

60. Keeton M, Eguchi Y, Swadey M, Ahn C, Loskutoff D. Cellular localization of type 1 plasminogen activator inhibitor messenger RNA and protein in murine renal tissue. Am J Pathol 1993; 142:59-70.

61. Saksela OD, Moscatelli D, Rifkin D. The opposing effects of basic fibroblast growth factor and transforming growth factor beta on the regulation of plasminogen activator activity in capillary endothelial cells. J Cell Biol 1987; 105:957-963.

62. Pepper MS, Ferrara N, Orci L, Montesano R. Vascular endothelial growth factor (VEGF) induces plasminogen activators and plasminogen activator inhibitor-1 in microvascular endothelial cells. Biochem Biophys Res Commun 1991; 181:902-906.

63. Pepper MS, Sappino A-P, Stocklin R, Montesano R, Orci L, Vassalli J-D. Upregulation of urokinase receptor expression on migrating endothelial cells. J Cell Biol 1993; 122:673-684.

64. Bikfalvi A, Sauzeau C, Moukadiri H, Maclouf J, Busso N, Bryckaert N, Plouet J, Tobelem G. Interaction of vasculotropin/vascular endothelial cell growth factor with human umbilical vein endothelial cells—Binding, internalization, degradation, and biological effects. J Cell Physiol 1991; 149:50-59.

65. Koolwijk P, van Erck MGM, de Vree WJA, Vermeer MA, Weich HA, Hanemaaijer R, van Hinsbergh VWM. Cooperative effect of TNFα, bFGF and VEGF on the formation of tubular structures of human microvascular endothelial cells in a fibrin matrix. Role of urokinase activity. J Cell Biol 1996; 6:1177-1188.

66. Mignatti P, Mazzieri R, Rifkin DB. Expression of the urokinase receptor in vascular endothelial cells is stimulated by basic fibroblast growth factor. J Cell Biol 1991; 113:1193-1201.

67. Mandriota S, Seghezzi G, Vassalli J-D, Ferrara N, Wasi S, Mazzieri R, Mignatti P, Pepper M. Vascular endothelial growth factor increases urokinase receptor expression in vascular endothelial cells. J Biol Chem 1995; 270:9709-9716.

68. Langer DJ, Kuo A, Kariko K, Ahuja M, Klugherz BD, Ivanics KM, Hoxie JA, Williams WV, Liang BT, Cines DB, Barnathan ES. Regulation of the endothelial cell urokinase-type plasminogen activator receptor—Evidence for cyclic AMP-dependent and protein kinase-C dependent pathways. Circ Res 1993; 72:330-340.

69. van Hinsbergh VWM. Impact of endothelial activation on fibrinolysis and local proteolysis in tissue repair. Ann NY Acad Sci 1992; 667:151-162.

70. Presta M, Maier JAM, Ragnotti G. The mitogenic signalling pathway but not the plasminogen activator-inducing pathway of basic fibroblast growth factor is mediated through protein kinase c in fetal bovine aortic endothelial cells. J Cell Biol 1989; 109:1877-1884.

71. Leibovich SJ, Polverini PJ, Shepard HM, Wiseman DM, Shively V, Nuseir N. Macrophage-induced angiogenesis is mediated by tumour necrosis factor-α. Nature 1987; 329:630-632.

72. Fràter-Schröder M, Risau W, Hallman R, Gautschi P, Böhlen P. Tumor necrosis factor type α, a potent inhibitor of endothelial cell growth in vitro, is angiogenic in vivo. Proc Natl Acad Sci USA 1987; 84:5277-5281.

73. Kirchheimer JC, Nong Y, Remold HG. IFN-γ, tumor necrosis factor-α, and urokinase regulate the expression of urokinase receptors on human monocytes. J Immunol 1998; 141:4229-4234.

74. Hanemaaijer R, Koolwijk P, Leclercq L, De Vree WJA, Van Hinsbergh VWM. Regulation of matrix metalloproteinase expression in human vein and microvascular endothelial cells—Effects of tumour necrosis factor-α, interleukin-1 and phorbol ester. Biochem J 1993; 296:803-809.

75. Cornelius LA, Nehring LC, Roby JD, Parks WC, Welgus HG. Human dermal microvascular endothelial cells produce matrix metalloproteinases in response to angiogenic factors and migration. J Invest Dermatol 1995; 105:170-176.

76. Sato H, Takin T, Okada Y, Cao J, Shinagawa A, Yamamoto E, Seiki M. A matrix metalloproteinase expressed in the surface of invasive tumour cells. Nature 1994; 370:61-65.

77. Foda HD, George S, Conner C, Drews M, Tomkins DC, Zucker S. Activation of human umbilical vein endothelial cell progelatinase a by phorbol myristate: A protein kinase c-dependent mechanism involving a membrane-type matrix metalloproteinase. Lab Invest 1996; 74:538-545.

78. Brooks PC, Strömblad S, Sanders LC, von Schalscha TL, Aimes RT, Stetler-Stevenson WG, Quigley JP, Cheresh DA. Localization of matrix metalloproteinase MMP-2 to the surface of invasive cells by interaction with integrin $\alpha_v\beta_3$. Cell 1996; 85:683-693.

79. Unemori EN, Bouhana KS, Werb Z. Vectorial secretion of extracellular matrix proteins, matrix-degrading proteinases, and tissue inhibitor of metalloproteinases by endothelial cells. J Biol Chem 1990; 265:445-451.

80. Fisher C, Gilbertson-Beadling S, Powers EA, Petzold G, Poorman R, Mitchell MA. Interstitial collagenase is required for angiogenesis in vitro. Dev Biol 1994; 162:499-510.

81. Karelina TV, Goldberg GI, Eisen AZ. Matrix metalloproteinases in blood vessel development in human fetal skin and in cutaneous tumors. J Invest Dermatol 1995; 105:411-417.

82. Galis ZS, Sukhova GK, Lark MW, Libby P. Increased expression of matrix metalloproteinases and matrix degrading activity in vulnerable regions of human atherosclerotic plaques. J Clin Invest 1994; 94:2493-2503.

83. Nikkari ST, O'Brien KD, Ferguson M, Hatsukami T, Welgus HG, Alpers CE, Clowes AW. Interstitial collagenase (MMP-1) expression in human carotid atherosclerosis. Circulation 1995; 92:1393-1398.

84. Rao JS, Yamamoto M, Mohaman S, Gokaslan ZL, Stetler-Stevenson WG, Roa VH, Liotta LA, Nicolson Gl, Sawaya RE. Expression and localization of 92 kDa type IV collagenase genatinase B (MMP-9) in human gliomas. Clin Exp Metastasis 1996; 14:12-18.

85. Liotta LA, Steeg PS, Stetler-Stevenson WG. Cancer metastasis and angiogenesis—An imbalance of positive and negative regulation. Cell 1991; 64:327-336.

86. Danø K, Andreasen PA, Grøndahl-Hansen J, Kristensen P, Nielsen LS, Skriver L. Plasminogen activators in tissue degradation and cancer. Adv Cancer Res 1985; 44:139-264.

87. Estreicher A, Mühlhauser J, Carpentier J-L, Orci L, Vassalli J-D. The receptor for urokinase type plasminogen polarizes expression of the protease to the leading edge of migrating monocytes and promotes degradation of enzyme inhibitor complexes. J Cell Biol 1990; 111:783-792.

88. Blasi F. Urokinase and urokinase receptor—A paracrine/autocrine system regulating cell migration and invasiveness. Bioessays 1993; 15:105-111.

89. Hébert CA, Baker JB. Linkage of extracellular plasminogen activator to fibroblast cytoskeleton: Colocalization of cell surface urokinase with vinculin. J Cell Biol 1988; 105:1241-1247.

90. Schleef RR, Birdwell CR. The effect of proteases on endothelial cell migration in vitro. Exp Cell Res 1982; 141:503-508.

91. Quax PHA, Koolwijk P, Verheijen JHM, Van Hinsbergh VWM. The role of plasminogen activators in vascular pericellular proteolysis. In: van Hinsbergh VWM, ed. Vascular Control of Hemostasis. Amsterdam: Harwood Academic Publishers, 1996:227-245.

92. Clowes AW, Clowes MM, Au YPT, Reidy MA, Belin D. Smooth muscle cells express urokinase during mitogenesis and tissue-type plasminogen activator during migration in injured rat carotid artery. Circ Res 1990; 67:61-67.

93. Carmeliet P, Collen D. Evaluation of the plasminogen/plasmin system in transgenic mice. Fibrinolysis 1994; 8:269-276.

94. Ploplis VA, Carmeliet P, Vazirzadeh S, Van Vlaenderen I, Moons L, Plow EF, Collen D. Effects of disruption of the plasminogen gene on thrombosis, growth, and health in mice. Circulation 1995; 92:2585-2593.

95. Bugge TH, Suh TT, Flick MJ, Daugherty CC, Rømer J, Solberg II, Ellis V, Danø K, Degen JJ. The receptor for urokinase-type plasminogen activator is not essential for mouse development or fertility. JBiol Chem 1995; 270:16886-16894.

96. Pepper MS, Vassalli J-D, Montesano R, Orci L. Urokinase-type plasminogen activator is induced in migrating capillary endothelial cells. J Cell Biol 1987; 105:2535-2541.

97. Sato Y, Rifkin DB. Autocrine activities of basic fibroblast growth factor: Regulation of endothelial cell movement,

plasminogen activator synthesis, and DNA synthesis. J Cell Biol 1988; 107:1199-1205.

98. Gualandris A, Presta M. Transcriptional and posttranscriptional regulation of urokinase-type plasminogen activator expression in endothelial cells by basic fibroblast growth factor. J Cell Physiol 1995; 162:400-409.

99. Franke RP, Gräfe M, Schnittler H, Seiffge D, Mittermayer C, Drenckhahn D. Induction of human vascular endothelial stress fibres by fluid shear stress. Nature 1984; 307:648-649.

100. Davies PF, Robotewsky A., Griem ML. Quantitative studies of endothelial adhesions: Directional modeling of focal adhesion sites in response to flow forces. J Clin Invest 1994; 93:2031-2038.

101. Ponfoort ED, van Bockel JH, van Hinsbergh VWM. Shear forces induce the synthesis of urokinase-type plasminogen activator in human iliac vein endothelial cells in vitro. Circulation 1995; 92(suppl.):3016.

102. Hobson B, Denekamp J. Endothelial proliferation in tumours and normal tissues: Continuous labelling studies. Br J Cancer 1984; 49:405-413.

103. Dvorak HF, Nagy JA, Berse B, Brown LF, Yeo K-T, Yeo T-K, Dvorak AM, Van De Water L, Sioussat TM, Senger DR. Vascular permeability factor, fibrin, and the pathogenesis of tumor stroma formation. Ann NY Acad Sci 1992; 667:101-111.

104. Folkman J. Tumor angiogenesis. In: Mendelsohn J, Howley PM, Israel MA, Liotta LA, eds. The Molecular Basis of Cancer. Philadelphia: WB Saunders Comp., 1995:206-232.

105. Burgess WH, Maciag T. The heparin-binding (fibroblast) growth factor family of proteins. Annu Rev Biochem 1989; 58:575-606.

106. Montesano R. Regulation of angiogenesis in vitro. European J Clin Invest 1992; 22:504-515.

107. Fong G-H, Rossant J, Gertsenstein M, Breitman ML. Role of the flt-1 receptor tyrosine kinase in regulating the assembly of vascular endothelium. Nature 1995; 376:66-70.

108. Shalaby F, Rossant J, Yamaguchi TP, Gertsenstein M, Wu X-F, Breitman ML, Schuh AC. Failure of blood-island formation and vasculogenesis in Flk-1-deficient mice. Nature 1995; 376:62-66.

109. Sato TN, Tozawa Y, Deutsch U, Wolburg-Buchholz K, Fujiwara Y, Gendron-Maguire M, Gridley T, Wolburg H, Risau W, Qin Y. Distinct roles of the receptor tyrosine kinases tie-1 and tie-2 in blood vessel formation. Nature 1995; 376:70-74.

110. Koch AE, Polverini PJ, Kunkel SL, Harlow LA, DiPietro LA, Elner VM, Elner SG, Strieter RM. Interleukin-8 as a macrophage-derived mediator of angiogenesis. Science 1991; 258:1798-1801.

111. Kwaan HC. Tissue fibrinolytic activity studied by a histochemical method, Fed Proc 1966; 25:52-56.

112. Pepper MS, Belin D, Montesano R, Orci L, Vassalli J. Transformtin growth factor-β-1 modulates basic fibroblast growth factor induced proteolytic and angiogenic properties of endothelial cells in vitro. J Cell Biol 1990; 111:743-755.

113. Pepper MS, Ferrara N, Orci L, Montesano R. Potent synergism between vascular endothelial growth factor and basic fibroblast growth factor in the induction of angiogenesis in vitro. Biochem Biophys. Res Commun 1992; 189:824-831.

114. Thompson JA, Anderson KD, DiPietro JM, Zwiebel JA, Zametta M, Anderson WF, Maciag T. Site-directed neovessel formation in vivo. Science 1988; 241:1349-1352.

115. Broadley KN, Aquino AM, Woodward SC, Buckley-Sturrock A, Sato Y, Rifkin D, Davidson JM. Monospecific antibodies implicate basic fibroblast growth factor in normal wound repair. Lab Invest 1989; 61:571-575.

116. Min HY, Doyle LV, Vitt CR, Zandonella CL, Stratton-Thomas JR, Shuman MA, Rosenberg S. Urokinase receptor antagonists inhibit angiogenesis and primary tumor growth in syngeneic mice. Cancer Res 1996; 56:2428-2433

117. Ausprunk D, Folkman J. Migration and proliferation of endothelial cells in preformed and newly formed blood vessels during tumor angiogenesis. Microvasc Res 1977; 14:52-65.

118. Dejana E, Lampugnani MG, Giorgi M, Gaboli M, Marchisio PC. Fibrinogen induces endothelial cell adhesion and spreading via the release of endogenous matrix proteins and the recruitment of more than one integrin receptor. Blood 1990; 75:1509-1517.

119. Thiagarajan P, Rippon AJ, Farrell DH. Alternative adhesion sites in human fibrinogen for vascular endothelial cells. Biochemistry 1996; 35:4169-4175.

120. Bunce LA, Sporn LA, Francis CW. Endothelial cell spreading on fibrin requires fibrinopeptide B cleavage and amino acid residues 15-42 of the β-chain. J Clin Invest 1992; 89:842-850.

121. Erban JK, Wagner DD. A 130-kDa protein on endothelial cells binds to amino acids 15-42 of the Bβ chain of fibrinogen. J Biol Chem 1992; 267:2451-2458.

122. Brooks PC, Clark RA, Cheresh DA. Requirement of vascular integrin $\alpha_v\beta_3$ for angiogenesis. Science 1994; 264:569-571.

123. Brooks PC, Montgomery AM, Rosenfeld M., Reisfeld RA, Hu T, Klier G, Cheresh DA. Intergrin $\alpha_v\beta_3$ antagonists promote tumor regression by inducing apoptosis of angiogenic blood vessels. Cell 1994; 79:1157-1164.

124. Hammes HP, Brownlee M, Jonczyk A, Sutter A, Preissner K. Subcutaneous injection of a cyclic peptide antagonist of vitronectin receptor-type integrins inhibits retinal neovascularization. Nature Medicine 1996; 2:529-533.

125. Friedlander M, Brooks PC, Shaffer RW, Kincais CM, Varner JA, Cheresh DA. Definition of two angiogenic pathways by distinct α_v integrins. Science 1995; 270:1500-1502.

126. Chang M-C, Wang B-R, Huang T-F. Characterization of endothelial cell differential attachment to fibrin and fibrinogen and its inhibition by Arg-Gly-Asp-containing peptides. Thromb Haemostas 1995; 74:764-769.

127. Pepper MS, Vassalli J-D, Wilks JW, Schweigerer L, Orci L, Montesano R. Modulation of bovine microvascular endothelial cell proteolytic properties of inhibitors of angiogenesis. J Cell Biochem 1994; 55:419-434.

128. Nehls V, Herrmann R. The configuration of fibrin clots determines capillary morphogenesis and endothelial cell migration. Microvascular Res 1996; 51:347-364.

129. Dvorak HF, Harvey S, Estrella P, Brown LF, McDonagh J, Dvorak AM. Fibrin containing gels induce angiogenesis. Implications for tumor stroma generation and wound healing. Lab Invest 1987; 57:673-686.

130. Fasol R, Schumacher B, Schlaudraff K, Hauenstein KH, Seitelberger R. Experimental use of a modified fibrin glue to induce site-directed angiogenesis from the aorta to the heart. J Thoracic Cardiovasc Surg 1994; 107:1432-1439.

Facilitation of Healing

Matrix Modulation

—————————————— CHAPTER 30 ——————————————

How Does Extracellular Matrix Control Capillary Morphogenesis?

Robert B. Vernon, E. Helene Sage

Angiogenesis: An Introduction

The blood vascular system has evolved a significant capacity for change. During embryonic and fetal life, the vasculature increases in quantity and complexity to serve developing tissues and organs. Vasculature of the adult is, in general, quiescent, yet it retains a capacity for growth, remodeling, and regression in response to the menstrual cycle, placentation, changes in adiposity, wound repair, and inflammation. During these processes, growth of new blood vessels is regulated and eventually ceases. In contrast, certain conditions such as tumor growth, diabetic retinopathies, arthritis, and psoriasis involve excessive proliferation of blood vessels that contributes directly to the pathological state.[1] Therefore, an understanding of the principles and mechanisms that direct the assembly new blood vessels, and the processes that start and stop vascular growth, are central to the development of agents and strategies to control vascularization in disease.[2]

Tissue engineering involves the fabrication of tissue or organ-like implants comprised of living cells in contact with a supportive matrix. Like cells of natural tissues and organs, cells associated with an implant must interface with the circulatory system for reception of oxygen and nutrients and removal of waste products. When implants are membranous, the metabolic needs of the resident cells can be met by simple diffusive exchanges with surrounding tissue fluids. However, a direct connection between the implant and the vascular system may be necessary when diffusion distances are long as a consequence of thickness or bulk of the implant. Moreover, in certain cases, resident cell types might require access to circulating blood so that they can sense and respond rapidly to changes in body chemistry and distribute their biosynthetic products (e.g., hormones) rapidly throughout the body. Exchanges between cells and blood in vivo are most efficient across blood vessels with small diameters and thin walls (e.g., capillaries); therefore, it would be desirable for implants to be invested by a microvasculature that is connected to the blood supply of the host via large-caliber arteries and veins. Artificial capillaries made from nonliving, semipermeable materials are likely to be occluded by thrombi and rendered impermeable by precipitated plasma proteins within a short period of time after exposure to flowing blood. Thus, it is likely that long term function of implants will require a microvasculature derived from the host. This microvasculature would be derived from the growth of extant blood vessels into the implant, a process termed neovascularization, that is typical of the vascularization of tumors. However, unlike the vasculature of a tumor, which grows and remodels continuously as the tumor grows, the vascular supply of an implant of finite mass must stop growing once a level of neovascularization sufficient to sustain the resident cell population has been achieved. Excessive and unceasing vascularization of the implant must be prevented, since an overexpression of some of the processes that mediate vascular growth (e.g., proteolysis or forces of cellular traction, which are discussed below) could compromise the function of the implant or destroy it altogether. Thus, the development of methods to control vascular growth will be an important goal for tissue engineers.

The sprouting of new blood vessels from extant vasculature, termed angiogenesis, is the principal form of vascular growth in the adult. Sprouts arise from endothelial cells (ECs) that line the lumens of capillaries and postcapillary venules—the smallest, most delicate branches of the vascular system where ECs are not confined by sheaths of smooth muscle or fibrous adventitia. The smallest capillaries are comprised of ECs alone and are capable of generating new capillary networks in the absence of other cell types. Although ECs contain all of the genetic information required for morphogenesis, their potential to organize into capillaries is realized only by interaction with a noncellular entity— the extracellular matrix (ECM). This review will discuss ways in which ECM mediates and modulates the behaviors of ECs that lead to the development of a capillary bed. Much of what we will relate is speculative, because mechanistic studies of the effects of ECM on vascular morphogenesis are in their infancy.

The Process of Angiogenesis

Angiogenesis is a complex, multistep process initiated in response to specific signals (e.g., diffusible, angiogenic proteins) that emanate from sites of potential vascularization. The stages of angiogenesis induced by solid tumors have been described[3,4] and can be summarized as follows:

1. Upon receipt of an angiogenic stimulus, ECs of the parent vessel degrade and penetrate the basement membrane that invests them, and subsequently migrate into the surrounding interstitial ECM as a knoblike or cone-shaped vascular sprout;
2. The invading ECs assume bipolar shapes and align behind one another in a follow-the-leader fashion;
3. ECs at the base or the middle of the sprout begin to divide and add to the population of migrating cells;
4. ECs organize into solid cords, which subsequently develop lumens;
5. Neighboring sprouts move toward one another and fuse to form vascular anastomoses;
6. Circulatory flow begins in the vascular anastomoses;
7. Pericytes emerge along the length of capillary sprouts, and a new basement membrane is synthesized.

It is likely that the above mentioned steps are typical of many forms of angiogenesis; however, solid cords of ECs may be absent from advancing sprouts in wounds and certain developing systems, such as the retina. Instead, nascent lumens form immediately behind the tips, which are comprised of one or two spindle-shaped ECs. Although specific elements of angiogenesis might vary, the molecular processes of capillary morphogenesis must mediate one or more of the following six individual or cooperative behaviors of ECs:

1. Migration—ECs must penetrate and move through interstitial ECM;
2. Cellular alignment—Unlike a migrating epithelium in which the cells move as a sheet, migrating ECs must follow one another in a "head-to-tail" orientation for nascent vessels to have a tubular form;
3. Cell division—ECs must increase in number to lengthen the nascent vessel;
4. Cell-cell adhesion—Migratory ECs must at some point make firm connections with one another to form a mechanically-integrated structure;
5. Formation of a lumen—Individual ECs must assume a curved shape to enclose a tubular space. Moreover, adjacent cells must join their individual tubular spaces to form a continuous lumen;
6. Branching and anastomosis—ECs must send off branches from the main sprout. These branches must find branches from other sprouts and fuse with them to form anastomoses (also referred to as vascular loops or arcades).

It is generally appreciated that genes regulate the activities of cells. Therefore, it has been proposed that the behaviors listed above are mediated and regulated by a specific "angiogenic program" or cascade that orchestrates the expression of EC gene products at specific times and in specific places.[5] This program is, in turn, controlled by a variety of soluble extracellular molecules ("growth factors") secreted by target tissues, organs, and tumors.[6,7] The role of growth factors in angiogenesis has been intensively studied: Much is known about the sources and structure of growth factors, receptors for growth factors on the surfaces of ECs, and signaling pathways within EC cytoplasm that are activated by growth factors. Moreover, the chemotaxis of EC sprouts in response to gradients of growth factors has been analyzed in detail.[8] What is not understood, however, is how regulation of expression of EC genes by growth factors specifies the actual *construction* of a capillary. Somehow, genetically programmed, quantitative changes in the synthesis of specific proteins by individual ECs are translated into spatial and vectorial information that directs the cooperative assembly of ECs into complex, three dimensional structures (Fig. 30.1). Studies of vascular development indicate that ECM plays a critical role in this translation. We will illustrate this concept by reviewing the development and characteristics of the most important models of angiogenesis— an exercise that will reveal the special relationship between ECs and ECM.

Models of Angiogenesis: The Essential Role of ECM

Windows In vivo

Angiogenesis is difficult to observe and manipulate in vivo because of the thickness and opacity of most tissues. Tissue sections offer only a static view and provide little information about the three dimensional structure of sprouting vasculature. Indeed, it is nearly impossible to identify the advancing fronts of sprouts (the critical areas of invasion and morphogenesis) in sectioned tissue. To circumvent these problems, investigators have attempted to find or make

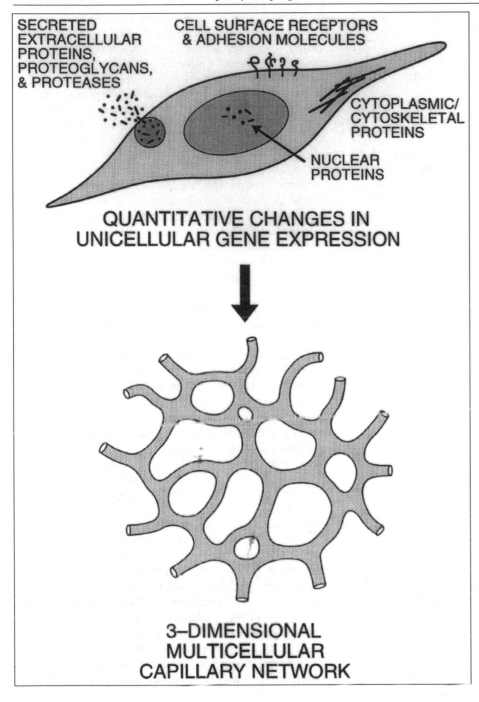

Fig. 30.1. ECs that initiate angiogenesis exhibit genetically derived, quantitative changes in the synthesis of specific proteins of the nucleus, cytoplasm, cell surface, and extracellular milieu. These changes, which constitute an "angiogenic program", are translated by poorly understood mechanisms into spatial and vectorial information that directs the assembly of ECs into a three dimensional capillary network.

windows into the living animal. In the late nineteenth and early twentieth centuries, angiogenesis had been observed directly in the thin, transparent tails of amphibian larvae (for references and description of early work, see ref. 10). In the 1930s, Clark and Clark[10] viewed the revascularization of wounds in rabbit ears through transparent chambers and made elegant drawings of the time course of angiogenic invasion, anastomosis, formation of lumens, and interaction of ECs with the ECM of the fibrin clot. Subsequent studies with the rabbit ear chamber and other window-type models (e.g., transparent chambers in mouse skin[11] and hamster cheek pouches,[12] rabbit corneal pockets,[13] and chick chorioallantoic membranes)[14] shifted the focus away from specific

details of vascular morphogenesis toward clinical investigations of the role of angiogenesis in the growth of tumors. From these largely descriptive studies came validation of the central paradigm of tumor-induced vascular chemotaxis and the corresponding discovery of diffusible, tumor-derived molecules that promoted vascular growth. An increasing interest in an understanding of angiogenesis at the molecular level led to the development of models in vitro, in which angiogenesis-related behaviors of ECs were studied under highly simplified, defined conditions. It was from such models that ECM was identified as a key element of vascular morphogenesis.

EC Monolayers In Vitro

In the 1970s, methods were developed to isolate ECs from large vessels and culture them in flat dishes for extended periods of time.[15,16] ECs grown under these conditions in vitro proliferated until they formed a confluent, pavement-like monolayer that simulated the endothelial lining of a blood vessel. It was appreciated that denuding injuries to the endothelium of large vessels induced ECs at the periphery of the wound to proliferate and migrate on the exposed ECM of the basement membrane until an unbroken endothelium was reestablished.[17,18] A similar progression of responses—proliferation, migration, re-establishment of integrity, quiescence—could be elicited in vitro from confluent monolayers of ECs "wounded" by removal of adherent cells with a scraper.[19,20] Thus, early studies of the relationship between ECs and ECM were designed in the context of re-endothelialization as comparisons between confluent monolayers and wounded (or simply subconfluent) ones. By this experimental approach, it was discovered that cultured bovine aortic ECs secreted fibronectin, laminin, heparan sulfate proteoglycan, and type I through V collagens;[20-22] moreover, they migrated better on a monomolecular coating of mixed type I and type III collagens than on a coating of fibronectin.[23] Studies of ECs (including ECs from capillaries) cultured as monolayers on molecular coatings of ECM have yielded important information; however, the migratory, chemotactic, proliferative, and synthetic responses of ECs that are elicited in these systems are not integrated in situ such that vessel-like structures are formed. For such an integration to occur in vitro, a significant quantity of malleable ECM is required.

Spontaneous Angiogenesis In Vitro

In 1980, following the successful, long term culture of capillary ECs,[24] Folkman and Haudenschild reported that 20-40 day cultures of bovine or human capillary ECs developed a two dimensional (planar) cellular network on top of the confluent cellular monolayer—a process they termed "angiogenesis in vitro".[25] By transmission electron microscopy, the ECs of the networks appeared to form tubes with lumens that were filled with variable amounts of fibrillar, membranous, and amorphous substances. This "string-like" extracellular material traversed the anastomoses between adjacent ECs and was proposed to act like a "mandril for the alignment of tubes from cell to cell".[25] Later studies showed that ECs from large vessels (e.g., human umbilical vein[26] and calf aorta[27]) could also form networks spontaneously in vitro. Here also, the lumens of the tubular ECs were filled with ECM that included fibronectin,[26,27] laminin, and type IV and V collagens.[28] Direct evidence of a morphogenetic role for ECM in what was now called "spontaneous angiogenesis in vitro" was provided by Ingber and Folkman,[29] who showed by time-lapse cinematography that the luminal ECM formed a "web" or "scaffold" on which the ECs organized themselves.

Traction, Tension, and Tessellation Mediate Spontaneous Angiogenesis In Vitro

A serious drawback of spontaneous angiogenesis in vitro was the length of time (up to six weeks) required for the formation of endothelial networks. In 1988, Kubota et al[30] reported that subconfluent ECs seeded on top of a malleable, hydrated gel of basement membrane ECM (Matrigel™) aligned in network-like patterns within one hour and formed a planar, capillary-like meshwork of cellular cords within eighteen hours. In later studies of this culture system,[30] we discovered that ECs formed networks as a consequence of the mechanical response of Matrigel to cellular tensile forces. The process (summarized in Fig. 30.2) begins as each EC continually pulls Matrigel toward itself by the motility-related phenomenon referred to as traction (described below). The centripetal movement of Matrigel toward ECs generates radiating fields of strain in the surrounding Matrigel (traction fields) that emanate from the ECs (which act as traction centers). Where adjacent fields of traction overlap, tension within the Matrigel is enhanced (the "two center effect"[32]) and causes fibers of ECM that comprise the Matrigel to align into narrow matrical tracks that connect the traction centers. The connection of neighboring traction centers soon establishes a tessellated (network-like) pattern on top of the flat field of Matrigel. ECs migrate along the network of matrical tracks by contact guidance and, with time, colonize the tracks to form a corresponding network of cellular cords. In situations where Matrigel is rendered highly malleable by a cycle of freezing and thawing, the centripetal movement of Matrigel to traction centers actually perforates the sheet of matrix and reorganizes it into a web of cables that subsequently become surrounded by cords of cells.[31] Matrical webs will form under variable circumstances in vitro, e.g., they can be generated from malleable layers of gelled, fibrillar type I collagen.[33] Moreover, the network of tension that tessellates a sheet of ECM can be developed by a confluent monolayer of ECs:[33] By this process, endogenously-synthesized ECM is organized into a web during spontaneous angiogenesis in vitro.[33]

Limitations of Planar Angiogenesis In vitro

The matrical scaffolds that arise in cultures that combine monolayers of ECs with sheets of ECM offer an attractive mechanism to explain how ECs orient themselves into networks in vivo. However, these planar models[33] lack certain defining characteristics of true angiogenesis:

1. Invasion—ECs in planar models form networks on top of ECM and show little propensity to burrow into the ECM;

2. Directionality—planar networks of ECs form in vitro by tessellation that is more or less simultaneous throughout a field of prepositioned cells, whereas angiogenesis in vivo involves the vectorial invasion of ECM by filamentous sprouts that arborize by multiple levels of branching;

3. Polarity—Although the ECs in planar models make unicellular tubes that markedly resemble capillaries,[26,27,34] they deposit basement membrane material on their luminal surfaces and have their thrombogenic surfaces facing outward to the surrounding culture media,[26,27] opposite to the situation in vivo.

Despite these deficiencies, the central characteristic of planar models—alignment of ECM in response to tension

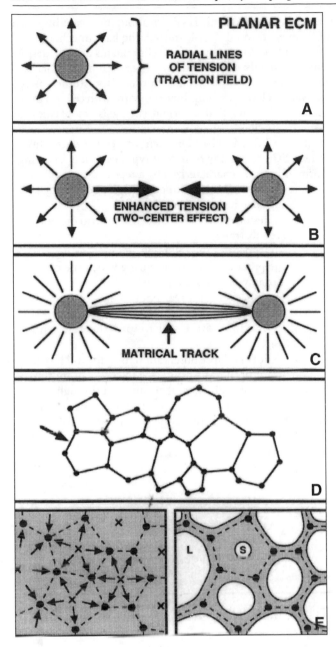

Fig. 30.2. Cellular traction generates patterns of order in planar ECM in vitro. (A) Viewed from above, a cellular traction center (shaded circle) in contact with malleable, planar ECM (rectangle) generates radial lines of tension (arrows) in the ECM that constitute a traction field. (B) Tension in ECM between adjacent traction centers is enhanced (large arrows) as a consequence of the two-center effect. (C) Fibers of ECM (black lines) align along the direction of principal stress. Fibers influenced by the two-center effect align to form a matrical track that connects the traction centers. (D) Traction centers (small black dots) arranged in a field on planar ECM become connected by matrical tracks (e.g., arrow) that form a network. (E) left panel: Where planar ECM (shaded) is highly malleable, centripetal movement (arrows) of ECM to traction centers (black dots) results in clearance of ECM from central areas (X) that are bordered by two-center effects (dotted lines). (E) right panel: Clearance process diagrammed in left panel is manifested as perforations (white areas) in the sheet of ECM (shaded). Perforations are small (S) initially but enlarge with time (L). ECM aligned by two-center effects (dotted lines) between traction centers (black dots) is resistant to cell-generated stresses. Reprinted from Vernon et al.[33] Copyright © 1995 by the Society for In Vitro Biology. Reproduced with permission of the copyright owner.

entation of ECs could be influenced significantly by the topology of their interaction with ECM. Although this particular three dimensional model lacks the characteristics of invasion (the ECs are pre-embedded in the ECM) and directionality (the ECs are evenly dispersed throughout the culture), it has proven useful in studies of lumen formation[37] and responses of ECs to growth factors.[38-41]

Three Dimensional Models with Invasive Characteristics

In 1982, Nicosia et al described the sprouting of ECs from sections of rat aorta ("aortic rings" one millimeter in thickness) embedded in a clot of chicken plasma.[42] Within 36 h, solid sprouts arose from the incised ends of the aorta and invaded the fibrin-rich ECM of the clot. Over a period of two weeks, ECs within sprouts migrated and proliferated to form branching, anastomosing cords that subsequently developed large, patent lumens. As in the three dimensional model with dispersed ECs, sprouts from aortic rings exhibited polarity like that in vivo. In addition, however, sprouts from aortic rings were truly invasive and exhibited a directional, branching morphogenesis. Aortic explants have been used to study the influence of tumors,[43] growth factors,[44,45] and various forms of ECM[46-50] on angiogenesis. Deficiencies in this model are typical of explant cultures, i.e., results can be influenced by non-EC types[51] and by growth factors that diffuse from the explant.[44] These problems are addressed by yet another model of vascular invasion in vitro. In 1985, Montesano and Orci[52] cultured confluent monolayers of bovine microvascular ECs on top of a layer of gelled type I collagen, and thereby generated an endothelium-like sheet of cells with a highly polarized morphology, i.e., the ECs possessed "luminal" surfaces that faced the overlying culture

generated by ECs—is likely to regulate the migration of ECs in vivo (discussed below). Fortunately, the problems of invasion, directionality, and polarity have been addressed by three dimensional models of angiogenesis, which are described below.

Angiogenesis in Three Dimensions

The recognition that capillary ECs are surrounded by ECM in vivo led to the development, in 1983,[35] of a three dimensional model of angiogenesis in which subconfluent bovine adrenal capillary ECs were embedded in a lattice of native type I collagen fibrils, commonly referred to as a collagen "gel".[36] Within two days, the ECs formed a network of cellular cords and tube-like structures with a polarity similar to that of capillaries in vivo, i.e., basal lamina-like material was deposited between the abluminal surfaces of the ECs and the collagen matrix. This result indicated that the ori-

medium, lateral surfaces that contacted adjacent ECs, and "abluminal" surfaces that faced the collagen substrate. This topology resulted in an angiogenesis-like response to the tumor-promoting ester phorbol myristate acetate: ECs penetrated the collagen as invaginations of the cellular sheet (much like the outpocketing that occurs during early stages of sprout formation in vivo) and formed branched, multicellular tubes with abluminal basal lamina-like material and patent, fluid-filled lumens similar to those of capillary sprouts in vivo[10] (Fig. 30.3). The induction of invasive sprouting by both micro- and macrovascular ECs[53-55] reinforces the notion that the structure of the parent vessel (i.e., a tube of mutually adherent cells with fluid plasma inside and ECM outside) provides vital cues and constraints that position ECs for correct orientative behaviors once their angiogenic programs are initiated.

Interactions Between ECs and ECM That Mediate Angiogenesis

As discussed above, differently-conceived models of angiogenesis all agree on the central role played by ECM in vascular morphogenesis. In the following section, we will move beyond descriptive studies to explore ways in which the behaviors of ECs and the structure of ECM interact mechanistically to promote the morphogenesis of capillaries.

Characteristics of EC Motility

Locomotion of ECs is a critical element of angiogenesis. A significant number of studies have examined the migration of ECs in response to various angiogenic molecules;

however, relatively little is known about the means by which ECs move through ECM. Indeed, the basic mechanism of ameboid movement by animal cells remains unclear, despite intensive study of selected cell types such as fibroblasts.[56] Moreover, almost all detailed mechanistic studies of cell movement have been conducted in vitro with cells on top of planar substrates that are rigid (i.e., glass or plastic), or semideformable (e.g., silicone rubber), and hence unlike malleable ECM in vivo. On such artificial surfaces, fibroblasts, ECs, and many other cell types exhibit a "crawling" form of motility characterized by a repeated cycle of:

1. Protrusion of lamellipodia or filopodia at the leading edge of the cell;
2. Adhesion of the protrusive structures to the supportive substrate;
3. Movement of the cell body and nucleus forward by the process of traction, during which the cell pulls strongly on the supportive substrate;
4. De-adhesion of the rear, pointed "tail" of the cell from the substrate; and
5. Retraction of the tail toward the cell center[56] (Fig. 30.4).

Classic time-lapse observations by Bard and Hay show chick corneal fibroblasts exhibiting this cycle of motility as they migrate through corneal stroma and through a gel of fibrillar type I collagen in vitro.[57] It is likely that ECs move through malleable three dimensional ECM in a similar manner.

Fig. 30.3. Vectorial invasion of type I collagen gels by confluent monolayers of ECs in vitro. In response to stimulatory molecules, such as phorbol esters, ECs of the monolayer penetrate the underlying collagen gel as invaginations of the cellular sheet. The invaginations elongate to form multicellular tubes with patent, fluid-filled lumens (L) that are continuous with the overlying culture medium. ECs that comprise the tubes deposit basal lamina-like material (BL) on their abluminal faces. It is likely that similar material is deposited underneath noninvasive ECs of the confluent monolayer (not shown).

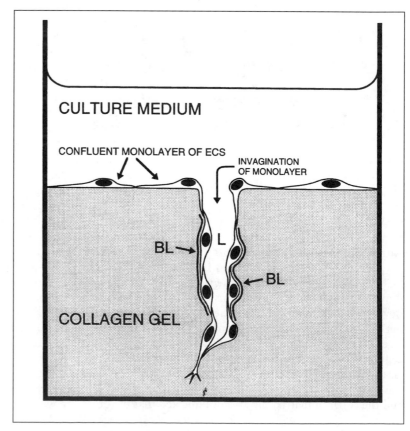

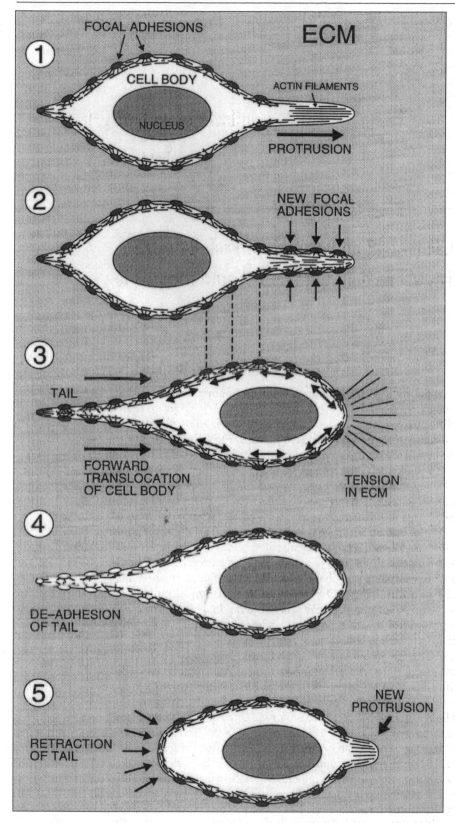

Fig. 30.4. Cycle of movement of an EC through three dimensional ECM. (1) The cycle begins with actin-mediated protrusion at the cell front. Focal adhesions (small gray ovals) anchor the cell body to the ECM (shaded background). (2) New focal adhesions anchor the protrusion to the ECM. (3) Cytoplasmic actin filaments and associated proteins generate traction forces (double-headed arrows) that pull on the ECM at the cell front and move the cell body forward past the focal adhesions, which remain fixed in position relative to the ECM (dotted lines). The rear of the cell remains attached to the ECM and is drawn out to form a pointed "tail". (4) Focal adhesions of the tail become altered (white ovals) and detach from the ECM. (5) The tail retracts into the cell body. At the cell front, a new protrusion begins the next cycle of forward progression.

Malleability of ECM as a Function of Its Composition

The migration of ECs and other cell types can be affected by the physical properties of the supportive ECM, notably malleability. In the context of angiogenesis, malleability is defined as the degree to which ECM deforms in response to forces generated by sprouting ECs. ECM is comprised of a hydrated gel of proteoglycans, glycoproteins, and hyaluronan in which fibrillar proteins (e.g., collagens and fibronectin) are embedded. The malleability of this mixture of macromolecules is significantly affected by the concentration and relative proportion of the major fibrillar proteins, such as type I and type III collagens that predominate in interstitial ECM. An additional element of physical heterogeneity involves the stiffness of individual protein fibrils, which depends in part on interactions with other components of ECM. For example, the polymerization of type I collagen in vitro yields thinner, more pliable fibrils in the presence of type III collagen,[58] the ECM protein TRAMP,[59] and the ECM proteoglycan decorin.[60] The malleability of ECM is decreased by increases in the physical entanglement of fibers (shear-drag) and by the presence of covalent crosslinks, such as the lysyl oxidase-catalyzed crosslinking of type I collagen fibers,[61] and the transglutaminase-catalyzed generation of fibronectin multimers.[62] The rigidifying effects of shear-drag and crosslinks are counteracted by specific molecular interactions (e.g., shear-drag between type I collagen fibers is reduced by the binding of type XII and type XIV collagens)[63] and by more general influences such as the reduction in fiber length and number by cell-mediated proteolysis. ECs within a vascular sprout influence the structural properties of ECM in their immediate vicinity by their synthesis of new forms of ECM and by chemical modification and/or degradation of extant ECM. These processes can be modulated to facilitate or inhibit vascular invasion, contingent upon the type of signals received by the ECs. Additional control over the rate, extent, and locale of vascular invasion resides with non-EC types (e.g., fibroblasts) that can control the composition of surrounding ECM via specific synthetic and degradative activities.

Malleability of ECM Influences the Motility of ECs

It is likely that the malleability of ECM directly influences the generation of protrusive structures by cells. Protrusion of filopodia and lamellipodia by crawling cells involves the polymerization of cytoplasmic actin that either pushes the plasma membrane forward or stabilizes bulges in the plasma membrane made by other means (e.g., via thermal movements or the local influx of water).[56] Counterforces exerted by ECM on the front of a cell (generated, for example, by the resistance of stiff, fibrillar ECM to bending or the resistance of charged, hydrated glycans to compression) would slow the rate or extent of protrusion by shifting the thermodynamic equilibrium in favor of actin depolymerization. Another consequence of ECM counterforces would be their effect on the shape of protrusions. For example, during progressive movement over rigid, planar substrates in vitro, during which viscous drag from the culture medium is negligible,[64] fibroblasts and ECs frequently project blunt or fan-shaped lamellipodia. In contrast, forward protrusions of ECs in ECM usually consist of one or more very thin, elongate filopodia that sometimes exhibit filamentous branches, i.e., structures with minimal frontal area that are thermodynamically favored in a viscous environment. The possibility that protrusive activity governs the rate of cell locomotion[65] might explain why movement of ECs into gelled collagen[66] or fibrin[67] is inhibited as the density of the ECM fibrils increases.

Traction of ECs as a Spatial Organizer of ECM

In crawling cells, actin filaments in the cytoplasmic cortex are driven rearward by association with other motive proteins, such as myosin.[56,68,69] Movement of actin is transduced into propulsive traction force by focal adhesions (Fig. 30.4), which are spot or bar-shaped specializations of the plasma membrane that adhere to the substrate (i.e., ECM) via their extracellular faces and connect to the actin via their cytoplasmic faces.[68-70] Traction is applied vectorially, and generates tension in malleable substrates in vitro (e.g., silicone rubber) that is directed parallel to the cellular axis of motion.[64,71] Remarkably, fibroblasts exert traction that is at least six orders of magnitude greater than is needed to propel the cell at a normal speed of 1 μm/sec against the viscous drag of aqueous medium.[64] It is important to realize that this magnitude of force and its vectorial application to the substrate are specialized features of crawling cells that are not intrinsic to ameboid locomotion. Neuronal growth cones and fish keratocytes that exhibit an alternative "gliding" form of ameboid motility[64] move 10-60 times faster than fibroblasts in vitro,[56] generate only 3-12% of the traction force,[64] and apply tension to the substrate at right angles to the direction of motion.[64,72]

It is thought that the "excessive" levels of traction developed by fibroblasts allow these cells to compress and align ECM in healing wounds[73] and within developing tendons, ligaments, and organ capsules.[74] The traction of ECs in vitro is similar in magnitude to that of dermal fibroblasts[75] and therefore is likely to serve a morphogenetic function. Traction at the advancing front of sprouts would tend to align ECM in the direction of invasion and thus would facilitate protrusion of filopodia from leading ECs. Moreover, elastic interactions among ECM fibrils allow them to be aligned over great distances (as much as one centimeter in vitro),[32,74] and to form pathways on which invading ECs would move by contact guidance.[76] Such matrical pathways mediate migration of ECs in planar angiogenesis in vitro and have been associated with the movement of endocardial cells into the endocardial cushions of the developing chicken heart.[77] Moreover, the existence of matrical pathways is consistent with the follow-the-leader behavior of ECs that migrate through three dimensional ECM in vitro[78] and in vivo.[3] Matrical pathways could also mediate the development of anastomoses between vascular sprouts. ECs at the tips of adjacent sprouts would align ECM between them by a traction-mediated two-center effect, approach one another via the matrical pathway, and fuse to establish a common lumen (Fig. 30.5).

Beyond the role of traction to facilitate vascular invasion and anastomosis of sprouts is the potential for traction

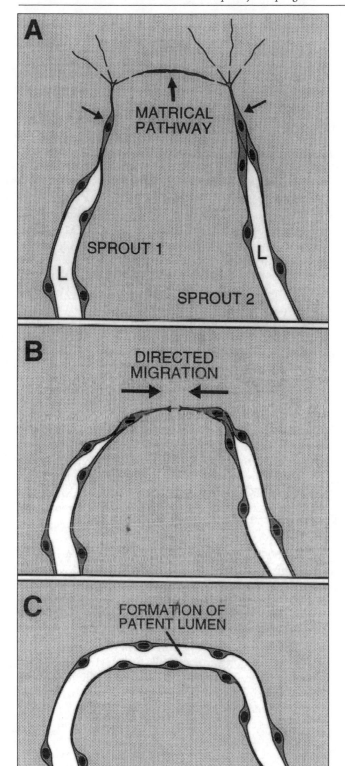

Fig. 30.5. Hypothetical role of matrical pathways in the anastomosis of angiogenic sprouts in vivo. (A) Migratory ECs (small arrows) at tips of adjacent sprouts create a connecting pathway of aligned ECM (matrical pathway) as a consequence of a traction-mediated two-center effect. Lumens (L) of sprouts are indicated. (B) Migratory ECs approach one another (arrows) via the matrical pathway. (C) The vascular loop is completed as ECs meet, adhere, and interact to form a patent lumen. Adapted from Vernon RB, Sage EH. Between molecules and morphology: Extracellular matrix and the creation of vascular form. Am J Pathol 1995; 147:873-883. Copyright © 1995 by the American Society for Investigative Pathology. Reproduced with permission of the copyright owner.

embryo,[33] capillary plexuses of acinar exocrine glands and pulmonary alveoli, and the microvasculature of the retina. For a given system of planar vasculature, the architecture of the cellular network and, indeed, whether such a network forms, are direct functions of the malleability of the ECM[31,79] and the levels of traction force generated by the component ECs[79]—parameters that are controlled by a multiplicity of regulatory signals.

Adhesion Between ECs and ECM as a Regulator of EC Migration

A crawling cell generates new focal adhesions at the front that persist and remain fixed to the substrate as the cell pulls itself over them.[80,81] Upon reaching the rear of the cell, the adhesions are released.[80] This dynamic circumstance suggests that an asymmetry of adhesive strength exists between the front and rear of the cell: Strong adhesion at the front enables the cell to pull itself forward and weaker adhesion at the rear allows the cell to free itself to begin the next cycle of movement. Mathematical models[82] predict that for a given level of cytoplasmic contractile force, the opposing force of substratum adhesion influences the rate of locomotion in a biphasic manner: Weak adhesion inhibits the conversion of cytoskeletal contractility into propulsive traction force, whereas excessive adhesion prevents the cell from freeing its rear from the substrate. Speed of migration is predicted to be maximal at an intermediate level of adhesion that allows dynamic making and breaking of cell contacts. This hypothesis is supported by studies in vitro that show biphasic relationships between the rate of cellular motility and the concentration of laminin,[83] laminin fragment E8,[83] fibronectin,[84] and type IV collagen[84] adsorbed to plastic.

ECs exhibit variable adhesion to different components of ECM in vitro: Bovine aortic ECs attach more avidly to type I collagen and fibronectin than to laminin and type III collagen.[85] Differential adhesion is correlated with varied rates of motility; for example, adhesion and migration of ECs on coatings of type IV collagen are higher than on coatings of laminin.[86] Thus, the composition of extant ECM could influence the migration of sprouting ECs, not only through mechanical resistance to cell protrusion, but also through adhesive control of traction. Moreover, migratory

to organize ECs into large-scale networks in vivo. This type of network organization has been modeled by planar angiogenesis in vitro and by a recent mathematical simulation.[79] A variety of network-like microvascular systems exhibit planar characteristics in vivo that render them amenable to morphogenesis via traction. Examples include the para-aortic and vitelline vascular plexuses of the early avian

ECs could control their adhesion directly by secretion of specific types of ECM in their immediate vicinity (referred to as pericellular matrix). For example, when stationary bovine aortic ECs are induced to migrate in vitro, they switch from synthesis of an ECM rich in heparan sulfate proteoglycan (which stabilizes the binding of focal adhesions to fibronectin and inhibits cell migration) to an ECM enriched in chondroitin/dermatan sulfate proteoglycans which destabilize adhesion sites and promote cell motility.[87,88]

Matricellular Proteins and Counteradhesion

In the context of EC adhesion, of particular relevance are matricellular proteins which reside (often transiently) in the ECM and influence adhesion between cells and their ECM ligands.[89,90] Unlike proteoglycans and other adhesion-modulating components of ECM, matricellular proteins do not contribute significantly to ECM structure. Matricellular proteins are secreted by many cell types and consist of three families exemplified by SPARC (*secreted protein, acidic and rich in cysteine*),[91] thrombospondin-1 (TSP),[90,92] and tenascin-C (TN).[93] Although SPARC, TSP, and TN are structurally unrelated, a commonality is their enhanced expression by migrating, dividing cells of subconfluent cultures and in tissues undergoing embryogenesis and wound repair.[94] Moreover, these proteins have similar effects on cells in culture: They inhibit attachment and spreading, and cause partial detachment and rounding of spread cells. In accordance with these counteradhesive properties, SPARC, TSP, and TN reduce the number of focal adhesions made by attached, subconfluent ECs.[94-96] Although these proteins are associated with capillaries in vivo,[97-99] their influence on angiogenesis remains unclear. Whereas SPARC itself has minimal effects on angiogenesis in vivo, specific peptide fragments of SPARC have angiogenic properties.[100] TSP is deposited in a trail behind migrating ECs[101] and promotes their chemotaxis in vitro.[102] It is also reported to inhibit the migration and sprouting of ECs in vitro.[103,104] TSP is generally believed to be anti-angiogenic in vivo;[98,103,105] however, it is proposed that TSP stimulates angiogenesis by indirect effects on non-EC types.[106] The association of TN with proliferating vessels in the vicinity of tumors[99,107,108] could indicate that it promotes angiogenesis. In accordance with this hypothesis, planar angiogenesis in vitro is inhibited by antibodies against TN.[104]

Matricellular proteins bind both to cells and to ECM. SPARC binds TSP[109] and type I through V collagens,[110,111] and also interacts with ECs via as yet uncharacterized binding proteins or receptors.[112] TSP binds collagen, fibronectin, laminin, fibrinogen,[89] and heparan sulfate proteoglycans of ECM or the cell surface.[92] Moreover, TSP binds to the cell surface integrin $\alpha_v\beta_3$,[92] an ECM receptor that is expressed on ECs and plays an important role in angiogenesis. TN has a low affinity for ECM proteins such as collagens, fibronectin, and laminin[113] but binds to several cell surface receptors, including integrins $\alpha_2\beta_1$ and $\alpha_v\beta_3$ on ECs,[114,115] integrin $\alpha_9\beta_1$,[116] proteoglycans,[117] and annexin II.[118] The cell and ECM-binding domains of matricellular proteins, either separately or in combination, could mediate counteradhesion by physical interference with the binding of cell surface ad-

hesive receptors (e.g., integrins) to their cognate ECM ligands. Alternatively, the cell-binding domains could interact with specific cell surface receptors to trigger counteradhesive responses through second messenger signaling pathways. In addition to matricellular proteins, investigators have identified other important classes and families of counteradhesive molecules, including some novel members.[119] It is likely that further study of counteradhesion will improve our understanding of how angiogenesis and other types of morphogenesis are regulated.

Integrins Mediate Adhesion to ECM and Signaling in Focal Adhesions

Integrins are a major class of transmembrane receptors that mediate the attachment of cells to ECM proteins via focal adhesions. They comprise a family of at least 16 α and 8 β subunits that associate noncovalently in over 20 different α/β combinations on the cell surface. Both α and β subunits are required for high-affinity binding to an ECM ligand: The specific ligand is determined by the combination of distinct α and β subunits. Some integrins recognize a single ECM protein (e.g., integrin $\alpha_5\beta_1$ recognizes only fibronectin); however, it is more common for an integrin to bind to two or more ligands. An ECM protein may be recognized by more than one integrin; for example, fibronectin and laminin are bound by the β_1 subunit in combination with one of four and five different α subunits, respectively. Different integrins that share an ECM ligand may bind to the ligand at the same site, as do $\alpha_5\beta_1$ and $\alpha_3\beta_1$, or they can recognize different regions of the ligand, as do the $\alpha_1\beta_1$ and $\alpha_6\beta_1$ laminin receptors, or the $\alpha_5\beta_1$ and $\alpha_4\beta_1$ fibronectin receptors.[120] ECs and other cell types typically express several different integrins on their surfaces concurrently and can alter the expression of one integrin or more in response to stimuli.

Unbound integrins are freely diffusive in the plane of the plasma membrane; however, binding to ECM or other ligands causes adjacent integrins to cluster, an event mediated by the cytoplasmic domains of the β subunits.[121] Clustering of unligated α/β heterodimers is prevented by the α subunit; however, this inhibition is removed following engagement of the ligand. Integrin clusters increase in size by further aggregation and eventually become large enough to be recognized as focal adhesions. As a focal adhesion grows, the clustering of the short cytoplasmic domains of the α and β integrin subunits nucleates the formation of large molecular complexes comprised of cytoskeletal linking proteins and a variety of catalytic signaling molecules. The cytoskeletal linking proteins, which include α-actinin, talin, vinculin, paxillin, and tensin, connect the clustered integrins to the actin cytoskeleton and thereby strengthen the focal adhesion mechanically and couple it to the motility apparatus. The catalytic signaling proteins (notably tyrosine kinases and their substrates) initiate cascades of molecular association and enzymatic activity in both the cytoplasm and the nucleus that regulate the cell cycle, responses to growth factors, and expression of specific gene products via several convergent pathways (see refs. 122-125 for general reviews of integrin-mediated signal transduction). The sequestration of signaling proteins in focal adhesions of ECs is rapid enough to play a role in integrin-mediated responses to cytokines. Fifteen to thirty minutes after bovine capillary ECs bind to fibronectin or the immobilized peptide Arg-Gly-Asp (the recognition site in fibronectin for integrin $\alpha_5\beta_1$) in vitro, their nascent focal adhesions are enriched in Flg (a high-affinity receptor for the angiogenic protein basic fibroblast growth factor [bFGF]), the tyrosine kinases pp60$^{c\text{-Src}}$ and pp125^{FAK}, and other signaling molecules including phosphatidylinositol-3-kinase, phospholipase C-γ, and the Na$^+$/H$^+$ antiporter.[126]

Functional Characteristics of Integrins Expressed by ECs

Human umbilical vein ECs in vitro express integrin α subunits 1-6[127,128] and β subunits 1 and 3,[127] with $\alpha_2\beta_1$ as the predominant combination. Integrin $\alpha_2\beta_1$ is present on capillaries in vivo,[129] and this integrin is responsible for most of the binding of ECs to type I and IV collagens in vitro.[128] Integrin $\alpha_2\beta_1$ promotes the migration of ECs on type I collagen[130] and mediates the reorganization of type I collagen by EC traction in vitro.[131] Although $\alpha_2\beta_1$ contributes significantly to the binding of human umbilical vein ECs to laminin-coated plastic,[127,128] it plays little or no role in the traction-mediated organization of ECs into networks on Matrigel in vitro[132]—a process dependent on the laminin-binding integrin $\alpha_6\beta_1$.[132,133] Despite the involvement of β_1 integrins in adhesion and traction-related processes in vitro, the role played by this integrin subfamily in vascular morphogenesis is unclear. A monoclonal antibody (CSAT) against the avian β_1 integrin subunit induced abnormalities of aortic vasculogenesis in the quail embryo that included inhibition of luminal development.[134] CSAT, however, does not inhibit angiogenesis in the chick chorioallantoic membrane despite the presence of β_1 integrins in nascent blood vessels.[135] In accordance with the effects of CSAT in the quail embryo, antibodies against the α_2 and β_1 integrin subunits inhibited development of lumen-like intracellular vacuoles within human ECs cultured in three dimensional type I collagen gels.[37] It is not known how the engagement of type I collagen by $\alpha_2\beta_1$ promotes the formation of lumens. Possible mechanisms include:

1. Induction of a "program for lumen formation" via intracellular signaling pathways;
2. Application of traction force to the collagen that causes distortion of cell structure (cavitation) rather than cell migration or reorganization of collagen; and
3. Clustering of $\alpha_2\beta_1$ at selected sites to provide cell-matrix anchor points for the development of pinocytotic membrane invaginations.[37]

Exposure of capillary ECs to bFGF augments their expression of integrin subunits α_2, α_3, α_5, α_6, β_1, β_3, β_4, and β_5 and results in a corresponding increase in adhesion of ECs to collagen, fibronectin, laminin, and vitronectin.[136,137] The anti-angiogenic transformtin growth factor-β (TGF-β) stimulates α_2, α_5, and β_1 in these cells;[137] the pattern of integrin expression by ECs is thus altered selectively by different cytokines.

Integrin $\alpha_v\beta_3$ binds to a variety of ECM proteins with an exposed tripeptide Arg-Gly-Asp moiety, such as vitronectin, fibronectin, fibrinogen, laminin, von willebrand factor, and denatured type I collagen. Thus, expression of this integrin enables a cell to adhere to, migrate on, or respond to almost any ECM protein it might encounter.[138] Integrin $\alpha_v\beta_3$ is expressed preferentially in angiogenic vessels[135,139] and is necessary for angiogenesis, since a monoclonal antibody (LM609) against this integrin blocked cytokine-induced angiogenesis in chick chorioallantoic membranes,[135] tumor-induced angiogenesis in human skin transplanted on severe combined immunodeficiency (SCID) mice,[140] and bFGF-induced angiogenesis in the rabbit cornea.[141] LM609 also disrupted vascular morphogenesis and lumen formation within vasculature of early quail embryos.[142] In the chick chorioallantoic membrane, antagonists of $\alpha_v\beta_3$ induced programmed cell death (apoptosis) of ECs in sprouting blood vessels. Engagement of $\alpha_v\beta_3$ with an ECM ligand might therefore provide a "survival signal" to ECs during angiogenesis.[143]

Integrins, Cell Shape, and Gene Expression

The genetic programs that mediate proliferation and differentiation of ECs and other cell types tend to be mutually exclusive in vitro; e.g., synthesis of cell-specific gene products diminishes when cells are stimulated to divide.[144] Since both programs are triggered by the binding of cell surface integrins to ECM, additional elements of control must exist to determine which program is selected. A variety of studies point to cell shape as an important element in the switch between proliferation and differentiation. In general, cells that assume rounded shapes exhibit a differentiated phenotype. For example, levels of synthesis of the milk protein β-casein by mouse mammary cells (induced by the binding of laminin to cell surface $\beta1$ integrins) are high in cells made round by culture on nonadhesive substrates, but are low in flattened, spread cells grown on surfaces that permit cell adhesion.[145] Spreading of cells facilitates proliferation: Ligand-induced clustering of integrins, in the presence of mitogenic factors, is sufficient to induce ECs and other cell types to exit from G_0 and progress into the late G_1-phase of the cell cycle in vitro;[146-149] however, the cells will not enter S-phase unless they are allowed to spread.[148,149] The pathways by which cell shape is coupled to proliferation and gene expression are not understood, although evidence points to involvement of the cytoskeleton. It is known that the network of actin filaments generates tension in the cytoplasm that promotes cell retraction and rounding. This tension is opposed both intracellularly by stiff, compression-resistant microtubules and extracellularly by the counteracting tension of ECM, which is coupled directly to the actin network through integrins within focal adhesions. It is hypothesized that the equilibrium between these forces places the cytoskeleton at a "setpoint" of stress which defines a specific pattern of gene expression via mechanically sensitive biochemical processes in the plasma membrane, cytoplasm, and nucleus.[150,151] It follows that a change in the setpoint of stress caused by alterations in:

1. Actin-generated forces;
2. Cytoskeletal structure;

3. Strength, number, or spatial arrangement of adhesive contacts to ECM; or

4. Malleability of ECM

would alter the biochemical equilibrium to favor expression of a different set of genes. Electron microscopic studies of resinless sections[152] reveal that tension applied to the cell surface could be transmitted first to the nuclear envelope, via bridges of intermediate filaments, and then into the nuclear interior, via nuclear fibrils that insert into the inner side of the nuclear envelope. In support of these observations, Maniotis et al have shown recently that a mechanical pull applied to integrins on the EC surface causes a physical distortion of the nucleus and a reorganization of nucleoli along the axis of applied tension.[153] The functional consequence of this chain of mechanical events might include control of DNA synthesis, since the degree to which ECs spread on coatings of ECM in vitro, the physical expansion of the nucleus, and the rate of DNA synthesis are closely correlated.[149]

During angiogenesis in vitro, ECs are likely to encounter a shifting pattern of external forces that are modulated by:

1. Cell-cell adhesion;

2. Enzymatic modification of extant vicinal ECM;

3. Synthesis of new ECM;

4. Changes in patterns of integrins or other cell-surface receptors that mediate adhesion to ECM; and

5. Restructuring of ECM by the traction of ECs and non-EC types.

Asymmetrical or focal application of forces to specific areas of a sprout could cause specific ECs to proliferate and/or express distinct gene products. Such localized behaviors could alter the morphology of the sprout—for example, the sprout could bend or branch. Clearly, much remains to be discovered regarding the complex role of biomechanical processes in vascular morphogenesis.

Angiogenesis Requires Proteolysis of ECM

At the site of a new vascular sprout, ECs of the parent vessel secrete proteases that effect a focal degradation of the basement membrane.[154] Proteolysis continues as the sprout invades the interstitial ECM: Clark and Clark observed that invasive capillaries within rabbit ear wounds dissolved fibrin in their immediate vicinity and thus created a "clear space" around each sprout.[10] Experimental studies have shown proteolysis is necessary for angiogenesis within the developing chorioallantoic membrane of the chicken[155] and for invasion of ECs into three dimensional ECM comprised of fibrin,[156] type I collagen,[55] and the amniotic basement membrane.[157] The basis of the permissive effect of proteolysis on angiogenesis is not fully understood. It is known that various angiogenic factors (e.g., bFGF) bound to the ECM are made available to ECs after the matrix is degraded. It is likely, however, that the most important effect of proteolysis is to alter the malleability and adhesivity of the ECM to facilitate the movement of ECs through it.

Two major groups of proteinases that regulate angiogenesis are the matrix metalloproteinases (MMPs) and the plasmin/plasminogen activator (PA) system. MMPs secreted by ECs include the interstitial collagenase MMP-1, which cleaves native type I, II, and III collagens at a single site;[158,159] gelatinases A (MMP-2) and B (MMP-9), which degrade denatured collagens (gelatins), type IV and V collagens, and elastin,[160,161] and stromelysin (MMP-3), which has a broad range of substrates that include laminin, fibronectin, the protein core of proteoglycans, and gelatin.[161,162] Recently, it has been demonstrated that MMP-2 is an interstitial collagenase with a specificity similar if not identical to those of MMPs-1 and -8.[163] Type I and type III collagens are highly resistant to proteolysis by trypsin, plasmin, and other members of the serine and sulfhydryl proteinase families. These collagens, however, are degraded by MMPs via a two-stage process involving initial cleavage by interstitial collagenases and subsequent digestion of the larger fragments by gelatinases.

Studies in vitro indicate a role for MMPs in angiogenesis. Exposure of ECs to phorbol esters and angiogenic growth factors in vitro induces production of MMPs-1, -2, -3, and -9.[164-167] MMPs are regulated in vivo by tissue inhibitors of metalloproteinases—a family of low molecular weight proteins (TIMPs-1, -2, and -3) that specifically block the catalytic activity of MMPs.[161] Inhibition of endogenous MMP activity of ECs in vitro, either by metal ion chelators or by TIMPs, suppresses traction-mediated reorganization of type I collagen gels[75] and the corresponding angiogenesis-like invasion of these gels.[52,55,168]

The inherent complexity of proteolysis and its regulation are well illustrated by the plasmin/PA system. PAs are serine proteinases that cleave the zymogen plasminogen (a plasma protein) to plasmin. Plasmin is itself a proteinase that degrades several components of ECM, such as fibronectin, laminin, the protein core of proteoglycans, and gelatins.[169] The tissue-type (tPA) form of PA is expressed by ECs of quiescent microvasculature and is neither modulated during angiogenesis nor expressed by sprouting ECs in vivo. In contrast, the urokinase (uPA) form of PA is expressed by angiogenic ECs associated with tumors, inflammation, hemangiomas, ovarian follicles, corpora lutea, and maternal decidua. Little or no uPA is expressed in quiescent vessels.[168]

Plasminogen is present in most tissues at high levels; therefore, its activation by PAs results in high local concentrations of plasmin. Moreover, plasmin-mediated, limited proteolysis activates latent elastase (a serine protease) and MMPs-1, -2, -3, and -9. Thus, small quantities of PA can generate significant levels of proteolytic activity with different substrate specificities.[169]

The position of uPA as the initiator of a proteolytic cascade dictates that its activity be strictly controlled during angiogenesis. Expression of uPA by ECs is modulated at the transcriptional level by a number of angiogenic growth factors. Moreover, angiogenic ECs in vitro and in vivo express high levels of PA inhibitor-1 (PAI-1),[170,171] a protein which blocks the formation of plasmin by PA and thereby inhibits the activation of elastase and MMPs. An additional element of control is the confinement of active uPA to the surface of ECs. uPA is secreted as a proenzyme (pro-uPA) that binds to uPA receptor (uPAR), a glycoprotein which is anchored to the surface of ECs at the site of focal adhesions.[172] The bound pro-uPA is subsequently activated by limited proteolysis.[173] The proteolytic function of uPA at the cell surface is facilitated by the binding of its substrate, plasminogen, to the plasma membrane by α-enolase-related proteins and cell-surface chondroitin-sulfate proteoglycans.[174,175] After a period of time (possibly several hours), active uPA is inactivated by binding to PAI-1, internalized, and rapidly degraded.[176] The importance of PAI-1 to the control of uPA activity is indicated by the effects of angiogenic growth factors on the expression of the two proteins. bFGF and vascular endothelial growth factor (VEGF) increase the ratio of uPA mRNA to PAI-1 mRNA in ECs, for a net increase in proteolysis. In contrast, TGF-β1 reduces the uPA:PAI-1 mRNA ratio for a net reduction in proteolysis—an effect consonant with its inhibition of angiogenesis and invasion of ECM by ECs in vitro.[168]

Migratory ECs exhibit increased expression of uPA and uPAR relative to nonmigratory ECs in confluent monolayers.[168] Nanomolar concentrations of uPA or of its noncatalytic A-chain stimulate motility of ECs.[177] Blockage of uPAR with monoclonal antibodies or a specific antagonist inhibits the migration of ECs on serum-coated substrates in vitro to a greater degree than has been observed after the inhibition of endogenous plasmin activity.[178] Moreover, uPAR binds to the ECM component vitronectin and inhibits its β1 integrin-dependent adhesion to fibronectin.[179] Collectively, these observations point to a direct involvement of the uPA/uPAR complex in the modulation of cell adhesion during motility by a mechanism independent from proteolysis. Since PAI-1 is also increased in migratory ECs,[168] it is possible that this inhibitor could influence adhesive interactions between uPA/uPAR and ECM ligands. A synergistic role for PAI-1 in counteradhesion would explain the finding that synthesis of PAI-1 by subconfluent, migratory ECs is increased in the presence of the counteradhesive, matricellular protein SPARC.[180]

The degree to which ECM must be degraded to facilitate angiogenesis in vivo is unclear; however, it appears that the range of optimal proteolysis has an upper limit. For example, the increased production of endogenous proteases by murine ECs that express the polyoma virus middle T oncogene is correlated with their organization into large, hollow cysts within fibrin clots in vitro.[181] In the presence of inhibitors of serine proteases, however, the cyst morphotype is replaced by capillary-like tubes that are generated by the invasion of ECs into the fibrin matrix. The fact that proteolysis of ECM inhibits the formation of endothelial tubes indicates that angiogenic sprouts are not elongated by forces derived solely from the parent vessel (e.g., by a hydraulic push). Alternatively, the sprouts pull themselves outward by a process (e.g., traction) that requires mechanical support from the ECM. Accordingly, excessive proteolysis of the ECM would disrupt its mechanical continuity to an extent that ECs would lack a fixed substrate against which they could pull.

Concluding Remarks

In this chapter we have introduced the fundamental characteristics of angiogenesis and have discussed the cell biology of this highly complex process. Given the necessity

of neovascularization for efficient healing of wounds, biointegration of prosthetic devices, functionality of the reproductive system, and regulation of tumor growth and metastasis, we could not overemphasize the need for a more complete and mechanistic understanding of angiogenesis as a therapeutic means for the prevention and treatment of human disease. In the field of tumor biology, for example, few would disagree that some form of anti-angiogenic therapy might be beneficial for the treatment of solid tumors. However, there is considerable debate regarding the type of intervention (i.e., which stage of blood vessel growth should be targeted), as well as the duration and route of administration of angiostatic drugs or compounds.

We have chosen to focus on questions and models that address the angiogenic process itself and have recapitulated the acknowledged stages of vascular sprout formation and progression—EC migration, alignment, proliferation, cohesion, lumen formation, and branching/anastomosis—in the context of cell adhesion, movement, and shape, molecular biology, receptor-ligand interactions, and extracellular proteolysis. To date, there are no "perfect" models in which to test angiogenic regulation, although much can be learned from culture systems in which ECs form capillary-like structures. At best, each of the models in vitro that were covered in this chapter appears optimal for one or more of the stages requisite to blood vessel formation. In contrast, tissues of living animals provide excellent examples of angiogenesis, but their disadvantages include the complex interactions among several types of cells and the limitations in visualization and quantification of blood vessel growth.

We have also stressed the importance of the ECM and its capacity for the regulation of EC behavior and vascular morphogenesis. Clearly, alteration of the properties of ECM through its molecular composition and/or proteolysis has profound effects on EC migration, proliferation, and biosynthetic capacity, all of which can be affected, in part, by changes in cell shape and adhesion. Both adhesive (e.g., collagen, fibronectin, laminin) and counteradhesive proteins (e.g., SPARC, TSP), as well as the integrins and other cell surface receptors for ECM macromolecules, are important in the regulation of EC shape and function.

There remain several unanswered questions that are currently receiving considerable attention in the field of vascular biology:

1. Which are the macromolecules that are truly critical for angiogenesis?
2. Is all angiogenesis the same (e.g., in a normal tissue versus a tumor, and in the endometrium versus the brain)?
3. What is the initiating stimulus for sprouting?
4. How is selective or focal proteolysis controlled?
5. What stage of angiogenesis provides the most reasonable site for intervention to effect either stimulation or stasis?

Reagents and methodology are largely in place to address these problems, although there is a continuing need for better quantitative models in vivo and in vitro. Within the next decade we should expect major and significant progress in basic research that will allow clinicians, bioengineers, and molecular/cellular biologists to develop and test novel strategies for the control of vascular growth.

References

1. Folkman J. Angiogenesis in cancer, vascular, rheumatoid and other disease. Nature Med 1995; 1:27-31.
2. Sage EH. Angiogenesis inhibition in the context of endothelial cell biology. Adv Oncol 1997; 12:17-29.
3. Folkman J. Tumor angiogenesis. Adv Cancer Res 1985; 43:175-203.
4. Paweletz N, Knierim M. Tumor-related angiogenesis. Crit Rev Oncol Hematol 1989; 9:197-242.
5. Folkman J. Angiogenesis: Retrospect and outlook. In: Steiner R, Weisz PB, Langer R, ed(s). Angiogenesis. Basel: Birkhäuser Verlag, 1992:4-13.
6. Zagzag D. Angiogenic growth factors in neural embryogenesis and neoplasia. Am J Pathol 1995; 146:293-309.
7. Fox SB, Gatter KC, Harris AL. Tumor angiogenesis. J Pathol 1996; 179:232-237.
8. Chaplain MAJ, Stuart AM. A model mechanism for the chemotactic response of endothelial cells to tumor angiogenesis factor. IMA J Math Appl Med Biol 1993; 10:149-168.
9. Omitted in proof.
10. Clark ER, Clark EL. Microscopic observations on the growth of blood capillaries in the living mammal. Am J Anat 1939; 64: 251-301.
11. Algire GH, Chalkley HW, Legallais FY et al. Vascular reactions of normal and malignant tissues in vivo. I. Vascular reactions of mice to wounds and to normal and neoplastic transplants. J Natl Cancer Inst 1945; 6:73-85.
12. Greenblatt M, Shubik P. Tumor angiogenesis:Transfilter diffusion studies in the hamster by the transparent chamber technique. J Natl Cancer Inst. 1968; 41:111-124.
13. Gimbrone MA, Cotran RS, Leapman S et al. Tumor growth and neovascularization: An experimental model using the rabbit cornea. J Natl Cancer Inst 1974; 52:413-427.
14. Ausprunk DH, Knighton DR, Folkman J. Differentiation of vascular endothelium in the chick chorioallantois:A structural and autioradiographic study. Dev Biol 1974; 38:237-248.
15. Jaffe EA, Nachman RL, Becker CG et al. Culture of human endothelial cells derived from umbilical veins. Identification by morphologic and immunologic criteria. J Clin Invest 1973; 52:2745-2756.
16. Gimbrone MA. Culture of vascular endothelium. In:Spaet TH, ed. Progress in Hemostasis and Thrombosis. Vol 3. New York:Grune and Stratton, 1976:1-28.
17. Fishman JA, Ryan GB, Karnovsky MJ. Endothelial regeneration in the rat carotid artery and the significance of endothelial denudation in the pathogenesis of myointimal thickening. Lab Invest 1975; 32:339-351.
18. Madri JA, Pratt BM. Endothelial cell-matrix interactions: In vitro models of angiogenesis. J Histochem Cytochem 1986; 34:85-91.
19. Gimbrone MA, Cotran RS, Folkman J. Human vascular endothelial cells in culture. Growth and DNA synthesis. J Cell Biol 1974; 60:673-684.
20. Madri JA, Stenn KS. Aortic endothelial cell migration I. Matrix requirements and composition. Am J Pathol 1982; 106:180-186.
21. Palotie A, Tryggvason K, Peltonen L et al. Components of subendothelial aorta basement membrane. Immunohistochemical localization and role in cell attachment. Lab Invest 1983; 49:362-370.
22. Sage H. Collagen synthesis by endothelial cells in culture. In:Jaffe EA, ed. Biology of Endothelial Cells. The Hague:Martinus Nijhoff, 1984:161-177.
23. Pratt BM, Harris AS, Morrow JS et al. Mechanisms of cytoskeletal regulation. Modulation of aortic endothelial cell spectrin by the extracellular matrix. Am J Pathol 1984; 117:349-354.
24. Folkman J, Haudenschild CC, Zetter BR. Long-term culture of capillary endothelial cells. Proc Natl Acad Sci USA 1979; 76:5217-5221.
25. Folkman J, Haudenschild C. Angiogenesis in vitro. Nature 1980; 288:551-556.
26. Maciag T, Kadish J, Wilkins L et al. Organizational behavior of human umbilical vein endothelial cells. J Cell Biol 1982; 94:511-520.
27. Feder J, Marasa JC, Olander JV. The formation of capillary-like tubes by calf aortic endothelial cells grown in vitro. J Cell Phys 1983; 116:1-6.
28. Madri JA. Endothelial cell-matrix interactions in hemostasis. In:Spaet TH, ed. Progress in Hemostasis and Thrombosis. Vol 6. New York:Grune and Stratton, 1982:1-24.
29. Ingber DE, Folkman J. Mechanochemical switching between growth and differentiation during fibroblast growth factor-stimulated angiogenesis in vitro: Role of extracellular matrix. J Cell Biol 1989; 109:317-330.
30. Kubota Y, Kleinman HK, Martin GR et al. Role of laminin and basement membrane in the morphological differentiation of human endothelial cells into capillary-like structures. J Cell Biol 1988; 107:1589-1598.
31. Vernon RB, Angello JC, Iruela-Arispe ML et al. Reorganization of basement membrane matrices by cellular traction promotes the formation of cellular networks in vitro. Lab Invest 1992; 66:536-547.
32. Harris AK, Stopak D, Wild P. Fibroblast traction as a mechanism for collagen morphogenesis. Nature (London) 1981; 290:249-251.
33. Vernon RB, Lara SL, Drake CJ et al. Organized type I collagen influences endothelial patterns during "spontaneous angiogenesis in vitro":Planar cultures as models of vascular development. In Vitro Cell Dev Biol 1995; 31:120-131.
34. Sage EH, Vernon RB. Regulation of angiogenesis by extracellular matrix: The growth and the glue. J Hypertension 1994; 12 (suppl 10):S145-S152.
35. Montesano R, Orci L, Vassalli P. In vitro rapid organization of endothelial cells into capillary-like networks is promoted by collagen matrices. J Cell Biol 1983; 97:1648-1652.
36. Elsdale T, Bard J. Collagen substrata for studies on cell behavior. J Cell Biol 1972; 54:626-637.
37. Davis GE, Camarillo CW. An $\alpha 2\beta 1$ integrin-dependent pinocytotic mechanism involving intracellular vacuole formation and coalescence regulates capillary lumen and tube formation in three-dimensional collagen matrix. Exp Cell Res 1996; 224:39-51.
38. Madri JA, Pratt BM, Tucker AM. Phenotypic modulation of endothelial cells by transformtin growth factor-β depends on the composition and organization of the extracellular matrix. J Cell Biol 1988; 106:1375-1384.
39. Merwin JR, Anderson JM, Kocher O et al. Transforming growth factor beta₁ modulates extracellular matrix orga-

nization and cell-cell junctional complex formation during in vitro angiogenesis. J Cell Phys 1990; 142:117-128.

40. Marx M, Perlmutter RA, Madri JA. Modulation of platelet-derived growth factor receptor expression in microvascular endothelial cells during in vitro angiogenesis. J Clin Invest 1994; 93:131-139.

41. Kuzuya M, Kinsella JL. Induction of endothelial cell differentiation in vitro by fibroblast-derived soluble factors. Exp Cell Res 1994; 215:310-318.

42. Nicosia RF, Tchao R, Leighton J. Histotypic angiogenesis in vitro:Light microscopic, ultrastructural, and radioautographic studies. In Vitro 1982; 18:538-549.

43. Nicosia RF, Tchao R, Leighton J. Angiogenesis-dependent tumor spread in reinforced fibrin clot culture. Cancer Res 1983; 43:2159-2166.

44. Villaschi S, Nicosia RF. Angiogenic role of endogenous basic fibroblast growth factor released by rat aorta after injury. Am J Pathol 1993; 143:181-190.

45. Nicosia RF, Nicosia SV, Smith M. Vascular endothelial growth factor, platelet-derived growth factor, and insulin-like growth factor-1 promote rat aortic angiogenesis in vitro. Am J Pathol 1994; 145:1023-1029.

46. Mori M, Sadahira Y, Kawasaki S et al. Capillary growth from reversed rat aortic segments cultured in collagen gel. Acta Pathol Jpn 1988; 38:1503-1512.

47. Nicosia RF, Ottinetti A. Modulation of microvascular growth and morphogenesis by reconstituted basement membrane gel in three-dimensional cultures of rat aorta:A comparative study of angiogenesis in matrigel, collagen, fibrin, and plasma clot. In Vitro Cell Dev Biol 1990; 26:119-128.

48. Nicosia RF, Bonanno E, Villaschi S. Large-vessel endothelium switches to a microvascular phenotype during angiogenesis in collagen gel culture of rat aorta. Atherosclerosis 1992; 95:191-199.

49. Nicosia RF, Tuszynski GP. Matrix-bound thrombospondin promotes angiogenesis in vitro. J Cell Biol 1994; 124:183-193.

50. Nicosia RF, Bonanno E, Smith M et al. Modulation of angiogenesis in vitro by laminin-entactin complex. Dev Biol 1994; 164:197-206.

51. Diglio CA, Grammas P, Giacomelli F et al. Angiogenesis in rat aorta ring explant cultures. Lab Invest 1989; 60:523-531.

52. Montesano R, Orci L. Tumor-promoting phorbol esters induce angiogenesis in vitro. Cell 1985; 42:469-477.

53. Montesano R, Orci L. Phorbol esters induce angiogenesis in vitro from large-vessel endothelial cells. J Cell Physiol 1987; 130:284-291.

54. Montesano R, Pepper MS, Orci L. Paracrine induction of angiogenesis in vitro by Swiss 3T3 fibroblasts. J Cell Sci 1993; 105:1013-1024.

55. Fisher C, Gilbertson-Beadling S, Powers EA et al. Interstital collagenase is required for angiogenesis in vitro. Dev Biol 1994; 162:499-510.

56. Mitchison TJ, Cramer LP. Actin-based cell motility and cell locomotion. Cell 1996; 84:371-379.

57. Bard JBL, Hay ED. The behavior of fibroblasts from the developing avian cornea. J Cell Biol 1975; 67:400-418.

58. Notbohm H, Mosler S, Müller PK. In vitro formation and aggregation of heterotypic collagen i and III fibrils. Int J Biol Macromol 1993; 15:299-304.

59. MacBeath JRE, Shackelton DR, Hulmes DJS. Tyrosine-rich acidic matrix protein (TRAMP) accelerates collagen fibril formation in vitro. J Biol Chem 1993; 268:19826-19832.

60. Vogel KG, Trotter JA. The effect of proteoglycans on the morphology of collagen fibrils formed in vitro. Coll Relat Res 1987; 7:105-114.

61. Siegel R. Lysyl oxidase. Int Rev Connect Tissue Res 1979; 8:73-118.

62. Fogerty FJ, Mosher DF. Mechanisms for organization of fibronectin matrix. Cell Differ Dev 1990; 32:439-450.

63. Nishiyama T, McDonough AM, Bruns RR et al. Type XII and XIV collagens mediate interactions between banded collagen fibers in vitro and may modulate extracellular matrix deformability. J Biol Chem 1994; 269:28193-28199.

64. Oliver T, Lee J, Jacobson K. Forces exerted by locomoting cells. Semin Cell Biol 1994; 5:139-147.

65. Keller HU, Bebie H. Protrusive activity quantitatively determines the rate and direction of cell locomotion. Cell Motil Cytoskel 1996; 33:241-251.

66. Vernon RB, Sage EH, unpublished observations.

67. Nehls V, Herrmann R. The configuration of fibrin clots determines capillary morphogenesis and endothelial cell migration. Microvasc Res 1996; 51:347-364.

68. Schmidt CE, Horwitz AF, Lauffenburger DA et al. Integrin-cytoskeletal interactions in migrating fibroblasts are dynamic, asymmetric, and regulated. J Cell Biol 1993; 123:977-991.

69. Felsenfeld DP, Choquet DP, Sheetz MP. Ligand binding regulates the directed movement of β1 integrins on fibroblasts. Nature 1996; 383:438-440.

70. Lauffenburger DA, Horwitz AF. Cell migration:A physically integrated molecular process. Cell 1996; 84:359-369.

71. Harris AK, Wild P, Stopak D. A new wrinkle in the study of locomotion. Science 1980; 208:177-179.

72. Oliver T, Dembo M, Jacobson K. Traction forces in locomoting cells. Cell Motil Cytoskel 1995; 31:225-240.

73. Reed MJ, Vernon RB, Abrass IB et al. TGF-β1 induces the expession of type I collagen and SPARC, and enhances contraction of collagen gels, by fibroblasts from young and aged donors. J Cell Physiol 1994; 158:169-179.

74. Stopak D, Harris AK. Connective tissue morphogenesis by fibroblast traction. Dev Biol 1982; 90:383-398.

75. Vernon RB, Sage EH. Contraction of fibrillar type I collagen by endothelial cells:A study in vitro. J Cell Biochem 1996; 60:185-197.

76. Guido S, Tranquillo RT. A methodology for the systematic and quantitative study of cell contact guidance in oriented collagen gels. J Cell Sci 1993; 105:317-331.

77. Markwald RR, Fitzharris TP, Bolender DL et al. Structural analysis of cell:matrix association during the morphogenesis of atrioventricular cushion tissue. Dev Biol 1979; 69:634-654.

78. Fournier N, Doillon CJ. In vitro angiogenesis in fibrin matrices containing fibronectin or hyaluronic acid. Cell Biol Int Rep 1992; 16:1251-1263.

79. Manoussaki D, Lubkin SR, Vernon RB et al. A mechanical model for the formation of vascular networks in vitro. Acta Biotheoret 1996; 44:271-282.

80. Izzard CS, Lochner LR. Formation of cell-to-substrate contacts during fibroblast motility: An interference reflexion study. J Cell Sci 1980; 42:81-116.

81. Regen CM, Horwitz AF. Dynamics of β1 integrin-mediated adhesive contacts in motile fibroblasts. J Cell Biol 1992; 119:1347-1359.

82. DiMilla PA, Barbee K, Lauffenburger DA. Mathematical model for the effects of adhesion and mechanics on cell migration speed. Biophys J 1991; 60:15-37.

83. Goodman SL, Risse G, von der Mark K. The E8 subfragment of laminin promotes locomotion of myoblasts over extracellular matrix. J Cell Biol 1989; 109:799-809.

84. DiMilla P, Stone JA, Quinn JA et al. Maximal migration of human smooth muscle cells on fibronectin and type IV collagen occurs at an intermediate attachment strength. J Cell Biol 1993; 122:729-737.

85. Macarak EJ, Howard PS. Adhesion of endothelial cells to extracellular matrix proteins. J Cell Physiol 1983; 116:76-86.

86. Herbst TJ, McCarthy JB, Tsilibary EC et al. Differential effects of laminin, intact type IV collagen, and specific domains of type IV collagen on endothelial cell adhesion and migration. J Cell Biol 1988; 106:1365-73.

87. Kinsella MG, Wight TN. Modulation of sulfate proteoglycan synthesis by bovine aortic endothelial cells during migration. J Cell Biol 1986; 102:679-687.

88. Wight TN, Kinsella MG, Quarnström EE. The role of proteoglycans in cell adhesion, migration, and proliferation. Curr Opin Cell Biol 1992; 4:793-801.

89. Sage EH, Bornstein P. Extracellular proteins that modulate cell-matrix interactions. SPARC, tenascin, and thrombospondin. J Biol Chem 1991; 266:14831-14834.

90. Bornstein P. Diversity of function is inherent in matricellular proteins:An appraisal of thrombospondin 1. J Cell Biol 1995; 130:503-506.

91. Lane TF, Sage EH. The biology of SPARC, a protein that modulates cell-matrix interactions. FASEB J 1994; 8:163-173.

92. Roberts DD. Regulation of tumor growth and metastasis by thrombospondin. FASEB J 1996; 10:1183-1191.

93. Erickson HP. Tenascin-C, tenascin-R, and tenascin-X: A family of talented proteins in search of functions. Curr Opin Cell Biol 1993; 5:869-876.

94. Murphy-Ullrich JE, Lane TF, Pallero MA et al. SPARC mediates focal adhesion disassembly in endothelial cells through a follistatin-like region of the Ca^{2+}-binding EF-hand. J Cell Biochem 1995; 57:341-350.

95. Murphy-Ullrich JE, Höök M. Thrombospondin modulates focal adhesions in endothelial cells. J Cell Biol 1989; 109:1309-1319.

96. Murphy-Ullrich JE, Lightner VA, Aukhil I et al. Focal adhesion integrity is downregulated by the alternatively spliced domain of human tenascin. J Cell Biol 1991; 115:1127-1136.

97. Iruela-Arispe ML, Lane TF, Redmond D et al. Expression of SPARC during development of the chicken chorioallantoic membrane:Evidence for regulated proteolysis in vivo. Mol Biol Cell 1995; 6:327-343.

98. Iruela-Arispe ML, Porter P, Bornstein P et al. Thrombospondin-1, an inhibitor of angiogenesis, is regulated by progesterone in the human endometrium. J Clin Invest 1996; 97:403-412.

99. Zagzag D, Friedlander DR, Dosik J et al. Tenascin-C expression by angiogenic vessels in human astrocytomas and by human brain endothelial cells in vitro. Cancer Res 1996; 56:182-189.

100. Jendraschak E, Sage EH. Regulation of angiogenesis by SPARC and angiostatin:Implications for tumor cell biology. Semin Cancer Biol 1996; 7:139-146.

101. Vischer P, Volker W, Schmidt A et al. Association of thrombospondin of endothelial cells with other matrix proteins, attachment sites and migration tracks. Eur J Cell Biol 1988; 47:36-46.

102. Taraboletti G, Roberts D, Liotta LA et al. Platelet thrombospondin modulates endothelial cell adhesion, motility, and growth:A potential angiogenesis regulatory factor. J Cell Biol 1990; 111 765-772.

103. Tolsma SS, Volpert OV, Good DJ et al. Peptides derived from two separate domains of the matrix protein thrombospondin-1 have antiangiogenic activity. J Cell Biol 1993; 122:497-511.

104. Canfield AE, Schor AAM. Evidence that tenascin and thrombospondin-1 modulate sprouting of endothelial cells. J Cell Sci 1995; 108:797-809.

105. Hsu SC, Volpert OV, Steck PA et al. Inhibition of angiogenesis in human glioblastomas by chromosome 10 induction of thrombospondin-1. Cancer Res 1996; 56:5684-5691.

106. Tuszynski GP, Nicosia RF. The role of thrombospondin-1 in tumor progression and angiogenesis. BioEssays 1996; 18:71-76.

107. Higuchi M, Ohnishi T, Arita N et al. Expression of tenascin in human gliomas:Its relation to histological malignancy, tumor dedifferentiation and angiogenesis. Acta Neuropathol 1993; 85:481-487.

108. Zagzag D, Friedlander DR, Miller DC et al. Tenascin expression in astrocytomas correlates with angiogenesis. Cancer Res 1995; 55:907-914.

109. Clezardin P, Malaval L, Ehrensperger A et al. Complex formation of human thrombospondin with osteonectin. Eur J Biochem 1988; 175:275-284.

110. Sage H, Vernon RB, Funk SE et al. SPARC, a secreted protein associated with cellular proliferation, inhibits cell spreading in vitro and exhibits Ca^{+2}-dependent binding to the extracellular matrix. J Cell Biol 1989; 109:341-356.

111. Maurer P, Hohenadl C, Hohenester E et al. The C-terminal portion of BM-40 (SPARC/osteonectin) is an autonomously folding and crystallisable domain that binds calcium and collagen iv. J Mol Biol 1995; 253:347-357.

112. Yost JC, Sage EH. Specific interaction of SPARC with endothelial cells is mediated through a carboxyl-terminal sequence containing a calcium-binding EF hand. J Biol Chem 1993; 268:25790-25796.

113. Lightner VA, Erickson HP. Binding of hexabrachion (tenascin) to the extracellular matrix and substratum and its effect on cell adhesion. J Cell Sci 1990; 95:263-277.

114. Joshi P, Chung C-Y, Aukhil I et al. Endothelial cells adhere to the RGD domain and the fibrinogen-like terminal knob of tenascin. J Cell Sci 1993; 106:389-400.

115. Sriramarao P, Mendler M, Bourdon MA. Endothelial cell attachment and spreading on human tenascin is mediated by α2-β1 and αv-β3 integrins. J Cell Sci 1993; 105:1001-1012.

116. Yokosaki Y, Palmer EL, Prieto AL et al. The integrin α9β1 mediates cell attachment to a non-RGD site in the third fibronectin type III repeat of tenascin. J Biol Chem 1994; 269:26691-26696.

117. Aukhil I, Joshi P, Yan Y et al. Cell- and heparin-binding domains of the hexabrachion arm identified by tenascin expression proteins. J Biol Chem 1993; 268:2542-2553.

118. Chung C-Y, Erickson HP. Cell surface annexin II is a high affinity receptor for the alternatively spliced segment of tenascin-C. J Cell Biol 1994; 126:539-548.

119. Chiquet-Ehrismann R. Inhibition of cell adhesion by antiadhesive molecules. Curr Opin Cell Biol 1995; 7:715-719.

120. Juliano RL, Haskill S. Signal transduction from the extracellular matrix. J Cell Biol 1993; 120:577-585.

121. Sastry SK, Horwitz AF. Integrin cytoplasmic domains:Mediators of cytoskeletal linkages and extra- and intracellular initiated transmembrane signaling. Curr Opin Cell Biol 1993; 5:819-831.

122. Schwartz MA, Schaller MD, Ginsberg MH. Integrins:Emerging paradigms of signal transduction. Annu Rev Cell Dev Biol 1995; 11:549-599.

123. Clark EA, Brugge JS. Integrins and signal transduction pathways:The road taken. Science 1995; 268:233-239.

124. Sastry SK, Horwitz AF. Adhesion-growth factor interactions during differentiation:An integrated biological response. Dev Biol 1996; 180:455-467.

125. Dedhar S, Hannigan GE. Integrin cytoplasmic interactions and bidirectional transmembrane signalling. Curr Opin Cell Biol 1996; 8:657-669.

126. Plopper GE, McNamee HP, Dike LE et al. Convergence of integrin and growth factor receptor signaling pathways within the focal adhesion complex. Mol Biol Cell 1995; 6:1349-1365.

127. Languino LR, Gehlsen KR, Wayner E et al. Endothelial cells use $\alpha_2\beta_1$ integrin as a laminin receptor. J Cell Biol 1989; 109:2455-2462.

128. Underwood PA, Bennett FA, Kirkpatrick A et al. Evidence for the location of a binding sequence for the $\alpha2\beta1$ integrin of endothelial cells, in the $\beta1$ subunit of laminin. Biochem J 1995; 309:765-771.

129. Zutter MM, Santoro SA. Widespread histologic distribution of the $\alpha2\beta1$ integrin cell-surface collagen receptor. Am J Pathol 1990; 137:113-120.

130. Leavesley DI, Schwartz MA, Rosenfeld M et al. Integrin $\beta1$- and $\beta3$-mediated endothelial cell migration is triggered through distinct signaling mechanisms. J Cell Biol 1993; 121:163-170.

131. Jackson CJ, Knop A, Giles I et al. VLA-2 mediates the interaction of collagen with endothelium during in vitro vascular tube formation. Cell Biol Internat 1994; 18:859-867.

132. Davis GE, Camarillo CW. Regulation of endothelial cell morphogenesis by integrins, mechanical forces, and matrix guidance pathways. Exp Cell Res 1995; 216:113-23.

133. Bauer J, Margolis M, Schreiner C et al. In vitro model of angiogenesis using a human endothelium-derived permanent cell line:Contributions of induced gene expression, G-proteins, and integrins. J Cell Physiol 1992; 153:437-449.

134. Drake CJ, Davis LA, Little CD. Antibodies to β_1-integrins cause alterations of aortic vasculogenesis, in vivo. Dev Dynam 1992; 193:83-91.

135. Brooks PC, Clark RAF, Cherish DA. Requirement of vascular integrin $\alpha_v\beta_3$ for angiogenesis. Science 1994; 264:569-571.

136. Klein S, Giancotti FG, Presta M et al. Basic fibroblast growth factor modulates integrin expression in microvascular endothelial cells. Mol Biol Cell 1993; 4:973-982.

137. Enenstein J, Walehm NS, Kramer RH. Basic FGF and TGF-β differently modulate integrin expression of human microvascular endothelial cells. Exp Cell Res 1992; 203:499-503.

138. Varner JA, Brooks PC, Cheresh DA. The integrin av$\beta3$: Angiogenesis and apoptosis. Cell Adhes Commun 1995; 3:367-374.

139. Enenstein J, Kramer RH. Confocal microscopic analysis of integrin expression on the microvasculature and its sprouts in the neonatal foreskin. J Invest Dermatol 1994; 103:381-386.

140. Brooks PC, Stromblad S, Klemke R et al. Antiintegrin av$\beta3$ blocks human breast cancer growth and angiogenesis in human skin. J Clin Invest 1995; 96:1815-1822.

141. Friedlander M, Brooks PC, Shaffer RW et al. Definition of two angiogenic pathways by distinct av integrins. Science 1995; 270:1500-1502.

142. Drake CJ, Cheresh DA, Little CD. An antagonist of integrin av$\beta3$ prevents maturation of blood vessels during embryonic neovascularization. J Cell Sci 1995; 108:2655-2661.

143. Brooks PC, Montgomery AMP, Rosenfeld M et al. Integrin $\alpha_v\beta_3$ antagonists promote tumor regression by inducing apoptosis of angiogenic blood vessels. Cell 1994; 79:1157-1164.

144. Vernon RB, Lane TF, Angello JC et al. Adhesion, shape, proliferation, and gene expression of mouse Leydig cells are influenced by extracellular matrix in vitro. Biol Reprod 1991; 44:157-170.

145. Roskelley CD, Bissell MJ. Dynamic reciprocity revisited:A continuous, bidirectional flow of information between cells and the extracellular matrix regulates mammary epithelial cell function. Biochem Cell Biol 1995; 73:391-397.

146. Schwartz MA, Lechene C, Ingber DE. Insoluble fibronectin activates the Na^+/H^+ antiporter by clustering and immobilizing integrin $\alpha5\beta1$, independent of cell shape. Proc Natl Acad Sci USA 1991; 88:7849-7853.

147. McNamee HP, Ingber DE, Schwartz MA. Adhesion to fibronectin stimulates inositol lipid synthesis and enhances PDGF-induced inositol lipid breakdown. J Cell Biol 1993; 121:673-678.

148. Hansen LK, Mooney DJ, Vacanti JP et al. Integrin binding and cell spreading on extracellular matrix act at different points in the cell cycle to promote hepatocyte growth. Mol Biol Cell 1994; 5:967-975.

149. Ingber DE, Prusty D, Sun Z et al. Cell shape, cytoskeletal mechanics, and cell cycle control in angiogenesis. J Biomechanics 1995; 28:1471-1484.

150. Ingber DE, Dike L, Hansen L et al. Cellular tensigrity:Exploring how mechanical changes in the cytoskeleton regulate cell growth, migration, and tissue pattern during morphogenesis. Int Rev Cytol 1994; 150:173-224.

151. Banes AJ, Tsuzaki M, Yamamoto J et al. Mechanoreception at the cellular level: The detection, interpretation, and diversity of responses to mechanical signals. Biochem Cell Biol 1995; 73:349-365.

152. Penman S. Rethinking cell structure. Proc Natl Acad Sci USA 1995; 92:5251-5257.

153. Maniotis AJ, Chen CS, Ingber DE. Demonstration of mechanical connections between integrins, cytoskeletal filaments, and nucleoplasm that stabilize nuclear structure. Proc Natl Acad Sci USA 1997; 94:849-854.

154. Liotta LA, Steeg PS, Stetler-Stevenson WG. Cancer metastasis and angiogenesis: An imbalance of positive and negative regulation. Cell 1991; 64:327-336.

155. Moses MA, Sudhalter J, Langer R. Identification of an inhibitor of neovascularization from cartilage. Science 1990; 248:1408-1410.

156. Montesano R, Pepper MS, Vassalli J-D et al. Phorbol ester induces cultured endothelial cells to invade a fibrin matrix in the presence of fibrinolytic inhibitors. J Cell Physiol 1987; 132:509-516.

157. Mignatti P, Tsuboi R, Robbins E et al. In vitro angiogenesis on the human amniotic membrane: Requirement of

basic fibroblast growth factor-induced proteinases. J Cell Biol 1989; 108:671-682.

158. Miller EJ, Harris ED, Chung E et al. Cleavage of type II and III collagens with mammalian collagenase:Site of cleavage and primary structure at the NH_2-terminal portion of the smaller fragment released from both collagens. Biochem 1976; 15:787-792.

159. Dixit SN, Mainardi CL, Seyer JM et al. Covalent structure of collagen:Amino acid sequence of $\alpha 2$-CB5 of chick skin collagen containing the animal collagenase cleavage site. Biochem 1979; 18:5416-5422.

160. Stetler-Stevenson WG. Type IV collagenases in tumor invasion and metastasis. Cancer Metast Rev 1990; 9:289-303.

161. Mignatti P, Rifkin DB, Welgus HG et al. Proteinases and tissue remodeling. In:Clark RAF, ed. Molecular and Cellular Biology of Wound Repair. Second Edition. New York:Plenum Press, 1996:427-474.

162. Wilhelm SM, Collier IE, Kronberger A et al. Human skin fibroblast stromelysin:Structure, glycosylation, substrate specificity, and differential expression in normal and tumorigenic cells. Proc Natl Acad Sci USA 1987; 84:6725-6729.

163. Aimes RT, Quigley JP. Matrix metalloproteinase-2 is an interstitial collagenase. J Biol Chem 1995; 270:5872-5876.

164. Moscatelli D, Jaffe E, Rifkin DB. Tetradecanoyl phorbol acetate stimulates latent collagenase production by cultured human endothelial cells. Cell 1980; 20:343-351.

165. Moscatelli D, Presta M, Rifkin DB. Purification of a factor from human placenta that stimulates capillary endothelial cell protease production, DNA synthesis, and migration. Proc Natl Acad Sci USA 1986; 83:2091-2095.

166. Herron GS, Werb Z, Dwyer K et al. Secretion of metalloproteinases by stimulated capillary endothelial cells. I. Production of procollagenase and prostromelysin exceeds expression of proteolytic activity. J Biol Chem 1986; 261:2810-2813.

167. Lewalle JM, Munaut C, Pichot B et al. Plasma membrane-dependent activation of gelatinase a in human vascular endothelial cells. J Cell Physiol 1995; 165:475-483.

168. Pepper MS, Montesano R, Mandriota SJ et al. Angiogenesis:A paradigm for balanced extracellular proteolysis during cell migration and morphogenesis. Enzyme Prot 1996; 49:138-162.

169. Mignatti R, Rifkin DB. Plasminogen activators and angiogenesis. Curr Topics Microbiol Immunol 1996; 213:33-50.

170. Hekman CM, Loskutoff DJ. Endothelial cells produce a latent inhibitor of plasminogen activators that can be activated by denaturants. J Biol Chem 1985; 260:11581-11587.

171. Pyke C, Kristensen P, Ralfkiaer E et al. The plasminogen activation system in human colon cancer: Messenger RNA for the inhibitor PAI-1 is located in endothelial cells in the tumor stroma. Cancer Res 1991; 51:4067-4071.

172. Conforti G, Dominguez-Jimenez C, Ronne E et al. Cell-surface plasminogen activation causes a retraction of in vitro cultured human umbilical vein endothelial cell monolayer. Blood 1994; 83:994-1005.

173. Vassalli J-D, Baccino D, Belin D. A cellular binding site for the M_r 55,000 form of the human plasminogen activator, urokinase. J Cell Biol 1985; 100:86-92.

174. Miles LA, Dahlberg CM, Plescia J et al. Role of cell-surface lysines in plasminogen binding to cells: Identification of alpha-enolase as a candidate plasminogen receptor. Biochem 1991; 30:1682-1691.

175. Plow EF, Miles LA. Plasminogen receptors in the mediation of pericellular proteolysis. Cell Differ Dev 1990; 32:293-298.

176. Cubellis MV, Wun TC, Blasi F. Receptor-mediated internalization and degradation of urokinase is caused by its specific inhibitor PAI-1. EMBO J 1990; 9:1079-1085.

177. Fibbi G, Ziche M, Morbidelli L et al. Interaction of urokinase with specific receptors stimulates mobilization of bovine adrenal capillary endothelial cells. Exp Cell Res 1988; 179:385-395.

178. Lu H, Mabilat C, Yeh P et al. Blockage of urokinase receptor reduces in vitro the motility and the deformability of endothelial cells. FEBS Lett 1996; 380:21-24.

179. Wei Y, Lukashev M, Simon DI et al. Regulation of integrin function by the urokinase receptor. Science 1996; 273:1551-1555.

180. Hasselaar P, Loskutoff DJ, Sawdey M et al. SPARC induces the expression of type I plasminogen activator inhibitor in cultured bovine aortic endothelial cells. J Biol Chem 1991; 266:13178-13184.

181. Montesano R, Pepper MS, Möhle-Steinlein U et al. Increased proteolytic activity is responsible for the aberrant morphogenetic behavior of endothelial cells expressing the middle T oncogene. Cell 1990; 62:435-445.

Facilitation of Healing

Matrix Modulation

--- CHAPTER 31 ---

Collagen Matrices Attenuate Fibroblast Response to TGF-β

Richard R. Clark, John M. McPherson

Modified with permission from J Cell Sci 1995; 108:1251-1261.

Introduction

Following loss of soft tissue, fibroblasts proliferate and produce an initially loose-weave provisional matrix which is heavily vascularized and which contains fibronectin, hyaluronate, and relatively little collagen.[1] Gradually this cell-rich granulation tissue becomes a predominantly collagen-rich tissue. The ultimate outcome of this biological process is an imperfect, yet expedient repair called scar formation. The rate and extent of repair depends, in part, on the net balance of negative and positive modulatory signals that impinge on fibroblasts at such sites.[2]

Fibroblasts' responses to various soluble mediators, e.g., growth factors and cytokines, have for the most part been studied with cells grown on tissue culture plastic.[2-5] However, in vivo fibroblasts are surrounded by an extracellular matrix (ECM), and ECM can have profound effects on cell function.[6-12] Thus the responsiveness of fibroblasts to growth factors and cytokines has been evaluated when the cells were cultured on or in various ECM components, especially collagen.[13] Such studies provide important insights into the integration of mediator and ECM signals on fibroblasts.[11-13]

Transformtin growth factor-β (TGF-β), a potent multifunctional cell regulatory protein factor,[5] induces increased fibroblast synthesis of collagen and fibronectin when the fibroblasts are grown on tissue culture plastic.[14-16] Since fibroblasts are usually surrounded by a collagen matrix in vivo, determination of the response of fibroblasts cultured in collagen gels to TGF-β would help elucidate the action of this factor in vivo.

It has become evident that the fibroblast phenotype that develops as a consequence of collagen matrix differs dramatically depending on whether the matrix is relaxed, as occurs in a floating collagen gel, or under tension, as occurs in an anchored collagen gel.[13] Cells in a relaxed collagen gel become stellate, mitogenically quiescent, and produce little collagen.[9,17-20] These are the morphological, proliferative and synthetic characteristics of normal dermal fibroblasts. In contrast, fibroblasts in an anchored collagen gel develop an elongated fusiform morphology as they attempt to contract the attached gel; furthermore, they actively proliferate and synthesize collagen.[19-21] These are the morphological, proliferative and synthetic characteristics of wound fibroblasts which have deposited substantial amounts of collagen in the granulation tissue, and which have begun to compact the collagen matrix and contract the wound.[1]

In this paper, we review evidence that type I procollagen and TGF-β are coexpressed in fibroblasts of early, collagen-poor granulation tissue, while fibroblasts in collagen-rich granulation tissue lack type I procollagen despite the persistence of TGF-β. Furthermore, human dermal fibroblasts cultured in stressed collagen matrices, an environment that simulates late collagen-rich granulation tissue, synthesize little collagen in response to TGF-β compared to fibroblasts cultured on tissue culture plastic, an environment that simulates early collagen-poor granulation tissue.

Results

Synchronous Expression of Type I Procollagen and TGF-β in Wound Fibroblasts of Early Collagen-Poor Granulation Tissue

Fibroblasts in 5 day full thickness porcine wounds were examined as noted in Figure 31.1 for expression of type I procollagen and TGF-β using a murine monoclonal anti-type I procollagen[22] or a polyclonal rabbit anti-TGF-β,[23] respectively. The two proteins demonstrated coordinate increasing expression from the wound edge to the wound center (Fig. 31.2). No type I procollagen or TGF-β appeared in cells near the wound edge (panels A and D, respectively), expression occurred in some fibroblasts between the wound edge and wound center (panels B and E, respectively), and in many fibroblasts at the wound center (panels C and F, respectively).

Discordant Expression of Type I Procollagen and TGF-β in Wound Fibroblasts of Late Collagen-Rich Granulation tissue

When day 7 and day 10 wounds were probed for type I procollagen and TGF-β (Fig. 31.3), both proteins appeared in most, if not all, wound fibroblasts at day 7 (panels A and B, respectively); however, type 1 procollagen was not apparent in day 10 fibroblasts despite the persistence of TGF-β (panels C and D, respectively). Collagen matrix density increased rapidly from day 5 to day 10 as judged by trichrome-stained histologic sections[1] and photometric analysis of Sirius red stained sections (Fig. 31.4). This led to the hypothesis that the rapidly accumulating collagen matrix markedly diminishes the ability of fibroblasts to produce additional collagen despite the presence of TGF-β.

To test this hypothesis, human dermal fibroblasts were cultured in conditions to simulate early, collagen-poor granulation tissue or late, collagen-rich granulation tissue. Fibroblasts cultured in plastic wells are closely juxtaposed to one another and produce abundant amounts of fibronectin, similarly to fibroblasts in early granulation tissue.[24] Fibroblasts cultured in a stressed collagen gel, i.e., the gel remains attached to a plastic well, simulate 10 day, collagen-rich granulation tissue, since in both situations fibroblasts form tension across a dense collagen matrix.[1,20]

Collagen Matrix Attenuates the Ability of TGF-β Stimulated Fibroblasts to Make Collagen

TGF-β stimulation of collagen synthesis was attenuated when neonatal human dermal fibroblasts were cultured in attached collagen gels compared to tissue culture plastic (Fig. 31.5A). In contrast, TGF-β stimulation of noncollagen synthesis was not substantially affected by the collagen matrix environment (Fig. 31.5B). The apparent TGF-β stimulation of noncollagen protein synthesis was largely attributable to a 2-fold increase in the specific activity of intracellular proline pools (control 19,900 dpm/nmole; 100 pM TGF-β,

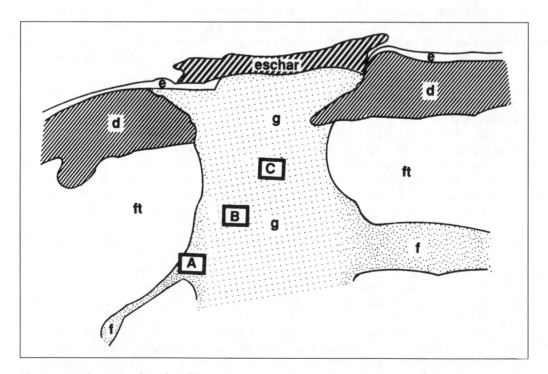

Fig. 31.1. A schematic of a 5 day old cutaneous wound in the flank of a Yorkshire pig. The boxes with capital letters represent the areas of the wound shown in the photomicrographs illustrated in Fig. 31.2. e = epidermis, d = dermis, g = granulation tissue, ft = fat, f = fibrous septa.

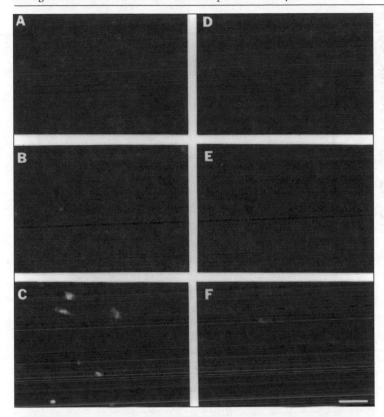

Fig. 31.2. Detection of procollagen and TGF-β in granulation tissue fibroblasts 5 days after excisional wounding of swine corium. (A)-(C): Photomicrographs taken from the edge (A), intermediate zone (B), and center (C) of wound granulation tissue stained with a monoclonal antibody specific for type I procollagen. Fibroblasts in the middle of granulation tissue stain strongly for procollagen (C), but this molecule was not detected in fibroblasts at the edge of the granulation tissue (A). Some but not all fibroblasts in the intermediate zone stained weakly positive (B). (D)-(F): Photomicrographs from the edge (D), intermediate zone (E), and center (F) of granulation tissue of adjacent sections of the same wound, stained with rabbit antibody to a synthetic polypeptide identical to the N-terminal 30 amino acids of TGF-β. Fibroblasts in the center of the granulation tissue stained for TGF-β (F). Some but not all fibroblasts in the intermediate zone stained weakly positive for TGF-β (E) while none of the fibroblasts at the periphery of the wound stained positive (D). Thus, the distribution of staining for TGF-β and procollagen in fibroblasts in granulation tissue in excisional swine skin wounds 5 days after wounding appeared similar. Bar = 20 μm.

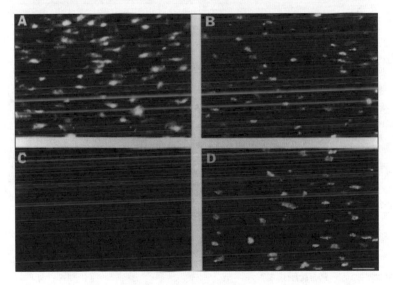

Fig. 31.3. Detection of procollagen (A,C) and TGF-β (B,D) in granulation tissue fibroblasts at 7 days (A,B) and 10 days (C,D) after wounding. All photomicrographs were taken at the center of the wound. Anti-type I procollagen antibodies reveal intense perinuclear fluorescence in day 7 fibroblasts (A) but not in day 10 fibroblasts (C). Anti-TGF-β antibodies reveal intense perinuclear fluorescence in day 7 fibroblasts (B) which persists in day 10 fibroblasts (D). Bar = 20 μm.

38,900 dpm/nmole) as previously reported.[15] Parenthetically, TGF-β did not increase the total intracellular proline pool (control, 1.62 nmole/μg DNA; 100 pM TGF-β, 1.68 nmole/μg DNA). Attached collagen matrix culture environment also consistently attenuated the collagen synthetic response of adult human dermal fibroblasts to TGF-β, while the noncollagen synthetic response was not affected (Table 31.1). Four strains of fibroblasts were examined, two in duplicate experiments. Although marked differences were noted in TGF-β response among these strains, all strains demonstrated attenuation of their TGF-β response when grown in collagen gels. In contrast, attached fibrin gels did not alter the collagen synthetic response to TGF-β (Table 31.2).

Five lines of evidence suggest that attenuation was not a trivial event. First, [14C]-labeled mixed amino acids and albumin freely diffused out of collagen gels, obtaining an equilibrium between the gels and the medium within 30 minutes. Second, total DNA of cells cultured for 3 days in collagen gels was not appreciably different than the DNA of cells cultured on plastic (Table 31.3). Third, LDH release from cells cultured 3 days on plastic or in collagen was not appreciably different and was always less than 5% of the total LDH. Fourth, basal collagen synthesis of fibroblasts cultured in collagen gels was usually similar to basal collagen synthesis of fibroblasts cultured on tissue culture plastic (Table 31.4). Fifth, TGF-β equally stimulated noncollagen synthesis of fibroblasts cultured in collagen gels or on tissue

Fig. 31.4. Increase of collagenous matrix in granulation tissue over time as determined by Sirius red birefringence. Acid-alcohol fixed specimens from 5, 7, 10, and 14 day wounds were stained with Sirius red and the birefringence of the central granulation tissue photometrically measured. Accumulation of wound collagen was then determined as the quotient of granulation tissue birefringence intensity divided by normal dermal collagen birefringence intensity x 100. The data points and brackets represent the means ± SEM, respectively, of three wound replicates at each time point.

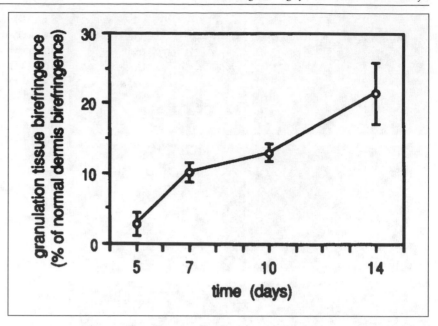

Table 31.1. Collagen matrices attenuate the collagen synthetic response of adult human dermal fibroblasts to TGF-β1.

Strain #	Condition	Collagen	Noncollagen
1	TC Plastic	2.1[a]	1.2
	Collagen gel	1.5	1.4
2	TC Plastic	4.6	3.0
	Collagen gel	2.7	2.5
3	TC Plastic	4.5	3.1
	Collagen gel	3.0	1.9
3	TC Plastic	5.0	3.0
	Collagen gel	3.8	2.1
4	Tc Plastic	9.1	3.4
	Collage Gel	1.8	3.6
4	TC Plastic	9.9	3.3
	Collagen gel	2.8	2.9
		p < 0.004[b]	NS

[a]Fold increase of fibroblasts stimulated with 100pM TGF-b over control
[b]Statistics were performed on the ranks by the Wilcoxon test

Table 31.2. Fibrin matrices do not attenuate the collagen synthetic response of adult human dermal fibroblasts to 100pM TGF-β.

	Collagen synthesis dpm/ug DNAx10^{-3}	Fold Increase with TGF-β	Noncollagen synthesis dpm/ug DNAx10^{-3}	Fold Increase with TGF-β
TC Plastic	16.24±3.03[a]		87.60±27.13	
TC Plastic +TGF-β	69.07±30.09	4.3x	314.37±76.75	3.6x
TC Plastic	15.78±9.78		157.14±11.35	
Fibrin gel +TGF-β	69.63±15.95	4.4x	539.30±96.25	3.4x

[a]Mean of 3 replicates ± standard deviations

Beta-aminoproprionitrile did not alter the collagen gel effect (data not shown).

Autoradiographic Analysis of TGF-β1-Stimulated Proteins

When equal aliquots of medium from each experimental condition shown in Figure 31.5 were analyzed on SDS-PAGE autoradiographs (Fig. 31.7A), most protein bands were notably increased by 100, 300, or 1000 pM TGF-β (lanes 2-4, respectively and lanes 6-8, respectively) compared to no TGF-β1 (lanes 1 and 5). Type I procollagen α1-and α2-chains and fibronectin (arrows) were increased to a greater degree than most other proteins. When fibroblasts were cultured in collagen gels, the TGF-β-induced increase of some protein bands was clearly attenuated (lanes 5-8) compared to cells cultured in tissue culture plastic (lanes 1-4). To resolve whether the attenuated TGF-β response involved mostly collagenous or noncollagen proteins, the newly synthesized proteins were digested with either pepsin or collagenase, respectively, prior to SDS-PAGE.

culture plastic (Table 31.1). In addition, nonspecific adsorption of TGF-β to the collagen matrix was not observed. TGF-β preincubated for 24 hours in collagen gels or in TC dishes stimulated collagen synthesis to the same extent when added subsequently to fibroblasts cultured on plastic.

TGF-β had no consistent effect on the proportion of collagen retained in the cell layers of neonatal or adult dermal fibroblasts whether the cells were cultured on plastic or in collagen gels (Fig. 31.6). For reasons that may be biologically important but are presently unclear, more collagen was retained in the cell layers of adult fibroblasts cultured in collagen gels regardless of whether TGF-β was added (Fig. 31.6).

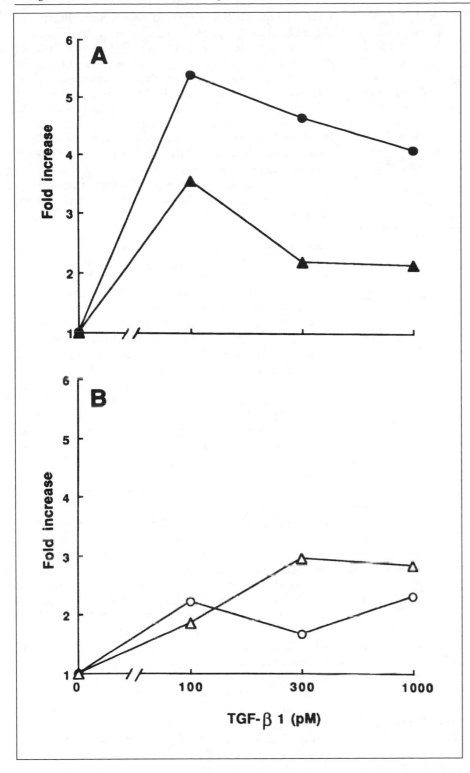

Fig. 31.5. Effect of collagen matrix environment on protein synthetic response of neonatal human dermal fibroblasts to TGF-β 1. (A) Collagen synthesis. (B) Noncollagen synthesis. Fibroblasts were plated at 5×10^5 cells/35 mm dish on TC plastic or suspended in 4 mg/ml collagen gels, treated with 0, 100, 300 or 1000 pM TGF-β1, and labeled with [14C] proline. Total collagen synthesis of fibroblasts on TC plastic (•) and in collagen gels (▲) was the sum of collagen in the medium and in the cell layer. Likewise, total noncollagen synthesis of fibroblasts on TC plastic (o) and in collagen gels (△) was the sum of values obtained for the medium and cell layer. The total [^{14}C]proline incorporation was normalized per μg DNA. Basal collagen synthesis in (A) was 30,130 dpm/μg DNA on TC plastic and 20,480 dpm/μg DNA in collagen gels. Basal noncollagen synthesis in (B) was 170,750 dpm/μg DNA on TC plastic and 95,420 dpm/μg DNA in collagen gels. Data shown is representative of three experiments with neonatal fibroblasts.

Increased collagen synthesis induced by TGF-β1 was best demonstrated by SDS autoradiography of medium samples that had been pepsin digested to remove noncollagen protein.[25] The major bands appearing on SDS-PAGE autoradiography after pepsin digestion were α1(I) and α1(III) chains (Fig. 31.7B, upper arrow), and α2(I) chains (Fig. 31.7B, lower arrow). These bands of collagen proteins were increased when fibroblasts were incubated with 100,

300, 1000 pM TGF-β1 (lanes 2-4 and lanes 6-8) compared to no TGF-β1 (lanes 1 and 5); however, the TGF-β response was markedly attenuated when fibroblasts were cultured in collagen gels (lanes 6-8) compared to fibroblasts in tissue culture plastic wells (lanes 2-4).

Using interrupted gel electrophoresis[26] and autoradiography on pepsin-digested samples, the TGF-β stimulation of α1(I) and α1(III) collagen chains was equally attenu-

Table 31.3. Total DNA of fibroblasts cultured on plastic or in collagen gels.

	DNA (ug)*	
TGF-B (pM)	TC Plastic	Collagen gel
0	4.8±1.2(9)	5.2±2.4(6)
100	5.4±1.0(9)	5.3±1.2(6)
300	4.5±0.7(2)	4.1±1.0(2)
1000	4.4±1.1(2)	4.0±1.2(2)

*Mean ± standard deviation of (n) replicates.

Table 31.4. Effects of attached collagen gels on basal collagen synthesis (DPM/μg DNA x 10⁻³) of human dermal fibroblasts.

Exp.#	Condition	Neonatal	Adult
1	TC Plastic	15.6	14.1
	Collagen gel	15.5	13.0
2	TC Plastic	30.1	8.3
	Collagen gel	20.5	10.6
3	TC Plastic	61.6	5.6
	Collagen gel	55.5	7.8
4	TC Plastic	8.4	13.1
	Collagen gel	12.9	11.9
5	TC Plastic	7.1	8.4
	Collagen gel	6.2	14.3
		NS	NS

Statistics were performed on the ranks by the Wilcoxon test

ated by collagen gels (data not shown). Thus, types I and III collagen are regulated synchronously under the conditions of these experiments.

Fibronectin was the major noncollagen band in autoradiographs of collagenase digested medium samples (Fig. 31.7C, arrow). Western blot analysis and immunoprecipitation with anti-fibronectin antibodies confirmed that the band was fibronectin (not shown). TGF-β markedly increased fibronectin synthesis as previously shown,[14] and collagen matrices appeared to have little effect on the TGF-β stimulation of fibronectin in either the medium (Fig. 31.7C, arrow) or cell layer (Fig. 31.7D, arrow). Unfortunately, synthesized proteins in the cell layers of fibroblasts grown in collagen gels could not be visualized by SDS-PAGE autoradiography except after collagenase treatment, since the large amount of collagen present caused distortion of the protein bands.

TGF-β Stimulation of Type I Procollagen as Visualized by Immunofluorescence Microscopy

Using a monoclonal antibody specific for the carboxy-terminal globular domain of type I procollagen,[22] we observed increased intensity and numbers of fluorescent, perinuclear granules in fibroblasts after stimulation with TGF-β

(Fig. 31.8, panels B and D) compared to unstimulated fibroblasts (Fig. 31.8, panels A and C), whether the fibroblasts were cultured on tissue culture plastic (Fig. 31.8, panels A and B) or in collagen gels (Fig. 31.8, panels C and D). However, whereas most fibroblasts on tissue culture plastic stained for type I procollagen after TGF-β1 treatment (> 90%) only a rare cell in collagen gels did so (< 10%). To maximize the observable response to TGF-β, strain #4 fibroblasts were utilized (see Table 31.1). These immunofluorescence data corroborated the biochemical data that TGF-β 1 stimulates fibroblasts to produce more collagen in tissue culture plastic conditions and that collagen gel matrices attenuate this response, apparently by inhibiting synthesis by most but not all cells.

Discussion

Fibroblasts undergo striking phenotypic modulation during tissue repair, embryogenesis and morphogenesis. Elucidating the controls of such phenotype switching will facilitate our ability to intercede when tissue development or repair goes awry. As a first step we designed a series of experiments to identify the temporal relationships of certain fibroblast phenotypic markers with ECM maturation and growth factor appearance. We observed that F-actin bundle formation and fibronectin receptor expression are coordinately regulated with fibronectin matrix assembly in wounds[1] as had been previously observed in cultured fibroblasts.[27-29] Here we review data demonstrating that type I procollagen expression and TGF-β are coordinately expressed in early stages of a healing wound (Figs. 31.2 and 31.3 A,B), however, by 10 days type I procollagen is no longer apparent while TGF-β expression persists (Fig. 31.3 C,D).

The coordinate expression of TGF-β in early wounds was not surprising since TGF-β is known to induce fibroblast production of types I and III collagen in vitro[14-16] and to induce a fibrotic reaction in vivo.[15,30-32] However, the disappearance of type I procollagen in fibroblasts that still expressed TGF-β was unanticipated. Although the antibody used for immunoprobing is specific for mature TGF-β,[33] the mature TGF-β may be latent or inactivated.[34-36] Alternatively, the fibroblasts may have become relatively refractory to TGF-β. Since the density of the collagen-rich ECM rapidly accumulated (Fig. 31.4) as type I procollagen expression disappeared (Fig. 31.3C), we hypothesized that collagen matrix might attenuate the fibroblasts' response to TGF-β.

Initially we were disturbed that there was a 40% increase in collagen density between days 10 and 14 (Fig. 31.4) despite the apparent absence of further collagen production (Fig. 31.3C); however, the wound area decreased by approximately 33% from day 10 to day 14,[1] presumably secondary to fibroblast-driven reorganization and compaction of wound matrix collagen bundles. Thus the increase in wound collagen density between days 10 and 14 is probably attributable to collagen compaction.

To test the hypothesis that collagen matrix attenuates fibroblasts' response to TGF-β, we assayed the ability of cultured human fibroblasts to respond to TGF-β in the presence of stressed collagen gels, a culture system in which fibroblasts are under tension similar to that of collagen-rich,

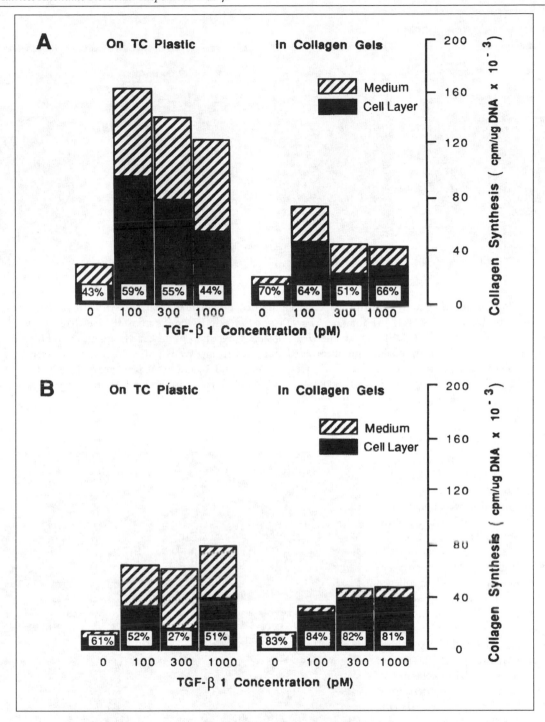

Fig. 31.6. Effect of TGF-β and collagen matrix on compartmentalization of newly synthesized collagen between the media and cell layers of neonatal (A) and adult (B) human dermal fibroblasts. Fibroblasts were cultured on TC plastic or in collagen gels and metabolically labeled with [¹⁴C]proline as described in Fig. 31.5. Collagen production in the culture medium and cell layer was determined using the modified Peterkofsky method. The amount of [14C]proline incorporated into newly synthesized collagen was normalized per μg DNA. The percent shown in each bar represents the percent collagen retained in the cell layer.

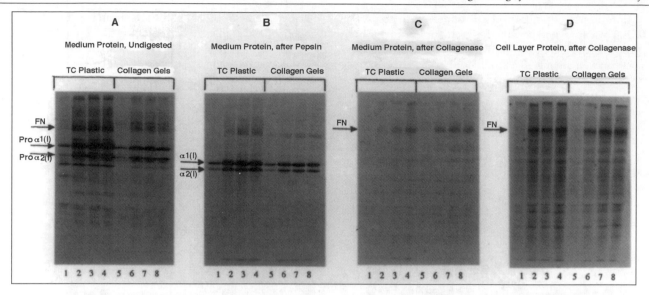

Fig. 31.7. SDS-PAGE autoradiography confirms that collagen matrices attenuate the collagen synthetic response of neonatal human dermal fibroblasts to TGF-β 1. (A) Total newly synthesized protein in the medium. (B) Newly synthesized pepsin-resistant protein in the medium. (C,D) Newly synthesized collagenase-resistant protein in the medium and in the cell layer, respectively. Medium samples from equal cell numbers based on DNA were analyzed by SDS-PAGE autoradiography. Samples were taken from fibroblasts cultured in the absence of TGF-β1 (lanes 1 and 5), and in the presence of TGF-β1 (100 pM, lanes 2 and 6; 300 pM, lanes 3 and 7; 1000 pM, lanes 4 and 8). Arrows indicate fibronectin (FN), type I procollagen α1 (pro α1) and α2 (pro α2) and type I collagen α1 and α2.

Fig. 31.8. Immunofluorescence staining for procollagen in cultured neonatal human dermal fibroblasts. Cultures containing 5 x 10^5 fibroblasts per 35 mm dish were prepared on tissue culture plastic (A and B) or suspended in 4 mg/ml hydrated collagen gels (C and D) and treated with 0 or 300 pM TGF-β 1 (A, C and B, D, respectively) for 22 hours. All cells were fixed with acid-alcohol. Cells in collagen gels were embedded in paraffin and sectioned. Cells on tissue culture plastic and in the sectioned collagen gels were immunostained for type I procollagen using an indirect avidin-biotin technique. Arrows indicate the areas of procollagen staining. Nuclei of cells in collagen gels (arrowheads) were counterstained by the 1% paraphenylenediamine used in the mounting medium. Bar = 20 μm.

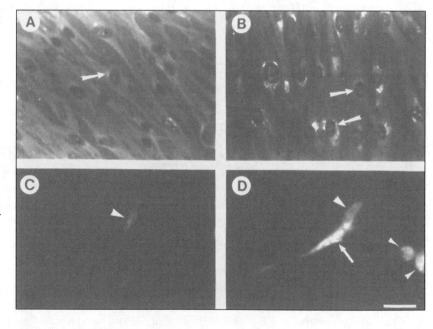

late (e.g., day 10), granulation tissue in which fibroblasts are under tension as they reorganize and compact the collagen matrix.[1,20] As shown in Figs. 31.4-31.7 and Table 31.1, such collagen gels consistently and significantly attenuated the collagen synthetic response of fibroblasts to TGF-β compared to fibroblasts cultured on plastic. When cultured on plastic, fibroblasts grow in close juxtaposition and deposit an abundance of fibronectin in the pericellular matrix, a situation that simulates early, fibronectin-rich and collagen-poor, granulation tissue. The attenuation by a collagen matrix

environment did not appear to be a trivial effect of the collagen gels on TGF-β or fibroblasts, as TGF-β was not bound by the collagen gels, and collagen gels did not cause nutrient deprivation or cell injury. Furthermore, TGF-β stimulation of noncollagen synthesis was usually not altered by the attached collagen gels used in these experiments (Table 31.1, Figs. 31.4 and 31.6). Specifically TGF-β stimulation of fibronectin synthesis appeared unaffected by stressed collagen gels. Biochemical results were confirmed by immunofluorescence studies of fibroblasts (Fig. 31.8). Most if not all fibroblasts cultured on plastic appeared to respond to TGF-β by expressing perinuclear granular staining for type I procollagen (Fig. 31.8B), while most cells in collagen were negative even after TGF-β stimulation (Fig. 31.8D). Nevertheless, an occasional cell in collagen stained at least as intense for type I procollagen as the TGF-β stimulated fibroblasts cultured on plastic (Fig. 31.8D). Thus, there appeared to be a marked heterogeneity of cultured fibroblasts in their ability to respond to collagen matrix.

The mechanism by which collagen matrix alters the responsiveness of fibroblasts to TGF-β is not known. One possibility is that the collagenous environment downregulates one or more of the three known cell surface receptors for TGF-β.[37,38] In fact, given that we have observed a differential effect of collagen gels on the biosynthesis of collagen and fibronectin in response to TGF-β (Fig. 31.6), collagen matrix may differentially affect these receptors. As a first step toward investigating these possibilities, we probed RNA extracts of human adult dermal fibroblasts for type II and type III TGF-β receptor expression when fibroblasts were grown in plastic tissue culture dishes verses collagen matrices. Using cDNA probes for the types II and III receptors obtained from Drs. Herbert Lin, Harvey Lodish, Robert Weinberg, and Xiao-Fan Wang,[39,40] we found no detectable differences in mRNA expression among these conditions. Nevertheless, at least one study has shown that the extracellular matrix environment can modulate TGF-β receptor expression with remarkable effects on cell responses to TGF-β.[41]

Alternatively, collagen matrix may influence signal transduction[42] and this may influence, perhaps differentially, the biosynthesis of ECM molecules. The pathway(s) through which collagen matrix transmits its effect on fibroblasts are currently a focus of study in our laboratory. It is clear that collagen matrix activates protein kinase-ζ (PKC-ζ) and Nf-κb, which leads to upregulation of α₂β₁ collagen receptors;[43,44] however, the relationship of these pathways to collagen matrix attenuation of TGF-β stimulated collagen synthesis is not known.

An interesting byproduct of this study was the failure of attached collagen gels to suppress basal collagen synthesis (Table 31.4). Previously, many investigators reported that basal collagen synthesis was suppressed by collagen gels.[17,18,20] However, in the studies reporting suppression of basal collagen synthesis, collagen gels were detached from the tissue culture dish, allowing the fibroblasts to isotropically contract the collagen matrix under relatively little tension. Ultimately the fibroblasts in floating collagen gels assume a stellate phenotype similar to fibroblasts in normal dermis.[20] Thus the released collagen gel model predicts that fibroblasts in normal skin may be maximally inhibited by their surrounding collagen matrix. In contrast, as fibroblasts in attached collagen gels attempt to contract the matrix under these anisotropic conditions, they generate increasing tension and assume a bipolar phenotype along the lines of maximum resistance.[20] A similar phenomenon occurs in 10 day collagen-rich, granulation tissue as wound contraction commences.[1] Thus, the attached collagen gels in our experiments kept the cells and collagen matrix under tension similar to 10 day, collagen-rich granulation tissue.[1] Our findings that basal collagen synthesis is depressed little,

if any, when fibroblasts are cultured in attached collagen gels confirm the studies from the Grinnell laboratory.[19-21] Although the attached collagen gel paradigm predicts that fibroblasts under tension as observed in 10 day, collagen-rich wounds would not show a decrease in basal collagen synthesis[1] (Fig. 31.1), our studies clearly demonstrate that fibroblasts in these conditions do lose their responsiveness to TGF-β. Recently we have found that while PKC-ζ and Nf-κb are activated by both stressed and relaxed collagen matrices, other signal transduction pathways are, however, affected differentially by these two physical forms of collagen matrix (unpublished data).

The concept of collagen matrix attenuation of fibroblast collagen synthesis to TFG-β is appealing and is consistent with previous results which showed that collagen matrices downregulated the responsiveness of fibroblasts to PDGF and other growth factors.[42,45] These data provide in some measure an explanation for the orderly progression of the wound repair process by a means of positive signals that stimulate cells to generate an environment that both provides for repair and establishes feed-back regulation of the process.

In contrast to the suppression effects of collagen gels on collagen synthesis, the permissive effects of fibrin gels are consistent with the role of this molecule in providing a provisional matrix during the early phases of the wound repair to support cell invasion, proliferation and matrix deposition. Thus the normal process of wound repair appears to be under the control of both soluble factors that stimulate certain events and the extracellular matrix, which can modulate the responsiveness of cells to these signals. It is likely that certain pathological fibrotic conditions develop when these feedback regulation systems become ineffective.

Acknowledgments
Funding for this work was provided by NIH grants HL27353 and AM31514 to Richard A. F. Clark.

References
1. Welch MP, Odland GF et al. Temporal relationships of F-actin bundle formation, collagen and fibronectin matrix assembly, and fibronectin receptor expression to wound contraction. J Cell Biol 1990; 110:133-145.
2. Clark RAF. Overview and general considerations of wound repair. In: Clark RAF, Henson PM, eds. The Molecular and Cellular Biology of Wound Repair. New York: Plenum Press, 1996:3-50.
3. Rifkin DB, Moscatelli D. Recent developments in the cell biology of basic fibroblast growth factor. J Cell Biol 1989; 109:1-6.
4. Ross RR, Raines EW. Platelet-derived growth factor and cell proliferation. In: Sara VR et al, eds. Growth Factors: From Genes to Clinical Application. New York: Raven Press, 1990; 193-199.
5. Sporn MB, Roberts AM. Transformtin growth factor-β: Recent progress and new challenges. J Cell Biol 1992; 119:1017-1021.
6. Gospodarowicz D, Delgado D, et al. Permissive effect of the extracellular matrix on cell proliferation in vitro. Proc Nat Acad Sci USA 1980; 77:4094-4098.

7. Sugrue SP, Hay ED. Response of basal epithelial cell surface and cytoskeleton to solubilized extracellular matrix molecules. J Cell Biol 1981; 91:45-54.

8. Wicha MS, Lowrie G et al. Extracellular matrix promotes mammary epithelial growth and differentiation in vitro. Proc Nat Acad Sci USA 1982; 79:3213-3217.

9. Mauch C, Adelmann-Grill B et al. Collagenase gene expression in fibroblasts is regulated by a three-dimensional contact with collagen. FEBS Lett 1989; 250:301-305.

10. Klein CE, Dressel D et al. Integrin α2β1 is upregulated in fibroblasts and highly aggressive melanoma cells in three demensional collagen lattices and mediates the reorganization of collagen i fibrils. J Cell Biol 1991; 115:1427-1436.

11. Damsky CH, Werb Z. Signal transduction by integrin receptors for extracellular matrix: Cooperative processing of extracellular information. Curr Opin Cell Biol 1992; 4:772-781.

12. Juliano RL, Haskill S. Signal transduction from the extracellular matrix. J Cell Biol 1992; 120:577-585.

13. Grinnell F. Fibroblasts, myofibroblasts, and wound contraction. J Cell Biol 1994; 124:401-404.

14. Ignotz RA, Massague J. Transformtin growth factor-β stimulates the expression of fibronectin and collagen and their incorporation into extracellular matrix. J Biol Chem 1986; 261:4337-4340.

15. Roberts AB, Sporn MB et al. Transforming growth factor beta: Rapid induction of fibrosis and angiogenesis in vivo and stimulation of collagen formation. Proc Natl Acad Sci USA 1986; 83:4167-4171.

16. Fine A, Goldstein RH. The effect of transformtin growth factor-β on cell proliferation and collagen formation by lung fibroblasts. J Biol Chem 1987; 262:3897-3902.

17. Nusgens B, Merrill C et al. Collagen biosynthesis by cells in a tissue equivalent matrix in vitro. Coll Relat Res 1984; 4:351-363.

18. Mauch C, Hatamochi A et al. Regulation of collagen synthesis in fibroblasts within a three-dimensional collagen gel. Exp Cell Res 1988; 178: 493-530.

19. Nakagawa S, Pawelek P et al. Extracellular matrix organization modulates fibroblast growth and growth factor responsiveness. Exp Cell Res 1989; 182:572-582.

20. Nakagawa S, Pawelek P et al. Long term culture of fibroblasts in contracted collagen gels: Effects on cell growth and biosynthetic activity. J Invest Dermatol 1989; 93:792-798.

21. Fukamizu H, Grinnell F. Spatial organization of extracellular matrix and fibroblast activity: Effects of serum, transforming growth factor β, and fibronectin. Exp Cell Res 1990; 190:276-282.

22. McDonald JA, Broekelmann TJ et al. A monoclonal antibody to the carboxyterminal domain of procollagen type I visualizes collagen-synthesizing fibroblasts. J Clin Invest 1986; 78:1237-1244.

23. Ellingsworth LR, Brennan JE et al. Antibodies to the N-terminal portion of cartilage-inducing factor A and transformtin growth factor-b. Immunohistochemical localization and association with differentiating cells. J Biol Chem 1986; 261:12362-12367.

24. Xu J, ClarkRAF. Extracellular matrix alters PDGF regulation of fibroblast integrins. J Cell Biol 1996; 132:239-249.

25. Leibovich SJ, Weiss JB. Electron microscope studies of the effects of endo and exopeptidase digestion on tropocollagen: A novel concept of role of terminal regions in fibrillogenesis . Biochim Biophys Acta 1970; 214:445-454.

26. Sykes B, Puddle B et al. The estimation of two collagens from human dermis by interrupted gel electrophoresis. Biochem Biophys Res Comm 1976; 72:1472-1480.

27. Hynes RO, Destree AT. Relationships between fibronectin (LETS) protein and actin. Cell 1978; 15:875-886.

28. Chen W-T, Wang J et al. Regulation of fibronectin receptor distribution by transformation, exogenous fibronectin, and synthetic peptides. J Cell Biol 1986; 103:1649-1661.

29. Roman J, LaChance RM et al. The fibronectin receptor is organized by extracellular matrix fibronectin: Implications for oncogenic transformation and for cell recognition of fibronectin matrices. J Cell Biol 1989; 108:2529-2543.

30. Sporn MB, Roberts AB et al. Polypeptide transforming growth factor isolated from bovine sources and used for wound healing in vitro. Science 1983; 219:1329-1331.

31. Mustoe TA, Pierce GF et al. Accelerated healing of incisional wounds in rats induced by transformtin growth factor-beta. Science. 1987; 237:1333-1336.

32. Sprugel KH, McPherson JM et al. Effects of growth factors in vivo. Am J Path 1987; 129:601-613.

33. Flanders KC, Thompson NL et al. Transformtin growth factor-β1: Histochemical localization with antibodies to different epitopes. J Cell Biol 1989; 108:653-666.

34. O'Connor-McCourt MD, Wakefield LM. Latent transformtin growth factor-b in serum. J Biol Chem 1987; 262:14090-14099.

35. Lyons RM, Keski-Oja J et al. Proteolytic activation of latent transformtin growth factor-β from fibroblast-conditioned medium. J Cell Biol 1988; 106:1659-1665.

36. Miyazono K, Heldin CH. Role for carbohydrate structures in TGF-β1 latency. Nature 1989; 338:158-160.

37. Chen R-H, Ebner R et al. Inactivation of the type II receptor reveals two receptor pathways for the diverse TGF-β activities. Science 1993; 260:1335-1338.

38. Lopez-Casillas F, Wrana JL et al. Betaglycan presents ligand to the TGF-β signaling receptor. Cell 1993; 73:1435-1444.

39. Wang XF, Lin HY et al. Expression cloning and characterization of the TGF-beta type III receptor. Cell 1991; 67(4):797-805.

40. Lin HY, Wang XF et al. Expression cloning of the TGF-beta type II receptor, a functional transmembrane serine/threonine kinase [published erratum appears in Cell Sep 18;70(6):following 1068]." Cell 68(4): 775-85.

41. Sankar S, Mahooti-Brooks N et al. Modulation of transforming growth factor β receptor levels on microvascular endothelial cells during in vitro angiogenesis. J Clin Invest 1996; 97(6):1436-46.

42. Lin Y-C, Grinnell F. Decreased level of PDGF-stimulated receptor autophosphorylation by fibroblasts in mechanically relaxed collagen matrice. J Cell Biol 1993; 122:663-672.

43. Xu J, Clark RAF. Collagen lattices stimulate fibroblast PKC-ζ activation: Role in α2 integrin subunit and collagenase-1 mRNA expression. J Cell Biol 1997; 136:473-483.

44. Xu J, Zutter MM et al. A three-dimensional collagen lattice activates Nf-κb in human fibroblasts: Role in integrin α2 gene expression and tissue remodeling. J Cell Biol in press. 1998; 140:709-719.

45. McPherson JM, Rhudy RW. Influence of the extracellular matrix on the proliferative response of human skin fibroblasts to serum and purified platelet-derived growth factor. J Cell Physiol. 1988; 137:185-191.

Facilitation of Healing

Matrix Modulation

─────────── CHAPTER 32 ───────────

Extracellular Matrix Proteins Are Potent Agonists of Human Smooth Muscle Cell Migration

Terry L. Kaiura, K. Craig Kent

Introduction

The current treatments of atherosclerotic occlusive disease are multiple and include bypass, endarterectomy, and angioplasty. Unfortunately, the long term success of these interventions is significantly jeopardized by a process known as intimal hyperplasia.[1,2] Tissue engineering and subsequent creation of a prosthetic graft that is resistant to the formation of an intimal plaque would be instrumental in improving the long term outcome of vascular reconstructions. In order to synthesize the "ideal" vascular graft, however, it is imperative that the critical cellular processes that precede the formation of intimal hyperplasia be understood.

The three essential components of intimal hyperplasia are smooth muscle cell (SMC) migration, proliferation, and extracellular matrix (ECM) production.[3] Although all three of these events are necessary for restenosis, their relative importance is not well understood. In normal human vasculature, the intima is almost completely devoid of SMCs. Thus, migration of SMC from the vessel media into the subintimal space is a critical initial step in the initiation of the restenotic process. Confirming the importance of SMC migration are studies that demonstrate that over 50% of the neointimal plaque is composed of nonproliferating SMC.[4]

Following vascular injury, SMC are exposed to a variety of growth factors, cytokines, and ECM proteins, all of which can potentially affect SMC migration. The role of growth factors in SMC chemotaxis has been studied in great detail and the platelet-derived growth factor BB homodimer (PDGF-BB) has been identified as an extremely potent agonist of SMC migration.[5] Moreover, a plethora of other growth factors including fibroblast growth factor (FGF), epidermal growth factor (EGF), and transformtin growth factor-β (TGF-β) have been found to affect SMC chemotaxis.[6,7] ECM proteins are also abundant in the arterial wall, and SMC are exposed to these proteins following vascular injury as well.[8] The role of ECM proteins in SMC migration, however, is less well understood, and is the focus of this chapter.

Cell Migration

Cell migration is a dynamic, complex process, the molecular biologic basis of which has not been fully described. The central component of the cellular apparatus that is necessary for migration is the actin cytoskeleton.[9] Actin is organized into stress fibers that create the framework of a cell. These filaments are anchored by actin binding proteins such as α-actinin[10] to the cell membrane via a series of proteins termed the focal adhesion complex.[11]

The focal adhesion complex itself is composed of clusters of proteins such as tensin, p125 focal adhesion kinase (FAK), paxillin, talin, and vinculin, that bind to transmembrane receptors called integrins (Fig. 32.1).[12] Integrin receptors in turn bind via their extracellular domains to surrounding matrix.[13]

Cellular migration is a cyclic process that initially requires detachment of the leading edge of a cell, reorganization of the actin filaments to allow forward movement, followed by reattachment of this "pseudopod" in a new location.[14] The body of the cell is then pulled forward to "catch up" with the leading edge, resulting in forward movement of the entire cell. This complex process requires that both focal adhesions and actin filaments be cyclically dissolved and then reformed.

The integrin receptor is central to the interaction between the cytoskeleton and the external cellular environment.[15] Integrin receptors have large extracellular domains, a single membrane-spanning domain and a short cytoplasmic domain. The extracellular domain attaches to matrix proteins that are specific for each integrin receptor and the cytoplasmic domain interacts with focal adhesions and actin filaments. It is increasingly recognized that integrin-matrix interactions are not purely structural or biomechanical, but that integrins transduce signals into cells which may be important in the regulation of multiple processes including cell motility.[16] Thus, integrins are similar to growth factor receptors in that ECM proteins can act as ligands that stimulate signaling events that ultimately influence cellular behavior. In the case of migration, integrins not only provide the structural mechanism that allows a cell to attach and migrate across ECM, but these same integrin receptors may transduce messages via ECM proteins into the cell that influence the propensity of a cell to migrate.[17]

Lysis of ECM may also be an important component of the process of migration. Lysis of these proteins allows a pathway to be created through which the cell can migrate.

Therefore, cellular secretion of proteolytic agents such as matrix metalloproteinase (MMP)-2, MMP-9, tissue type plasminogen activator, and urokinase plasminogen activator appear to be necessary for cell locomotion.[18,19] It has been demonstrated that PDGF increases the expression of several proteases found in the ECM;[20] therefore PDGF may contribute to cellular migration by acting directly on the cytoskeleton or also by modifying the environment that surrounds a cell. Heparin, for example, which is a known deterrent of intimal hyperplasia inhibits expression of tissue type plasminogen activator and collagenase.[21]

The migratory response of SMC to an agonist can assume three different patterns, depending upon the state and solubility of the stimulatory protein. Chemokinesis describes random cellular migration in response to a soluble factor, chemotaxis refers to directed migration toward a positive gradient of soluble attractant, and haptotaxis defines directed cellular migration toward a positive gradient of an insoluble agonist such as a substrate bound matrix protein.[21] Whether or not matrix proteins are in a soluble or insoluble form at the time of vascular injury is not clear. This may be an important distinction, since the magnitude of the migratory response may vary depending upon whether the stimulus is that of haptotaxis or chemotaxis. Moreover, it has been shown that the signaling pathways that mediate these two responses are distinct.[22] Possibly all three stimuli have the potential to influence vascular SMCs during the repair and remodeling process that follows vascular injury.[3]

Extracellular Matrix Proteins

ECM proteins are ubiquitous in the normal vessel wall. Endothelial cells manufacture an underlying basement membrane that is superficial to the internal elastic lamina. This layer is composed primarily of type IV collagen, laminin, and heparan sulfate proteoglycan.[23] The media is composed of smooth muscle cells that are surrounded by a plethora of ECM proteins that include fibronectin,[24] types I, III, and V

Fig. 32.1. The focal adhesion complex, illustrating clusters of proteins including paxillin, tensin, vinculin, p125[FAK], and talin which interact with both actin filaments and integrins.

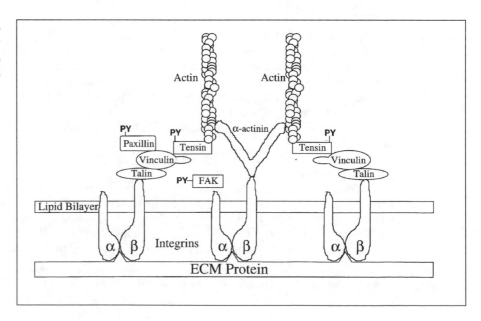

collagen,[25] as well as elastin,[26] and proteoglycans.[27] The adventitia, which consists mainly of collagen, is bound on its outer aspect by loose connective tissue that includes collagen type I and proteoglycans.[23]

ECM comprises as much as 60-80% of a mature intimal plaque.[28,29] The predominant proteins are collagen types I and III,[30] elastin,[31] fibronectin,[32,33] and proteoglycans such as versican-like chondroitin sulfate.[34] Two weeks following vessel injury and after the period of maximal SMC proliferation and migration, cell numbers in the intima reach a maximum. The continued expansion of intimal plaque is then due to the synthesis of the ECM proteins previously mentioned.[28] A variety of less predominant proteins have also been identified in intimal plaque including osteopontin,[35] vitronectin,[36] thrombospondin,[37] and tenascin.[38] These proteins are synthesized and secreted primarily by SMC. The prevalence of ECM in the normal and pathological vessel has spurred our investigation into the effect of these proteins on SMC migration.

Extracellular Matrix Protein and Migration

In recent years, the effect of a number of ECM proteins on SMC migration has been investigated. In the following paragraphs, the results of these investigations will be reviewed.

Osteopontin has been widely studied because of its expression in tissues that undergo remodeling, such as the smooth muscle layer of the intestinal tract and the normal intima of the ductus arteriosus.[20] Liaw et al have demonstrated that osteopontin is dramatically elevated in the rat carotid artery and aorta following balloon injury.[39] Studies of human vascular tissue have revealed focal expression of osteopontin in atherosclerotic plaques but not in normal human arteries.[40] Osteopontin, in vitro, has a strong stimulatory effect on SMC chemotaxis.[41] Moreover, antibodies directed against osteopontin inhibit SMC migration and also neointima thickening in the injured rat carotid artery.[42] It is likely that osteopontin works in conjunction with other ECM proteins, integrins, and matrix proteases to promote adhesion and migration of SMCs.

Chen et al has shown that the large ECM glycoprotein, tenascin, is distributed throughout the neointima of hyperplastic lesions derived from human arteriovenous polytetrafluoroethylene grafts that have been removed for revision.[43] Tenascin has also been found in the intimal layer of injured rat aorta and carotid arteries.[38] This glycoprotein, which has been reported to have both adhesive and antiadhesive domains, is a mediator of focal adhesion disassembly as well.[44] As such, Majesky has speculated that this disbursement of focal adhesions, or sites of cellular attachment to the ECM, may facilitate the transition of a cell from a nonmotile to a migrating state.[45] Accordingly, there is evidence that tenascin supports the migration of rat aortic smooth muscle cells, although the effect of this ECM on human SMC migration has not been investigated.[46]

Similarly to tenascin, thrombospondin (TSP) possesses both adhesive and counteradhesive properties and is a prominent facilitator of focal adhesion disassembly.[44] TSP is present in the ECM of the normal arterial wall; however,

following vascular injury, its expression rapidly increases.[45] Yabkowitz et al have found that TSP is a potent mediator of calf pulmonary artery SMC migration.[47] Either inhibition of TSP synthesis or TSP-SMC interactions decreased in response to SMC migration. Interestingly, SMC migration to the combination of TSP and PDGF was greater than the maximal response observed with PDGF alone.[47]

The glycosaminoglycan hyaluronan (HA) is synthesized and deposited in the neointima soon after vascular injury.[48] Riessen et al found through histological analyses of both rat and human vascular tissues that HA is a predominant component of the early vascular lesion.[48] Savani et al demonstrated that HA stimulated the migration of arterial bovine SMCs, and that an antibody to the HA-binding RHAMM receptor blocked migration.[49] CD44 is another HA binding receptor that is upregulated in the neointima and may also play a role in SMC migration.[20] Moreover, the ability of HA to bind to large amounts of water and to create a gel-like environment may also potentially facilitate SMC migration.[48]

Vitronectin, otherwise known as the serum-spreading factor or S-protein is present as an ECM protein in the circulation, as well as in the vessel wall.[36] This ECM protein is also increased in atherosclerotic tissues.[50] Vitronectin is involved in the adhesion of cells to the ECM and in the regulation of complement and coagulation pathways.[51] Naito et al found that vitronectin invoked SMC haptotaxis and postulated that vitronectin, which is found in the subendothelial matrix, may stimulate migration of SMCs from the media to the intima.[52] Moreover, Brown et al have shown that vitronectin induces human aortic SMC migration via the $\alpha_v\beta_3$ integrin to an extent that is comparable to that of the growth factor PDGF-BB.[53]

Although all of the above described proteins are expressed following arterial injury and promote SMC migration, these proteins constitute a relatively small portion of the total ECM within both normal and diseased vessels. More predominant components of normal artery and vein and intimal plaque include proteins such as collagen types I and IV, fibronectin, and laminin.[24] The effect of these ECM proteins on SMC migration has been less well investigated. As a result, our group has recently studied the effect of these four proteins on all three mechanisms of migration (namely chemokinesis, chemotaxis, and haptotaxis) using human smooth muscle cells derived from saphenous veins.

We found that collagen types I and IV, fibronectin, and laminin were all very potent agonists of SMC migration.[54] In our initial studies, we determined the concentration of each matrix protein that produced maximal cell movement. Maximal migration was achieved with intermediate concentrations of fibronectin and laminin. Higher concentrations of these two proteins did not produce a further increase in the migratory response. Type I and IV collagen similarly produced maximal migration at intermediate concentrations of protein; however, higher concentrations of both collagens led to a decrease in SMC migration. Corroborating our findings, DiMilla et al found that high concentrations of type IV collagen increased SMC attachment, but decreased SMC migration.[55] These authors concluded that cell migration on a matrix protein may be inversely related to the ability of a cell to attach this protein.

To determine the relative potency of these proteins as stimulants of migration, we studied SMC chemotaxis, haptotaxis, and chemokinesis in response to optimal concentrations of each matrix protein.[54] We also compared the relative effect of these matrix proteins to the prototypical migratory stimulus, PDGF. Collagen types I and IV produced the most significant increase in chemotaxis, with a respective increase of approximately 17- and 21-fold in the rate of migration compared to control. Providing less of a stimulatory effect was fibronectin (5-fold increase), followed by PDGF-AB (3-fold increase) and finally laminin (2-fold increase). This same hierarchy was demonstrated for both chemokinesis and haptotaxis as well.

Thus, despite the previous focus on growth factors as stimulants of SMC migration, our findings suggest that matrix proteins, which are plentiful in the vessel wall after arterial injury, are as a group more potent stimuli of SMC migration.[54] Although PDGF-BB is a stronger stimulant for migration than PDGF-AB, neither of these growth factors could produce a migratory response that equaled that of collagen type I or type IV.[54] We and others have also previously demonstrated that soluble growth factors such as EGF and bFGF are less potent agonists of SMC migration than PDGF-AB.[56] These findings imply that matrix proteins may be the predominant "in vivo" stimulus for SMC migration following arterial injury.

In these studies, we consistently found that haptotaxis (SMC migration toward a gradient of insoluble matrix protein) was the most profound stimulus of human SMC migration.[54] These findings were reproducible for all four matrix proteins; the SMC response to haptotaxis was on average 33% greater than the response of SMC to chemotaxis for the same agonist. Haptotaxis of neoplastic cells has been previously studied in some detail and is thought to play a significant role in the invasion and spread of metastatic tumor cells.[57] It appears that haptotaxis and chemotaxis are in fact very distinct processes rather than an extension of the same process.[58] In studies with thrombospondin, haptotaxis and chemotaxis were found to be mediated by completely separate peptide domains of the thrombospondin molecule and the signaling pathways activated by these two processes were also very different.[59]

After investigating the influence of individual growth factors and ECM proteins on SMC migration, we next studied the chemotactic response of SMC to combinations of these proteins.[60] At the time of arterial injury, SMCs are exposed to a plethora of growth factors and ECM proteins. Presumably these proteins can act in concert to influence SMC migration. Possible interactions include:

1. One factor may mask the other, with the combined response being equivalent to that of the more potent agonist;
2. The two factors may have an additive response;
3. The two factors may act in a synergistic manner in which the sum of both factors is greater than the sum of their individual effects.[60]

We found that simultaneous stimulation of SMC with PDGF-AB and collagen type I or IV, fibronectin, or laminin synergistically enhanced SMC migration to a level that was greater than the addition of their individual effects.[60] At both low and high concentrations of the collagens, the chemotactic response was enhanced 20-60% by the simultaneous stimulation of SMC with PDGF and collagen. Alternatively, with low concentrations of laminin or fibronectin the response with PDGF was additive, whereas, at higher concentrations, laminin and fibronectin produced a 40-70% enhancement of PDGF-induced migration compared to what would be anticipated by the addition of these two proteins. Surprisingly, we did not find synergy between the growth factors EGF or bFGF and any of the ECM proteins.[60]

Synergism between growth factors and ECM proteins has been previously observed in other cell types. As previously mentioned, Yabkowitz et al, who studied the effect of TSP on PDGF-dependent migration of calf pulmonary artery SMCs, noted a 60% increase in PDGF-induced migration with concentrations of TSP that alone had no effect on SMC migration.[47] Vitronectin and type IV collagen have also been noted to synergistically increase chemotaxis induced by insulin-like growth factor I in a human breast cancer cell line.[61]

Integrins

The above outlined effect of matrix proteins on SMC locomotion are mediated largely through activation of integrin receptors.[62] It is through these receptors that matrix proteins are able to influence the intracellular machinery that is necessary to initiate the migratory response. Identification of the integrin receptors that are required for matrix protein-driven SMC migration is critical to the understanding of this complex process.

Integrins are a family of heterodimeric cell surface receptors composed of α and β subunits.[63] Approximately 17 different α subunits and 8 β subunits and over 20 different $\alpha\beta$ pairings have been identified. Three families of integrins have been designated according to their β subunits, which include β_1, β_2, or β_3. Beta $_2$ is localized largely in platelets; however, β_1 and β_3 have been detected in vascular SMCs.[15] A single ECM protein is able to bind multiple integrin receptors and a single integrin receptor is able to bind multiple ligands.[64] In this way, the same ECM protein can mediate different cellular responses via a variety of integrin receptors. Therefore, past associations of a single integrin and receptor such as the designation of $\alpha_5\beta_1$ as the "fibronectin" receptor and $\alpha_v\beta_3$ as the "vitronectin" receptor are too restrictive, since both $\alpha_5\beta_1$ and $\alpha_v\beta_3$ are able to be affected by multiple ECM proteins. Thus, the control over cellular function exerted via integrin receptors is complex and critically important to normal and abnormal cellular function. Although there has been extensive investigation of integrins and their importance in vascular biology, here we will discuss the different integrins involved in matrix protein driven SMC migration.

Choi et al explored the role of the $\alpha_v\beta_3$ integrin in human and rabbit PDGF-AB stimulated SMC migration.[65] These investigators chose to study $\alpha_v\beta_3$ because of its ability to bind to several ECM proteins by its RGD-containing binding site, making it a possible candidate as a mediator of cell motility. Antibodies to $\alpha_v\beta_3$, as well as an RGD peptide antagonist of this same integrin, both inhibited PDGF-AB stimulated SMC migration in vitro, albeit incompletely, implicating involvement of other integrins in this process. They did not assess the in vitro role of $\alpha_v\beta_3$ in matrix protein driven SMC migration. In a rabbit carotid injury model, these same investigators found that a monoclonal antibody to $\alpha_v\beta_3$ did not inhibit intimal hyperplasia, although a specific RGD peptide antagonist did. Further supporting the role of $\alpha_v\beta_3$ in SMC migration, Clyman et al studied migration in fetal lamb ductus arteriosus SMC and found that SMC migration on type I and IV collagen, fibronectin, and laminin was mediated predominantly by the $\alpha_v\beta_3$ integrin.[66] The importance of the $\alpha_v\beta_3$ integrin in SMC migration, however, remains controversial. Recent immunocytochemical studies by Hosiga et al revealed that the $\alpha_v\beta_3$ was localized only in the media and not the neointima of rat aortic tissue following injury.[67] Skinner et al were not able to identify the $\alpha_v\beta_3$ integrin in an arterial SMC line.[64] In immunohistochemical studies from this laboratory, cultured human saphenous vein SMC stained only weakly positive for the $\alpha_v\beta_3$ integrin and only after permeabilization.[68] We were not able to identify the $\alpha_v\beta_3$ integrin in the intima or media of hyperplastic lesions excised from patients following saphenous vein bypass grafting (despite positive staining for this integrin in the microvessels of the adventitia of these same lesions), nor was $\alpha_v\beta_3$ present in atherosclerotic plaque removed at the time of carotid endarterectomy. Using SMC derived from human saphenous vein and blocking antibodies, we found that $\alpha_v\beta_3$ was not required for ECM protein (collagen type I or IV, laminin, fibronectin, or vitronectin) stimulated SMC migration; however $\alpha_v\beta_3$ did play a role in PDGF mediated chemotaxis.[68]

Our studies and those of others suggest that the β_1 integrin subunit has a more dominant role in SMC migration.[68] Skinner et al studied several β_1 integrin combinations and demonstrated that $\alpha_1\beta_1$, but not $\alpha_2\beta_1$, was expressed in vivo in normal intact human arterial tissue; however in cell culture the expression of α_1 was downregulated and $\alpha_2\beta_1$ was upregulated.[64] These authors postulated that $\alpha_1\beta_1$ may be present in normal venous tissue, but that hyperplastic plaque might then preferentially express $\alpha_2\beta_1$, and that this conversion might contribute to the pathophysiology of intimal hyperplasia. In immunohistochemical studies of normal human saphenous vein and specimens of intimal hyperplasia derived from excised vein grafts, we found the β_1 subunit to be homogeneously distributed throughout both normal and abnormal tissues.[68] Similarly, the α_1 integrin was found in normal human saphenous vein as well as hyperplastic tissue from saphenous vein grafts. Interestingly, the α_2 integrin was only identified in specimens of intimal hyperplasia, corroborating the hypothesis proposed by Skinner et al that the $\alpha_2\beta_1$ integrin is expressed only following arterial injury.

We conducted further studies which verified the physiologic importance of the $\alpha_2\beta_1$ integrin in human SMC migration. We found that a blocking antibody to the β_1 integrin subunit produced an inhibitory effect on chemotaxis and haptotaxis to type I and IV collagen, fibronectin, and laminin.[68] This effect was consistently greater for type I collagen and laminin versus type IV collagen and fibronectin. Moreover, a blocking antibody to the α_2 integrin subunit inhibited chemotaxis and haptotaxis to type I and IV collagen and laminin, though these effects were less than those observed with the β_1 antibody.[68] In similar experiments, Skinner et al found that a blocking antibody to the $\alpha_2\beta_1$ integrin also inhibited migration of cultured human SMCs on type I collagen.[64]

There is some evidence that the $\alpha_1\beta_1$ integrin might also be involved in SMC migration. Clyman et al detected $\alpha_1\beta_1$ in cultured rat vascular SMC.[69] Moreover, Gotwals et al, again using rat SMC, found that $\alpha_1\beta_1$ is the primary facilitator of SMC migration on collagen.[70] It is possible that the findings of the latter two studies were related to the use of rat SMC, and the critical integrin necessary for SMC migration may differ between human and rat.

In our immunohistochemical studies, the α_5 subunit was found homogeneously distributed throughout normal human saphenous vein vascular SMCs and in hyperplastic plaques from saphenous vein grafts; however, a blocking antibody to the α_5 integrin subunit had no effect on chemotaxis or haptotaxis of saphenous vein SMC following their stimulation with any of the ECM proteins.[68] Though the $\alpha_5\beta_1$ has been reported by other investigators to be the prototypical integrin for fibronectin,[21] our results suggest that this integrin does not mediate fibronectin migration of human saphenous vein SMC.

It is important to note that there is tremendous variation in the distribution and function of integrins from one tissue to another (animal versus human, primary versus cultured cells, artery versus vein). Therefore, it is necessary to critically analyze data from the appropriate cell type before making conclusions about the importance of integrins in remodeling after vascular injury. In studies of SMC derived from human saphenous vein, we and Skinner et al have found the α_2 and β_1 subunits to be the most critical receptors required for ECM protein stimulated chemotaxis and haptotaxis.[64,68] Thus, modulating the $\alpha_2\beta_1$ integrin may be a potentially effetive method for controlling intimal hyperplasia.

Cell Signaling

We and others have extensively evaluated the intracellular signaling pathways associated with PDGF-induced cell migration. A variety of signaling proteins and ions appear to be involved, including phosphatidylinositol-3-OH kinase (PI3K),[71] phospholipase C (PLC),[72] MAPK,[73] Src,[74] calcium,[75] calmodulin-dependent protein kinase II (CamKII),[76] and the small G-protein rho.[77] The intracellular signaling events that mediate matrix protein-induced SMC migration have been less well studied. Our early investigations suggest that at least some of these pathways may be distinct from those used by growth factor receptors.

Matrix protein-driven signaling events are initiated through activation of integrin receptors.[62] As previously mentioned, matrix proteins attach to the extracellular domain of integrin receptors, and the short cytoplasmic domains of both the α and β integrin subunits allow transfer of messages to the intracellular environment.[15] These cytoplasmic domains have direct access to the signaling machinery in the cell, and studies have demonstrated that mutations or truncations of the distal end of both the α and the β cytoplasmic tail can interfere with integrin signaling and cytoskeletal organization.[78] Further evidence of the importance of the β subunit in intracellular signaling can be derived from studies where overexpression of a single β cytoplasmic tail leads to inhibition of tyrosine phosphorylation of intracellular proteins such as FAK,[79] whereas overexpression of multiple β subunits configured in clusters results in an increase in tyrosine phosphorylation.[80] Through these and similar studies, the concept has evolved that integrin clustering is a prerequisite for the initiation of intracellular signalling.[81] In in vitro studies, the α and β cytoplasmic domains have been found to couple with a variety of cytoplasmic proteins such as p125[FAK], α-actinin, talin, vinculin and paxillin.[17] It is activation of these proteins that allows for the induction of intracellular signaling pathways that lead to migration.

Focal adhesion kinase (FAK) is a nonreceptor tyrosine kinase that has been found to be activated by both ECM and soluble signaling factors.[81] Ligand attachment leads to direct phosphorylation of FAK by the β subunit of the integrin receptor.[16] FAK can then interact with Src, another nonreceptor tyrosine kinase, which is localized to focal adhesions by its SH2 domain.[82] Src in turn can activate the Ras/MAPK signaling pathways,[83] both which have been previously implicated in SMC migration.[73,84] MAPK may promote migration either through the phosphorylation and activation of transcription factors which regulate integrin gene expression, or by phosphorylating and activating cytoplasmic phospholipase A2 (cPLA2), which hydrolyzes glycerophospholipids to produce arachidonic acid.[16] It has been previously demonstrated that inhibition of cPLA2 prevents cell migration, an effect that can be reversed by the readdition of arachidonic acid.[16]

We and others have shown a relationship between levels of intracellular calcium and PDGF-induced SMC migration.[75,76] We postulated that a rise in intracellular calcium might also be required for SMC migration in response to matrix proteins.[60] Despite the potent stimulatory effect of collagen types I and IV, fibronectin, and laminin on SMC migration, none of the matrix proteins produced a sustained or prolonged rise in intracellular calcium.[60] This was true even if calcium measurements were carried out for more than 30 minutes after stimulation. This finding was surprising, since activation of the $\alpha_v\beta_1$ integrin by fibronectin has been shown to produce a persistent rise in intracellular calcium in endothelial cells.[85] These findings imply that calcium plays little if any role in matrix protein stimulated SMC locomotion. We did find that fibronectin, laminin, and type I and IV collagen augmented the early peak in intracellular calcium produced by PDGF.[60] Although it is possible that this augmentation provides at least a partial explanation for the synergistic enhancement by matrix proteins of PDGF-induced SMC migration, the physiologic relevance of this finding is still unclear.

We have also studied the role of large G-proteins (Gs) in the intracellular signaling pathways involved in matrix protein-driven SMC migration.[54] Cholera toxin, which leads to constitutive activation of Gs,[21] profoundly inhibited SMC migration in response to collagen types I and IV, fibronectin, and laminin and even eliminated baseline migration in unstimulated cells.[54] Activation of Gs increases levels of cAMP through stimulation of adenylate cyclase, and agonists of cAMP such as forskolin and 8-bromo-cAMP have been found to inhibit SMC migration.[86] Thus, the inhibitory effect of Gs activation with cholera toxin may be due to elevated levels of cAMP.[87] Surprisingly, pertussis toxin, which inhibits the Gi subtypes, including Gi1, Gi2, and Gi3, and thereby releases the inhibitory effect that Gi has on adenylate cyclase,[21] had no effect on chemotaxis or haptotaxis to fibronectin, type I or type IV collagen.[54] However, pertussis toxin did partially inhibit haptotaxis and completely eliminated chemotaxis to laminin.[54] Similarly, Aznavoorian et al found that pertussis toxin decreased chemotactic migration of A2058 human melanoma cells when stimulated with laminin; however, with these same cells there was no inhibition of fibronectin-induced chemotaxis.[88] Although Gi proteins can influence adenylate cyclase, the multiple Gi subtypes can also interact with enzymes such as phospholipase A2, C, and D, and ion transporters such as potassium and calcium channels.[89] Thus, the varying role that pertussis toxin has on SMC migration may be due to either inhibition of the inhibitory influence of Gi on cAMP or perhaps the lack of interaction of Gi with one or more of these other signaling substrates.

ECM proteins are known to play a role in the turnover of phospholipids. In fibroblasts, fibronectin increased the production of phosphatidylinositol 4,5 bisphosphate (PIP_2) and dissociation of these same cells from fibronectin resulted in a rapid decrease in cellular PIP_2.[90] PIP_2, in turn, has been implicated in cellular migration[91] and this effect may be mediated by several pathways. It has been speculated that the upregulation of the production of PIP_2 may facilitate the polymerization of actin because of a regulatory effect of PIP_2 on actin binding proteins such as profilin.[16] PIP_2 is also an important substrate for the enzyme PLC.[63] PLC hydrolyzes PIP_2 into the active second messengers diacylglycerol (DAG) and inositol trisphosphate (IP3), which then respectively activate protein kinase C (PKC) and the release of intracellular calcium. Both PKC and calcium have been implicated in the signaling pathways for cell migration.[75,92]

We have previously demonstrated that growth factors and matrix proteins act synergistically to promote SMC migration.[60] The mechanism through which these two agonists might interact is not clear; however, the point of intersection may be either at the level of the receptor or at a mutual downstream signaling pathway. There is some evidence that ECM activation of integrins can up or downregulate growth factor receptors. The term "crosstalk" has been used to describe such interactions between growth factor receptors and integrins.[93] We have recently reported that type I collagen enhances clustering and activation of the PDGF-β receptor.[94] Tyrosine phosphorylation by growth factor receptors of the cytoplasmic domains of integrins, or of proteins associated with the focal adhesion complex is an additional mechanism by which these two ligands/receptors might interact.[60] Other potential sites of interaction are at the level of the proteins, MAPK, PI3K and/or PIP_2. It is important that we investigate the synergistic interactions between matrix proteins and growth factors, since these points of interaction may represent exceedingly effective targets for inhibitors of intimal hyperplasia.

Conclusion

In this chapter, we have reviewed the effect of the numerous matrix components of the vessel wall on SMC migration. It is clear that many of these proteins produce a strong stimulus for migration. Moreover, the effect of these matrix proteins on SMC migration may be more profound than that of many of the growth factors that have been traditionally studied. We have also shown that these matrix proteins can interact with growth factors to provide a synergistic stimulus for SMC locomotion. The chemotaxic effect of matrix proteins is mediated through integrin receptors of which, at least for human venous SMC, $\alpha_2\beta_1$ appears to be the most critical. The signaling pathways that mediate matrix-induced migration have not been fully elucidated but appear to be distinct from those that mediate migration of SMC in response to growth factors.

Vascular disease remains a major cause of morbidity and mortality in the United States. Treatment is often palliative because of the frequent occurrence of recurrent disease at sites of vascular reconstruction. Engineering of an "ideal" vascular graft that is not affected by intimal hyperplasia would prolong life and reduce morbidity. Matrix proteins must be an essential component of this engineered conduit, and the proteins that are included should be chosen based not only on their structural characteristics but also on their effect on SMC physiology and pathophysiology. Moreover, with the realization that ECM proteins and integrins play an important role in SMC migration, pharmacological agents such as integrin inhibitors may be developed and integrated into vascular grafts to prevent the formation of intimal hyperplasia. The development of an ideal prosthesis is an onerous task but before this goal can be realized, there must be a thorough understanding of the pathophysiology of restenosis in vascular reconstructions.

References

1. Chervu A, Moore WS. An overview of intimal hyperplasia. Surg Gynecol Obstet 1990; 171:433-40.
2. Donaldson MC, Mannick JA, Whittemore AD. Causes of primary graft failure after in situ saphenous vein bypass grafting. J Vasc Surg 1992; 15:113-20.
3. Casscells W. Migration of smooth muscle and endothelial cells. Critical events in restenosis. Circ 1992; 86:723-9.
4. Clowes AW, Schwartz SM. Significance of quiescent smooth muscle cell migration in the injured rat carotid artery. Circ Res 1985; 56:139-45.
5. Ross R. The pathogenesis of atherosclerosis: A perspective for the 1990s. Nature 1993; 362:801-9.
6. Mii S, Ware JA, Kent KC. Transformtin growth factor-β inhibits human vascular smooth muscle cell growth and migration. Surgery 1993; 114:464-70.

7. Chen P, Gupta K, Wells A. Cell movement elicted by epidermal growth factor receptor requires kinase and autophosphorylation but is separable from mitogenesis. J Cell Biol 1994; 124:547-555.
8. Madri JA, Bell L, Marx M et al. Effects of soluble factors and extracellular matrix components on vascular behavior in vitro and in vivo: Models of de-endothelialization and repair. J Cell Biochem 1991; 45(2):123-30.
9. Stossel TP. From signal to pseudopod. J Biol Chem 1989; 264:18261-18264.
10. Vandekerckhove J. Actin-binding proteins. Curr Opin in Cell Biol 1990; 2:41-50.
11. Burridge K, Fath K, Kelly T et al. Focal adhesions: Transmembrane junctions between the extracellular matrix and the cytoskeleton. Ann Rev Cell Biol 1988; 4:487-525.
12. Luna EJ, Hitt AL. Cytoskeleton-plasma membrane interactions. Science 1992; 258:955-964.
13. Huttenlocher A, Ginsberg MH, Horwitz AF. Modulation of cell migration by integrin-mediated cytoskeletal linkages and ligand-binding affinity. J Cell Biol 1996; 134(6);1551-62.
14. Stossel TP. On the crawling of animal cells. Science 1993; 260(5111):1086-94.
15. Hynes RO. Intergrins: Versatility, modulation and signalling in cell adhesion. Cell 1992; 68:11-25.
16. Clark EA, Brugge JS. Integrins and signal transduction pathways: The road taken. Science 1995; 268:233-238.
17. Shattil SJ, Ginsberg MH. Integrin signaling in vascular biology J Clin Invest 1997; 100(1):1-5.
18. Bendeck MP, Irvin C, Reidy MA. Inhibition of matrix metalloproteinase activity inhibits smooth muscle cell migration but not neointimal thickening after arterial injury. Circ Res 1996; 78::38-43.
19. Kenagy RD, Vergel S, Mattsson E et al. The role of plasminogen, plasminogen activators, and matrix metalloproteinases in primate arterial smooth muscle cell migration. Arterioscler Throm Vasc Biol 1996; 16(11):1373-82.
20. Schwartz SM. Smooth muscle migration in atherosclerosis and restenosis. J Clin Invest 1997; 99(12):2814-2817.
21. Zetter BR, Brightman SE. Cell motility and the extracellular matrix. Curr Opin Cell Biol 1990, 2:850-856.
22. Taraboletti G, Roberts DD, Liotta LA. Thrombospondin induced tumor cell migration: Haptotaxis and chemotaxis are mediated by different molecular domains. J Cell Biol 1987; 105:2409-15.
23. Ruoslahti E, Engvall E. Integrins and vascular extracellular matrix assembly. J Clin Invest 1997; 99(6):1149-52.
24. Carey DJ. Control of growth and differentiation of vascular cells by extracellular matrix proteins. Annu Rev Physiol 1991; 53:161-77.
25. Murata K, Motayama T, Kotake C. Collagen types in various layers of the human aorta and their changes with the atherosclerotic process. Athero 1986; 60:251-62.
26. Ross R, Klebanoff SJ. The smooth muscle cell: In vivo synthesis of connective tissue proteins. J Cell Biol 1971; 50:159-171.
27. Wight TN, Ross R. Proteoglycans in primate arteries: Synthesis and secretion of glycosaminoglycans by arterial smooth muscle cells in culture. J Cell Biol 1975; 67:675-686.
28. Kraiss LW, Kirkman TR, Kohler TR et al. Shear stress regulates smooth muscle proliferation and neointimal thickening in porous polytetrafluoroethylene grafts. Arterio and throm 1991; 11:1844-1852.

29. Geary RL, Kohler TR, Vergel S et al. Time course of flow-induced smooth muscle cell proliferation and intimal thickening in endothelialized baboon vascular grafts. Circ Res 1993; 74:14-23.

30. Barnes M. Collagens in atherosclerosis. Collagen Rel Res 1985; 5:65-97.

31. Snow AD, Bolender RP, Wight TN, Clowes AW. Heparin modulates the composition of the extracellular matrix domain surrounding arterial smooth muscle cells. Am J Pathol 1990; 137:313-330.

32. Bjorkerud S. Cultivated human arterial smooth muscle displays heterogeneous pattern of growth and phenotypic variation. Lab Invest 1985; 53(3):303-310.

33. Van Zanten GH, de Graaf S, Slootweg PJ et al. Increased platelet deposition on atherosclerotic coronary arteries. J Clin Invest 1994; 93(2):615-32.

34. Wolf YG, Rasmussen LM, Ruoslahti E. Antibodies against transforming growth factor β-1 suppresses intimal hyperplasia in a rat model. J Clin Invest 1994; 93:1172-1178.

35. O'Brien ER, Garvin MR, Stewart DK et al. Osteopontin is synthesized by macrophage, smooth muscle, and endothelial cells in primary and restenotic human coronary atherosclerotic plaques. Arterioscler Throm 1994; 14(10):1648-56.

36. Van Aken BE, Seiffert D, Thinnes T et al. Localization of vitronectin in the normal and atherosclerotic human vessel wall. Histochem Cell Biol 1997; 107(4):313-20.

37. Patel MK, Clunn GF, Lymn JS et al. Thrombospondin-1 induces DNA synthesis and migration in human vascular smooth muscle cells. Biochem Soc Trans 1996; 24(3):446

38. Hedin U, Holm J, Hansson GK. Induction of tenascin in rat arterial injury. Relationship to altered smooth muscle cell phenotype. Am J Path 1991; 139(3):649-56.

39. Liaw L, Almeida M, Hart CE et al. Osteopontin promotes vascular cell adhesion and spreading and is chemotactic for smooth muscle cells in vitro. Circ Res 1994; 74:214-224.

40. Fitzpatrick LA, Severson A, Edwards WD et al. Diffuse calcification in human coronary arteries: Association of osteopontin with atherosclerosis. J Clin Invest 1994; 94:1597-1604.

41. Yue T, McKenna PJ, Ohlstein EH et al. Osteopontin-stimulated vascular smooth muscle cell migration is mediated by β3 integrin. Exp Cell Res 1994; 214:459-464.

42. Liaw L, Lombardi DM, Almeida SM et al. Neutralizing antibodies directed against osteopontin inhibit rat carotid neointimal thickening following endothelial denudation. Arterioscler Thromb Vasc Biol 1997; 17:188-193.

43. Chen C, Ku DN, Kikeri D et al. Tenascin: A potential role in human arteriovenous PTFE graft failure. J Surg Res 1996; 60(2):409-16.

44. Murphy-Ullrich JE, Pallero MA, Boerth N et al. Cyclic GMP-dependent protein kinase is required for thrombospondin and tenascin mediated focal adhesion disassembly. J Cell Sci 1996; 109(10):2499-508.

45. Majesky MW. Neointima formation after acute vascular injury. Role of counteradhesive extracellular matrix proteins. Tex Heart Inst J 1994; 21(1):78-85.

46. Hahn AW, Jonas U, John M et al. Functional aspects of vascular tenascin-c expression. J Vasc Res 1995; 32(3):162-74.

47. Yabkowitz R, Mansfield PJ, Ryan US et al. Thrombospondin mediates migration and potentiates platelet-derived growth factor-dependent migration of calf pulmonary artery smooth muscle cells. Jour Cell Physio 1993; 157:24-32.

48. Riessen R, Wight TN, Pastore C et. al. Distribution of hyaluron during extracellular matrix remodeling in human restenotic arteries and balloon-injured rat carotid arterties. Circ 1996; 93:1141-1147.

49. Savani RC, Wang C, Yang B et al. Migration of bovine aortic smooth muscle cells after wounding injury: The role of hyaluronan and RHAMM. J Clin Invest 1995; 95:1158-1168.

50. Niculescu F, Rus HG, Porutiu D et al. Immunoelectron-microscopic localization of S-protein/vitronectin in human atherosclerotic wall. Athero 1989; 78(2-3)197-203.

51. Preissner KT. Structure and biological role of vitronectin. Annu Rev Cell Biol 1991; 7:275-310.

52. Naito M et al. Vitronectin-induced haptotaxis of vascular smooth muscle cells in vitro. Exp Cell Research 1991; 194:154-156.

53. Brown SL, Lundgren CH, Nordt T et al. Stimulation of migration of human aortic smooth muscle cells by vitronectin: Implications for atherosclerosis. Cardiovas Research 1994; 24:1815-1820.

54. Nelson PR, Yamamura S, Kent CK. Extracellular matrix proteins are potent agonist of human smooth muscle cell migration. J Vasc Surg 1996; 24:25-33.

55. DiMilla PA, Stone JA, Quinn JA et al. Maximal migration of human smooth muscle cells on fibronectin and collagen iv occurs at an intermediate attachment strength. J Cell Biol 1993; 122:729-37.

56. Mii S, Ware JA, Kent KC. Transformtin growth factor-β inhibits human vascular smooth muscle cell growth and migration. Surgery 1993; 114:464-470.

57. Tsuruoka T, Azetaka M, Iizuka Y et al. Inhibition of tumor cell haptotaxis by sodium D-glucaro-delta-lactam. Jpn J Cancer Res 1995; 86(11):1080-5.

58. Keller UH, Wissler JH, Ploem J. Chemotaxis is not a special case of haptotaxis. Experienta 1979; 35:1669-71.

59. Taraboletti G, Roberts DD, Liotta LA. Thrombospondin-induced tumor cell migration: Haptotaxis and chemotaxis are mediated by different molecular domains. J Cell Biol 1987; 105:2409-15.

60. Nelson PR, Yamamura S, Kent CK. Platelet-derived growth factor and extracellular matrix proteins provide a synergistic stimulus for human vascular smooth muscle cell migration. J Vasc Surg 1997; 26:104-12.

61. Doerr ME, Jones JI. The roles of integrins and extracellular matrix proteins in the insulin-like growth factor I-stimulated chemotaxis of human breast cancer cells. J Biol Chem 1996; 271:2443-47

62. Clark EA, Brugge JS. Integrins and signal transduction pathways: The road taken. Science 1995; 268:233-238.

63. Schwartz MA. Transmembrane signaling by integrins. Trends Cell Biol 1992; 2:304-8.

64. Skinner MP, Raines EW, and Ross R. Dynamic expression of $\alpha_1\beta_1$ and $\alpha_2\beta_1$ integrin receptors by human vascular smooth muscle cells. Am J Pathol 1994; 145:1070-1081.

65. Choi ET, Engel L, Callow A et al. Inhibition of neointimal hyperplasia by blocking $\alpha_v\beta_3$ integrin with a small peptide antagonist GpenGRDSPCA. J Vasc Surg 1994; 19:125-34.

66. Clyman RI, Mauray F, Kramer RH. β_1 and β_3 integrins have different roles in the adhesion and migration of vascular smooth muscle cells on extracellular matrix. Exp Cell Res 1992; 200:272-284.

67. Hosiga M, Alpers CE, Smith LL. $\alpha_v\beta_3$ integrin expression in normal and atherosclerotic artery. Circ Res 1995; 77:1129-1135.

68. Itoh H, Nelson PR, Mureebe L et al. The role of integrins in saphenous vein vascular smooth muscle cell migration. J Vasc Surg 1997; 25:1061-9.

69. Clyman RI, Turner DC, Kramer RH. An $\alpha_1\beta_1$-like integrin receptor on rat aortic smooth muscle cells mediates adhesion to laminin and collagen types I and IV. Arterio 1990; 10:402-409.

70. Gotwals PJ, Chi Rosso G, Lindner V et al. The $\alpha_1\beta_1$ integrin is expressed during neointima formation in rat arteries and mediates collagen matrix reorganization. J Clin Invest 1996; 97:2469-2477.

71. Yamamura S, Derman MP, Cantly LG et al. The role of phosphatidylinositol 3-kinase in proliferation and migration of human vascular smooth muscle cells. Book of Abstracts, Annual Meeting of the Society for Vascular Surgery, 1995, p.53

72. Yamamura S, Nelson PR, Mureebe L, Kent KC. Proliferation and migration of vascular smooth muscle cells are mediated by distince signaling pathways involving phospholipase C. Surgical Forum Volume 1996; 47:362-64.

73. Nelson PR, Mureebe L, Itoh H, Kent KC. Smooth muscle cell migration and proliferation are mediated by distinct phases of activation of the intracellular messenger mitogen-activated protein kinase. Submitted J Vasc Surg. 1997.

74. Mureebe L, Nelson PR, Yamamura S, Kent KC. Activation of pp60^{c-src} is necessary for human smooth muscle cell migration. In Press, Surgery 1997.

75. Yamamura S, Nelson PR, Kent KC. The role of intracellular calcium in migration of human vascular smooth muscle cells. Surgical Forum Volume 1995; 46:386-389.

76. Pauly RR, Bilato C, Sollott SJ. Role of calcium/calmodulin-dependent protein kinase II in the regulation of vascular smooth muscle cell migration. Circ 1995; 91(4):1107-1115.

77. Jiang B, Ware JA, Mallette SA, Kent KC. Migration and proliferation of vascular smooth muscle cells are mediated by distinct signal transduction pathways. Circ 1994; 90:1190.

78. Ylanne J, Huuskonen J, O'Toole TE et al. Mutation of the cytoplasmic domain of the integrin β3 subunit: Differential effects on cell spreading and migration, and matrix assembly. J Cell Biol 1994; 270:9550-9557.

79. Chen YP, O'Toole TE, Shipley T et al. "Inside-out" signal transduction inhibited by isolated integrin cytoplasmic domians. J Biol Chem 1994; 269:18307-18310.

80. Lukashev ME, Sheppard D, Pytela R. Disruption of integrin function and induction of tyrosine phosphorylation by the autonomously expressed β1 integrin cytoplasmic domain. J Biol Chem 1994; 269:18311-18314.

81. Illic D, Damsky CH, Yamamoto T. Focal adhesion kinase: At the crossroads of signal transduction. J Cell Sci 1997; 110:401-407.

82. Calalb MB, Polte TR, Hanks SK. Tyrosine phosphorylation of focal adhesion kinase at sites in the catalytic domain regulates kinase activity: A role for Src family kinases. Mol Cell Biol 1995; 15:954-63.

83. Schlaepfer DD, Hanks SK, Hunter T et al. Integrin-mediated signal transduction linked to Ras pathway by GRB2 binding to focal adhesion kinase. Nature 1995; 372:786-791.

84. Irani K, Herzlinger S, Finkel T. Ras proteins regulate multiple mitogenic pathways in A10 vascular smooth muscle cells. Biochem Biophys Res Commun 1994; 202(3):1252-8.

85. Schwartz MA, Denninghoff K. Alpha v integrins mediate the rise in intracellular calcium in endothelial cells on fibronectin even though they play a minor role in adhesion. J Biol Chem 1994; 269(15):11133-7.

86. Horio T, Kohno M, Kano H et al. Arenomedulin as a novel antimigration factor of vascular smooth muscle cells. Circ Res 1995; 77:660-4.

87. Gilman AG. G-proteins: Transducers of receptor-generated signals. Annu Rev Biochem 1987; 56:615-49.

88. Aznavoorian S, Stracke ML, Krutzch H et al. Signal transduction for chemotaxis and haptotaxis by matrix molecules in tumor cells. J Cell Biol 1990; 110:1427-1438.

89. Lester BR, McCarthy JB, Sun Z. G-protein involvement in matrix-mediated motility and invasion of high and low experimental metastatic B16 melanoma clones. Can Res 1989; 49:5940-5948.

90. McNamee HP, Ingber DE, Schwartz MA. Adhesion to fibronectin stimulates inositol lipid synthesis and enhances PDGF-induced inositol lipid breakdown. J Cell Biol 1993; 121:673-8.

91. McNamee HP, Liley HG, Ingber DE. Integrin-dependent control of inositol lipid synthesis in vascular endothelial cells and smooth muscle cells. Exp Cell Res 1996; 224(1):116-22.

92. Vuori K and Ruoslahti E. Activation of protein kinase C precedes alpha 5 beta 1 integrin-mediated cell spreading on fibronectin. J Biol Chem 1993; 268(29):21459-2.

93. Seki J, Koyama N, Kovach NL et al. Regulation of β1 integrin function in cultured human vascular smooth muscle cells. Circ Res 1996; 78:596-605.

94. Itoh H, Mureebe L, Kubaska S, Kent KC. Type I collagen enhances phosphorylation of the PDGF receptor and acts synergistically to augment PDGF-induced vascular smooth muscle cell proliferation. Surgical Forum Volume XLVIII 1997:406-408.

Facilitation of Healing

Matrix Modulation

──────────────── CHAPTER 33 ────────────────

Extracellular Matrix Effect on Endothelial Control of Smooth Muscle Cell Migration and Matrix Synthesis

Richard J. Powell

Introduction

Intimal hyperplasia remains the most common cause of early failure following angioplasty and bypass surgery.[1,2] Intimal hyperplasia is a particularly prevalent problem in small diameter synthetic grafts used for extremity bypasses performed to tibial and peroneal targets.[3] The development of intimal hyperplasia following smooth muscle cell (SMC) injury is characterized by SMC dedifferentiation from a contractile to synthetic phenotype.[4,5] Following phenotypic modulation, SMCs migrate into the subintimal space, proliferate and secrete extracellular matrix. For the first several weeks following injury the intimal hyperplastic lesion is predominantly cellular. However, as the lesion continues to enlarge, extracellular matrix gradually becomes the predominant component.[1,4-7] Several months following injury, extracellular matrix comprises 80% of the mature intimal hyperplastic lesion.[8]

In several recent studies, endothelial cell (EC) seeding of injured arterial wall segments and synthetic grafts has been shown to limit the development of intimal hyperplasia. Bush and co-workers have shown that EC seeding of endarterectomized canine arteries decreased the intimal hyperplastic response.[8,9] Conte has shown that EC seeding of injured hypercholesterolemic rabbit femoral arteries also limits the intimal hyperplastic response.[10] In addition, several in vivo human studies have shown improved patency of endothelial sodded synthetic grafts when compared to unsodded grafts.[11-14] The improved patency has been attributed to decreased thrombogenicity and increased resistance to intimal hyperplasia in the sodded grafts. Zilla and co-workers have recently shown that EC lined synthetic grafts have a 73%, 5 year primary patency rate in the below knee position compared to 31% for unlined grafts.[12] They now have follow up data out to 6.5 years with a patency rate of 71% in the EC lined grafts and 0% in the controls.[11] However, not all studies of EC sodded grafts have shown improved patency rates. A report by Herring and co-workers failed to show any improvement in EC sodded graft patency when compared to control grafts.[3] One explanation for the lack of effect of EC sodding was thought to be the low EC seeding density used to line the grafts, which resulted in an incomplete coverage of the graft lumen.

Extracellular matrix profoundly affects both endothelial and smooth muscle cell function. Following arterial wall injury, not only is extracellular matrix quantity increased but alterations in matrix composition occurs as well. Matrix composition can affect SMC functions such as migration and proliferation, and may also affect matrix synthesis.[15] For instance, following vascular wall injury there is an increase in type I collagen present within the restenotic lesion. Type I collagen has been shown to stimulate smooth muscle cell

Tissue Engineering of Prosthetic Vascular Grafts, edited by Peter Zilla and Howard P. Greisler.
©1999 R.G. Landes Company.

dedifferentiation and increase SMC proliferation.[16] In addition, type I collagen has been shown to upregulate the expression of the growth factor TGF-β1.[17] TGF-β1 is a potent stimulant of extracellular matrix synthesis and inhibits matrix degradation.[18] TGF-β1 has been shown to potentiate the development of intimal hyperplasia in animal models following arterial injury.[19] In similar studies, neutralizing antibodies to TGF-β1 have been shown to inhibit the development of intimal hyperplasia following arterial injury. Transcripts to TGF-β1 are upregulated in intimal hyperplastic human coronary lesions retrieved by coronary atherectomy.[20] TGF-β1 appears to be an important mediator of the increased extracellular matrix deposition which occurs during vascular wall remodeling.

The effects of various extracellular matrix proteins on endothelial cell control of smooth muscle cell function is unknown. This information is important in the study of tissue engineering of prosthetic grafts. To which particular matrix protein endothelial cells and smooth muscle cells are exposed will determine what effect ECs have on such SMC functions as phenotype expression, proliferation, migration and matrix synthesis. This could obviously affect the patency of EC sodded prosthetic grafts. The purpose of the work performed in our laboratory is to define the effect of matrix composition on the ability of ECs to regulate smooth muscle cell functions. In particular, we are interested in the matrix effect on EC control of SMC migration and extracellular matrix synthesis. To study this we have developed a coculture model in which ECs are cultured opposite SMCs on a semipermeable membrane.

Model

Bovine aortic ECs and SMCs are harvested using the collagenase method for ECs and the explant method for SMCs. Cells are grown for 3-5 passages from primary cultures in Dulbecco's Modified Eagles Media/10% calf serum (DMEM/10% CS). ECs are identified by their cobblestone morphology and positive uptake of di-I-acetylated ldl. SMCs are identified using an anti-α-actin antibody (Sigma A-2547, Sigma Chemical, St. Louis, MO). For each component of these studies, SMC cultures are established by plating cells on a 13 μm thick polyethylene terapthalate (PET) membrane with 0.45 μm pores configured at a density of 1.6 million pores/cm² (Cyclopore membrane, Falcon cell culture insert, Becton Dickinson, Lincoln Park, NJ). EC/SMC cocultures

are established by plating ECs on the outer side of the membrane and grown to confluence over 3-5 days. Once the ECs are confluent (2-3 days, as determined by phase contrast microscopy), SMCs are plated on the opposite side of the PET membrane (see Fig. 33.1). After 24 h both cell types are placed in DMEM/2.5% CS for the duration of each experiment.

This coculture model allows for the diffusion of soluble factors across the membrane, yet the two cell types remain separated for examination. Previous work has shown that ECs maintain SMCs in a more differentiated contractile phenotype when compared to SMCs cultured alone, which exhibit a synthetic phenotype.[21,22] There is limited physical contact across the membrane during the first 4-6 days following coculture; after which, however, SMC cytoplasmic projections begin to cross the membrane and contact the ECs.[23]

Effect of Matrix on Endothelial Cell Control of Smooth Muscle Cell Migration

Migration of SMCs into the anastomotic site following bypass grafting is an early and important event in the development of intimal hyperplasia.[24] SMC migration occurs following phenotypic modulation to a synthetic phenotype and prior to SMC proliferation and extracellular matrix synthesis. The process of migration is distinct from cellular proliferation. Soluble factors such as bFGF, PDGF and extracellular matrix are involved in the control of SMC migration and appear to play a role in the intimal hyperplastic response.[24,25]

The role of ECs in modulating the SMC response to injury is unclear. Previous work evaluating the effect of ECs on SMC proliferation have yielded controversial results and have not directly addressed the effect of ECs on SMC migration. In vivo studies by Fingerle and co-workers have demonstrated that the loss of ECs from the arterial intima results in the development of an intimal hyperplastic lesion and that this lesion formation can be limited by rapid re-endothelialization.[26] Although this is suggestive of the important role of ECs in limiting this process, these authors have not identified an EC released substance which might account for this phenomenon. Conte and co-workers failed to show any attenuation of the intimal hyperplastic response following early luminal EC seeding of balloon catheter injured arterial wall segments in rabbits with normal choles-

Fig. 33.1. Diagram of the coculture model consisting of a Falcon coculture insert shown in plate (A). This cell insert is placed in a six well tissue culture plate as shown in plate (B). Endothelial cells (ECs) are plated on

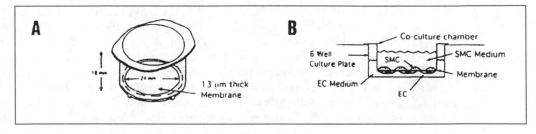

the under surface of the membrane and smooth muscle cells (SMCs) are plated on the upper surface. The membrane contains 0.45 μm pores configured at a density of 1.6 million pores/cm².

terol levels, but did show a reduction in intimal hyperplasia in a hypercholesterolemic model.[10] In addition, Reidy and Silver failed to show any increase in SMC replication following gentle denudation of ECs from the intimal surface as long as there was no injury to the underlying SMCs.[27] Several reports describing the increased resistance of EC sodded grafts to the development of intimal hyperplasia have been previously mentioned. More recently, synthetic graft seeding studies performed by Lewis and co-workers have shown that EC sodded grafts produce EC-derived vasoactive factors which could limit SMC proliferation and migration.[28] Thus it is unclear how important the role of the EC is in controlling SMC, migration and proliferation following vascular wall injury *in-vivo.*

In vitro cell culture studies by Castellot and co-workers have shown that ECs can inhibit SMC proliferation as a result of secreted heaprin sulfates from the abluminal endothelial cell surface.[29] These results conflict with studies performed by Fillinger and co-workers as well as from our own laboratory which have shown that ECs stimulate SMC proliferation when these two cell types were cocultured on opposite sides of a semipermeable membrane.[22,30] Since proliferation and migration are unassociated processes, these above studies cannot be used to address what effect ECs have on SMC migration. Using a steel fence assay our laboratory has previously demonstrated that ECs stimulate SMC migration in vitro and that this process can be mediated by a secreted soluble factor.[15] Possible factors involved include PDGF and endothelin-1, growth factors which have been shown to be secreted by cultured ECs. In addition, we have previously shown that ECs may regulate TGF-β1 activation in coculture.[22] Changes in TGF-β1 levels could as a result alter SMC migration. Finally, ECs may secrete extracellular matrix proteins which could deposit on the opposite side of the membrane and subsequently affect SMC migration.

Previous investigators have shown that SMC migration can be modulated by the extracellular matrix substrate composition. Our laboratory has shown that shown that fibronectin decreases the migration of SMCs cultured alone when compared to cells cultured on plastic (see Fig. 33.2).[15] The presence of ECs stimulated SMC migration on both plastic and fibronectin coated membranes. This finding was different when SMCs were cultured on type I collagen which stimulated migration in SMCs cultured alone compared to SMCs cultured on plastic or fibronectin. In addition, the presence of type I collagen significantly inhibited the ability of ECs to stimulate SMC migration such as that observed on plastic and fibronectin (see Fig. 33.2). Thus, matrix composition affected the EC ability to modulate SMC migration.

Cell matrix interactions which allow the cell to attach and detach from the extracellular matrix are also important in the migration process.[31] It has been shown that there is an intermediate cell attachment strength at which cell migration rate is optimized. Altering either the expression or organization of cell surface integrin and nonintegrin attachment molecules will subsequently affect cell migration, as will altering extracellular matrix composition. In support of this hypothesis are the recent reports which demonstrate that following dedifferentiation SMCs alter their expression of cell surface integrins, upregulating $\alpha_2\beta_1$ integrin and decreasing $\alpha_1\beta_1$ integrin expression.[32]

Basson and co-workers have shown that the growth factor TGF-β1 alters integrin expression, whereas matrix composition can change the cell surface integrin organization.[33] Our laboratory has shown that adhesion molecule expression and/or organization as determined by cell adhesion is altered by the presence of ECs.[15] This is true regardless of whether SMCs are cultured on fibronectin, type I collagen or plastic. The mechanism by which this occurs is

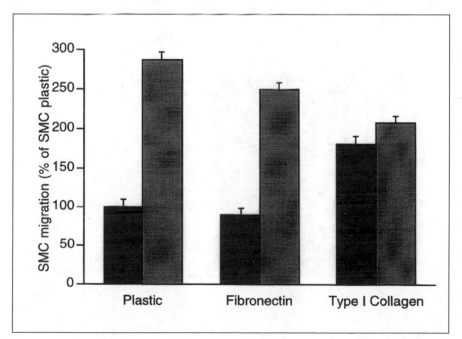

Fig. 33.2. Migration of SMCs cultured alone (Black bars) compared to SMCs cocultured with ECs (gray bars) on different extracellular matrices. ECs increased SMC migration on plastic and fibronectin (p < 0.01, SMC vs. EC/SMC). Type I collagen stimulated migration in SMCs cultured alone (p < 0.01, SMC type I collagen vs. SMC plastic and fibronectin). In addition, the presence of ECs resulted in only a minimal increase in migration on type I collagen. Results are expressed as the mean ± standard error of the mean (SEM).

unclear, but is likely related to the EC release of a soluble factor. At present antibodies specific for various bovine integrins are not available; however, future studies need to be performed to identify the specific integrin compositional and organizational changes in integrin expression that occur in SMCs as a result of ECs.

Cell spreading has been shown to correlate more closely with migration rate than cell attachment.[34] Whereas cell attachment is likely to be primarily integrin mediated, cell spreading appears to involve nonintegrin matrix binding proteins as well.[34] Differences in cell spreading on various matrix types were similar to those seen in SMC migration (plastic<fibronectin<type I collagen).[15] We have shown that ECs increase SMC cell spreading. SMC cell spreading was increased in SMCs cocultured as a bilayer with ECs compared to SMCs cultured alone. Thus, ECs may alter SMC matrix adhesion molecule expression or organization to account for the increased migration in cocultured SMCs. However, this is indirect evidence and does not exclude the possibility that ECs may stimulate SMC migration by other mechanisms as well. For example, cultured ECs have been shown to secrete PDGF, a factor which stimulates SMC migration. This may be an alternative or additional mechanism by which ECs stimulate SMC migration in vitro.

EC stimulation of SMC migration is counterintuitive to what one would expect. However migration is just one process in the restenotic process. As we will see in the upcoming section of this monograph, ECs may limit the development of intimal hyperplasia by affecting other mechanisms in the process, namely by inhibiting SMC matrix production.

Matrix Effect on Endothelial Cell Control of Smooth Muscle Cell Matrix synthesis

The continued accumulation of extracellular matrix forms the bulk of the mature intimal hyperplastic lesion.[1,7] For the most part, the origin of extracellular matrix is differentiated SMCs which have migrated into the subintimal space following vessel wall injury. In addition to increased matrix deposition, the matrix composition of the fibroproliferative vascular lesion is altered, containing increased amounts of the fibrillar collagens such as type I collagen (8). We have shown that ECs can inhibit both SMC collagen protein synthesis and type I collagen gene expression in bilayer coculture (see Fig. 33.3). It is interesting to note that in these studies, ECs inhibited SMC type I collagen RNA levels by 50%, which is similar to the 40% EC inhibition of SMC collagen protein synthesis. The ability of

Fig. 33.3. (A) Representative Northern blot which shows a decrease in transcripts for type I collagen in cocultured SMCs compared to SMCs cultured alone. Densitometry for three experiments shows a 60% reduction in type I collagen transcripts in SMCs cultured opposite ECs (*p < 0.01). (B) Compared to SMCs cultured alone (black bars), ECs cocultured with SMCs(hatched bars) inhibited SMC collagen synthesis measured as trichloroacetic acid precipitatable tritiated proline counts per ug of DNA in SMC conditioned media by 50% (*p < 0.01).

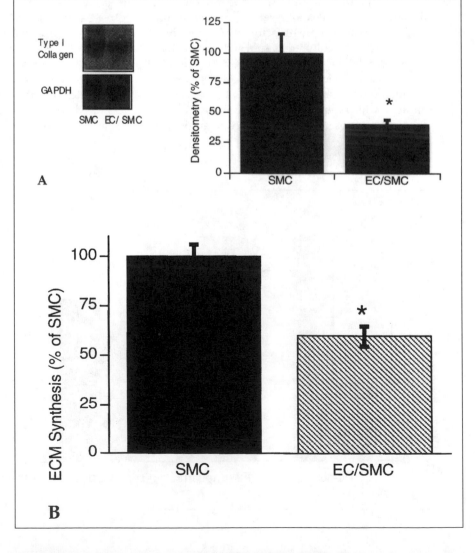

ECs to inhibit SMC collagen synthesis in vitro suggests that this may be one mechanism by which ECs may alter vascular wall remodeling and smooth muscle cell function following vascular wall injury in vivo.

The mechanism by which ECs inhibit SMC collagen synthesis in bilayer coculture is unclear. TGF-β1 is upregulated in the injured arterial wall.[19,20] It is a potent stimulant for extracellular matrix synthesis, and antibodies against TGF-β1 have been shown to limit the fibroproliferative response following balloon angioplasty in animal models.[19] However, in our coculture studies the addition of TGF-β1 antibody and aprotinin (a plasmin inhibitor which prevents the activation of TGF-β1) did not inhibit SMC extracellular matrix in SMCs cultured alone. This suggests that, at least in this in vitro coculture model, EC effects on TGF-β1 activation do not play a major role in this process (see Fig. 33.4). Though we did not perform a dose response curve using the TGF-β1 antibody, our studies indicate that the antibody did at the least partially inhibit TGF-β1 based on the diminished SMC hill and valley growth seen in these cultures. Hill and valley growth has been shown to occur as a result of active TGF-β1.[35] The plasmin inhibitor aprotinin completely suppressed hill and valley growth, suggesting complete inhibition of TGF-β1 activation.

Endothelial cells have been shown to secrete various extracellular matrix proteins which could cross the semipermeable membrane and as a result affect SMC function. Endothelial cells are typically seeded on the membrane for 4-6 days (to allow the ECs to grow to confluence), prior to adding SMCs. This allows ample opportunity for ECs to coat the opposite surface of the membrane with matrix proteins. Previous investigators have shown that extracellular matrix composition strongly influences SMC integrin expression, organization and cytoskeletal structure.[36] In order to determine the effect of extracellular matrix composition on EC inhibition of SMC collagen synthesis coculture, we repeated experiments on various matrix proteins. The extracellular matrix proteins studied were types I and IV collagen, Matrigel and fibronectin. Type I collagen is a fibrillar collagen which is increased in intimal hyperplasia and has been shown to increase SMC proliferation. Fibronectin is a high molecular weight glycoprotein which is also present in the extracellular matrix of restenotic lesions and affects SMC proliferation and migration. Type IV collagen is a constituent of the normal EC basement membrane and has been shown to maintain ECs in a more differentiated state. Matrigel is a reconstituted composition of basement membrane proteins laminin and type IV collagen. Laminin is a component of the EC basement membrane and has been shown to maintain ECs in a differentiated state. We have found that type IV collagen and Matrigel decreased collagen synthesis in SMCs cultured alone (see Fig. 33.5). These data demonstrate that matrix proteins which normally reside in the EC basement membrane can inhibit SMC matrix synthesis. In addition, the data indirectly support the concept that EC synthesized matrix proteins could be a possible mechanism by which ECs inhibit SMC matrix synthesis.

In contrast to the effects of the EC basement membrane matrix proteins, type I collagen, a fibrillar collagen, actually increased collagen synthesis of SMCs cultured alone to the greatest degree. In other studies, type I collagen has been shown to potentiate SMC dedifferentiation to a synthetic phenotype and is abundant in fibroproliferative vascular lesions.[16]

To determine if differences in cell proliferation and thus cell density could account for the differences in collagen

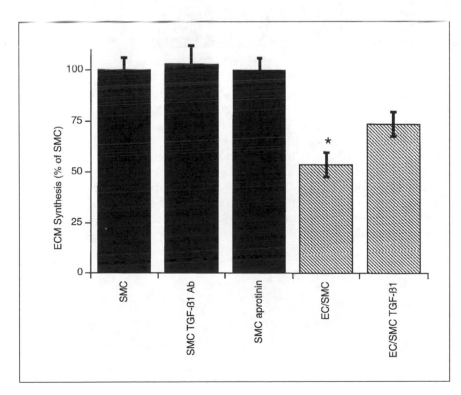

Fig. 33.4. Inhibition of TGF-β1 activity either with TGF-β1 neutralizing antibody (TGF-β1 Ab, 25 µg/ml) or with aprotinin (plasmin inhibitor which prevents the plasmin-mediated activation of TGF-β1, SMC aprotinin, 200 µg/ml) did not inhibit SMC collagen synthesis when compared to SMCs cultured alone. ECs inhibited collagen synthesis in cocultured SMCs (EC/SMC)(*p < 0.01 vs. all SMC groups). The addition of 5 ng/ml TGF-β1 had a modest stimulatory effect on SMC collagen synthesis (EC/SMC TGF-β1, p=NS).

synthesis observed in this study, we examined cell density at the completion of each experiment. As shown in Figure 33.4, the cell density (cell number after three days in culture) of SMCs cultured alone was greatest in cells cultured on Matrigel. There was no difference in cell density when fibronectin, type I collagen, and type IV collagen were compared; however, collagen synthesis was significantly less in the type IV collagen group. This suggests that the matrix protein effect on SMC collagen synthesis is due not only to changes in cell proliferation and cell density, but is extracellular matrix specific. We have not as yet explored the mechanisms by which matrix proteins effect SMC collagen synthesis. As is the case with the effect of matrix proteins on proliferation and migration, it is likely that specific extracellular matrix proteins interact with cell membrane adhesion molecules and as a result activate various intracellular signaling pathways.

Matrix substrate composition can also affect the ability of ECs to inhibit SMC collagen synthesis.[37] We have shown that ECs decrease smooth muscle cell collagen synthesis when these cells are cocultured together on type I and IV collagen and Matrigel (see Fig. 33.6). Fibronectin prevented the EC inhibition of SMC collagen synthesis, and in fact actually increased collagen synthesis. Thus, the ability for grafts sodded with ECs to resist the development of intimal hyperplasia may depend upon the matrix substrate the ECs are cultured on.

In conclusion, using an in vitro coculture model, we have shown that ECs stimulate SMC migration but inhibit SMC collagen synthesis and transcripts for type I collagen gene expression. The effect of ECs does not appear to be mediated through changes in active TGF-β1 levels but may be due to secreted matrix proteins. Extracellular matrix proteins have a profound effect on SMC collagen synthesis and on the ability of ECs to modulate SMC functions such as migration and matrix synthesis.

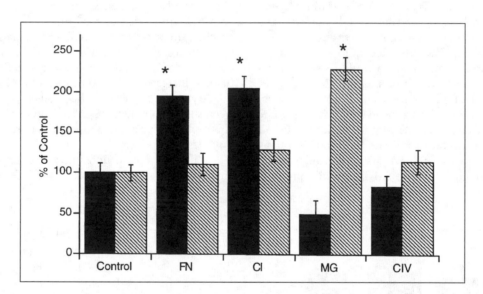

Fig. 33.5. Collagen synthesis (tritiated proline counts per µg DNA in conditioned media; black bars) of SMCs cultured alone on Matrigel (MG) and type IV collagen (CIV) was decreased when compared to plastic (Control). Fibronectin (FN) and type I collagen (CI) both significantly increased SMC collagen synthesis when compared to SMCs cultured on plastic (*p < 0.01 vs. other groups). SMC density is shown in the hatched bars. Cell density (cell number after three days in culture) was greatest in the SMCs cultured on MG. There was no difference in cell density when FN, CI and CIV were compared; however, collagen synthesis was significantly less in the CIV group. This suggests that matrix effects on SMC collagen synthesis are due not only to changes in cell proliferation and cell density but are extracellular matrix specific.

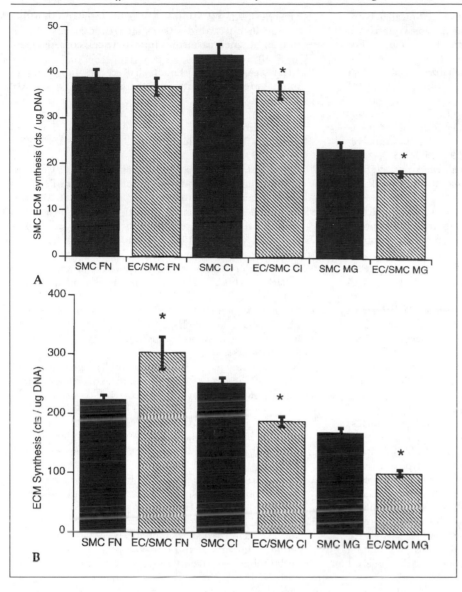

Fig. 33.6. (A) ECs inhibited soluble tritiated proline levels in the conditioned media of cocultured SMCs (hatched bars) on type I collagen (EC/SMC CI) and Matrigel (EC/SMC MG) when compared to SMCs cultured alone (black bars). Fibronectin prevented the EC effect on SMCs (EC/SMC FN vs. SMC FN). (B) ECs inhibited cell-associated tritiated proline levels in cocultured SMCs (hatched bars) on type I collagen (EC/SMC CI) and Matrigel (EC/SMC MG) when compared to SMCs cultured alone (black bars). ECs stimulated collagen synthesis in cocultured SMCs on fibronectin(EC/SMC FN) when compared to SMCs cultured alone.

References

1. Clowes AW, Reidy MA, Clowes MM. Mechanisms of restenosis after arterial injury. Lab Invest 1983; 49:208-215.
2. Liu MW, Roubin GS, King SB. Restenosis after coronary angioplasty: Potential biologic determinants and role of intimal hyperplasia. Circulation 1989; 79:1374-1387.
3. Herring M, Smith J, Dalsing M et al. Endothelial cell seeding of polytetrafluoroethylene femoral popliteal bypasses: The failure of low-density seeding to improve patency. J Vasc Surg 1994; 20:650-655.
4. Kocher O, Gabbiani F, Gabbiani G et al. Phenotypic features of smooth muscle cells during the evolution of experimental carotid artery intimal thickening. Lab Invest 1991; 65(4):459-470.
5. Mosse PRL, Campbell GR, Wang ZL et al. Smooth muscle cell expression in human carotid arteries. Lab Invest 1985; 53(5):556-562.
6. MacLeod DC, Strauss BH, DeLong M et al. Proliferation and extracellular matrix synthesis of smooth muscle cells cultured from human coronary atherosclerotic and restenotic lesions. J Am Coll Cardiol 1994; 23:59-65.
7. Rasmussen LM, Wolf YG, Ruoslahti E. Vascular smooth muscle cells from injured rat aortas display elevated matrix production associated with transformtin growth factor-b activity. Am J Path 1995; 147:1041-1048.
8. Mesh CL, Majors A, Mistele D et al. Graft smooth muscle cells specifically synthesize increased collagen. J Vasc Surg 1995; 22:142-149.
9. Bush HJ, Jakubowski JA, Sentissi JM et al. Neointimal hyperplasia occurring after carotid endarterectomy in a canine model: Effect of endothelial cell seeding vs perioperative aspirin. J Vasc Surg 1987; 5:118-125.
10. Conte MS. Endothelial cell resurfacing improves remodeling of balloon-injured arteries in the hypercholesterolemic rabbit. Surg Forum 1996; 47:333-336.
11. Zilla P. Long term effects of clinical in-vitro endothelialization on grafts. Research Initiatives in Vascular Disease 1997:82-85.

12. Zilla P, Deutsch M, Meinhart J et al. Clinical in vitro endothelialization of femoropopliteal bypass grafts: An actuarial follow-up over three years. J Vasc Surg 1994; 19:540-548.

13. Zilla P, Fasol R, Callow A. Endothelialization of vascular grafts. Applied Cardiovascular Biology 1990-1991 1992;:78-131.

14. Magometschnigg H, Kadletz M, Vodrazka M et al. Prospective clinical study with in vitro endothelial cell lining of expanded polytetratfluoroethylene grafts in crural repeat reconstruction. J Vasc Surg 1992; 15:527-535.

15. Powell R, Carruth J, Basson M et al. Matrix specific effect of endothelial cell control of smooth muscle cell migration. J Vasc Surg 1996.

16. Yamamoto M, Yamamoto K, Noumura T. Type I collagen promotes modulation of cultured rabbit arterial smooth muscle cells from a contractile to a synthetic phenotype. Exp Cell Res 1993; 204:121-129.

17. Streuli CH, Schmidhauser C, Kobrin M et al. Extracellular matrix regulates expression of the TGF-β1 gene. J Cell Biol 1993; 120(1):253-260.

18. Penttinen RP, Kobayashi S, Bornstein P. Transformtin growth factor-β increases mRNA for matrix proteins both in the presence and in the absence of changes in mRNA stability. Proc Natl Acad Sci 1988; 85:1105-1108.

19. Majesky MW, Lindner V, Twardzik DR et al. Production of transforming growth factor β_1 during repair of arterial injury. J Clin Invest 1991; 88:904-10.

20. Nikol S, Isner JM, Pickering JG et al. Expression of transformtin growth factor-b$_1$ is increased in human vascular restenosis lesions. J Clin Invest 1992; 90:1582-92.

21. Powell RJ, Cronenwett JL, Wagner RJ et al. Endothelial modulation of smooth muscle cell phenotype and macroscopic growth pattern. Surg Forum 1993; 44:380-384.

22. Powell RJ, Cronenwett JL, Fillinger MF et al. Effect of endothelial cells and TGF-β1 on cultured vascular smooth muscle cell growth patterns. J Vasc Surg 1994; in press.

23. Fillinger MF, Sampson LN, Cronenwett JL, Powell RJ, Wagner RJ. Coculture of endothelial cells and smooth muscle cells in bilayer and conditioned media models. J Surg Res 1997; 67:169-178.

24. Casscells W. Migration of smooth muscle and endothelial cells. Circulation 1992; 89:723-729.

25. Bell L, Madri J. Effect of platelets on migration of cultured bovine aortic endothelial and smooth muscle cells. Circ Res 1989; 65:1057-1065.

26. Fingerle J, Au YP, Clowes AW et al. Intimal lesion formation in rat carotid arteries after endothelial denudation in absence of medial injury. Arteriosclerosis 1990; 10(6):1082-87.

27. Reidy MA, Silver M. Endothelial regeneration: Lack of intimal proliferation after defined injury to rat aorta. AJP 1985; 118(2):173-177.

28. Lewis DA, Lowell RC, Cambria RA et al.. Production of endothelium-derived factors from sodded expanded polytetrafluoroethylene grafts. J Vasc Surg 1997; 25:187-197.

29. Castellot J, Addonizio ML, Rosenberg R et al. Cultured endothelial cells produce a heparin like inhibitor of smooth muscle cell growth. J Cell Biol 1981; 90:372-379.

30. Fillinger MF, O'Conner S, Wagner RJ et al. The effect of endothelial cell coculture on smooth muscle cell proliferation. J Vasc Surg 1993; 17(6):1058-1067.

31. DiMilla P, Stone J, Quinn J et al.. Maximal migration of human smooth muscle cells on fibronectin and type IV collagen occurs at an intermediate attachment strength. J Cell Biol 1993; 122:729-737.

32. Skinnere M, Raines E, Ross R. Dynamic expression of alpha 1 beta 1 and alpha 2 beta 2 integrin receptors by human vascular smooth muscle cells. Am J Path 1994; 145:1070-1081.

33. Basson C, Kocher O, Basson M et al.. Differential modulation of vascular cell integrin and extracellular matrix expression in vitro by TGF-β1 correlates with reciprocal effects on cell migration. J Cell Phys 1992; 153:118-128.

34. Basson C, Knowles W, Bell L et al.. Spatiotemporal segregation of endothelial cell integrin and nonintegrin extracellular matrix-binding proteins during adhesion events. J Cell Biol 1990; 110:789-801.

35. Majack RA. Beta-type transforming growth factor specifies organizational behavior in vascular smooth muscle cell cultures. J Cell Biol 1987; 105:465-71.

36. Madri JA, Bell L, Marx M et al. Effects of soluable factors and extracellular matrix components on vascular cell behavior in-vitro and in-vivo: Models of de-endothelialization and repair. J Cell Biochem 1991; 45:123-130.

37. Powell RJ, Hydowski J, Frank O et al.. Endothelial cell effect on smooth muscle cell collagen synthesis. Accepted for publication.

Facilitation of Healing

Cell Entrapment from the Circulation

—————————————— CHAPTER 34 ——————————————

Circulating Stem Cells: A Fourth Source for the Endothelialization of Cardiovascular Implants

Willie R. Koen

Introduction

An endothelialized blood-contacting surface remains the key to long term cardiovascular implants. The source for this endothelium could be either the intima of the adjacent artery or perigraft capillaries. Accordingly, the mode of endothelialization would either be through transanastomotic outgrowth or transmural ingrowth.[1-4] However, certain devices such as artificial hearts cannot rely on either form of ingrowth, due to device isolation from adjacent tissue. Therefore, the only means of obtaining an endothelium on these surfaces is either by seeding,[5-10] or by capturing from the blood. The latter possibility of a blood borne source of endothelial cells has been postulated and debated for the past three decades.[11-15] However, in the last few years enough data was produced to confirm that this fourth source of endothelium is no longer a myth but a fact. As a logical consequence, the question arose as to whether circulating cells could be harnessed in the development of a long lasting tissue engineered cardiovascular implant.

The History of Spontaneously Healing Surfaces

In 1963 Stump et al noticed that a 4.5 cm Dacron vascular implant was fully endothelialized after 7 days of implantation into a pig. Since this short period of implantation could not be explained with transanastomotic pannus ingrowth, it was speculated that a different cell source, such as the circulating blood, could have been responsible for this spontaneous endothelialization. To further elucidate this possibility, a cell trapping device was constructed which included a small square Dacron hub suspended in the center of the lumen of a Dacron prosthesis. This hub was anchored with stitches, which prevented it from coming into contact with the graft wall. After a 4 week period of canine implantation, silver nitrate stain demonstrated an endothelial coverage of the entire hub surface. Although the conclusion of a circulating cell source was drawn from these experiments, explanations for this phenomenon remained vague.[11]

To shed some light onto the chronology of events taking place in a spontaneous endothelialization of grafts, Mackenzie (1968) implanted into dogs 20 crimped terylene vascular grafts which were isolated with a surrounding Nylon sheath. After two and four weeks, patches of silver-stained round cells were found on the luminal side, lining the underlying amorphous protein mass. By four weeks these patches were composed of cells that looked like endothelial cells.[12]

Later on, spontaneous endothelialization was also observed on other cardiovascular implants such as ventricular assist devices. In 1982 Bossart[13] described a pseudo-neointoma (PNI) consisting of mainly myofibroblasts and endothelial cells on a textured surface of an assist device after two years of implantation. This PNI consisted of a matrix layer of collagen bundles embedded in proteinaceous material and interspersed with myofibroblasts. Furthermore, this layer was covered by a monolayer of cells with electron microscopic characteristics of endothelial cells. Based on these findings as well as literature evidence that similar fibrous plaques can arise from cultured guinea pig bone marrow, Bossart postulated that the source of PNI cells could be multipotential bone marrow stem cells.[13] This hypothesis of circulating cells as a source for spontaneously endothelializing grafts was once again brought up by Feigel in 1985[14] after a series of experiments investigating the process of intravascular thrombus organization. He summarized clot organization as a chronological sequence of events which starts off with activation of the mononuclear/macrophage system. Large numbers of early monocytic cells are noted in the thrombus, which he subscribed to chemotactic mechanisms as well as the ability of monocytic cells to adhere to surfaces. This event of macrophage activation is then followed by the elongation of monocyte nuclei, the appearance of myofibroblastic cells and eventually endothelial cell formation, suggesting a transformation of mononuclear cells into endothelial cells.[14,16] In 1994 distinct evidence in favor of a circulating endothelial cell source was brought forward by Shi et al,[15] which he referred to as fallout endothelialization. By using impervious Dacron grafts implanted into different anatomic positions in dogs, a healed surface could be demonstrated as early as four weeks after implantation. Furthermore, endothelial cell presence was for the first time confirmed by using immunohistochemistry, which included von Willebrandt factor staining.

With enough evidence at hand that a synthetic surface does have the ability to spontaneously endothelialize simply by being exposed to the circulating blood, the question remains concerning the origin of these cells. Over the years two basic theories evolved: The first theory is that the source of fallout endothelialization is cells that detached from the vascular wall in areas of high shear stress. This explanation has also been supported by the observation that in dynamic tissue culture studies endothelial cells are most prone to detach at the time of mitotic division.[17] The second theory is that the fallout endothelial cells arise from circulating precursor cells which eventually differentiate into mature endothelial cells.[13-15,18] Although this source has been speculated on for many years, it was only recently that published data confirmed that isolated putative progenitor endothelial cells from the human circulation were able to differentiate in vitro into endothelial cells.[19] If this differentiation phenomenon is to be the link to a nonthrombogenic tissue engineered synthetic cardiovascular implant, one needs to understand stem cell physiology to identify aspects which could be exploited for facilitated surface endothelialization.

Properties of Hematopoietic Stem Cells and Progenitor Cells

A hematopoietic stem cell can be defined as a cell with self-renewal proliferative potential, coupled with the potential to differentiate into progenitor cells of all blood lineages. Furthermore, a stem cell is typically not terminally differentiated and can divide without limit. However, when it divides, each daughter cell has a choice either to remain a stem cell, or embark on a course leading irreversibly to terminal differentiation. Therefore, the pluripotent stem cell normally generates either more pluripotent stem cells (with self-renewal potential), or committed progenitor cells (also referred to as colony forming cells—CFC). Committed progenitor cells are irreversibly determined to produce only one or a few types of blood cells.[20] Moreover, committed progenitor cells divide rapidly (amplification divisions) for only a limited number of times, and at the end of this series of divisions they develop into terminally differentiated cells. These terminally differentiated cells usually have a limited number of divisions and eventually die after several days. Other properties frequently ascribed to stem cells include the ability to undergo asymmetric cell divisions as well as the ability to exist in a mitotically quiescent form.[21] During asymmetrical division, the stem cells divide into two daughter cells, of which one remains a stem cell and the other becomes a differentiated (progenitor) daughter cell. However, during symmetrical division of stem cells, the stem cell divides into two daughter cells, both of which either remain stem cells or become differentiated progenitor cells. Therefore, symmetrical divisions allow the size of the stem cell pool to be regulated.[22] Yet, stem cells can also enter a mitotic quiescent stage where the divisions take place very slowly or rarely. This feature of mitotic quiescence is thought to be true for stem cells in the skin and bone marrow. In contrast, stem cells in the mammalian intestinal crypts have been estimated to divide every 12 h.[22]

The Location of Hematopoietic Progenitor Cells

The main source of pluripotential hematopoietic stem cells is the bone marrow microenvironment. This complex space is occupied by hematopoietic cells at all different stages of differentiation. In addition to the hematopoietic cells, stroma cells account for the rest of the bone marrow content. Stroma cells consist of fibroblasts, endothelial cells, adipocytes, monocytes and osteoclasts and can be regarded as the backbone of the marrow microenvironment. The function of the stroma is 3-fold namely:

1. The production of extracellular matrix;
2. The secretion of cytokines, and
3. The mediation of direct cellular contacts regulating hematopoiesis.[23]

From the bone marrow, hematopoietic cells enter the blood stream via the bone marrow endothelium (BMEC), which also acts as a gatekeeper in regulating this passage.[24] Furthermore, it has been hypothesized that BMEC is a unique endothelium that may regulate hematopoiesis by direct cellular contact and/or expression and secretion of specific cytokines.[25]

Apart from the bone marrow, a second source of hematopoietic stem cells is the peripheral blood. Mature peripheral blood cells are derived from a small pool (1-3%) of primitive precursor cells in the bone marrow that bear a unique surface glycoprotein, CD34 (Fig. 34.1). Furthermore, CD34+ cells are also found at lower concentrations in peripheral blood, where they are capable of reconstituting hematopoiesis.[26] As a result of this feature, transplantation of allogeneic peripheral blood stem cells has become a successful and common modality of treatment in clinical practice.[27]

Recognition of Stem Cells

The direct microscopic recognition of stem cells is very intricate and unreliable for various reasons, namely:

1. In bone marrow samples, it is basically impossible to distinguish between distinct precursor cells in their different stages of differentiation; and also

2. In peripheral blood, the concentration of stem cells is simply too low.

However, this dilemma has been overcome by the detection of specific surface markers on hematopoietic stem cells that can be harnessed for cell recognition. Probably the most prevalent surface antigen in stem cell isolation at present is cluster derivative 34 (CD34). This glycosylated protein has a molecular weight of 115 kDa and is expressed on human hematopoietic stem and progenitor cells as well as on vascular endothelial cells.[26] During vasculogenesis, hematopoietic stem cells form clusters with angioblasts and share common antigenic determinants such as CD34 and fetal liver kinase-1 receptor (Flk-1).[28] Furthermore, the CD34 surface antigen is also detected in peripheral blood cells, but only on 0.03-0.09% of circulating hematopoietic cells.[16] Compared to peripheral blood, the fallout cells noticed on explanted ventricular assist device surfaces express a 100-fold

increase in CD34 cell concentration, suggesting surface colonization with hematopoietic precursor cells.[16] Therefore, should these CD34 hematopoietic precursor cells possess the ability to mature and differentiate into endothelial cells, then the answer to the origin of fall-out endothelialization becomes more unclouded. The speculation that circulating hematopoietic precursor (CD34+) cells possess the ability to differentiate into endothelial cells was eventually answered by Asahara et al (1997).[19] In his study, mononuclear cells were isolated from human peripheral blood by magnetic bead selection on the basis of cell surface antigen expression. In vitro, cells isolated with anti-CD34 or anti-Flk-1 antibodies differentiated into endothelial cells. This was confirmed by the expression of ecNOS, Flk-1/KDR and CD31 mRNA by using the reverse transcription-polymerase chain reaction (RT-PCR).

Control of Stem Cells

The ligand-receptor mechanism remains the most commonly researched topic in the control of stem cell differentiation. In general, a receptor can be defined as a structure (generally a protein) located on or in a cell, which specifically recognizes a binding molecule, a ligand, and thereby initiates either a specific biological response (the wide sense of receptor) or the transduction of a signal (the narrow sense of receptor). Furthermore, receptors can be situated in the plasma membrane (receptors for neurotransmitters, growth factors, sensory stimulants and most circulating hormones), in an organelle membrane (e.g., Ca^{2+} release transduction) or in the cytosolic solution (as for the receptors for steroid and thyroid hormones). A receptor of particular interest in the field of tissue engineering as well as stem cell biology involves the growth factor receptor. By definition, a growth factor receptor is a cell surface protein whose purpose is to

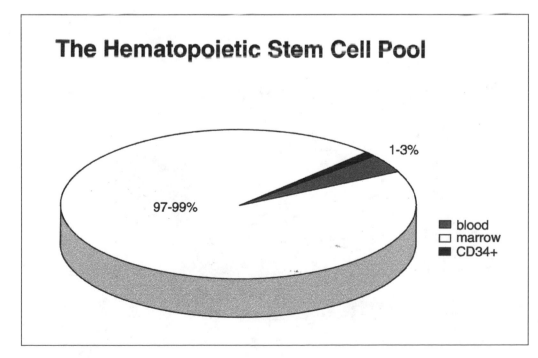

Fig. 34.1. The main source of pluripotent hematopoetic stem cells is the bone marrow microenvironment, which forms 97-99% of the total stem cell pool. Ther peripheral blood contributes to the remaining 1-3%. Of this peripheral pool, opnly 0.03-0.09% are CD34 positive cells.

receive information from outside cells and convey it across the cell membrane. It binds to a receptor and converts the receptor to an active state which then interacts with proteins on the inner surface of the membrane. This interaction consequently stimulates a program of events leading, amongst other effects, to cell division.[29-31]

Growth factor receptors can be classified into three groups, namely:

1. The tyrosine kinase receptors.
2. Seven transmembrane domain receptors; and
3. The nontyrosine kinase receptors.

The tyrosine kinase receptors have been grouped into families on the basis of kinase domains, general structure and ligand structure similarities. Among tyrosine kinase receptors, the type I receptor family includes the receptors for epidermal growth factor as well as transformtin growth factor-β (TGF-β). The type II receptors include insulin-like receptors and the type III receptors consist of the platelet-derived growth factor (PDGF) receptors A and B, c-Kit as well as c-Fms (also known as colony-stimulating factor). Finally, the type IV family is a group of receptors whose ligands are not yet known (Eph, Elk, Eck, Eek and Erk).[29-31]

The most commonly used ligands in stem cell research as well as in clinical practice are the colony stimulating factors (CSF). In bone marrow transplantation, CSF have been used to mobilize hematopoietic stem cells to optimize the harvest of peripheral blood stem cells. CSF were first defined by the stimulation of granulocyte/macrophage colo-

nies in soft agar culture. Currently, four major colony-stimulating molecules are known, namely:

1. Granulocyte/macrophage colony-stimulating factor (GM-CSF);
2. Granulocyte colony-stimulatin factor (G-CSF);
3. Colony-stimulating factor-1 (CSF-1) or macrophage colony stimulating factor (M-CSF); and
4. Multi-colony stimulating factor (multi-CSF) or interleukin-3 (IL-3).

Interleukin-3 (IL-3) is primarily an activated T cell-derived pleiotropic factor (Fig. 34.2) that can stimulate the proliferation and differentiation of pleuripotent hematopoietic stem cells as well as various lineage-committed progenitors. Following the purification and cloning of IL-3, it became apparent that this same protein had been studied under different names, including mast cell growth factor, P cell stimulating factor, burst promoting activity, multi-colony stimulating factor, Thy-1 inducing factor and WEHI-3 growth factor.[32-34]

However, more specific growth factor receptors are now known to be present on stem cells. For example, the fetal liver kinase-1 receptors (Flk-1 in mouse, also known as KDR in human) are expressed by both the vasculogenic angioblasts and the hematopoietic stem cells as well as vascular endothelial cells. Yet, although this receptor is specific for vascular endothelial growth factor (VEGF) (Fig. 34.3), it ceases to be expressed during hematopoietic differentiation.[28,35] Furthermore, it has been demonstrated in

Fig. 34.2. A summary of the control and regulation of hemotopoietic stem cells in their differentiation towards the mature endothelial cell.

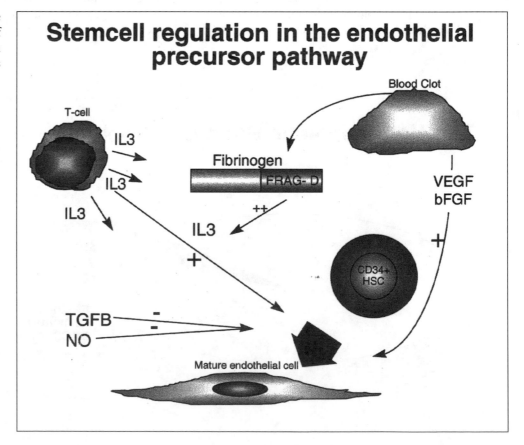

Flk-1/KDR knockout mice that few, if any, vascular endothelial cells are present.[36] Moreover, Asahara et al (1997) demonstrated the differentiation of Flk-1 positive precursor cells into VEGF producing vascular endothelial cells, thereby underlining once again the theory of a circulating endothelial cell source. In contrast to the stimulation of stem cells, there are also known factors that inhibit the differentiation and proliferation of stem cells. So far, such inhibiting factors include nitric oxide (NO) and transformtin growth factor-β (TGF-β).

Speculative Application

In summary, our knowledge of specific surface markers for circulating progenitor endothelial cells is at this stage limited to the CD34 antigen as well as the Flk-1/KDR receptor. Furthermore, VEGF is a specific ligand for the Flk-1/KDR receptor, as opposed to the less specific ligands for the CD34 antigen (including β-selectins) (Fig. 34.3). Therefore, circulating progenitor endothelial cells could be addressed by targeting the Flk-1 receptor.

In summary, it seems as if in our striving toward a spontaneously healing, long lasting cardiovascular implant, we could rely on circulating endothelial progenitor cells. Our optimism is based on two key facts, namely:

1. The proof of the presence of circulating progenitor endothelial cells which have the potential to differentiate into functioning endothelial cells[19]; and
2. Available receptors on these precursor cells making manipulation with specific ligands possible.

However, a number of questions still remain open before one can exploit circulating stem cells for the spontaneous endothelialization of synthetic impermeable implants.

Do Precursor Endothelial Cells Have Self-Renewal Potential?

Per definition, a stem cell has the potential to renew itself. From experiments carried out in baboons it could be demonstrated that highly enriched populations of autologous CD34+ marrow cells can restore hematopoiesis and lead to a long term recovery of bone marrow function in lethally irradiated baboons.[37] Furthermore, it has been known for more than 20 years that, after chemotherapy, circulating myeloid progenitor cells are recruited from the bone marrow to the periphery. This recruitment can be further enhanced by using colony stimulating factors to produce a more profound mobilization of CD34+ cells. Today, peripheral blood stem cell (CD34+) transplantation is regarded as equivalently successful, even superior in certain cases, to bone marrow transplantation.[38-42] Yet, can we assume that the self-renewal of CD34+ stem cells also applies to the precursor endothelial cell? This question was addressed by Hammond et al: Pigs were lethally irradiated and subsequently transplanted with sibling bone marrow cells. After 6 weeks of implantation, hematopoiesis was restored and the explanted vascular grafts showed the presence of donor related endothelial cells staining positive for factor VIII. Therefore, this study suggests that peripheral blood stem cells exert self-renewal potential to eventually restore hematopoiesis as well as graft endothelialization.[43]

To What Extent Are Circulating Endothelial Precursor Cells Committed?

Using fluorescence-activated cell sorting (FACS) the CD45 leukocyte common antigen could be demonstrated on 94% of freshly isolated CD34+ mononuclear blood cells.

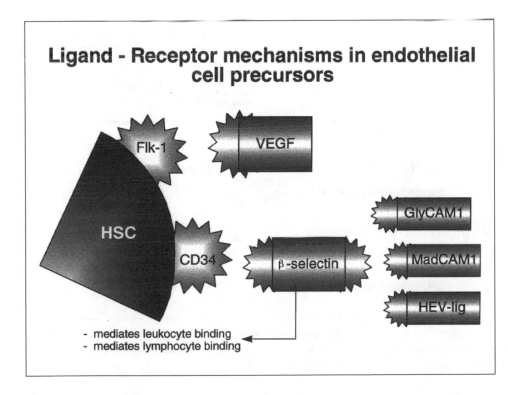

Fig. 34.3. The hematopoietic stem cell has two well known surface antigens, namely CD34 and Flk-1. The Flk-1 receptor has a specific ligand, namely VEGF. The ligands for the Cd34 surface antigen are the β-selecings, which have a less specific binding.

However, attached CD34$^+$ cells, after being in culture for a week on a fibronectin-coated surface, expressed the CD45 antigen on only 27% of cells.[19] Therefore, it seems that endothelial precursor cells circulate as CD34 and CD45 positive without being finally committed. After attachment, these noncommited cells become CD45 negative (after a week) and are then committed to further differentiate into endothelial cells. This CD34$^+$CD45$^+$ circulating cell stage reminds us of the burst forming cell unit (BFU) in erythropoiesis that differentiates into colony forming cell units (CFU) or, in our case, CD34$^+$CD45$^-$ cells. The colony forming cells in turn differentiate into erythrocytes, or in our scenario, endothelial cells. Furthermore, it is well described that erythropoietin does not act on burst forming unit-erythroid (BFU-E) alone, but in concert with other growth factors. The formation of BFU-E necessitates the presence of other bioactive molecules, originally termed burst-promoting activities, of which IL-3 was the first to be well characterized. Interleukin-3 acts synergistically with erythropoietin to induce proliferation of BFU-E,[44] but does not appear to augment the effect of erythropoietin on CFU-E.[45] Therefore, with IL-3 also stimulating the formation of circulating hematopoietic stem cells (CD34$^+$CD45$^+$), it might well be that

the further differentiation into CD34$^+$CD45$^-$ cells and eventually endothelial cells could be more specifically addressed, for instance with VEGF.

At What Stage of Differentiation Do Endothelial Precursor Cells Attach to a Surface?

Freshly isolated CD34$^+$ cells attach to a fibronectin coated culture flask as early as on day 3 and express at that stage the CD45 antigen in 94% of cells (Fig. 34.4). After a week in culture, the CD45 antigen practically disapears.[19] Therefore, these cells attach at the CD34$^+$CD45$^+$ stage, the burst-forming stage. From here, they could then further differentiate into CD34$^+$CD45$^-$ cells, the colony-forming stage, and eventually endothelial cells, or they can remain CD34$^+$CD45$^+$ cells and further differentiate into myeloid leukocytes. This decision could well be influenced by fibronectin and/or VEGF.

A Practical Vision for Future Cardiovascular Implants

Tissue engineering can be defined as the application of engineering disciplines to either maintain existing tissue structures or to facilitate tissue growth. From the materials

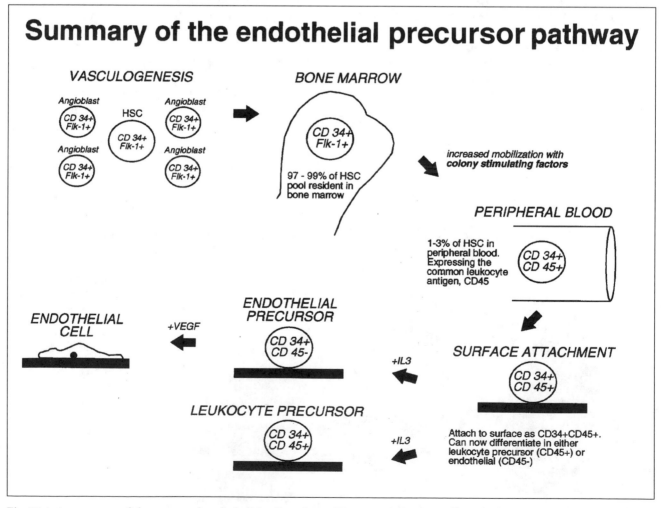

Fig. 34.4. A summary of the proposed endothelial cell pathway. Hematopoietic stem cell in the bone marrow enters the blood stream and changes its surface status after a) surface attachment as well as b) the presence of IL3, to form a committed endothelial precursor cell. This precursor differentiates into an endothelial cell in the presence of VEGF.

engineering point of view, tissues are considered to be cellular composites representing multiphase systems.[46] In order to support tissue engineered tissue, researchers used scaffolds made of various absorbable as well as materials including polidioxanone, polyglycolic acid, polyesther (Dacron), ePTFE, polyurethanes and collagen.[47-49] Today, scaffold research plays a major role in the overall drive towards tissue engineered vascular implants. Furthermore, the technology of covalent bonding of certain peptides, including cytokines, to polymeric surfaces holds the promise that scaffolds may play a much more bioactive role in tissue engineering in the future. It may well be possible to produce a synthetic polymeric scaffold for a cardiovascular implant with specific ligands within or on the surface of the structure which elicits a specific biological response. Such a response, in our vision, will be the spontaneous endothelialization of the blood-contacting surface from recruited circulating precursor cells. Therefore, one could hypothesize that the immobilization of VEGF onto a synthetic surface could be one possible step towards spontaneous endothelialization, as it may promote stem cell attachment and differentiation, as well as maintenance.

However, since surface endothelialization will eventually need a mature underlying connective tissue matrix, the wide open question regarding the existence of circulating cells promises the next exciting chapter in this field.

References

1. Berger K, Sauvage LR, Rao AM, Wood SJ. Healing of arterial prostheses in man: Its incompleteness. Ann Surg 1972; 175:118-127.
2. Greisler HP. Arterial regeneration over absorbable prostheses. Arch Surg 1985; 120:315-323.
3. Greisler HP, Ellinger J, Schwartz TH, Golan J, Raymond RM, Kim DU. Arterial regenration over polydioxanone prosthesis in the rabbit. Arch Surg 1987;122:715-721.
4. Greisler HP, Schwartz TH, Ellinger J, Kim DU. Dacron inhibition of arterial regenerative activity. J Vasc Surgery 1986; 3:747-756.
5. Zilla P, Fasol R, Dudeck U, Siedler S, Preiss P, Fischlein T, Muller-Glauser W, Baitella G, Sanan D, Odell J, Reichart B. In-situ cannulation, microgrid follow up and low density plating provide first passage endothelial cell mass-cultures for in-vitro lining. J Vasc Surg 1990; 12:180-89.
6. Kadletz M, Moser R, Preiss P, Deutsch M, Zilla P, Fasol R. In vitro lining of fibronectin coated PTFE grafts with cryopreserved saphenous vein endothelial cells. Thorac Cardiovasc Surgeon 1987; 35:143-147.
7. Fasol R, Zilla P, Deutsch M, Grimm M, Fischlein T, Laufer G. Human endothelial cell seeding: Evaluation of its effectiveness by platelet parameters after one year. J Vasc Surg 1989; 9:432-436.
8. Zilla P, Deutsch M, Meinhart J, Eberl T, Puschmann R, Minar E, Dudczak R, Lugmaier H, Schmidt P, Fischlein T. In vitro endothelialization of femoro-popliteal bypass grafts: An actuarial follow up after 3-years J Vasc Surg 1994; 19:540-548.
9. Fasol R, Zilla P, Deutsch M, Fischlein T, Kadletz M, Griesmacher A, Mller MM. Endothelialization of artificial surfaces: Does surface tension determine in vitro growth of HSVEC? J Tex Heart Inst 1987; 14:119-126.
10. Zilla P, Grimm M, Fasol R, Eberl T, Fischlein T, Preiss P, Krupicka O, Deutsch M, vonOppell U. Growth properties of cultured human endothelial cells on differently coated artificial heart materials. J Thorac Cardiovasc Surg 1991; 101:671-680.
11. Stump MM, Jordan GJ, De Bakey, Halpert B. Endothelium grown from circulating blood on isolated intravascular dacron hub. Am J Path 1963; 43:361-367.
12. Mackenzie JR, Hackett M, Topuzlu C, Tibbs DJ. Origin of arterial prosthesis lining from circulating blood cells. Arch Surg 1968; 97:879-886.
13. Bossart MI, Turner SA, Milam JD, Connor DJ, Urrutia CO, Frazier OH. Multipotential cells in the circulating blood: Ultrastructural evidence in the calf. Trans Am Sac Artif Intern Organs 1982; 28:185-189.
14. Feigl W, Susani M, Ulrich W, Matejka M, Losert U, Sinzinger H. Organization of experimental thrombosis by blood cells. Virchows Arch (Path Anat) 1985; 406:133-148.
15. Shi Q, Wu M, Hayashida N, Werchezac AR, Clowes AW, Sauvage LR. Proof of fallout endothelialization of impervious Dacron grafts in the aorta and inferior vena cava of the dog. J Vasc Surg 1994; 20:546-547.
16. Rafii S, Oz MC, Seldomridge JA, Ferris B, Asch A, Nachman RL, Shapiro F, Rose EA, Levin HR. Characterization of haematopoietic cells arising on the textured surface of ventricular assist devices. Ann Thorac Surg 1995; 60:1627-32.
17. Werchezac AR, Viggers RF, Coan DE, Savauge LR. Mitosis and cytokinesis in subconfluent endothelial cells exposed to increasing levels of shear stress. J Cell Physiol 1994; 159:83-91.
18. Dasse KA, Chipman SD, Sherman CN, Levine AH, Frazier OH. Clinical experience with textured blood contacting surfaces in ventricular assist devices. Trans Am Sac Artif Intern Organs 1987; 33:428-425.
19. Asahara T, Murohara T, Sullivan A, Silver M, van der Zee R, Li T, Witzenbichler B, Schatteman G, Isner JM. Isolation of putative progenitor endothelial cells for angiogenesis. Science 1997; 275:964967.
20. The Cell differentiated cells and the mainteninace of tissue.
21. Hall PA, Watt FM. Stem cells: The generationand maintenance of cellular diversity. Development 1989; 106:619-633.
22. Potten CS, Loeffler M. Stem cells: Attributes, cycles, spirals, pitfalls and uncertainties. Lessons for and from the crypt. Development 1990; 110:1001-1020.
23. Wichkramasinghe. Observations on the ultrastructure of sinusoids and reticular cells in human bone marrow. Clin Lab Haematol 1991; 13:263-269.
24. Weiss L, Chen LT. The organization of haematopoietic cords and vascular sinusses in bone marrow. Blood Cells 1975; 1:617.
25. Rafii S, Shapiro F, Rimarachin J, Nachman RL, Ferris B, Weksler B, Moore M, Asch A. Isolation and characterization of human bone marrow microvascular endothelial cells: Hematopoietic progenitor cell adhesion. Blood 1994; 84(1):10-19.
26. Sutherland DR, Stewart AK, Keating A. CD34 antigen: Molecular features and potential clinical applications. Stem Cells; 1993; 11(suppl 3):50-57.
27. Besinger WI, Appelbaum FA, Demirer T, Torok-Storb B, Storb R, Buckner CD. Transplantation of allogeneic peripheral blood stem cells. Stem Cells 1995; Dec 13 suppl 3:63-70.

28. Matthews W, Jordan CT, Gavin M, Jenkins NA, Copeland NG, Lemischka IR. A receptor tyrosine kinase cDNA isolated from a population of enriched primitive hemaropoietic cells and exhibiting close genetic linkage to c-kit. Proc Natl Acad Sci USA 1991; 88:9026.

29. Albert B, Bray D, Lewis J, Raff M, Roberts K, Watson JD. Cell signaling In: Albert B, Bray D, Lewis J, Raff M, Roberts K, Watson JD, eds. Molecular Biology of the Cell, 2nd edition. New York & London: Garland Publishing, Inc., 1989:681.

30. Lodish H, Baltimore D, Berk A, Zipursky SL, Matsudaira P, Darnell J. Cell-to-cell signalling: Hormones and receptors In: Lodish H, Baltimore D, Berk A, Zipursky SL, Matsudaira P, Darnell J. Molecular cell biology, 3rd edition. New York: Scientific American Books, Inc., 1995:853.

31. Kendrew J. Receptor In: The Encyclopedia of Molecular Biology Oxford,: Blackwell Science Ltd., 1994:939.

32. Quesenberry PJ. Hemopoietic stem cells, progenitor cells, and cytokines. 211.

33. Bagley CJ, Woodcock JM, Stomski FC, Lopez AF. The structural and functional basis of cytokine receptor activation: Lessons from the common beta subunit of the granulocyte-macrophage-colony-stimulating factor, interleukin-3 and interleukin-5 receptors. Blood 1997; 89(5):1471.

34. Hara T, Miyajima A. Function and signal transduction mediated by interleukin-3 receptor system in hematopoiesis. Stem Cells 1996; 14(6):605-618.

35. Millauer B, Longhi MP, Plate KH, Shawver LK, Risau W, Ullrich A, Strawn LM. Dominant-negative inhibition of Flk-1 suppresses the growth of many tumor types in vivo. Cancer Research 1996; 56(7):1615-20.

36. Fong GH, Rossant J, Gertsenstein M, Breitman ML. Role of Flt-1 receptor tyrosine kinase in regulating the assembly of vascular endothelium. Nature 1995; 367:66-70.

37. Berenson RJ, Andrews RG, Bensinger WI et al. Antigen CD34+ marrow cells engraft lethally irradiated baboons. J Clin Invest 1988; 81:951.

38. Shpall EJ, Jones RB, Franklin W et al. CD 34+ marrow and/or peripheral blood progenitor cells (PBPCs) provide effective hematopoietic reconstitution of breast cancer patients following high-dose chemotherapy with autologous hematopoietic progenitor cell support. Blood 1992; 80(suppl 1):24.

39. Shpall EJ, Jones RB, Franklin W et al. Transplantation of CD34+ marrow and/or peripheral blood progenitor cells (PBPC) into breast cancer patients following high dose chemotherapy. Blood 1994; 84(suppl 1):396.

40. Shpall EJ, Jones RB, Franklin W et al. Transplantation of enrichedCD34+ autologousmarrow into breast cancer patients following high-dose chemotherapy: Influence of CD34+ peripheral blood progenitors and growth factors on engraftment. J Clin Oncol 1994; 12:28.

41. Jones HM, Jones SA, Watts MJ et al. Development of a simplified single apheresis approach for peripheral blood progenitor cell transplantation in previously treated patients with lymphoma. J Clin Oncol 1994; 12:661.

42. Pettengell R, Morgenstern GR, Woll PJ et al. Peripheral-blood progenitor cell transplantation in lymphoma and leukemia using a single apheresis. Blood 1993; 82:3770.

43. Hammond W. NAVBO Satelite Symposium on fallout healing. Seattle, WA Sept 1996 [ABS].

44. Migliaccio G, Migliaccio AR, Visser JW. Synergism between erythropoietin and IL-3 in the induction of hematopoietic stem cell proliferation and erythroid burst colony formation. Blood 1988; 72:944.

45. Umemura T, Papayannopoulou T, Stamatoyannopoulos G. The mechanism of expantion of late eryhtroid progenitors during erythroid generation: Target cells and the effect of IL-3 and erythropoietin. Blood 1989; 73:1993.

46. Wintermantel E, Mayer J, Blum J, Eckert KL, Lusher P, Mathey M. Tissue engineering scaffolds using superstructures. Biomaterials 1996; 17(2):83-91.

47. Greisler HP. Arterial regeneration over absorbable prostheses. Arch Surg 1985; 120:315-323.

48. Greisler HP, Ellinger J, Schwartz TH, Golan J, Raymond RM, Kim DU. Arterial regeneration over polydioxanone prosthesis in the rabbit. Arch Surg 1987; 122:715-721.

49. Greisler HP, Schwartz TH, Ellinger J, Kim DU. Dacron inhibition of arterial regenerative activity. J Vasc Surg 1986; 3:747-756.

Facilitation of Healing

Cell Entrapment from the Circulation

―――――――――――――――――― CHAPTER 35 ――――――――――――――――――

Surface Population with Blood-Borne Cells

William P. Hammond

Background

The developmental biology of blood vessels has long been believed to consist of two phases. The first, vasculogenesis, is the development during embryologic life of the original precursors to all vessels.[1] Our understanding of this phenomenon has been built around detailed studies of the development of chick and quail embryos, and the elegant tracing of cellular movement during early development. Angiogenesis, on the other hand, is the term applied to development of new blood vessels during adult life, which largely serves a reparative function.[2] In addition to wound healing, this form of new blood vessel formation by sprouting from existing blood vessels is believed to explain the development of vessels to feed growing tumor cell masses. The understanding of regulatory factors for this form of new vessel growth in the adult has been a principal theoretical model for the last few decades.

The introduction of vascular prostheses prompted study of the basic biology through which these grafts maintain patency and integrity as blood conduits. As early as 1955, Sauvage and Wesolowski had noted the apparent importance of tissue ingrowth to prosthesis performance.[3] Wesolowski's experimental studies convinced him of the importance of porosity to tissue ingrowth and prompted him to develop a high porosity knitted prosthesis.[4,5] In 1962, Florey et al observed islands of endothelium around mouths of vascular channels seen on the flow surface of knitted Dacron grafts implanted in the baboon.[6] Although they could not determine the origin of these channels, they noted that they appeared to connect with perigraft vessels. In 1985 Greisler et al demonstrated arterial regenerative activity in polyglycolic acid absorbable aorta replacements in the rabbit,[7] and in 1986, Clowes and colleagues demonstrated in the baboon the capacity of a special porous form of PTFE, with an internodal distance of 90 μm, to admit the development of transmural microvessels from the perigraft tissue;[8] this suggested that the usual tissue response to the placement of vascular prostheses involves a local variant of angiogenesis, which subsequently leads to endothelial resurfacing of the graft, thereby contributing to its patency. In 1989 Kogel et al studied transprosthetic vascularization in the dog, using a polyester-based resin to make three dimensional casts, and concluded that midgraft endothelialization in PTFE grafts with 60 μm internodal distances was attributable to ingrowth of microvessels from the perigraft tissue through the graft and into the lumen; this phenomenon was not observed in microporous polyurethane grafts.[9] In 1990 Golden and Clowes et al reported the importance of graft porosity to healing of PTFE prostheses in the baboon; they found that a 60 μm internodal distance produced optimal endothelial coverage.[10] In 1995, Bull et al also reported midgraft endothelialization of 60 μm internodal distance PTFE grafts implanted in the dog carotid, and attributed it to microvessel ingrowth to the flow surface; they also noted that an external jugular vein wrap around the grafts produced endothelialization as early as 7 days.[11] In 1996 our center reported histological demonstration of the continuity of a microvessel between the perigraft vessels and flow surface microostia in a porous Dacron prosthesis; however, we were unable to determine whether its origin was in the outer wall or on the inner flow surface of the graft.[12]

In 1963, Stump et al described the presence of endothelium on Dacron hubs suspended in the descending thoracic aorta of young pigs, and cited this as evidence for formation of endothelium from circulating cells in the blood.[13] More recently, Scott et al found endothelium on the surfaces of pledgets of vascular graft material implanted in dog aortas.[14] A direct demonstration of endothelium in the blood stream was developed by Sbarbati et al using an endothelial-specific monoclonal antibody to analyze patients' arterial and venous blood before and after heart catheterization,[15] and in the following year George et al identified postangioplasty circulating human endothelial cells with S-Endo1 coupled to immunomagnetic beads.[16] Further evidence of circulating endothelium has been supplied by Frazier's[17] and Rafii's[18] studies of human endothelial cells found on the lining of ventricular assist devices.

Previous Studies

The following studies have produced data that, taken together, strongly support the concept of a circulating endothelial precursor cell and suggest several implications for the engineering of vascular prostheses in the future.

Impervious Grafts

In 1994, Shi and Sauvage et al reported the results of a study designed to demonstrate unequivocally that perigraft tissue ingrowth is the sole source of healing beyond the pannus areas.[19] Dacron grafts were made impervious by a coating of silicone rubber and shielded from pannus ingrowth (which is very limited in humans and dogs)[20] by 2.5-6 cm lengths of microporous (30 μm internodal distance) PTFE at each end. Suitable lengths of this composite graft were implanted in the descending thoracic aorta, abdominal aorta and inferior vena cava of the same dog. At the end of the implant periods, light microscopy study confirmed that there was no perigraft tissue ingrowth (Fig. 35.1). Instead of the expected unhealed flow surface, by 4 weeks all these impervious grafts had scattered islands of endothelialization (Fig. 35.2). We named this phenomenon "fall-out" healing, because the only possible source appeared to be the blood flowing through the graft.

The experimental study was extended to include 70 cm long impervious grafts implanted in the carotid-femoral position in dogs.[21] At 3 months, each of the 5 extra-anatomic grafts that remained patent had results similar to the aorta and inferior vena cava grafts, with scattered endothelial islands in the midgraft area despite a lack of ingrowth from the outer wall.

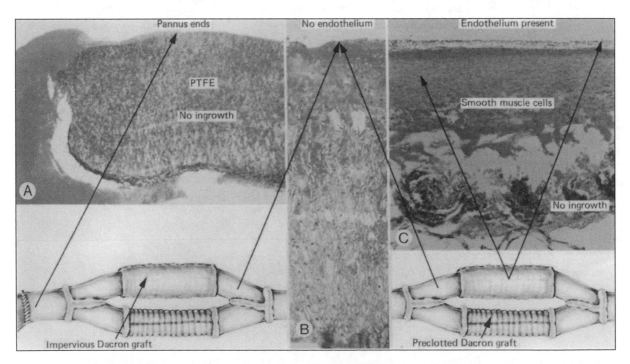

Fig. 35.1. NOTE: See color insert for color representation. Blockage of pannus and transmural ingrowth for study of fallout endothelialization of isolated central Dacron limb of a prosthesis made impervious by a coating of silicone rubber and implanted for 8 weeks in the descending thoracic aorta of a dog. (A) No transmural ingrowth from perigraft tissues and limited pannus from native aorta onto PTFE (LM, x50). (B) PTFE graft, beyond the pannus zone, showing no perigraft tissue growth into the graft (LM, x25). (C) No perigraft tissue ingrowth into the impervious Dacron graft, but presence of endothelial-like cells on flow surface, with α-actin positive smooth muscle cells beneath (H&E; LM, x50). Reprinted with permission from Shi et al. Proof of fallout endothelialization of impervious Dacron grafts in the aorta and inferior vena cava of the dog. J Vasc Surg 1994; 20:549.

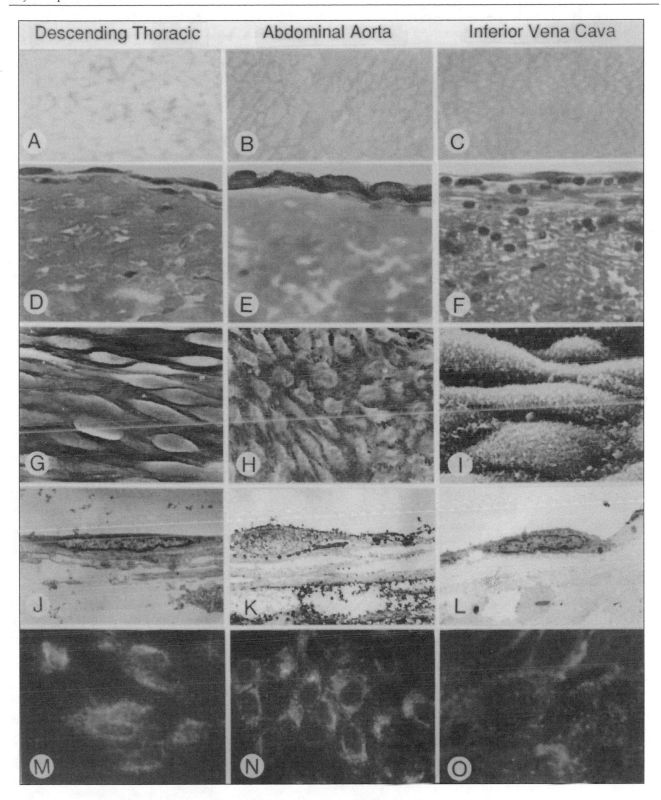

Fig. 35.2. NOTE: See color insert for color representation. Findings for specimens taken from areas beyond the pannus zone of Dacron grafts made impervious to perigraft tissue ingrowth by a silicone rubber coating and implanted in the dog. (A)-(L) Endothelial-like cells on flow surfaces of Dacron prostheses implanted in the descending thoracic aorta, abdominal aorta and inferior vena cava of the dog: (A)-(C) LM, AgNO$_3$, x70; (D)-(F) LM, x500; (G) SEM, x1000; (H) SEM, x500; (I) SEM, x3000; (J)-(L) TEM, x4000. (M)-(O) Proof of endothelium by FVIII/vWF positivity on flow surface of isolated Dacron grafts: (M)-(N) x500; (O) x1000. Reprinted with permission from Shi et al. Proof of fallout endothelialization of impervious Dacron grafts in the aorta and inferior vena cava of the dog. J Vasc Surg 1994; 20:550.

Porous Grafts, Using Early Implantation Periods

My colleagues have also demonstrated the phenomenon we refer to as fall-out healing in porous grafts by using early implant periods.[22-24] In 2 studies, they accelerated endothelialization by wrapping a resected segment of the autogenous inferior vena cava around knitted Dacron grafts implanted in the abdominal aorta of dogs. In the first study, at 2 weeks they found active angiogenesis between the wrap and the outer graft wall, regardless of whether the intima or adventitia of the inferior vena cava was placed against the graft (Fig. 35.3).[22] Endothelialization and ostia formation occurred on some flow surface areas at 2 weeks, either before the tissue ingrowth had reached into the graft wall, or before it had grown close to the lumen (Fig. 35.4). In a second study of this accelerated endothelialization model, BrdU staining revealed endothelial cells and increased cellular proliferation near the flow surface as early as 7 days, with no associated tissue ingrowth from the outer wall.[23] Porous grafts without inferior vena cava wraps were then studied for short periods ranging from 7-14 days in the dog's descending thoracic aorta: At 7 and 10 days, endothelial cells were found on the midgraft area of the flow surface, with no connection to pannus or perigraft tissue ingrowth.[24]

Substrate Observations

We have seen three basic types of substrates beneath single-layer endothelium in impervious grafts:

1. A fibrin matrix layer;
2. A fibrin matrix layer topped with a thin layer of macrophages and leukocytes;
3. Multiple layers of α-actin positive cells; in a few instances, microvessels were associated with the latter (Fig. 35.1C).[19]

It is possible that this manifestation was time dependent: It was seen in descending thoracic aorta grafts at 8 and 12 weeks, but not in 4 week descending thoracic aorta, abdominal aorta and inferior vena cava grafts (all carotid-femoral grafts were implanted for 3 months).

Human Grafts

In 1975 Sauvage et al reported endothelium on the flow surface of a human axillofemoral graft; unfortunately, their analysis was limited because the only technique available to them was silver nitrate staining for morphology.[25] However, in 1995 we observed a patch of endothelium far from areas of pannus ingrowth on a woven Dacron human axillofemoral bypass graft, and endothelial factor VIII/von Willebrand factor and *Ulex europaeus* agglutinin were available to confirm this finding (Fig. 35.5).[26] This graft had no perigraft tissue attachment due to serous fluid that had surrounded it for two years,[26] a factor that suggested fall-out healing was the endothelial source, as did microscopic evidence that there was no tissue in the interstices.

Fig. 35.3. NOTE: See color insert for color representation. Ostia and microvessels in knitted Dacron grafts wrapped in segments of the inferior vena cava and implanted in the abdominal aorta of dogs. (A) At 2 weeks, flow surface microostia identified by AgNO₃ stain (LM, x74). (B) At 2 weeks, flow surface microostium (SEM, x444). (C) Microvessels in the flow surface lining at 2 weeks (H&E; LM, x486). (D) A 4 week serial section showing a large microvessel between the flow surface and the perigraft tissue (H&E; LM, x108). Reprinted with permission from Onuki et al. Accelerated endothelialization model for the study of Dacron graft healing. Ann Vasc Surg 1997; 11:147.

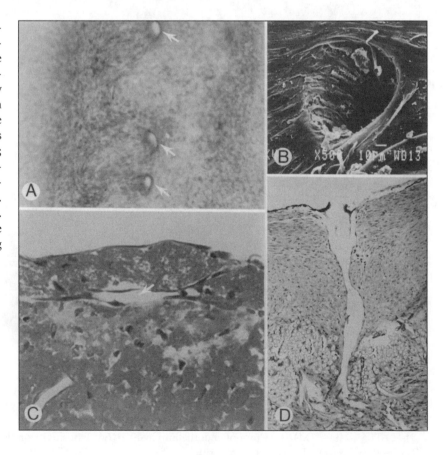

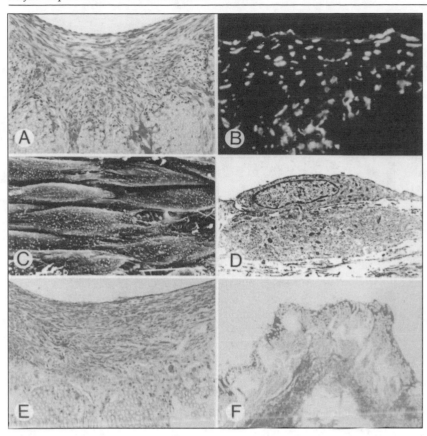

Fig. 35.4. NOTE: See color insert for color representation. Two week specimens from knitted Dacron grafts wrapped in autogenous inferior vena cava and implanted in dogs. (A) A monolayer of endothelial-like cells on the flow surface (H&E; LM, x108). (B) Proof of endothelium (FVIII/vWF; x460). (C,D) SEM and TEM, respectively, showing morphology typical of endothelium (SEM, x1918; TEM, x4640). (E) α-actin stained smooth muscle cells in the neointima (LM, x108). (F) Control graft, which was not wrapped in inferior vena cava, showing incomplete healing (H&E stain; LM, x42). Reprinted with permission from Onuki et al. Accelerated endothelialization model for the study of Dacron graft healing. Ann Vasc Surg 1997; 1:146.

Present Studies

Ontogeny of Endothelial Cells Observed on the Flow Surface of Impervious Grafts

Sbarbati's and George's direct demonstrations of circulating endothelial cells dislodged from the vascular tree by heart catheterization and angioplasty indicate one possible source for fall-out endothelialization.[15,16]

We are currently testing the hypothesis that the cell of origin is a primitive mesenchymal cell, possibly related to hematopoietic cell populations, and is not derived from adjacent existing blood vessels. One possibility is that hematopoietic progenitor, or "stem", cells can differentiate into endothelial cells. Our experimental in vivo studies are continuing, with implantation of impervious Dacron grafts in the descending thoracic aorta of beagles that have received bone marrow transplants, and in which the DNA of donor marrow cells can be distinguished from the DNA of host tissue cells.

Character of Other Cells Lining Impervious Grafts

In our studies we have demonstrated the presence of smooth muscle cells and microvessels beneath endothelium on the flow surface of completely impervious Dacron grafts, or porous grafts retrieved before transmural angiogenic ingrowth could traverse the wall.[19,21,23] At 14 days we observed unconnected microvessels in the intima and perigraft areas of the graft, suggesting that microvessel ingrowth also occurs from the flow surface.[24] The microvessels may have

developed as a result of fall-out endothelialization, a concept that is supported by the 1983 report of tube formation from a monolayer of endothelium in a collagen matrix.[27] The presence of smooth muscle cells in the neointima of the graft surface beneath the fall-out endothelium may also be attributed to cells from the blood stream, because there seems to be no other source; however, unlike endothelial cells, smooth muscle cells have not been observed in circulating blood, although Stump reported elongated cells resembling smooth muscle cells on isolated Dacron hubs,[13] and in Scott's study of suspended PTFE and Dacron pledgets smooth muscle cells also were observed.[14] Recently, a clinical case report from Deutsch et al reported a matrix containing cells between a PTFE graft and an endothelial monolayer, which resulted from preoperative lining with autologous cultures of cephalic vein endothelial cells.[28] Many of the cells in this matrix were actin and desmin positive, resembling smooth muscle cells; this group also mentions the blood as a possible source, in addition to coseeding or pannus migration.

Related Findings

Until our report in 1995,[26] it was believed that endothelium did not appear on the flow surfaces of artificial vascular grafts implanted in humans. However, we have now demonstrated endothelium on the flow surface of three additional Dacron arterial prostheses explanted from humans.[29] As discussed earlier, one of these grafts was surrounded by seroma, which prevented any perigraft tissue ingrowth into the graft.[26] Of the remaining 3, 2 bifurcated

Fig. 35.5. NOTE: See color insert for color representation. Sections taken from the midgraft area of a woven Dacron axillofemoral bypass graft explanted from a patient during redo surgery after an implant period of 26 months. (A) TEM showing typical endothelial-cell morphology (x3050). (B) Positive factor VIII/vWF staining confirms endothelium (x485). (C) Confirmation of endothelium by positive *Ulex europaeus* agglutinin staining (x1210). (D) HAM 56 staining confirms presence of macrophages (x485). Reprinted with permission from Wu et al. Definitive proof of endothelialization of a Dacron arterial prosthesis in a human being. J Vasc Surg 1995; 21:865.

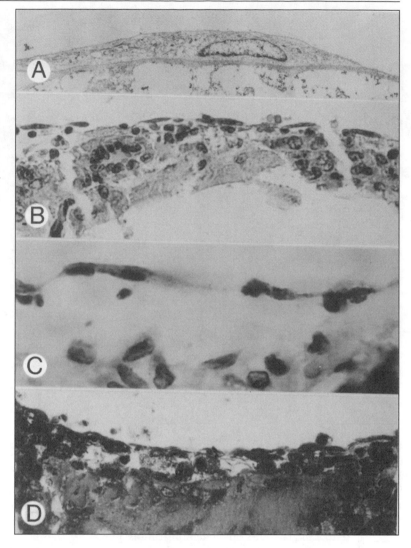

woven grafts had endothelium in areas with no tissue ingrowth.[29] The endothelium in all 4 instances was located in the midgraft area, far from any possible extension of pannus ingrowth from the native vessel.

The occurrence rate for endothelialization of human vascular grafts is, of course, impossible to estimate. However, the usual failure to find it in explanted specimens may be due more to the amount of elapsed time after death before removal and preservation than to the actual frequency: The 3 specimens we have reported were all fixed either immediately or within 5 hours after death.

The possibility of clinical graft endothelialization raises the question of whether it would be possible to encourage this phenomenon, either through treatment of the graft or the patient.

Recently, Asahara et al reported in vitro magnetic bead studies in which they isolated putative endothelial cell progenitors from human peripheral blood.[30] They then injected DiI-labeled CD34 positive mononuclear blood cells into the tail veins of mice with unilateral ischemia of a hind limb; later examination demonstrated proliferative DiI-labeled cells in the reparative vascularization of the ischemic area. Similar results were obtained in rabbits. Although they refer to this process as "therapeutic angiogenesis", it suggests a form of vasculogenesis, as do our experimental and clinical findings of endothelialization of synthetic flow surfaces in the absence of blood vessel ingrowth. If hematopoietic progenitor cells can be shown to differentiate into endothelial cells, the case for an adult form of vasculogenesis will be strengthened.

Implications

The implications of these findings are potentially far reaching. In basic science our understanding of the development of new blood vessels, and in particular their endothelial cell linings, would be transformed by a new understanding of the origins of these cells. The existence of a circulating "angioblast" would significantly alter how one approaches disorders of new blood vessel formation, including the management of tumor metastases. Should we discover the existence of a true multipotential "hemangioblast", it would be necessary to dramatically reshape our concepts of angiogenesis and vasculogenesis. In fact, definitive proof of the presence of a mesenchymal precursor for both hematopoietic cells and vascular cells would suggest an adult version of vasculogenesis which would profoundly alter the view of both normal physiology of the vasculature as well as pathologic changes in blood vessels.

In the clinical realm the application of these concepts could be very important. Many efforts over the past decade or so employing techniques for "seeding" of vascular grafts would have to be rethought in light of new concepts in stem cell biology applied to endothelium, and possibly smooth muscle cells as well. The potential for specific identification of cells giving rise to new endothelial surfaces could significantly alter the basic approaches to design of experiments using seeding. A second clinical implication is that the evolution of design concepts in vascular prostheses has moved from "bioinert" to "biocompatible" materials,[31] and will almost surely need to evolve further to a concept of "biospecific" materials. For example, where a goal in the past may have been the synthesis of biopolymers that failed to activate coagulation processes of blood and subsequently moved toward materials that are capable of passive, nonactivating interactions with their surroundings, the present studies suggest a need to develop materials with specific affinities for the circulating cells, which would also promote both their landing and growth in situ on the appropriate graft materials. If circulating endothelial progenitor cells truly exist, the clinical approach to accelerated healing of prostheses will be totally transformed, and the tissue engineering required for vascular graft prostheses will be entirely different in the future.

References

1. Risau W, Flamme I. Vasculogenesis. Ann Rev Cell Dev Biol 1995; 11:73-91.
2. Folkman J, Shing Y. Angiogenesis. J Biol Chem 1992; 267:10931-10934.
3. Sauvage LR, Wesolowski SA. The healing and fate of arterial grafts. Surgery 1955; 38:1090-1131.
4. Wesolowski SA, Fries CC, McMahon JD, Martinez A. Evaluation of a new vascular prosthesis with optimal specifications. Surgery 1966; 59:40-56.
5. Wesolowski SA, Sauvage LR, Golaski WM, Komoto Y. Rationale for the development of the gossamer small arterial prosthesis. Arch Surg 1968; 97:864-871.
6. Florey HW, Greer SJ, Kiser J, Poole JCF, Telander R, Werthessen NT. The development of the pseudointima lining fabric grafts of the aorta. Br J Exp Pathol 1962; 43:655-60.
7. Greisler HP, Kim DU, Price JB, Voorhees AB Jr. Arterial regenerative activity after prosthetic implantation. Arch Surg 1985; 120:315-323.
8. Clowes AW, Kirkman TR, Reidy MA. Mechanisms of arterial graft healing. Rapid transmural capillary ingrowth provides a source of intimal endothelium and smooth muscle in porous PTFE prostheses. Am J Pathol 1986; 123:220-230.
9. Kogel H, Amselgruber W, Frosch D, Mohr W, Cyba-Altunbay S. New techniques of analyzing the healing process of artificial vascular grafts, transmural vascularization, and endothelialization. Res Exp Med 1989; 189:61-68.
10. Golden M, Hanson SR, Kirkman TR, Schneider PA, Clowes AW. Healing of polytetrafluoroethylene arterial grafts is influenced by graft porosity. J Vasc Surg 1990; 11:838-845.
11. Bull DA, Hunter GC, Holubec H, Aguirre ML, Rappaport WD, Putnam CW. Cellular origin and rate of endothelial cell coverage of PTFE grafts. J Surg Res 1995; 58:58-68.
12. Wu MH-D, Shi Q, Onuki Y et al. Histologic observation of continuity of transmural microvessels between the perigraft vessels and flow surface microostia in a porous vascular prosthesis. Ann Vasc Surg 1996; 10:11-15.
13. Stump MM, Jordan GL Jr, De Bakey ME, Halpert B. Endothelium grown from circulating blood on isolated intravascular Dacron hub. Am J Pathol 1963; 43:361-367.
14. Scott SM, Barth MG, Gaddy LR, Ahl ET Jr. The role of circulating cells in the healing of vascular prostheses. J Vasc Surg 1994; 19:585-593.
15. Sbarbati R, deBoer M, Marzilli M, Scarlattini M, Rossi G, van Mourik JA. Immunologic detection of endothelial cells in human whole blood. Blood 1991; 4:764-769.
16. George F, Brisson C, Poncelet P et al. Rapid isolation of human endothelial cells from whole blood using S-Endo1 monoclonal antibody coupled to immuno-magnetic beads: Demonstration of endothelial injury after angioplasty. Thromb Haemost 1992; 67:147-53.
17. Frazier OH, Baldwin RT, Eskin SG, Duncan JM. Immunochemical identification of human endothelial cells on the lining of a ventricular assist device. Texas Heart Inst J 1993; 2:78-82.
18. Rafii S, Oz MC, Seldomridge JA, Ferris B, Asch AS, Nachman RL, Shapiro F, Rose EA, Levin HR. Characterization of hematopoietic cells arising on the textured surface of left ventricular assist devices. Ann Thorac Surg 1995; 60:1627-1632.
19. Shi Q, Wu MH-D, Hayashida N et al. Proof of fallout endothelialization of impervious Dacron grafts in the aorta and inferior vena cava of the dog. J Vasc Surg 1994; 20:546-57.
20. Sauvage LR, Berger KE, Wood SJ et al. Interspecies healing of porous arterial prostheses. Observations, 1960 to 1974. Arch Surg 1974; 109:698-705.
21. Kouchi Y, Onuki Y, Wu MH-D et al. Apparent blood stream origin of endothelial and smooth muscle cells in the neointima of long, impervious carotid-femoral grafts in the dog. Ann Vasc Surg, in press.
22. Onuki Y, Hayashida N, Wu MH-D et al. Accelerated endothelialization model for the study of Dacron graft healing. Ann Vasc Surg 1997; 11:141-48.
23. Onuki Y, Kouchi Y, Yoshida H et al. Early flow surface endothelialization before microvessel ingrowth in accelerated graft healing, with BrdU identification of cellular proliferation. Ann Vasc Surg, 1998; 12:207-215.
24. Onuki Y, Kouchi Y, Yoshida H et al. Early presence of endothelial-like cells on the flow surface of porous arterial prostheses implanted in the descending thoracic aorta of the dog. Ann Vasc Surg, 1997; 11:604-11.
25. Sauvage LR, Berger K, Beilin LB, Smith JC, Wood SJ, Mansfield PB. Presence of endothelium in an axillary-femoral graft of knitted Dacron with an external velour surface. Ann Surg 1975; 182:749-753.
26. Wu MH-D, Shi Q, Wechezak AR et al. Definitive proof of endothelialization of a Dacron arterial prosthesis in a human being. J Vasc Surg 1995; 21:862-67.
27. Montesano R, Orci L, Vassalli P. In vitro rapid organization of endothelial cells into capillary-like networks is promoted by collagen matrices. J Cell Biol 1983; 97:1648-52.

28. Deutsch M, Meinhart J, Vesely M et al. In vitro endothelialization of expanded polytetrafluoroethylene grafts: A clinical case report after 41 months of implantation. J Vasc Surg 1997; 25:757-63.

29. Shi Q, Wu MH-D, Onuki Y et al. Endothelium on the flow surface of human aortic Dacron vascular grafts. J Vasc Surg 1997; 25:736-42.

30. Asahara T, Murohara T, Sullivan et al. Isolation of putative endothelial cells for angiogenesis. Science 1997; 275:964-67.

31. Hubbell JA. Engineering the cellular-synthetic substrate interface. How to build a blood vessel; Lifeline Foundation Research Initiatives in Vascular Disease Conference, Bethesda, February 27, 1997, Program Book, abstract 94.

Facilitation of Healing

Cell Entrapment from the Circulation

─────────────── CHAPTER 36 ───────────────

Cellular Population of the Textured-Surface Left Ventricular Assist Devices Leads to Sustained Activation of a Procoagulant and Proinflammatory Systemic Response

Talia B. Spanier, Ann Marie Schmidt, Mehmet C. Oz

Overview

The use of LVAD technology has a potentially critical role in the management of patients with end-stage cardiac failure.[1-6] The ability of this device to enhance left ventricular function as a bridge to transplantation or for longer periods is well established. However, as with any foreign material implanted into a host, the issue of host-graft interaction becomes an integral part of LVAD biology, beyond its mechanical function as a pump. Compared with early design LVADs, whose surface was mainly of smooth contour, the Thermocardiosystems HeartMate LVAD™ was designed with a textured surface polyurethane diaphragm, intended to minimize the potential for thromboembolic complications by facilitating the formation of a tightly adherent "pseudoneointima" on the blood-contacting surface[7-12] (Fig.36.1). The goal of this strategy was to reduce the risk of development of thromboemboli by eliminating direct contact between the device and circulating blood.[11] The apparent success of this modification in LVAD design was suggested by studies which reported a thromboembolic rate of < 2% associated with use of this modified surface.[12] Furthermore, patients receiving this device were apparently safely maintained with no or minimal forms of systemic anticoagulation.

The implantation of this device with its subsequent cellular population and creation of a biological lining, however, has significant impact on its host, with both procoagulant and proinflammatory consequences. Of considerable interest, we believe that so few instances of clinically apparent thromboembolic phenomena are seen because of the creation of a delicate balance between the generation of thrombin and activation of fibrinolytic pathways which occurs as a result of device implantation. Furthermore, it is tempting to speculate that perturbations of vascular homeostasis associated with infection, inflammation or surgery, for example, might easily tip the balance of hemostatic mechanisms to formation of thrombi or consumptive coagulopathy. Thus, dissecting the mechanisms by which prothrombotic tendencies, anticoagulant defenses and fibrinolysis are balanced in this LVAD environment become essential for understanding clinically relevant prothrombotic disorders in these patients.

The development of clinically important immune alterations in patients related to the implantation of the textured surface LVADs also is of significant interest. It has been observed that LVAD patients develop increased levels of anti HLA antibodies[13-15] in a time-dependent manner over the course of LVAD implantation.[15] In our own experience, the

Tissue Engineering of Prosthetic Vascular Grafts, edited by Peter Zilla and Howard P. Greisler.
©1999 R.G. Landes Company.

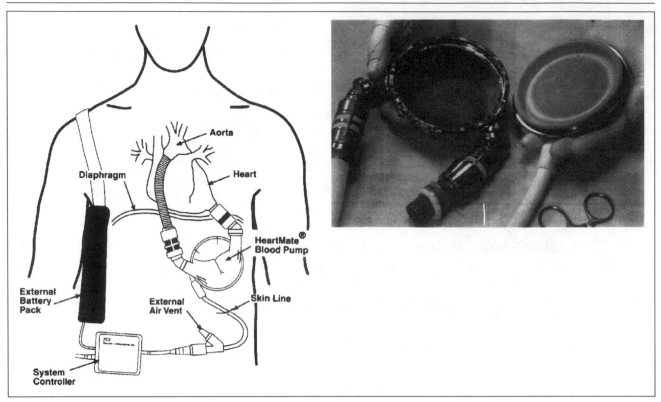

Fig. 36.1. LVAD. Left Panel. Schematic illustration of the LVAD implanted in a patient. The pump is positioned intraperitoneally in the upper left quadrant of the abdomen. Dacron conduits are used to connect the pump between the apex of the left ventricle and the ascending thoracic aorta. The LVAD is either pneumatically or electrically driven via a percutaneous drive line powered by an external console or battery pack, respectively. Porcine valves placed in the inflow and outflow conduits ensure the unidirectional flow of blood. Right Panel. The blood-contacting surfaces of both the titanium housing component and the flexible polyurethane diaphragm are textured to encourage the formation and adherence of a biological lining. The flexible diaphragm consists of a fibrillar surface integral with the base material to eliminate detaching of fibrils. The individual fibrils measure approximately 18 μm in diameter to 300 μm in length. The nonflexible housing surface is fabricated from titanium microspheres sintered together to form a porous nonpermeable topography. The diameter of the spheres ranges from 50-75 μm, with a resultant pore size ranging from 25-50 μm.

clinical consequences of these antibodies are significant and unique to each class of antibody produced. Anti-MHC class I antibodies, measured in the panel reactive antibody assay (PRA), are associated with a prolonged waiting time to transplantation because of difficulty in finding a negative crossmatched donor organ. Anti-MHC class II antibodies are associated with increased severity and frequency of cellular rejection episodes after transplantation. Of note, our data do not suggest that these findings are related to such factors as number of blood transfusions, use of filtered blood, age or gender. However, we propose that one potential perturbant in this setting may be the presence of CD34 positive cells and other activated inflammatory cells populating the LVAD. We believe, in fact, that interactions between the LVAD surface and host mononuclear cells leads to a Th2 pattern of cytokine expression by activated T cells, which contributes to B cell hyperreactivity in vivo (Fig.36.2). These interactions ultimately culminate in immune alterations in the host, further emphasizing the necessity of understanding the identity and functional significance of the cellular populations of the LVAD surface.

Thrombin Generation and Fibrinolysis

In order to better understand the hematologic profile which underlies the low thromboembolic risk associated with the textured surface LVAD, and to more fully understand the long term physiologic implications of its use, we analyzed measurements of thrombin generation and fibrinolysis in patients supported by the TCI LVAD. Our data indicate that despite both apparent clinical stability and "normal" screening values of routine hemostatic parameters such as platelet count, prothrombin and activated partial thromboplastin times, patients with textured surface LVADs nevertheless demonstrate significant activation of coagulation with secondary fibrinolysis.[16] The etiology (ies) underlying these hemostatic and immune abnormalities are of considerable interest. Such LVAD-specific etiologies as the textured polyurethane surface, the titanium housing, and the dacron inflow / outflow lines need to be considered. Other etiologies, such as altered flow characteristics and the presence of preexisting clots in the failed ventricles, must also be investigated (Fig. 36.3). Our data do not suggest that these findings are a direct result of the surgical implantation proce-

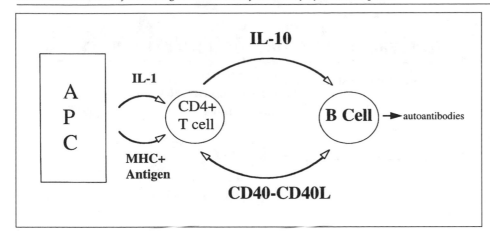

Fig. 36.2. B cell antibody production results from antigen driven CD4 positive Th2 T cell activation: B cell antibody production results from the following complex pathway. First: Macrophages on the LVAD surface activate CD4 positive T cells by presenting antigen in the context of MHC class II molecules together with IL-1 production. The subsequent activation of Th2 T cells leads to production of IL-10 and CD40-CD40L interactions, which act on B cells to induce antibody production.

dure of the LVAD, as hemostatic findings remain abnormal at least up to the 335th day of LVAD therapy. Jeevanandam and colleagues have shown that in the perioperative period, compared with coronary artery bypass graft (CABG) patients, LVAD patients consistently demonstrate significantly higher markers of thrombin generation (TAT and F_{1+2}) and fibrinolysis (D-dimers and FDPs).[17] Our studies examining LVAD patients in this regard do not, however, demonstrate that these perioperative findings are sustained, as the overt indices of thrombin generation and fibrinolysis are acute and procedure-related. In fact, prospective analysis of 20 LVAD patients from the time of LVAD insertion for up to 335 days revealed an initial rise in markers of thrombin generation as measured by elevated levels of prothrombin fragment 1+2 (F_{1+2}) and thrombin-antithrombin III complex (TAT). The data demonstrated an increase in each of these parameters in the immediate perioperative period which declined progressively by days 5-7. Subsequently, indices of thrombin generation and fibrinolysis rose in a time-dependent manner, reaching an apparent maximum by day 35 which was sustained through at least day 335 (Fig 36.4A,B). Similar results were observed for levels of D-dimers (Fig. 36.4C).

These data suggest that activation of coagulation in LVADs is biphasic. Initial / immediate activation of coagulation and fibrinolysis in the perioperative period is likely secondary to acute contact activation of the blood with the extensive foreign surfaces of the cardiopulmonary bypass and with the LVAD itself, as well as perioperative surgical response. Later, a second, sustained phase of activation of coagulation/fibrinolysis is created in these LVAD patients, which is caused by the progressive cellular population of the LVAD surface with cellular entrapment, activation and enhanced procoagulant activity. Furthermore, although we found no evidence of increased IL-1 β or TNF-α in the peripheral plasma of LVAD patients over the time course of LVAD implantation, sustained elevations in levels of tissue factor antigen were present in LVAD patients compared to normal controls (Fig 36.5A). This, together with the finding of increased tissue factor activity as reflected by enhanced

macrophage procoagulant activity (Fig. 36.5B), is consistent with the hypothesis that the microenvironment created by the LVAD was indeed reflective of a systemic prothrombotic effect.

LVAD Surface Cellularization

Indeed, these data suggest that a specific characteristic of the LVAD textured surface itself is, at least in part, responsible for these observations. The blood contacting surfaces of both the titanium housing component and the flexible polyurethane diaphragm are textured to encourage the formation and adherence of a biological lining (Fig. 36.1, right panel). The flexible diaphragm consists of a fibrillar surface integral with the base material to eliminate detaching of fibrils. The individual fibrils measure approximately 18 μm in diameter to 300 μm in length. The nonflexible housing surface is fabricated from titanium microspheres sintered together to form a porous nonpermeable topography. The diameter of the spheres ranges from 50-75 μm, with a resultant pore size ranging from 25-50 μm.[9]

Although either the sintered titanium surface or the polyurethane diaphragm should in theory be capable of cellular entrapment, we and others have demonstrated in studies of explanted LVADs considerable cellular entrapment specifically by the polyurethane diap-Bposits on the sintered titanium housing.[18-22] Flow cytometry studies have demonstrated that the majority of these diaphragm cells are myeloid/monocytic in origin. In addition, a smaller percentage of the cells are pluripotential hematopoietic cells which can be induced to differentiate in culture to mature hematopoietic cells.[22] Menconi and colleagues[21] found that the surface of explanted LVADs contained adherent mononuclear cells, platelets, and myofibroblasts intermingled with areas of compact fibrinous material, as well as areas of collagenous tissue. Similarly, Salih and colleagues[18] found the surface of the explanted LVAD polyurethane membrane to consist of fibrinous and cellular layers. The immediate layer atop the membrane was composed of a compact fibrin coating as well as numerous mononuclear cells and spindle-shaped cells. This was followed by an intermediate middle layer consisting

Fig. 36.3. Activation of coagulation and fibrinolysis. As demonstrated by our studies, evidence exists for significant thrombin generation (as reflected by increased levels of thrombin-ANTITHROMBIN COMPLEX (TAT) and prothrombin activation peptide (F_{1+2})) and fibrinolysis (increased levels of D-dimers and fibrinogen (fibrin) degradation products (FDPs)) in patients with TCI LVAD compared with normal control population values and patients with end-stage heart failure not supported by LVAD or anticoagulant therapy. The mechanism (s) underlying the generation of a procoagulant state are not yet clear since, for example, it is not known if activation of the intrinsic and/or extrinsic pathways of coagulation underlie these findings. Closed arrows are indicative of the procoagulant pathway resulting in the formation of a fibrin clot. Open arrows follow the fibrinolytic pathway. Dotted arrows and bold font signify the markers of these pathways reported in this study.

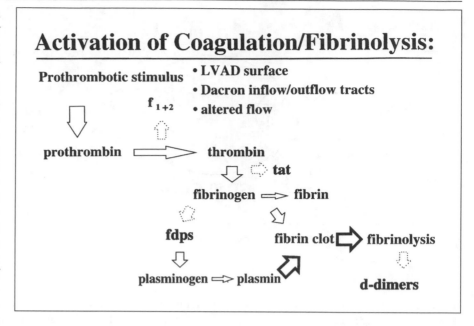

Activation of Coagulation/Fibrinolysis:

Prothrombotic stimulus

- **LVAD surface**
- **Dacron inflow/outflow tracts**
- **altered flow**

f₁₊₂

prothrombin ⟹ **thrombin**

tat

fibrinogen ⟹ **fibrin**

fdps

fibrin clot ⟹ **fibrinolysis**

plasminogen ⟹ **plasmin**

d-dimers

of cells resembling fibroblasts and fewer mononuclear cells than in the immediate inner layer, and the outermost layer, at the biomaterial/tissue interface, contained a foreign body type reaction with numerous multinucleated giant cells. Sections of tissue islands removed from the titanium surface revealed organized fibrous and collagenous tissue with few cellular areas, except for occasional mononuclear cells. While Salih and colleagues found no evidence of endothelial cells on the surface of the LVAD, other studies have disputed this. Specifically, Frazier and colleagues[19] found evidence for the presence of endothelial cells on the pseudointimal lining of the textured LVAD surface. Using antibodies to von Willebrand factor, they demonstrated positive immunoreactivity in certain cells on the lining, suggestive of the presence of endothelial cells. (Of course, platelet material may also be responsible for this positive immunostaining for von Willebrand factor). The significance of defining the presence of endothelial cells in this setting cannot be overstated, since their presence may suggest the potential for restoration of normal control of the vascular pro- and anticoagulant pathways.

In an attempt to more clearly delineate the cellular content of the LVAD surface, we began to try to more definitively define the phenotypes of cells which are adsorbed to the LVAD surface.

Our demonstration of CD34 positive cells on the LVAD surface (Fig. 36.6) confirms the results of Rafii and colleagues.[22] Such cells, likely to be derived from the bone marrow, are progenitor cells which under normal conditions differentiate into red blood cells, myeloid cells and platelets. Under homeostatic conditions, their numbers in the periphery are quite low (0.01-0.1%).[23] This suggests the presence

of a stimulus releasing increased numbers of dendritic cells into the blood of patients with LVAD and/or the presence of highly efficient mechanisms capable of trapping them on the LVAD surface. In the first context, the presence of significant hemolysis in LVAD patients (as defined by elevated plasma free hemoglobin and absent haptoglobin) suggests a possible mechanism underlying bone marrow stress. The presence of activated macrophages on the LVAD surface provides an environment potentially enhancing recruitment of CD34 positive and other cells, such as lymphocytes. In this context, the work of Browning, Gallo and colleagues[24] concerning Kaposi's sarcoma-like spindle cells (derived from the peripheral blood of HIV-1-infected individuals) is especially of interest. They found that such cells expressed markers found on both activated cells of monocyte/macrophage and endothelial lineage, similar to what we have observed in cells populating the LVAD. The authors speculated that a likely origin of Kaposi's spindle cells would be a circulating bone marrow progenitor cell. The finding that culturing of these spindle cells required the presence of conditioned medium from activated lymphocytes suggested the requirement for an additional stimulus to promote differentiation and proliferation of Kaposi's cells. By analogy with the situation in LVAD, we propose that the initial recruitment of immune/inflammatory cells to the LVAD surface establishes a local milieu facilitating recruitment of CD34 positive cells from the blood. This further promotes the establishment of the LVAD as an organ with impact on diverse host response mechanisms.

Until future studies identify whether there are elevated levels of CD34 positive cells in the periphery and whether there are specific stimuli recruiting them to the LVAD in these patients, an alternate explanation must be considered.

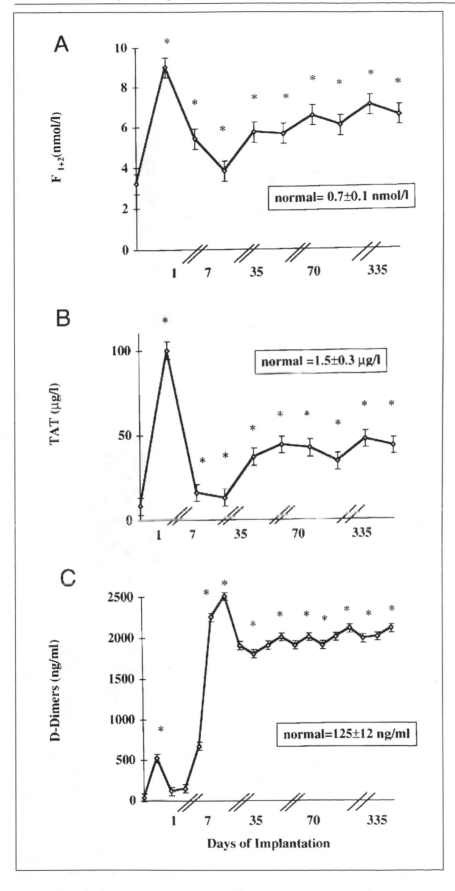

Fig. 36.4. Prospective analysis of hemostatic parameters obtained from patients with textured surface LVAD. Twenty patients with LVAD as described above were examined at various time points as indicated for levels of: (A) prothrombin fragment 1+2 [F_{1+2}] (nmol/ml); (B) thrombin-antithrombin III complex [TAT] (µg/ml); and (C) D-dimers (ng/ml). Each point represents the mean of duplicate values ± standard error. Normal values for each parameter are indicated in the inset of each figure. * denotes $p < 0.01$ compared with normal values by analysis of variance (ANOVA)

Fig. 36.5. (A) Analysis of systemic inflammatory/procoagulant mediators in the peripheral blood of LVAD patients. Peripheral blood was obtained from 11 LVAD patients at random times during LVAD implantation (but at least at or beyond 35 days). Plasma was prepared by centrifugation and assayed by ELISA for IL-1β, TNF-α or tissue factor as described above. Data from LVAD patients are reported as % above normal population values as reported by the manufacturer. Each point represents the mean of duplicate determinations per patient (reported as mean ± SE). * denotes $p < 0.001$ compared to normal values by ANOVA. Open bars represent normal values, and black bars represent values obtained from LVAD patients. (B) Enhanced tissue factor activity in peripheral blood monocytes of patients with LVADs. Peripheral blood mononuclear cells were isolated from LVAD patients (n = 5) or normal controls (n = 3) and tissue factor activity assays performed. TF activity was then performed as described in triplicate and reported as the mean ± SE. * indicates $p < 0.05$ by ANOVA.

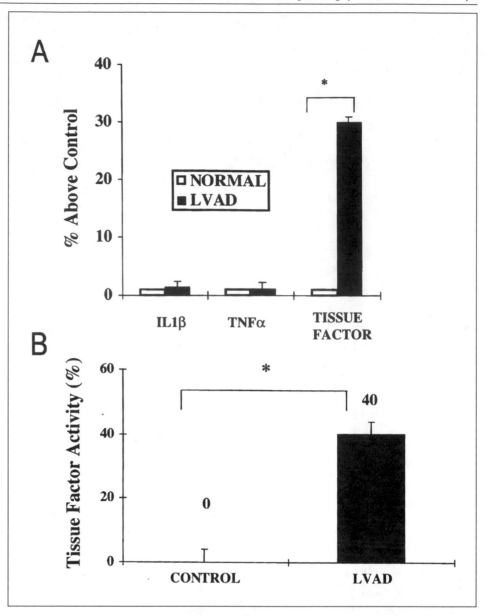

Fig. 36.6. Immunohistochemical analysis of cells derived from the LVAD surface: CD34. A distinct cellular population was found to be positive for CD34, a marker of pluripotent hematopoietic stem cells.

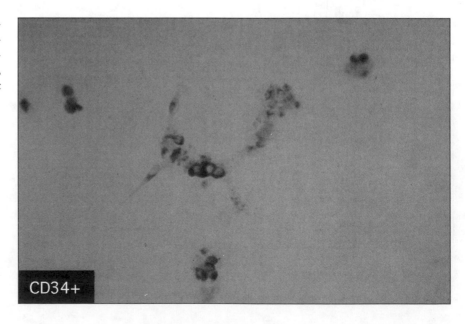

Previous studies have suggested that bone marrow transplanted onto vascular prostheses (composed of polytetrafluoroethylene, PTFE), results in complete endothelialization by three weeks. Such graft areas populated with a confluent layer of cells were completely patent and without evidence of thrombotic occlusion. In contrast, control grafts (without bone marrow transplantation) were covered by thrombi, as expected. Despite the fact that these authors did not immunotype the cells transplanted onto the prostheses, it is likely that the complex mixture contained multiple hematopoietic precursor CD34 positive-like cells. While it is possible that the LVAD surface-derived cells have the capacity to form a confluent monolayer, potentially explaining why frank thromboses are not often observed, there is a critical distinction between the experimental previous results on PTFE and our data on the LVAD surface. Overwhelming evidence of angiogenesis was evident on the vascular PTFE prostheses, manifested by new capillary formation.[25] In contrast, our study of multiple explanted LVAD surfaces has not shown angiogenesis, evidence of crude capillary formation or continuous cell monolayers covering the LVAD surface. Rather, we consistently observe that there are patches of discrete cells (data not shown). Therefore, at this time, we conclude that it is less likely that the cells on this surface are directed toward the formation of discrete vascular, confluent, nonthrombogenic structures or monolayers.

Further immunophenotypic characterization of cellular populations on the LVAD surface suggested that interactions among different lineages of cells was likely occurring. Quiescent round monocyte lineage cells expressing CD14 were present (Fig. 36.7, right panel). In addition, numerous larger cells with prominent cytoplasmic processes and multinucleated morphology were present which express the macrophage marker CD68, not CD14, and are therefore most likely activated macrophage lineage cells. (Fig. 36.7,

left panel). Suggestive of enhanced macrophage procoagulant activity of these cells was the presence of increased immunostaining for tissue factor (Fig. 36.8). And, the cells which were phenotypically similar to the population of CD34 positive cells appeared to bear markers suggestive of endothelium, such as thrombomodulin (Fig. 36.9, left panel) and von Willebrand factor (Fig. 36.9, right panel).

Since CD34 positive cells are known to express adhesion molecules, we postulated that such cells on the LVAD surface might express vascular cell adhesion molecule-1 (VCAM-1) and intercellular adhesion molecule-1 (ICAM-1), thereby favoring the recruitment and adherence of further mononuclear/inflammatory cells. Immunocytochemistry revealed immunoreactivity for both of these adhesion molecules (Fig. 36.10, right and left panels, respectively). In the context of the LVAD surface, this is likely to be significant, since the presence of adhesion molecules provides a mechanism for triggering the further recruitment of inflammatory/immune effector cells, thus propagating cellular activation on the LVAD. In contrast to the presence of cells bearing dendritic and monocytic markers, there was no staining with antibody to smooth muscle actin or nonimmune IgG (Fig. 36.11 right and left panels, respectively).

Finally, the presence of proinflammatory leukocytes was confirmed in the abundance of T lymphocytes which expressed strong immunoreactivity for CD3/CD4 and CD25 (Fig. 36.12), consistent with activated helper T cells.

There was also a distinct B cell population immunoreactive for CD20 (Fig. 36.13).

The presence of dendritic type CD34 positive cells with a procoagulant phenotype, as well as activated macrophages surrounded by proinflammatory leukocytes, certainly set the stage to explain the proinflammatory/procoagulant phenotype created as a result of device implantation.

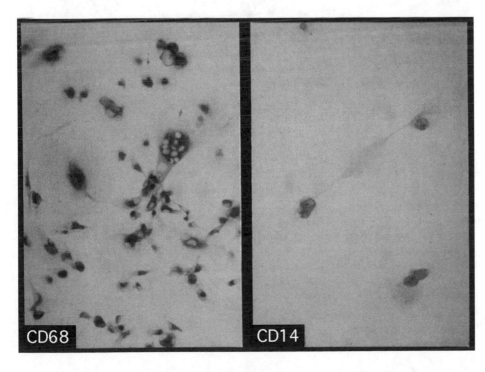

Fig. 36.7. CD14/CD68. Immunophenotypic characterization of the cellular populations on the LVAD surface demonstrated that the most prominent cell types were a population of quiescent monocytic cells bearing the marker CD14 (right panel) as well as activated macrophages bearing the marker CD68 (left panel).

Fig. 36.8. Procoagulant TF: Tissue factor on the surface of these cells confirms their procoagulant phenotype.

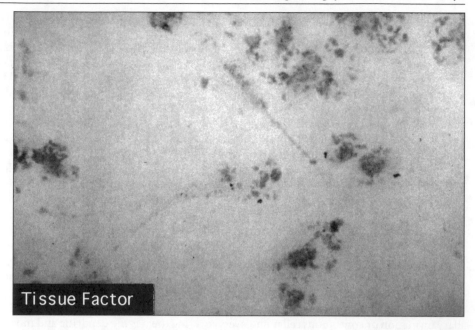

Fig. 36.9. Endothelial markers: TM and vWB. These cells express typical endothelial type markers like thrombomodulin (sTM, left panel) and von Willebrand factor (vWB, right panel).

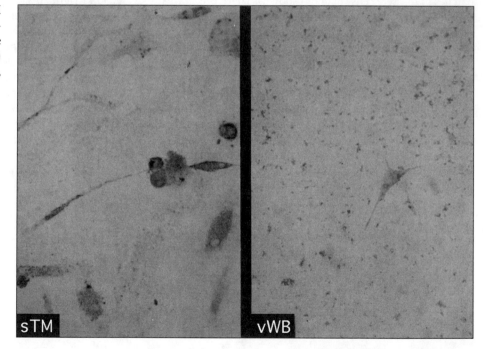

Cellular Activation

Consistent with the hypothesis that the LVAD surface itself contributes to the multiple biologic phenomena observed in the course of its use, studies have revealed that this lining is metabolically active. Menconi et al[20] showed by RNA hybridization analysis that the colonizing cells actively expressed genes encoding proteins for cell proliferation markers, cell adhesion molecules, cytoskeletal structures and extracellular matrix components.

Evidence for immunological cellular activation on the LVAD surface was confirmed by evaluating the presence of transcripts for inflammatory mediators. RT-PCR of RNA prepared from the cells harvested from the LVAD surface demonstrated amplicons of the appropriate size for the proinflammatory cytokines IL-1, IL-2 and TNF as well as the proinflammatory adhesion molecules VCAM-1 and ICAM-1 (Fig. 36.14). RT-PCR for β-actin was utilized as the positive control.

To specifically demonstrate interactions between macrophages and T cells, our results were consistent with macrophage driven T cell activation as evidenced by the presence of mRNA for macrophage derived IL-1 and T cell derived IL-2R and IL-2 (Fig. 36.15). To determine whether there was a predominance of Th1 or Th2 T cell activation and to evaluate potential T cell/B cell interactions, we looked at cytokine gene expression for IFN-γ, IL-4 or IL-5 which was

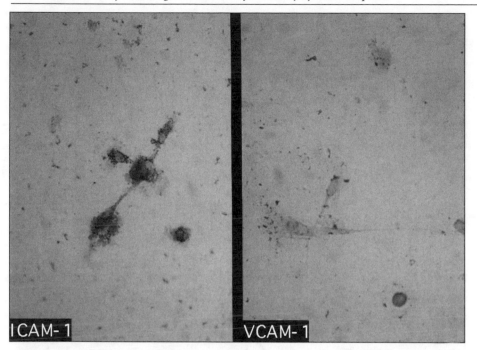

Fig. 36.10. Inflammatory cell recruitment: Cell adhesion molecules. These cells strongly express intercellular adhesion molecule (ICAM-1, left panel) and vascular cell adhesion molecule (VCAM-1, right panel) consistent with their capacity to recruit other circulating cells thereby sustaining the inflammatory phenotype.

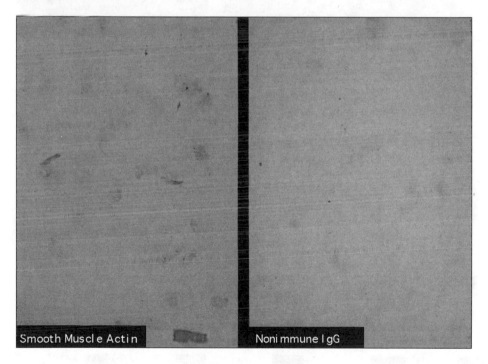

Fig. 36.11. Smooth muscle actin and nonimmune IgG. There was no staining with antibodies to smooth muscle actin (left panel) or nonimmune IgG(right panel).

found to be absent. In contrast, prominent expression of IL-10 mRNA was detected. Importantly, the production of IL-10 is known to have a stimulatory effect on B cells and has been reported to be increased in SLE and implicated in the pathogenic mechanism of autoantibody production in this disease. Evidence for T cell / B cell interactions involved in B cell hyperreactivity was shown by the presence of mRNA for CD40 ligand. (CD40 on B cells and CD40 ligand on T cells are the principal molecules involved in T cell contact-mediated B cell stimulation.)(Fig. 36.16) Together these findings led us to our supposition, as described earlier, that acti-

vated macrophages on the LVAD surface activate CD4 positive T cells by presenting antigen in the context of MHC class II molecules together with IL-1 production. The subsequent activation of a Th2 subset of T cells leads to production of IL-10 and CD40-CD40L interactions, which act on B cells to induce antibody production (Fig. 36.2).

LVAD as Inflammatory/Immune Organ

Taken together, these data suggest that considerable interactions between the LVAD surface cells and the host are occurring throughout the time course of LVAD

Fig. 36.12. Activated T cells. There was an abundance of T lymphocytes which expressed strong immunoreactivity for CD3/CD4 and CD25, consistent with activated helper T cells.

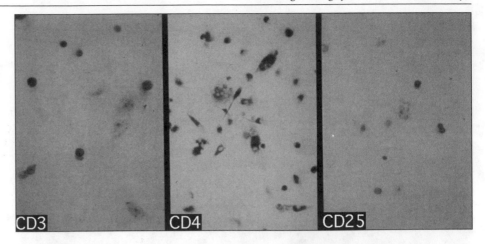

Fig. 36.13. Antibody-producing B cells. There was also a distinct B cell population which was immunoreactive for CD20.

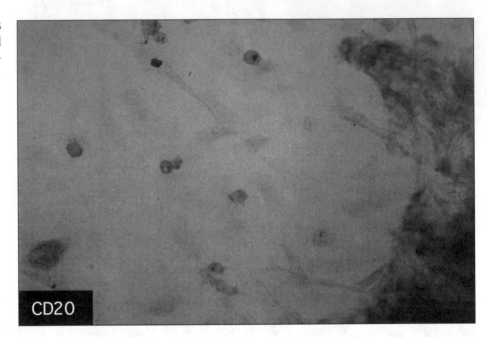

Fig. 36.14. Activated cells are present on the LVAD surface: Examination by RT-PCR. RT-PCR was performed from material directly removed from the LVAD surface at the time of explantation as described above using specific primers. Positive amplicons for the following were identified: (A) interleukin-1β, (B) interleukin-2, (C) TNF-α, (D) Vascular cell adhesion molecule-1 and (E) intercellular adhesion molecule-1. Markers are indicated on the right hand side of each panel.

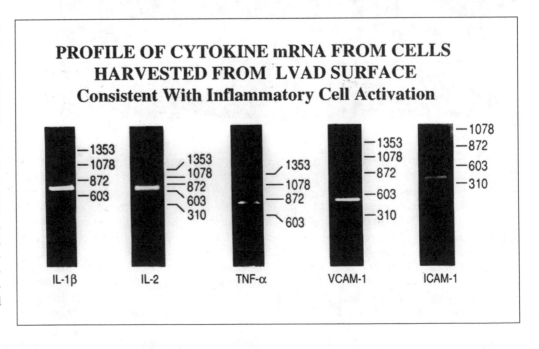

implantation. We postulate that the mononuclear cells, platelets and pluripotential stem cells initially trapped by the polyurethane surface, not the titanium housing or Dacron grafts, become activated, thus leading to the generation of a local proinflammatory/procoagulant state, and that this mechanism is, at least in part, responsible for triggering and subsequently sustaining the systemic activation of the coagulation and fibrinolytic cascades. Furthermore, inflammatory cells present on the LVAD surface appear to demonstrate production of proinflammatory cytokines and expression of adherence molecules which promote cell activation, as well as facilitate recruitment of other cell types from the circulating blood, thereby sustaining the immune alterations (Fig. 36.17). Our observation that monocyte-derived macrophages seeded on the LVAD surface generate tissue factor,

a cell-associated and released form, suggests a direct mechanism for activation of coagulation. This is consistent with the presence of tissue factor antigen in the plasma of patients with LVADs,[16] and suggests a mechanism for disseminating the locally intense inflammatory and procoagulant stimuli in the LVAD milieu. Furthermore, when monocytes were placed onto the LVAD surface in tissue culture, their capacity to respond to exogenously added LPS was enhanced (unpublished observation). This supports the concept that the LVAD primes adherent cells for heightened responsiveness to superimposed inflammatory stimuli.

We believe, therefore, that the biology of cells in the LVAD resembles a two-hit model in which the initial placement of the device within the circulation results in recruitment of adherent cells, initially likely to be CD34 positive

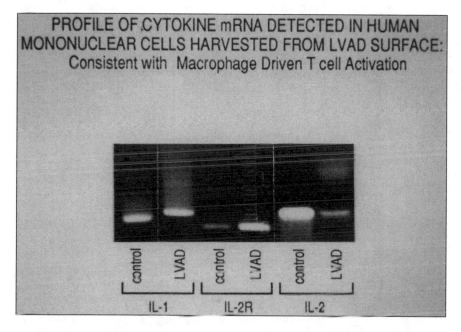

Fig. 36.15. Macrophage-driven T cell activation. To demonstrate interactions between macrophages and T cells we evaluated cytokine gene expression by mononuclear cells harvested from the LVAD surface. Our results were consistent with macrophage-driven T cell activation as evidenced by the presence of mRNA for macrophage derived IL-1 and T cell derived IL-2R and IL-2. Positive controls for each gene product were supplied by the manufacturer. (As shown by the lanes marked 'control').

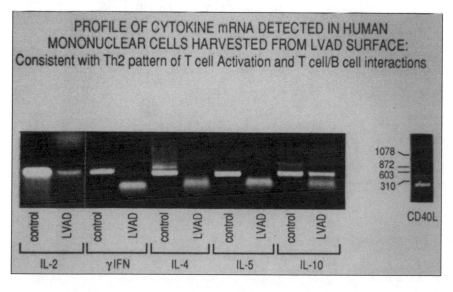

Fig. 36.16. Th2 pattern of T cell activation. To determine whether there was a predominance of Th1 or Th2 T cell activation and to evaluate potential T cell/B cell interactions, we looked at cytokine gene expression by mononuclear cells derived from the LVAD surface. As shown in this representative individual, no messenger RNA for IFN-γ, IL-4 or IL-5 was present. In contrast, prominent expression of IL-10 mRNA was detected. Importantly, the production of IL-10 is known to have a stimulatory effect on B cells and has been reported to be increased in SLE and implicated in the pathogenic mechanism of autoantibody production in this disease. Evidence for T cell/B cell interactions was shown by the presence of mRNA for CD40 ligand. CD40 on B cells and CD40 ligand on T cells are the principal molecules involved in T cell contact-mediated B cell stimulation.

pluripotent hematopoietic cells and monocytes, which then undergo subsequent differentiation and activation with the capacity to recruit other cells, such as dendritic-type cells and lymphocytes, consequently sustaining and expanding the local host response. From such a view, the LVAD emerges as an immune/inflammatory organ which redirects the host response, modulating multiple effector systems such as coagulation and immune mechanisms.

NF-κB Is a Marker of Cellular Activation in the LVAD Surface Milieu and a Target for Anti-Inflammatory Intervention

An important goal of our studies in attempting to understand the intricate interactions between the populated LVAD surface and the host was to determine if therapeutic strategies might be designed to limit the generation of proinflammatory and prothrombotic mediators that appear to be central to the activation of coagulation/immune pathways observed in the setting of the textured surface LVAD. We therefore sought evidence that the generation of cytokines and tissue factor reflected ongoing cellular stimulation and activation of cell signaling pathways in the cells populating the diaphragm. A potential culprit in this setting is the nuclear transcription factor NF-κB, an inducible transcription factor of the Rel family which is known to have a central role in the inflammatory response. Specifically, in endothelial cells, NF-κB is required for the transcriptional activation of VCAM-1, ICAM-1 and E-selectin in response to TNF-α, thus contributing to the expression of cell adhesion molecules involved in the recruitment of leukocytes to an inflammatory nidus. And, in proinflammatory leukocytes

NF-κB is involved in the transcriptional activation of inflammatory cytokines such as IL-1, IL-2, IL-6 and IL-8 in response to LPS or TNF, thereby facilitating the further propagation of the inflammatory response. Electrophoretic mobility shift assays using nuclear extracts prepared from cells removed from the LVAD surface[26-27] as well as a [^{32}P]-radiolabeled consensus probe for NF-κB demonstrated a marked gel band shift, confirming NF-κB activation in this setting (Fig. 36.18). This finding, in addition to lending further support to the concept that the cells colonizing the surface of the LVAD are activated with respect to the generation of a proinflammatory/procoagulant environment, also provided a potential target for therapeutic anti-inflammatory intervention in LVAD patients. In this context, a number of studies have suggested that NF-κB's role as a central regulator of the inflammatory response can be downregulated by anti-inflammatory agents such as high dose salicylates (ASA).[28-33] The specific cellular mechanism of ASA seems to be dependent on its ability to act as an antioxidant and free radical scavenger, thereby preventing the inducible decay of I-κB and therefore the subsequent activation of NF-κB. This effect has been shown to be independent of the cycloxygenase pathway, as agents such as indomethacin are ineffective in blocking I-κB-NF-κB signaling.

To test this hypothesis, we began a prospective evaluation of ASA (325 mg PO/PR QD) started in LVADs within three days of implantation. Markers of thrombin generation (TAT and F_{1+2}) and fibrinolysis (D-dimers) were significantly reduced compared to untreated LVADs (n = 20), as were peripheral TF antigen and macrophage procoagulant activity (p < 0.05). Inflammatory cell activation was also

Fig. 36.17. LVAD surface cellularization by circulating blood elements promotes proinflammatory/procoagulant environment. To explain our findings, we propose that the textured surface LVAD selectively adsorbs and activates dendritic type cells and macrophages from the circulating blood, allowing them to create a proinflammatory/procoagulant microenvironment with the expression of cell adhesion molecules and cytokines which favor the further recruitment and activation of T cells and B cells, as well as the expression of procoagulant tissue factor. Together, these forces contribute to the activation of both the coagulation and immune pathways associated with the implantation of this device.

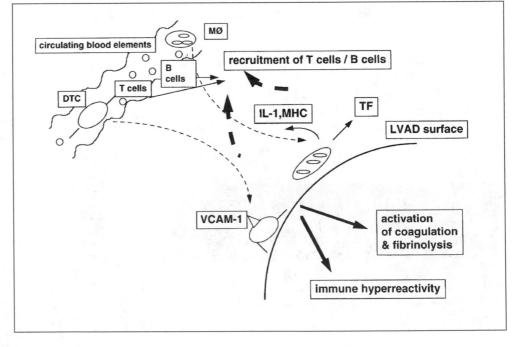

abated, as none of the treated LVADs developed elevated PRAs up to 90 days post implantation. Analysis of cells on the LVAD surface at explant (n = 3) compared to untreated LVADs (n = 6) confirmed marked downregulation of the inflammatory response:

1. Markers of macrophage activation (CD68) were distinctly absent;
2. Cells did not express procoagulant TF or vascular cell adhesion molecule-1; and
3. There was a marked absence of B cells (CD20) and T cells (CD3/4/25)—

all consistent with a primary decrease in inflammation at the LVAD surface as well as diminished ability to further recruit inflammatory cells. Taken together, these data suggest that targeted anti-inflammatory intervention with ASA may be an effective means to diminish cellular adsorption/ activation by the textured surface LVAD, thereby attenuating the associated inflammatory response and improving long term tolerance and eventual clinical outcome (Fig. 36.19).

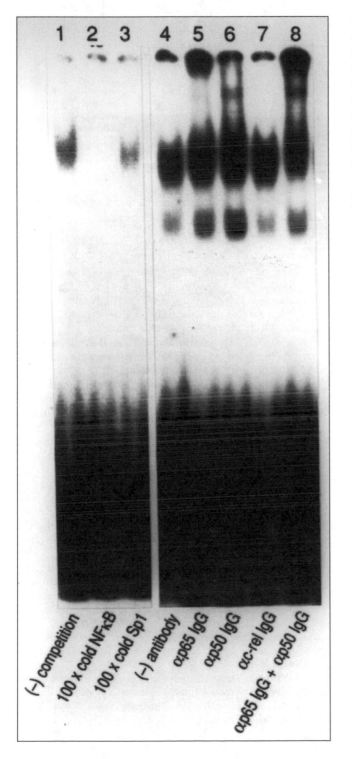

Fig. 36.18. Binding of nuclear proteins derived from LVAD cells to NF-κB consensus probe: Analysis by electrophoretic mobility shift assay. Cells were harvested from the LVAD surface and immediately frozen in liquid nitrogen. Nuclear extracts were subsequently prepared as described. Nuclear protein (10 μg) was incubated with [^{32}P]-labeled consensus probe for NF-κB alone (lane 1 and 4) or in the presence of an 100-fold molar excess of unlabeled NF-κB (lane 2) or unleveled Sp1 (lane 3). In certain experiments, nuclear protein was preincubated with anti-p65 IgG (lane 5), anti-p50 IgG (lane 6), anti-p50 and anti-p65 IgG together (lane 8) or anti-c-Rel IgG (lane 7). In all supershift assays, IgG (7.5 μg/ml) was utilized. This experiment was performed from cells obtained from two different LVAD surfaces, with identical findings. A representative assay is demonstrated.

Fig. 36.19. Anti-inflammatory intervention with ASA
attenuates the proinflam-
matory/procoagulant re-
sponse created by LVAD implantation. These encouraging results support our hypothesis that indeed the critical phenotype defining the
textured surface LVAD is its
ability to selectively trap and
adsorb dendritic and monocytic cells from the circulating blood elements. Activation of these cells, however, is
clearly dependent on the interactions between the host
and the cellular population of
the LVAD surface and is critically linked to activation of
the NF-κB signal transaction
pathway. Inhibition of this
mechanism, therefore, does
appear to quiet these

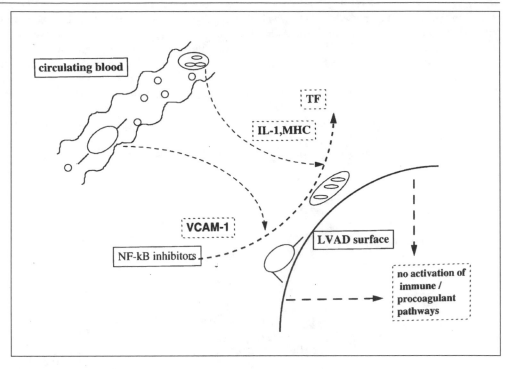

adsorbed cells, inhibiting the production of cytokines and adhesion molecules necessary for the further recruitment and activation
of circulating B cell and T cells. NF-κB inhibitors, therefore, do appear to be effective in downregulating the proinflammatory/
procoagulant systemic milieu associated with LVAD implantation.

Conclusion

We propose that the textured surface LVAD microenvironment presents a prototypic model for the study of
cellular mechanisms that underlie the pathogenesis of
prothrombotic/proinflammatory disorders caused by
implantation of foreign devices. These data suggest that
modification of the present LVAD surface might be
warranted to minimize cellular entrapment and activation.
The activation of NF-κB in this setting provides insight into
a possible target of anti-inflammatory intervention in patients with LVADs (especially as the success of this device
has prompted moves toward its use as a permanent form of
cardiac replacement), and also an excellent setting in which
to delineate the intricate molecular mechanisms that underlie the potent proinflammatory/ prothrombotic environment created by this device. Future studies designed to address the role of both anti-inflammatory intervention in
LVAD patients, as well as modifications in LVAD surface
design and composition as a means of maximizing host-
device compatibility and long term tolerance, are under active investigation.

References

1. McCarthy PM, Portner PM, Tabler CH et al. Clinical experience with the Novacor ventricular assist system. Bridge
   to transplantation and the transition to permanent application. J Thorac Cardiovasc Surg 1991; 102:578-87.
2. Frazier OH, Rose EA, Macmanus Q et al. Multicenter
   clinical experience with the Heartmate 1000 IP LVAD.
   Ann Thorac Surg 1992; 53:1080-1090.
3. Burton NA, Lefrac E, Macmanus Q et al. A reliable bridge
   to cardiac transplantation: The TCI left ventricular assist
   device. Ann Thorac Surg 1995; 55:1425-30.
4. Frazier OH, Macris MP, Myers TJ et al. Improved survival after extended bridge to cardiac transplantation. Ann
   Thorac Surg 1994; 57:1416-1422.
5. McCarthy PM, James KB, Savage RM et al. Implantable
   left ventricular assist device. Approaching an alternative
   for end-satge heart failure. LVAD study group. Circulation 1994; 90(5 pt 2):II83-6.
6. Pennington DG, McBride LR, Peigh PS et al. Eight years
   experience with bridging to cardiac transplantation. J
   Thorac Cardiovasc Surg 1994; 107:472-80.
7. Bernhard WF, Lafarge CG, Robinson et al An improved
   blood pump interface for left ventricular bypass. Ann Surg
   1968; 168:750.
8. Clark R, Boyd J, Moran J. New principles governing the
   tissue reactivity of prosthetic materials. J Surg Research
   1974; 16:510-522.
9. Dasse KA, Chipman S, Sherman C et al. Clinical experience with textured blood contacting surfaces in ventricular assist devices (VADs). Trans Am Soc Artif Intern Organs 1987; 33:418-425.
10. Rose EA, Levin HR, Oz MC et al. Artificial circulatory
    support with textured interior surfaces. A counterintuitive
    approach to minimize thromboembolism. Circulation
    1994; 90(5pt 2):II87-91.
11. Graham TR, Dasse K, Coumbe A et al. Neointimal devel-
    opment on textured biomaterial surfaces during clinical
    use of an implantable left ventricular assist device. Eur J
    Cardio Thoracic Surg 1990; 4:182-190.

12. Slater JP, Rose EA, Levin HR et al. Low thromboembolic risk without anticoagulation using advanced design left ventricular assist devices. Ann Thorac Surg 1996; 62:1321-8.

13. Lavee J, Kormos RL, Duquesnoy RJ et al. Influence of panel-reactive antibody and lymphocytoxic crossmatch on survival after heart transplantation. J. Heart Lung Transplant 1991; 10:921-930.

14. Smith JD, Danskine AJ, Laylor RM et al. The effect of panel reactive antibodies and the donor specific crossmatch on graft survival after heart and heart-lung transplantation. Transplant Immunol 1993; 1:60-65.

15. Massad MG, Cook DJ, Vargo R et al. Factors influencing HLA-sensitization in implantable LVAD recipients. Intl Soc Heart & Lung Transplantation 1996; Abstract #109.

16. Spanicr TB, Oz MC, Levin HR et al. Activation of coagulation and fibrinolytic pathways in patients with left ventricular assist devices. J Thorac Cardiovasc Surg 1996; 112:1090-7.

17. Bibiokis EJ, Livingston AS, Pethak CD et al. The biochemical basis of bleeding during left ventricular assistance. Intl Soc for Heart & Lung Transplantation. 1996; Abstract #110.

18. Salih V, Graham TR, Berry CL et al. The lining of textured surfaces in implantable left ventricular assist devices: An immunocytochemical and electronmicroscopic study. Am J Cardiovasc Pathol 1993; 4:317-325.

19. Frazier OH, Baldwin RT, Eskin SG et al. Immunochemical identification of human endothelial cells on the lining of a ventricular assist device. Texas Heart Inst J 1993; 20:78-82.

20. Menconi MJ, Owen T, Dasse KA et al. Molecular approaches to the characterization of cell and blood/biomaterial interactions. J Cardiac Surg 1992; 7(2):177-187.

21. Menconi MJ, Prockwinse S, Owen TA et al. Properties of blood-contacting surfaces of clinically implanted cardiac assist devices: Gene expression, matrix composition, and ultrastructural characterization of cellular linings. J Cell Biochem 1995; 57:557-573.

22. Rafii S, Oz MC, Seldomridge JA et al. Characterization of human hematopoietic cells arising on the textured surface of left ventricular devices. Ann Thorac Surg 1995; 60:1627-1632.

23. Stella CC, Cazzola M, De Fabritiis P et al. CD34-positive cells: Biology and clinical relevance. Haematologica 1995; 80:367-387.

24. Browning PJ, Sechler JMG, Kaplan M et al. Identification and culture of Kaposi's sarcoma-like spindle cells from the peripheral blood of human immunodeficiency virus-1 infected individuals and normal controls. Blood 1994; 84:2711-2720.

25. Noishiki Y, Tomizawa Y, Yamane Y et al. Autocrine angiogenic vascular prosthesis with bone marrow transplantation. Nat Med 1996; 2:90-92.

26. Leonardo MJ, Fen CM, Baltimore D. The involvement of Nf-κb in interferon gene regulation reveals its role as a widely-inducible mediator of signal transduction. Cell 1989; 57:287-294.

27. Baeuerle PA, Henkel T. Function and activation of NF-κB in the immune system. Ann Rev Immunol 1994; 12:141-179.

28. Nolan G, Ghosh S, Liou HC et al. DNA binding and IkB inhibition of the cloned p65 subunit of Nf-κb: A rel-related polypeptide. Cell 1991; 64:961-969.

29. Manning AM, Anderson DC. Transcription factor Nf-κb: An emerging regulator of inflammation. Annu Rep Med Chem 1994; 29:241.

30. Weber C, Wolfgang E, Pietsch A et al. Aspirin inhibits Nf-κb mobilization and monocyte adhesion on stimulated human endothelial cells. Circulation 1995; 91:1914-1917.

31. Chen CC, Rosenbloom CL, Anderson DC et al. Selective inhibition of E-selectin, vascular cell adhesion molecule-1 and intercellular adhesion molecule—1 expression by inhibitors of IkB-α phosphorylation. J Immunol 1995; 155:3538-3545.

32. Koop E, Ghosh S. Inhibition of Nf-κb by sodium salicylate and aspirin. Science 1994; 265:956-958.

33. Pierce JW, Read MA, Ding H et al. Salicylates inhibit IkB-a phosphorylation, endothelial leucocyte adhesion molecule expression, and neutrophil transmigration. J Immun 1996; 156:3961-3969.

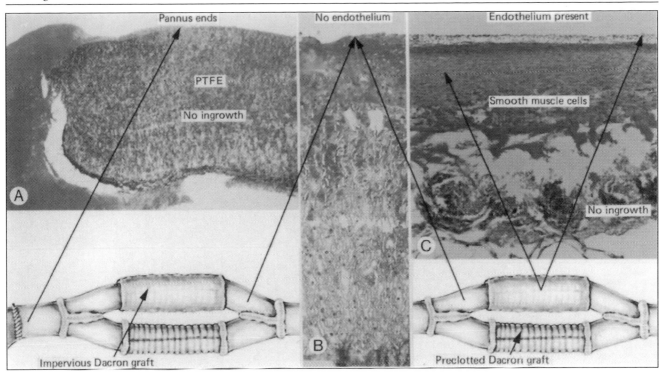

Fig. 35.1. Blockage of pannus and transmural ingrowth for study of fallout endothelialization of isolated central Dacron limb of a prosthesis made impervious by a coating of silicone rubber and implanted for 8 weeks in the descending thoracic aorta of a dog. (A) No transmural ingrowth from perigraft tissues and limited pannus from native aorta onto PTFE (LM, x50). (B) PTFE graft, beyond the pannus zone, showing no perigraft tissue growth into the graft (LM, x25). (C) No perigraft tissue ingrowth into the impervious Dacron graft, but presence of endothelial-like cells on flow surface, with α-actin positive smooth muscle cells beneath (H&E; LM, x50). Reprinted with permission from Shi et al. Proof of fallout endothelialization of impervious Dacron grafts in the aorta and inferior vena cava of the dog. J Vasc Surg 1994; 20:549.

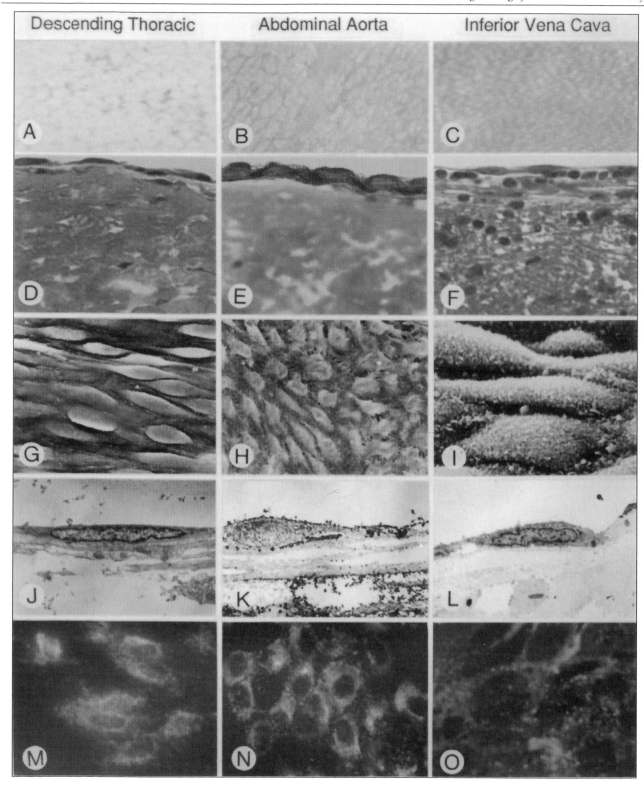

Fig. 35.2. Findings for specimens taken from areas beyond the pannus zone of Dacron grafts made impervious to perigraft tissue ingrowth by a silicone rubber coating and implanted in the dog. (A)-(L) Endothelial-like cells on flow surfaces of Dacron prostheses implanted in the descending thoracic aorta, abdominal aorta and inferior vena cava of the dog: (A)-(C) LM, AgNO$_3$, x70; (D)-(F) LM, x500; (G) SEM, x1000; (H) SEM, x500; (I) SEM, x3000; (J)-(L) TEM, x4000. (M)-(O) Proof of endothelium by FVIII/vWF positivity on flow surface of isolated Dacron grafts: (M)-(N) x500; (O) x1000. Reprinted with permission from Shi et al. Proof of fallout endothelialization of impervious Dacron grafts in the aorta and inferior vena cava of the dog. J Vasc Surg 1994; 20:550.

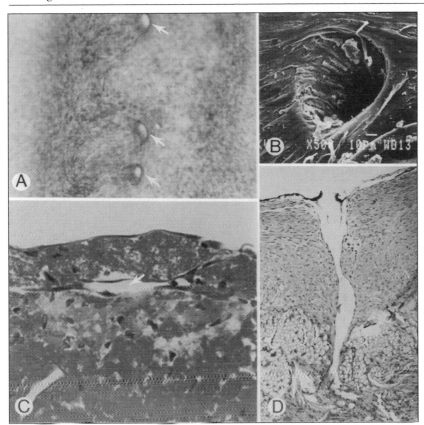

Fig. 35.3. Ostia and microvessels in knitted Dacron grafts wrapped in segments of the inferior vena cava and implanted in the abdominal aorta of dogs. (A) At 2 weeks, flow surface microostia identified by AgNO₃ stain (LM, x74). (B) At 2 weeks, flow surface microostium (SEM, x444). (C) Microvessels in the flow surface lining at 2 weeks (H&E; LM, x486). (D) A 4 week serial section showing a large microvessel between the flow surface and the perigraft tissue (H&E; LM, x108). Reprinted with permission from Onuki et al. Accelerated endothelialization model for the study of Dacron graft healing. Ann Vasc Surg 1997; 11:147.

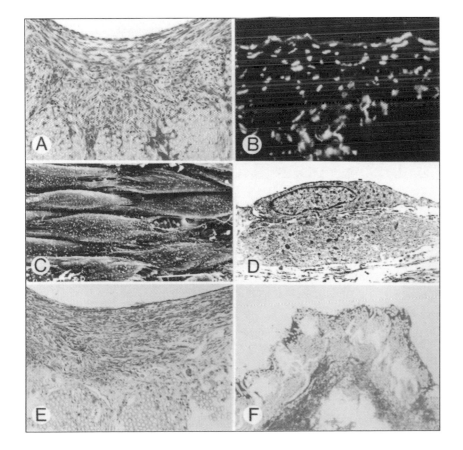

Fig. 35.4. Two week specimens from knitted Dacron grafts wrapped in autogenous inferior vena cava and implanted in dogs. (A) A monolayer of endothelial-like cells on the flow surface (H&E; LM, x108). (B) Proof of endothelium (FVIII/vWF; x460). (C,D) SEM and TEM, respectively, showing morphology typical of endothelium (SEM, x1918; TEM, x4640). (E) α-actin stained smooth muscle cells in the neointima (LM, x108). (F) Control graft, which was not wrapped in inferior vena cava, showing incomplete healing (H&E stain; LM, x42). Reprinted with permission from Onuki et al. Accelerated endothelialization model for the study of Dacron graft healing. Ann Vasc Surg 1997; 1:146.

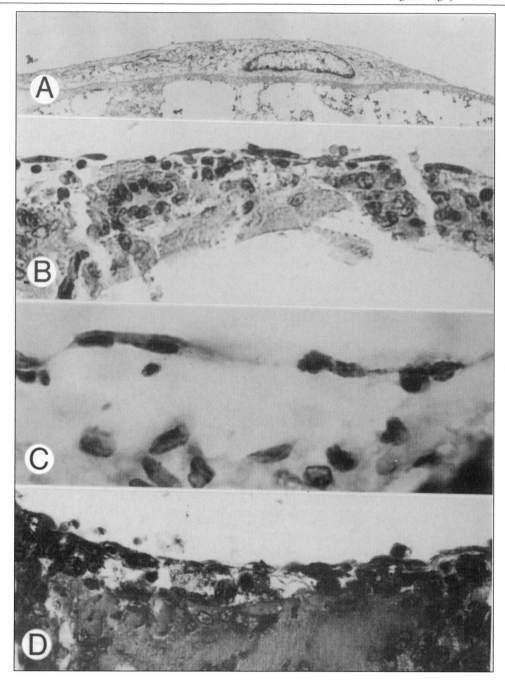

Fig. 35.5. Sections taken from the midgraft area of a woven Dacron axillofemoral bypass graft explanted from a patient during redo surgery after an implant period of 26 months. (A) TEM showing typical endothelial-cell morphology (x3050). (B) Positive factor VIII/vWF staining confirms endothelium (x485). (C) Confirmation of endothelium by positive *Ulex europaeus* agglutinin staining (x1210). (D) HAM 56 staining confirms presence of macrophages (x485). Reprinted with permission from Wu et al. Definitive proof of endothelialization of a Dacron arterial prosthesis in a human being. J Vasc Surg 1995; 21:865.

Facilitation of Healing

Transdifferentiation

——————————— CHAPTER 37 ———————————

Transdifferentiation and the Vascular Wall

William A. Beresford

The solidity of the idea of a continent hindered accepting that continents move and change. Likewise, the long-accumulated robust bases for defining tissue and cell identities obliged one to doubt that the occasional clearcut switches in character by mature, differentiated cells—transdifferentiations[1-3]—were typical of cells in general and had far-reaching significance. But today, such 'plasticity', although a vogue word, demands the attention of surgeons and bioengineers if they are to understand their live working materials. For instance, has what one grows in culture for grafting the phenotype one wants? Will this introduced tissue be stable, and how will it interact with other tissues to maintain or alter their characters? Will reactions to foreign materials or viral vectors for gene transfer[4] encourage cells to take on undesirable phenotypes? Can new and beneficial phenotypes be created in vitro or in animals, for example, cells resistant to rejection or lacking dangerous cytokines? The de novo generation of cardiac myocytes by transdifferentiation is a recent proposal.[5] Certain smooth muscle cells and fibroblasts can become epithelial and glandular. Hence, can one graft to a vascular site cells transfected for long term prolific liberation of a therapeutic substance, but which still have a sufficiently 'vascular' nature to be properly integrated? Or which might also be regulated or transfected to express adhesion molecules to hold the cells in place? Answers lie in seeing how each cell type of the many vascular walls can change its phenotype (Figs. 37.1 and 37.2), uncovering the stimuli and their sources, and tracking the regulatory pathways and interactions.

Endothelial Cells

Endothelial cells (ECs) have multiple personalities, recognized as their many responsibilities at any particular site,[6] and their different properties and responses at various locations[7,8] and in the regions of a vascular bed.[9] Examples are urea transport in the renal medulla,[10] and directing T lymphocyte homing to superficial rather than deep vessels of the dermis.[11] ECs' biochemical profiles must reflect this diversity, but the transdifferentiations detected thus far are mainly morphological.

To further aid lymphocyte homing and emigration, ECs in venules of nodes, tonsils, and mucosal lymphoid organs become cuboidal, quite rich in organelles, and express discernible antigens—high endothelial venules (HEVs).[12] Coagulating and severing the afferent lymphatic vessels to rat popliteal nodes causes the high endothelium to flatten and lose its secretory ultrastructure by three weeks. Injecting sheep erythrocyte antigen into such a node rapidly restores some of the high ECs and the lymphocyte traffic; thus the conversion is reversible.[13]

HEVs develop from normal endothelium in chronically inflamed synovium, both human and experimental animal.[14,15] Other experiments demonstrate the role of an

Tissue Engineering of Prosthetic Vascular Grafts, edited by Peter Zilla and Howard P. Greisler.
©1999 R.G. Landes Company.

Fig. 37.1. Transdifferentiations of vascular grafts.

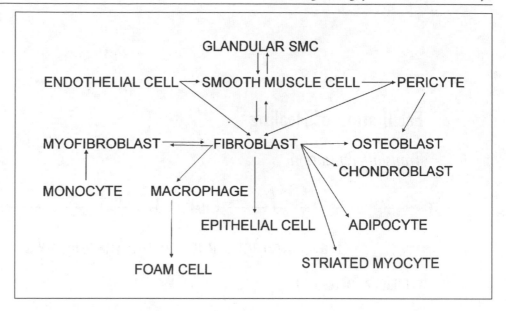

Fig. 37.2. Less gene-flexing transdifferentiations.

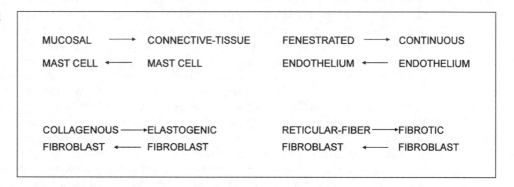

immunoreactive environment and the generality of the transdifferentiation. An immune mediator—gamma-interferon—induces expression of an HEV antigen in cultured nonlymphoid ECs from mouse lung and marrow.[16] Interferon-β, IL-2, and mitogens for ECs did not result in HEV-marker expression. The HEV marker and plumper ECs appeared in dermal venules where sheep red blood cells in Freund's adjuvant had been injected. Subcutaneous implants of sponges loaded with splenic lymphocytes acquire vessels which display a high endothelium, if the lymphocytes are allogeneic.[17]

The second and also reversible EC transdifferentiation is between fenestrated and continuous endothelium. The change may come about rapidly, within 10 minutes,[18] on a physiological time scale (Fig. 37.3), or be slow and enduring. Cirrhosis of the liver in man[19] and in rats injected with CCl$_4$[20] is accompanied by the fenestrated sinusoids acquiring a basement membrane and a continuous endothelium: a capillarization. If the cirrhotic liver progresses to hepatocellular carcinoma, the tumor cells appear to cause the development of a basement membrane and endothelial CD34 expression in the sinusoids of the tumor.[21,22] ECs of these capillary-like tumor vessels are peculiar in having so many

microfilaments with focal densities as to lead some authors to term them 'myoendothelial'.[23]

The contrary phenomenon—an induction of fenestrae in continuous ECs—also occurs in vivo:

1. During regrowth of capillaries in wounded guinea-pig cremaster muscle;[24]
2. In vessels growing into the rat retinal pigment epithelium after urethane-induced loss of the photoreceptors;[25] and
3. In human dermal papillary vessels affected by psoriasis.[26]

Experimental instances are in:

1. The new capillaries of hypertrophied guinea pig gut muscle;[27]
2. Rabbit lingual microvessels a few hours after destruction of the animal's platelets by anti-serum;[28] and
3. Rat cremasteric and dermal capillaries treated locally with vascular endothelial growth factor (VEGF).[29]

A month of continuous infusion of retinoic acid or phorbol acetate into the rat cortex[30] results in fenestrated vessels in cerebral cysts. After cessation of the infusion and removal of the cannula, the vessels in the cystic cavity slowly become continuous, despite the absence of astrocytes. There

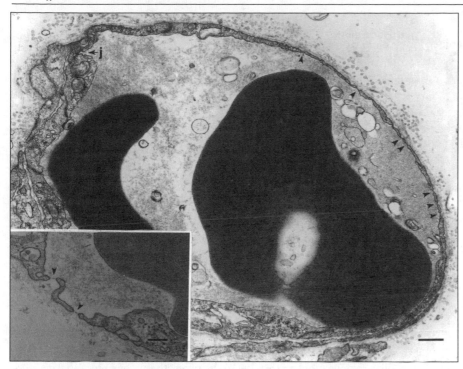

Fig. 37.3. Electron micrographs depicting acute effects of hu rVEGF on the microvasculature. After topical application of VEGF-165 for 10 minutes, the rat cremaster muscle was processed for EM (inset: topically applied VEGF-121). The cremaster muscle is supplied with a continuous (nonfenestrated) endothelium, but within 10 minutes of exposure to VEGF, fenestrations (arrowheads) are formed in the microvascular endothelium. Another effect of VEGF is the loosened interendothelial junction (j). Both fenestrations and open/loose junctions contribute to the permeability-enhancing properties of VEGF. Bar: 500 nm; inset bar: 200 nm. Figure kindly provided by Dr. W Gregory Roberts, University of California, San Diego.

is other evidence in vivo[31] that coculture work may have been misleading as to the importance of astrocytes in regulating how brain ECs create the blood-brain barrier. However, factors in the neural environment are significant, since local chick vessels growing into intracoelomically grafted embryonic quail brain acquire morphological and histochemical features of brain capillaries, with their special variety of continuous endothelium.[32]

For an analysis of factors controlling transdifferentiations, we note that ECs are a form of epithelium, and epithelial-mesenchymal interactions are well investigated, and slowly making sense, in a variety of organs. Similar work in vitro on ECs indicates that fenestrated adrenal capillaries lose their pores unless cultured on basement membrane, newly formed by MDCK cells,[33] or reconstituted as Matrigel. However, the same MDCK-derived matrix was unable to switch continuous capillary ECs to fenestrated.[34] Two specific differentiative agents, having opposite effects on fenestrae of adrenal ECs, were retinoic acid, increasing their number, and TGF-β, causing a marked reduction.[35]

A different and more comprehensive approach in vivo is to examine markers of continuous endothelium and of sinusoids, along with changes in the molecular composition of the adjacent matrix, as human liver sinusoids develop.[36] After an early phase of matrix and cellular structural change (and the loss of capillary markers), the sinusoidal EC markers (CD4, ICAM-1, CD32, and CD14) appeared. Unexpectedly, tenascin, although present, seemed not to regulate EC development, but laminin probably does.[37] The influence of adjacent tissue stands out in the rabbit's nose, where the endothelium of the capillaries and venous sinuses is fenestrated only on the side of the vessel facing the nasal epithelium.[38]

A differentiative role for basement membrane and neighboring tissue[39] is clear in the conversion of embryonic cardiac endothelium of the atrioventricular canal to the mesenchymal cells that will form the cardiac cushion, from which the AV valves and septa develop (Fig. 37.4).[40] This transdifferentiation, in keeping with certain others of embryonic, but partly differentiated, cells is termed an 'epithelial-mesenchymal transition/transformation'. It appears to require specific matrix glycoproteins[41,42] and, in the chick, TGF-β3,[43] but in mouse the TGF isoform responsible and whether it comes from the myocardium are uncertain.[44] Preliminary evidence suggests that, in the earliest development of the avian dorsal aorta, the first SMCs may be derived from the endothelium in chick[45] and quail,[46] from the sharing of endothelial and smooth muscle markers. The endothelial-mesenchymal conversion may not be restricted to embryonic times. Human foreskin microvessel ECs grown in cyclic AMP-deficient medium lose their epithelial and EC characteristics and become mesenchyme-like,[47] as do dermal ECs exposed to interleukin-1β.[48] That this was more than an in vitro dedifferentiation needs evidence that the resulting cells have true mesenchymal potential, but there are other instances of possible EC to SMC conversions.[49]

The localized cardiac loss of endothelial character early in development raises the issue of homeobox phenotype determining genes and their products. Receptors for the vascular endothelial growth factor (VEGF) family are the tyrosine kinases Flk-1 and Flt-1. Two related receptors, also almost restricted to endothelial cells, are Tie and Tek, but their ligand is unknown. Working upstream of the genes for these receptors is the product of a gene altered in the *cloche* mutation in zebrafish.[50] This mutation causes the developing heart to lack endothelial cells. Here one can ask a question

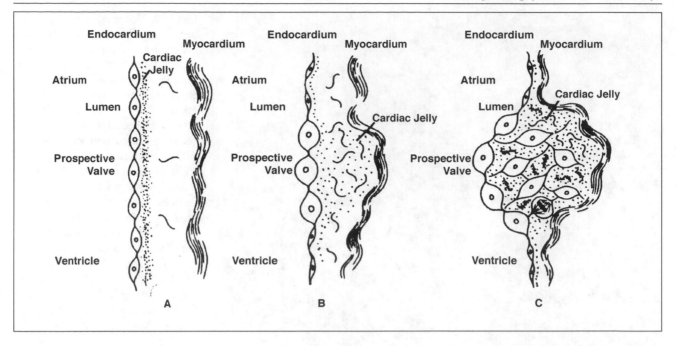

Fig. 37.4. Diagrammatic summary of endocardial cytodifferentiation. In (A) the endocardium of an 8 somite embryo is shown as consisting of uniformly similar cell types in all areas of the simple tubular heart. In (B) the two pathways of endocardial development are shown as they first occur in 16-18 somite embryos: In the atrium and ventricle, the endocardium becomes attenuated with reduced secretory potential and acquires an "endothelial look". Trabeculation brings the myocardium in close proximity to the endocardium (B) and (C) and appears to be temporally related to "endothelization" of atrial and ventricular endocardium. Conversely, in sites where prospective valvular and septal primordia (cushion tissue) will form, the endocardium hypertrophies and acquires and amplifies secretory potential. The initial formation of cushion tissue cells (C) beneath the endocardium, and their morphologic similarity to the latter, suggest that valvular and septal primordia are endocardial derivatives. Reprinted from Markwald G et al. Devel Biol 1975; 42:160-180, with kind permission from Academic Press Inc., Orlando, Florida.

basic to any transdifferentiation, of whether in the endothelial to mesenchymal switch the cell type specific *cloche, Flk-1, flk-2, tie* and *tek* genes stop expression. If so, one asks, 'When?' since there is a sequence to gene activation during embryonic endothelial differentiation. Secondly, are the *Hox* and other genes needed to generate a cell type in normal development (better understood in blood cell lineages[51,52]) again required when that type derives later from a transdifferentiation? If so, this would offer an opportunity for experimental influences on mature cells.

Fibroblasts

The tantalizing variety of site-related fibroblastic phenotypes[53] extends to several kinds of transdifferentiation—glandular, skeletal, and muscular, for example. Stromal fibroblasts of the rodent endometrium become glandular epithelial decidual cells in normal physiology, and in response to various experimental provocations.[54] Stromal cells of the human uterus, tube, and ovary behave similarly. Renal medullary interstitial fibroblasts are laden with lipid droplets and may be endocrine,[55] but in anemia the cortical fibroblasts also acquire significant lipid[56] and are recruited to produce erythropoietin (Fig. 37.5).[57,58] Fibroblasts from somatic rather more than visceral sources become chondroblasts and/or osteoblasts, depending on the stimulus and the animal species,[59,60] but ectopic cartilage and bone

can develop in vascular walls.[61] Phagocytic cells removing surplus collagen from the tadpole's degenerating tail are adapted local fibroblasts.[62]

When the bladder outlet is partially obstructed, submesothelial fibroblasts of the rabbit's urinary bladder proliferate and thicken the serosa. The proliferating cells progress from expressing keratin-18 to become myofibroblasts, and finally resemble fetal smooth muscle cells,[63] based on their immunoreactive cytoskeletal profiles. The authors suggest that the keratin positivity indicates that some of the proliferating fibroblasts become mesothelial cells to replace lost mesothelium. A dual potency of submesothelial fibroblasts is further indicated by the mixture of smooth muscle cells (SMCs) and decidua-like cells in the guinea pig peritoneum, resulting from giving progesterone after three months of estrogen priming.[64]

In vitro studies mirror most of the above transdifferentiations in vivo, and add more. Notable is the conversion of the fibroblast-like 3T3 cell line to adipocytes.[65] Blocking mitosis with relaxin does not prevent the adipogenic conversion,[66] giving further evidence that transdifferentiation can be direct,[67] i.e., not dependent on cell division. A mesenchymal to epithelial switch is demonstrated by 3T3 cells transfected with hepatocyte growth factor (HGF/SF) and the human Met receptor.[68] The cells become epithelial-like in vitro and tumorigenic in nude mice.

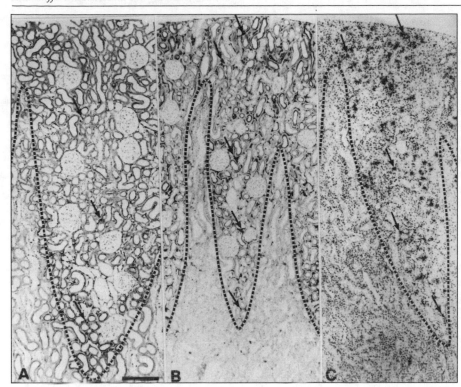

Fig. 37.5. Distribution of interstitial ecto-5'-nucleotidase activity (ena) (A,B) and of mRNA of erythropoietin (C) in cortex of rat kidney. (A) In normemic rats interstitial staining for ena (arrows) is strong only in deep levels of the cortical labyrinth (above broken line); extent and intensity of staining decease toward superficial labyrinth (bar = 200 μm). (B) In an anemic rat the extent of superficial staining is increased, and staining intensity is strong; (C) In situ hybridization of mRNA for erythropoietin in same animal as in (B), showing same distribution pattern as for ena. Reprinted from Hir ML, Kaissling B. Am J Physiol 1993; 264:F377-F387, with kind permission of the American Physiological Society, Bethesda, Maryland.

Taxol treatment of mouse embryonic fibroblasts makes them adopt an epithelial morphology.[69]

Hypoxic pulmonary vasoconstriction and hypertension result from keeping newborn calves at simulated high altitude. Among the structural remodelings is the switch of adventitial fibroblasts of the pulmonary arteries to making elastin.[70] Medium from culturing SMCs from hypoxic arteries brings about an elastogenic response in cultured adventitial fibroblasts from normal pulmonary arteries. In general, the role of adventitial fibroblasts in vessel-wall remodeling may have been underestimated.[71]

The 'myofibroblast'[72]—the cell combining features of fibroblast and SMC—is a practical and theoretical challenge. Uncovering and understanding transdifferentiations of fibroblasts to or towards muscle cells stumble on six issues:

1. How does one know that the starting cell was a fibroblast, since many organs normally contain myofibroblasts, including aortic valves?[73]
2. Somatic connective tissues by and large lack myofibroblasts, unless disturbed or diseased,[74,75] and help with this problem;
3. How easily are SMCs, fibroblasts, and myofibroblasts to tell apart? They are distinguished by certain definitive ultrastructural features, such as microfilament bundles and dense bodies which got the myofibroblast idea started, but mostly by quantitatively different profiles[76] rather than by specific markers, although α-smooth muscle actin has been the main standby, signifying a shift towards muscle. (Specific cell type markers now exist only as smoothelin for smooth muscle[77] and certain mAbs for fibroblast surface epitopes.[78])

4. Myofibroblasts occur as subtypes based on how far they share other cytoskeletal components, such as desmin with smooth muscle,[79] and there are species differences;[80]
5. Some myofibroblasts may be caught part way though a fibroblast to smooth muscle conversion;[81] many others seem to be a stable endpoint of a transdifferentiation, although still able to revert to fibroblasts;[82]
6. Study of the production of extracellular matrix by myofibroblasts has focused on collagen until recently;[83]
7. The organ diversity of fibroblastic forms brings variety to the starting cell: How fibroblastic are hepatic stellate cells,[84] renal mesangial cells,[85] and renal interstitial fibroblasts?[86]

The bulky literature on myofibroblasts concentrates on visceral fibrosis and dermal wound healing, but some of the experiments are exciting, with new stimuli acting on the usual cells, and old stimuli provoking newly examined cells. The general phenotype-altering agent 5-azacytidine confers an SMC-like phenotype on mouse mesangial cells.[87] Exposing mouse dermal fibroblasts continuously to culture medium from growing C2C12 skeletal myoblasts causes the fibroblasts to express a skeletal muscle-specific transcription factor—MyoD—and desmin.[88] And the differentiation-perturbing factor TGF-β1 similarly has cardiac fibroblasts in culture becoming like cardiac myocytes.[89] Intriguingly, striated muscle, smooth muscle, and fibroblasts are already linked in that all three, and endothelium, synthesize a special collagen—type XV.[90]

The cells involved in colonizing and incorporating a Dacron graft to the canine aorta imply a similar connection. The graft becomes lined with collagen-synthesizing myofibroblasts, with a gradation of phenotype from fibroblasts in the pseudointima. Filaments in the early central endothelioid cells indicated that some of the endothelial cells might derive from the adjacent myofibroblasts,[91] a counterpoint to embryonic aortic endothelial cells being a source of VSMCs. However, fibroblasts and endothelial cells are not directly tied to muscular phenotypes in that it is only the three muscle varieties that share use of the Gax homeodomain protein during mouse embryogenesis.[92] Lastly, angioplastic balloon injury elicits proliferation and a myofibroblastic reaction from adventitial fibroblasts in porcine coronary arteries.[93]

Analyzing how cytokines influence the phenotypic conversions is of general interest. Four experiments point the way. Fibrosis is an end result requiring adequate numbers of myofibroblasts, so which cytokines promote proliferation? And which cause transdifferentiation? When TGF-β1 induces quiescent normal human breast fibroblasts to express α-smooth muscle actin in culture without dividing, this shows the differentiative role of TGF-β, and that the phenotype does not arise by selection of a subpopulation.[74] This is, incidentally, another example of a direct transdifferentiation. Overexpression of GM-CSF in the rat lung in vivo expands and activates the macrophage population, which then provides the TGF-β causing the myofibroblasts to develop and make collagen.[94] Detection of levels of, and relations between, cytosolic signal-transduction molecules, such as Ras and MAPK, in cells responding to TGF-β can rule out the involvement of certain other cytokines in myofibroblast activity.[84] Lastly, as rat cardiac fibroblasts convert to myofibroblasts in response to injury, they express angiotensin-converting enzyme (ACE) on their surface. The resulting angiotensin ii may stimulate the release of TGF-βl by autocrine and paracrine modes from the myofibrolasts themselves and macrophages, respectively (Fig. 37.6).[95]

Smooth Muscle Cells

The diversity of smooth muscle phenotypes expresses different embryological germ layer origins, locations, changed physiological demands, pathological effects, and species. Ectodermal neural crest gives rise to smooth muscle of great arteries, but, if ablated, is replaced inadequately by mesodermal SMCs.[96] Lineage maintains its influence on the thoracic versus abdominal aortic SMCs in their adult behavior. Vascular smooth muscle cells (VSMCs) are distinct from gastrointestinal, uterine and tracheal smooth muscles, and experience most of the known transdifferentiations. In the kidney, the afferent arterioles become glandular and secrete renin in response to a variety of stimuli,[67] including an inhibitor of angiotensin I converting enzyme.[97] SMCs of some muscular arteries become fibroblastic in situ, producing excessive collagen and other ECM materials in medial fibromuscular dysplasia,[98,99] a condition reproduced in dogs after several months by blocking the vasa vasorum with a mixture of thrombin and gelatin.[100] A more physiological phenomenon is the remodeling and increase in medial collagen in mesenteric arteries of spontaneously hypertensive rats,[101] although the changes precede the increase in blood pressure,[102] so that what prompts the response is unclear.

Fig. 37.6. A theoretical model depicting inflammatory and postinflammatory phases of tissue repair. Reprinted from Weber KT et al. Int J Biochem Cell Biol 1997; 29:31-42, with kind permission from Elsevier Science Ltd., Kidlington OX5 1GB, UK.

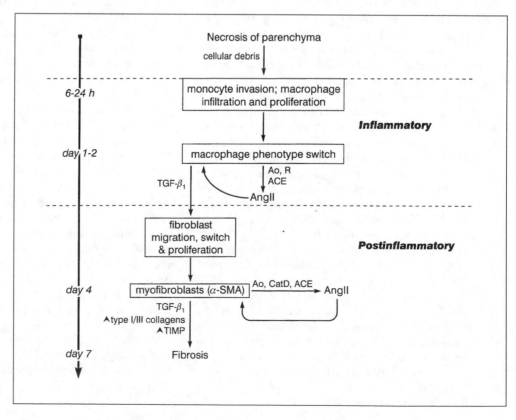

Knowing the ontogeny of the cells, migratory possibilities, and the actual state of the tissue believed to undergo conversion is essential for accurate interpretation. For example, veins grafted in place of arteries are thought to undergo 'arterialization'. But the smooth muscle of the neointima may have migrated from host arterial wall,[103] or come in as myofibroblasts from the remodeling venous perivascular tissue,[104] or even have been present before grafting.[105]

Intense clinical interest focuses on atherosclerosis-mimicking fibroblastic behaviors of VSMCs, which include proliferation and migration—striking changes in the normally quiescent contractile cells. Circumstances evoking a contractile to synthetic arterial VSMC transition (Fig. 37.7) include: culturing in serum;[106] luminal injury;[107] intraperitoneal injections of benzo[*a*]pyrene;[108] uremia from subtotal nephrectomy;[109] adjacent mesenteric fibrosis;[110] giant-cell arteritis;[111] immune injury from allogeneic transplantation;[112] and, perhaps closer to etiological mechanisms, topical application of cytokines.[113] The examples show that VSMCs from both muscular and elastic arteries execute the switch.

How much of a change is it for VSMCs to become fibroblastically 'synthetic'?[106] First, the cells in development are substantial synthesizers of ECM, while acquiring contractility. Secondly, normal human aortic VSMCs contain the synthetic organelles—granular endoplasmic reticulum and a Golgi complex, in addition to the contractile machinery,[114] whereas those of the usual experimental animals are far fewer. In some species the media includes 'nonmuscle' cells.[115-117] Thirdly, VSMCs becoming synthetic in culture can be returned to a contractile state.[118-120] Some would question whether the acquisition of a phenotype by a reversion to embryonic behavior, or by boosting existing activi-

ties, qualifies as a transdifferentiation. An eclectic lumping of all such phenomena is justified, since so little is known of what aspects of phenotype are significant, and any rules of regulation learned in a suspect transdifferentiation illuminate differentiation mechanisms in general. The contractile to synthetic shift is reflected in abundantly altered gene expressions, with activation or reactivation for cytokeratins 8 and 18,[121] tenascin,[122] collagen type VIII,[123] α_3 integrin,[124] nonmuscle myosin heavy chain,[93] platelet-derived growth factor A chain,[125] and the related transmembrane proteoglycans, syndecans 1 and 4,[126] with changed balances of alternative RNA-splicing,[127] a marked downregulation of 'contractile' genes, and upregulation for collagen,[128] c-*myc*,[129] sulfated proteoglycans,[130] and matrix metalloproteinases.[131,132] Caveolin is not reduced, but is redistributed internally.[133]

Analysis of phenotypic regulation has penetrated to the coordination of gene transcriptions and the search for shared type-specific transcription factors.[134] The control of key cytokines occurs both by the sequestration by binding in the ECM[135] and by localization to cell surface proteoglycan modulators.[136] Signals come via cell-matrix binding from the ECM made by the cells themselves[137] and by adjacent cells.[124] The confirmation and stabilization of phenotype also derive from the linking of cells by cell-cell junctions, including the innervation.[138] For the earliest establishment of vascular smooth muscle, tissue factor (used later to help initiate clotting) is needed, as shown by a gene inactivation experiment in mice,[139] but homeotic gene expression patterns specific for VSMC precursors at this stage are not yet known.

Other smooth muscles than vascular resemble VSMCs in their heterogeneity[140] and plasticity: Tracheal SMCs become 'synthetic' in culture;[141] gut SMCs make more ECM material, if the ileum is partially obstructed in guinea-pigs;[27]

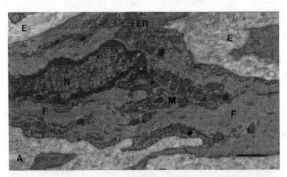

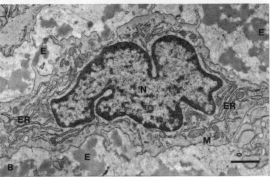

Fig. 37.7. (A) shows a contractile smooth muscle cell from the media of the rat carotid artery, and (B) a synthetic smooth muscle cell from the neointima two weeks after balloon injury. E, elastic fibers; ER, endoplasmic reticulum; F, myofilaments; M, mitochondria; N, nucleus. Magnification x15,000; bar = 1 μm. Reprinted from Thyberg J et al. Cell Tissue Res 1995; 281:421-433, with kind permission from Springer-Verlag GmbH, Heidelberg, Germany.

and TGF-β1 stimulates collagen production by human gut SMCs in vitro.[142] However, the different layers of smooth muscle in the gut require independent developmental control, including neural and epithelial influences, and the major lability is back and forth between an α-SM actin-expressing smooth muscle myoblast and a γ-SM actin-endowed SMC.[143]

Pericytes

Pericytes resemble smooth muscle cells in their contractile proteins, membrane receptors, and membrane properties,[144,145] but junctions between pericytes are lacking.[146] Pericytes attach to endothelial cells, but whether there are gap junctions between endothelial cells and SMCs is controversial.[147] Pericytes bind a specific antiganglioside antibody.[144] A transdifferentiation related to their probable function of contraction is from pulmonary arteriolar pericytes to SMCs in rats kept for several days in hypobaric chambers.[148] Also, cells already intermediate in ultrastructure between SMCs and pericytes became SMCs. The idea of a stable, normal, intermediate pericyte phenotype[149] is met elsewhere as the myofibroblast of normal tissues, renal cells expressing both myoid and renin-secreting properties, and normal VSMCs with dual synthetic and contractile roles.

Other pericyte transdifferentiations include cultured bovine retinal pericytes becoming bone-forming osteoblasts,[150,151] and a fibroblastic conversion in excessive human dermal scarring.[152] Based on double immunofluorescent reactivities for indicators of collagen synthesis and a pericyte marker, a switch of pericytes to perivascular fibroblasts takes place in the scarring.

Mast Cells

Mast cells of rats and mice express distinct phenotypes related to where they are located—the gastrointestinal mucosae versus connective tissue and the peritoneum (MMCs vs. CTMCs). The cell types are well delineated by granule and mediator chemistry and responses.[153] By contrast, the two main types of human mast cell (MC) usually occur together, but may work with different ends in mind,[154] which locally influences the balance of numbers. Mucosae and immune defense require the MC_T, whereas the MC_{TC} is active in connective tissues, fibrosis, and atherosclerosis.[155]

The phenotypic distinction is based on the MC_{TCS} having chymase, carboxypeptidase, and cathepsin G, in addition to mast cell tryptase. Furthermore, the granule ultrastructure also does not completely distinguish the two.[156] The clearer cut phenotypes of murine mast cells, mast cell-deficient mutant mice, and the ability of mouse precursor cells to differentiate in culture render convincing the evidence for transdifferentiations in rodents. MMCs become CTMCs when injected intraperitoneally[157] or into the skin,[158] and a CTMC introduced into gastric mucosa gave rise to MMCs.[159] More elaborate experiments indicate that the switches are reversible.[160] Helping to pinpoint how their environment switches mast cell types was the conversion of mucosal-like MCs to CTMCs by coculture with 3T3 fibroblasts,[161] and a variety of studies on how cytokines affect mast cell differentiation.[153]

Macrophages

The working macrophage has already experienced two profound changes of phenotype, which are, in a sense, transdifferentiations: from circulating monocyte to tissue macrophage;[162,163] and from quiescent macrophage to activated macrophage.[164] An activation step, under the prompting of cytokines, happens to endothelial[165] and other cells, and is not peculiar to leukocytes. These conversions are relevant to transdifferentiation,[166] but will be set aside for more extreme changes of macrophage phenotype.

Surface and other markers indicated that most of the foam cells of atherosclerotic lesions are modified macrophages.[167] Providing modified cholesterol to macrophages in culture turns them into foam cells,[168] a process accompanied by changes in the expression of many genes.[169] Circulating monocytes might convert to myofibroblasts organizing thromboses[170] and intraperitoneal blood clots,[171] but an origin from fibroblasts has not totally been excluded. Macrophages may become producers of collagen, while creating a capsule around implanted mammary tumor cells.[172] In the developing chick optic nerve, some of the macrophages disposing of dying redundant neurons elongate and become like microglia.[173] Embryonic macrophages give rise to the Hofbauer cells of the placental villi,[174] yet another example where organ-specific circumstances fine tune and stabilize cell phenotypes.

Two proposed additional origins for macrophages also rest on transdifferentiations: Coculturing mouse B lymphocytes with splenic fibroblasts confers some macrophage properties on the B cells;[175] and renal glomerular podocytes become macrophage-like in rat cell culture, and perhaps in human crescentic glomerulonephritis.[176] A fair conclusion from this miscellany of phenomena is that the macrophage bears close watching and is more experimentally challenging because of its undoubted heterogeneity,[177] functional plasticity, and metaplastic potential. Quickly aroused at the scene of injury and a potent source of cytokines, the macrophage and its characteristics must be known for its conduct to be steered.

Conclusions

The lessons apply to transdifferentiation generally, and to any organ, because it will have vessels with cells exquisitely adapted to serve that organ's tasks. For cell phenotype, location is almost everything. Knowing very few of the elements of phenotype, one can still experiment fruitfully using the shorthand of organ and site, e.g., renal medullary interstitial fibroblasts. The picture one thereby builds of the human body is not like the four entities (tissues) of the United Kingdom, but rather the astounding patchwork of 18th century Germany, with autonomous parts ranging from the Margraviate of Braunschweig-Luneburg to the imperial cities of Schweinfurt and Wangen.

Cell lineage and current local microenvironment specify what cells are and do within a normal physiological range. For convenience, one speaks of 'modulations' of activity and characteristics within this range, but excursions beyond enter into the territory of transdifferentiation, but not necessarily immediately, in the sense that there is implicitly, and often overtly, an intermediate zone—reflected in the myofibroblast, epithelioid SMC, and such others. However, as the investigation probes phenotype more deeply, the extent of molecular change involved in, say, a contractile SMC becoming a synthetic SMC may amount to a transdifferentiation. Differential gene and protein analysis and display will help define exactly how related cell types differ.[178]

Progress requires that the differentiated state and its conversions be understood in terms of cell structure, behavior (including polarity, proliferation, migration, adhesion,[179] and inclination to apoptosis[180]) the distinctive working molecules, the transcriptional and translational regulators producing those molecules, the receptors and transduction mechanisms controlling the production and deployment of the principal molecules, the external relations of the cell with signals, cells, and matrix, and what the cell 'remembers' of its lineage, i.e., its precursor states. Relative to what should be known, transdifferentiations are testified to by a very few structural and chemical markers, expressing what available technique, curiosity, current concerns, and often chance happened upon in regeneration and disease. Routes to a more systematic study include such questions as: Can cells return along lineage pathways that they have traversed? (Osteoblasts and mast cells may be more terminal than fibroblasts and pericytes.) And, if reversion occurs, what is the story of homeodomain genes and 'master' transcriptional factors, and of signaling mechanisms? Answers learned from the classic transdifferentiations in amphibia, worms, hydra, plants, and other mammalian systems[2,3] remain pertinent.

The question of what restrains adult cell phenotype received new impetus from the cloning of a lamb from a ewe's mammary epithelial cell nucleus.[181] The lineage of the mammary cells of the lamb is extraordinary, but highlights what was already evident from experiments with hybrid fused cells, transplanted differentiated embryonic cells, and gene transfections,[182] namely that mature cells remain able to become vastly different cell types. This potential lies fallow for the bioengineer's cultivation, but within many constraints, some of which have emerged during the look at vascular transdifferentiations.

If any cell can transdifferentiate, this clouds cell responsibility. For example, the matrix-depositing atherosclerotic intimal cell could derive from SMCs—the customary view—or endothelial cells,[46] or adventitial fibroblasts,[93] or from more than one source. Which choice is correct informs the steps to therapy and prevention. Lineage has to do not only with specific expressions, e.g., of major determinants of phenotype, such as NeuroD,[183] but with their timing, to which controlled useful transdifferentiations will have to pay heed.

There is an enduring consistency of cell behavior and matching phenotype, but experimental and pathological perturbation shows this calm harmony is precarious and the product of ceaseless communication between cells and their milieu. Transdifferentiations often happen because of disruption. The inherent contradiction is in seeking what confirms and stabilizes cell phenotype from studies of brief provocation. To be useful a new phenotype must integrate harmoniously over the longer term. The invasive growth within the brain of fibroblasts expressing a transgene for tyrosine hydrolase[184] illustrates the danger of modifying only one aspect of phenotype. Fortunately, cell proliferation is not a prerequisite for a switch of phenotype, making it easier to aim for a new cell type while taking steps to prevent runaway growth in vivo.

Another route to sufficient cells of a desired type is to steer stem cells to differentiate while they proliferate, but again the problem arises of matching in vitro cell type to host organ locale. Can one achieve sufficient refinement in this before grafting? Detection of the critical environmental factors, along with coculture or transfer of medium, may be an avenue.

The paucity of known controlling factors constitutes another obstacle—TGF-β and retinoic acid influence the differentiation of several different, but in vivo adjacent, cell types. For selectivity, much more needs to be known of how such factors are released, bind, are activated, work in sequence and combination, and affect the transduction systems. Beyond the signals are the transcriptional controls, where the complexity multiplies almost by the month for any given cell type specific gene, including sometimes the discovery that the gene is expressed in cell types not conventionally thought to be related, such as prostate-specific antigen in the female breast. Nevertheless, cures can be effective without one knowing how, and induced bone for skeletal repair[60,185] shows that transdifferentiations[186] can be applied to healing before they are satisfactorily understood at cellular and molecular levels.

References

1. Beresford WA. Chondroid Bone, Secondary Cartilage, and Metaplasia. Munich & Baltimore: Urban & Schwarzenberg, 1981:1-454.
2. Okada TS, Kondoh H. Transdifferentiation and Instability in Cell Commitment. Kyoto: Yamada Science Foundation, 1986:1-433.
3. Reyer RW, Lion W, Pinkstaff CA. Ultrastructure and glycoconjugate histochemistry of the lens capsule during lens regeneration from the iris in the newt. Exp Eye Res 1994; 58:315-329.
4. Arnold TE, Gnatenko D, Bahou WF. In vivo gene transfer into rat arterial walls with novel adeno-associated virus vectors. J Vasc Surg 1997; 25:347-355.
5. Olson EN. Things are developing in cardiology. Circ Res 1997; 80:604-606.
6. Shireman PK, Pearce WH. Endothelial cell function: Biologic and physiologic functions in health and disease. AJR 1996; 166:7-13.
7. Fajardo LF. The complexity of endothelial cells. Am J Clin Pathol 1989; 92:241-250.
8. Garlanda C, Dejana E. Heterogeneity of endothelial cells. Specific markers. Arterioscler Thromb Vasc Biol 1997; 17:1193-1202.
9. Spanel-Borowski K. Diversity of ultrastructure in different phenotypes of cultured microvessel endothelial cells isolated from bovine corpus luteum. Cell Tissue Res 1991; 266:37-49.

10. Xu Y, Olives B, Bailly P et al. Endothelial cells of the kidney vasa recta express the urea transporter HUT11. Kidney Int 1997; 51:138-146.

11. Kunstfeld R, Lechleitner S, Groger M et al. HECA-452+ T cells migrate through superficial vascular plexus but not through deep vascular plexus endothelium. J Invest Dermatol 1997; 108:343-348.

12. Kraal G, Duijvestijn AM, Hendriks HH. The endothelium of the high endothelial venule: A specialized endothelium with unique properties. Exp Cell Biol 1987; 55:1-10.

13. Hendriks HR, Eestermans IL. Disappearance and reappearance of high endothelial venules and immigrating lymphocytes in lymph nodes deprived of afferent lymphatic vessels: A possible regulatory role of macrophages in lymphocyte migration. Eur J Immunol 1983; 13:663-669.

14. Miller JJ III. Studies of the phylogeny and ontogeny of the specialized lymphatic vessels. Lab Invest 1969; 21:484-490.

15. Freemont AJ, Jones CJP, Bromley M et al. Changes in vascular endothelium related to lymphocyte collections in diseased synovia. Arthr Rheum 1983; 26:1427-1433.

16. Duijvestijn AM, Schreider AB, Butcher EC. Interferon-gamma regulates an antigen specific for endothelial cells involved in lymphocyte trafficking. Proc Natl Acad Sci USA 1986; 83:9114-9118.

17. Bishop DK, Sedmak DD, Leppink DM et al. Vascular endothelial differentiation in sponge matrix allografts. Hum Immunol 1990; 28:128-133.

18. Roberts WG, Palade GE. Increased microvascular permeability and endothelial fenestration induced by vascular endothelial growth factor. J Cell Sci 1995; 108:2369-2379.

19. Schaffner F, Popper H. Capillarization of hepatic sinusoids. Gastroenterology 1963; 44:239-242.

20. Martinez-Hernandez A, Martinez J. The role of capillarization in hepatic failure: Studies in carbon tetrachloride-induced cirrhosis. Hepatology 1991; 14:864-874

21. Cui S, Hano H, Sakata A et al. Enhanced CD34 expression of sinusoid-like vascular endothelial cells in hepatocellular carcinoma. Pathol Int 1996; 46:751-756.

22. Nakamura S, Muro H, Suzuki S et al. Immunohistochemical studies on endothelial cell phenotype in hepatocellular carcinoma. Hepatology 1997; 26:407-415.

23. Haratake J, Scheuer PJ. An immunohistochemical and ultrastructural study of the sinusoids of hepatocellular carcinoma. Cancer 1990; 65:1985-1993.

24. McKinney RY, Singh BB, Brewer PD. Fenestrations in regenerating skeletal muscle capillaries. Am J Anat 1977; 150:213-218.

25. Burns MS, Hartz MJ. The retinal pigment epithelium induces fenestration of endothelial cells in vivo. Current Eye Res 1992; 11:863-873.

26. Braverman IM, Yen A. Ultrastructure of the capillary loops in the dermal papillae of psoriasis. J Invest Dermatol 1977; 68:53-60.

27. Gabella G. Hypertrophic smooth muscle. V. Collagen and other extracellular materials. Vascularization. Cell Tissue Res 1984; 235:275-283.

28. Kitchens CS, Weiss L. Ultrastructural changes of endothelium associated with thrombocytopenia. Blood 1975; 46:567-578.

29. Roberts WG, Palade GE. Neovasculature induced by vascular endothelial growth factor is fenestrated. Cancer Res 1997; 57:765-772.

30. Kaya M, Chang L, Truong A et al. Chemical induction of fenestrae in vessels of the blood-brain barrier. Exp Neurol 1996; 142:6-13.

31. Krum JM. Effect of astroglial degeneration on neonatal blood-brain barrier marker expression. Exp Neurol 1996; 142:29-35.

32. Stewart PA, Wiley MJ. Developing nervous tissue induces formation of blood-brain barrier characteristics in invading endothelial cells: A study using quail-chick chimeras. Devel Biol 1981; 84:183-192.

33. Milici AJ, Furie MB, Carley WW. The formation of fenestrations and channels by capillary endothelium in vitro. Proc Natl Acad Sci USA 1985; 82:6181-6185.

34. Carley W, Milici AJ, Madri JA. Extracellular matrix specificity for the differentiation of capillary endothelial cells. Exp Cell Res 1988; 178:426-434.

35. Lombardi T, Montesano R, Furie MB et al. In vitro modulation of endothelial fenestrae: Opposing effects of retinoic acid and transforming growth factor β. J Cell Sci 1988; 91:313-318.

36. Couvelard A, Scoazec J-Y, Dauge M-C et al. Structural and functional differentiation of sinusoidal endothelial cells during liver organogenesis in humans. Blood 1996; 87:4568-4580.

37. Couvelard A, Scoazec J-Y, Feldmann G. Expression of cell-cell and cell-matrix adhesion proteins by sinusoidal endothelial cells in the normal and cirrhotic liver. Am J Pathol 1993; 143:738-752.

38. Grevers G. The role of fenestrated vessels for the secretory process in the nasal mucosa: A histological and transmission electron microscopic study in the rabbit. Laryngoscope 1993; 103:1255-1258.

39. Beresford WA. A stromal role in epithelial metaplasia and cancer. Cancer J 1988; 2:145-147.

40. Markwald RR, Fitzharris TP, Adams Smith WN. Structural analysis of endocardial differentiation. Devel Biol 1975; 42:160-180.

41. Sinning AR, Krug EL, Markwald RR. Multiple glycoproteins localize to a particulate form of extracellular matrix in regions of the embryonic heart where endothelial cells transform into mesenchyme. Anat Rec 1992; 232:285-292.

42. Zhang H-J, Kluge M, Timpl R et al. The extracellular matrix glycoproteins BM-90 and tenascin are expressed in the mesenchyme at sites of endothelial-mesenchymal conversion in the embryonic mouse heart. Differentiation 1993; 52:211-220.

43. Nakajima Y, Mironov V, Yamagishi T et al. Expression of smooth muscle alpha-actin in mesenchymal cells during formation of avian endocardial cushion tissue: A role for transforming growth factor β3. Devel Dynam 1997; 209:296-309.

44. Nakajima Y, Miyazono K, Kato M et al. Extracellular fibrillar structure of latent TGFβ binding protein-1: Role in TGFβ-dpendent endothelial-mesenchymal transformation during endocardial cushion formation in mouse embryonic heart. J Cell Biol 1997; 136:193-204.

45. Bergwerff M, DeRuiter MC, Poelman RE et al. Onset of elastogenesis and downregulation of smooth muscle actin as distinguishing phenomena in artery differentiation in the chick embryo. Anat Embryol 1996; 194:545-557.

46. DeRuiter MC, Poelmann RE, VanMunsteren JC et al. Embryonic endothelial cells transdifferentiate into mesenchymal cells expressing smooth muscle actins in vivo and in vitro. Circ Res 1997; 80:444-451.

47. Lipton BH, Bensch KG, Karasek MA. Microvessel endothelial cell transdifferentiation: Phenotypic characterization. Differentiation 1991; 46:117-133.

48. Romero LI, Zhang D-N, Herron GS et al. Interleukin-1 induces major phenotypic changes in human skin microvascular endothelial cells. J Cell Physiol 1997 173:84-92.

49. Majesky MW, Schwartz SM. An origin for smooth muscle cells from endothelium. Circ Res 1997; 80:601-603.

50. Liao W, Bisgrove BW, Sawyer H et al. The zebrafish gene *cloche* acts upstream of a *Flk-1* homologue to regulate endothelial cell differentiation. Development 1997; 124:381-389.

51. Shivdasani RA, Orkin SH. The transcriptional control of hematopoiesis. Blood 1996; 87:4025-4039.

52. Bijl J, van Oostveen JW, Kreike M et al. Expression of HOXC4, HOXC5, and HOXC6 in human lymphoid cell lines, leukemias, and benign and malignant lymphoid tissue. Blood 1996; 87:1737-1745.

53. Komuro T. Re-evaluation of fibroblasts and fibroblast-like cells. Anat Embryol 1990; 182:103-112.

54. Abrahamsohn PA, Zorn TMT. Implantation and decidualization in rodents. J Exp Zool 1993; 266:603-628.

55. Kaissling B, Hegyi I, Loffing J et al. Morphology of interstitial cells in the healthy kidney. Anat Embryol 1996; 193:303-318.

56. Kaissling B, Spiess S, Rinne B et al. Effects of anemia on morphology of rat renal cortex. Am J Physiol 1993; 264:F608-F617.

57. Koury ST, Koury MJ, Bondurant MC et al. Quantitation of erythropoietin-producing cells in kidneys of mice by in situ hybridization: correlation with hematocrit, renal erythropoietin mRNA, and serum erythropoietin concentration. Blood 1989; 74:645-651.

58. Maxwell PH, Ferguson DJP, Nicholls LG et al. Sites of erythropoietin production. Kidney Int 1997; 51:393-401.

59. Mizuno S, Glowacki J. Chondroinduction of human dermal fibroblasts by demineralized bone in three-dimensional culture. Exp Cell Res 1996; 227:89-97.

60. Herr G, Hartwig C-H, Boll C et al. Ectopic bone formation by composites of BMP and metal implants in rats. Acta Orthop Scand 1996; 67:606-610.

61. Beresford WA. Ectopic cartilage, neoplasia, and metaplasia. In: Hall BK, ed. Cartilage, vol 3. New York: Academic Press, 1983:1-48.

62. Kinoshita T, Takahama H, Sasaki F. Changes in the function of dermal fibroblasts in the tadpole tail during anuran metamorphosis. J Exp Zool 1991; 257:166-177.

63. Pampinella F, Roelofs M, Castellucci E et al. Proliferation of submesothelial mesenchymal cells during early phase of serosal thickening in the rabbit bladder is accompanied by transient keratin 18 expression. Exp Cell Res 1996; 223:327-339.

64. Fuji S, Nakashima N, Okamura H et al. Progesterone-induced smooth-muscle-like cells in subperitoneal nodules produced by estrogen. Am J Obstet Gynecol 1981; 139:164-172.

65. Green H, Kehinde O. Spontaneous heritable changes leading to increased adipose conversion in 3T3 cells. Cell 1976; 7:105-113.

66. Pawlina W, Larkin LH, Ogilvie S et al. Human relaxin inhibits division but not differentiation of 3T3-L1 cells. Mol Cell Endocrinol 1990; 72:55-61.

67. Beresford WA. Direct transdifferentiation: Can cells change their phenotype without dividing? Cell Different Devel 1990; 29:81-93.

68. Tsarfaty I, Rong S, Resau JH et al. The Met protooncogene mesenchymal to epithelial cell conversion. Science 1994; 263:98-101.

69. Pletjushkina OJ, Ivanova OJ, Kaverina IN et al. Taxol-treated fibroblasts acquire an epithelioid shape and a circular pattern of actin bundles. Exp Cell Res 1994; 212:201-208.

70. Mecham RP, Whitehouse LA, Wrenn DS et al. Smooth muscle-mediated connective tissue remodeling in pulmonary hypertension. Science 1987; 237:423-426.

71. Arribas SM, Hillier C, Gonzalez C et al. Cellular aspects of vascular remodeling in hypertension revealed by confocal microscopy. Hypertension 1997; 30:1455-1464.

72. Gabbiani G, Majno G. Dupuytren's contracture: Fibroblast contraction? Am J Pathol 1972; 66:131-146.

73. Messier RH Jr, Bass BL, Aly HM et al. Dual structural and functional phenotypes of the porcine aortic valve interstitial population: Characteristics of the leaflet myofibroblast. J Surg Res 1994; 57:1-21.

74. Ronnov-Jessen L, Petersen OW. Induction of α-smooth muscle actin by transformtin growth factor-β1 in quiescent human breast gland fibroblasts. Lab Invest 1993; 68:696-707.

75. Nakanishi I, Kajikawa K, Okada Y et al. Myofibroblasts in fibrous tumors and fibrosis in various organs. Acta Pathol Jpn 1981; 31:423-437.

76. Hebda PA, Collins MA, Tharp MD. Mast cell and myofibroblast in wound healing. Dermatologic Clinics 1993, 11.685-696.

77. Wehrens XHT, Mies B, Gimona M et al. Localization of smoothelin in avian smooth muscle and identification of a vascular-specific isoform. FEBS Lett 1997; 405:315-320.

78. Saalbach A, Anderegg U, Bruns M et al. Novel fibroblast-specific monoclonal antibodies: Properties and specificities. J Invest Dermatol 1996; 106:1314 1319.

79. Gabbiani G. The biology of the myofibroblast. Kidney Int 1992; 41:530-532.

80. Kapanci Y, Ribaux C, Chaponnier C et al. Cytoskeletal features of alveolar myofibroblasts and pericytes in normal human and rat lung. J Histochem Cytochem 1992; 40:1955-1963.

81. Buoro S, Ferrarese, Chiavegato A et al. Myofibroblast-derived smooth muscle cells during remodelling of rabbit urinary bladder wall induced by partial outflow obstruction. Lab Invest 1993; 69:589-602.

82. Oda D, Gown AM, Vande Berg JS et al. Instability of the myofibroblast phenotype in culture. Exp Mol Pathol 1990; 52:221-234.

83. Berndt A, Kosmehl H, Katenkamp D et al. Appearance of the myofibroblastic phenotype in Dupuytren's disease is associated with a fibronectin, laminin, collagen type IV and tenascin extracellular matrix. Pathobiology 1994; 62:55-58.

84. Reimann T, Hempel U, Krautwald S et al. Transformtin growth factor-β1 induces activation of Ras, Raf-1, MEK and MAPK in rat hepatic stellate cells. FEBS Lett 1997; 403:57-60.

85. Iehara N, Takeoka H, Tsuji H et al. Differentiation of smooth muscle phenotypes in mouse mesangial cells. Kidney Int 1996; 49:1330-1341.

86. Hewitson TD, Becker GJ. Interstitial myofibroblasts in IgA glomerulonephritis. Am J Nephrol 1995; 15:111-117.

87. Grupp C, Lottermoser J, Cohen DI et al. Transformation of rat inner medullary fibroblasts to myofibroblasts in vitro. Kidney Int 1997; 52:1279-1290.

88. Wise CJ, Watt DJ, Jones GE. Conversion of dermal fibroblasts to a myogenic lineage is induced by a soluble factor derived from myoblasts. J Cell Biochem 1996; 61:363-374.

89. Eghbali M, Tomek R, Woods C et al. Cardiac fibroblasts are predisposed to convert into myocyte phenotype: Specific effect of transforming growth factor β. Proc Natl Acad Sci USA 1991; 88:795-799.

90. Kivirikko S, Saarela J, Myers JC et al. Distribution of type XV collagen transcripts in human tissue and their production by muscle cells and fibroblasts. Am J Pathol 1995; 147:1500-1509.

91. Sottiurai VS, Batson RC. Role of myofibroblasts in pseudointima formation. Surgery 1983; 94:792-801.

92. Skopicki HA, Lyons GE, Schattemann G et al. Embryonic expression of the Gax homeodomain protein in cardiac, smooth, and skeletal muscle. Circ Res 1997; 80:452-462.

93. De Leon H, Scott NA, Martin F et al. Expression of nonmuscle myosin heavy chain-B isoform in the vessel wall of porcine coronary arteries after balloon angioplasty. Circ Res 1997; 80:514-519.

94. Xing Z, Tremblay GM, Sime PJ et al. Overexpression of granulocyte-macrophage colony-stimulating factor induces pulmonary granulation tissue formation and fibrosis by induction of transformtin growth factor-β1 and myofibroblast accumulation. Am J Pathol 1997; 150:59-66.

95. Weber KT, Sun Y, Katwa LC. Myofibroblasts and local angiotensin ii in rat cardiac tissue repair. Int J Biochem Cell Biol 1997; 29:31-42.

96. Thieszen SL, Dalton M, Gadson PF et al. Embryonic lineage of vascular smooth muscle cells determines responses to collagen matrices and integrin receptor expression. Exp Cell Res 1996; 227:135-145.

97. Gomez RA, Chevalier RL, Everett AD et al. Recruitment of renin-expressing cells in adult rat kidneys. Am J Physiol 1990; 259:F660-F665.

98. Lin WW, McGee GS, Patterson BK et al. Fibromuscular dysplasia of the brachial artery: A case report and review of the literature. J Vasc Surg 1992; 16:66-70.

99. Stanley JC, Gewertz BL, Bove EL et al. Arterial fibrodysplasia. Histopathologic character and current etiologic concepts. Arch Surg 1975; 110:561-566.

100. Sottiurai V, Fry WJ, Stanley JC. Ultrastructural characteristics of experimental arterial medial fibroplasia induced by vasa vasorum occlusion. J Surg Res 1978; 24:169-177.

101. McGuffee LJ, Little SA. Tunica media remodeling in mesenteric arteries of hypertensive rats. Anat Rec 1996; 246:279-292.

102. Dickhout JG, Lee RMKW. Structural and functional analysis of small arteries from young spontaneously hypertensive rats. Hypertension 1997; 29:781-789.

103. Tennant M, McGeachie JK. Adaptive remodelling of smooth muscle in the neo-intima of vein-to-artery grafts in rats: A detailed morphometric analysis. Anat Embryol 1993; 187:161-166.

104. Shi Y, O'Brien JE, Mannion JD et al. Remodeling of autologous saphenous vein grafts. The role of perivascular myofibroblasts. Circulation 1997; 96:2684-2693.

105. Milroy CM, Scott DJA, Beard JD et al. Histological appearances of the long saphenous vein. J Pathol 1989; 159:311-316.

106. Chamley-Campbell J, Campbell GR, Ross R. The smooth muscle cell in culture. Physiol Rev 1979; 59:1-61.

107. Chen Y-H, Chen Y-L, Lin S-J et al. Electron microscopic studies of phenotypic modulation of smooth muscle cells in coronary arteries of patients with unstable angina pectoris and postangioplasty restenosis. Circulation 1997;95:1169-1175.

108. Zhang Y, Ramos KS. The induction of proliferative vascular smooth muscle cell phenotypes by benzo[a]pyrene does not involve mutational activation of ras genes. Mutation Res 1997; 373:285-292.

109. Amann K, Wolf B, Nichols C et al. Aortic changes in experimental renal failure. Hyperplasia or hypertrophy of smooth muscle cells? Hypertension 1997; 29:770-775.

110. Wagenaar SS, Wagenvoort CA. Experimental production of longitudinal smooth muscle in the intima of muscular arteries. Lab Invest 1978; 39:370-374.

111. Shiiki H, Shimokama T, Watanabe T. Temporal arteritis: Cell composition and possible pathogenetic role of cell-mediated immunity. Hum Pathol 1989; 20:1057-1064.

112. Amano J, Ishiyama S, Nishikawa T et al. Proliferation of smooth muscle cells in acute allograft vascular rejection. J Thorac Cardiovasc Surg 1997:113:19-25.

113. Fukumoto Y, Shimokawa H, Ito A et al. Inflammatory cytokines cause coronary arteriosclerosis-like changes and alterations in the smooth-muscle phenotypes in pigs. J Cardiovasc Pharmacol 1997; 29:222-231.

114. Dingemans KP, Jansen N, Becker AE. Ultrastructure of the normal human aortic media. Virchows Arch Pathol Anat 1981:392:199-216.

115. Bergwerff M, DeRuiter MC, Poelmann RE et al. Onset of elastogenesis and downregulation of smooth muscle actin as distinguishing phenomena in artery differentiation in the chick embryo. Anat Embryol 1996; 194:545-557.

116. Frid MG, Dempsey EC, Durmowicz AG et al. Smooth muscle heterogeneity in pulmonary and systemic vessels. Arterioscler Thromb Vasc Biol 1997; 17:1203-1209.

117. Seidel CL. Cellular heterogeneity of the vascular tunica media. Implications for vessel wall repair. Arterioscler Thromb Vasc Biol 1997; 17:1868-1871.

118. Campbell GR, Chamley-Campbell JH. Invited review: The cellular pathobiology of atherosclerosis. Pathology 1981; 13:423-440.

119. Pauly RR, Passaniti A, Crow M et al. Experimental models that mimic the differentiation and dedifferentiation of vascular cells. Circulation 1992; 86[suppl III]:III68-III73.

120. Aikawa M, Sakomura Y, Ueda M et al. Redifferentiation of smooth muscle cells after coronary angioplasty determined via myosin heavy chain expression. Circulation 1997; 96:82-90.

121. Jahn L, Franke WW. High frequency of cytokeratin-producing smooth muscle cells in human atherosclerotic plaques. Differentiation 1989; 40:55-62.

122 Hedin U, Holm J, Hansson GK. Induction of tenascin in rat arterial injury. Relationship to altered smooth muscle cell phenotype. Am J Pathol 1991; 139:649-656.

123. MacBeath JR, Kielty CM, Shuttleworth CA. Type VIII collagen is a product of vascular smooth-muscle cells in development and disease. Biochem J 1996; 319:993-998.

124. Yamamoto M, Nakamura H, Yamato M et al. Retardation of phenotypic transition of rabbit arterial smooth muscle cells in three-dimensional primary culture. Exp Cell Res 1996; 225:12-21.

125. Sjolund M, Hedin U, Sejersen T et al. Arterial smooth muscle cells express platelet-derived growth factor (PDGF) A chain mRNA, secrete a PDGF-like mitogen, and bind exogenous PDGF in a phenotype- and growth state-dependent manner. J Cell Biol 1988; 106:403-413.

126. Cizmeci-Smith G, Langan E, Yuokey J et al. Syndecan-4 is a primary-response gene induced by basic fibroblast growth factor and arterial injury in vascular smooth muscle cells. Arterioscler Thromb Vasc Biol 1997; 17:172-180.

127. Nakasaki Y, Iwamoto T, Hanada H et al. Cloning of the rat aortic smooth muscle Na^+/Ca^{2+} exchanger and tissue-specific expression of isoforms. J Biochem 1993; 114:528-534.

128. Kato S, Stanley JR, Fox JC. Serum stimulation, cell-cell interactions, and extracellular matrix independently influence smooth muscle cell phenotype in vitro. Am J Pathol 1996; 149:687-697.

129. Miano JM, Vlasic N, Tota RR et al. Smooth muscle immediate-early gene and growth factor activation follows vascular injury. Arterioscler Thromb Vasc Biol 1993; 13:211-219.

130. Merrilees MJ, Campbell JH, Spanidis E et al. Glycosaminoglycan synthesis by smooth muscle cells of differing phenotype and their response to conditioned medium. Atherosclerosis 1990; 81:245-254.

131. Bendeck MP, Zempo N, Clowes AW et al. Smooth muscle cell migration and matrix metalloproteinase expression after arterial injury in the rat. Circ Res 1994; 75:539-545.

132. Shofuda K-i, Yasumitsu H, Nishihashi A et al. Expression of three membrane type matrix metalloproteinases (MT-MMPs) in rat vascular smooth muscle cells and characterization of MT3-MMPs with and without transmembrane domain. J Biol Chem 1997; 272:9749-9754.

133. Thyberg J, Roy J, Tran PK et al. Expression of caveolae on the surface of rat arterial smooth muscle cells is dependent on the phenotypic state of the cells. Lab Invest 1997; 77:93-101.

134. Gadson PF Jr, Dalton ML, Patterson et al. Differential response of mesoderm- and neural crest-derived smooth muscle to TGF-β1: regulation of c-myb and α1(I) procollagen genes. Exp Cell Res 1997; 230:169-180.

135. Lee SH, Yan H, Reeser JC et al. Proteoglycan biosyntheis is required in BC3H1 myogenic cells for modulation of vascular smooth muscle α-actin gene expression in response to microenvironmental signals. J Cell Physiol 1995; 164:172-186.

136. Sklaletz-Rorowski A, Schmidt A, Breithardt G et al. Heparin-induced overexpression of basic fibroblast growth factor, basic fibroblast growth factor receptor, and cell-associated proteoheparan sulfate in cultured coronary smooth muscle cells. Arterioscler Thromb Vasc Biol 1996; 16:1063-1069.

137. Sibinga NES, Foster LC, Hsieh C-M et al. Collagen VIII is expressed by vascular smooth muscle cells in response to vascular injury. Circ Res 1997; 80:532-541.

138. Kacem K, Bonvento G, Seylaz J. Effect of sympathectomy on the phenotype of smooth muscle cells of middle cerebral and ear arteries of hyperlipidaemic rabbits. Histochem J 1997; 29:279-286.

139. Carmeliet P, Mackman N, Moons L et al. Role of tissue factor in embryonic blood vessel development. Nature 1996; 383:73-75.

140. Halyko AJ, Rector E, Stephens NL. Characterization of molecular determinants of smooth muscle heterogeneity. Can J Physiol Pharmacol 1997; 75:917-929.

141. Tom-Moy M, Madison JM, Jones CA et al. Morphologic characterization of cultures of smooth muscle cells isolated from the tracheas of adult dogs. Anat Rec 1987; 218:313-328.

142. Graham MF, Bryson GR, Diegelmann RF. Transforming growth factor β1 selectively augments collagen synthesis by human intestinal smooth muscle cells. Gastroenterology 1990; 99:447-453.

143. McHugh KM. Molecular analysis of gastrointestinal smooth muscle development. J Ped Gastroenterol Nutrit 1996; 23:379-394.

144. Anderson DR, Davis EB. Glaucoma, capillaries, and pericytes. 2. Identification and characterization of retinal pericytes in culture. Ophthalmologica 1996; 210:263-268.

145. Schor AM, Canfield AE, Sutton AB et al. Pericyte differentiation. Clin Orthop Rel Res 1995:313:81-91.

146. Schulze C, Firth JA. Junctions between pericytes and the endothelium in rat myocardial capillaries: A morphometric and immunogold study. Cell Tissue Res 1993; 271:145-154.

147. Christ GJ, Spray DC, El-Sabban M et al. Gap junctions in vascular tissues. Circ Res 1996; 79:631-646.

148. Meyrick B, Reid L, The effect of continued hypoxia on rat pulmonary arterial circulation. Lab Invest 1978; 38:188-200.

149. Nehls V, Drenckhahn D. The versatility of microvascular pericytes: From mesenchyme to smooth muscle? Histochemistry 1993; 99:1-12.

150. Canfield AE, Sutton AB, Hoyland JA et al. Association of thrombospondin-1 with osteogenic differentiation of retinal pericytes in vitro. J Cell Sci 1996; 109:343-353.

151. Doherty MJ, Ashton BA, Grant ME et al. Vascular pericytes express osteogenic markers in vitro and form bone in vivo. Int J Exp Pathol 1996; 77:32A.

152. Sundberg C, Ivarsson M, Gerdin B et al. Pericytes as collagen-producing cells in excessive scarring. Lab Invest 1996:74:452-466.

153. Galli SJ. New insights into "The Riddle of the Mast cells": Microenvironmental regulation of mast cell development and phenotypic heterogeneity. Lab Invest 1990; 62:5-33.

154. Church MK, Levi-Schaffer F. The human mast cell. J Allergy Clin Immunol 1997; 99:155-160.

155. Jeziorska M, McCollum C, Wooley DE. Mast cell distribution, activation, and phenotype in atherosclerotic lesions of human carotid arteries. J Pathol 1997; 182:115-122.

156. Weidner N, Austen KF. Evidence for morphologic diversity of human mast cells. An ultrastructural study of mast cells from multiple body sites. Lab Invest 1990; 63:63-72.

157. Otsu K, Nakano T, Kanakura Y et al. Phenotypic changes of bone marrow-derived mast cells after intraperitoneal transfer into W/Wᵛ mice that are genetically deficient in mast cells. J Exp Med 1987; 165:615-627.

158. Yamamura T, Nakano T, Fukuzumi T et al. Electron microscopic changes of bone-marrow derived cultured mast cells after injection into the skin of genetically mast cell-deficient W/Wᵛ mice. J Invest Dermatol 1988:91:269-273.

159. Sonoda S, Sonoda T, Nakano T et al. Development of mucosal mast cells after injection of a single connective tissue-type mast cell in the stomach mucosa of genetically mast cell-deficient W/Wᵛ mice. J Immunol 1986; 137:1319-1322.

160. Kanakura Y, Kuriu A, Waki N et al. Multiple bidirectional alterations of phenotype and changes in proliferative potential during the in vitro and in vivo passage of clonal mast cell populations derived from mouse peritoneal mast cells. Blood 1988; 72:877-885.

161. Dayton ET, Pharr P, Ogawa M et al. 3T3 fibroblasts induce cloned interleukin 3-dependent mouse mast cells to

resemble connective tissue mast cells in granular constituency. Proc Natl Acad Sci USA 1988; 85:569-572.

162. Brugger W, Reinhardt D, Galanos C et al. Inhibition of in vitro differentiation of human monocytes to macrophages by lipopolysaccharides (LPS): Phenotypic and functional analysis. Int Immunol 1991; 3:221-227.

163. Ring WL, Riddick CA, Baker JR et al. Human monocytes lose 5-lipoxygenase and FLAP as they mature into monocyte-derived macrophages in vitro. Am J Physiol 1996; 271:C372-C377.

164. Polverini PJ. How the extracellular matrix and macrophages contribute to angiogenesis-dependent diseases. Eur J Cancer 1996; 32A:2430-2437.

165. Anrather J, Csizmadia V, Brostjan C et al. Inhibition of bovine endothelial cell activation in vitro by regulated expression of a transdominant inhibitor of NF-kappaB. J Clin Invest 1997; 99:763-772.

166. De Meyer GRY, Herman AG. Vascular endothelial dysfunction. Progr Cardiovasc Dis 1997; 39:325-342.

167. Fowler SD, Mayer EP, Greenspan P. Foam cells and atherogenesis. Ann NY Acad Sci 1985; 454:79-90.

168. Greenspan P, Yu H, Mao F et al. Cholesterol deposition in macrophages: Foam cell formation mediated by cholesterol-enriched oxidized low density lipoprotein. J Lipid Res 1997; 38:101-109.

169. Wang N, Winchester R, Ravalli S et al. Interleukin 8 is induced by cholesterol loading of macrophages and expressed by macrophage foam cells in human atheroma. J Biol Chem 1996; 271:8837-8842.

170. Feigl W, Susani M, Ulrich W et al. Organisation of experimental thrombosis by blood cells. Virchows Arch Pathol Anat 1985; 406:133-148.

171. Campbell GR, Ryan GB. Origin of myofibroblasts in the avascular capsule around free-floating intraperitoneal blood clots. Pathology 1983; 15:253-261.

172. Vaage J, Harlos JP. Collagen production by macrophages in tumour encapsulation and dormancy. Br J Cancer 1991; 63:758-762.

173. Moujahid A, Navascues J, Marin-Teva JL et al. Macrophages during avian optic nerve development: Relationship to cell death and differentiation into microglia. Anat Embryol 1996; 193:131-144.

174. Takahashi K, Naito M, Katabuchi H et al. Development, differentiation, and maturation of macrophages in the chorionic villi of mouse placenta with special reference to the origin of Hofbauer cells. J Leukocyte Biol 1991; 50:57-68.

175. Borello MA, Phipps RP. Fibroblasts support outgrowth of splenocytes simultaneously expressing B lymphocyte and macrophage characteristics. J Immunol 1995; 155:4155-4161.

176. Orikasa M, Iwanaga Y, Takahashi-Iwanaga H et al. Macrophagic cells outgrowth from normal rat glomerular culture: Possible metaplastic changes from podocytes. Lab Invest 1996; 75:719-733.

177. Takahashi K, Naito M, Takeya M. Development and heterogeneity of macrophages and their related cells through their differentiation pathways. Pathol Int 1997; 46:473-485.

178. Niwa H, Harrison LC, DeAizpurua HJ et al. Identification of pancreatic β cell-related genes by representational difference analysis. Endocrinology 1997; 138:1419-1426.

179. Yeh H-I, Dupont E, Coppen S et al. Gap junction localization and connexin expression in cytochemically identified endothelial cells of arterial tissue. J Histochem Cytochem 1997; 45:539-550.

180. Desmouliere A, Badid C, Bochaton-Piallat M-L et al. Apoptosis during wound healing, fibrocontractive diseases and vascular wall injury. Int J Biochem Cell Biol 1997; 29:19-30.

181. Wilmut I, Schnieke AE, McWhir J et al. Viable offspring derived from fetal and adult mammalian cells. Nature 1997; 385:810-813.

182. van Neck JW, Medina JJ, Onnekink C et al. Basic fibroblast growth factor has a differential effect on MyoD conversion of cultured aortic smooth muscle cells from newborn and adult rats. Am J Pathol 1993; 143:269-282.

183. Lee JE. NeuroD and neurogenesis. Dev Neuroscience 1997; 19:27-32.

184. Fisher LJ, Jinnah HA, Kale LC et al. Survival and function of intrastriatally grafted primary fibroblasts genetically modified to produce l-DOPA. Neuron 1991; 6:371-380.

185. Urist M. Bone morphogenetic protein: The molecularization of skeletal system development. J Bone Mineral Res 1997; 12:343-346.

186. Okada TS. Transdifferentiation. Oxford: Clarendon Press, 1991:1-233.

Facilitation of Healing

Transdifferentiation

―――――――――――――――― CHAPTER 38 ――――――――――――――――

Endothelial Cells Transformed from Fibroblasts During Angiogenesis

Takashi Fujiwara, Kazunori Kon

Introduction

Angiogenesis, the formation of new blood vessels, is of fundamental importance for several physiological and pathological processes. It occurs, as is well known, during organ development, wound healing and tumor growth.[1-6] Endothelial cells of newly formed blood vessels are widely believed to derive from preexisting blood vessels. According to Furcht,[7] and Rhodin and Fujita,[8] the process of angiogenesis can be broken down into a number of discrete yet overlapping steps:

1. Increase of vessel permeability;
2. Dissolution of basal lamina caused by a variety of enzymes and penetration of basal lamina by endothelial projections;
3. Matrix 'channel' formation in the interstitial connective tissue and migration of endothelial cells from the preexisting vessel;
4. Proliferation of endothelial cells;
5. Sprout and loop formation;
6. Canalization of the loops; and
7. Association of pericytes and fibroblasts with the newly formed blood vessels.

In such an angiogenic process, endothelial cell migration from preexisting vessels and its proliferation is requisite. However, questions have been addressed to this current angiogenic mechanism[9] because of several puzzling phenomena outlined as follows:

1. Nonendothelial cells are integrated into the linings of newly formed blood vessels;[10-12]
2. Angiogenesis takes place without apparent endothelial cell proliferation[13] and without endothelial cell migration from preexisting blood vessels;[10] and
3. Factors inhibiting in vitro proliferation of endothelial cells, tumor necrosis factor-α (TNF-α)[14] and transformtin growth factor-β (TGF-β),[15] stimulate in vivo angiogenesis.[16]

Therefore, we aimed to examine whether endothelial cells of preexisting blood vessels are the only origin of endothelial cells of newly formed blood vessels.

Angiogenesis in Rabbit Ear Chamber

Ultrastructure of the Tips of Newly Formed Blood Vessels

A transparent rabbit ear chamber (REC), 6 mm in diameter and 100 µm in depth, was implanted into an ear of an adult rabbit under anesthetization with pentobarbital sodium

―――

Tissue Engineering of Prosthetic Vascular Grafts, edited by Peter Zilla and Howard P. Greisler.

(40 mg/kg body weight).[17] Newly formed blood vessels appeared in the chamber space about one week after the chamber implantation. The newly formed vessels invaded the space which extravasated fibrin and red blood cells filled. For mapping the network of newly formed blood vessels, invaginated red cells prepared by treating with trifluoperazine were perfused through the ear artery, enabling us to detect tips of blood vessels growing among numerous extravasated red cells in the REC. After fixation, newly formed blood vessels were processed for electron microscopy in usual way and observed with an electron microscope.

Some newly formed blood vessels containing invaginated red cells were lined with partially discontinuous endothelium (Fig. 38.1). Endothelial cells of the blood vessel were provided with well developed rough ER and many mitochondria, morphologically resembling fibroblasts in the interstitium. This phenomenon suggests that endothelial cells may derive from fibroblasts. Then we paid particular attention to the possible role of fibroblasts as progenitors of endothelial cells, since mesenchymal cells are known to be the origin of vascular endothelial cells in fetal tissue, and fibroblasts function as embryonic mesenchymal cells in some circumstances in adult tissue.[18]

To give an insight into the transformation of fibroblasts into endothelial cells, transplantation of cultured fibroblasts into the space of REC was designed. For this purpose, the fibroblasts were marked so as to trace them. We used two methods for marking fibroblasts, carbon particle ingestion and [³H]thymidine uptake of fibroblasts.

Transformation of Fibroblasts Marked with Carbon Particles into Endothelial Cells

Fibroblasts were separated from rabbit ear skin as reported previously[19] and were cultured in Eagle's minimal essential medium (MEM). The identification of fibroblasts was confirmed by their spindle shape and by the inhibitory effect of cis-hydroxyl proline on fibroblast proliferation.[20] When 100 mg/ml of cis-hydroxyl proline was added to the cultures, the cellular number decreased as shown previously.[20] Furthermore, no contamination of endothelial cells in culture was ascertained by the negative uptake to fluorescence labeled acetyl low density lipoprotein by the cultured cells.[21] During the fifth passage, fibroblasts were cultured in MEM containing India ink particles for 10 h to mark fibroblasts by their ingestion of India ink particles.[22] Fibroblasts contain India ink particles in the cytoplasm for as long as 9 months, enabling us to keep fibroblasts marked with India ink particles for a long time. The marked fibroblasts, about 1×10^4 cells, were washed to remove free carbon particles from the suspension, with MEM solution two times and with Hanks' solution three times, and then transplanted autologously into the space between protective covers of the chamber with a fine needle at 2 days after the chamber implantation. On 8 days after the autologous transplantation of the marked fibroblasts into REC, growing vessels in the REC were fixed and cut into sections for light microscopy.

Newly formed blood vessels of various diameters were found in the connective tissue, identified as venules, capillaries and arterioles by their morphological characteristics.[23-25] Endothelial cells containing carbon particles in the cytoplasm were, though only occasionally, found to line newly formed blood vessels (Fig. 38.2), indicating that the transplanted fibroblasts transformed into the endothelial cells. Extravasation of red cells from the openings of newly formed blood vessels was sometimes observed in the specimens prepared after autologous transplantation of carbon-marked fibroblasts (Fig. 38.2). This is consistent with the well known high permeability and fragility of newly formed blood vessels.[26]

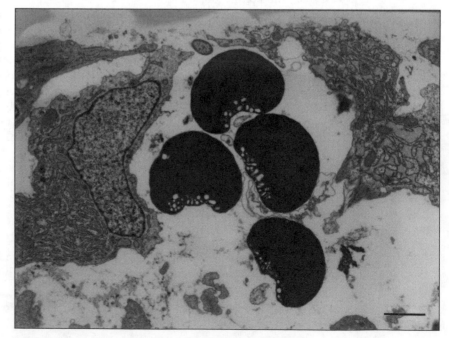

Fig. 38.1. Ultrastructure of newly formed blood vessel in the rabbit ear chamber. The presence of invaginated red cells which were infused through the ear artery show that the structure is a vessel. The endothelial cells have well developed rough ER in the thick cytoplasm, suggesting a close resemblance to fibroblasts in the interstitial space. Note a large intercellular gap between adjacent endothelial cells. x5400: Bar = 2 μm.

Transformation of Fibroblasts Labeled with [³H]Thymidine into Endothelial Cells

We labeled fibroblasts with [³H]thymidine to confirm the result obtained by fibroblasts marked with carbon particles.

Fibroblasts were separated from rabbit ear skin and cultured as mentioned above. During the fifth passage, the fibroblasts were cultured in MEM containing [³H]thymidine (185 Kbq/ml) for 6 days for labeling. To remove free [³H]thymidine, the fibroblasts were washed twice with MEM solution, then with Hanks' solution three times. Two days after the chamber implantation, the labeled fibroblasts, about 1×10^4 cells, were autologously transplanted into the space between protective covers of the chamber with a fine needle. Tissues of the proximal part of the vascular bed were prepared for light microscopic autoradiography on days 7, 9, 12 and 23 and for electron microscopic autoradiography on day 12 after the chamber implantation.

Capillaries (Figs. 38.3A,B), arterioles (Figs. 38.3C,D) and venules (Figs. 38.3E,F) were found in autoradiographic preparations. Numerous autoradiographic silver grains were frequently observed over the endothelial cell nuclei of these newly formed blood vessels.[27] There were also many fibroblasts labeled with silver grains in the connective tissue (Figs. 38.3A,D). In our experiments, it could not be excluded that endothelial cells took up radioactive compounds which might be released from degenerated fibroblasts and diffused toward the endothelial cells. If so, however, the concentration of [³H]thymidine in the interstitium surrounding endothelial cells of newly formed blood vessels must be lower than that in our culture medium, predicting that silver grain density on endothelial cell nucleus must be lower than that of fibroblasts. Furthermore, if diffusion of [³H]thymidine from degenerated fibroblasts occurred in the interstitium, almost all of the endothelial cells and fibroblasts should be more or less labeled. In our experiment, the silver grain density on each nucleus of endothelial cells was very similar to that of fibroblasts, and not all of the endothelial cells and fibroblasts were labeled: The percentage of labeled cells was 66.8 ± 8.1 for endothelial cells and 55.9 ± 4.5 for fibroblasts in 10 preparations examined, indicating that the radioactive labels are not transmitted to the endothelial cells by uncontrolled uptake from degenerating transplanted fibroblasts.

In electron microscope autoradiography, a few silver grains were found over the nuclei of the endothelial cells of capillaries, arterioles (Fig. 38.4A) and venules (Fig. 38.4B). The labeled cells were joined together by intercellular junctions and were surrounded by a basal lamina on their abluminal surface, provided with some of the morphological characteristics of endothelial cell. These data also indicate that fibroblasts transform into endothelial cells of newly formed blood vessels.

Silver grains were observed over the nuclei of the pericytes of capillaries (Fig.38.3A) and venules (Fig. 38.3F), and the nuclei of arteriolar smooth muscle cells (Figs. 38.3C,D, 38.4A), suggesting that both pericytes and vascular smooth muscle cells are derived from fibroblasts.

Discussion

Endothelial Cell Origin and Formation of New Blood Vessels

Endothelial cells of newly formed blood vessels are generally believed to derive from preexisting blood vessels. Pioneering studies on transformation of nonendothelial cells, such as mesenchymal cells[10] and tumor cells,[11] into endothelial cells have been carried out. These studies, however, have not attracted general notice, probably because their evidence is indirect. Here, we clearly showed by tracing cultured fibroblasts marked with carbon particles that fibroblasts transform into endothelial cells of newly formed blood vessels, challenging the general agreement on angiogenic mechanism. The transformation of fibroblasts into endothelial cells has been supported by an experiment with quail chick chimeras. Stein et al[28] transferred limb buds of three day old quail embryos to the chorioallantoic membrane of 10 to 14 day old chick embryos. Six days after grafting, several quail-derived capillaries were found in each of the

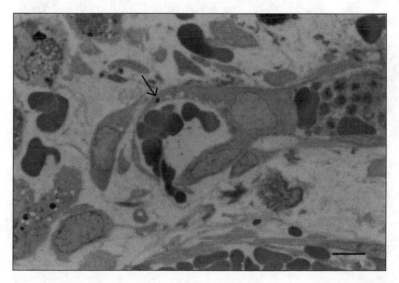

Fig. 38.2. A microphotograph of newly formed blood vessels in the rabbit ear chamber. Cultured fibroblasts marked with India ink carbon particles were transplanted into the ear chamber two days after the implantation of the chamber. Eight days after the transplantation of the fibroblasts, the tissue was fixed and processed for light microscopy. A carbon particle (arrow) is observed in the cytoplasm of an endothelial cell. Red blood cells extravasate from the gap of endothelium. x1700: Bar = 5 μm.

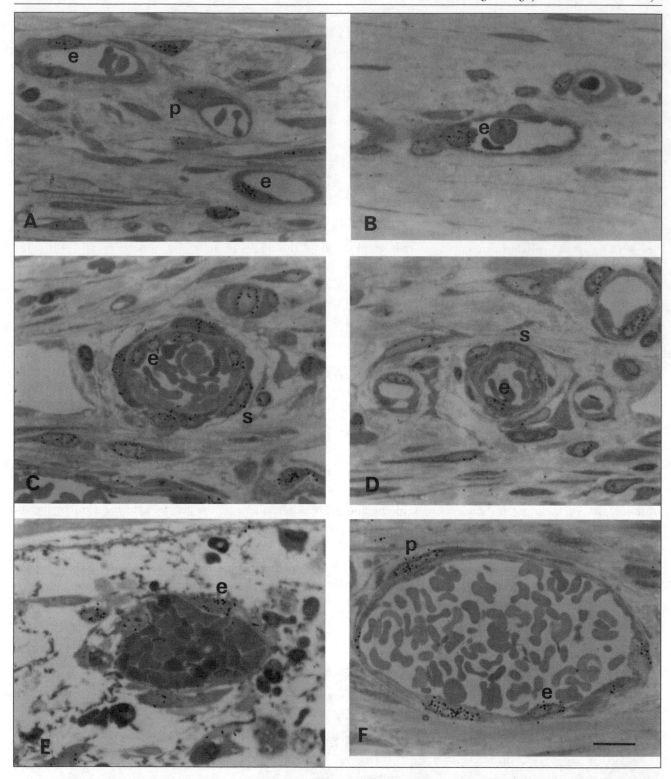

Fig. 38.3. Light microscopic autoradiography. Autoradiographic silver grains are found over the nuclei of the endothelial cells of capillaries (A, B), arterioles (C,D) and venules (E,F). Silver grains are also observed over the nuclei of the pericytes of capillaries (A) and venules (F) and over the nuclei of the smooth muscle cells of arterioles (C, D). Fibroblasts labeled with silver grains are distributed in the connective tissue (A, D). Tissues were prepared on days 7 (E), 9 (A), 12 (C,D and F) and 23 (B), after chamber implantation. e: endothelial cell; p: pericyte; s: smooth muscle cell. x930: Bar = 10 μm.

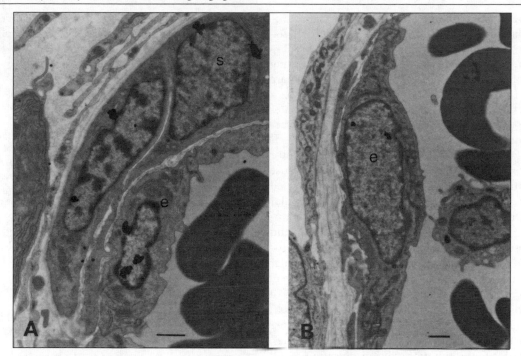

Fig. 38.4. Electron microscopic autoradiography. The endothelial cells of an arteriole (A) and a venule (B) and the smooth muscle cell of an arteriole are labeled with silver grains over their nuclei. The endothelial cells are joined together with intercellular junctions and surrounded by a basal lamina, exhibiting typical features of endothelial cells. The specimens were prepared on day 12 after chamber implantation. e: endothelial cell; s: smooth muscle cell (A) x7600: Bar = 1 μm; (B) x5400: Bar = 1 μm.

transplanted limb buds, suggesting that quail fibroblasts, better to say mesenchymal cells, participate in new blood vessel formation. Similar findings that some mesenchymal cells have an ability to transform into endothelial cells have been reported by several studies on quail chick transplantation in the embryonic stage,[29-31] and on mammalian embryos.[32] These studies indicate that the endothelial cells from preexisting blood vessels are not the only origin of endothelial cells of newly formed blood vessels. Recently Asahara et al[12] have clearly demonstrated that putative endothelial cell progenitors in circulating blood differentiated into endothelial cells in vitro and incorporated into sites of active angiogenesis in vivo.

We observed that endothelium of newly formed vessels was occasionally discontinuous and that blood cells circulating in the vessels extravasated into interstitial space through the gaps of endothelium. This extravasated blood may flow back and forth in the interstitium and show only oscillatory movements as described by Hadlicka,[33] forming a matrix channel in the interstitial space.[8] Fibrin deposits in the interstitial space are supposed to play a critical role in providing a matrix channel, from our experimental finding that fibrinosis of accumulated fibrin in REC by plasminogen activator causes complete inhibition of new vessel formation. Fibroblasts in the interstitium may find an opportunity to face and directly contact flowing blood in the matrix channel. Then they may come to line the luminal surface of the channel in place of normal endothelial cells, form-

ing a new blood vessel. Such an incorporation of cells from the abluminal side into newly formed blood vessels has been drawn schematically.[29]

Origin of Pericytes and Vascular Smooth Muscle Cells from Fibroblasts

Fibroblasts have also been clearly demonstrated here to be the origin of both pericytes and smooth muscle cells of blood vessels, as shown previously.[8,28,34,35] Accordingly, these results indicate that fibroblasts can be the common origin for all cellular elements of blood vessels, i.e., endothelial cells, pericytes and smooth muscle cells. A similar phenomenon of cell origin is known in fetal vasculogenesis, in which mesenchymal cells are the common origin for these three cellular elements.[36] This is consistent with the view that fibroblasts function in adult tissue as embryonic mesenchymal cells in some aspects.[18]

Possible Contribution of Fibroblasts to Angiogenesis

From our experiments, an increase in fibroblast density can be expected to promote angiogenesis. This view is supported by the experimental evidences that activated fibroblasts are associated with angiogenesis in electrically stimulated skeletal muscle[37] and that inhibition of fibroblast proliferation by proline analogs,[20] on the contrary, inhibits angiogenesis.[38] The puzzling phenomenon of TNF-α and TGF-β promoting in vivo angiogenesis, in spite of their inhibitory effect on endothelial cell proliferation, has previously been rationalized by the suggestion that stimulated secondary cells produce angiogenic factors.[4,16] Based on our data, however, we suggest that TNF-α and TGF-β contribute to promoting angiogenesis by the increasing population of fibroblasts.[39,40] Both TNF-α[39] and TGF-β[41] are mitogens for fibroblasts, and TGF-β is also a chemoattractant[40,42] for fibroblasts. Fibrin also stimulates angiogenesis[43,44] through its proliferative[43] and chemotactic[44] effects on fibroblasts. Fibroblast-dependent angiogenesis is quite favorable for wound healing tissues and tumor tissues where rapid blood vessel growth is needed, because the proliferation rate of endothelial cells has been reported to be too slow to account for rapid growth of the vascular network.[45] Our data suggest that angiogenesis can be modulated by manipulating fibroblast density and activity[9] and that fibroblast transformation into endothelial cells can provide a benefit on clinical applications, in prosthetic vascular grafts and gene therapy.

When arterial reconstruction is required in cases of arterial stenosis or occlusion, such as ischemic heart disease, autologous veins or arteries or prosthetic vascular grafts are used for the replacement of stenotic or occluded arteries. Graft failures due to thrombotic occlusion, however, are still serious complications.[46,47] One of the various methods to reduce the thrombogenicity of prosthetic grafts is to line the luminal surface with endothelial cells.[48,49] As an attempt at lining the lumen of synthetic vascular prostheses, microvascular endothelial cells[50] and large vessel endothelial cells[51] have been seeded and cultured on them.[50,51] Recently Noishiki et al[52] have completely endothelialized the luminal surface of a vascular prosthesis by infiltration of bone marrow cells and kept patency of the vascular prosthesis for longer than three weeks after the implantation of the vascular prosthesis.

It has also been considered whether the performance and versatility of prosthetic vascular grafts might be improved by lining the luminal surface with endothelial cells genetically modified to prevent thromboses.[49] Furthermore, the endothelial cells have recently been paid attention, since endothelial cells may serve as vehicles for the introduction in vivo of functioning recombinant genes because of their proximity to the blood stream.[53,54] Endothelial cells expressing recombinant genes have been introduced into denuded arteries of syngeneic animals.[55] Because fibroblasts, in general, can more feasibly be isolated from patients, are more easily cultured and proliferate more quickly than endothelial cells, they may be more appropriate for lining the luminal surface of prosthetic vascular grafts or for transferring genes into arteries than endothelial cells.

Concluding Remarks

We here described transformation of fibroblasts into endothelial cells of newly formed blood vessels based on our study on angiogenesis during wound healing in the rabbit ear chamber. This gives us an another idea of the origin of endothelial cells of newly formed blood vessels and of the mechanism of angiogenesis than the idea which is widely believed. The transformation of fibroblasts into endothelial cells accounts for some puzzling phenomena on angiogenesis and provides a benefit on clinical applications. However, we need further studies to reveal whether transformation of fibroblasts into endothelial cells generally takes place in angiogenesis.

References

1. Blood CH, Zetter BR. Tumor interactions with the vasculature: Angiognesis and tumor metastasis. Biochem Biophys Acta 1990; 1032:89-118.
2. Liotta LA, Steeg PS, Stetler-Stevenson WG. Cancer metastasis and angiogenesis: An imblance of positive and negative regulation. Cell 1991; 64:327-336.
3. Risau W. Vasculogenesis, angiogenesis and endothelial differentiation during embryonic development. In: Feinberg RN, ed. The Development of the Vascular System, Issues Biomed Volume 14. Basel: Karger, 1991:58-68.
4. Folkman J, Brem H. Angiogenesis and inflammation. In: Gallin JI, ed. Inflammation: Basic Principles and Clinical Correlates, 2nd edition. New York: Raven Press, 1992:821-839.
5. Folkman J, Shing Y. Angiogenesis. J Biol Chem 1992; 267:10931-10934.
6. Fidler IJ, Ellis LM. The implications of angiogenesis for the biology and thereapy of cancer metastasis. Cell 1994; 79:185-188.
7. Furcht LT. Critical factors controlling angiogenesis: Cell products, cell matrix and growth factors. Lab Invest 1986; 55:505-509.
8. Rhodin JAG, Fujita H. Capillary growth in the mesentery of normal young rats. Intravital video and electron microscope analyses. J Submicrosc Cytol Pathol 1989; 21:1-34.
9. Arnold F, West DC. Angiogenesis in wound healing. Pharmac Ther 1991; 52:407-422.
10. Aloisi M, Giacomin C, Tessari R. Growth of elementary blood vessels in diffusion chambers. I. Process of formation and conditioning factors. Virchows Arch B Cell Pathol 1970; 6:350-364.
11. Hammersen F, Endrich B, Messmer K. The fine structure of tumor blood vessels. Int J Microcirc Clin Exper 1985; 4:31-43.
12. Asahara T, Murohara T, Sullivan A et al. Isolation of putative progenitor endothelial cells for angiogenesis. Science 1997; 257:964-967.
13. Sholley MM, Ferguson GP, Seibel HR et al. Mechanisms of neovascularization. Vascular sprouting can occur without proliferation of endothelial cells. Lab Invest 1984; 51:624-634.
14. Fajardo LF, Kwan HH, Kowalski J et al. Dual role of tumor necrosis factor-α in angiogenesis. Amer J Pathol 1992; 140:539-544.
15. Heimark RL, Twardzik DR, Schwartz SM. Inhibition of endothelial regeneration by type-beta transforming growth factor from platelets. Science 1986; 233:1078-1080.
16. Klagsbrun M, D'Amore PA. Regulators of angiogenesis. Annu Rev Physiol 1991; 53:217-239.
17. Asano M, Yoshida K, Tatai K. Observations of the behavior of microcirculation by rabbit ear chanmber technique. I. On a modification of rabbit ear chamber, development of microphotoelectric plethysmography, and rythmic fluctuation of microcirculation. Bull Inst Publ Health 1963; 12:34-44.
18. Alberts B, Bray D, Lewis J et al. Fibroblasts and their transformations: The connective-tissue cell family. In: Molecular Biology of The Cell, 3rd edition. New York and London: Garland Publishing, 1994:1179-1187.

19. Schneider E, Mitsui Y. The relationship between in vitro cellular aging and in vivo human age. Proc Natl Acad Sci USA 1976; 73:3584-3588.

20. Kao WW-Y, Prockop DJ. Proline analogue removes fibroblasts from cultured mixed cell populations. Nature 1977; 266:63-64.

21. McGuire PG, Orkin RW. Methods in laboratory investigation. Isolation of rat aortic endothelial cells by primary explant techniques and their phenotypic modulation by defined substrata. Lab Invest 1987; 57:94-105.

22. Fujita H, Nishii Y, Yamashita K et al. The uptake and long-term storage of India ink particles and latex beads by fibroblasts in the dermis and subcutis of mice, with special regard to the non-inflammatory defense reaction by fibroblasts. Arch Histol Cytol 1988; 51:285-294.

23. Rhodin JAG. The ultrastructure of mammalian arterioles and precapillary sphincters. J Ultrastruc Res 1967; 18:181-223.

24. Rhodin JAG. Ultrastructure of mammalian venous capillaries, venules and small collecting veins. J Ultrastruc Res 1968; 25:452-500.

25. Fujiwara T, Uehara Y. The cytoarchitecture of the wall and the innervation pattern of the microvessels in the rat mammary gland: A scanning electron microscopic observation. Amer J Anat 1984; 170:39-54.

26. Majno G. Ultrastructure of the vascular membrane. In: Hamilton WF, Dow P, eds. Handbook of Physiology. Circulation III. Washington, DC: Amer Physiol Soc, 1965:2293-2375

27. Kon K, Fujiwara T. Transformation of fibroblasts into endothelial cells during angiogenesis. Cell Tissue Res 1994; 278:625-628.

28. Stein J, Drenckhahn D, Nehls V. Development of pericyte-like cells during anbgiogenesis in quail chick chimeras as detected by combined Feulgen reaction and immunohistochemistry. Ann Anat 1996; 178:153-158.

29. Noden DM. Embryonic origins and assembly of blood vessels. Amer Rev Respir Dis 1989; 140:1097-1103.

30. Pardanaud L, Yassine F, Dieterlen-Lievre F. Relatioship between vasculogenesis, angiogenesis and heamopoiesis during avian ontogeny. Development 1989; 105:473-485.

31. Wilms P, Christ B, Wilting J et al. Distribution and migration of angiogenic cells from grafted avascular intraembryonic mesoderm. Anat Embryol 1991; 183:371-377.

32. Hara K Doi Y Nagata N et al. Role of mesenchymal cells in the neovascularization of the rabbit phallus. Anat Rec 1994; 238:15-22.

33. Hudlická O, Tyler KR. Growth of vessels under pathological conditions. In: Angiogenesis The growth of the vascular system. London: Harcourt Brace Jovanovich, 1986:115-149.

34. Cliff WJ. Observations on healing tissue: A combined light and elctron microscopic investigation. Phil Trans Roy Soc London Ser B 1963; 246:305-325.

35. Nehls V, Denzer K, Drenckhahn D. Pericyte involvement in capillary sprouting during angiogenesis in situ. Cell Tissue Res 1992; 270:469-474.

36. Demir R, Kaufmann P, Castellucci M et al. Fetal vasculogenesis and angiogenesis in human placental villi. Acta Anat 1989; 136:190-203.

37. Hansen-Smith FM, Hudlicka O, Egginton S. In vivo angiogenesis in adult rat skeletal muscle: Early changes in cappillary network architecture and ultrastructure. Cell Tissue Res 1996; 286:123-136.

38. Ingber D, Folkman J. Inhibition of angiogenesis through modulation of collagen metabolism. Lab Invest 1988; 59:44-51.

39. Piguet PF, Grau GE, Vassalli P. Subcutaneous perfusion of tumor necrosis factor induces local proliferation of fibroblasts, capillaries, and epidermal cells, or massive tissue necrosis. Amer J Pathol 1990; 136:103-110.

40. Yang EY, Moses HL. Transforming growth factor β1-induced changes in cell migration, proliferation, and agiogenesis in the chicken chorioallantoic membrane. J Cell Biol 1990; 111:731-741.

41. Roberts AB, Sporn MB, Assoian RK et al. Transformtin growth factor type b: Rapid induction of fibrosis and angiogenesis in vivo and stimulation of collagen formation in vitro. Proc Natl Acad Sci USA 1986; 83:4167-4171.

42. Pierce GF, Mustoe TA, Lingelbach J et al. Platelet-derived growth factor and transformtin growth factor-b enhance tissue repair activities by unique mechanisms. J Cell Biol 1989; 109:429-440.

43. Dvorak HF, Harvey VS, Estrella P et al. Fibrin containing gels indue angiogenesis. Implications for tumor stroma generation and woulnd healing. Lab Invest 1987; 57:673-686.

44. Brown LF, Dvorak AM, Dvarak HF. Leaky vessels, fibrin deposition, and fibrosis: A sequence of events common to solid tumors and to many other types of disease. Amer Rev Respir Dis 1989; 140:1104-1107.

45. Fujimoto S, Yamamoto K, Kagawa H et al. Neovascularization in the pre- and postnatal rabbit corpora cavernosa penis: Light and elctron microscopy and autoradiography. Anat Rec 1987; 218:30-39.

46. Rutherford RB, Jones DN, Bergentz S-E et al. Factors affecting the patency of infrainguinal bypass. J Vasc Surg 1988; 8:236-246.

47. Schuman ES, Gross GF, Hayes J F et al. Long-term patency of polytetrafluoroethylene graft fistulas. Amer J Surg 1988; 155:644-646.

48. Williams SK, Jarrell BE, Friend L et al. Adult human endothelial cell compatibility with prosthetic graft material. J Surg Res 1985; 38:618-629.

49. Wilson JM, Birinyi LK, Salomon RN et al. Implantation of vascular grafts lined with genetically modified endothelial cells. Science 1989; 244:1344-1346.

50. Park PK, Jarrell BE, Williams SK et al. Thrombus-free, human endothelial surface in the midregion of a Dacron vascular graft in the splanchnic venous circuit—Observations after nin months of implantation. J Vasc Surg 1990; 11:468-475.

51. Radomski JS, Jarrell BE, Pratt KJ et al. Effects of in vitro aging on human endothelial cell adherence to Dacron vascular graft material. J Surg Res 1989; 47:173-177.

52. Noishiki Y, Tomizawa Y, Yamane Y et al. Autocrine angiogenic vascular prosthesis with bone marrow transplantation. Nature Medicine 1996; 2:90-93.

53. Zwiebel JA, Freeman SM, Kantoff PW et al. High-level recombinant gene expression in rabbit endothelial cells transduced by retroviral vectors. Science 1989; 243:220-222.

54. Yao S-N, Wilson JM, Nabel EG et al. Expression of human factor IX in rat capillary endothelial cells: Toward somatic gene therapy for hemophilia B. Proc Natl Acad Sci USA 1991; 88:8101-8105.

55. Nabel EG, Plautz G, Boyce FM et al. Recombinant gene expression in vivo within endothelial cells of the arterial wall. Science 1989; 244:1342-1344.

Facilitation of Healing

Transdifferentiation

--------------------- CHAPTER 39 ---------------------

Mechanical Forces and Cell Differentiation

Ira Mills, Bauer E. Sumpio

Introduction

Our laboratory and others have been rigorously studying the influence of mechanical forces on vascular cell biology. It has been our contention that static conditions commonly utilized to study vascular cells in culture may not reflect their in vivo milieu. Vascular cells in vivo are subjected to a variety of flow-related forces including shear stress, hydrostatic pressure, and cyclic strain[1,2] (see Fig. 39.1, ref. 3). Shear stress is the tangential stress applied across the endothelial cell surface due to the bulk flow of blood. Hydrostatic pressure is the normal stress acting radially on the vessel wall due to the propagation of the pressure wave. Cyclic strain represents the stress acting along the vessel wall due to circumferential deformation. Endothelial cells are exposed to all three forces, whereas the underlying smooth muscle cells are exposed to hydrostatic pressure and cyclic strain. There are a number of recent reviews of the effects of shear stress on endothelial cells.[3-5] Therefore, we will mention but not provide details for shear studies. We will not consider the effect of shear stress on smooth muscle cells, since this force is considered insignificant as compared to cyclic strain.[3]

Cyclic strain, along with the other forces listed above, plays an important role in the regulation of vascular tone, remodeling, and the genesis of atherosclerosis in vivo.[6,7] The mechanism by which cultured vascular endothelial cells and smooth muscle cells perceive cyclic strain, utilizing in vitro devices to model this force, is the subject of this chapter.[1,2] The strains described for the in vitro studies herein (~10% strain) are functionally significant based on in vivo models that replicate the major geometric features of blood vessels. These studies report a 5-6% wall excursion at peak systole under normal conditions, which can increase to 10% in the hypertensive state.[8-10]

Several recent studies in the literature suggest that the study of mechanical forces on vascular cell biology may have fruitful applications in the field of tissue engineering of prosthetic vascular grafts.[11] In one such study, Ott and Ballerman[12] found that shear stress preconditioning of endothelial cells led to an improved tolerance (i.e., cell adherence) of endothelialized grafts to acute shear stress. Assessment of endothelial cell tolerance was determined by counting the number of dislodged cells, examining the grafts by light and scanning electron microscopy and by measurement of whole blood clotting time. Shear stress preconditioned grafts, as compared to control grafts, showed fewer numbers of dislodged cells, the presence of an intact monolayer, and a prolonged clotting time. Thus, this study provides evidence to suggest that preconditioning by shear stress leads to amelioration of the poor retention of endothelial cells, as well as the thrombogenicity of prosthetic vascular grafts.

Tissue Engineering of Prosthetic Vascular Grafts, edited by Peter Zilla and Howard P. Greisler.
©1999 R.G. Landes Company.

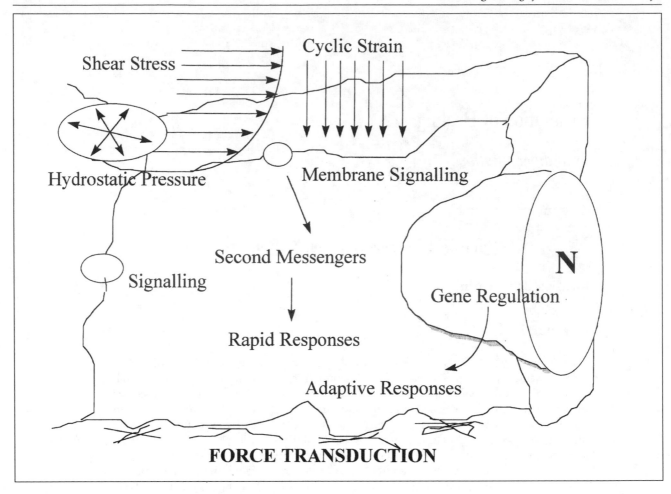

Fig. 39.1. Schematic showing mechanical forces of shear stress, cyclic strain, and hydrostatic pressure and associated signalling pathways that occur in vascular cells. Adapted from ref. 3.

The mechanism responsible for the improved status of the shear stress-preconditioned prosthetic grafts remains unclear, but Ballermann and Ott[11] suggest that a shift of endothelial cells towards a more differentiated state may be involved. Endothelial cells cultured under normal conditions tend to become dedifferentiated. In the presence of shear stress, they observed the appearance of more differentiated features, including a tighter adherence to the substratum that resembled in vivo endothelial cells displaying an organized cytoskeleton, Weibel-palade bodies and basal stress fibers with focal adhesion plaques.

Clowes and colleagues[13-15] have characterized the effects of blood flow and shear stress on subendothelial smooth muscle cell proliferation in baboon prosthetic grafts. They have found that neointimal hyperplasia in endothelialized grafts is inhibited by increased blood flow. In the presence of a distal arteriovenous fistula that caused nearly 3-fold elevations in flow and shear stress, smooth muscle cell number was reduced with a consequent reduction in the cross-sectional area of the neointima at 3 months. Moreover, ligation of the fistula after 2 months caused a rapid increase in neointimal thickness,[13] showing a strong association between blood flow and the smooth muscle cell response in vascular grafts.

In a recent study, Kraiss et al[15] have provided mechanistic data to explain the smooth muscle cell proliferation associated with abrupt reductions in fluid shear stress. They found that PDGF-A gene expression in both subluminal endothelium and subadjacent smooth muscle cells is increased in low flow grafts. This was convincingly shown by Northern blot analysis, in situ hybridization studies and immunohistochemical studies. Increases in the PDGF-A transcript of 2.9-fold were noted in neointimal areas in the presence of reduced shear stress. Even greater changes were indicated by in situ studies, presumably due to the predominance of upregulated message in the luminal surface of the neointima. This study emphasizes the need to delineate the responsiveness of vascular cells to mechanical perturbation to better understand their behavior in situations such as tissue engineering of vascular grafts.

The complexity of the nature of the forces perceived by grafts was illustrated by Dobrin et al,[16] who subjected autogenous vein grafts to a variety of conditions of pressure and flow including three static deformations, three static stresses, increased pulsatile deformations, pulsatile stresses, and altered shear stress at the blood-intima interface. Three sequential experiments were performed to sequentially determine the role of nine factors. In agreement with Clowes' work,[13-15] low flow velocity was associated with intimal hyperplasia. Moreover, medial thickening of autogenous vein grafts was observed with increased deformation of the vein wall in the circumferential direction, which mimics clinical findings.

Over the years, we have acquired a large body of data to suggest that the study of vascular cells challenged with mechanical stimuli is indeed a more appropriate method for studying their biology.[17-32] This chapter represents an update of an earlier review of the literature describing the effect of cyclic strain on vascular cell biology.[22] Data obtained from our laboratory and that of others have begun to delineate the signaling pathways that may be involving in affecting vascular cell phenotype and is commented on in great detail in this review. We also discuss the recent discovery of strain-sensitive genes that appear to be finely tuned in their ability to distinguish mechanical perturbations based on unique strain sensitive or shear sensitive cis-elements in their promoter regions that respond to unique strain-activated or shear-activated transcriptional factors that either induce or repress gene induction.

Recent studies suggest that the state of differentiation of vascular cells in culture is fluid,[33-35] and a novel stimulus for controlling the phenotypic state of these cells is mechanical strain.[36] As described below, recent studies suggest that cyclic strain may direct endothelial cells to a more differentiated state as evidenced by phosphorylation of focal adhesion proteins.[37] However, the state of differentiation of endothelial cells as well as smooth muscle cells in response to cyclic strain is complex, since many other responses indica-

tive of a dedifferentiated state occur, such as elevated proliferation.[38] For example, recent work by Reusch et al[39] suggests that smooth muscle cells become more differentiated upon cyclic strain as evidenced by the upregulation of myosin heavy chain expression. As described in greater detail below, other responses of smooth muscle cells to cyclic strain portend a dedifferentiated state such as enhanced proliferation.[24,40] It is clear that much work needs to be done in characterizing the modulation of cyclic strain on vascular cell biology before any mechanistic significance can be ascribed to its role in advancing tissue engineering of prosthetic grafts.

As recently reviewed by Zilla et al,[41] "manipulation of the endothelium might provide the next major advancement for therapeutic and preventive measures for cardiovascular disease". It is with this objective that the following studies are outlined that characterize the mechanical manipulation of both endothelial cells and smooth muscle cells. It is hoped that a greater delineation of the mechanisms involved in the strain-induced modulation of vascular cell phenotype will lead to better diagnosis and treatment of vascular disease and the implementation of improvements in tissue engineering of prosthetic grafts.

Effect of Cyclic Strain on Endothelial Cell Biology

General Phenotype

Previous studies in our and others' laboratories have shown that cyclic strain can alter the general phenotype of

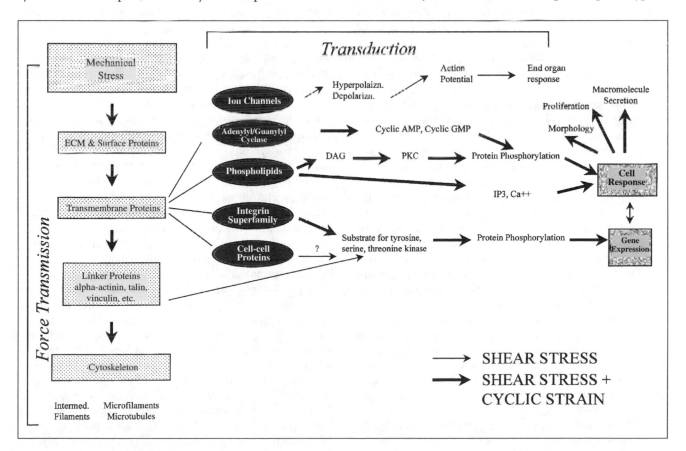

Fig. 39.2. Schematic showing mechanical force transmission and transduction pathways in vascular cells. Adapted from ref. 47.

Table 39.1. Effect of cyclic strain and shear stress on endothelial cell phenotype. (Adapted from ref. 3)

Response	Cyclic Strain	Ref. #	Shear Stress	Ref. #
Proliferation	Increase	27,38	Increase; Turbulent flow	52
Alignment	Perpendicular	18,42, 43	Parallel	53,54
F-Actin Redistribution	Yes	18	Yes	48,55
Focal Adhesion Site Modification	Yes	37,50, 56	Yes	49,55
Macromol: PG12	Increased	29,57	Increased	58
NO	Increased	44,45	Increased	59
tPA	Increased	20,32	Increased	60
Endothelin-1	Decreased	(Koo, unpublished data)	Increased/ Decreased	61,62

endothelial cells, including their proliferative rate,[27,38] morphology[18,42,43] and the secretion of macromolecules such as prostacyclin,[29] endothelin,[30] nitric oxide,[44,45] tissue plasminogen activator[20] and plasminogen activator inhibitor-1 (PAI-1)[46] (see Fig. 39.2, see ref. 47).

Changes in endothelial cell phenotype are also modulated by shear stress (see Table 39.1). Changes include alterations in proliferation, morphology and the synthesis and secretion of many of the same proteins influenced by cyclic strain.[3-5] However, the nature of the changed phenotype can be markedly different, whether the perturbation is either shear stress or cyclic strain. For example, the orientation of endothelial cells in response to shear stress is parallel to the direction of flow.[48] In contrast, cyclic strain causes a perpendicular alignment of endothelial cells in relationship to the strain vector.[18]

More recent studies performed in our laboratory support the involvement of focal adhesion plaques in the transmission of cyclic strain to the cell. Yano et al[37] demonstrated phosphorylation of cytoskeletal proteins that reside at the cytoplasmic face of the focal adhesion plaques, namely pp125[FAK] and paxillin. The strain-induced phosphorylation of these proteins occurs on tyrosine residues and can be inhibited by specific tyrosine kinase inhibitors. The tyrosine phosphorylation of pp125[FAK] occurs earlier and is more robust than that observed with paxillin. However, after a four hour exposure to strain, both cytoskeletal proteins were found to align as shown by confocal microscopy.[37] This observation was in sharp contrast to their random distribution found in stationary controls. Tyrphostin A25, a tyrosine kinase inhibitor, is blocked by the strain-induced phosphorylation of pp125[FAK] and paxillin as well as by their strain-induced alignment. Moreover, the importance of focal adhesion proteins on the mechanically induced gross morphological changes of endothelial cells was implied by the ability of tyrphostin A25 to reverse both cellular alignment and migration caused by strain.

Davies et al[49] have studied the effect of shear stress on focal adhesion sites in bovine aortic endothelial cells. By tandem scanning confocal microscopy and digitized image

analysis, they found a remodeling of focal adhesion sites in the direction of flow. In addition to this response, shear stress caused a redistribution of intracellular stress fibers, alignment of individual focal adhesion sites, and the coalescing of smaller sites to larger, and fewer, focal adhesions per cell.

Yano et al[50] recently studied the involvement of different integrins in signaling induced by cyclic strain, since integrins have been localized to focal adhesion sites. Furthermore, these focal adhesion sites are known to exhibit pp125[FAK] phosphorylation by cyclic strain as well as by integrins. Cyclic strain of 4 h led to a redistribution of α and β integrins in human umbilical vein endothelial cells.[50] In addition, β_1 integrin reorganized in a linear pattern parallel with the long axis of the elongated cells, creating a fusion of focal adhesion plaques in cells plated on fibronectin (a ligand for $\alpha_5\beta_1$) or collagen (a ligand for $\alpha_2\beta_1$) coated plates. In contrast, the vitronectin receptor, β_3 integrin, failed to redistribute in endothelial cells subjected to cyclic strain. Cyclic strain also caused a reorganization of α_5 and α_2 integrins in a linear pattern on cells seeded on fibronectin and collagen-coated plates, respectively. However, the expression of α_5, α_2, and β_1 was not influenced by 24 h of cyclic strain as assessed by immunoprecipitation of these integrins. Strain-induced phosphorylation of pp125[FAK] occurred concomitantly with the reorganization of β_1 integrin. Thus, $\alpha_5\beta_1$ and $\alpha_2\beta_1$ integrins may play an important role in transducing mechanical stimuli into intracellular signals.[50]

Thoumine et al[51] demonstrated effects on the organization and composition of the extracellular matrix upon subjecting endothelial cells to shear stress. They examined the pattern and levels of various extracellular matrix proteins including fibronectin, laminin, type IV collagen, and vitronectin. Of these, fibronectin was found to be the most affected by shear stress, with a thickening and alignment of its fibril tracts. Moreover, the level of fibronectin increased after 1 or 2 days of shear stress after an earlier reduction at 12 h. The extracellular matrix response to shear was found to be specific for fibronectin, since both laminin and type IV collagen showed thickening of fibrils, but no alignment. Vitronectin was unaffected in any respect.

Table 39.2A. Effect of cyclic strain on second messenger pathways in endothelial cells. (Adapted from ref. 3)

Effect	Strain	Cell Type	Response Time	Significance	Reference Number
↑ [Ca^{2+}]	10% avg., 60 cpm	BAEC	12 s, initial peak: 2nd phase sustained, 15-35 s	Activation of Ca^{2+} sensitive pathways	63
↑ IP$_3$	10% avg., 60 cpm	BAEC	10 s peak	Phosphoinositide sensitive pathways	74
↑ Diacylglycerol	10% avg., 60 cpm	BAEC	d10 s, initial peak, 2nd phase sustained to 500 s	Activation of the PKC pathway	65,74
↑ PKC	10% avg., 60 cpm	BAEC	10 s initial peak, 2nd phase from 100 s sustained to 8 min	Phosphoinositide sensitive pathways	74
↑ Adenylyl cyclase	10% avg., 60 cpm	BAEC	5-60 min	Activation of the cAMP pathway	68
↑ cAMP	10% avg., 60 cpm	BAEC	15-30 min	Activation of the cAMP pathway	68
↑ PKA	10% avg., 60 cpm	BAEC	10-60 min	Activation of the PKA pathway	68

Table 39.2B. (Adapted from ref. 3)

Effect	Shear	Cell Type	Response Time	Significance	Reference Number
↑ [Ca^{2+}]	0.2-4.0 dynes/cm^2	BAEC	15-40 sec	Activation of Ca^{2+} sensitive pathways	64
↑ IP$_3$	30 and 60 dynes/cm^2	BAEC, HUVEC	10 sec peak	Phosphoinositide sensitive pathways	66, 75
↑ cGMP	0-40 dynes/cm^2	BAEC	60 sec	Vasoregulation Mechanisms	76
↑ MAP kinase	3.5-117 dynes/cm^2	BAEC	5 min peak, 20-30 min	Involvement of membrane mitogen receptor-like pathway	77

Cell Signaling

Second Messenger Pathways (See Table 39.2A, B)

[Ca^{2+}]$_i$, Inositol Phosphates and Diacylglycerols

Previous studies have demonstrated that cyclic strain causes a rapid but transient generation of 1,4,5 inositol trisphosphate (IP$_3$), which peaked by 10 seconds of cyclic strain. To address the effect of cyclic strain on intracellular [Ca^{2+}] and its temporal relationship to IP$_3$ generation, bovine aortic endothelial cells were grown on flexible membranes, loaded with aequorin and the membranes placed in a custom designed flow through chamber.[63] The chamber was housed inside a photo multiplier tube and vacuum was utilized to deform the membranes. The initiation of strain caused a rapid increase in intracellular calcium of two components. The first component was a large initial peak 12 seconds after the initiation of stretch that closely followed the IP$_3$ peak. The second component was a subsequent lower, but sustained, phase. Pretreatment with 5 µM gadolinium for 10 minutes or nominally calcium-free medium for 3 minutes reduced the magnitude of the initial rise and abolished the sustained phase.

Shear stress has been demonstrated to induce calcium transients in single endothelial cells as measured by fura-2.[64] Geiger et al[64] studied the effect of shear stress at 30 dynes/cm^2 in endothelial cells subjected to flow in parallel plate flow chambers and glass capillary tubes. They found a rapid increase in [Ca^{2+}] that peaked by 30 seconds and decreased slowly to a plateau that persisted for greater than 5 minutes.

Recent studies performed in our laboratory show that cyclic strain causes a biphasic increase in diacylglycerol.[65] These data support a mechanism of phosphatidylcholine hydrolysis and diacylglycerol generation at both an early and late phase. Cyclic strain was shown to stimulate phospholipase C acutely and phospholipase D activity in an immediate and sustained manner.[65] Bhagyalakshmi et al[66] also showed stimulation of DAG by shear stress. In another study of shear stress-activated platelets, pathological levels of shear (i.e., 90 dynes/cm^2) failed to elevate DAG despite increased PKC activity.[67]

Adenylyl Cyclase

Cyclic strain causes activation of the adenylyl cyclase/ cyclic AMP/protein kinase a pathway in bovine aortic endothelial cells.[68] In membranes deformed with 150 mm Hg (average 10% strain) vacuum at 60 cycles per minute (0.5 sec strain; 0.5 sec relaxation) for 15 minutes, there was a 1.5- to 2.2-fold increase in adenylyl cyclase, cAMP and PKA activity as compared to unstretched controls. The strain-induced activation of this pathway appears to occur by exceeding a strain threshold, since no change in adenylyl cyclase, cyclic AMP or PKA was observed in cells subjected to 37.5 mm Hg (average 6% strain). Further studies demonstrated an increase in cAMP response element activity as shown by gel shift analysis. Thus, cyclic strain may stimulate the expression of genes containing cAMP-responsive elements.

We next tested the hypothesis that cyclic strain modulates G protein function, since G proteins are intimately involved in the activation of adenylyl cyclase (Mills, unpublished observations). To test this hypothesis, we examined the effect of acute cyclic strain on the immunoreactivity of the alpha subunits of the heterotrimeric G proteins, Gs and Gi, that promote stimulation and inhibition of AC activity, respectively. We observed a transient decrease in the immunoreactivity of the inhibitory G protein alpha subunits (Giα1,2).In contrast, immunoreactivity of Gs in bovine aortic endothelial cells and Giα1,2 and Gs in bovine aortic smooth muscle cells were unaffected by cyclic strain.

Frangos and colleagues have shown shear stress activation of G proteins, particularly Gαq/α11 and Gαi3/αo.[69] This was determined by labelling of flow-stimulated G proteins with a nonhydrolyzable GTP photoreactive analog. The rapidity by which this response is obtained (1 sec) suggests a key role of G proteins in the mechanotransduction of shear stimuli. Previous studies by the same group further established a role of G proteins in the responsiveness of endothelial cells to shear stress. Both shear stress mediated prostacyclin and nitric oxide production were found to be mediated by pertussis-toxin sensitive and insensitive G proteins, respectively.[70,71]

Protein Phosphatase Activity

As described above, we have reported previously that PKC in the membrane fraction of endothelial cell lysates is activated in response to cyclic strain.[72] To better understand cellular responses that are dependent on the phosphorylated state of proteins, it is also important to study the role of protein phosphatases. In a recent study,[73] we examined the effect of cyclic strain on protein phosphatase-1 and -2A activity in bovine aortic endothelial cells. Protein phosphatase-2A activity in the cytosol was decreased by 36.1% in response to 60 minutes of cyclic strain, whereas activity in the membrane was unchanged. Furthermore, treatment with a low concentration of okadaic acid (0.1 nM) enhanced proliferation of both static and stretched endothelial cells in 10% fetal bovine serum. These data suggest that protein phosphatase-2A acts as a growth suppresser, and cyclic strain may enhance cellular proliferation by inhibiting protein phosphatase-2A.[73]

Transcriptional Factor Activation (See Table 39.3B)

In a recent study, Cheng et al[46] demonstrated strain-induced activation of PAI-1 secretion. Although this effect could be accomplished directly on the secretory process, the authors postulate the upregulation of the PAI-1 gene via a

Table 39.3A. Effect of cyclic strain on transcription factor activation in endothelial cells. (Adapted from ref. 3)

Effect	Strain	Cell Type	Response Time	Significance	Reference Number
↑ AP-1	10% avg., 60 cpm	HUVEC	4 h	Activation of genes w/AP-1 binding sites	78
↑ AP-1	10% avg., 60 cpm	HAEC	2 h	Activation of genes w/AP-1 binding sites	78
↑ CRE	10% avg., 60 cpm	HUVEC	Biphasic; 15 min, 24 h	Activation of genes w/CRE binding sites	78
↑ CRE	10% avg., 60 cpm	HAEC	Biphasic; 2-4 h 24 h	Activation of genes w/CRE binding sites	78
↑ Nf-κb	10% avg., 60 cpm	HUVEC	4 h	Activation of genes w/Nf-κb binding sites	78
↑ Nf-κb	10% avg., 60 cpm	HAEC	By 2 h, peak at 4 h	Activation of genes w/Nf-κb binding sites	78

Table 39.3B. Effect of shear stress on transcription factor activation in endothelial cells. (Adapted from ref. 3)

Effect	Shear	Cell Type	Response Time	Significance	Reference Number
↑ AP-1	12 dyn/cm^2	BAEC	Biphasic, 20 min and 2 h	Activation of genes w/AP-1 binding sites	79
↑ Nf-κb	10% avg., 60 cpm	HUVEC	30 min-2 h	Activation of genes w/Nf-κb binding sites	79
↑ Nf-κb	10% avg., 60 cpm	BAEC	1 h	Activation of genes w/Nf-κb binding sites	5, 81

functional AP-1 binding site in its promoter regions. Interestingly, the strain-induced secretion of PAI-1 was shown to involve reactive oxygen species, a known activator of both AP-1 and NF-κB transcription factors. Further studies will be required to test this hypothesis. However, studies performed in our laboratory support the hypothesis of increased activity of transcriptional activators in endothelial cells subjected to cyclic strain.[78]

Since previous studies demonstrated that cyclic strain stimulates protein kinase c activity in endothelial cells,[72] we tested the hypothesis that downstream induction of the *fos* and *jun* genes and the transcription factor activator protein-1 (AP-1) were also activated by strain. Sumpio et al[31] showed that human umbilical vein endothelial cells subjected to cyclic strain for as short a duration as 30 minutes leads to the induction of *c-fos*, *fosB* and *c-jun* genes. In contrast, *junB* and *junD* were not altered by cyclic strain under identical conditions. We did detect an increase in AP-1 binding activity as measured by EMSA conducted after 2 h of cyclic strain. It may be concluded that cyclic strain may be coupled to the endothelial cell response via activation of protein kinase c and elevated steady state levels of different Fos and Jun products, which may enhance the activity of the transcriptional activator AP-1.[31]

In more rigorous studies performed to characterize the induction of transcriptional factor activation, AP-1, CRE binding protein and NF-κB were examined in endothelial cells obtained from a variety of beds and species.[78] These include endothelial cells obtained from human umbilical vein, human aorta and bovine aorta. In human umbilical vein endothelial cells subjected to cyclic strain, AP-1 activity was elevated as compared to unstretched controls.[31] The onset of strain-induced AP-1 activity was at 2 h, peaked by 4 h, and returned to baseline levels by 24 h. Similar findings were obtained in human aortic endothelial cells but not in bovine aortic endothelial cells.[78] A more pronounced retardation indicative of a supershift was noted in the presence of antibodies to c-Jun in HUVECs.

CRE binding activity was also influenced by cyclic strain in a species and vascular bed-dependent manner.[78] CRE levels were significantly stimulated in human umbilical vein endothelial cells in a biphasic manner with a 2-fold increase at 15 minutes and a nearly 5-fold increase at 24 h. Similar trends and kinetics were found in endothelial cells derived from bovine aorta. Similar to what is described above for AP-1, we failed to detect a change in CRE binding activity in this study.[78]

NF-κB binding activity in response to cyclic strain was also dependent on the vascular bed and species under study. NF-κB binding activity was stimulated in a monophasic manner in endothelial cells obtained from umbilical vein with a 4.6-fold increase at 4 h. As observed for AP-1, NF-κB was stimulated earlier by 2 h in human aortic endothelial cells, with a peak observed at 4 h. NF-κB binding activity, as shown above for AP-1 and CRE, was not altered by cyclic strain in bovine aortic endothelial cells in this study.[78]

However, in a later study we did show evidence for strain-induced stimulation of CRE binding activity in bovine aortic endothelial cells.[68] In this study, CRE binding activity was found by 30 minutes and diminished by 4 h.

Selective seeding of the endothelial cells to the high strain region (7-24% strain) led to a greater response than found in those cells grown in the central, low strain region (0-7%). An increase in CRE binding activity was not observed in cells subjected to an average 6% strain. The reasons for observation of a strain response in stimulation of CRE binding activity of bovine aortic endothelial cells in this study,[68] but not the earlier one,[78] is unclear and may suggest other variables aside from species and vascular bed diversity that remain to be uncovered. The nature of the mechanical force may also be critical in activating a particular transcription factor. For example, Lan et al[79] and Resnick et al[80] have both shown NF-κB activation in bovine aortic endothelial cells subjected to shear stress; a finding we have not been able to replicate in response to cyclic strain.

Gene Expression

Endothelin

Cyclic strain stimulates endothelin-1 secretion and mRNA levels in human umbilical vein endothelial cells.[82] Elevated expression of endothelin-1 mRNA was detected in cells subjected to 2 h or longer duration of cyclic strain. This was abolished by treatment with actinomycin D. The strain-induced elevation of ET-1 mRNA synthesis was found to be mediated by the activation of the PKC pathway and was shown to require extracellular Ca^{2+}. Involvement of the PKC pathway was determined since the PKC inhibitor calphostin C prevented strain-induced entothelin-1 expression. In contrast, the cAMP-dependent protein kinase inhibitors KT5720 or KT5823 only partially blocked endothelin-1 expression stimulation by cyclic strain. A requirement of extracellular Ca^{2+} was determined by blockade of strain-induced endothelin-1 mRNA by EGTA as well as a lesser effect by BAPTA/AM, an intracellular calcium chelator.[82] In our hands, we have observed strain-dependent reduction in ET-1 (Koo J et al, unpublished data).

Similar contradictory effects of shear stress have also been detected in measurements of ET-1.[61,62,83] Malek et al[83] have shown shear stress-mediated downregulation of ET-1 expression in bovine aortic endothelial cells conferred by a cis-element between -2.5 kb and -2.9 kb of the 5'-upstream promoter region that does not involve the AP-1 or GATA-2 factor binding site. In contrast, Morita et al[61,84] have shown shear stress-induced ET-1 expression in porcine aortic endothelial cells that appears to be related to cytoskeletal disruption.

Prostacyclin

Previous studies indicate that cyclic strain[29] and shear stress[58,85] can increase PGI_2 secretion by endothelial cells, but the effect of these forces on prostacyclin synthase (PGIS) gene expression remains unclear. In a recent study, we examined this question by studying PGIS gene expression by Northern blot analysis and protein level by Western blot analysis.[57] In addition, the effect of cyclic strain on the PGIS promoter was determined by the transfection of a 1 kb human PGIS gene promoter construct coupled to a luciferase reporter gene into EC, followed by determination of luciferase activity.

PGIS gene expression increased 1.7-fold in EC subjected to cyclic strain for 24 h.[57] Likewise, EC transfected with a pGL3B-PGIS(-1070/-10) construct showed an approximate 1.3-fold elevation in luciferase activity in EC subjected to cyclic strain for 2, 4, 8 and 12 h. The weak stimulation of PGIS gene expression by cyclic strain was reflected in an inability to detect alterations in PGIS protein levels in EC subjected to cyclic strain for as long as 5 days. These data suggest that strain-induced stimulation of PGIS gene expression plays only a minor role in the ability of cyclic strain to stimulate PGI2 release in EC. These findings, coupled with our earlier demonstration of a requisite addition of exogenous arachidonate in order to observe strain-induced PGI2 release,[29] implicates a mechanism that more likely involves strain-induced stimulation of PGIS activity.

Tissue Plasminogen Activator (tPA)

Previous studies showed an increase in tPA mRNA, immunoreactive tPA protein and tPA activity in the medium of cultured bovine aortic endothelial cells exposed to 10% average strain.[19,20] Previous studies documented that tPA expression is upregulated by shear stress.[60] We have more recently examined the regulation of tPA gene expression in endothelial cells by cyclic strain.[32] A functional analysis of the tPA promoter was performed by transfecting bovine aortic endothelial cells with a 1.4 kb construct of the human tPA promoter coupled to CAT. After 4 h of cyclic strain, a nearly 3-fold increase in the activity of the 1.4 kb tPA promoter was detected.[32] A 60% drop off in activity was found between position -145 and -105 by analysis of deletion mutants. DNase I protection analysis of the segment downstream of position -196 suggested involvement of AP-2 or CRE-like regions, which was confirmed by EMSA analysis. Site directed mutants of either the AP-2 or CRE-like regions resulted in a 65% decrease in activity compared to the wild type. In addition, double mutations abolished basal transcription and any strain-induced activity. A SSRE binding site was found to be present at -945, but site directed mutants failed to show any drop in strain-induced activity as compared to the wild type. Overall, our studies demonstrate that cyclic strain regulates tPA gene transcription in bovine aortic endothelial cells by a mechanism similar to that shown previously for phorbol ester.

Nitric Oxide

Awolesi et al[45] demonstrated that cyclic strain can upregulate the expression of endothelial nitric oxide synthase (eNOS) in bovine aortic endothelial cells. At an average strain of 10%, eNOS expression in these cells was shown to be increased as compared to unstretched controls as determined by Northern blot analysis. A milder elevation in eNOS expression was measured in cells exposed to a lesser degree of strain of 6%. The strain-induced activation of eNOS expression was attributed to stimulation of transcriptional activity as shown by nuclear runoff assays. Western blot analysis and immunochemistry confirmed that eNOS protein levels were similarly increased in response to strain; again 10% strain led to a heightened response as compared to 6% strain.

Awolesi et al[44] showed that the strain-induced upregulation of eNOS expression in bovine aortic endothelial cells translates into an increase in functional activity. In this study, 10% cyclic strain for 24 h led to an increase in both citrulline production and accumulated nitrite (Greiss reaction) as indices of eNOS activity. Specificity of this response was confirmed by blockade with EDTA and L-NAME. As is the case for strain-induced expression, strain-induced eNOS functional activity was more pronounced at 10% average strain as compared to 6% strain. The effect of 10% strain was as potent as that observed with the calcium ionophore, A23187.[44]

Shear stress has also been shown to increase nitric oxide gene expression in endothelial cells.[59,86,87] In a recent study, Uematsu et al[59] reported 2 to 3-fold elevations in eNOS by shear stress of 15 dynes/cm^2 for up to 1 day. The involvement of K$^+$ channels was suggested, since shear stress induction of nitric oxide mRNA was blocked by tetraethylammonium chloride, a K$^+$ channel antagonist.

MCP-1

Wang et al[88] studied the effect of cyclic strain on monocyte chemotactic protein-1 (MCP-1) expression in cultured human umbilical vein endothelial cells (HUVECs). They found a two-fold enhancement in MCP-1 expression as early as one hour after the initiation of strain. This response was maintained for at least 24 h in the presence of strain, but was restored to baseline levels 3 h after its release. Calphostin C was able to abolish strain-induced MCP-1 expression, implicating a role of PKC as a mediator of this response. In addition, a strong Ca^{2+} requirement for strain-induced, as well as basal, expression of MCP-1 was determined by blockade with either EGTA pretreatment, BAPTA/AM chelation, or verapamil addition to HUVECs.[88]

Shear stress-induced expression of MCP-1 has been shown to involve a cis-acting TRE-responsive element in its promotor.[89] A construct of multiple copies of the TRE-responsive element coupled to a prolactin minimal reporter and luciferase gene was found to be sufficient to confer shear sensitivity in transfected bovine aortic endothelial cells.

ICAM/VCAM

In recent studies conducted in our laboratory, we have obtained evidence to suggest that ICAM and VCAM expression are downregulated by cyclic strain in human umbilical vein endothelial cells (Lee et al, unpublished observations). In contrast ICAM-1 expression is upregulated in the same cell type under conditions of shear stress.[87,90]

Effect of Cyclic Strain on Vascular Smooth Muscle Cell Biology

General Phenotype

Smooth muscle cells are known to exist in two classic phenotypic states.[26] In vivo, under normal conditions, smooth muscle cell proliferation is slow and the contractile or differentiated phenotype predominates. The differentiated phenotype is characterized by a heterochromatic nucleus, abundant actin and myosin filaments. The contractile smooth muscle cells contract in response to both chemical and mechanical stimulation. In vivo counterparts of the contractile phenotype are smooth muscle cells from media of vessels of normal adults.

However, the smooth muscle cell is not terminally differentiated and is able to undergo phenotypic modulation under a variety of circumstances. This phenotypic modulation occurs upon vessel injury and is characterized by a reduction in smooth muscle contractile proteins such as α-actin and smooth muscle myosin heavy chain, and by a shift toward a synthetic state accompanied by the laying down of extracellular matrix molecules.[35] Such changes can be mimicked in vitro by growing smooth muscle cells in a serum-fed preconfluent condition. Morphological characteristics of the synthetic smooth muscle cell phenotype include a euchromatic nucleus as well as a prominent endoplasmic reticulum and Golgi complex. These smooth muscle cells resemble those found in diffuse intimal thickenings of atherosclerotic lesions.[91]

However, the identification of smooth muscle cells as belonging to either a contractile or synthetic phenotype may be a gross simplification.[92,93] Rather, the behavior of smooth muscle cells is not locked into a particular phenotype such that those classified as belonging to the "synthetic" phenotype are not able to contract and vice versa. For example, Chamley and Campbell[94] found that single smooth muscle cells from newborn guinea pig vas deferens underwent mitosis (as observed by time-lapse photography) despite the fact that the cells were in a morphologically-defined differentiated state. This finding emphasized the need to examine biochemical parameters, in addition to morphology, in order to better define the phenotypic state of smooth muscle cells in culture.[93]

As described recently by Owens,[36] the factors that normally control the differentiation of the smooth muscle cell are not understood. However, a recent paper by Reusch et al[39] is lauded as providing the most definitive study to date identifying a positive differentiation influence/factor in smooth muscle cells. The work by Reusch et al[39] describes cyclic strain as the factor. Notably, the story as described below is most complex, as strain has been shown to not only upregulate markers of differentiation (i.e., SM-1, SM-2) but also to stimulate smooth muscle cell growth. Whether this represents an artifact of the system due to its heterogeneous strain gradient, is due to distinct subpopulations of smooth muscle cells, or reflects the fact that growth and differentiation are not necessarily exclusive properties remains to be established.[36]

Since previous studies had shown that PDGF secretion is elevated by cyclic strain,[40] the authors examined whether secreted PDGF affects the strain-induced changes in contractile protein expression. Interestingly, PDGF-AB was shown to cause a qualitatively opposite change in myosin isoform expression, decreasing smooth muscle myosin by greater than half. Moreover, neutralization of PDGF-AB with neutralizing antibodies led to a strain-induced increase in SM-1 that was enhanced 10-fold. Thus, PDGF fails to mediate the effect of cyclic strain on smooth muscle myosin isoform distribution. Instead, it is concluded that cyclic strain

is mediating opposing activities; PDGF secreted in response to cyclic strain opposes the effect of strain to upregulate smooth muscle heavy chain isoforms.

The findings of Reusch et al[39] also confirm the earlier work of Birukov et al[95] who showed a dual effect of cyclic strain in modulating rabbit aortic smooth muscle cell phenotype. Cyclic strain was found to both increase proliferation and also increase expression of markers of smooth muscle cell differentiation, in this case h-caldesmon. Common attributes of these studies included a dependence on quiescent conditions to observe many of their effects (i.e., strain-induced myosin heavy chain expression and proliferation), as well as modulation by extracellular matrix proteins that served as a substratum for the smooth muscle cells. In the study by Birukov et al,[95] smooth muscle myosin heavy chain was increased in the presence of 0.5% serum, but not observed at concentrations of 2, 5 and 10%. However, strain-induced h-caldesmon expression was less dependent on serum levels. Laminin was a preferred substrate for detection of strain-induced h-caldesmon levels[95] and was also a preferable substrate, along with type I collagen, in promoting differentiation of smooth muscle cells in the study by Reusch et al.[39]

The authors also studied the effect of extracellular matrix molecules on strain-induced SM-1 expression,[39] since earlier studies indicated its modulation of strain responsiveness.[96] In this study, matrix was again found to be an important factor in how SMCs transduce the strain stimuli. The ability of cyclic strain to increase SM-1 was 2-fold in SMCs grown on type I collagen, 3-fold on laminin, and absent in fibronectin-coated wells. It was concluded that mechanical strain can alter myosin isoform expression to a more differentiated state in a matrix-dependent manner.[96]

The findings of Reusch et al[39] confirmed earlier observations of Kanda and Matsuda[97] that indicated stress-induced differentiation of bovine aortic smooth muscle cells. In their study, Kanda examined smooth muscle cells cultured in a three dimensional type I collagen gel. Smooth muscle cells were exposed to 3 conditions including isotonic control, isometric stress or static stress and dynamic stress consisting of periodic stretching and recoiling of 5% above and below the resting tissue length at 60 cycles per minute. After 4 weeks of this regimen, smooth muscle cell morphology was examined by light microscopy and transmission electron microscopy. Smooth muscle cells subjected to the dynamic regimen were unique in exhibiting a more differentiated state as shown by increased fractions of contractile apparatus. Over time on stress, the content of myofilaments, dense bodies and extracellular filamentous basement membrane-like materials increased. This was an indication that dynamic stress in cells laid down in a 3-dimensional collagen matrix inclines them toward a more differentiated state.[97]

The effect of cyclic strain on smooth muscle cell proliferation is predominantly stimulatory[40,95,98,99] Davis[99] observed strain-induced cell proliferation of 33% in serum-starved rat aortic smooth muscle cells supplemented with insulin and transferrin. Although significant, this response was only one fifth that observed in the presence of repleted calf serum of 10%. Likewise, Yang et al[98] showed a significant increase, albeit slight (13%), by 6 days of cyclic strain exposure in cultured smooth muscle cells obtained from the media of human left descending coronary artery. In neonatal rat smooth muscle cells grown to quiescence, Wilson et al[40] observed a similar 40% increase in the proliferative response to cyclic strain as compared to static controls. In rabbit aortic smooth muscle cells, cyclic strain also caused an increase in cell number.[95] Interestingly, the ability to detect an increase in cell proliferation induced by cyclic strain was dependent on the cells being serum activated. In quiescent cultures, smooth muscle cells failed to respond to cyclic strain. In this study, Birukov et al[95] also showed that the number of detached cells (i.e., an index of cell attachment to membranes) was unaffected by cyclic strain. In another control experiment, motion effects of circulating medium in response to cyclic strain was ruled out as a contributory factor to the stretch-induced increase in smooth muscle cell proliferation, since no difference was noted in control versus nutational conditions.

The effect of cyclic strain on DNA synthesis in smooth muscle cells is more pronounced than for proliferation. In coronary artery smooth muscle cells obtained from human left descending coronary arteries, Yang et al[98] found that cyclic strain stimulates DNA synthesis greater than 2-fold after 24 h. In rat aortic smooth muscle cells, Davis et al[99] showed a 2-fold increase in [³H]thymidine incorporation by cyclic strain. In smooth muscle cells obtained from newborn rat, Wilson et al[40] demonstrated a nearly 3-fold increase in [³H]thymidine incorporation by cyclic strain of -20 kPa at 60 cycles/min for 48 h. This elevation afforded by strain was less potent as compared to that observed with 1 U/ml thrombin or 5 ng/ml platelet derived growth factor (PDGF). Further study showed that combinatorial addition of strain and thrombin led to even greater stimulation of DNA synthesis. However, strain and PDGF did not exhibit significantly greater stimulation of [³H]thymidine as compared to that observed with PDGF alone. The authors suggest that this observation may be explained by strain itself acting via autocrine production of PDGF.[40]

Wilson et al[96] further studied the matrix dependence of the strain-induced mitogenic response in rat vascular smooth muscle cells. They found that cyclic strain increased DNA synthesis in SMCs grown not only on type I collagen, but also fibronectin or vitronectin. However, on plates coated with elastin or laminin, strain induction of DNA synthesis was not observed. The integrin binding peptide GRGDTP was shown to block the mitogenic response of SMCs to strain in cells seeded on type I collagen. Specificity of this response was noted by the inability of the inactive peptide GRGESP to also block strain-induced mitogenesis. In addition, strain-induced expression of a PDGF-A chain promoter-CAT construct transiently transfected into SMCs was blocked by the integrin binding protein GRGDTP. A role for specific integrins involved in sensing mechanical strain in SMCs was shown by studies with antibodies to both β_3 and $\alpha_v\beta_5$ integrins, which also blocked the mitogenic response to strain.

However, there are conflicting reports in the literature regarding the effect of mechanical strain on smooth muscle cell proliferation, depending on the exact source of tissue and the regimen under study. For example, Sumpio and Banes[28] showed that the proliferative response of porcine aortic smooth muscle cells is inhibited by cyclic strain. In another study using early passaged smooth muscle cells from lamb pulmonary artery, Kulik and Alvarado[100] failed to detect any increase in cell number after 24 h of 20% stretch. Similarly, DNA synthesis as measured by [³H]thymidine incorporation was unaffected by stretch. In the same study, a passaged clonal line of rat cells (PAC1) did show a modest elevation (17% increase) in the percentage of [³H]thymidine-labeled cells. However, TCA-precipitated [³H]thymidine was unaffected by cyclic strain.

In a follow up study to the earlier work of Kulik and Alvarado[100] failing to demonstrate an effect of mechanical forces on the growth of smooth muscle cells from pulmonary artery, Kolpakov et al[101] reexamined this finding in a whole vessel model. Interestingly, they found that subjecting rabbit pulmonary arteries to varying magnitudes of stretch led to an increased rate of protein synthesis (as measured by quantitative autoradiography) and replication of smooth muscle cells. Moreover, synthesis of extracellular matrix proteins, elastin and collagen, were elevated in 4 day stretched segments as compared to static controls. The authors also showed that these effects were independent of endothelium interaction, as its removal did not prevent the aforementioned changes.

This study illustrates the caution that should be exercised in interpretation of in vitro experiments that may not be analogous to the condition in vivo or even in an ex vivo model. The authors rightly assert that their earlier negative findings of in vitro studies could be attributed to cell shape, its orientation relative to the applied strain, matrix substratum, and of course, the cell culture milieu.[101]

Cell Signaling

Second Messenger Pathways

Adenylyl Cyclase

In bovine aortic smooth muscle cells, we have demonstrated strain-induced activation of the adenylyl cyclase/cyclic AMP/protein kinase a pathway.[24] Basal adenylyl cyclase was elevated nearly 2-fold in SMC subjected to 150 mm Hg vacuum deformation for 30 min and returned to basal levels by 60 min. Likewise, cyclic AMP accumulation was also stimulated by cyclic strain at 30 min and returned to basal values by 60 min. Protein kinase a activity was also stimulated by cyclic strain. The activation of this pathway was strain specific, such that cells subjected to low strain (0-7%) in the center of the well were found to significantly stimulate PKA activity, as compared to cells in the peripheral, high strain (7-24%) region of the well. Similar findings of an elevated response from cells obtained from the center region were observed for CRE binding protein levels as measured by gel shift analysis.

The relationship between strain-activated signaling events and downstream responses is complex. This is exemplified by our inability to demonstrate any effect of

Rp-cAMP, a PKA inhibitor, on strain-induced proliferation or alignment.[24] Thus, although strain activated the adenylyl cyclase signaling pathway, the lack of an effect of PKA inhibition suggests either the lack of involvement of this pathway or the multifactorial nature of these responses.

Tyrosine Kinase

Davis et al[99] showed that cyclic strain stimulates the phosphotyrosine accumulation in smooth muscle cells obtained from rat aorta. Proteins with upregulated phosphotyrosine content in response to cyclic strain included species of 110-130 kDa and 70-80 kDa as determined by Western blot analysis. The identity of these proteins was not ascertained, but ascribed to proteins of corresponding molecular weight, including GTPase and p74^{Raf}, respectively. Specificity of tyrosine kinase activity induced by cyclic strain was shown by blockade with the phosphotyrosine kinase inhibitor herbimycin A. Moreover, both herbimycin A and genistein, another tyrosine kinase inhibitor, were found to have cyclic strain-induced DNA synthesis as measured by incorporation of [^{3}H]thymidine. Thus, it was concluded that cyclic strain stimulates vascular smooth muscle cell proliferation through activation of tyrosine kinases.[99]

Phosphatases

Phosphorylation of the 20 kDa regulatory myosin light chain (MLC20) is the seminal event in the initiation of vascular smooth muscle cell contraction. We sought to determine whether cyclic strain affects MLC20 phosphorylation in bovine aortic smooth muscle cells. We studied the effect of cyclic strain on serum-fed SMCs already displaying a high level of MLC20 phosphorylation. Confluent SMCs were subjected to 10% average strain at 60 cycles per minute for 30 and 60 minutes. Basal MLC20 phosphorylation (N=non, M=mono, D=di) of serum-fed SMC was as follows: N=34%: M=27%: D=39%. After 60 minutes of cyclic strain, both the mono and diphosphorylated species of MLC20 were decreased by 21% and 15%, respectively. The strain-induced dephosphorylation of MLC20 was partially inhibited by the protein phosphatase 1/2A inhibitor calyculin A. However, phosphorylase A phosphatase activities in Triton-soluble and insoluble fractions of SMCs were unaffected by cyclic strain.

Our data suggested that cyclic strain causes dephosphorylation of MLC20 in SMCs, which may be partially due to the activation of MLC20 phosphatase and/or inhibition of MLC20 phosphorylation.

Gene Expression

PDGF

PDGF-AA and -BB secretion and PDGF-A expression were stimulated in smooth muscle cells subjected to cyclic strain.40 Moreover, neutralizing antibodies to both PDGF-AA and -AB were found to block strain-induced stimulation of DNA synthesis. In contrast, bFGF antibody failed to prevent the mitogenic response to cyclic strain.[40]

Myosin Heavy and Light Chain

Reusch et al[39] recently examined the effect of mechanical strain on the expression of myosin heavy chain isoform expression in neonatal rat vascular smooth muscle cells. As a marker of differentiation, they studied expression of the smooth muscle myosin heavy chain isoforms, SM-1 and SM-2 (see Fig. 39.7 in ref. 39). These isoforms are well characterized markers of differentiation expressed at high levels in postconfluent, quiescent SMC.[102] In quiescent smooth muscle cells grown in 0.5% fetal bovine serum, SM-1 and SM-2 protein content was elevated by 4.5- and 3.5 fold, respectively, after 72 h of cyclic strain. In addition, nonmuscle myosin A (NM-A) protein content decreased to 30% of control levels. Cyclic strain was also found to increase gene expression of SM-1 and decrease that of NM-A, with peak changes occurring at 12 h and 3 h, respectively.

Summary

In summary, recent data support the hypothesis that vascular endothelial and smooth muscle cells are keenly sensitive to mechanical perturbation such as cyclic strain. Our group and others have characterized changes in the phenotype of both cell types and have begun to delineate the relevant signaling pathways and strain-sensitive genes. Continued advances in this field may prove beneficial in developing novel approaches to improve tissue engineering of prosthetic grafts.

Table 39.4. Effect of cyclic strain on smooth muscle cell signaling pathways

Effect	Strain	Cell Type	Response Time	Significance	Reference Number
↑ PKC	10% avg., 60 cpm	BASMC	10 sec	Activation of the PKC pathway	24
↑ Adenylyl cyclase	10% avg., 60 cpm	BASMC	30 min	Activation of the cAMP pathway	24
↑ cAMP	10% avg., 60 cpm	BASMC	30 min	Activation of the cAMP pathway	24
↑ PKA	10% avg., 60 cpm	BASMC	30 min	Activation of the PKA pathway	24
↑ Tyrosine Phosphorylation	10% avg., 15 cpm	RASMC	10 min	Role in SMC growth	99

References

1. Panaro NJ, McIntire LV. Flow and shear stress effects on endothelial cell function. In: Sumpio BE, ed. Hemodynamic Forces and Vascular Cell Biology. Austin: R.G. Landes Co., 1993:47-65.

2. Oluwole BO, Du W, Mills I, Sumpio BE. Gene regulation by mechanical forces. Endothelium 1997; 5:85-93.

3. Davies PF. Flow-mediated endothelial mechanotransduction. Physiol Rev 1995; 75:519-560.

4. Nerem RM, Harrison DG, Taylor WR, Alexander RW. Hemodynamics and vascular endothelial biology. J Cardiovasc Pharm 1993; 21(S1):S6-S10.

5. Resnick N, Gimbrone MA Jr. Hemodynamic forces are complex regulators of endothelial gene expression. FASEB J 1995; 9:874-882.

6. Thubrikar MJ, Robicsek F. Pressure-induced arterial wall stress and atherosclerosis. Ann Thorac Surg 1995; 59:1594-1603.

7. Langille BL. Chronic effects of blood flow on the artery wall. In: Frangos JA, ed. Physical forces and the mammalian cell. San Diego: Academic Press, 1993:249-274.

8. Patel DJ, Greenfield WG, Austen WG, Fry DL. Pressure flow relationships in the ascending aorta and femoral artery of man. J Appl Physiol 1965; 20:459-463.

9. Bergel DH. The static elastic properties of the arterial wall. J Physiol 1961; 156:445-457.

10. Steinman DA, Ethier CR. The effect of wall distensibility on flow in a two-dimensional end-to-side anastomosis. J Biomech Eng 1994; 116:294-301.

11. Ballermann BJ, Ott MJ. Adhesion and differentiation of endothelial cells by exposure to chronic shear stress: A vascular graft model. Blood Purification 1995; 13:125-134.

12. Ott MJ, Ballermann BJ. Shear stress-conditioned, endothelial cell-seeded vascular grafts: Improved cell adherence in response to in vitro shear stress. Surgery 1995; 117:334-339.

13. Kohler TR, Kirkman TR, Kraiss LW, Zierler BK, Clowes AW. Increased blood flow inhibits neointimal hyperplasia in endothelialized vascular grafts. Circ Res 1991; 69:1557-1565.

14. Geary RL, Kohler TR, Vergel S, Kirkman TR, Clowes AW. Time course of flow-induced smooth muscle cell proliferation and intimal thickening in endothelialized baboon vascular grafts. Circ Res 1993; 74:14-23.

15. Kraiss LW, Geary RL, Mattsson EJR, Vergel S, Au YPT, Clowes AW. Acute reductions in blood flow and shear stress induce platelet-derived growth factor-A expression in baboon prosthetic grafts. Circ Res 1996; 79:45-53.

16. Dobrin PB, Littooy FN, Endean ED. Mechanical factors predisposing to intimal hyperplasia and medial thickening in autogenous vein grafts. Surgery 1989; 105:393-400.

17. Mills I, Cohen CR, Sumpio BE. In: Sumpio BE, ed. Hemodynamic Forces and Vascular Cell Biology. Austin: R.G. Landes Co., 1993; 5:66-89.

18. Iba T, Sumpio BE. Morphological response of human endothelial cells subjected to cyclic strain in vitro. Microvasc Res 1991; 42:245-254.

19. Iba T, Shin T, Sonoda T, Rosales OR, Sumpio BE. Stimulation of endothelial secretion of tissue-type plasminogen activator by repetitive stretch. J Surg Res 1991; 50:457-460.

20. Iba T, Sumpio BE. Tissue plasminogen activator expression in endothelial cells exposed to cyclic strain in vitro. Cell Transplantation 1991; (1):43-50.

21. Iba T, Mills I, Sumpio BE. Intracellular cyclic AMP levels in endothelial cells subjected to cyclic strain in vitro. J Surg Res 1992; 52(6):625-30.

22. Mills I, Cohen CR, Sumpio BE. Cyclic strain and vascular cell biology. In: Sumpio BE, ed. Hemodynamic Forces and Vascular Cell Biology. Austin: R.G. Landes Co., 1993:66-89.

23. Mills I, Murata K, Packer CS, Sumpio BE. Cyclic strain stimulates dephosphorylation of the 20kDa regulatory myosin light chain in vascular smooth muscle cells [published erratum appears in Biochem Biophys Res Commun 1995 Feb 27; 207(3):1058]. Biochem Biophys Res Commun 1994; 205(1):79-84.

24. Mills I, Cohen CR, Kamal K, Li G, Shin T, Du W, Sumpio BE. Strain activation of bovine aortic smooth muscle cell proliferation and alignment: Study of strain dependency and the role of protein kinase a and C signaling pathways. J Cell Physiol 1997; 170:228-234.

25. Mills I, Cohen CR, Kamal K, Sumpio BE. Cyclic strain stimulates ADP-ribosylation of the inhibitory G protein, $G_{i\alpha}$, in bovine aortic endothelial cells. 1998; in press.

26. Mills I, Sumpio BE. Vascular smooth muscle cells. In: Sidawy AN, Sumpio BE, DePalma RG, eds. The Basic Science of Vascular Disease. Armonk: Futura Publishing Company, Inc., 1997:187-226.

27. Sumpio BE, Banes AJ, Levin LG, Johnson G. Mechanical stress stimulates aortic endothelial cells to proliferate. J Vasc Surg 1987; 6:252-256.

28. Sumpio BE, Banes AJ. Response of procine aortic smooth muscle cells to cyclic tensional deformation in culture. J Surg Res 1988; 44:696-701.

29. Sumpio BE, Banes AJ. Prostacyclin synthetic activity in cultured aortic endothelial cells undergoing cyclic mechanical deformation. Surgery 1988; 104:383-389.

30. Sumpio BE, Widmann MD. Enhanced production of an endothelium derived contracting factor by endothelial cells subjected to pulsatile stretch. Surgery 1990; 108:277-282.

31. Sumpio BE, Du W, Xu W-J. Exposure of endothelial cells to cyclic strain induces c-fos, fosB and c-jun but not jun B or jun D and increases the transcription factor AP-1. Endothelium 1994; 2:149-156.

32. Sumpio BE, Chang R, Xu W-J, Wang X-J, Du W. Regulation of tissue plasminogen activator in bovine endothelial cells exposed to cyclic strain: The functional significance of the CRE, AP-2 and SSRE sites. Am J Physiol 1997; 42:C1441-C1448.

33. Augustin HG, Kozian DH, Johnson RC. Differentiation of endothelial cells: Analysis of the constitutive and activated endothelial cell phenotypes. Bioessays 1994; 16(12):901-6.

34. Risau W. Differentiation of endothelium. FASEB Journal 1995; 9(10):926-33.

35. Thyberg J, Hedin U, Sjolund M, Palmberg L, Bottger BA. Regulation of differentiated properties and proliferation of arterial smooth muscle cells. Arteriosclerosis 1990; 10:966-990.

36. Owens GK. Role of mechanical strain in regulation of differentiation of vascular smooth muscle cells. Circ Res 1996; 79:1054-1055.

37. Yano Y, Geibel J, Sumpio BE. Tyrosine phosphorylation of pp125[FAK] and paxillin in aortic endothelial cells induced by mechanical strain. Am J Physiol 1996; 271:C635-C649.

38. Li G, Mills I, Sumpio BE. Cyclic strain stimulates endothelial cell proliferation. Characterization of the strain requirements. Endothelium. 1994; 2:177-181.

39. Reusch P, Wagdy H, Reusch R, Wilson E, Ives HE. Mechanical strain increases smooth muscle and decreases nonmuscle expression in rat vascular smooth muscle cells. Circ Res 1996; 79:1046-1053.

40. Wilson E, Mai Q, Sudhir K, Weiss RH, Ives HE. Mechanical strain induces growth of vascular smooth muscle cells via autocrine action of PDGF. Journal of Cell Biology 1993; 123(3):741-7.

41. Zilla P, von Oppell U, Deutsch M. The endothelium: A key to the future. J Card Surg 1993; 8:32-60.

42. Ives CL, Eskin SG, McIntire LV. Mechanical effects on endothelial cell morphology: In vitro assessment. In Vitro Cell Dev Biol 1986; 22:500-507.

43. Shirinsky VP, Antonov AS, Birukov KG. Mechanochemical control of human endothelium orientation and size. J Cell Biol 1989; 109:331-339.

44. Awolesi MA, Widmann MD, Sessa WC, Sumpio BE. Cyclic strain increases endothelial nitric oxide synthase activity. Surgery 1994; 116(2):439-44; discussion 444-5.

45. Awolesi MA, Sessa WC, Sumpio BE. Cyclic strain upregulates nitric oxide synthase in cultured bovine aortic endothelial cells. J Clin Invest 1995; 96(3):1449-54.

46. Cheng JJ, Chao YJ, Wung BS, Wang DL. Cyclic strain-induced plasminogen activator inhibitor-1 (PAI-1) release from endothelial cells involves reactive oxygen species. Biochem Biophys Res Commun 1996; 225(1):100-5.

47. Davies PF, Tripathi SC. Mechanical stress mechanisms and the cell. An endothelial paradigm. Circ Res 1993; 72:239-245.

48. Dewey CF Jr, Bussolari SR, Gimbrone MA Jr, Davies PF. The dynamic response of the vascular endothelial cells to fluid shear stress. J Biomech Eng 1981; 103:177-188.

49. Davies PF, Robotewskyj A, Griem ML. Quantitative studies of endothelial cell adhesion. Directional remodeling of focal adhesion sites in response to flow forces. J Clin Inv 1994; 93:2031-2038.

50. Yano Y, Geibel J, Sumpio BE. Cyclic strain induces reorganization of integrin $\alpha_2\beta_1$ in human umbilical vein endothelial cells. J Cell Biochem 1997; 64:505-513.

51. Thoumine O, Nerem RM, Girard PR. Changes in organization and composition of the extracellular matrix underlying cultured endothelial cells exposed to laminar steady shear stress. Lab Invest 1995; 73:565-576.

52. Davies PF. Flow-mediated signal transduction in endothelial cells. In: Bevan J, Kaley G, Rubanyi G, eds. Flow dependent regulation of vascular function in health and disease. New York: Academic Press, 1984:46-61.

53. Eskin SG, Ives CL, McIntire LV, Navarro LT. Response of cultured endothelial cells to steady flow. Microvasc Res 1984; 28:87-93.

54. Levesque MJ, Nerem RM. The study of rheological effects on vascular endothelial cells in culture. Biorheology 1989; 26:345-357.

55. Girard P, Nerem RM. Shear stress modulates endothelial cell morphology and F-actin organization through the regulation of focal adhesion-associated proteins. J Cell Physiol 1995; 163:179-193.

56. Yano Y, Saito Y, Narumiya S, Sumpio BE. Involvement of rho p21 in cyclic strain-induced tyrosine phosphorylation of focal adhesion kinase (pp125[FAK]), morphological changes and migration of endothelial cells. Biochem Biophys Res Commun 1996; 224(2):508-15.

57. Segurola RJ, Oluwole B, Mills I, Yokoyama C, Tanabe T, Kito H, Nakajima N, Sumpio BE. Cyclic strain is a weak inducer of prostacyclin synthase expression in bovine aortic endothelial cells. J Vasc Res 1997; 69:135-138.

58. Frangos JA, Eskin SG, McIntire LV, Ives CL. Flow effects on prostacyclin production by cultured endothelial cells. Science 1985; 27:1477-1479.

59. Uematsu M, Ohara Y, Navas JP, Nishida K, Murphy TJ, Alexander RW, Nerem RM, Harrison DG. Regulation of endothelial cell nitric oxide synthase mRNA expression by shear stress. Am J Physiol 1995; 269:C1371-C1378.

60. Diamond SL, Sharefkin JB, Diefenbach C, Frazier-Scott K, McIntire LV. Tissue plasminogen activator mRNA levels increase in cultured human endothelial cells exposed to laminar shear stress. J Cell Physiol 1990; 143:364-371.

61. Morita T, Kurihara H, Maemura K, Yoshizumi M, Yazaki Y. Disruption of cytoskeletal structures mediates shear stress-induced endothelin-1 gene expression in cultured porcine aortic endothelial cells. J Clin Inv 1993; 92:1706-1712.

62. Malek A, Izumo S. Physiological fluid shear stress causes down-regulation of endothelin-1 mRNA in bovine aortic endothelium. Am J Physiol 1992; 263:C389-C396.

63. Rosales OR, Isales CM, Barrett PQ, Brophy C, Sumpio BE. Exposure of endothelial cells to cyclic strain induces elevations of cytosolic calcium through mobilization of intracellular and extracellular pools. Biochem J 1997; 326:385-392.

64. Geiger RV, Berk BC, Alexander RW, Nerem RM. Flow-induced calcium transients in single endothelial cells: Spatial and temporal analysis. Am J Physiol 1992; 262:C1411-C1417.

65. Evans L, Frenkel L, Brophy CM, Rosales O, Sudhaker S, Li G, Du W, Sumpio BE. Activation of diacylglycerol in cultured endothelial cells exposed to cyclic strain. Am J Physiol 1997; 41:C650-C659.

66. Bhagyalakshmi A, Berthiaume F, Reich KM, Frangos JA. Fluid shear stress stimulates membrane phospholipid metabolism in cultured human endothelial cells. J Vasc Res 1992; 29:443-449.

67. Kroll MH, Hellums JD, Guo Z, Durante W, Razdan K, Hrbolich JK, Schafer AI. Protein kinase c is activated in platelets subjected to pathological shear stress. J Biol Chem 1993; 268:3520-3524.

68. Cohen CR, Mills I, Du W, Kamal K, Sumpio BE. Activation of the adenylyl cyclase/cyclic AMP/protein kinase a pathway in endothelial cells exposed to cyclic strain. Expt Cell Res 1997; 231:184-189.

69. Gudi SRP, Clark CB, Frangos JA. Fluid flow rapidly activates G proteinse in human endothelial cells. Involvement of G proteins in mechanochemical signal transduction. Circ Res 1996; 79:834-839.

70. Kuchan MJ, Jo H, Frangos JA. Role of G proteins in shear stress-mediated nitric oxide production by endothelial cells. Am J Physiol 1994; 267:C753-C758.

71. Berthiaume F, Frangos JA. Flow-induced prostacyclin production is mediated by a pertussis toxin-sensitive G protein. FEBS Lett 1992; 308:277-279.

72. Rosales OR, Sumpio BE. Protein kinase c is a mediator of the adaptation of vascular endothelial cells to cyclic strain in vitro. Surgery 1992; 112(2):459-66.

73. Murata K, Mills I, Sumpio BE. Protein phosphatase 2A in stretch-induced endothelial cell proliferation. J Cell Biochem 1996; 62:1-9.

74. Rosales OR, Sumpio BE. Changes in cyclic strain increase inositol trisphosphate and diacylglycerol in endothelial cells. Am J Physiol 1992; 262(4 Pt 1):C956-62.

75. Nollert MU, Eskin SG, McIntire LV. Shear stress increases inositol trispohosphate levels in human endothelial cells. Biochem Biophys Res Comm 1990; 170:281-290.

76. Ohno M, Cooke JP, Dzau VJ, Gibbons GH. Fluid shear stress induces endothelial TGF-β1 transcription and production. Modulation by potassium channel blockade. J Clin Inv 1995; 95:1363-1369.

77. Tseng H, Peterson TE, Berk BC. Fluid shear stress stimulates mitogen-activated protein kinase in endothelial cells. Circ Res 1995; 77:869-878.

78. Du W, Mills I, Sumpio BE. Cyclic strain causes heterogeneous induction of transcription factors, AP-1, CRE binding protein and Nf-κb, in endothelial cells: Species and vascular bed diversity. J Biomech 1995; 28(12):1485-91.

79. Lan Q, Mercurius KO, Davies PF. Stimulation of transcription factors Nf-κb and AP1 in endothelial cells subjected to shear stress. Biochem Biophys Res Comm 1994; 201:950-956.

80. Resnick N, Collins T, Atkinson W, Bonthron DT, Dewey CF Jr, Gimbrone MA. Platelet-derived growth factor B chain promoter contains a cis-acting fluid shear-stress-responsive element. Proc Natl Acad Sci 1993; 90:4591-4595.

81. Khachigian LM, Resnick N, Gimbrone MA Jr, Collins T. Nuclear factor-κB interacts functionally with the platelet-derived growth factor B-chain shear-stress response element in vascular endothelial cells exposed to fluid shear stress. J Clin Inv 1995; 96:1169-1175.

82. Wang DL, Wung BS, Peng YC, Wang JJ. Mechanical strain increases endothelin-1 gene expression via protein kinase c pathway in human endothelial cells. J Cell Physiol 1995; 163(2):400-6.

83. Malek AM, Greene AL, Izumo S. Regulation of endothelin 1 gene by fluid shear stress is transcriptionally mediated and independent of protein kinase c and cAMP. Proc Natl Acad Sci USA 1993; 90:5999-6003.

84. Morita T, Kurihara H, Maemura K, Yoshizumi M, Nagai R, Yazaki Y. Role of Ca2+ and protein kinase c in shear stress-induced actin depolymerization and endothelin 1 gene expression. Circ Res 1994; 75:630-636.

85. Grabowski EF, Jaffe EA, Weksler BB. Prostacyclin production by cultured endothelial cell monolayers exposed to step increases in shear stress. J Lab Clin Med 1985; 105:36-43.

86. Norris M, Morigi M, Donadelli R, Aiello S, Foppolo M, Todeschini M, Orisio S, Remuzzi G, Remuzzi A. Nitric oxide synthesis by cultured endothelial cells is modulated by flow conditions. Circ Res 1995; 76:536-543.

87. Topper JN, Cai J, Falb D, Gimbrone MA Jr Identification of vascular endothelial genes differentially responsive to fluid mechanical stimuli: Cyclooxygenase-2, manganese superoxide dismutase, and endothelial cell nitric oxide synthase are selectively up-regulated by steady laminar shear stress. Proc Natl Acad Sci USA 1996; 93:10417-10422.

88. Wang DL, Wung BS, Shyy YJ, Lin CF, Chao YJ, Usami S, Chien S. Mechanical strain induces monocyte chemotactic protein-1 gene expression in endothelial cells. Effects of mechanical strain on monocyte adhesion to endothelial cells. Circulation Research. 1995; 77(2):294-302.

89. Shyy YJ, Lin MC, Han J, Lu Y, Petrime M, Chien S. The cis-acting phorbol ester "12-O-tetradecanoylphorbol 13-acetate"-responsive element is involved in shear stress-induced monocyte chemotactic protein 1 gene expression. Proc Natl Acad Sci 1995; 92:8069-8073.

90. Nagel T, Resnick N, Atkinson WJ, Dewey CF Jr, Gimbrone MA Jr. Shear stress upregulates intercellular adhesion molecule-1 expression in cultured human vascular endothelial cells. J Clin Inv 1994; 94:885-891.

91. Moose PRL, Campbell GR, Wang ZL, Campbell JH. Smooth muscle phenotypic expression in human carotid arteries. I. Comparison of cells from diffuse intimal thickenings adjacent to atheromatous plaque, and cultured rat aortic media. Lab Inv 1985; 53:556-562.

92. Campbell JH, Campbell GR. Methods of growing vascular smooth muscle cells in culture. In: Campbell JH, Campbell GR, eds. Vascular smooth muscle in culture. Boca Raton: CRC Press, 1987:15-21.

93. Gordon D, Schwartz SM. Arterial smooth muscle differentiation. In: Campbell JH, Campbell GR, eds. Vascular smooth muscle in culture. Boca Raton: CRC Press, 1987:1-14.

94. Chamley JH, Campbell GR. Mitosis of contractile smooth muscle cells in tissue culture. Expt Cell Res 1974; 84:105-110.

95. Birukov KG, Shirinsky VP, Stepanova OV, Tkachuk VA, Hahn AWA, Resink TJ, Smirnov VN. Stretch affects phenotype and proliferation of vascular smooth muscle cells. Mol Cell Biochem 1995; 144:131-139.

96. Wilson E, Sudhir K, Ives HE. Mechanical strain of rat vascular smooth muscle cells is sensed by specific extracellular matrix/integrin interactins. J Clin Inv 1995; 96:2364-2372.

97. Kanda K, Matsuda T. Mechanical stress-induced orientation and ultrastructural change of smooth muscle cells cultured in three-dimensional collagen lattices. Cell Transplant 1994; 3(6):481-92.

98. Yang Z, Noll G, Luscher TF. Calcium antagonists differently inhibit proliferation of human coronary smooth muscle cells in response to pulsatile stretch and platelet-derived growth factor. Circ 1993; 88:832-836.

99. Davis MG, Ali S, Leikauf GD, Dorn. GWI Tyrosine kinase inhibition prevents deformation-stimulated vascular smooth muscle growth. Hypertension 1994; 24:706-713.

100. Kulik TJ, Alvarado AP. Effect of stretch on growth and collagen synthesis in cultured rat and lamb pulmonary arterial smooth muscle cells. J Cell Physiol 1993; 157:615-624.

101. Kolpakov V, Rekhter MD, Gordon D, Wang WH, Kulik TJ. Effect of mechanical forces on growth and matrix protein synthesis in the in vitro pulmonary artery. Analysis of the role of individual cell types. Circ Res 1995; 77:823-831.

102. Rovner AS, Murphy RA, Owens GK. Expression of smooth muscle and nonmuscle myosin heavy chains in cultured vascular smooth muscle cells. J Biol Chem 1986; 261:14740-14745.

PART III

Biointeractive Prostheses: Complete Healing

Engineering Components

Scaffold Engineering

Structural Designs

---------------------- CHAPTER 40 ----------------------

An Integral Mathematical Approach to Tissue Engineering of Vascular Grafts

Greg R. Starke, A.S. Douglas, D.J. Conway

Introduction

The development of neointimal hyperplasia near the anastomosis of small diameter grafts has been positively linked to changes in the arterial fluid dynamics. Graft materials such as woven Dacron or polytetrafluoroethylene (PTFE) are relatively rigid when compared to the native artery. The implantation of these less compliant grafts causes a considerable alteration in the fluid flow patterns of the arterial system. Altered flow patterns result in high shear stresses on the vessel wall[1,2] and turbulence downstream of the anastomosis,[3] possibly causing endothelial cell damage.[4-6] Several studies[7-10] have shown a positive correlation between compliance matching and graft patency.

Other mechanical issues, apart from altered blood flow, have also been implicated in the formation of intimal hyperplasia. Various research groups[11,12] have suggested that the development of hyperplasia is a consequence of the normal remodelling response, as a result of the stress concentrations that will occur around the individual sutures. They argued that the proliferation of smooth muscle cells, and the deposition of extracellular matrix around the suture line, is a process which increases the amount of load bearing material in an attempt to reduce the strain to more physiological levels. Finite element models of a bypass graft have been used to investigate the stress distribution in the region of the anastomosis.[11] This study showed that the presence of the graft resulted in stress magnitude of approximately 1.5 times the normal value. Increasing the amount of tissue in the region, to reproduce the experimentally observed geometry, resulted in a reduction in stress to 1.2 times the normal value. In a subsequent study[12] the same research group examined the development of cellular hyperplasia around individual sutures and showed that thickening was more pronounced around the sutures. In a corresponding finite element model they showed that, in the early post-operative period, stresses were concentrated around the sutures—which were subsequently dispersed once healing had progressed. However, it may be argued that the observed remodelling was a response to the surgical injury—although it is likely that both mechanisms play a role.

Minimising the stress gradient at the anastomosis requires the correct sizing of the graft in relation to the host artery. To predict the size of the vessels during diastole and systole requires the accurate characterisation of the materials and the loading. Paasche et al[13] investigated the choice graft sizes in an effort to minimise suture line stresses. In this investigation they assumed that the graft could be regarded as rigid when compared to the host. They found that the suture line stresses were at a minimum when the ratio between the

---

graft and the host artery sizes was approximately 1.45. However, in a polymeric tissue engineered graft the implant should not be assumed to be rigid. Therefore the optimal size of the graft in relation to the host needs to be investigated in the light of graft compliance. In addition, the presence of soft tissue within the graft structure will alter the compliance, and will also alter the suture line stresses at the anastomosis. Therefore the compliance matching and graft size selection needs to consider the evolutionary nature of the implant compliance. Reproducing the stress/strain behavior of the native artery also means that diameter compatibility can be examined. If diameter matching is achieved in the long term, then stress concentrations at the anastomosis will be kept to a minimum and thus progressive remodelling will not be necessary to reach a homeostatic state.

A tissue engineered vascular graft is intended to provide a scaffold for the development of tissue; therefore, the structure has to be sufficiently porous, with interconnectivity, so as to allow for vascularization and the subsequent infiltration of cells. However, in the early post-operative period, before tissue ingrowth has taken place, the scaffold needs to have sufficient structural integrity to withstand the applied loads, without leading to excessive deformation or rupture. Greer et al[14] investigated the material properties of a collagen/smooth muscle cell gel and found that the stress/strain characteristics, as well as the stress relaxation, were both strongly dependent on the extent of cell seeding. This preliminary study shows how the biological features of a tissue-engineered graft can alter the mechanics of the graft. Furthermore, the development of tissue may depend on the loading environment. Therefore, the graft structure needs to create optimal strain conditions, during both diastole and systole, that will facilitate the development and maintenance of smooth muscle cells within the porous structure.

Mathematical modelling provides a means for characterizing the mechanical response to loading of the native artery, as well as the structured polymer from which a tissue engineered graft might be constructed. Such models allow for the investigation of compliance, remodelling, sizing and failure prediction. This approach offers the potential for aiding the design process by allowing the developer to test design concepts and parameters without the time consuming, and costly, process of prototyping. Furthermore, it is often difficult—if not impossible—to measure quantities such as stress, strain or displacement. These quantities can, however, be readily calculated from mathematical models of the loaded implant. Accurate predictions require sound constitutive (material) laws describing the behavior of the intact artery as well as the proposed graft material. Analytical solutions of arterial systems are rarely possible because of the complexity of the material formulations, structures, boundary conditions and initial loading conditions. However, making use of sophisticated numerical techniques such as the finite element method can approximate solutions.

Many of the mechanical design requirements can, however, be derived from the mechanics of the intact artery—as the success of the graft will depend in part on recreating the mechanics of the natural vessel. However, the mechanics of the native vessel needs to be reproduced in a synthetic material with a highly porous structure. In addition, the process of tissue infiltration and development will alter the mechanical properties of the graft. The remainder of this chapter is therefore concerned with the development of a numerical formulation for mechanics of the native artery as well as a polymer graft.

The Mechanics of Arteries

The flow of blood can be related to the elasticity of an artery by considering the feedback loop shown in Figure 40.1. The bottom block shows the artery as a rigid conduit allowing blood flow. A pulsating pressure results from this flow. If the artery is treated as an elastic body, as shown in the top block, the pressure will then act to deform the conduit, which in turn will affect the nature of the flow. The flow characteristics can then be analyzed assuming that the vessel is rigid, and has a diameter that has been altered by the flow pressure. The deformation of the artery can then be determined using the laws of elasticity assuming a constant pressure and determining the nature of the deformation. In this way the flow of blood is coupled to the elasticity of the vessels.

Fig. 40.1. Interaction between the flow of blood and the mechanical deformation of an artery, adapted from Fung, 1996.

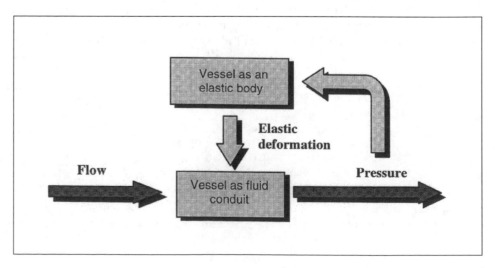

Structural Morphology

The structural characteristics of arteries arise from the tissue composition of the media and the adventitia. The media is made up of smooth muscle cells and bundles of collagen fibrils which are layered between a number of elastic sheets. The structure of the adventitia results from collagen fibres, fibroblasts and ground substance. A relatively thick layer of elastin separates the media and adventitia. The endothelial cells of the intima do not have any significant influence on the artery mechanics, and therefore the intima and media can essentially be grouped together in so far as the elastic response is concerned. In the low strain region (near zero stress) the stiffness of the intima-media layer is almost an order of magnitude greater than that of the adventitia. However, at larger strains the collagen bundles begin to straighten and then stretch, which increases the stiffness contribution from the adventitia. The relative thickness of the intima-media/adventitia varies as a function of the position in the body and therefore so too does the elastic response.[15] The walls of the artery are structurally anisotropic, incompressible and highly deformable, exhibiting non-linear stress/strain characteristics.

Non-Linear Elastic Response

The most striking aspect of the mechanical response of arteries is the non-linear relation between the pressure acting within an artery and the resulting change in diameter. Experimental evidence[16-18] has shown that as the pressure increases, and hence the stress within the arterial walls, the change in diameter is initially rapid, but as the stress increases the change in strain becomes smaller until increases in stress are accompanied by only very small increases in strain. This high degree of non-linearity is illustrated in Fig-ure 40.2, which shows experimentally determined and numerically predicted stress/strain relationships for the arterial walls of four normal rabbit arteries.[17] The effective Young's modulus of the material can be viewed as the slope of the stress/strain curve. Since the modulus increases with strain, arterial stiffness is a non-linear function of strain. The stiffening of the arterial wall, which occurs when the collagen bundles become straightened and go into tension, is observed in the region of 150 mm Hg pressure. This behavior protects the arteries from excessive dilation and therefore offers protection against the development of aneurysms.

The complex composition and structure of arteries means that the material properties of the wall are not the same in all directions (the material is therefore anisotropic). Several research studies have shown that the stiffness of the arterial wall in the circumferential direction is greater than in the axial direction.[19,20] However, this result is by no means conclusive, as previously Tanaka and Fung[21] found the opposite result. The are many factors, including the specimen, species and testing methodology, to which the difference in results may be attributed.

As a result of the high fluid content in the arterial wall tissue, the material is often assumed to be incompressible—hence volume is preserved during deformation. Such an assumption considerably simplifies the mechanics of the walls, as the deformation in the radial direction can be directly related to the deformation in the longitudinal and circumferential directions. The assumption of incompressibility has been validated by Choung and Fung[23] who found that the percentage of fluid extrusion of the undeformed tissue was between 0.5 and 1.26% as a result of radial compression of rabbit aortic tissue. This result showed that, while the arterial tissue is slightly compressible, it would suffice to assume incompressibility.

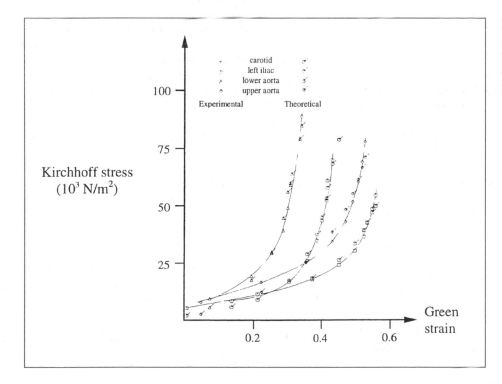

Fig. 40.2. True stress plotted against true strain for arteries from the canine coroid, left iliac as well as the lower and upper aorta, adapted from Fung et al 1979.

Viscoelasticity

Thus far the non-linear large strain elastic behavior typically exhibited by arteries has been discussed. However, no mention has been made of a further (often very typical) material characteristic of soft tissues, namely their time-dependent nature. In such materials, the current stress is dependent not only on the current strain but also on the strain history. Since no materials respond truly instantaneously to a load (indeed, neither can loading be applied instantaneously without inducing large inertia effects), the response is always delayed to some degree, and in so-called viscoelastic materials this delay is significant enough to necessitate quantification and modelling. Typically the elastic response to a sudden stress is characterized by an equally sudden strain (the glassy response) followed by a gradual increase in the strain (the rate of which decays exponentially). The simplest model of such a material is one which is described by one time scale, τ, and one elastic modulus, G. Typically, τ is defined as the time it takes for a material to reach a set factor (approximately 0.37) of the asymptotic, long term elastic response to a step load (force or displacement). Real viscoelastic materials may have infinitely many time scales (ranging from milliseconds to days and longer), each with its own associated elastic modulus. These parameters are defined by way of a continuum modulus function that must be determined experimentally. Details of these continuum functions and the salient aspects of viscoelastic constitutive modelling are presented later.

Depending on the type of loading conditions experienced by a viscoelastic material, it will display one of the following responses:

1. Delayed elastic (deformation, strain) response to a constant, suddenly applied load
2. Stress relaxation under a constant strain;
3. Delayed recovery on removal of all loads.

These responses are all illustrated in Figure 40.3. If, in addition to all these fully reversible responses, a material exhibits gradually increasing permanent deformation under a constant load, the material is said to creep. This is not a property of purely viscoelastic materials since creep is not recoverable, and hence not elastic. However, some viscoelastic materials do have very large time constants with associated moduli that are large enough so that the material ap-

pears to deform indefinitely under a constant load, and the recovery is so slow that the material appears to have crept.

There have been a number of important studies over the last 40 years that have contributed greatly to our understanding of the specific viscoelastic behavior of arterial wall tissue and biological soft tissues in general. Fung[24] found that while arterial tissue does indeed exhibit a delayed response to loading and increased stiffness with increased loading rate, the amount of lag is fairly insensitive to strain rate. This result allowed Fung to postulate a fairly simple continuous modulus function from which he found model parameters using canine aortas. Some detail on this approach is given in the viscoelastic properties subsection of the section "Materials Testing". Fung's models assume linear viscoelastic behavior—an assumption that was consistent with the results of some later animal studies by Hutchinson,[25] Newman[26] and Greenwald.[27] In contrast, however, work done by Langewouters et al[28,29] has shown that human arterial wall tissue has a non-linear viscoelastic response (i.e., the viscoelastic parameters vary significantly with varying strain). There now appears to be consensus in the literature that the true viscoelastic behavior of biological soft tissues (including arterial tissue) is indeed non-linear,[16,30-35] and the reason for this phenomenon has been explained with reference to the ultrastructure of the tissue. The two major stress-bearing constituents in arterial tissue are elastin, which maintains a fairly constant Young's modulus over the range of physiological strains, and collagen, whose stiffness increases considerably with increased stretch. The exponential stiffening with increased strain is attributed to the straightening out and tensioning of the wavy collagen strands as they appear in an unstretched state.[36,37] This process is referred to as collagen recruitment. Thus the purely elastic behavior of arterial tissue is almost always modelled non-linearly. It has been shown[38] that collagen exhibits double the amount of stress relaxation as that of elastin, but at a fifth of the rate of elastin relaxation at room temperature (assuming simple rheological models with only one relaxation time constant per material). Collagen recruitment means that collagen takes up proportionally more of the load as the artery wall dilates and so its viscoelastic properties also become increasingly predominant—which explains the non-linear viscoelastic behavior.

Fig. 40.3. Schematic illustration of delayed elastic response, stress relaxation, and delayed recovery of viscoelastic materials.

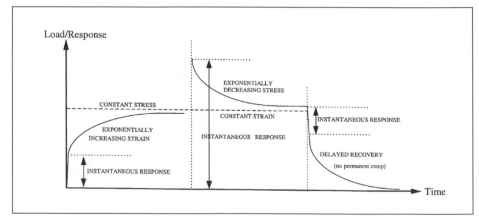

In spite of this evidence, most research in this field still assumes quasi-linear viscoelasticity (i.e., non-linear in the elastic deformation response but linear in the history of deformation). This approach avoids difficulties associated with implementing non-linear viscoelasticity numerically, and the more complex materials testing that would be required for the constitutive characterisation. Huyghe et al[39] implemented a quasi-linear viscoelastic formulation for passive heart muscle tissue. They found that all the mechanical characteristics of tissue—which are essentially the same for arterial wall tissue (including the weak frequency dependency of the dissipation energy during cyclic loading (i.e., lag time))—were accommodated by their model. However, when they set the relaxation parameters in order to correctly predict the dissipation energy, they found that the model overpredicted the amount of stress relaxation by over 100%. This discrepancy they attributed to the non-linear viscoelasticity of true cardiac tissue.

Young et al,[16] Decraemer et al,[32] Wu and Lee[33] and Johnson et al[35] have all incorporated non-linear viscoelasticity in their constitutive models for soft biological tissues. These laws were reported to predict results that correlate fairly well with existing experimental test data for tissues such as human patellar tendon, canine collateral ligament and canine arterial wall tissue. Such models do have potential to make more accurate predictions in the design process than the simpler quasi-linear laws. However, the experimental determination of the constitutive parameters is necessarily a far more complex task with these more realistic models. Until accurate and accessible experimental methods are developed which enable such parameterization, it can be argued that the simpler, numerically more robust quasi-linear laws are sufficient. Myers et al[40] discuss the limitations of quasi-linear theory and suggest methods for reducing the effects of this simplifying assumption.

Pre-Stress

In a thick walled cylinder under internal pressure the distribution of the circumferential strain through the wall varies considerably, with a peak at the inner surface which decays exponentially towards the outer surface. It has been shown that several tissue types, including bone, will remodel so as to reach a homeostatic strain condition. In order to moderate the peak strain, and produce a more uniform distribution through the thickness, the artery walls are pre-stressed. This pre-stressing is evident by the way an artery will spring open if a transverse section is removed and cut radially along the longitudinal axis. Pre-stressing has been investigated by several researchers,[41,42] resulting in the "uniform strain" hypothesis.

Fung et al[42] examined the no load and no stress state of the pulmonary and ileac arteries of rats. Figure 40.4a shows the cross section of the pulmonary artery at a blood pressure of 15 mm Hg. In the no load state (Fig. 40.4b) the artery has reduced considerably in diameter and has therefore increased in wall thickness. Figure 40.4c shows the section of the artery following the radial cut that has removed the pre-stress. In order to quantify the extent of pre-stressing within the wall, the angle to which the artery opens is measured. This angle determines the amount of displacement caused by the pre-stress and can therefore be related to the magnitude of pre-stress.[41]

In a further study, Greenwald et al[43] measured the opening angle of rat aortic arteries following the removal of various of the structural components. They found that the removal of smooth muscle and collagen had no effect on the opening angle, while the removal of elastin had a significant effect, resulting in a decrease in the opening angle. This study concluded that the residual stresses are stored in the elastic component of the media.

The opening of the artery shows that the pre-stressing puts the internal surface of the wall into a state of compression and the external surface into tension. Subsequently, the tensile stresses that are experienced during normal loading are reduced by the initial compressive component, resulting in a more uniform distribution of stress, as is shown schematically in Figure 40.5.

Material Laws for the Native Artery and Graft Materials

The extent of the porosity of a polymeric graft, as well as the nature of the structure, requires careful engineering design which will consider not only the mechanical aspects, but also the coupling with the biological design. In designing an artery graft, many of the design objectives can be learned from studying the mechanics of the intact vessel. Also, failures of grafts typically occur in the region of the anastomosis, and a mechanical model of the interaction between the graft and the host is therefore needed for graft design. Since any mechanical model will require the constitutive response of both the graft and the natural artery, the fundamentals of the mechanical response of compliant materials are reviewed.

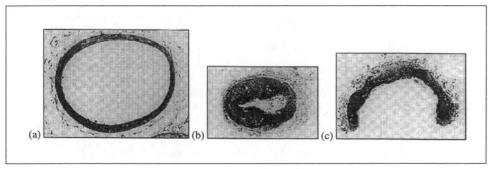

Fig. 40.4. Sectional geometry of the rat pulmonary artery at (a) in vivo loading of 15mmHg, (b) no-load and (c) no stress. Reproduced with permission from Fung et al 1992.

Fig. 40.5. Schematic representation of the influence of artery pre-stressing on the resultant stress distribution through the artery wall.

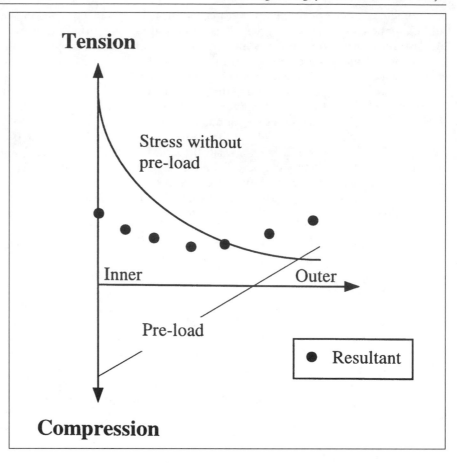

Compliant engineering materials (such as polymers) and soft tissues deform appreciably under load and care must be taken to describe their behavior. Most soft tissues sustain large strains, are generally non-linear in their constitutive response (see Fig. 40.2), exhibit either transverse isotropy or anisotropy and are either incompressible or nearly so. Compliant materials, or rubber-elastic materials, also sustain large strains, may be anisotropic and are often incompressible.

To describe the mechanical behavior of both soft tissues and compliant engineering materials, researchers usually use a hyperelastic (Green elastic) strain energy function of the local deformation or strain, W. The existence of a strain energy function for a material implies that it is hyperelastic and that, regardless of deformation path, equal work is done in going from one deformation (or strain) state to another. In order to characterize compliant graft materials and the natural artery, we need to formulate appropriate strain energy functions W. To do this we must first develop a framework with which to describe the deformations, strains and stresses required. Note that, since soft tissue is not strictly hyperelastic, it is characterized by a pseudostrain energy function.

Characterizing Finite Deformation

The motion of a compliant material can be described as a mapping, χ, which defines the deformed position, $\mathbf{x}$, of a particle which occupied the position, $\mathbf{X}$, in the reference configuration; thus $\mathbf{x} = \chi(\mathbf{X})$. We can also relate the motion,

$\chi(\mathbf{X})$, to the displacements of each material point, $\mathbf{u}(\mathbf{X})$, if we note that the deformed position is merely the sum of the reference position and the displacement of that point, viz. $\mathbf{x} = \mathbf{X} + \mathbf{u}(\mathbf{X})$. To characterize the deformation of this material we need to examine how the deformed position or the displacements change spatially. Both the deformation gradient tensor, $\mathbf{F}$, the components of which are given by

$$F_{ij} = \frac{\partial \chi_i}{\partial X_j} \qquad (1)$$

where $i, j = 1,2,3$, and the displacement gradient tensor, $\mathbf{H}$, with components given by

$$H_{ij} = \frac{\partial u_i}{\partial X_j} \qquad (2)$$

characterize the deformation at the point $\mathbf{X}$. The deformation gradient tensor $\mathbf{F}$ also contains information about the local rotation. However, since we would like to relate the strain energy function, W, to deformation alone, we define the right and left Cauchy-Green deformation tensors, $\mathbf{C} = \mathbf{F}^T\mathbf{F}$ and $\mathbf{B} = \mathbf{F}\mathbf{F}^T$, respectively, which depend only on the deformation (not the rotation) at any point in the material. Strain is also a measure of deformation, independent of rotation, and used to characterize the strain energy function. The Lagrangian strain, $\mathbf{E}$, is defined by

$$\mathbf{E} = \tfrac{1}{2}\left[\mathbf{F}^T\mathbf{F} - \mathbf{I}\right] = \tfrac{1}{2}\left[\mathbf{H} + \mathbf{H}^T + \mathbf{H}^T\mathbf{H}\right] \qquad (3)$$

where $\mathbf{I}$ is the identity tensor (Note that $\mathbf{F} = \mathbf{H} + \mathbf{I}$).

In soft tissue mechanics, since deformations and rotations are finite, we need to be precise about the definitions of stress. The true, or Cauchy, stress is the symmetric second-rank tensor, σ, (with components σ_{ij}) which relates the actual loads to the current deformed configuration. Since the Second Piola-Kirchhoff stress, $\mathbf{S}$, considers the reference configuration, it is more easily measured in experiments and is related to the Cauchy stress by

$$\sigma_{ij} = \left(\frac{\rho}{\rho_0}\right) F_{ik}\, S_{kl}\, F_{jl}, \qquad (4)$$

where ρ and ρ_0 are the current and reference tissue densities, respectively, and repeated indices imply a summation from 1 to 3.

Hyperelasticity

The mechanical constitutive description of both soft tissues and compliant engineering materials assumes that these materials are hyperelastic. Tests therefore need to be conducted to determine the functional form and parameters which define the strain energy (or pseudo-strain energy) function, W. The simplest strain energy functions describe isotropic materials. Since the behavior of these materials is independent of orientation, the strain energy is a function of the three invariants of the Cauchy-Green deformation tensor, viz.,

$$W = W\left(I_1, I_2, I_3\right), \qquad (5)$$

where

$$I_1 = \mathrm{tr}(\mathbf{C}),\, I_2 = \tfrac{1}{2}[(\mathrm{tr}\mathbf{C})^2 - \mathrm{tr}(\mathbf{C}^2)],\, \text{ and } I_3 = \det \mathbf{C}. (6)$$

If the material is incompressible, then $I_3=1$ and $W=W(I_1,I_2)$ only.

For transversely isotropic (these have a single preferred orientation defined by the unit vector $\mathbf{N}$ in the reference configuration) and incompressible materials, the strain energy is dependent on four invariants,

$$W = W\left(I_1, I_2, I_4, I_5\right), \qquad (7)$$

where

$$I_4 = \mathbf{N}\cdot\mathbf{C}\mathbf{N} = \alpha^2 \text{ and } I_5 = \mathbf{N}\cdot\mathbf{C}^2\,\mathbf{N}. \qquad (8)$$

Note that, in Equation (8), α is the stretch in the direction $\mathbf{N}$, so that if $\mathbf{N}$ is the muscle fibre orientation, α is the muscle fibre stretch.

If the material is incompressible, the hydrostatic stress is not determined by the material deformation, but is set by the boundary conditions and the equations of equilibrium. The constitutive response must therefore introduce a Lagrange multiplier to accommodate this hydrostatic stress. The deviatory stress is determined by the strain energy, so that the Cauchy stress, for a material with a strain energy function dependent on three invariants, $W=W(I_1,I_2,\alpha)$, is given by Humphrey et al,[44,45]

$$\sigma = -p\mathbf{I} + 2W_1\,\mathbf{B} - 2W_2\,\mathbf{B}^{-1} + \tfrac{1}{\alpha}W_\alpha\,\mathbf{F}\left(\mathbf{N}\otimes\mathbf{N}\right)\mathbf{F}^T$$

$$(9)$$

where W_1, W_2 and W_α are the derivatives of the strain energy function with respect to its arguments and $\mathbf{N}\otimes\mathbf{N}$ is the tensor product of the two unit vectors.

We can also cast the strain energy functions in terms of the Lagrangian strain components, E_{ij}, since these are easy to measure in experiments. Using the notation of Fung,[22] if W is the strain energy per unit mass of the tissue, then ρ_0 is the strain energy per unit volume in the zero stress (reference) state (ρ_0 is the density in the reference state). The Second Piola-Kirchhoff stress is then given by

$$S_{ij} = \frac{\partial\left[\rho_0\,W(\mathbf{E})\right]}{\partial\,E_{ij}} \qquad (10)$$

for compressible materials, and by

$$S_{ij} = -p\,F_{ik}^{-1}\,F_{jk}^{-1} + \frac{\partial\left[\rho_0\,W(\mathbf{E})\right]}{\partial E_{ij}} \qquad (11)$$

for incompressible materials.

For the special case in which the strain energy function is quadratic in strain, or $\rho_0\,W = \tfrac{1}{2}D_{ijkl}\,E_{ij}\,E_{kl}$, there is a linear relationship between the Piola-Kirchhoff stress, S_{ij}, and the Lagrangian strain, E_{ij}, given by

$$S_{ij} = D_{ijkl}\,E_{kl}. \qquad (12)$$

For any non-linear material, the increment in stress, dS_{ij}, is related to the increment in strain, dE_{ij} through

$$dS_{ij} = \frac{\partial^2 W}{\partial\,E_{ij}\,\partial\,E_{kl}}\,dE_{kl} = D_{ijkl}\,dE_{kl}, \qquad (13)$$

where D_{ijkl} is the incremental material modulus.

Viscoelasticity

Thus far we have outlined constitutive modelling of the time independent elastic response of soft tissues materials and described how a postulated strain energy function is used to calculate the stress for any given strain state. As discussed earlier, both arterial wall tissue and many elastomeric materials exhibit significant viscous behavior at strain rates typical of heart rates. Since the concern in the design of artery grafts is to construct the graft so that it closely matches the instantaneous compliance of the native artery, we need to include the viscoelastic nature of both the arterial tissue and the graft material in our constitutive law.

Fortunately, the addition of viscoelasticity in the material model does not mean that we have to discard our statically determined hyperelastic strain energy function. A finite strain viscoelastic material law still requires the strain energy function, W, for the long-term modulus.

The description of viscoelasticity that follows is restricted to linear (or quasi-linear) viscoelasticity—where the rate of the delayed response to a given load is only a function of time (not of the magnitude of load). Recall that quasi-linear viscoelasticity does allow for non-linear long term hyperelastic behavior.

Spring and dashpot models are a good analogy for modelling material viscoelastic behavior, since they allow the characterisation of the material both qualitatively and quantitatively. The simplest model for the elastic behavior of a material is the linear spring where stress, σ, is simply proportional to the strain, ε,

$$(\sigma = k\varepsilon)_{spring}, \qquad (14)$$

where k is the spring constant. The spring element stores elastic energy. The lagging component of a material response to an applied load can be modelled with a dashpot (which dissipates energy), where the stress is proportional to the strain rate ε:

$$(\sigma = \eta\dot{\varepsilon})_{dashpot} \qquad (15)$$

where η is the viscosity constant. The two simplest viscoelastic models are the Kelvin-Voigt and Maxwell models, illustrated in Figure 40.6.

In the Kelvin-Voigt model, the strain is the same in both the spring and the dashpot, and the stresses in each element add to balance the applied load. Thus the equilibrium equation is:

$$\sigma = k\varepsilon + \eta\dot{\varepsilon} \qquad (16)$$

In the Maxwell model, the strains are additive, while the stress is constant throughout, thus:

$$\dot{\varepsilon} = \frac{1}{k}\dot{\sigma} + \frac{1}{\eta}\sigma \qquad (17)$$

(The Maxwell equilibrium is written in terms of strain rate since the dashpot equilibrium is defined in terms of strain rate). Solving these two differential equations yields:
1. The retarded strain at time, t, for a constant stress applied at time, $t = 0$

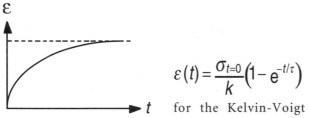

$$\varepsilon(t) = \frac{\sigma_{t=0}}{k}\left(1 - e^{-t/\tau}\right)$$

for the Kelvin-Voigt

2. The relaxation stress at time, t, for a constant strain applied at time, $t = 0$ model where t = h/k;

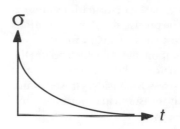

$s(t) = ke_{t=0}e^{-t/t}$ for the Maxwell Model. The relaxation time, t, is the time taken for the stress to relax by a factor $e^{-1} \approx 0.37$ of the initial value.

A true viscoelastic material will exhibit a delayed elastic response, stress relaxation and strain recovery (i.e., a gradual return to the original undeformed configuration on the removal of all applied loads). Neither the Kelvin-Voigt nor the Maxwell model adequately represents all these characteristics. However, a combination of the two models, giving the 3-element or standard linear models shown in Figure 40.7, will accommodate all the required characteristics.

In order to capture the full range of time scales (i.e., a continuous spectrum) that typically exist in a true viscoelastic material, one would need to assemble an infinite number of these 3-element units in series or parallel. However, the major viscoelastic trends can usually be satisfactorily characterized with only a few such units. Langewouters et al[29] found good correlation to human aortic creep curves for their 5-element model (i.e., with only two time scales). van Dijk[46] also characterized smooth muscle cell stress relaxation with two time constants. These models are parameterized by curve fitting to delayed elastic or stress relaxation experimental data.

For a multi-element Maxwell model (with N units), the stress relaxation under a constant strain is:

$$\sigma(t) = \varepsilon_0 G(t) \text{ where } G(t) = G_\infty + \sum_{n=1}^{N} G_n e^{-t/\tau} \qquad (18)$$

where G_∞ is the long term modulus—calculated from the hyperelastic strain energy function, and G_η is the instantaneous modulus of element n. For a continuous spectrum of relaxation times, the relaxation modulus can be written:

$$G(t) = \int_0^\infty S(\tau)e^{-t/\tau} d\tau \qquad (19)$$

where $S(\tau)$ is the relaxation spectrum. Experimentally, the determination of this S(τ) is perhaps easier than finding discrete time scales and moduli from creep test data. The methodology for finding such a relaxation spectrum is described in the section "Materials Testing".

Fig. 40.6. Simple Kelvin-Voigt and Maxwell vscoelastic models.

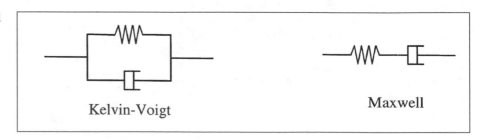

Kelvin-Voigt   Maxwell

Thus far we have only considered the time-varying response to a constant load applied at some time in the past. Assuming linear viscoelastic behavior, we can use the principle of linear superposition to calculate the response to a time-varying load. Casting the problem into an incremental form, an increment in strain for the function, $\varepsilon(t)$, over a small time increment Δt is written as

$$\Delta\varepsilon(\tau) = \frac{d\varepsilon_\tau}{dt}\Delta t \text{ at time, } t = \tau. \qquad (20)$$

Thus from Equation (18) the stress response at time t (where $t > \tau$) to this strain increment (held constant after its application) is

$$\sigma(t)_{\Delta\varepsilon(\tau)} = G(t-\tau)\frac{d\varepsilon_\tau}{dt}\Delta t. \qquad (21)$$

Now, the principle of linear superposition allows us to sum the elastic responses to all the past increments in load from time $-\infty$ to t. By taking infinitesimal increments in time we can write Equation (21) in integral form as

$$\sigma(t) = \int_{-\infty}^{t} G(t-\tau)\frac{d\varepsilon}{dt}d\tau. \qquad (22)$$

Integrating by part yields

$$\sigma(t) = G(0)\varepsilon(t) - \int_{-\infty}^{t} \frac{dG(t-\tau)}{dt}\varepsilon(\tau)d\tau \qquad (23)$$

where $G(0)$ is the so called glassy or instantaneous modulus.

Similarly, the delayed strain response to a smooth stress function of time is

$$\varepsilon(t) = J(0)\sigma(t) - \int_{-\infty}^{t} \frac{dJ(t-\tau)}{d\tau}\sigma(\tau)d\tau \qquad (24)$$

where $\qquad J(t) = \int_{0}^{\infty} T(\tau)\left(1-e^{-t/\tau}\right)d\tau,\qquad$ and

$T(\tau)$ is the retardation spectrum.

Equations (23) and (24) are constitutive laws for a linear viscoelastic material. They can be implemented in a numerical algorithm, such as the finite element method, to predict the history of any geometry with a continuum viscoelastic material behavior subjected to a time-varying stress or strain.

Modeling Microstructure

It was noted earlier that the complete geometry of the structure must be fully characterized. However, in the case of a porous material, it would neither be possible, nor desirable, to model precisely the structure of each pore. There-

fore, in this case it would be advantageous to include information about the microstructure in the description of the material behavior. The porous microstructure is then modeled as a continuum (solid) region that has the apparent (or effective) properties of the porous material. This idea can be taken one step further by including structural properties, such as porosity, as variables in the material formulation. Obviously the relation between the material behavior and the structural property needs to be determined. But once this has been achieved, it becomes a simple matter to examine the influence of changes in material microstructure on the structural response of the component without having to undertake complex geometrical modeling.

In most porous materials the single most important parameter in determining the mechanical properties is the relative density ρ/ρ_s, where ρ is the apparent density while ρ_s is the density of the structural members. The porosity is therefore defined as $1-\rho/\rho_s$. It turns out that cell size is generally far less important in the determination of material properties; however, cell shape will have a notable influence. The distinction needs to be made between open and closed cells: In an open configuration, the cells are interconnected, whereas in a closed cell arrangement each cell is isolated from its neighbor. As interconnectivity is vital in a tissue-engineered graft, only the mechanics of open celled structures will be considered. Most porous structures are anisotropic to a greater or lesser extent. Anisotropy arises from the shape of the cells, and is characterized by the ratio of the largest to the smallest cell dimension (R). Typically in a foam that is considered to be isotropic, $R \approx 1.3$; however, values in the range from one to ten are not uncommon.

For most linear-elastic, isotropic, cellular structures the apparent material modulus E can be related to the apparent density by

$$E/E_s \propto (\rho/\rho_s)^M \qquad (25)$$

where E_s is the elastic modulus of the solid material, and M is a constant which is generally greater than one. However, if the material structure is anisotropic, and therefore the stiffness cannot be represented by a scalar quantity, a more complex description is required. Common porous materials have distinct directionality and can be regarded as either transversely isotropic or orthotropic. A transversely isotropic material has one preferred direction and any transverse plane will be isotropic. An orthotropic material will have three orthogonal planes of symmetry. For these materials the moduli in the preferred directions will be a function of the density as well as the anisotropy ratio. For most porous materials the elastic modulus is approximately proportional to R^2 while the strength is typically proportional to R.[47]

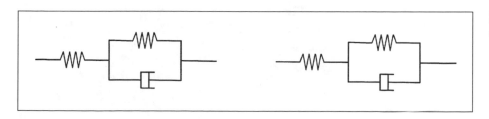

Fig. 40.7. Standard linear viscoelastic models.

Based on analytical and experimental studies,[47] parameters such as the yield strength and the compressive collapse load of a porous material can also be determined as a function of relative density and material structure. However, these investigations are limited to the case where the material comprising the structure of a foam is operating in the linear elastic regime. In a highly porous material subjected to large forces this would not be the case, and therefore other means of characterizing the material response are required. One approach for determining the apparent properties of a material is to develop numerical models of the microstructure under investigation. If the behavior of the material from which the structure is made has been completely characterized, and if the material has a uniform structure, then a single structural unit can be tested in order to obtain the apparent properties of the material.

An example of this approach is shown in Figure 40.8. The polyurethane microstructure (Fig. 40.8a) has been idealized and modeled using the finite element method (Fig. 40.8b). This model is then subjected to a range of numerical tests, from which the apparent material behavior can be determined. This approach has great flexibility, as it makes possible the investigation of the influence of relative density, cell shape and size. It also becomes a relatively simple matter to distort the cells so as to create an anisotropic structure and then quantify the structural response. Once the nature of the apparent material has been determined this information can be used to model a complete implant (Fig. 40.8c) without having to consider the geometry of the internal microstructure.

The presence of a viscous fluid within a porous material will have a considerable influence on the strength. When the material is compressed the fluid will be squeezed out, while it will be drawn in when the material is extended. As the fluid has viscosity, work is done during material deformation. The higher the loading rate the greater will be the amount of work, and therefore a strong dependence on strain rate exists. In the early postoperative stages of a tissue-engineered graft, the graft material will contain fluid. In addition, the normal loading rate of approximately one cycle per second will likely be high enough to make the influence of loading rate noticeable. For these reasons the fluid phase of the porous structure needs to be given consideration. The foam can be treated as a porous material with an absolute permeability K. The velocity of the fluid v within the porous material can then be determined from Darcy's law

$$v = -\frac{K}{\mu}\frac{dp}{dx}, \qquad (26)$$

where μ is the dynamic viscosity of the fluid and dp/dx is the pressure gradient within the porous structure. The permeability can be determined from the relative density and the pore structure, while the pressure gradient can be related to the applied stress. After some mathematical manipulation the strength of the porous material can be related to the viscosity of the fluid, the strain rate and some geometrical information.

Material Testing

Material testing forms the basis of the characterization of the mechanical properties of the native artery and the graft material. The material morphology and the extent to which the material needs to be characterized determine the complexity of the testing. For isotropic materials, simple uniaxial extension tests may be sufficient to obtain the necessary information for characterizing the material. However, for transversely isotropic and orthotropic materials, biaxial testing is required.

Hayashi et al[9] developed a highly elastic, blood compatible, small diameter vascular graft fabricated from segmented polyurethane. Introducing porosity into the material, which also allowed for possible tissue ingrowth, created

Fig. 40.8. (a) Micrograph of a polyurethane microstructure and (b) and idealized model of the microstructure which is then used (c) for the determination of an equivalent material for the properties of a porous structure.

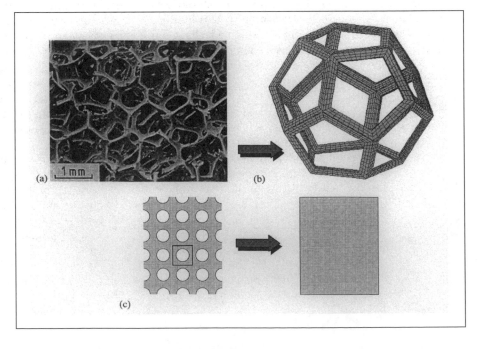

a physiologically realistic compliance for the graft. Electron microscopy revealed the graft material to be approximately isotropic, and therefore the mechanical properties were determined using simple uniaxial tests. Their strength tests revealed the importance of pretreatment of the material prior to mechanical testing. They found that the material became stable, in terms of mechanical properties, after having been immersed in a saline solution for 30 minutes.

They compared the stress/strain characteristics of their graft material to those of traditional grafts as well as the natural artery (Fig. 40.9). In order to present excessive dilation, the graft was coated with a woolly polyester net. However, such a net will reduce the compliance of the graft. The mechanical test results showed that the porous polyurethane exhibited an almost linear stress/strain response (KP), with a slight tendency to strain more at higher stresses. This result is in contrast to the highly non-linear behavior of the calf's thoracic aorta (Ao) which shows a very strong decline in the amount of strain at elevated stresses. However, in the low strain region (up to approximately 30%) the stiffness of the polyurethane graft is very similar to the thoracic aorta. This result further shows the considerable difference in stiffness between the compliant polyurethane graft and the more stiff traditional Dacron grafts (CW, GT, CV and DB).

Although the material developed for this graft is very compliant and exhibits strain of over 200% before failure, it does not show the stiffening behavior normally associated with polymeric materials. The slight softening at high strains may be a result of the failure of the woolly coating. Further-more, the time dependent behavior (viscoelasticity) of the material will influence the sizing of the graft, and therefore needs to be considered in the design of the implant.

Hyperelastic Properties

In order to develop the constitutive models for soft tissues and compliant engineering materials, the general form of the strain energy function must be postulated. This should be as simple and convenient as possible, as laboratory tests will be required to set the relevant parameters in the strain energy function. These energy functions are based on qualitative observations of the material behavior and on prior testing of similar materials. The functional form of the strain energy function is subject to much debate and both polynomial and exponential forms are in current use.

The development of sound constitutive laws to describe the mechanical behavior of arterial vessels has been the focus of numerous research efforts.[17,48-50] Since these constitutive laws are set out in terms of large strain hyperelasticity, experiments are required to determine both the functional form and the coefficients defining the strain energy function, W.

Essentially three forms of strain energy functions are used to describe arterial walls: polynomial, exponential and logarithmic. The polynomial function of Vaishnav et al,[51] which was used to describe a cylindrical vessel subject to internal pressure, is the simplest; in general it has seven coefficients and is given as follows:

$$W = aE_{\theta\theta}^2 + bE_{\theta\theta}E_{zz} + cE_{zz}^2 + dE_{\theta\theta}^3 + eE_{\theta\theta}^2E_{zz} + fE_{\theta\theta}E_{zz}^2 + gE_{zz}^3 \quad (27)$$

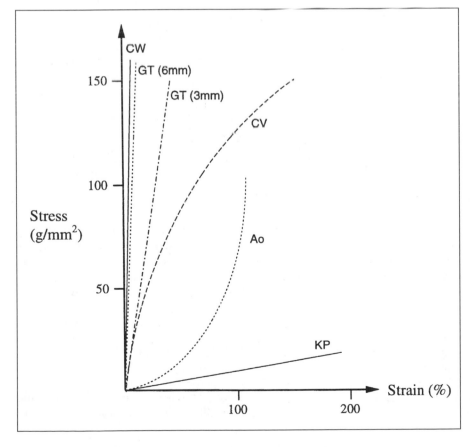

Fig. 40.9. Comparison of stress—strain characteristics for a porous polyurethane graft (KP) with other traditional graft materials (CW—Cooley low porosity woven Dacron, GT—Gore-Tex thin walled EPTFE, CV—Cooley double velour knitted Dacron) as well as the thoracic aorta (Ao). Adapted from Hayashi et al 1989.

where *a, b, c, d, e, f, g* are material constants, and $E_{\theta\theta}$ and E_{zz} are the longitudinal strain components in the circumferential and axial directions, respectively.

Fung et al[17] proposed an exponential function of the form

$$W - C \exp\left(a_1 E_{\theta\theta}^2 + a_2 E_{zz}^2 + a_4 E_{\theta\theta} E_{zz}\right) \quad (28)$$

where c, α_1, α_2 and α_4 are the material constants. Experimental data was determined from the cardiac, left iliac, lower aorta and upper aortic arteries of rabbits, which was used to determine the coefficients defining the strain energy functions. The comparison of the experimental and theoretical results, using Equation (10), are shown in Figure 40.2.

Lastly, Takamizawa and Hayashi[18] proposed a logarithmic function that again has four coefficients

$$W = -C \ln\left[1 - \tfrac{1}{2}a_{\theta\theta} E_{\theta\theta}^2 - \tfrac{1}{2}a_{zz}E_{zz}^2 - a_{\theta z} E_{\theta\theta} E_{zz}\right] (29)$$

where C, a_{qq}, a_{zz} and a_{qz} are material constants.

The different layers and components making up the arterial wall result in an inhomogenous structure—that is to say, the properties of the material change through the thickness of the wall.[52] The models that have been previously discussed have not included the different layers when analyzing the mechanical response. To address this limitation, von Maltzahn et al[53] modeled the artery using two layers, each having different properties. The arterial wall is generally considered to be anisotropic; however, this does not necessarily mean that each layer within the wall is anisotropic. Their model consisted of a transversely isotropic media and an anisotropic adventitia. This two layer model was compared to the single layer model of Vaishnav et al,[51] and it was found that it more accurately predicted the experimental data. This was the case even when the fourth order terms were included into the polynomial function. The model also had the advantage that the material parameters could be related to specific mechanical properties within the artery.

Viscoelastic Properties

The appropriate choice of experiment for the determination of viscoelastic properties depends on a number of factors. If the modulus or compliance function is to be approximated with only a few relaxation times, then either a stress relaxation or a retarded strain test would suffice. The time constants and associated moduli or compliance coefficients would be found by curve fitting to the assumed form of the rheological model. To characterize the full constitutive behavior, tensile, shear and volumetric (if the material is compressible) testing must be done. Such time-history tests are problematic in practice because they require the application of sudden large stresses or strains without inducing significant inertial effects. This means that the loading cannot be applied too quickly and so very small relaxation time scales cannot be measured with such tests. The determination of very large time constants—longer than a few days—is also impractical. The long term behavior of materials which do creep (such as non-crosslinked polymers) can thus not realistically be fully characterized.

Dynamic testing with sinusoidal loading over a large range of frequencies will provide data for the determination of the continuous spectrum functions $S(\tau)$ and $T(\tau)$. The viscoelastic strain response to a sinusoidal stress,

$$\sigma(t) = \sigma_0 \sin \omega t, \quad (30)$$

at frequency ω, and amplitude σ_0 is

$$\varepsilon(t) = \varepsilon_0 \sin(\omega t - \delta) \quad (31)$$

where the peak strain ε_0 lags the peak stress by δ—the loss angle. These relations can be written in complex form as

$$\sigma(t) = \sigma_0^* e^{i\omega t} \text{ and } \varepsilon(t) = \varepsilon_0^* e^{i(\omega t - \delta)} \quad (32)$$

where ρ_0^* and ε_0^* are the complex amplitudes.

The complex modulus, made up of a real (stiffness) and complex (damping) part, is

$$G^* = \frac{\sigma_0}{\varepsilon_0} e^{i\delta} = G_1 + iG_2 \quad (33)$$

with an amplitude ε_0 lagging the stress. The loss tangent is the ratio of the complex to real parts of G^*, viz.

$$\tan \delta = \frac{G_2}{G_1}. \quad (34)$$

Thus, measuring ρ_0, ε_0, and δ for a range of frequencies and using Equations (33) and (34), we can plot G_1 and G_2 as functions of frequency. An appropriate continuous relaxation spectrum $S(\tau)$ is chosen based on the form of these curves. Fung[22] describes this procedure in detail. See also Ferry[54] for a comprehensive treatise on this topic.

Fung[24] found that for a wide range of frequencies, the damping modulus is constant for biological soft tissues. This result allows for a very simple relaxation spectrum, $S(\tau)=c/\tau$. Lockett[55] reported the same result for polymethylmethacrylate (PMMA). However, he found a considerable frequency dependency above 1 Hz for a lightly crosslinked amorphous polymer.

One other important consideration when undertaking materials testing is the fact that viscoelastic properties tend to be highly temperature dependent. There are established, proven laws which allow one to simply shift the compliance/time curve for a particular material up or down the time line if the temperature is decreased or increased respectively. In the case of tissue engineered products this is not an issue for developing a constitutive model. However, it is vital that all materials tests are done at normal core body temperature.

A detailed treatment on the issues involved in viscoelastic materials testing is given by Lockett.[55] Other useful literature includes Christensen[56] and Sternstein.[57]

Finite Element Implementation

General Outline

The finite element method is a numerical procedure frequently used for analyzing complex deformable bodies subjected to mechanical loading. The finite element procedure essentially involves discretizing a component into a number of small (finite size) regions called the elements, (which are defined by nodes—or nodal points), and approximating the mechanical response in each element by assuming that the local deformation can be represented by low-order polynomials.

For time independent linear problems, the potential energy of the entire system can be minimized in one step that produces a large number of algebraic simultaneous equations in the nodal displacements, which are solved using a computer. The results obtained using this method are not exact but with increased model refinement, and subsequently more computational effort, solutions to the approximated displacement field of the desired resolution may be obtained.

For the non-linear and time-dependent problems presented in the design of artery grafts, the problem is broken down into a number of linearized increments. The method therefore requires repeated solution of simultaneous equations to solve for increments in nodal displacements. However, to illustrate the finite element method here, we limit the discussion to the linear, time independent problem.

The finite element method requires:

1. That the behavior of the component material be precisely defined;
2. That the geometry of the component in the unloaded state be known; and
3. That the boundary conditions, which include the mechanical loading, the supports or restraints holding the structure and, for time dependent problems, the initial velocities, are fully characterized.

From this problem definition the finite element procedure will be able to analyze the structure and calculate the design parameters, such as the deformations and stresses over the entire component domain. These results will allow decisions on the appropriate material choice and component geometry to be made. The flexibility and predictive power of the finite element method allows engineers the ability to test various design parameters. In the case of a porous graft, for example, the finite element method is an efficient way to examine the effect on overall component compliance of changes in the graft diameter, thickness, material stiffness, porosity, pre-stress, etc.

Minimizing the Potential Energy

In the continuum description of hyperelastic material behavior, it was most convenient to use tensor notation to describe the field quantities (stresses, strains and displacements) in a deformable body. However, since the finite element method describes these fields with their values at discrete points (for example, at the nodes for the displacements) it is most effective to use matrix notation for the finite element equations.

Since the finite element method computes the displacement field that minimizes the potential energy, the primary variables are the displacements of the nodes. The vector $\{u\}$ represents these displacements. The finite element method seeks to minimize the potential energy by selecting the values of $\{u\}$ which minimize

$$U(\{u\}) = \int_V W(E(\{u\}))dV - \{f\}^T\{u\} \qquad (35)$$

for all kinematically admissible $\{u\}$, where V is the volume of the body and $\{f\}$ is the vector of nodal loads.

Element Behavior

To calculate elastic strain energy in the body, the material domain is discretized into small regions called elements (see, for example, Fig. 40.10). The geometry of each element is described by the location of a set of nodes (different element types have different numbers of nodes) which also serve as inter-element connections.

Within each element the displacement field is approximated by low-order piecewise continuous polynomials, specially chosen such that their coefficients are the nodal displacement components for that element, $\{\alpha^e\}$, which is a subset of the global displacements, $\{u\}$. In each element, the element strains, $\{E\}$, are obtained from the displacements of the nodes in that element $\{\alpha^e\}$, by writing Equation (3) as the compatibility requirement

$$\{E\} = [B(\{a^e\})]\{a^e\}. \qquad (36)$$

The Piola-Kirchhoff stress components in each element are written as a vector $\{S\}$, so that the constitutive relation, Equation (10), which accounts for all of the interactions between the stress and strain components in a linear elastic body, can now be written as

$$\{S\} = [D]\{E\} \qquad (37)$$

where $[D]$ is the square matrix of coefficients representing the tensor D_{ijkl} in Equation (12). Essentially, the matrix $[D]$ describes the stresses required to produce the given strains in the material, and is determined by the strain energy function, W, using Equation (12). The strain energy W is determined by laboratory testing on the material of interest.

Materials such as soft tissue exhibit non-linear time dependent behavior and Equation (13) must be written in an incremental form

$$\{dS\} = [D(\{E\}, \{\dot{E}\})]\{dE\}. \qquad (38)$$

Therefore the components of $[D]$ depend on the strain $\{E\}$ and the strain rate $\{\dot{E}\}$. Materials of this type can cause significant computational difficulties, but the general procedures are the same as in the linear case.

For time-independent hyperelastic materials, the elastic strain energy in each element, W^e, is computed by integrating the hyperelastic strain energy potential W over the volume of the element, V^e, viz.,

$$W^e = \int_{V^e} W \, dV^e$$

$$= \frac{1}{2} \int_{V^e} \{S\}^T \{E\} dV^e$$

$$= \frac{1}{2} \{a\}^T \int_{V^e} [B]^T [D][B] dV^e \{a\} \qquad (39)$$

where we have used both the material constitutive equation (37) and the compatibility relationship (36) for that element (note that the superscript $(\,)^T$ denotes the transpose of the vector or matrix). It is convenient to define the element stiffness matrix [ke], by

$$\left[k^e\right] = \int_{V^e} [B]^T [D][B] dV^e \qquad (40)$$

so that the elastic potential energy (or strain energy) for a single element is given by

$$W^e\left(\{a^e\}\right) = \frac{1}{2} \{a^e\}^T \left[k^e\right]\{a^e\} \qquad (41)$$

Element Assembly

To compute the strain-energy for the entire structure, $W^\Sigma(\{u\})$, the element strain energies, $W^e(\{\alpha^e\})$, are summed. This is done by summing the element stiffness matrices, $[k^e]$, for each element. Since each set of element displacements, $\{\alpha^e\}$, is a different subset of the global displacements, $\{u\}$, we must relate the local to the global displacements, which can be done by defining a locator matrix for each element, from which $\{\alpha^e\} = [P^e]\{u\}$. This allows us to compute a global stiffness matrix, which represents the structural stiffness of the entire component. Mathematically,

$$\mathbf{W}^\Sigma(\{u\}) = \sum_e \mathbf{W}^e(\{\alpha\}) = \frac{1}{2}\{u\}^T [K]\{u\}$$

$$= \frac{1}{2}\sum_e [\{\alpha\}^T [k^e]\{\alpha\}]$$

$$= \frac{1}{2}\{u\}\sum_e [[P^e]^T [k^e][P^e]]\{u\}$$

$$\qquad (42)$$

Problem Solution

To compute the total energy of the system, $U(\{u\})$, we require the work done by the loads on the component, which is merely the inner product of the loads at each node, $\{f\}$, and the nodal displacements, $\{u\}$. Thus, the total energy of the system

$$U\left(\{u\}\right) = \frac{1}{2}\{u\}^T [K]\{u\} - \{u\}^T \{f\}. \qquad (43)$$

Minimizing the total energy requires the solution of the (usually large) system of simultaneous linear equations

$$[K]\{u\} - \{f\} = \{0\}, \qquad (44)$$

for which modern computers are highly effective. The displacements, $\{u\}$, which are an approximation to the true displacement field, can be used to compute the nodal displacements, $\{\alpha^e\}$, from which the strains, $\{E\}$, and the stresses, $\{S\}$, can be computed within each element. Hence the distribution of stress and strain can be found over the region of interest.

Examples of Artery Graft Modeling

Once the mechanics of a material has been fully characterized, the geometry of the graft can be modeled using the finite element method. To complete the modeling process, the loading and boundary conditions need to be described in terms of the finite element modeling. In the case of the natural artery, or a vascular graft, the loading magnitudes are easily quantified from blood pressures. In addition, the time dependence of the loading pulse can also be determined and used as input to the numerical model.

In order to illustrate some aspects of the mechanical design process, a few examples of artery graft modeling are presented. Figure 40.10 shows the displaced shape of a simple finite element model of the anastomosis region of the natural artery and a porous polyurethane graft. The artery (shaded) is modeled as a single layer, using the simple hyperelastic material model proposed by Fung et al,[17] and does not include any pre-stress. The graft is modeled as a hyperelastic and isotropic material, using the experimental data from the uniaxial tensile test data of the porous polyurethane. The graft is analyzed for a range of relative porosities. The different porosities were created by altering the ratio of the salt to polymer concentration in the manufacturing process (values of 1:1, 3:1, 5:1 and 7:1 have been investigated). Both the native artery and the graft are assumed to have an internal diameter (D) of 6 mm and a wall thickness of 1 mm. The model was loaded with an internal pressure, which is initially set to 70 mm Hg, and then increased linearly to 120 mm Hg—thus ΔP is 50 mm Hg.

The resultant compliance of the artery and the graft, as a function of the axial distance, is shown in Figure 40.11. A simple measure of vascular compliance[58]

$$C_v = \left(\frac{2}{D}\right)\left(\frac{\Delta D}{\Delta P}\right), \qquad (45)$$

which relates the change in graft diameter ΔD to the change in pressure, is used to compare the compliance of the native artery to the porous graft. This relation is chosen, as it does not contain any information about the properties of the two materials, which are non-linear and therefore cannot be characterized with a single constant parameter. The compliance of the native artery was predicted to be 0.273%/mm Hg (or 13.65% for a pulse pressure of 50 mm Hg), which was greater than any of the four grafts analyzed. In the region of the anastomosis the compliance of the artery is affected by the presence of the graft and therefore reduces towards the junction, which is halfway (5 mm) along the length. The lowest porosity graft (1:1) results in the smallest compliance, which is 0.05%/mm Hg. As the porosity increases to 7:1, the graft compliance increases to approximately 80% that of the host. It is interesting to see that with this more compliant graft material a hyper-compliant zone of about 2 mm, on the arterial side of the anastomosis, is predicted. In this region the compliance of the artery is increased by approximately 0.4%. A similar zone of hyper-compliance was predicted by Chandan et al[59] and observed in vivo by Hasson et al.[60] However, in the in vivo study the extent of hyper-compliance was more dramatic, with a localized increase in compliance of up to 50%.

The graft compliance as a function of the porosity is shown in Figure 40.12. The result shows that the percentage compliance increases exponentially as the porosity increases. However, increase in porosity will also be accompanied by a decrease in yield strength of the material.

The results of the proceeding example are based on a static analysis and do not show the influence of the time dependent behavior of the material. The viscoelasticity of the polyurethane will result in a gradual increase in the graft diameter, as a result of strain accumulation during cyclic loading. The increase in diameter will reach a steady state after some time. Therefore the inclusion of viscoelasticity is important in determining the final size of the graft after implantation.

The flexibility of the modeling approach means that complex geometrical features, with a host of different interacting materials, can be simulated. Figure 40.13 shows

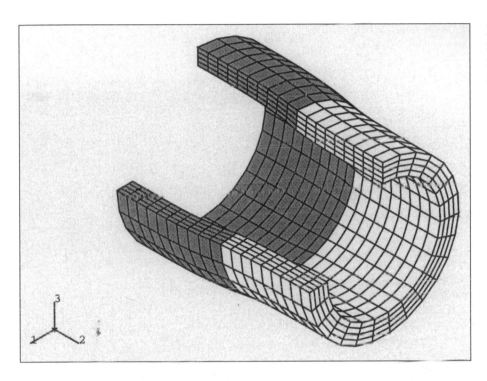

Fig. 40.10. Simple axisymmetric finite element model of anastomosis region of the native artery and the polyurethane graft.

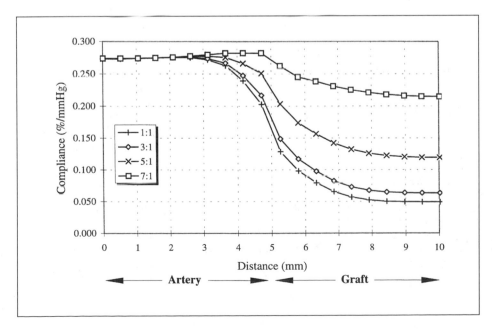

Fig. 40.11. Compliance (%/mmHg) of the native artery and the polyurethane graft for various porosity's of the graft material shown as a function of the axial distance.

a finite element model of a graft that has been reinforced with two spiral wound fibres. This type of model can be used to determine the compliance and the stresses within the reinforcing fibres, as well as the local strain distribution through the wall of the graft material.

Conclusions

The design of a tissue-engineered vascular graft involves mechanical issues that are ideally suited to sophisticated analysis methods such as the finite element method. However, the mechanics of both the intact artery and the graft materials is extremely complex. The complexities arise from the many different characteristics that the materials exhibit, such as the non-linearity, hyperelasticity, viscoelasticity, anisotropy. Combining all these three characteristics, while also introducing the effect of the microstructure, results in an involved material formulation. However, once the materials involved have been adequately characterized, a host of design issues can be examined with relative ease. The finite element method is therefore an ideal tool for aiding the development of the mechanical aspects of a tissue-engineered vascular graft.

References

1. Rodgers VGJ, Teodori MF, Borovetz HS. Experimental determination of mechanical shear stress about an anastomotic junction. J Biomech 1987; 20:795-803.
2. Weston MW, Rhee K, Tarbell JM. Compliance and diameter mismatch affect the wall shear rate distribution near an end-to-end anastomosis. J Biomech 1996; 29:187-198.
3. Stewart SFC, Lyman DJ. Effects of vascular graft/natural artery compliance mismatch on pulsatile flow. J Biomech 1992; 25:297-310.
4. Fry DL. Acute vascular endothelial changes associated with increased blood velocity gradients. Circ Res 1968; 22:165-197.
5. Wong AJ, Pollard TD, Herman IM. Actin filament stress fibres in vascular endothelial cells in vivo. Science 1983; 219:867-869.
6. Ishibashi H, Park H, Ojha M, Langdon S, Langille L. Shear-intimal thickening on the bed of an end-to-end anastomosis model. Advances in Bioengineering ASME BED- 1996; 33:475-476.
7. Lyman DJ, Fazzio FJ, Voorhees H, Robinson G. Compliance as a factor affecting the patency of a copolyurethene vascular graft. J Biomed Mater Res 1978; 12:337-345.
8. Seifert KB, Albo D, Knowlton H, Lyman DJ. Effect of elasticity of prosthetic wall on patency of small-diameter arterial prostheses. Surg Forum, 1979; 30:206-208.

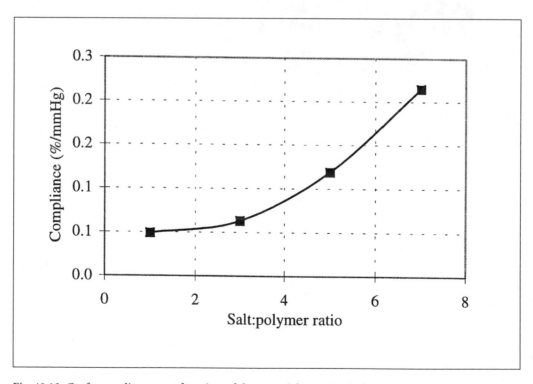

Fig. 40.12. Graft compliance as a function of the material porosity (salt:polymer ratio).

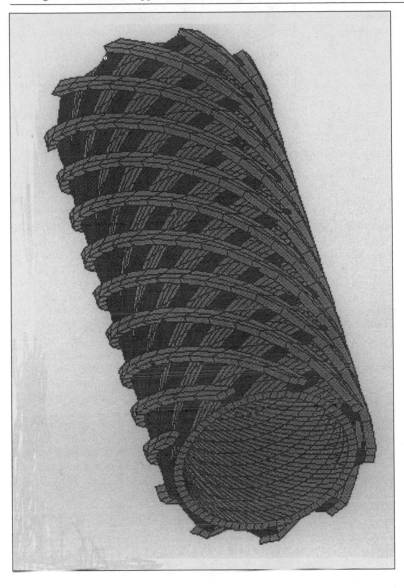

Fig. 40.13. Finite element model of a possible graft structure showing an underlying porous graft material surrounded by a reinforcing weave.

9. Hayashi K. Elastic properties and strength of a novel small-diameter compliant polyurethane vascular graft. J Biomed Mater Res 1989; 23:229-244.

10. Deweese JA. Anastomotic neointimal fibrous hyperplasia. In: Complications in vascular surgery, 2nd edition. Orlando: Grune and Stratton, 1985:157-170.

11. Ballyk PD, Ojha M, Walsh C, Butany J. Suture-induced intramural stresses and intimal hyperplasia. Advances in Bioengineering ASME BED- 1996; 33:213-214.

12. Ballyk PD, Walsh C, Ojha M. Effect of intimal thickening on the stress distribution of an end-to-side graft-artery junction. Advances in Bioengineering ASME BED- 1995; 31:327-328.

13. Paasche PE, Kinley CE, Dolan FG, Gonza ER, Marble AE. Consideration of suture line stresses in the selection of synthetic grafts for implantation. J Biomech 1973; 6:253-259.

14. Greer LS, Vito RP, Nerem RM. Material property testing of a collagen-smooth muscle cell lattice for the construction of a bioartificial vascular graft. Advances in Bioengineering ASME BED 1994; 28:69-70.

15. Fung YC, Biomechanics: Circulation 2nd Edition, Springer,1996.

16. Young JT, Vaishnav RN, Patel DJ. Non-linear anisotropic viscoelastic properties of canine arterial segments. J Biomech 1977; 10:549-559.

17. Fung YC, Fronek K, Patitucci P. Pseudoelasticity of arteries and the choice of its mathematical expression. Am J Physiol 1979; 237:H620-H631.

18. Takamizawa K, Hayashi K. Strain energy density function and uniform strain hypothesis for arterial mechanics. J Biomech 1987; 9:293-300.

19. Cox RH. Anisotropic properties of the canine carotid artery in vitro. J Biomech 1975; 8:293-300.

20. Dobrin PB. Biaxial anisotropy of dog carotid artery: Estimation of circumferential elastic modulus. J Biomech 1986; 19:351-358.

21. Tanaka TT, Fung YC. Elastic and inelastic properties of the canine aorta and the variation along the aortic tree. J Biomech 1974; 7:357-370.

22. Fung YC. Biomechanics: Mechanical properties of living tissue 2nd Edition, Springer,1993.

23. Chuong CJ, Fung YC. Compressibility and constitutive equations of arterial wall in radial compression experiments. J Biomech 1984; 17:35-50.

24. Fung YC. Stress-strain history relations of soft tissues in simple elongation. In: Fung YC, Perrone N, Anliker M, eds. Biomechanics: Its foundations and objectives Englewood Cliffs: Prentice-Hall, 1972.

25. Hutchinson KJ. Effect of variation of transmural pressure on the frequency response of isolated segments of canine arotid arteries, Cirulation Res 1974; 35:742-751.

26. Newman DL, Bowden NLR, Gosling RG. The dynamic and static elastic properties of the aorta of the dog. Cardiovasc Res 1975; 9:679-684.

27. Greenwald SE, Newman DL, Denyer HT. Effect of smooth muscle activity on the static and dynamic elastic propertries of the rabbit carotid artery. Cardiovasc Res 1982; 16:86-94.

28. Langewouters GJ, Wesseling KH, Goedhard WJA. The static elastic properties of 45 human thoracic and 20 abdominal aortas in vitro and the parameters of a new model. J Biomech 1984; 17:425-435.

29. Langewouters GJ, Wesseling KH, Goedhard WJA. The pressure dependent dynamic elasticity of 35 thoracic and 16 abdominal human aortas in vitro described by a five component model. J Biomech 1985; 18:613-620.

30. Haut RC, Little RW. A constitutive equation for collagen fibres. J Biomech 1972; 5:423-430.

31. Dehoff PH. On the nonlinear viscoelastic behavior of soft biological tissues. J Biomech 1978; 11:35-40.

32. Decraemer WF, Maes MA, Van Huyes VJ, Van Peperstraete P. A non-linear viscoelastic constitutive equation for soft biological tissues. J Biomech 1980; 13:559-564.

33. Wu SG, Lee GC. On nonlinear viscoelastic properties of arterial tissue. ASME J Biomech Eng 1984; 106:42-47.

34. Demiray H. A quasi-linear constitutive relation for arterial wall materials. J Biomech 1996; 29:1011-1014.

35. Johnson GA, Livesay GA, Woo SL-Y, Rajagopal KR. A single integral finite strain viscoelastic model of ligaments and tendons. J Biomech Eng 1996; 118:221-226.

36. Lanir Y. A microstructural model for the rheology of mammalian tendon. J Biomech Eng 1980; 102:332-339.

37. Lanir Y. Constitutive equations for fibrous connective tissue. J Biomech 1983; 16:1-12.

38. Minns RJ, Soden PD, Jackson DS. The role of the fibrous components and ground substance in the mechanical properties of biological tissues: A preliminary investigation. J Biomech 1973; 6:153-165.

39. Huyghe JM, Van Campen DH, Arts T, Heethaar RM. The constitutive behavior of passive heart muscle tissue: A quasi-linear viscoelastic formulation. J Biomech 1991; 24:841-849.

40. Myers BS, McElhaney JH, Doherty BJ. The viscoelastic responses of the human cervical spine in torsion: Experimental limitations of quasi-linear theory, and a method for reducing these effects. J Biomech 1991; 24:811-817.

41. Chuong CJ, Fung YC. On residual stresses in arteries. J Biomech Eng 1986; 108:189-192.

42. Fung YC, Liu SQ. Strain distribution in small blood vessels with zero stress state taken into consideration. Am J Physiol 1992; 264:H544-H552.

43. Greenwald SE, Rachev A, Moore JE, Meister JJ. The contribution of the structural components of the arterial wall to residual strain. Advances in Bioengineering ASME BED 1994; 28:63-64.

44. Humphrey JD, Strumpf RK, Yin FCP. Determination of a constitutive relation for passive myocardium: I. A new functional form. J Biomech Eng 1990; 112:333-339.

45. Humphrey JD, Strumpf RK, Yin FCP. Determination of a constitutive relation for passive myocardium: II.—Parameter estimation. J Biomech Eng 1990; 112:340-345.

46. Van Dijk AM. Vascular single smooth muscle cells and whole tissue. Mechanical properties and response of stimuli. PhD Thesis University of Leiden, Netherlands: 1983.

47. Gibson LJ, Ashby MF. Cellular solids: Structure and properties, Pergamon Press, 1988.

48. Carmines DV, McElhaney JH, Stack R. A piece-wise nonlinear elastic stress expression of human and pig coronary arteries tested in vitro. J Biomech 1991; 24:899-906.

49. Hayashi K. Experimental approaches on measuring the mechanical properties and constitutive laws of arterial walls. J Biomech Eng 1993; 115:481-487.

50. McAfee MA, Kaufmann MV, Simon BR, Baldwin AL. Experimental/numerical approach to the determination of material properties of large arteries. Advances in Bioengineering ASME BED 1994; 28:111-112.

51. Vaishnav RN, Young JT, Patel DJ. Distribution of stresses and of strain-energy-density through the wall thickness in a canine aortic segment. Circ Res 1973; 32:577-583.

52. von Maltzahn WW, Warriyar RG, Kietzer WF. Experimental determination of the elastic properties of media and adventitia of bovine carotid arteries. J Biomech 1984; 17:839-847.

53. von Maltzahn WW, Besdo D, Wiemer W. Elastic properties of arteries: A non-linear two-layer cylindrical model. J Biomech 1981; 14:389-397.

54. Ferry JD. Viscoelastic properties of polymers. New York: Wiley and Sons, 1961.

55. Lockett FJ. Nonlinear Viscoelastic Solids. New York: Academic Press, 1972.

56. Christensen RM. Theory of Viscoelasticity: An Introduction, New York: Academic Press, 1971.

57. Sternstein SS. Mechanical properties of glassy polymers: Treatise on Materials Science and Technology. In: Schultz JM, ed. Volume 10, part B, New York: Academic Press

58. Gow BS, Taylor MG. Measurement of viscoelastic properties of arteries in the living dog. Circ Res 1968; 23:111-122.

59. Chanran KB, Gao D, Han G, Baraniewski H, Corson JD. Finite element analysis of arterial anastomoses with vein, Dacron and PTFE grafts. Med Biol Eng Comp 1992; 30:413-418.

60. Hasson JE, Megerman J, Abbott WA. Increased compliance near vascular anastomosis. J Vasc Surg 1985; 2:419-423.

Scaffold Engineering

Material Aspects

――――――――――――――――――― CHAPTER 41 ―――――――――――――――

Bioinertness: An Outdated Principle

David F. Williams

The Convention of Inertness

Biomaterials have been with us for the majority of the twentieth century. Their nature has evolved during this time, and the applications for which they have been used have increased in complexity and diversity. However, for much of this time, the functions required of these materials and the performance parameters of the medical devices in which they have been used have been relatively straightforward and largely confined to mechanical and physical characteristics. The selection and design of biomaterials have therefore been similarly constrained by the conventional engineering concepts underlying these applications. During the last few years the situation has changed quite radically as new concepts and new treatment modalities have required a fundamental reappraisal of the scientific principles upon which biomaterials science are based. Nowhere is this seen more vividly than in the use of biomaterials for implantable devices within the cardiovascular system, and specifically in relation to the application of tissue engineering concepts in reconstructive vascular surgery. In this chapter we attempt to provide a rationale for this fundamental change and to demonstrate the pivotal role of surface reactivity in the products and devices of the future.

If we consider the historical role of biomaterials in implantable devices we can identify several clinical conditions that underlie their use, including congenital and developmental defects and trauma, but must recognize that it is in the treatment of diseases which have caused irreversible changes in tissues and organs that biomaterials play their biggest part. Thus, we see the widespread use of total joint replacements associated with the very widespread incidence of osteoarthritis, of intraocular lenses necessitated by cataracts, of prosthetic heart valves in the treatment of valvular disease, of dental implants following tooth and periodontal destruction, and of vascular prostheses and devices used for the prosthetic reconstruction of arteries.

In all of these situations the functional requirements of the materials are simple and essentially nonbiological. The major implantable devices of the twentieth century either transmit loads, facilitate sliding motion, passively direct fluid flow, control fluid flow or simply fill a space. The materials that permit the devices to perform these functions need to have the appropriate mechanical properties and little else. Indeed, in the majority of these cases, the mechanical and physical requirements are not themselves very onerous, and a wide range of materials is theoretically available for the construction of these devices.

In reality, of course, the situation is not quite so straightforward, since the devices usually have to perform their function for a long period of time within the confines of the human body. This implies that the materials have to supply these mechanical or physical characteristics without interference from the hostile physiological environment and without

Tissue Engineering of Prosthetic Vascular Grafts, edited by Peter Zilla and Howard P. Greisler.
©1999 R.G. Landes Company.

causing any untoward or adverse effects in the patient. The latter two aspects are subsumed within the phenomenon of biocompatibility, and it has been a combination of the mechanical and physical properties together with biocompatibility considerations that have determined the selection of materials available for implantable medical devices at the present time.

The term biocompatibility sounds simple to interpret since, as alluded to above, it implies compatibility or harmony with living systems. This concept, however, is too simple to be useful and the meaning of compatibility has to be explored further, both to understand the real logic of today's material selection and the opportunities for the future. It is intuitively obvious that a biomaterial or an implanted medical device should cause no harm to the recipient. This is the underlying principle of biological safety, and it is this rather than the totality of biocompatibility which has shaped the historical evolution of biomaterials. Most crucially, the requirements of biomaterials have been dominated by the perceived necessity to be safe, which has usually been interpreted as a requirement that a biomaterial should be totally inert in the physiological environment and should itself exert no effect on that environment. In other words, there should be no interaction between biomaterials and their host, implying that the material should be nontoxic, nonirritant, nonallergenic, noncarcinogenic, nonthrombogenic and so on.

This concept of biocompatibility which equates "biological performance" to inertness and biological indifference has resulted in the selection of a portfolio of acceptable or standard biomaterials that have widespread usage in applications such as those mentioned above. These range from the passive alloys such as stainless steel and titanium alloys, the noble metals of gold and platinum, some oxide ceramics such as alumina and zirconia, various forms of carbon and a range of putatively stable polymeric materials including silicone elastomers, polyolefins, fluorocarbon polymers and some acrylics and polyesters. The precise material chosen for an application from this type of list would depend on the precise mechanical or physical property specifications.

It cannot be denied that this approach has led to the successful deployment of many types of prostheses in wide-ranging clinical areas, and, apart from a few notable and controversial situations, such implantable devices rarely impact adversely on the health of the patient. The concept of bioinertness has therefore served a useful purpose. Even when we look at these generally successful areas, however, it can be seen that there are significant limitations to their performance and to the type of patient in which they can be used with confidence. Total joint replacements are generally contra-indicated in the younger, more active patient; the performance of vascular prostheses decreases as the devices are used more distally; bioprosthetic heart valves give greater cause for concern in very young patients; and intraocular lenses may not give satisfactory results in patients with underlying inflammatory conditions. Questions may be raised, therefore, as to whether bioinertness is the most acceptable principle underpinning material selection or whether alternative concepts would be preferable.

There are three fundamental reasons why bioinertness may not necessarily be the sensible choice. The first is that complete inertness is unachievable, so that any strategy predicated on this quality is ultimately doomed to fail. Secondly, if a device is made from materials which are inert and which do not interact with the body in any way, then it is unlikely that it can be truly incorporated into the body. For effective, long term performance in the dynamic tissue environment, it is usually preferable for there to be functional incorporation, which implies that the device should be stimulating the tissues to react to it positively rather than permitting them to ignore it. Thirdly, the emergence of tissue engineering principles, in which biomaterials are usually seen to act in a supporting role to biological components, has placed a very considerable emphasis on the utilization of intentionally degradable materials. These three features, which are determining the changing emphasis away from bioinertness, are explained below.

The Impossibility of Inertness

The convention described above is based on the assumption that a prosthetic device replaces, augments or modifies tissues or organs and is intended to remain within the patient for the length of time that the function is required, typically for the natural lifetime of that patient. The inertness was considered to be of crucial importance, both to allow the device to retain its structural integrity and thereby maintain its performance, and to prevent or at least limit the release of any substance or component from the material which would have some toxicological or other adverse biological consequence. In the vast majority of circumstances, sufficient control has been exercised over the chemical stability of biomaterials to ensure that no catastrophic loss of that integrity occurs as a result of compromised bioinertness. There have been some exceptions and there are no grounds for undue complacency in this respect, but this is generally not the most important of considerations. On the other hand, the potential to initiate harmful biological processes in the host will always be finite as long as there are structures capable of degradation or components free to be released.

Several features of the inherent structure of materials and of the complex nature of the tissue environment aggravate this situation. In particular, inertness in the physiological sense requires a great deal more than resisting degradation at the atomic or molecular level and, furthermore, even if it were that straightforward it would be extremely difficult to achieve. Indeed, it is now recognized that no material is totally inert in the body. Even those very stable materials mentioned earlier will interact to some extent with tissues. Titanium, although one of the most corrosion-resistant engineering alloys, corrodes in the body, judging by the presence of the metal in surrounding tissues. Gold and platinum will interact electrochemically with the saline-based extracellular fluid. For reasons not entirely understood, the most inert of the oxide ceramics suffer some long term changes within the body, and almost all known polymers will undergo oxidation, hydrolysis or other changes upon implantation.

With many materials, while the main component itself may be exceptionally inert, there are often minor components, perhaps impurities or additives, which can be released under some circumstances. The leaching of plasticizers and other additives from plastics provide good examples of interactions which are not necessarily related to the molecular breakdown of the material, but which nevertheless confer a degree of instability to the product.

It should also be noted that descriptions of material degradation mechanisms have to take into account the special and indeed, unique, features of the tissue environment. Whatever its location, a biomaterial will continuously encounter an aqueous environment during its use. This is not simply a saline solution, however, but a complex solution containing a variety of anions and cations, a variety of large molecules, some of which are very reactive chemically, and a variety of cells. There are occasions when a degradation process can be explained, mechanistically and qualitatively, by the presence of electrolyte. This is the situation with most metals when they suffer from corrosion in a physiological environment. Even here, however, it is known that the kinetics of corrosion may be influenced by the organic species present, especially the proteins, and it is indeed possible for the corrosion mechanism to be somewhat different from that found in nonbiological situations.

This phenomenon is even more pronounced with other groups of materials and it is clear that with polymers the kinetics and mechanism of degradation are fundamentally related to the precise details of the environment. Although hydrolysis remains the substantive mechanism for degradation of most heterochain polymers, including polyamides and polyesters, this hydrolysis may be profoundly influenced by the active species present in the tissue. In particular, the lysosomal enzymes synthesized and released from cells of the inflammatory response to biomaterials may influence the degradation process. Moreover, the hydrolysis may be supplemented by oxidative degradation, again occurring not only by virtue of passively dissolved oxygen in body fluids, but by active oxidative species such as superoxides, peroxides and free radicals generated by activated inflammatory cells such as macrophages. It is thus possible for homochain polymers not particularly susceptible to hydrolysis and not normally oxidized at room temperature to undergo oxidative degradation upon implantation. Polyolefins such as polyethylene and polypropylene come into this category.

On the basis of a vast amount of experimental work and clinical experience, it is now clear that all biomaterials are inherently susceptible to some degradation process within the physiological environment. It is equally clear that although a variety of surface treatment methodologies are available to reduce or ameliorate the degradation, none of these are entirely effective and their availability does not negate the now accepted principle that complete inertness cannot be achieved. Moreover, in the context of interactions which affect the overall performance of the material in the physiological environment, it is important to note that an interfacial reaction involving a physicochemical process such as protein adsorption will inevitably take place, further emphasizing the fact that inertness is a very relative term and

that there is no such thing as an inert biomaterial. It is never a question of whether a biomaterial will interact with the body but rather when and how. Under these circumstances, the preferred alternative strategy is to accept that such interactions take place and to attempt to control these interactions proactively and to incorporate these interactions into the design specifications.

The Requirement for Controlled Reactivity

The above arguments indicate that complete inertness may not be possible, but still do not indicate that it is undesirable. The possibility that the products of any interaction between a biomaterial and its physiological environment could be released into the host has generally been considered a sufficient deterrent to utilizing any material that was significantly reactive in that environment. This logic is clearly only valid if those products were going to initiate an undesirable response from the host, either locally or systemically. If interactions took place whereby the products were totally harmless, then there would be less cause for concern over the inability to achieve inertness. More importantly, if the nature of the interaction were one which produced a more appropriate response from a tissue, then a positive virtue could be made of this lack of inertness.

This quite different thinking is now enshrined in the current concepts and definition of biocompatibility. Instead of biocompatibility being equated with inertness, it is now recognized that it should encompass a wide range of reactivity, with the caveat that any reactivity is beneficial rather than harmful. On the basis of these ideas biocompatibility was redefined a few years ago as "the ability to perform with an appropriate host response in a specific application". It is apparent that this definition still encompasses the situation where inertness is required, since the most appropriate response in some situations is indeed no response. A traditional bone fracture plate is most effective when it is attached mechanically to the bone and does not corrode. No response of the tissue to the material is required under these circumstances.

In the type of device mentioned earlier in this chapter, in which the performance is dependent upon its physical replacement of diseased tissues and its incorporation into the structure of the body, inertness of all of the components may prevent optimal performance from being achieved. In particular, if a material is inert and unreactive within tissues, the long term host response will be associated with a lack of recognition and a lack of functional incorporation. An inert polymer such as polyethelyne or PTFE will induce the formation around it of a thin layer of collagenous fibrous tissue which can neither facilitate incorporation of the device into the tissue nor assist the device in achieving any of its functions. Moreover, this fibrous layer is unlikely to be stable and may alter its characteristics over time, this often being the ultimate cause of the device failure. In such circumstances, the biocompatibility characteristics of the materials in contact with their host tissues should be those which favor a positive interaction between the molecules of the material and the relevant molecules of that tissue, such that there is a functional attachment between the two. A total joint replacement which has the nonarticulating surfaces composed of materials or substances that are able to interact with the cellular components that promote bone regeneration at the interface should yield a more appropriate host response in the context of the long term mechanical stability of the joint. Similar arguments could be put forward for many of today's implantable devices that are used in reconstructive surgery.

This concept may be extended to many other types of implantable device, including those which function through an intervention in healing processes. For example, whilst it was noted before that conventional fracture plates need to be inert, on the basis that degradation or corrosion products could be harmful to the local tissue, it is not impossible for such devices to be made with surfaces that interact with osteoblasts, thus actively promoting or accelerating the healing process. Similarly, while many intravascular stents are fabricated from alloys chosen on the basis of their corrosion resistance and general inertness, the application of substances to the surfaces of these alloys which potentially have an ability to interact at the molecular level with those agents that are responsible for restenosis provides a new concept of bioreactivity rather than bioinertness for these devices.

Almost every type of implantable device which has hitherto been associated with materials chosen for their apparent inertness may now be reconsidered in this light. This applies equally to devices where active surface molecules can control thrombogenicity, to devices which are able to encourage tissue repair and to devices which are able to minimize the undesirable consequences of inflammation.

The Essential Requirement of Reactivity in Tissue Engineering

The desirability of some degree of reactivity in conventional implantable devices can be seen as a precursor to the essentiality of reactivity associated with the concepts and products of tissue engineering. It is important to remember here that the underlying principle of tissue engineering involves the combination of biological principles and substances with medical engineering principles and devices in order to provide products that are able to persuade the body to heal itself. In this rapidly emerging field, the major products utilize some material structure as a support, matrix or vehicle for the delivery of active biological molecules or cellular species to a target site in the host where repair or reconstruction is to be effected. Important as these material structures are, they do not normally constitute a component that is intended to remain in the body for very long, and certainly their function is incompatible with the characteristic of total inertness.

There are several different levels at which reactivity is desirable or essential. As alluded to above, the most obvious of these is the desirability for intentional biodegradation in the polymeric support structures that form the basis of tissue-engineered reconstruction devices. Whether this is concerned with the repair of cartilage defects, of nerve tissue, of damaged skin or diseased tissue within the vascular system, the template of a device usually involves a polymer that can degrade over a period of time ranging from a few weeks to a few years and where the degradation profile is consistent with the delivery of active tissue repair promoting molecules and with the physical support necessary for the developing tissue structure. It goes without saying of course that such a material should not degrade to produce harmful side effects, which could be associated with either the chemical characteristics of any degradation products or their physical morphology. Although this is not a trivial matter, such that inflammatory reactions associated with the degradation cannot be ruled out, there are several biodegradable polymers which may now be used with reasonable confidence in these situations.

Tissue engineering products should, however, involve more than a degradable structural polymer. The real essence of such a product is the biological activity which it imparts to the host site. A simple, empty, porous scaffold of a degradable polymer implanted within connective tissue may become infiltrated with repair tissue and may ultimately degrade to leave an area of reconstituted tissue derived from that infiltration. This, however, is not tissue engineering, since the tissue will not have been directed or controlled in terms of its structure and nature. In order to be really useful, this product would have to incorporate the appropriate cellular components, normally previously derived from the hosts, or certain molecules that are able to signal to the host cells the appropriate instructions to produce the desired tissue morphology and function. Under these circumstances, the biodegradable polymer has to be chosen very carefully, such that at the very least it will be compatible with the desired cell function in its vicinity or, preferably, such that it is capable of delivering these cell signaling molecules with the desired activity and in the desired manner. Inherent inertness is therefore unacceptable in these tissue-engineered products. The challenge is to introduce the desired level of reactivity without compromising the biological safety of the material.

Conclusions

For all the reasons outlined above, bioinertness can be considered as an outdated principle. Although there are some types of implantable device which are still better served by inert materials, the majority should preferably incorporate intentionally interactive materials, whilst others, especially in this new area of tissue engineering, positively demand this characteristic.

It has to be said, however, that academic arguments in favor of replacing a concept that is perceived to be out of date with a new principle cannot be sustained unless this new principle can be verified and reduced to practice. In view of the fact that bioinertness has never produced any harm, it is indeed a brave new world which is predicated on the availability of biomaterials that are both functionally interactive with their host and intrinsically safe. Many might argue that these in fact are contradictory requirements. Clearly that need not be the case, but the whole future of tissue engineering products that are able to demonstrate efficacy and safety is dependent on the development of the appropriate materials. However outdated bioinertness may be, it should not be replaced by materials based upon hope rather than scientific reality.

Scaffold Engineering

Material Aspects

──────────────── CHAPTER 42 ────────────────

Bioinert Biomaterials: Are Their Properties Irreplaceable?

Patrick T. Cahalan

In 1955 Sewell and colleagues[1] performed a study comparing ovine and bovine sources of catgut sutures in three animal models. The objective of the study was to quantitatively compare the tissue response to the implanted material, and this event is often cited as the beginning of biocompatibility testing. Coincident to this was the rapidly expanding postwar technology in high performance plastics, with mounting evidence that biological grafts, even homografts, were not going to survive the challenges in vascular graft applications.[2] Voorhees' observations in 1952 of a neointima free of thrombi on a silk thread, and his later experiments with Vinyon "N" cloth in dog aortas, clearly showed that a synthetic material could serve as a conduit, and be accepted by the tissue.[3] Studies would follow showing the merits of other materials, particularly Teflon and Dacron.[4] The paradigm was set, and materials were classified as very reactive to inert.

What followed was once described as "20 years of frustration".[5] During this period commercial efforts were driven by the promise of a very large market, estimated between 0.6 to 1 billion dollars annually. Scientific efforts were focused on comparing properties of materials with limited physiological markers, primarily the occurrence of thrombi on the material surface. An example of surface property concepts that were hypothesized to be beneficial are seen in Figure 42.1.[6] The majority of the surfaces listed are in essence attempts to create surfaces with minimal effect, whether it be termed low protein or platelet adhesion. In the same 1972 article, Baier refers to much of the individual surface property characterization towards blood compatibility as people working in a maze within a maze.

Hydrophilic surfaces, for example, while showing low platelet adhesion and therefore thought to be blood compatible, when tried in a vascular graft position did not prove to provide patency. Thus, researchers thinking they had found a way out of the blood compatibility maze found themselves in another maze with new barriers to solve. Baier's representation of the surface properties compared to the living blood vessel intima serves to highlight the focus of blood compatibility to the vascular application. This narrow focus, plus the lack of clearer understanding of cellular and molecular biology, helped continue the quest for the "holy grail" of inert materials.

Not until it was shown in the late 1970s that endothelial cells were more active in maintaining blood compatibility[7] did the paradigm begin to change. Until this time it was even possible to hypothesize that endothelial cells were the perfect inert surface. The emergence of RIA and ELISA in the mid-70s opened up the possibilities of looking at the molecular and cellular aspects involved at the surface. The common use of these tools did not make its way into blood compatibility research until well into the 1980s, and today a significant number of papers are still offered that rely largely on platelet adhesion alone to determine blood compatibility of surfaces. The increase in understanding of reactions between coagulation factors and formed elements of the blood has led to a change in thinking that

Tissue Engineering of Prosthetic Vascular Grafts, edited by Peter Zilla and Howard P. Greisler.
©1999 R.G. Landes Company.

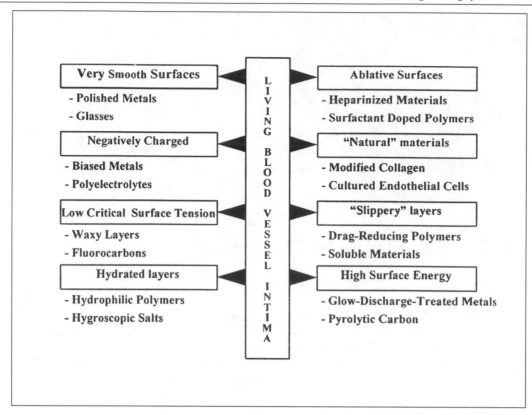

Fig. 42.1. General approaches to improve blood compatibility: early years (70s).

previously focused on the bulk reactions in blood to the realization that these critical reactions "occur almost exclusively on surfaces".[8] The formerly thought to be inert endothelial cell has been shown to have as many procoagulant properties as anticoagulant.[9] The pat answer for years to the question, "What is the perfect surface?" was: "An endothelialized surface." The fact that an endothelialized surface can be thrombogenic opens up a new maze. It also begs the question, "Bioinert biomaterials: Are their properties irreplaceable?"

"The long sought after biologically inert material has not as yet been developed, and the realization of the inherent 'biointeractivity' of all implanted polymers has led many investigators to pursue strategies aimed at optimizing the biological interactions with the synthetic polymer rather than to minimize all biological interaction."[10] This statement would seem to put an end to the question, "Is there a need for bioinert materials?" Unfortunately, vascular grafts and other biomedical devices still use synthetic materials of construction, and their replacement with other biological materials or repair therapies is not on the very near horizon. The great promise of biodegradable materials has not been realized, and attempts at endothelialization of synthetic materials, while showing promise, have not consistently exceeded the performance of autologous tissue. Preadsorption of synthetic vascular grafts with cellular adhesive proteins tends to enhance the short term attachment of endothelial cells, but platelet adhesion, and therefore increased thrombogenicity, typically increases with time.[11] A possible

explanation for this failure may be the nondiscriminatory nature of some of the cell adhesion receptors to adhesion proteins. Some new approaches to deal with the nondiscriminatory cell receptor binding to adhesion proteins attempt to attach peptide adhesion ligands to surfaces.[12] A critical requirement stated by Hubbell in such attachment is to render the surfaces resistant to protein adsorption by first grafting with a hydrophilic nonionic polyethylene oxide (PEO) chain to which the peptide ligand could be tethered.

The latter stated requirement could serve to finally propose a more pragmatic application of the "inert" concept. Inertness with respect to a nonionic hydrophilic spacer that is resistant to protein adhesion permits a selectivity or control of molecular and cellular events at surfaces. The challenges left with this approach are to achieve the proper density of ligands on the surface, their orientation, and the ability to accomplish this on synthetic substrates in the geometric configuration of a biomedical device such as a vascular graft, artificial heart, heart valve, or ventricular assist device. While this elegant concept represents a major advance in the effort to make an endothelialized and hopefully long term blood-compatible surface on a vascular graft, it is not certain whether another maze will not open up, such as continued hyperplasia. Due to noncompliance of synthetic structures, some might argue that a truly new totally functioning vascular tissue might not be possible, and that even though there is an endothelial layer on the lumen, the structure will succumb to other mechanisms of failure. More optimistically, it could be hoped that compliant structures could be engineered that also could be modified to promote spatially correct cellularization of smooth muscle cells, and even include neovascularization. The progress made by persistent researchers[10,12] in the vascular graft field suggests that the latter possibility is not out of the question.

As mentioned earlier, the vascular graft focus may have actually been in part responsible for a lack of more rapid progress in understanding the cellular and molecular events at the surface, particularly in development of more blood-compatible surfaces. Other application areas such as dialysis and cardiopulmonary bypass (CPB) have created a strong research effort in providing surfaces with enhanced blood compatibility, and in this effort industry, academia, and clinicians have invested large amounts of time and capital in investigating improved biocompatible surfaces on devices not necessarily designed for permanent implant. From a strictly clinical perspective, the ability to monitor coagulation and inflammatory responses to foreign surfaces during CPB, and evaluate devices after use, has created a plethora of scientific publications involving measurement of molecular and cellular events on blood-contacting surfaces. This has also created a commercial stimulus for funding research on blood materials interactions and research in surface modification of biomedical devices.

In our laboratory, surfaces deemed "inert" have been studied using multiple ELISA markers such as TAT, F1.2, elastase, and SC5b-9 (terminal complement complex) in addition to measuring platelet adhesion and activation. The most often cited inert molecule is poly(ethylene glycol) or (PEG). It has been suggested by some that a PEG surface has little or no protein adsorption or interaction.[13,14] This premise has also been challenged by some researchers.[15,16] It has further been suggested that PEG surfaces may serve to delay rather than reduce protein adsorption and activation.[17] With respect to blood compatibility, we found that while a PEG surface does in fact show lower protein adsorption and platelet adhesion, it does not show any improvement in TAT, complement (SC5b-9), or elastase. These studies used a blood loop system that contained a valve to effect physiological flow, and human blood containing 1 U/ml of heparin. While PEG surfaces have been studied and widely reported to approach inertness, it is obvious that there is yet much to be learned before this technology is optimized. Nevertheless, the suggested use of this molecule to tether a peptide, or possibly a specific adhesion molecule, may in the end prove to be the best application of PEG.

Another molecule that is receiving considerable attention for its low protein and platelet adhesion is phosphatidylcholine (PC). Methacrylate copolymers with pendant PC groups (MPC) have been coated with a facile process to polymers, and the PC moiety is expressed to a high degree on the uppermost surface.[18] Conceptually, the MPC coating is said to mimic the natural phosphatidylcholine present on the surface of nonactivated platelets. In testing in our laboratory, this surface does show reduced platelet adhesion and less TAT formation. Additional testing needs to be completed to evaluate the complement and white cell response to this surface. In our hands this polymer has shown material-dependent coating characteristics, and evaluation is tedious,

as optimal pretreatments followed by confirming XPS and TofSIMS data is required to assure optimal presentation of PC moieties on the surface before testing. There is supporting evidence for the inertness of a pure PC surface.[19] Studies performed at the University of Maastricht have demonstrated that a phospholipid bilayer of pure dioleoyl-phosphatidylcholine (DOPC) on an ellipsometry plate is indeed an inert surface, and assembly of the prothrombinase complex requires the addition of dioleoyl-phosphatidylserine (DOPS) in significant amounts.[28] DOPS is present on the internal surface of the platelet membrane, and platelet activation causes a flip-flop of the DOPS to the external surface of the membrane. When DOPS is on the surface, the prothrombinase complex can be assembled and thrombin generation can take place. Unfortunately, the stability of a DOPC bilayer is very poor, and at this time has not been attained with consistency on a polymeric surface. The MPC polymer approach would be to assure uniformity and density of the PC moiety on the surface, and thus impart through mimicry an inertness to the surface.

While the DOPC surface appears to be the closest thing to an inert surface, the actual surface of the plasma membrane is in fact made of more than just DOPC. Transmembrane proteins assure that platelets in the end are very reactive with their environment. It is perhaps appropriate to reflect back to the comments of Spaet[8] with respect to all important reactions in the body taking place on surfaces, and that these surfaces we have learned to be anything but inert.

In the end, one of the roles or properties of inert biomaterials that is needed is their ability to enhance the expression of another molecule, such as a peptide as suggested by Hubbell. This may be accomplished by minimizing competing phenomena such as protein adsorption, as well as presenting a molecule in a conformation more accessible to its target receptor. This property is indeed possibly irreplaceable. Our studies specific to the attachment of heparin to surfaces clearly indicates that the bioactivity of an attached molecule is dependent on its ability to interact with target molecules, and the ability to control the loading and the reactivity of the attached molecules is critical to achieve optimal functioning on the surface.[20] Heparin on these surfaces was tethered to a nonionic hydrogel that was derivatized to achieve different loadings of heparin. Here the surface is certainly not inert, but it is designed to optimally compete with the undesirable physiological mechanisms of coagulation and platelet adhesion. These surfaces do not prevent protein adhesion, but the proteins that have adhered show different relative concentrations to control surfaces, and the performance of the surfaces correlates with these adhesion profiles.[21] In nature, a denuded endothelial lining exposes a procoagulant surface, yet this surface can rapidly passivate without excessive thrombin formation. Fibrinolysis, controlled inflammation and, finally, remodeling give a normal healing response that restores the tissue to a functional state, barring the introduction of complications of a biomaterial, ongoing disease state or flow restrictions. A normal healing response replaces inertness with spatially correct signals via the subendothelial extracellular matrix and thus controls the first step of repair, which is platelet adhesion and coagulation. A naturally formed and controlled hemostatic response (clot) presumably is resolved without the excessive inflammatory reactions associated with the presence of foreign materials. If those foreign materials possess an inert surface, the resultant histology should resemble that of a injury without the presence of a foreign material. Since injury exposes the blood to nonendothelialized surfaces, and these surfaces do bind plasma proteins, it might be a better approach to attempt to modify a surface to have a similar protein adsorption profile. Implants of biomaterial surfaces modified with collagen (data to be published) after 10 weeks show minimal capsule formation with microvascular structures within two fibroblast layers of the biomaterial surface. The control biomaterial surface (polyurethane) has macrophage and foreign body giant cells (two layers) followed by 12-15 layers of densely packed fibroblasts adjacent to the material surface (a typical fibrotic response). The attachment of the collagen to the above mentioned surface was not simple adsorption, but rather a covalent attachment with isolation of the collagen layer to the uppermost layer (70 Å).[22] XPS data showed a pure surface of collagen, and this was attainable based on the inherent properties of the grafted surface beneath. This should be a target for modification of surfaces whether inert or interactive, and that being complete and uniform coverage without influence from intermediate chemistries used to couple the molecules to the surface.

In addition to the property of inertness being used to enhance the presentation of molecular species to the physiological environment, there is another possibly irreplaceable property of inertness. That is the relative chemical inertness of biomaterials. In addition to finding the optimal protein adhesion mosaic on a surface, the biomaterial of construction of a device must withstand the degradative environment of the body. Numerous attempts have been made, for example, to fabricate vascular prostheses using polyurethane, when several instances of urethane degradation in vivo have been documented.[23,24] Attempts to mimic the in vivo response in an in vitro system have shown that adsorption of the plasma protein α_2-macroglobulin could play a role in biodegradation of the urethane.[25] It might be hypothesized that a surface modification that could isolate the biomaterial surface from protein and cell attachment could serve to protect its stability. Those who would choose to continue the use of polyurethanes for vascular grafts will need to deal with the potential degradation mechanisms demonstrated. An alternative approach to elastomeric materials may be fabricated grafts using very stable materials such as PTFE and PET that have mechanical properties created by the bulk design of the device.

Biodegradable materials have boasted the promise of ultimate inertness in that they are not left behind for reaction with the body. While very impressive advances are being made in resorbable polymers,[26] their application at this time may still be limited by the need for mechanical properties that are best met with traditional biomaterials. An additional issue with resorbable materials is the control of the rate and type of resorption, ablative or eroding. It is also somewhat taken for granted that the inflammatory responses of these materials can easily be controlled by coupling the release of anti-inflammatory drugs; this may possibly open up yet another maze.

In summary, the 20 years of frustration[27] to which Andrade referred have been replaced by numerous multidisciplined efforts, aided by a much better understanding of molecular and cellular events at surfaces. The knowledge gained has opened up many approaches to finding the holy grail, and also created a number of positive spin-offs in therapies apart from vascular grafts. The concept of bioinert materials still persists, not as an end in itself, but rather as a tool to enhance positive mechanisms or to retard undesirable competing mechanisms. In the quest for new biomaterials, and for tissue engineering to replace diseased tissue with new functioning tissue, we will surely progress in an iterative manner. Mundane issues such as sterilization may render new concepts nonfunctional, but may stimulate new sterilization technology in order to bring them to market. Mechanical property limitations may require creative processing or fabrication advances. Promising surface modifications may first produce composite hybrid structures with traditional materials that can later be replaced by resorbable materials. What in the end is probably irreplaceable is the learning process involved in trying to find inert biomaterials.

References

1. Sewell WR, Wiland J, Craver BN. A new method of comparing suture of ovine catgut with sutures of bovine catgut in three species. Surg Gynecol Obstet 1955; 100:483.
2. Szilagyi DD, McDonald RT, Smith RF et al. Biological fate of human arterial homografts. Arch Surg 1957; 75:506.
3. Voorhees AB, Jaretski A, Blakemore AH. The use of tubes constructed from Vinyon "N" cloth in bridging arterial defects. Ann Surg 1952; 135:332.
4. Deterling RA, Bhonslay SB. An evaluation of synthetic materials and fabrics suitable for blood vessel replacement. Surgery 1955; 38:71.
5. Andrade JD, Nagaoka S, Cooper S, Okano T, Kim SW. Surfaces and blood compatibility: Current hypotheses. Vol XXXIII Trans Am Soc Artif Organs 1987.
6. Baier RE. The role of surface energy in thrombogenesis, Bulletin of The NY Academy of Medicine 1972; 48(2):257-272.
7. Weskler BB, Marcus AJ, Jaffe EA. Synthesis of prostaglandin 12 (prostacyclin) by cultured human and bovine endothelial cells. Proc Natl Acad Sci USA 1977; 74: S.3922-3926.
8. Spaet TH. Blood in contact with artificial surfaces: Where have we been and where are we going. Annals of The New York Academy of Sciences, 1987; 516.
9. Gimbrone Jr MA. Vascular endothelium: Nature's blood container. Vascular Endothelium in Hemostasis and Thrombosis. Gimbrone Jr MA, Ed. Edinburgh: Churchill Livingstone, 1986; 1-13.
10. Greisler HP, Gosselin C, Ren D, Kang SS, Kim DU. Biointeractive polymers and tissue engineered blood vessels. Biomaterials 1996; 17:329-336.
11. Seeger JM, Klingman N. Improved endothelial cell seeding with cultured cells in fribronection-coated grafts. J Surg Res 1985; 38:641-647.
12. Massia SP, Hubbell JA. Tissue engineering in the vascular graft. Cytotechnology 1992; 10:189-204.

13. Merrill EW, Salzman EW. Polyethylene oxide as a biomaterial. Am Soc Artif Intern Organs 1993; 6:60.

14. Harris JM. Poly(ethylene glycol) Chemistry: Biotechnical and Biomedical Applications. New York: Plenum Press, 1992:15.

15. Llanos G, Sefton MV. J Biomater Sci Polymer Edn, 1993; 4:381-400.

16. Sheth SR, Leckband D. Measurements of attractive forces between proteins and end-grafted poly(ethylene glycol) chains.

17. Kulik E et al. Poly(ethylene glycurface: Reduced vs delayed protein adsorption and activation. Abstract from Firth World Biomaterials Congress, Toronto, Canada. 1996; 29 May-2 June.

18. Ishihar K, Nakabayashi N. Part A: Polymer Chemistry: Specific interaction between water-soluble phospholipid polymer and liposome. J Poly Sci 1991; 29:831-835.

19. Andree HAM. Phospholipid binding and anticoagulant action of annexin V. Ph.D. thesis at the University of Maastricht, The Netherlands 1992.

20. Lindhout T et al. Antithrombin activity of surface-bound heparin studied under flow conditions. J Biomed Mater Res 1995; 29:1255-1266.

21. Sapatnekar et al. Blood-biomaterial interactin in a flow system in the presence of bacteria: Effect of protein adsorption. J Biomed Mater Res, 1995; 29:247-256.

22. HendriksM. A study on the covalent surface-immobilization of collagen. Ph.D. thesis, Development of biomaterials with enhanced infection resistance. University of Eindhoven, The Netherlands. 1996:127-148.

23. Stokes K. Environmental stress cracking in implanted polyether-polyurethanes. Polyurethanes in Biomedical Engineering. Plank H, Egbccrs G, Syre I, eds. Amsterdam: Elsevier, 1984:243.

24. Takahara A, Hergenrother RW, Coury AJ, Cooper SL. Effect of soft segment chemistry on the biostability of segmented polyurethanes. II. In vitro hydrolytic degradation and lipid adsorption. J Biomed Mater Res 1992; 26:801-818.

25. Schubert MA, Wiggins MJ, Schaefer MP, Hiltner A, Anderson J. Oxidative biodegradation mechanisms of biaxially strained poly(etherurethane urea) elastomers. J Biomed Mater Res 1995; 29:337-347.

26. Sawhney AS, Pathak CP, Hubbell JA. Bioerodible hydrogels based on photopolymerized poly(thylene glycol)-co-poly(α-hydroxy acid) diacrylate macromers. Macromolecules 1993; 26:581-587.

27. Andrade JD, Coleman DL, Didisheim P, Hanson SR, Mason R, Merrill E. Blood-materials interactions: 20 years of frustration. Trans Am Soc Artif Intern Organs 1981; 27:659-662.

28. Smeets E. Scrambling of Membrane Phospholipids in Platelets and Erythrocytes. Ph.D. Thesis, University of Maastricht, The Netherlands, 1996.

Scaffold Engineering

Material Aspects

--------- CHAPTER 43 ---------

Biostable Polymers as Durable Scaffolds for Tissue Engineered Vascular Prostheses

Arthur J. Coury

Introduction

The successful implementation of any medical device requires a systematic development process from concept through use in humans. Rigorous quality systems and design controls are now mandated by law,[1] and the framework they provide[2] is especially relevant to the development of systems as complex as tissue engineered vascular prostheses.

The selection of polymeric materials to serve as structural scaffolds for the vascular prostheses should only be made in the context of the design intent of the device. In the spirit of design control, this chapter begins with a concept statement—the first stage of the design process. The intent is not to completely design the device but to provide a minimum set of characteristics which will set rather loose boundaries, to allow a range of prosthetic materials to be considered in this chapter.

Design Concept

The product is a vascular prosthesis intended to address the unmet medical need for functional replacement of small ($\leq$ 6 mm) and medium (6-12 mm) diameter arterial segments.[3-4] The device consists of a structural matrix (scaffold) of available synthetic biomaterials and possibly other components assembled prior to implantation. The scaffold promotes and retains attachment and/or ingrowth of biological tissues. The synthetic scaffold is biostable, that is, resistant to excessive structural deterioration for the projected lifetime of the device, which is considered to be a "permanent" implant. The synthetic components of the device elicit an acceptable host response alone or through pharmacologic intervention. The device can be produced by available techniques into configurations which provide adequate hemodynamic flow. It may be packaged, sterilized, stored and implanted by accepted processes. It is amenable to any special techniques (e.g., in vitro cell seeding or surface modification) which are required for its proper function.

Material Requirements and Limitations

Given the design intent of the device, specific material requirements for the structural matrix are discussed as subtopics of this section. It must be stated at the outset that no material is optimal in all of the requirements. The final selection of a material will involve compromises from the ideal, but demonstration of acceptable characteristics by appropriate testing is required.

Tissue Engineering of Prosthetic Vascular Grafts, edited by Peter Zilla and Howard P. Greisler.
©1999 R.G. Landes Company.

Availability by Purchase or Synthesis

Particular attention should be paid to long term availability of the polymer. In recent years, major suppliers of polymers have withdrawn their products from consideration for implantable devices, [5-6] chiefly for liability reasons. In the United States, several legislative initiatives have led to the passage of the Biomaterials Access Assurance Act on July 30, 1998 (Public Law 105-230) which offers protection to biomaterials suppliers. The effect of this legislation will likely take several years to be fully realized. The supply problem is especially serious for stable biomaterials which often require capital-intensive processes available only to large chemical companies—the sources of highest liability exposure. This problem has led device manufacturers to search internationally for biomaterial equivalents or to work with smaller companies with limited manufacturing capability, but lower potential liability consequences.

Fabricable into Intended Configuration

Reasonable mechanical characteristics of the tubular device include flexural compliance, kink resistance and suturability. While materials with a wide range of physical properties can achieve these goals, there are property-dependent limitations on the configurations of these materials that can be used. Fiber-based or expanded wall configurations are probably required if the material has a relatively high to medium modulus (e.g., poly(ethylene terephthalate), polypropylene, polytetrafluoroethylene). Low modulus compositions such as elastomers (e.g., polyurethanes) can be considered as solid-wall, porous-wall or fiber-based tubes. Extrusion, molding or casting processes must be available to produce the base configuration. If surface modification is required, acceptable processes must be applicable to the material.

Stable to Processing, Storage and Use Conditions

Maintenance of structural integrity by the biomaterial scaffold is the main requirement of this chapter and is addressed in the sections on degradation mechanisms and discussions of individual materials. The major point to make here is that there are stability considerations at each of the many stages of processing and storage of the biomaterial, not just during residence in vivo.[8] The material, at the time of implant, is the product of its prior history and attention to preserving its integrity throughout can assure stability of the implant.

Elicits Acceptable Host Response for Life of Device

Inherent nonthrombogenicity of the biomaterial is not likely and is not assumed to be required. A biological response will be induced, and control of that response is the function of the tissue engineering component of the vascular product. It is assumed that the matrix material has passed a standard biocompatibility protocol[2] and that control of other responses can be achieved by mechanical design, local or systemic drug delivery, surface or bulk modification. Any additives used for processing, stabilizing or effecting biological responses are likewise assumed to be nontoxic.

Modes of Polymer Degradation

The requirement of biostability does not imply that the biomaterial is inert in the medium under consideration. It must be appreciated that a polymer, and all materials, respond continuously to changes in environment before and during the implantation period.[8] All polymers are permeable to gases and liquids. They absorb, transmit and desorb components. Their surface and bulk properties change with time and the imposition of external forces, sometimes reversibly, other times irreversibly. The changes can be favorable or unfavorable.[8] Degradation leading to compromised performance of a scaffold in vivo can be physical, chemical, or a combination of both. Both types of degradation can also necessitate rejection of a component or device prior to use.[9]

Physical changes may include swelling, plasticization, crystallization, decrystallization, fatigue fracture, creep, simple stress cracking and kinking, among others.[10] Chemical degradation generally consists of covalent bond cleavage, but, in some cases, covalent crosslinking or ionic bond transformations are involved. Variables such as heat, moisture, oxygen, light, radiation, even mechanical stress, induce chemical degradation.[10] Many or all of these factors may be encountered by a biomaterial prior to its implantation. Each of these destructive agents is generally manageable to acceptable levels by process and exposure control and the use of additives[10] if the material is inherently stable in the body.

The longest intended phase in the lifetime of a "permanent" implant is residence in the body. The polymeric scaffold for a tissue engineered vascular prosthesis is subject to all of the forces listed above which may induce physical degradation. Appropriate device design and processing (e.g., to provide burst strength and minimize residual stress) and proper implantation techniques (e.g., to minimize kinking and applied stress) must be implemented to minimize physical degradation.[10]

Chemical degradation forces are also encountered at every phase of the biomaterial scaffold's lifetime. The objective is to understand these forces and the material's susceptibility to them and to protect against their effects. For example, antioxidants can protect polymers such as polypropylene and polyurethanes from thermooxidative, photooxidative and autooxidative (oxygen induced) degradation.[10]

In the body environment, modes of chemical degradation consist of three major types: hydrolysis, oxidation and mineralization (calcification). The latter mode may or may not induce significant covalent bond cleavage, but does involve chemical transformations that cause structural damage to the polymer and will be treated as one of the three subtopics discussed next.

Hydrolysis

Hydrolysis is the cleavage of susceptible chemical bonds with water. Simple hydrolysis can be catalyzed by acid or base and occurs as a consequence of the number and reactivity of the cleavable bonds. Enzyme-catalyzed hydrolysis (e.g., by esterases, proteases) has been reported[9,11-14] but, for most synthetic polymers, enzymatic effects are superficial and minor and will not be further discussed here.

Hydrolytically susceptible bonds generally consist of carbonyl groups with a heteroatom (O,N,S) on one or both sides of it. These structures and several other hydrolyzable groups are listed in Figure 43.1.

Hydrolysis rates differ among the susceptible groups. For example, carbonyl group reactivity decreases in the order: anhydride > ester > urethane > amide. Ethers, ketals and acetals are labile to acidic pH but stable to basic conditions.

Backbone structure and intermolecular interactions of hydrolyzable polymers also affect degradation rate. Factors such as crystallinity, hydrophobicity and crosslink density tend to decrease hydrolysis rate[9] and render polymers based on hydrolytically labile groups potentially viable candidates for long term implant.

Polymer structures that resist hydrolysis include hydrocarbons, silicones, sulfones, halocarbons and isolated carbonyl-containing molecules (i.e., ketones).

Oxidation

Oxidative degradation of polymers involves destruction or modification of molecular structure via electron transfer reactions.[9] The polymers to be considered have varying degrees of susceptibility to oxidation. Prior to implantation, specific operations such as melt processing, radiation sterilization or exposure to light containing ultraviolet wavelengths can promote oxidative degradation. Autooxidation involves reaction with molecular oxygen and is a likely mechanism of many oxidative events.[15] Other oxidants (e.g., metal ions, hypochlorite, hydroperoxides)[16] are also effective in causing degradation.

Inside the body, biomaterials are subject to oxidative insult as a consequence of inflammation due to the foreign body reaction (phagocytic attack).[9,17] Powerful oxidative products result from phagocyte activation (e.g., hydroxyl radical, peroxynitrite, hypochlorite), which can attack oxidizable bonds. Susceptible sites generally are those that can stabilize a free radical (Figure 43.2).[9]

Oxidatively stable structures include straight-chain hydrocarbons, halocarbons and fully-oxidized groups (e.g., ketones, sulfones, carbonates, esters, urethanes). We have, however, produced some evidence that the carbon atom next to the heteroatom of the latter carbonyl groups may be amenable to oxidation.[17]

Evidence for direct (receptor-ligand) enzymatic catalysis of oxidation is limited and inidcative of minor consequences.[12,18]

In vivo oxidation of polymers has been most extensively studied for polyurethanes and polyethylenes.[9,15-24] Structural degradation due to oxidation is usually manifest as surface fissuring, deep crack formation, fragmentation or wear, often in zones of applied stress. Radiation sterilization (e.g., of polyethylene) can produce long-lived radicals with autooxidation and embrittlement leading to increased wear and fragmentation in use.

Mitigation of structural degradation due to oxidation can be accomplished by minimizing residual and applied stress, controlling exposure to destructive radiation, use of antioxidants, isolating susceptible polymers in a device from direct attack by phagocytes or soluble oxidants and, finally, by the use of oxidation resistant materials.[9,10,15,16]

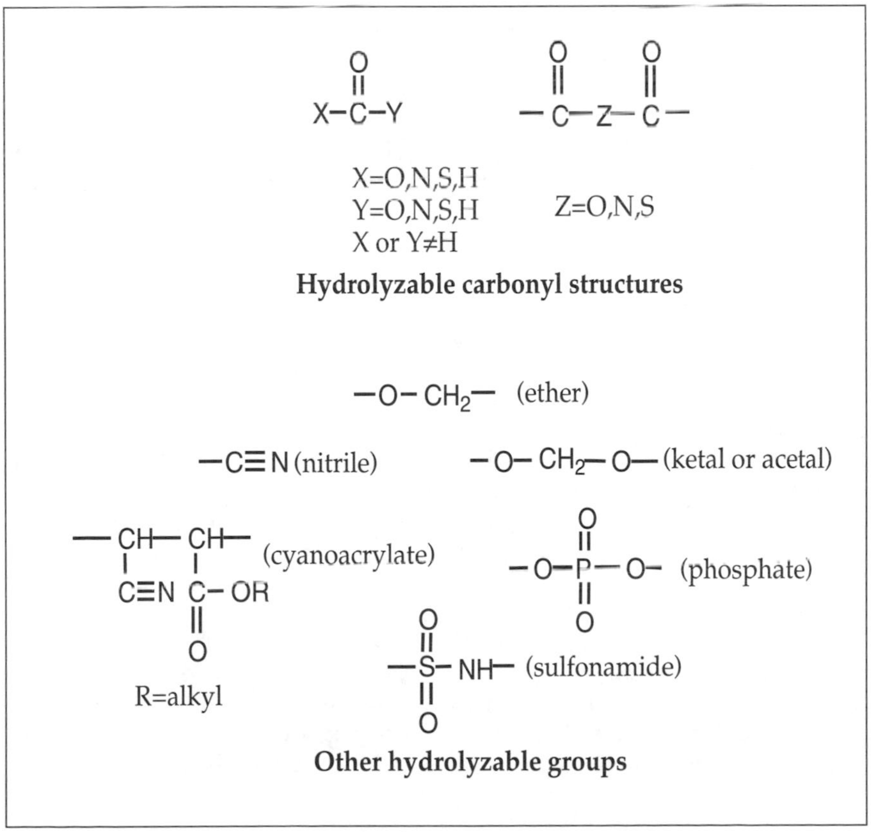

Fig. 43.1. Hydrolytically susceptible groups.

Fig. 43.2. Oxidatively susceptible groups.

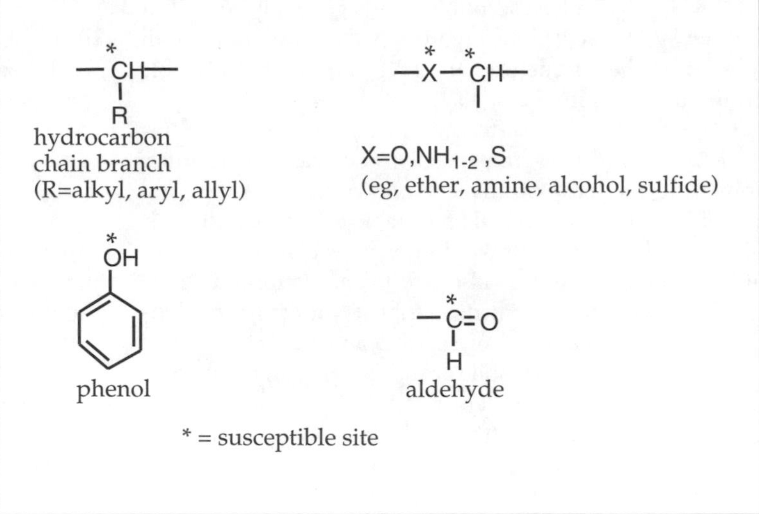

hydrocarbon chain branch (R=alkyl, aryl, allyl)

X=O,NH$_{1-2}$,S (eg, ether, amine, alcohol, sulfide)

phenol

aldehyde

* = susceptible site

Calcification

Calcification or mineralization involves the deposition of calcium phosphate salts on or within implanted structures. These phenomena are termed extrinsic and intrinsic calcification respectively. Extent of calcification is related to the level of soluble calcium and the device function, more than the chemical composition of the material.[25,26] Calcification has been reported to occur with synthetic vascular prostheses, causing stiffening and obstruction.[25] The most prominent effects of calcification occur, however, in devices that undergo extensive cyclical deformations in vivo (e.g., prosthetic heart valves, heart assist devices).[25] Generation of microscopic defects in the polymer may produce nucleation sites for the initiation of crystal formation, which can lead to extensive mineralization and, ultimately, mechanical failure of the device. Chemical degradation of the biomaterials has not yet been implicated in initiating or promoting calcification. Anticalcification additives have been applied to synthetic biomaterials with some success.[26] Vascular implants that undergo moderate deformation should present a relatively low risk for calcification.

Polymers with Potential to Serve as Biostable Scaffolds

This section describes polymers with potential for use as scaffolds for permanent tissue engineered vascular prostheses. Commercial polymers used in existing prostheses will be described first. Polymers that may not have been commercialized but have been described in the literature for use in medical devices will be briefly described. Finally, commercial polymers that have not been reported in vascular prosthesis literature, but may satisfy the design requirements for scaffolds listed above, will be mentioned.

All of the polymers to be described are assumed to contain additives such as processing aids and stabilizers. Different grades, lots or brands of polymers with the same generic structure may be more or less stable as a result of additives, processing conditions, molecular weight differences, crystallinity differences and other variables.

The emphasis of this section is primarily on biostability, although product design and biocompatibility are not ignored. The general assumption is that the latter two requirements can be met by approaches described in this book if the scaffold can perform its function for the intended period.

Poly(Ethylene Terephthalate)(PET)

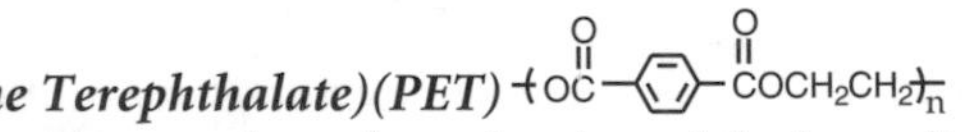

PET vascular prostheses have dominated the large diameter field since their introduction in 1957.[27] PET displays several advantages in its "standard" or "micro-denier" fiber form. It is a strong material having a tensile strength in oriented form of 170-180 MPa and a tensile modulus of about 14,000 MPa.[28] It is readily fabricable into woven or knitted textile or mesh form. It can be crimped to enhance kink resistance. It is relatively stable. Although it is based on the hydrolytically susceptible ester group, it is highly crystalline (MP ~ 265°C) because of its ordered chain structure and deep drawing during fiber formation.[9] Implant durability studies have shown or estimated progressive deterioration of physical properties over decades as a consequence of hydrolysis, and, possibly, some oxidation induced by activated phagocytes.[29-31] In vivo studies have projected approximately 30 years to full resorption in humans.[29,30]

PET is relatively stable to sterilization by ethylene oxide and ionizing radiation;[32,33] however, techniques involving steam, dry heat or chemically reactive sterilants[32-34] may cause deformation or degradation.

Mitigating against the use of PET for small diameter prostheses is the high reactivity of blood and vascular tissue toward the implant with consequent high inflammation, neointimal proliferation and inhibition of cellular regeneration. This response to PET has been demonstrated with textile vascular prostheses[35-39] and vascular stents in open mesh configuration.[40,41] The blood and vascular tissue reactivity of PET can vary with the proprietary additives and treatments applied to the individual manufactured devices.[42]

PET has successfully served as the structural matrix for composite vascular devices. Albumin, collagen or gelatin impregnation of PET textile prostheses is performed to seal them against blood leakage.[38-43] Healing responses of the composite are comparable to the unsealed PET.[44] The Omniflow Vascular Prosthesis (Bio Nova, International) is formed from PET mesh placed on a silicone mandrel and implanted in sheep to produce a collagen-PET composite device. It has been used successfully for peripheral vascular replacement.[45] Other modifications, such as incorporation of bioactive molecules[46,47] and surface modification for blood compatibility[48] have shown promise.

In sum, PET should be considered a highly credible candidate for biostable vascular scaffolds.

Polytetrafluoroethylene(PTFE) $+CF_2CF_2\frac{}{n}$

PTFE is a member of the fluorocarbon class of polymers. It is, by far, the most commonly used fluorocarbon[49] in implants because of its demonstration of long term biostability and biocompatibility in vivo. PTFE vascular prostheses are prominent in the medium diameter (~7-9 mm) and dialysis access markets.[27]

The polymer is prepared in powdered form from tetrafluoroethylene monomer. The product is a highly crystalline material (> 90% crystallinity) which is not completely fusible, but is formed into shapes by sintering.[49] A densely sintered configuration approaches the intrinsic properties of the material and gives a moderate stiffness (tensile modulus of elasticity = 0.5 GPa) and tensile strength (14 MPa).[49]

Implantable forms of the material of interest for vascular prostheses include the "expanded" and textile products.[50] Expanded PTFE (ePTFE) is made by an extrusion, drawing and sintering process[50] to produce a tube with a porous wall consisting of fibrils and nodules which is controllable to different pore sizes (e.g., 30 and 60 μm). The porosity can be used advantageously to promote ingrowth of tissue and formation and retention of an endothelial layer in vascular prostheses.[51,52]

Knitted PTFE cloth is effectively used as sewing rings for heart valve prostheses,[53,54] and should be considered when a textile configuration for a biostable scaffold is preferred. It should be noted here that the preparation of PTFE fibers requires the use of sizing agents which must be removed by vigorous (and proprietary) cleaning processes.

PTFE has a notable shortcoming—its susceptibility to degradation by ionizing radiation as experienced during gamma sterilization.[32,33] It is completely stable to other forms of sterilization, however.

Another potential issue with PTFE concerns the adherence of other materials to its surface. The polymer is noted for its release properties, and this is an advantage for declotting vascular access prostheses.[27] However, if a hybrid bio-artificial device requires the bonding of a substantial amount of tissue to the PTFE surface (i.e., without complete mechanical interlock), a potential for delamination may exist. This factor has been recognized and promising approaches to enhance the binding of, for example, endothelial cells are being developed. These include denucleation of ePTFE by saturating its pores with water, use of surfactants and treatment with adhesion molecules (e.g., fibronectin) or adhesion peptides.[52,55]

Polypropylene(PP) $+CH-CH_2\frac{}{n}$ with CH_3

PP has considerable appeal as a biostable scaffold. It is a relatively strong (tensile strength = 400 MPa), crystalline, high modulus (tensile modulus = 2.6 GPa) thermoplastic in its isotactic form.[56] Its hydrocarbon structure renders PP insensitive to hydrolytic attack. However, since every other atom on the polymeric chain is a tertiary carbon, it is susceptible to oxidation during processing, storage and implantation.[57] This type of degradation can be effectively countered by the use of antioxidants, which are universally used in PP products.[57,58] Consequently, stabilized PP is considered a "permanent" implant material.

Biostability, strength, and durability combined with a relatively low inflammatory tendency[59-61] make stabilized PP the material of choice for vascular anastomotic sutures,[59-61] certain ligament augmentation devices[58,62] and mesh for surgical repair.[63]

PP yarns have been woven into multifilament tubes for investigation as single component vascular prostheses[59] or as the reinforcing matrix for partially absorbable composite devices.[64] Chronic animal implant studies indicated that PP offered potential advantages in efficacy over expanded PTFE and PET in small diameter vascular applications.[59] Biomechanical behavior, which could be readily modulated by varying fiber diameter and weaving conditions, was shown to have a significant effect on tissue ingrowth and the resulting hybrid bio-artificial composite.[64,65]

PP is one of the least resistant structural polymers to sterilization by ionizing radiation.[32,33] However, it is safely sterilized by chemical agents and autoclaving.[32-34]

Recent innovations in the technology of PP include a syndiotactic product and an ionomer (ion-containing polyethylene)-modified isotactic PP which produce lower moduli (0.5 GPa) than isotactic PP (2.6 GPa).[56] Finally, a formulation of polypropylene rendered radiation resistant by the incorporation of hindered amine light stabilizers and a plastomeric ethylene polymer has been described.[66]

PP is normally considered a low surface energy, hydrophobic material to which surface bonding is difficult. However, certain highly hydrophobic cellular strains adhere strongly to PP.[67] This suggests that the adherence of tissue generated on PP scaffolds should be studied on a case by case basis with consideration of the possibility surface modification to control delamination.

Polypropylene should be considered in the top tier of candidates for biostable vascular matrices.

Polyurethanes(PUR) $-NHCO-$ with O double bond

PURs comprise a large family of polymers which is notable for its diversity. The only required attribute that individual members have in common is the presence of the urethane [-NH(CO)O-] group in some repeating sequence on the main chain, from the reaction of an isocyanate group with an alcohol group. Most likely, however, there are other functional groups which make up the soft segment of the PUR, which is generally a copolymer consisting of hard and soft segments. The hard segment generally consists of the

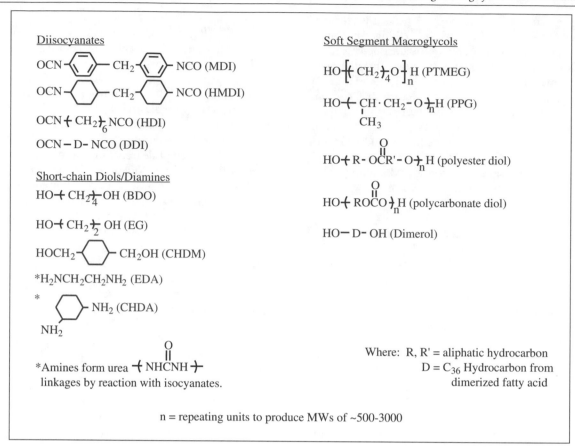

Fig. 43.3 Monomers for polyurethanes.

reaction product of a diisocyanate and a diol or diamine. The soft segment is derived from a macromonomer ranging from several hundred to several thousand in molecular weight.[10] Typical monomers for polyurethanes which have been used as "permanent" implants are listed in Figure 43.3.[10] Most of the polyurethanes used in medical devices are based on difunctional monomers.

Commercial PURs usually contain additives such as catalyst residues, processing aids and stabilizers. These additives often migrate to the surface of the PUR part and serve as the material in contact with blood or soft tissue.[10] Certain PURs have demonstrated relatively low thrombogenicity.[10]

PURs range in physical properties from soft, tough elastomers to strong, rigid structural polymers (e.g., tensile strength = 20-50 MPa, tensile modulus = 5-1150 MPa).[10] As a result, PURs have been considered for soft, flexible implantable device components such as pacemaker lead insulation[15] tubing and compliant vascular prostheses[68-70] as well as hard, rigid components such as pacemaker lead connectors.[10] The polyurethanes used in medical devices are usually formed into shapes by solution or melt processes[10] and can be solution or melt spun into fibers, cast into porous or solid-wall structures, or extruded into solid-wall tubing.

The record for PURs in "permanent" implants is mixed, because of hydrolytic and oxidative degradative mechanisms that may come into play. Generally, the site of

biodegradation is the soft segment (ester, ether, carbonate). While hydrolysis of the urethane (or urea) hard segment linkages is possible, those groups are relatively stable and do not comprise the primary mode of biodegradation.

Polyester soft segments have generally degraded quickly and severely by hydrolysis.[16] Polyether urethanes are susceptible to oxidative degradation as described in the "Modes of Polymer Degradation" section, above.[71,72] Since oxidative susceptibility is generally proportional to ether content,[9,10,15,16] relatively hard (low ether content) PURs have performed with minimal degradation for periods as long as the lifetime of pacemakers (8-10 yr). Even soft polyether urethanes are capable of performing as intended for years in the absence of high stress or strong oxidative attack.[15,16]

Over the past few years, several industrial concerns have reported on the development of polyurethanes based on polycarbonate soft segments.[69,73-75] These have shown very high resistance to degradation in short term studies, although minor hydrolytic effects have been noted on the implant surfaces.[69,76] However, in vascular implants approaching one year, structural degradation of the poly(carbonate urethane) fibers was detectable.[69] This is predictive, in my opinion, of a progressive hydrolytic degradation that should make a device designer very wary of choosing poly(carbonate urethanes) as "permanent" scaffolds until long term (> 5 years) studies have confirmed their stability.

An approach to polyurethane design that uses soft segments composed entirely of hydrocarbon molecules (i.e., a 36 carbon structure derived from dimerized fatty acids) with no ether, ester or carbonate groups to degrade[77,78] has theoretical appeal. However, this concept must also pass the test of long term implant stability before it may be used with confidence.

Polyurethanes are generally resistant to sterilization of all types except steam and, possibly, dry heat.[10] They are susceptible to calcification, especially in highly dynamic applications such as leaflet heart valves.[25]

Although polyurethanes display some of the most favorable mechanical properties for compliant grafts, no composition has yet demonstrated dependable long term stability in vivo, especially as a fibrous vascular implant.

Polyethylene(PE) $+CH_2\text{-}CH_2+_n$

PE is produced in several forms including very low density (VLDPE), low density (LDPE), medium density (MDPE), high density (HDPE), linear low density (LLDPE) and ultra high molecular weight (UHMWPE), each with different thermal and mechanical characteristics.[49] The variations in density and physical properties result from differences in polymerization conditions or the use of other olefinic hydrocarbon comonomers.[49] All of these molecular structures are amenable to fabrication into fibers or cellular structures, which are the forms most likely to meet the requirements of the "design concept."

Although PE has been reported as being used in vascular prostheses[40] and is regularly used in several forms of permanent implants,[79] recent literature describing its use in vascular prostheses is sparse. More commonly reported is the use of solid-wall polyethylene tubing with or without coatings for thrombogenicity studies.[80-82] The studies show that PE can be modified to improve surface wetability for binding of coatings (e.g., heparin)[81] and, potentially, other components for tissue engineered prostheses. Structurally, PE compositions range from relatively low to medium modulus when thermally processed (Table 43.1).[83]

PE in its various structural forms is stable to hydrolytic media and resistant to oxidation in proportion to its ratio of linear to branched chain structure and crystallinity. PE is susceptible to the phenomenon of environmental stress cracking (ESC) produced by exposure of stressed specimens to aggressive media such as detergents (and, possibly, blood). Cracking occurs because of stress relaxation of "tie mol-

ecules" in the zones between crystalline regions in these semi-crystalline polymers.[84] ESC is reduced in PE with lower crystallinity (LLDPE) or higher molecular weight (UHMWPE) because of higher concentrations of tie molecules relative to crystalline regions.[84] Therefore, two forms of PE, LLDPE[85] and UHMWPE, have theoretical appeal for ESC resistant fiber-based prostheses. The latter has been used as fibers for sutures.[86] The LLDPE is reported to be resistant to cracking.[85] A previously unmentioned form of PE deserves mention—gel-spun UHMWPE. These fibers achieve levels of tensile strength (2-4 GPa) and tensile modulus (125-175 GPa) that are multiples of the PE levels reported above.[87] Their high stability and strength at very low fiber diameters are potentially useful design features for scaffolds.

PE is resistant to chemical sterilization and susceptible to degradation by ionizing radiation.[22] Most forms of thermal sterilization would warp the relatively low melting PE (MP 104-135°C).[83]

The PE family, in my opinion, has not received adequate consideration for use in filament-based vascular prostheses.

Polydimethylsiloxane (PDMS) $+O\text{-}\underset{\underset{CH_3}{|}}{\overset{\overset{CH_3}{|}}{Si}}+_n$

The PDMSs comprise a family of thermoset elastomers with a long history of successful use in implantable devices.[79,88] Structural devices are usually produced by crosslinking 2-part systems at room temperature or higher. The crosslinked products are highly elastic and extensible. The tensile modulus (2-9 MPa) and ultimate tensile strength (2-10 MPa) are relatively low compared to other polymers considered in this chapter.[10] However, excellent flex fatigue resistance and tear resistance of some compositions,[10] combined with high biostability,[88,89] make PDMS a worthy contender for compliant vascular prosthesis scaffolds.

PDMS has been studied in vascular prostheses. Because of its low modulus, porous-wall structures have been favored over filamentous configurations. The "Replamineform" process uses sea urchin spine machined into tubular shape as template for fabrication of porous PDMS vascular devices.[90,91] The spine, consisting of microporous calcite, is dissolved in acid, leaving behind an open-cell PDMS structure with adequate strength and the potential for tissue ingrowth.[90]

PDMS derives much of its strength from silica filler. The filler is actively thrombogenic; however, PDMS without filler can be used as a less thrombogenic coating.[82] PDMS has been used as a surface for endothelial cell growth;[82] however, it is a relatively low energy surface and the authors caution that resistance to cell detachment under conditions of blood flow must be verified before a hybrid device based on PDMS is deemed suitable for long term function.[82]

PDMS can be sterilized under relatively mild ionizing radiation conditions and by heat or chemical sterilants.[32]

A final note on PDMS is in order. The PDMS class of elastomers has come under severe scrutiny in recent years because of its use in mammary prostheses. Reports of autoimmune responses to implanted devices have focused

Table 43.1. Properties of PE compositions[83]

2	Tensile Strength (MPa)	Tensile modulus (MPa)
LDPE	15-80	55-170
MDPE	10-20	170-380
HDPE	15-35	415-1035

on PDMS oil-filled PDMS shell designs. Leakage of the oil is alleged to cause systemic responses to PDMS.[92] However, decades of successful use of PDMS in solid form[79,93] provide a massive body of evidence that these materials are chemically stable and safe as implants. The list of suppliers of PDMS for "permanent" implants is currently short, but PDMS raw materials are available[93] and these elastomers merit serious consideration as scaffolds for "permanent" hybrids.

Other Polymer Scaffold Materials

This subsection speculates briefly on polymers that have not received much reported consideration for vascular prostheses, but are judged to have the potential to meet the design criteria for a tissue engineered device. The selection is based on my experience in working with or considering the materials for use in "permanent" implants. The sparseness of available information offers the opportunity for technical advancement associated with several risks. At best, there will be substantial development expense to assure successful implementation. There will likely be increased regulatory complexity for new vascular materials. A new vascular material is riskier, because an established clinical history would have revealed characteristics of a material that might not be anticipated in the development plan. Finally, there is the risk that some of these materials have been studied by others and rejected for good cause without the results being published.

The subsection is now separated into two parts, the first listing high-modulus linear polymers which are best utilized in fiber form, the second listing low-modulus elastomers which may be fabricated into fiber-based, solid-wall or porous devices.

High Modulus Polymers

PTFE is just one of several polymers which belong to the fluoropolymer category. It also includes: poly(ethylene tetrafluoroethylene), poly(ethylene chlorotrifluoroethylene), poly(vinylidine fluoride), fluorinated ethylene propylene, perfluoroalkoxy resin, polychlorotrifluoroethylene and others.[49,94] They all offer exceptional resistance to hydrolysis and oxidation. Just as with PTFE, they are sterilizable by all common means except, possibly, ionizing radiation.[32] The "other" fluoropolymers are worth considering as an alternative to PTFE because most are more readily proccessable by melt or solution techniques. They also offer a broad range of modulus characteristics to choose from.[94]

Several rigid polyamides should have the chemical resistance to provide long term service in vivo. These include Nylon 11, Nylon 12[95] and aromatic polyamides (Aramids).[96,97] Their stability arises either from hydrophobicity of the backbone (Nylon 11, 12) or high crystallinity (Aramid). Braided Aramid fiber prostheses have been studied for artificial ligaments.[96,97] While mechanical degradation was observed under dynamic conditions,[96] long term chemical stability in human plasma was confirmed.

Certain aromatic polyesters and poly(ester amides) belong to a class of polymers called liquid crystalline polymers (LCPs). They are so named because of their high degree of order in the liquid phase. Upon cooling, these polymers solidify to structures with anisotropic skin-core morphologies and tensile properties among the highest of known polymers (i.e., tensile strengths to 240 MPa, tensile moduli to 32 GPa).[98] Chemical degradation resistance is also exceptionally high. The materials can be readily extruded into tubing and fibers.[99] If the fibers are not too stiff, LCPs may be worth considering as structural matrices for hybrid vascular prostheses.

A group of rigid thermoplastics having amorphous or semicrystalline morphologies and superior resistance to chemical degradation includes the polysulfones (polysulfone, polyethersulfone, polyarylsulfone) the polyketones (PEK, PEEK, PAEK, PEKK, where P=poly; A=aryl; E=ether; K=ketone), poly(ether imide), polyimide, poly(methyl methacrylate) and others.[98,100-104] The stated polymers normally would comprise the nonfibrous component of a fiber-reinforced composite used, for example, in orthopedic devices.[100-104] Investigation of fibrous forms of these materials is a worthwhile undertaking, in my opinion. This is being done with poly(methyl methacrylate) currently, and the results are impressive.[103] For example, the ultimate tensile strength of PMMA can be increased from 25-50 MPa to as high as 220 MPa while enhancing ultimate elongation from 5-35% with fiber drawdown ratios of ~20.[103,104] Tensile moduli increase from ~2 GPa in castings to ~8 GPa in the fibers, which would suggest the use of very thin fiber diameters in vascular scaffolds.

Poly(acrylonitrile-co-vinyl chloride) has been fabricated into hollow fiber form as a cell encapsulation membrane for hybrid bio-artificial organs and hemo-filtration membranes. It has been shown to be stable in long term implants and can likely be extruded or solution spun into fibers suitable for consideration for vascular scaffolds.[105]

Low Modulus Elastomers

Elastomers meriting consideration in this subsection, in addition to the ones already considered, may be either thermoplastic or thermoset. Both types may be fabricated into fibrous, porous or solid wall form. Thermoset rubbers are often prepared from prepolymers ("millable gums") by hot molding processes. In such cases, residues from the "vulcanization" (crosslinking) process may need to be removed by extraction to make the scaffold nontoxic. The elastomers are often compounded with fillers, stabilizers, processing aids and other ingredients to control physical and chemical properties of the final product.

Certain of the compositions to be described may not be available in prepolymer form for fabrication into desired shapes, but are sold in finished form by the materials manufacturer. Therefore, any evaluation of a scaffold configuration would require the approval and fabrication by the material supplier. In these times of high liability risk, some elastomer suppliers may not approve the use of their product as "permanent" implants.

Nonetheless, elastomers offer the potential advantage of radial compliance and deserve consideration. This section provides a very brief overview, but recent reviews of elastomers are more detailed and comprehensive.[106,107]

Polyolefins include rubbers synthesized from olefinic hydrocarbons, generally crosslinked with dienes. Rubbers of ethylene, propylene, isobutylene and higher olefins are included here. They may be compounded to various ranges of strength, hardness and elongation. They are highly resistant to hydrolysis, and have low residual olefin content for oxidation stability (in contrast to rubbers from dienes such as butadiene). However, they have branched-chain sites which may be susceptible to irradiation and thermooxidative degradation, similar to polypropylene. One polyolefin, poly(1-hexene) crosslinked with methyl hexadiene, has enjoyed special success in implantable devices (finger joints, artificial heart pumps, compliance chambers, intervetrebral discs).[106] It has excellent biocompatibility (after solvent extraction), fatigue resistance and biostability.

Fluoroelastomers and fluorosilicone elastomers should have excellent resistance to processing, storage and biological media while retaining low modulus and resilience of true elastomers.[106,107]

Polychloroprene, a diene rubber, will not hydrolyze and has much greater resistance to oxidation than other diene rubbers (e.g., natural rubber, butadiene rubber). It should be quite biocompatible if extracted after vulcanization.

Many other elastomers are available commercially which may be worth considering as scaffolds.[106,107] The ones selected for discussion are the ones I might select in a first round of testing. All of those listed in this subsection would require substantial process development and validation before clinical studies would be justified.

Concluding Comments

The extensive list of polymers suggested as potential scaffolds for hybrid bio-artificial vascular prostheses was feasible because the "design concept" was rather broad and limited in detail. With a more stringent set of design criteria in place, some of the polymer candidates should be eliminated. The strategy of this chapter was to be inclusive, so that the major categories of relatively stable polymers were captured. One category and one polymer within that category will be the best one. The search for that biomaterial offers certain challenge but great potential reward.

Finally, I offer a biased opinion about the hybrid device discussed in this chapter. Ideally, the permanent scaffold is an interim solution on the road to a resorbable scaffold which would produce a completely biological, fully functional neo-artery. My personal experience with a degradable cellular polyurethane vascular prosthesis was that a biological conduit indeed was generated. It had many of the structural elements of natural artery, but they were not organized in the same way. The conduit dilated to unacceptable levels over several months. Dilatation was also observed by other investigators using this type of material.[108]

A successful result requires guided tissue regeneration which withstands the pressures of the arterial system for the long term. The answer will likely lie in the structural design of the temporary scaffold, its mechanical properties and its degradation characteristics. The pursuit of this design is,

indeed, a worthy one which I believe will ultimately be successful.

Acknowledgments

The literature provided by Drs. Giovani Galletti, Robert Guidoin, Howard Greisler, Vince Medenhall, Colin Pitt and J. Paul Santerre is gratefully acknowledged. I sincerely thank Mrs. Sandra Brigham for her expert preparation of this manuscript.

References

1. Stoeger KJ. Implementing the new quality system requirements. Design controls. Biomed Instrum Technol 1997; 31(2):119-127.
2. AAMI Standards and Recommended Practices. Biological evaluation of medical devices. Washington, D.C.: Assoc for the Advancement of Med Instrumentation, 1996:4.
3. Graham L, Whittlesey D, Bevacqua B. Cardiovascular implantation: Vascular grafts. In: Ratner B et al, eds. Biomaterials Science, An Introduction to Materials in Medicine. San Diego: Academic Press, 1996:420-422.
4. Kantor C. Biological small diameter vascular grafts. AAMI Medical Device Research Report 1996; 3(1):8-11.
5. Galletti PM. Biomaterials availability in the U.S. J Biomed Mater Res 1996; 32(3):289-291.
6. Citron P. Medical devices: Factors adversely affecting innovation. J Biomed Mater Res 1996; 32(1):1-2.
7. O'Connor KW. Biomaterial bill passes Congress, signed into law. The AIMBE News, Fall, 1998; 6(3):1,2.
8. Coury AJ. Preparation of specimens for blood compatibility testing. Cardiovasc Pathol 1993; 2(3) (Suppl):1015-1105.
9. Coury AJ. Chemical and biochemical degradation of polymers. In: Ratner B et al, eds. Biomaterials Science, An Introduction to Materials in Medicine. San Diego: Academic Press, 1996; 243-260.
10. Coury AJ, Slaikeu P, Cahalan P et al. Factors and interactions affecting the performance of polyurethane elastomers in medical devices. J Biomater Appl 1988; 3:130-179.
11. Zhu KJ, Hendren RW, Jensen K et al. Synthesis, properties and biodegradation of poly(1,3-trimethylene carbonate). Macromolecules (1991); 24:1736-1740.
12. Santerre JP, Labow RS, Adams GA: Enzyme-biomaterial interactions: Effect of biosystems on degradation of polyurethanes. J Biomed Mater Res 1993; 27:97-109.
13. Ratner BD, Gladhill KW, Horbett TA. In vitro studies of the enzymatic biodegradation of polether urethanes. Trans 12th Ann Mtg Soc Biomater 1986; 9:190.
14. Ratner BA, Tyler BJ. Variations between biomer lots 2: The effect of differences between lots on in vitro enzymatic and oxidative degradation of a commercial polyurethane. J Biomed Mater Res 1993; 27:327-334.
15. Stokes K, Coury A, Urbanski P. Autooxidative degradation of implanted polyether polyurethane devices. J Biomater Appl 1987; 1:412-448.
16. Coury AJ, Stokes KB, Cahalan PT et al. Biostability considerations for implantable polyurethanes. Life Support Systems 1987; 5:25-39.
17. Sutherland K, Mahoney JR, Coury AJ et al. Degradation of materials by phagocyte-derived oxidants. J Clin Invest 1993; 92:2360-2367.
18. Santerre JP, Labow RS, Duguay DG et al. Biodegradation evaluation of polyether- and polyester-urethanes with

oxidative and hydrolytic enzymes. J Biomed Mater Res 1994; 28:1187-1199.

19. Taylor G, Gsell R, King R et al. Stability of N_2 packaged gamma irradiated UHMWPE. Trans 23rd Ann Mtg Soc Biomater 1997; 20:421.

20. Furman BD, Reish TG, Li S. The effect of implantation on the oxidation of ultra high molecular weight polyethylene. Trans 23rd Ann Mtg Soc Biomater 1997; 20:427.

21. Wang A, Polineni VK, Essner A et al. Effect of radiation dosage on the wear of stabilized UHMWPE evaluated by hip and knee joint simulators. Trans 23rd Ann Mtg Soc Biomater 1997; 20:394.

22. Premnath V, Harris WH, Jasty M et al. Gamma sterilization of UHMWPE articular implants: An analysis of the oxidation problem. Biomaterials 1996; 17:1741-1753.

23. del Prever EB, Crova M, Costa L et al. Unacceptable biodegradation of polyethylene in vivo. Biomaterials 1996; 17:873-878.

24. Lewis G. Polyethylene wear in total hip and knee arthroplasties. J Biomed Mater Res 1997; 38(1):55-75.

25. Pathak Y, Schoen FJ, Levy RJ. Pathologic calcification of biomaterials. In: Ratner B et al, eds. Biomaterials Science, An Introduction to Materials in Medicine. San Diego: Academic Press, 1996; 272-281.

26. Joshi RR, Frautschi JR, Phillips RE. Immobilized heparin and heparin-bisphosphonate prevent polyurethane calcification and thrombosis: In vitro and in vivo studies. 5th World Biomater Congress 1996; May 29-June 2: 610.

27. Ku DN, Allen RC. Vascular grafts. In: Bronzino JD, ed. The Biomedical Engineering Handbook. Boca Raton: CRC Press, Inc 1995; 1871-1878.

28. Lawton EL, Ringwald EL. Physical constants of Poly(oxyethylene oxyterephthaloyl)[poly(ethylene terephthalate)]. In: Brandrup J., Immergut EH, eds, Polymer Handbook. 3rd Ed, New York: John Wiley & Sons, 1989:V101-V105.

29. Williams DF. Review: Biodegradation of surgical polymers. J Mater Sci 1982; 17:1239-1240.

30. Kopecek J, Ulbrich K. Biodegradation of biomedical polymers. Prog Polym Sci 1983; 9:31.

31. Ambrosio L, Apicella A, Mensitieri M et al. Physical and chemical decay of prosthetic ACL after in vivo implantation. Clin Mater 1994; 15:29-36.

32. Lee HB, Kim SS, Khang G. Polymeric biomaterials: Sterilization. In: Bronzino JD, ed. The Biomedical Engineering Handbook. Boca Raton: CRC Press, Inc 1995; 581-592.

33. Kowalski JB, Morrissey RF. Sterilization of implants. In: Ratner, B et al, eds. Biomaterials Science, An Introduction to Materials in Medicine. San Diego: Academic Press 1996; 415-420.

34. Booth AE. Industrial sterilization technologies: New and old trends shape manufacturer choices. Med Device Diagn Industry; 1995; Feb: 64-72. **Author: Please provide volume number rather than month.**

35. Zenni GC, Ellinger J, Lam T et al. Biomaterial-induced macrophage activation and monokine release. J Invest Surg 1994; 7:135-141.

36. Greisler HP, Petsikas D, Cziperle DJ et al. Dacron stimulation of macrophage transformtin growth factor-β release. Cardiovasc Surg 1996; 4(2):169-173.

37. Greisler HP, Dennis JW, Endean ED et al. Derivation of neointima in vascular grafts. Circ 1988; 78(Suppl 1):I-6 to I-12.

38. Swartbol P, Truedsson L, Parsson H et al. Tumor necrosis factor-α and interleukin-6 release from white blood cells induced by different graft materials in vitro are affected by pentoxifylline and iloprost. J Biomed Mater Res 1977; 36: 400-406.

39. Greisler HP, Schwarcz TH, Ellinger J et al. Dacron inhibition of arterial regenerative activities. J Vasc Surg 1986; 3(5):747-756.

40. Peng T, Gibula P, Yao K et al. Role of polymers in improving the results of stenting in coronary arteries. Biomaterials 1996; 17(7):685-694.

41. Murphy JG, Schwartz RS, Edwards WD et al. Percutaneous polymeric stents in porcine coronary arteries. Circ 1992; 86:1596-1604.

42. Marois Y, Guidoin R, Roy R et al. Selecting valid in vitro biocompatibility tests that predict in vivo healing response of synthetic vascular prostheses. Biomaterials 1996; 17:1835-1842.

43. Marois Y, Chakfe N, Guidoin R et al. An albumin-coated polyester arterial graft: In vivo assessment of biocompatibility and healing characteristics. Biomaterials 1996; 17:3-14.

44. Cziperle DJ, Joyce KA, Tattersall CW et al. Albumin impregnated vascular grafts: Albumin resorption and tissue reactions. J Cardiovasc Surg 1992; 33:407-414.

45. White JE, Werkmeister JA, Edwards GA et al. Structural analysis of a collagen-polyester composite vascular prosthesis. Clin Mater 1993; 14:271-276.

46. Fournier N, Doillon CJ. Biological molecule-impregnated polyester: An in vivo angiogenesis study. Biomaterials 1996; 17:1659-1665.

47. Greisler HP, Klosak I, Dennis JW et al. Endothelial cell growth factor attachment to biomaterials. Trans Am Soc Artif Intern Organs 1986; XXXII:346-349.

48. Phaneuf MD, Quist WC, Bide MJ et al. Modification of polyethylene terephthalate (Dacron) via denier reduction: Effects on material tensile strength, weight, and protein binding capabilities. J Appl Biomater 1995; 6:289-299.

49. Lee HB, Kim SS, Khang G. Polymers used as biomaterials. In: Bronzino JD, ed. The Biomedical Engineering Handbook. Boca Raton: CRC Press, Inc 1995; 580-591.

50. Shalaby S. Classes of materials used in medicine: Fabrics. In: Ratner B et al, eds. Biomaterials Science, An Introduction to Materials in Medicine. San Diego: Academic Press 1996; 118-124.

51. Greisler HP. Growth factor release from vascular grafts. J Controlled Release 1996; 39:267-280.

52. Greisler HP, Johnson S, Joyce K et al. The effects of shear stress on endothelial cell retention and function on expanded polytetrafluoroethylene. Arch Surg 1990; 125:1622-1625.

53. Changdran KB. Blood-interfacing implants. In: Bronzino JD, ed. The Biomedical Engineering Handbook. Boca Raton; CRC Press, Inc 1995; 648-655.

54. Yoganathan AP. A brief history of heart valve prostheses. In: Bronzino JD, ed. The Biomedical Engineering Handbook. Boca Raton: CRC Press, Inc 1995; 1848-1853.

55. Wigod MD, Klitzman B. Quantification of in vitro endothelial cell adhesion to vascular graft material. J Biomed Mater Res 1993; 27:1057-1062.

56. Liu CK. Medical fibers spun from polypropylene. Proc 13th Southern Biomed Eng Conf 1994; 748-751.

57. Williams DF. Review: Biodegradation of surgical polymers. J Mater Sci 1982; 17:1233-1237.

58. Gibbons DF, Mendenhall HV, Van Kampen CL et al. The effect of motion on the tissue response to polymeric fiber implants. Clin Mater 1994; 15:37-41.

59. Greisler HP, Tattersall CW, Henderson SC et al. Polypropylene small-diameter vascular grafts. J Biomed Mater Res 1992; 26:1383-1394.

60. Bakkum EA, Dalmeijer RAJ, Verdel MJC et al. Quantitative analysis of the inflammatory reaction surrounding sutures commonly used in operative procedures and the relation of postsurgical adhesion formation. Biomaterials 1995; 16:1283-1289.

61. Faulkner BC, Tribble CG, Thacker JG et al. Knot performance of polypropylene sutures. J Biomed Mater Res (Appl Biomater) 1996; 33:187-192.

62. McPherson GK, Mendenhall HV, Gibbons DF et al. Experimental mechanical and histologic evaluation of the Kennedy ligament augmentation device. Clin Orthop 1985; 196:186-195.

63. Bellon JM, Contreras LA, Bujan J et al. Effect of phosphatidyl choline on the process of peritoneal adhesion following implantation of a polypropylene mesh prosthesis. Biomaterials 1996; 17:1369-1372.

64. Greisler HP. Effects of polypropylene's mechanical properties on histological and functional reactions to polyglactin 910/polypropylene vascular prostheses. Am Coll Surg Surg Forum 1987; XXXVIII:323-326.

65. Zenni GC, Gray JL, Appelgren EO et al. Modulation of myofibroblast proliferation by vascular prosthesis biomechanics. ASAIO J (1993); Vol. 39, No. 3:M496-M500.

66. Portnoy R. Clear, radiation-tolerant, autoclavable polypropylene. Med Plast Biomater 1997; 4(1):40-48.

67. Kiremitci-Gumusderelioglu M, Pesmen A. Microbial adhesion to ionogenic PHEMA, PU and PP implants. Biomaterials 1996; 17:443-449.

68. DeCossart L, Annis D. An assessment of rigidly controlled technique for the implantation in dogs of a new microfibrous 3.8 mm I.D. polyurethane arterial prosthesis. Proc 2nd Ann Scientific Session, Acad Surg Res 1986; Oct. 31-Nov. 1, Clemson SC: 36.

69. Zhang Z, Marois Y, Guidoin RG et al. Vascugraft® polyurethane arterial prosthesis as femoro-popliteal and femoro-peroneal bypasses in humans: Pathological, structural and chemical analyses of four excised grafts. Biomaterials 1997; 18:113-124.

70. Doi K, Matsuda T. Enhanced vascularization in a microporous polyurethane graft impregnated with basic fibroblast growth factor and heparin. J Biomed Mater Res 1997; 34:361-370.

71. Zhao QH, McNally AK, Rubin KR et al. Human plasma α_2-macroglobulin promotes in vitro oxidative stress cracking of Pellethane 2363-80A: In vivo and in vitro correlations. J Biomed Mater Res 1993; 27:379-389.

72. Schubert MA, Wiggins MJ, Anderson JA. Role of oxygen in biodegradation of poly(etherurethane urea) elastomers. J Biomed Mater Res 1997; 34:519-530.

73. Szycher M, Edwards A, Carson RJ. In vivo testing of a biodurable polyurethane. Trans 23rd Ann Mtg Soc Biomater 1997; 296.

74. Ward RS, White KA, Gill RS. Development of biostable thermoplastic polyurethanes with oligomeric polydimethylsiloxane end groups. Trans 21st Ann Mtg Soc Biomater 1995; 18:268.

75. Kato YP, Dereume JP, Kontges H et al. Preliminary mechanical evaluation of a novel endoluminal graft. Trans 21st Ann Mtg Soc Biomater 1995; 18:81.

76. Mathur AB, Collier TO, Kao W et al. In vivo biocompatibility and biostability of modified polyurethanes. J Biomed Mater Res 1997; 36:246-257.

77. Coury AJ, Hobot CM, Iverson VB. Novel soft segment approaches to implantable biostable polyurethanes. Trans 4th World Biomater Cong 1992; 661.

79. Visser SA, Hergenrother RA, Cooper SL. Classes of materials used in medicine: Polymers. In: Ratner B et al, eds. Biomaterials Science, An Introduction of Materials in Medicine. San Diego: Academic Press 1996; 50-60.

80. Rubens FD, Weitz JI, Brash JL et al. The effect of antithrombin III-independent thrombin inhibitors and heparin on fibrin accretion onto fibrin-coated polyethylene. Thromb Hemost 1993; 69(2):130-134.

81. Evangelista RA, Sefton MV. Coating of two polyether-polyurethanes and polyethylene with a heparin-poly(vinyl alcohol) hydrogel. Biomaterials 1986; 7:206-211.

82. Keough FM, Mackey WC, Connolly R et al. The interaction of blood components with PDMS [polydimethylsiloxane and LDPE (low-density polyethylene)] in a baboon ex vivo arteriovenous shunt model. J Biomed Mater Res 1985; 19:577-587.

83. Quirk RP, Alsamarraie MAA. Physical constants of poly(ethylene). In: Brandrup J and Immergut EH, eds. Polymer Handbook. 3rd Ed. New York: John Wiley & Sons, 1989:V15-V26.

84. Lustiger A. Understanding environmental stress cracking in polyethylene. Med Plast Biomaterials 1996; 3(4):12-18.

85. Thermoplastic Processes, Inc. LLDPE tubing resists cracking. Med Plast Biomater 1996; 3(3):61.

86. Tomita N, Tamai S, Morihara T et al. Handling characteristics of braided structure materials for tight tying. J Appl Biomater 1993; 4:61-65.

87. Prevorsek DC. Preparation, structure, properties and applications of gel-spun ultrastrong polyethylene fibers. Trends Pol Sci 1995; 3(1):4-11.

88. McMillin CR. An assessment of elastomers for biomedical applications. In: Szycher, M, ed. High Performance Biomaterials. Lancaster: Technomic Publishing Co, Inc 1991; 37-49.

89. Chawala AS, Hinber I. Laboratory evaluation of explanted gel filled silicone breast implants. Trans World Biomater Cong 1996:300.

90. Tizian C, Salyer KE. Production process of a microvascular prosthesis using the "replamineform" principle. Int J Artif Organs 1980; 6:364-465.

91. Hiratzka LF, Goeken JA, White RA et al. In vivo comparison of replamineform silastic and bioelectric polyurethane arterial grafts. Arch Surg 1979; 114(6):698-702.

92. Nicholson J III, Hill SL, Frondoza CG et al. Silicone gel and octamethylcyclotetrasiloxane [D4] enhances antibody production to bovine serum albumin in mice. Trans 5th World Biomater Cong 1996; 304.

93. Winn A. Factors in selecting medical silicones. Med Plast Biomater 1996; 3(2):16-19.

94. Resins and compounds: Fluoroplastics. In: Kaplan WA, managing ed. Modern Plast Encyclopedia '97. New York: McGraw-Hill Co's., Inc., 1996:B158-B160.

95. Resins and compounds: polyamides. In: Kaplan WA, ed. Modern Plast Encyclopedia, '97. New York: McGraw-Hill Co., Inc., 1996:B175.

96. Durselen L, Claes L, Ignatius A et al. Comparative animal study of three ligament prostheses for the replacement of the anterior cruciate and medical collateral ligament. Biomaterials 1996; 17(10):977-982.

97. Wening JV, Lorke DE. A scanning electron microscope (SEM) investigation of Aramid (Kevlar) fibers after incubation in plasma. Clin Mater 1992; 9:1-5.

98. Canale B, Hanley S, Braeckel M. New possibiliities for liquid crystal polymers. Med Plast Biomater 1995; 2(3):24-31.

99. ACT Medical, Inc. Liquid crystal polymer tubing. Med Device Diagn Industry 1997; 19:211.

100. Moore R, Beredjiklian P Rhoad R et al. A comparison of the inflammatory potential of particulated derived from two composite materials. J Biomed Mater Res 1997; 34:137-147.

101. Zhang G, Latour Jr RA, Kennedy JM et al. Long-term compressive property durability of fiber reinforced polyetheretherketone composite in physiological saline. Biomaterials 1996; 17(8):781-789.

102. Barton AJ, Sagers RD, Pitt WG. Bacterial adhesion to orthopedic implant polymers. J Biomed Mater Res 1996; 30:403-410.

103. Gilbert JL, Ney DS, Lautenschlager EP. Self-reinforced composite poly(methyl methacrylate): static and fatigue properties. Biometerials 1995; 16:1043-1055.

104. Lewis G. Properties of acrylic bone cement: state of the art review. J Biomed Mater Res (Appl Biomater) 1997; 38:155-182.

105. Shoichet MS, Rein DH. In vivo biostability of a polymeric hollow fiber membrane for cell encapsulation. Biomaterials 1996; 17(3):285-290.

106. McMillin CR. An assessment of elastomers for biomedical applications. In: Szycher M, ed. High Performance Biometerals. Lancaster: Technomic Publishing Co., Inc., 1991:37-49.

107. Courtney PJ, Sevenson JA, Verosky C. Bonding elastomers with adhesives. Med Plast Biomater 1997; 4(3):60-68.

108. Galletti G, Farruggia F, Baccarini E et al. Prevention of platelet aggregation by dietary polyunsaturated fatty acids in the biodegradable polyurethane vascular prosthesis: An experimental model in pigs. Ital J Surg Sci 1989; 19(2):121-130.

Scaffold Engineering

Material Aspects

---------------------- CHAPTER 44 ----------------------

Biophilic Polymers: What's on the Horizon?

Patrick T. Cahalan

This chapter was outlined for a section of this book entitled 'Bio-Interactive' Prostheses, and was further subdivided to a section including biostable polymers/materials. The other chapter in this subsection, titled "Biostable Polymers as Durable Scaffolds for Tissue Engineered Vascular Prostheses" is being written by a dear colleague, Art Coury, who shares this author's sense of trepidation as to achieving substance in the context of the remaining chapters of the overall section. It is hoped that, although this chapter will be written from an industrial perspective, it will have some practical value for the reader.

The word biophilic cannot be found in the dictionary, but then neither can the word biocompatible. In the early 1980s materials were placed in four basic groups:

1. Bioinert;
2. Biocompatible;
3. Bioactive; and
4. Biointeractive.

Bioinert surfaces were hypothesized to be "invisible" to the body, and to have little or no interaction. Proposed early examples were negative surface charge to repel cell adhesion,[1] high surface energy materials[2] such as pyrolytic carbon and low critical surface tension materials[3] such as fluoropolymers, which also claimed low protein and platelet adhesion. Also in the early 1980s, hydrophilic materials were suggested to be low protein adsorbing and platelet adhering,[4] and in particular PEG-like surfaces were claimed to have increased surface motion (flagella-like activity) that served to decrease protein adsorption and denaturation.[5] The term biocompatible could be applied to any material that when implanted showed an equal or better tissue response compared to a control material, such as polypropylene, that was accepted as biocompatible. Bioactive surfaces were surfaces designed to promote an advantageous effect such as preferential adsorption of albumin by C-18 alkylated surfaces.[6] Finally, biointeractive surfaces were those designed to interact with a specific physiological mechanism such as coagulation; an early example is ionically bound heparin for local release to decrease coagulation.[7,8] Heparin was finally covalently immobilized and shown to have bioactivity without releasing by Larm;[9] this surface has been shown in vitro to bind ATIII to produce a catalytic rate of thrombin deactivation. These categories were arrived at largely from the perspective of the empirical surface response, and arguably need some revaluation with more instrument-intensive analytical methods now available to properly order them by rank in a new era of tissue engineered materials.

The editors have chosen new labels, and have done so with the healing response in mind. Thus they have set the stage for the conceptual advantages of tissue engineering. In labeling bio-inert materials as those exhibiting insufficient healing, biolized (endothelialized surfaces) as surface healing, and bio-interactive as complete healing, they have set the goal to incorporate all that has been learned to date towards designing materials and structures

---

Tissue Engineering of Prosthetic Vascular Grafts, edited by Peter Zilla and Howard P. Greisler.
©1999 R.G. Landes Company.

that should more closely approximate naturally functioning tissue. In the early years of vascular graft implantation, Voorhees' observations with Vinyon "N" cloth in dog aortas clearly showed that a synthetic material could serve as a conduit, and be accepted by the tissue.[10] Tissue engineering, or the integration of biology and biomaterials, holds out the promise of producing more than an accepted conduit, and obviating all the problems associated with the current commercial products such as thrombotic occlusion, anastomotic hyperplasia, aneurysmal dilatation, and infection. Presumably, bio-interactive prostheses are the desired approach to achieving this goal.

During the period between 1982 and 1988, this author was involved with research to find a small diameter (4 mm or less) vascular graft that could exhibit patency at least equivalent to that of autologous saphenous vein. In reality the effort was more a development, or an evaluation exercise, that included animal implantation of numerous technology platforms to include:
1. Biodegradable polyurethane-PLLA grafts;
2. Biostable polyurethane grafts made by phase inversion, electrostatic spinning, and spray techniques;
3. Alternatively (non glutaraldehyde) fixed heterografts;
4. Plasma TFE coated Dacron prostheses;
5. Silicone replamarinaform porous conduits; and
6. Dacron and PTFE control grafts from commercial sources.

Predominant modes of failure were: aneurysmal dilatation (1 and 2); in vivo degradation across species (3); rejection by surgeons at the need to cut the prostheses with an electrical device (the flaming graft), and undesirable suture characteristics (4); poor crush resistance leading to thrombotic occlusions, and poor suture pull out properties (5). The Dacron and PTFE grafts had patency rates not competitive with autologous vein, and in general showed a fibrotic nonintegrated histology. Fabricating prostheses for implantation gives one an appreciation for necessary mechanical properties such as suture strength, ease of suture, burst strength, porosity, and wall thickness for matching vessel anastomosis. Since these properties have been achieved for the most part in commercially available materials, it was felt that applying surface modification technologies to existing materials might be able to control problems such as thrombosis and anastomotic hyperplasia, and possibly achieve a healing response that would result in neovascularization, endothelialization, and a tissue response that was not primarily a fibrotic or a chronic inflammatory response. The latter could help a graft towards long term patency and infection resistance.

If one defines biophilic polymers as those specifically synthesized to interact in an advantageous manner with the body, there are many claims, but few real candidates are on the near horizon for application. There are numerous claims for heparinoid polymers.[21] These polymers often have carboxyl and sulfate functionality approximating the ratio contained in heparin. Studies showing less adhered platelets, or changing clotting times, are generally used as proof of heparin-like activity. In light of studies demonstrating the unique pentasaccharide sequence required for activation of ATIII, and slight changes in this structure resulting in 90% to complete loss of heparin activity, it is highly optimistic to hope for a synthetic anionic polymer with heparin properties.[22] Studies in our laboratory with compounds reported as heparinoid or anticoagulant fail to produce heparin-like activity when measured in solution with ATIII and thrombin. Surfaces with immobilized cationic or anionic character can adsorb ATIII and thrombin respectively, and give false positives for heparin activity. An amine functional surface can show binding of ATIII that is resistant to extensive 0.15 ionic strength rinsings, and if given time will deactivate thrombin, though not in a catalytic fashion. An anionic surface can bind thrombin that does not rinse off in the normal rinse steps used before difference measurement using chromogenic substrate, giving a false measure of thrombin deactivated. Active thrombin can be witnessed by adding substrate back to the surface and obtaining a color change in the substrate. Since it is well known that anionic surfaces are contact activating, it is of concern to have an anionic surface present that does not have high heparin activity. Since coagulation is so dependent on platelets, it is hypothesized that by using a polymer that mimics the nonactivated platelet membrane, namely phosphatidylcholine, it would be possible to prevent platelet interaction with the polymer surface (Fig. 44.1).

Phosphatidylcholine in the form of commercially available lecithin can coat surfaces of hydrophobic polymers, but is easily removed with flowing plasma. In attempt to remedy this problem, commercial efforts have given rise to a network polymer with strong adhesive properties to polymers, and containing pendant phosphorylcholine moieties as seen in Figure 44.2.[23]

The most common network polymer is an acrylate backbone that has good adhesive properties for PVC and polyurethanes. The polymer gives excellent wetting properties to the surfaces it coats, and has very low platelet adhesion. Human blood testing in our laboratories show this polymer to be promising, but material-dependent.

Perhaps the most innovative biophilic polymer synthesis to date is the work of David Tirrell in recombinant artificial structural proteins. These polymers hold out the potential of engineering proteins with controlled crystallinity and expression of specific peptide sequences at surfaces. If desirable mechanical properties can be engineered into the protein polymers, and if processing methods are devised to make fibers, extrusion, or coating possible, then these polymers can make their way into devices.

There has been somewhat of a rebirth in surface modifying additives (SMAs). If a commercial group could blend in additives to polymers that would express themselves on surfaces of devices that their customers manufacture, and demonstrate enhanced biological response, then a premium price could be charged for such materials. To date, because of the lack of tonnage of polymers used in biomaterials, it has been less than attractive for larger chemical companies to specifically manufacture biomaterials. That, together with the liability issues surrounding medical devices, makes it difficult to see new formulations coming from the larger chemical companies. SMA technology is particularly being

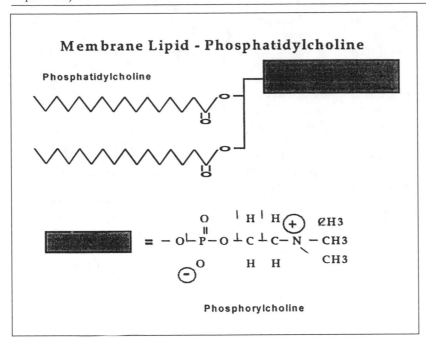

Fig. 44.1. Membrane lipid—phosphatidylcholine.

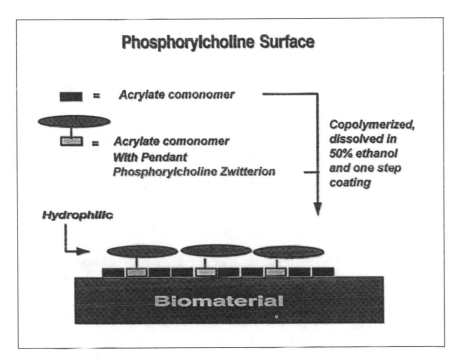

Fig. 44.2. Phosphorylcholine surface.

applied for blood-contacting surfaces for short term use, such as cardiopulmonary bypass circuits.

For the most part, biophilic polymers on the near horizon are going to be polymers that have been surface modified. Simple adsorbed coatings will be problematic from the standpoint of assuring stability for permanent implants, and there continues to be a quest for the universal biophilic polymer that can coat all materials. It was the choice of our group to attempt to comprehensively evaluate methods to covalently couple molecules to the surfaces of common polymeric biomaterials in hopes of creating new modified biophilic polymers that are stable and have controlled loading of bioactive molecules. If we achieve covalent and stable

attachment, then, with some license in nomenclature, we have created new polymers. In light of later chapters on surface modification for specific surfaces, we hope that it is appropriate in this chapter to discuss the more general methods of surface modification that can be used to get to the biophilic surface, and point to critical concerns and opportunities that may be afforded from our experiences.

In 1989 we created a biomaterials laboratory in Maastricht, The Netherlands. The main objective was to focus on surface modification technologies to improve the biocompatibility of materials used to construct biomedical devices. The industrial laboratory was ideally situated 100 meters from the Biomedical Research Institute of The

University of Maastricht, and the group of Professor Coen Hemker, an experienced and respected expert in thrombosis and hemostasis. A partnership was established between the University of Maastricht (RL), The Bakken Research Center (BRC) and The Center for Surface and Materials Analysis (CSMA), in Manchester, England. The BRC was to provide modified biomaterials for characterization by CSMA, using predominantly XPS and TofSIMS, and biocompatibility testing by RL. The partnership received a three year research subsidy from the EC in the form of a Brite EuRam grant (BE 5972). In this project a broad survey of physical and chemical methods to modify biomaterials was performed (Table 44.1), and these methods were evaluated on seven common biomaterials for feasibility.[11] Equipped in our laboratory with a plasma reactor, corona treater, ozone generator, UV photopolymerization equipment, and a nearby gamma-beta commercial irradiation source, we were prepared to generate many of the surfaces proposed to be more biocompatible for head to head comparisons with our partners' assistance. What will be presented in this chapter are our somewhat narrow perspectives on making polymers biophilic; our experience with synthesis is limited to modifying the surface of biomaterials, and does not include creating new bulk polymers. With respect to the latter, we maintain surveillance of the literature and sample new materials through our testing schemes when available from the developers.

The processes mentioned in Table 44.1, although not complete, represent treatments that were performed on at least 3-7 common materials for each method. Some brief comments will be given here that are felt to be important concerning these surface modification methods and their applicability to biomaterials and biomedical devices.

Physical Methods

Irradiation

Early work by Ratner and Hoffman[4] showed the potential of grafting biomaterials with irradiation sources. Our efforts included irradiation using electron beam sources to successfully graft to polyolefins. E-beam or gamma radiation can introduce several functionalities to polymeric materials, such as free radicals, vinyl bonds and, in the presence of oxygen, hydroperoxides, carbonyls, aldehydes and carboxyl groups. This can also be accompanied by crosslinking or chain scission, the former leading to increase in tensile properties and the latter to polymer degradation. The first consideration on the use of irradiation should be if the polymer to be modified is predominantly a crosslinking or chain scission polymer. Some common chain scission polymers are polymethylmethacrylate (PMMA), polytetrafluoroethylene (PTFE), poly(vinylidene chloride), polyisobutylene (and copolymers) and polypropylene. Attempting to modify these materials with irradiation may give a surface modification, but on a degraded material. Recent high voltage accelerators with high penetration potential have been suggested as an alternative, because relatively low total dosage is required. It has also been suggested that total devices can be modified.[12] The listed materials that are claimed to have been successfully modified include in particular the scission polymer PMMA. These irradiation techniques, particularly when grafting is performed in situ, require near oxygen free environments and thus create some problems for ease of manufacture. Nevertheless, irradiation is a very effective method for covalently grafting molecules to biomaterial surfaces.

Plasma

Plasma polymerization has been touted as the most exact method to modify biomaterial surfaces; this is in a large part due to the control over the plasma gases, and the thickness and uniformity of the modified surface. Some drawbacks to plasma are:

1. Requirement for reactor specific design based on geometry and materials of construction;
2. In almost all cases the process will be a batch operation; and
3. Contamination of the reactor and thus the requirement for cleaning cycles and for single process dedication of reactors. Several investigators have proposed simple plasma treatment to make materials more hydrophilic and thus more blood compatible.[13] Plasma treatments may show initial lowering of contact angle, and will follow with an inversion within hours back to a hydrophobic surface. The latter is particularly true of elastomers.

Plasma polymerized surfaces can be directly deposited on a surface, or plasma can be used to activate a surface for subsequent grafting of molecules. The latter is difficult, as the surface generally requires a short plasma discharge time, or pulsed plasma discharge. It has been hypothesized that free radicals are short lived on the surface of plasma treated materials, due largely to the rapid termination by vicinal radicals.[14] A final observation on plasma-modified surfaces is that the reactivity in terms of coupling further biomolecules has been less than expected. Evaluation of coupling to plasma functionalized surfaces based on the results of XPS data suggests that a significant portion of the functional groups do not react. One possible explanation is that organic chemistry, and particularly biomolecules, react in three dimensions, and the plasma surface is highly ordered and rather two dimensional in its ability to enter into reactions.[15] If one sees new biophilic surfaces as containing high

Table 44.1. Methods to functionalize/activate surfaces (Brite EuRam)

Physical	Chemical
Irradiation	Oxidation
Plasma	Reduction
Corona	Hydrolysis
CVD and PVD	Ozonization
"Simple" Coating	Silanization
Entanglement	Grafting
Textruing	Photocuping
Ion Beam Implant	Add'n/Subst'n

density biomolecules such as heparin, proteins and/or growth factors, they will have to be coupled postplasma treatment and the ability to control the quantity and density of coupling may prove to be a challenge.

Corona

Corona treatment has been used extensively in industry for improvement of adhesion. It is also the subject of several papers on surface activation to effect grafting to surfaces.[16-18] Several affinity schemes can be used to attach biomolecules to the grafted surfaces. Corona treatment is a rough process compared to plasma discharge, and takes place in an air atmosphere. This results in a highly oxidized surface, to include sufficient free radicals to effect grafting of vinyl monomers. It can be used to graft to most polymers, but does not work for most fluoropolymers. Corona and plasma can be used to make surfaces more wettable for simple adsorptive coating approaches. There are several suggested universal adsorptive coating schemes that often require a pretreatment such as corona to improve the uniformity of coating as well as the adhesive strength of the coating to the base material.

CVD and PVD

Chemical vapor deposition (CVD) and physical vapor deposition (PVD) have long been used in industry as barrier coatings. In the European food industry, PVD has been used to apply a layer of SiO to packaging material to prevent moisture transmission through wrapping. CVD has been used in electronics to provide moisture barriers and insulative coatings. It was hoped that these methods could be used as a base for engineering biologically active surfaces. The ability to deposit a metallic surface such as gold would give a base for self assembled surfaces.[19] It has also been suggested that a ceramic based PVD surface could be activated to produce functionality (carboxyl groups) to which biomolecules could be coupled.[20]

Simple Coatings

We define simple coatings as those that are designed to be applied by simple dipping, spraying, or by pumping solutions through devices. There is a plethora of coatings of this nature offered for short term blood compatibility. All of these coatings have performance that is material dependent; this problem is often overcome by a pretreatment such as corona. Special attention should be paid to devices made from materials that undergo bending and flexing, as these coatings may have a tendency to crack. Dislodgement of the coating may cause a problem, depending on the application. Most manufacturing engineers of biomedical devices will require a battery of tests to assure integrity of the coating, especially if the device is to be a permanent implant such as a vascular graft. While the list of short term coatings is long, the list for permanent implants is very limited.

Entanglement

In the late 70s and early 80s the wide acceptance of Biomer as a blood compatible material led to several applications where the device was simply coated with the polyurethane polymer. This was best effected by finding a solvent that could attack the surface of the material to be coated and result in a mixing of polymer chains that would give a mechanical bond upon solvent removal. The same method has been used to imbrue drugs into polymers using solvents that could swell the polymer, taking in the drug and leaving it upon solvent evaporation. The latter method has been used for introducing antimicrobial agents to polymers. The same principle applies for SMAs or blooming agents. Addition of amphipathic molecules to polymers can result in the more hydrophilic portion being expressed on the polymer surface, anchored by the more hydrophobic end entangled in the polymer surface. In the case of polyurethanes, most contain processing waxes that migrate to the surface and prevent the polymer from being tacky during extrusion. One such additive, ethylene bis-stearamide wax, has been reported to be in part responsible for improved blood compatibility. Studies in our laboratory of such additives reveal that performance in blood is optimal immediately after thermal processing, but changes with time. XPS shows considerable increase over time in amide functionality, which may be less effective than the long fatty chain in improving blood compatibility. It appears that perhaps entanglement or SMAs may be difficult to control at the surface, and thus present some challenges to be solved.

Texturing

Professor Andreas von Recum has been one of the leading researchers in the field of tissue response to textured surfaces. He has demonstrated that textured implants with internodal distances of approximately 1-3 microns appear to have much thinner capsules, indicating less fibrotic response.[38,39] One of the hypotheses offered in explanation is that the textured surface allows for more stable anchorage of fibroblasts, and less destruction of these cells due to microvibration that can lead to further inflammatory response. A possible further explanation is that the microtextrue allows for an improved production and attachment of extracellular matrix on the material surface. Research on immunoisolation membranes by Becton Dickinson presented at an ACS workshop indicated that optimal surface texture could result in minimal capsule formation and vascular structures present very close to the material surface. The latter was independent of the material of construction for the membrane. Applying microtextrue to devices is a developing technology, and one promising approach is the use of photopolymerization. This technique holds out the promise of introducing texture and chemistry to surfaces, plus the ability to use photo resists or screening techniques to pattern the sights for cellular attachment to surfaces. Application of this technology to vascular grafts will be more complicated than simply applying this technique to the inside of a polymeric tube that has laser drilled holes for porosity if one hopes to maintain other important features for grafts such as porosity for ingrowth, kink resistance, compliance, and suture characteristics.

Ion Beam Implantation

Ion beam has been used to impart surface texture in addition to surface chemistry. In the orthopedic area it is useful in improving fixation of prostheses to tissue. The Spire Corporation offers ion beam treated surfaces for improved slip properties and antimicrobial surfaces, and has made claims to improved blood compatibility.[24] As with PVD, a metallic surface could provide advantages for further surface modification using self assembling techniques. Ion beam implantation can result in crosslinking the surface, and impart mechanical properties to the material. The tendency for cracking of the surface on elastomers and materials that will see chronic flexing should be considered. For elastomeric materials, and in particular silicone, the resultant surface may still present the elastomer chemistry primarily.

Chemical Methods

Oxidation, Reduction, Hydrolysis

Most synthetic polymers do not possess functionality to perform coupling reactions. Several of the physical methods mentioned can oxidize the surface and produce radicals, hydroxyl, carboxyl, and carbonyl groups. This oxidation can also be induced by chemical means such as acid etching or treatment with peroxides.[25] For fluoropolymers that are oxidation resistant, reduction by exposure to sodium metal in napthalene can produce unsaturation in the polymer, and subsequent direct grafting of hydrogels can be effected.[26] Hydrolysis, particularly of esters, can introduce functional groups such as carboxyls to surfaces. All these methods involve degradation of the polymer, and it is necessary to control or limit the degradation to have stable surfaces, as well as to prevent degradation of the mechanical properties of the base material.

Addition/Substitution

Some polymers such as polyurethane have sites that can be attacked by proton extracting bases such as sodium hydride. The reduced urethane group can then undergo alkyl substitution using alkyl halides such as octadecyl iodide.[27] An impressive body of work has been documented by the group of Cooper, showing improvement in blood compatibility and the ability to control the loading of alkyl groups on the surface. This method of introducing alkyl groups to the surface may provide better and more stable performance than previously mentioned methods using SMAs.

Ozonization

Treatment of materials by exposure to ozone has proven effective in activating surfaces for subsequent grafting reactions.[28] Ozone can be applied as a gas or dissolved in water, which gives very attractive manufacturing features for devices with complex geometry and multiple materials, as ozone is effective on almost all polymers save fluoropolymers. Ozone is primarily an oxidative approach, and can produce peroxy radicals, but also can introduce functionality from oxidative degradation. Because it can result in degradation, care needs to be taken to control the exposure time, concentration of ozone, and temperature. These can be done fairly easy in aqueous solutions. The ozone penetrates materials at different rates and this can be measured using colorimetric methods.[29] Materials modified by ozone may need final reduction to assure that radicals are not present, and should undergo rigorous mechanical testing to assure no loss in durability of the native polymer substrate.

Silanization

Silanization is most frequently used for coupling to metal surfaces. The use of organofunctional silanes allows the addition of reactive organofunctional groups to the metal oxide surface. These groups can the be used to directly couple biomolecules. The most common mistake made with silanization treatments is improper application and cure methods. Excessive coating with silanes results in weak surfaces that will delaminate, and failure to properly hydrolyze the silane before drying will fail to create enough reactive silanol groups to couple during the dehydration and final formation of the polysiloxane network. Covalently attached heparin via silane activation has been released for commercial application to intravascular stents in Europe.[30]

Photocoupling

In 1969 Knowles demonstrated the effectiveness of 2-nitro-4-azidobenzene in forming a nitrene radical upon exposure to UV that could extract a proton directly from a polymeric backbone and substitute the organo group to which it was attached directly to the polymer.[31] Application of this method to the biological field was pioneered by Patrick Guire,[32] leading eventually to commercialization by the BSI (Biometric Systems Inc.) Corporation.[33] Numerous applications are envisioned by BSI to include enhancement of endothelial cell attachment, blood compatible surfaces, and infection resistant surfaces. While photocoupling appears to be a facile process of direct coupling to polymers, it is also material dependent, and often requires a pretreatment of the surface to remove contaminants or promote better wetting of the coupling reagents. It also often requires repeated coatings and light exposures to effect a uniform and dense coupling. This latter process can result in crosslinking of photobiomolecules within a matrix and somewhat diminish their activity. Careful cleaning of these surfaces is required to remove any unreacted or leachable species, as is the case with almost all surface modification approaches. Nevertheless, this method is receiving very favorable attention as a commercially feasible method to modify biomaterials, especially for short term use.

Grafting

Direct grafting of hydrogels to surfaces is only possible on a limited number of materials. The best know material is polyurethane, where the carbamate group can be activated using ceric ion initiation.[34] Another material also shown many years ago to undergo direct grafting is dialysis membrane.[35] Early studies on hydrogel grafted surfaces showed promises of being cell friendly.[36] Ratner and Hoffman, using a baboon shunt model, later showed that hydrogel surfaces may produce emboli and, while not being thromboadherent, were in fact capable of being thrombogenic. Attempts to utilize the positive aspects of grafted hydrogels by coupling bioactive agents is now commonplace. A possible advantage of this approach is lower protein adsorption and nonspecific cell adhesion. Grafted hydrogels do not require crosslinking and when coupled with biomolecules can express more bioactivity of the attached molecule. For most grafted hydrogels some sort of activation of the base polymer is required, such as plasma, corona, irradiation, or ozonization. Depending on the grafted species, additional functionalization may be required to provide optimal control of coupling with respect to loading and spacing chemistry. A good stable grafted hydrogel allows for numerous coupling strategies available from affinity chromatography techniques. Some affinity schemes have unstable bonds that are allowable for chromatographic application, but not desirable for biological application. The coupling scheme should be tested rigorously to assure that there is no leaching. In our laboratory we have found that grafting followed by intermediate functionalization allows for easier control and clean up of the grafted surface, as well as optimal loading of biomolecules, even to the point of presenting the biomolecule in high purity at the uppermost layers of the hydrogel.[37]

Summary

The horizon for biophilic polymers was discussed in this chapter with an obvious bias toward surface modification of polymers to make them biointeractive. Our efforts have led to covalent grafted surfaces on almost all common biomaterials including metals, and stable covalent biomolecules coupled to these surfaces. In our opinion, the closest thing to a biophilic commercially available polymer in the near future would be one that maintains high mechanical performance characteristics of existing polymers and contains pendant reactive groups that can have biomolecules coupled to these functionalities in an economic process. It is doubtful that a biomolecule could be reacted into a material and still maintain its activity through processing. It would be also difficult to expect optimal presentation of the biomolecule to the blood or tissue. It may be possible for certain molecules or drugs that are targeted for release, but probably not for scaffolding applications.

It is hoped that this chapter gives some useful information regarding several of the methods employed to make surfaces more biocompatible, and some appreciation for problems and opportunities that are attendant upon these methods. Knowledge of several techniques can allow for a number of combined processes that can bring optimal performance as well as economic reality to creating biocompatible surfaces.

References

1. Sawyer PN. Surface charge and thrombosis. Ann NY Acad Sci 1984; 416: 561-584.
2. Chin TH, Nyilas E, Turcotte LR. Microcalorimetric and electrophoretic studies of protein sorption. Trans Am SocArtif Intern Organs 1978; 24:389-402.
3. Andrade JD. Interfacial phenomena and biomaterials. Med Instrum 1976; 7:110-120.
4. Ratner BD, Weathersby P, Hoffman AS, Kelly MA, Scharpen LH. Radiation-grafted hydrogels for biomaterial applications as studied by the ESCA technique. J Appl Polym Sci 1978; 22:643-664.
5. Merrill EW, Salzman EW. Polyethylene oxide as a biomaterial. ASAIO Journal 1983; 6:60-64.
6. Munro MS, Eberhart RC, Make NJ, Brink BE, Fry WJ. Thromboresistant alkyl-derivatized polyurethanes. J Am Soc Artif Int Organs 1982; 6:65-75.
7. Leininger RI. Polymers as surgical implants. CRC Critical Reviews in Bioengineering 1972; 1:333-381.
8. Gott VL, Koepke DE, Daggett RL, Zarnstorff W, Young WP. The coating of intravascular plastic prostheses with colloidal graphite. Surgery 1961; 50:382.
9. Larm O, Larsson R, Olsonn P. A new nonthrombogenic surface prepared by selective covalent binding of heparin via a modified reducing terminal residue. Biomat Med Dev Art Org 1983; 11:161-173.
10. Voorhees AB, Jaretski A, Blakemore AH. The use of tubes constructed from Vinyon "N" cloth in bridging arterial defects. Ann Surg 1952; 135:332.
11. Cahalan PT. Brite EuRam Final Technical Report, Contract Number: BREu-336, Project Number BE-5972-92.Title: Surface modification of Biomaterials for Biomedical Devices. European research subsidy granted in Nove. 1992 running until Nov. 1995. Report available through European Commission, Director General XII, Science, Research, and Development, Rue de la Loi 200, B-1049 Brussels, Wetstraat 200, Brussels, Belgium Office: M075 1/5.
12. Goldberg et al. Surface modified surgical instruments, devices, implants, contact lenses and the like. U.S. Patent 5,100,689, Assignee: University of Florida, Gainesville March 31, 1992.
13. Andrade JD, Triolo PM. Surface modification and evaluation of some commonly used catheter materials. I. J Biomed Mater Res 1983; 17:129-247.
14. Suzuke M, Kishida A, Iwata H, Ikada Y. Graft copolymerization of acrylamide onto a polyethylene surface pre treated with a glow discharge. Macromolecules 1986; 19.1804-1808.
15. Dias AJ, McCarthy TJ. Synthesis of a two-dimensional array of organic functional groups: Surface-selective modifications of poly(vinylidene). Macromolecules 1984; 17:2529-2531.
16. Okada T, Ikada Y. Tissue reactions to subcutaneously implanted, surface modified silicones. J Biomed Mater Res 1993; 27:1509-1518.
17. Okada T, Ikada Y. In vitro and in vivo digestion of collagen covalently immobilized onto the silicone surface. J Biomed Mater Res 1992; 26:1569-1581.
18. Okada T, Tamada Y, Ikada Y. Surface modification of silicone for tissue adhesion. Biomaterials and Clinical Applications, 1987.
19. Whiteside et al. Langmuir, 1988; 4:365.
20. Gauckler L. Personal communication at The Monte Verita Conference on Biocompatible Materials Systems. Ascona, Switzerland, 1993: October 11.
21. Csomor K, Karpati E, Nagy M, Gyorgyi-Edeleny J, Machovich R. Blood coagulation is inhibited by sulphated copolymers of vinyl alcohol and acrylic acid under in vitro as well as in vivo conditions. Thrombosis Research, 1994; 74(4):389-398.

22. van Boeckel CAA. From heparin to a synthetic drug: A multi-disciplinary approach. Trends in Receptor Research. Elsevier Publishers B.V. 1993.

23. Ishihara K, Nakabayashi N, Nishida K, Sakakida M, Shchiri M. Designing biocompatible materials. Chemtech, 1993.

24. Sioshansi P. Ion beam modification of materials for biomedical application. Seminar; Biomaterials: Medical and Pharmaceutical Applications, sponsored by Technomic Publishing Company, Inc, 851 New Holland Ave., Lancaster, PA: 1990.

25. Larsson N, Senius P, Eriksson JC, Maripuu R, Lindberg B. J Colloid Interface Sci, 1982; 90:127-136.

26. Yun JK, DeFife K, Colton E, Stack S, Azeez A, Cahalan L, Verhoeven M, Cahalan PL, Anderson JM. Human monocyte/macrophage adhesion and cytokine production on surface-modified poly(tetrafluoroethylene/ hexafluoropropylene) polymers with and without protein preadsorption. J Biomed Mater Res, 1995; 29:257-268.

27. Pitt WG, Cooper SL. Albumin adsorption on alkyl chain derivatized polyurethanes: I. The effect of C-18 alkylation. J Biomed Mater Res 1988; 22:359-382.

28. Yamauchi J, Yamaoka A, Ikemoto K, Matsui T. J Appl Polym Sci 1991; 43:1197-1203.

29. Kulik E et al. Poly(ethylene glycol) enriched surface: Reduced vs delayed protein adsorption and activation. Abstract from Firth World Biomaterials Congress. Toronto, Canada: 1996:May 29-June 2.

30. Cahalan L et al. Biocompatible medical article and method. U.S. Patent 5,607,475. Assignee: Medtronic Inc. 1997:March 4.

31. Knowles JR. Accounts of Chemical Research 1972; 5:90-119.

32. Guire P, Fliger D, Hodgson J. Photochemical coupling of enzymes to mammalian cells. Pharmacological Research Communications, 1977; 9(2).

33. Guire PE. Binding reagents and methods. U.S. Patent 4,722,906, Assignee: Bio-Metric Systems Inc. 1988:Feb. 2.

34. Annual Report (July 1, 1971-June 30, 1972), Medical Devices Applications Program of the National Heart & Lung Institute, Bethesda, MD.

35. Luttinger M, Cooper CW. J Biomed Mater Res 1967; 1:67.

36. Ratner BD, Horbett T, Hoffman AS. Cell adhesion to polymeric materials: Implications with respect to biocompatibility. J Biomed Mater Res, 1975; 9:407-422.

37. Hendriks M. A study on the covalent surface-immobilization of collagen. Development of biomaterials with enhanced infection resistance; a surface modification approach, Ph.D. Thesis from University of Eindhoven, 1966.

38. von Recum AF, Park JDB. Permanent percutaneous devices, CRC Crit Rev Bioeng 1981; 5:37-77.

39. von Recum AF, van Kooten TG. The influence of microtopography on cellular response and the implications for silicone implants. J Biomater Sci Polymer Edn 1995; 7:181-198.

Scaffold Engineering

Material Axpects

――――――――――――――――――――― CHAPTER 45 ―――――――――――――――――――――

Bioresorbable Grafts: A Counterintuitive Approach

David Fox, David A. Vorp, Howard P. Greisler

Overview

This chapter reviews the use of bioresorbable materials in vascular grafting. First, the theoretical basis for the use of bioresorbable materials is presented. Next, the various materials and the results of experimental work with them are discussed. Bioresorbable materials have been incorporated into vascular prostheses in a number of novel ways. Accordingly, the chapter is organized primarily by the manner in which bioresorbable materials have been incorporated. These include the bioresorbable material as a stand-alone graft, in combination with nonresorbable materials as a partially resorbable bi-component, or compound graft, and finally as a supportive scaffold over a biological graft. The chapter also discusses the use of biological grafts that have been chemically modified so as to be at least partially resorbable.

Definitions

The terms biodegradable, bioresorbable and bioabsorbable have been used relatively interchangeably in the literature reporting this heterogeneous class of biomaterials. An attempt was made to reach a consensus on precise definitions at The First International Scientific Consensus Workshop on Degradable Materials held in Toronto in 1989. Biodegradation was defined as "loss of a property (of a biomaterial) caused by a biological agent." The Workshop was unable, however, to agree on definitions of degradation, bioabsorption and bioresorption.[1] Therefore, in this chapter the terms biodegradable, bioresorbable and bioabsorbable are in general applied in accordance with the original authors, without implication of specific mechanisms of degradation.

Introduction

Despite the successful application of prosthetic grafts in the replacement of large arteries, the performance of prosthetics as medium and small caliber replacements has been less than satisfactory, resulting in both early and late graft failures, increasing the need for reoperation and limb loss. Factors contributing to these failures include thrombogenicity, inadequate tissue ingrowth and hyperproliferation of tissue with deposition of extracellular matrix resulting in myointimal hyperplasia.[2]

Biodegradable grafts have been investigated as a potential alternative to conventional biostable prosthetic grafts. The concept of a biodegradable graft emerged from the work of Arthur Voorhees' group at Columbia University. In 1954 Voorhees reported the first truly successful clinical application of prosthetic arterial prostheses, replacing 17 abdominal aortas and 1 popliteal aneurysm with grafts composed of Vinyon-N cloth tubes.[3] The success of the Vinyon-N fabric prostheses was in large part a function of its porosity, which allowed the ingress of capillaries and fibroblasts. This granulation tissue served as the nidus for the formation of an organized inner surface of flattened cells.[4] Thus, it became apparent that the graft material itself may be needed only transiently, to function as a scaffolding for regeneration of the vascular wall rather than as a permanent conduit.

After Voorhees' success, many other materials were proposed. Sigmund Wesolowski and his co-workers, working at Walter Reed, evaluated 45 prospective materials and confirmed the concept that the porosity of a graft material and not its inertness determined the success of a prosthetic vascular graft.[5] Prior to this time, the prevailing concept was that the biological inertness of a prosthetic material was the critical determinant of its clinical success as a vascular graft.[6] Wesolowski determined that grafts constructed of materials of relatively high porosity were resistant to late calcification and occlusion. The problem of hemorrhage during implantation, however, remained an important obstacle. To overcome this problem, the concept of constructing a composite graft emerged. The ideal composite graft would exhibit the property of low porosity at implantation, by virtue of a degradable component combined with a permanent component of high porosity. Over time, the degradable component would be depleted, leaving a high porosity graft capable of being incorporated by tissue.[7]

The feasibility of incorporating absorbable collagen and gelatin components into Dacron grafts had been reported by Humphries and Bascon in 1961.[8,9] Weselowski took a different approach, suggesting the use of a temporary scaffold fabricated from a slowly absorbable polymeric material as a vascular graft.[5] This scaffold would enable the arterial wall to reorganize by virtue of natural repair processes.[7] The American physiologist Claude Guthrie has been credited with the origin of this concept. In 1919 he wrote, "To restore and maintain mechanical function an implanted segment only temporarily restores mechanical continuity and serves as a scaffolding or bridge for the laying down of an ingrowth of tissue derived from the host."[10]

Since Wesolowski's report, many additional biodegradable materials have been proposed for use as components in the fabrication of vascular prostheses. These materials have been incorporated into grafts in a number of interesting and novel ways that will be described in this chapter. The majority of investigators have used the biodegradable material as a stand-alone graft. Others have constructed compound grafts wherein the degradable material is combined with a nonabsorbable prosthetic or biological graft. The degradable materials have been applied as a lining or wrap and in some cases have been interweaved with the prosthetic.

The biomaterials used in the fabrication of bioresorbable vascular grafts have a unique dual function. They serve as temporary vascular conduits while simultaneously inducing the regeneration of the arterial wall. As will be elaborated, complex interactions between the bioresorbable material and host macrophages are a critical step in the process of arterial regeneration.

Single Component Resorbable Grafts

The materials most commonly used in the fabrication of resorbable grafts have been synthetic polymers based upon naturally occurring hydroxy acids such as lactic and glycolic acid.[11] The rate of resorption of these copolymers is determined to a degree by the ratio of lactide to glycolide rings and decreases as the percentage of lactide component increases.[12] The primary mechanism of resorption is by the hydrolytic cleavage of ester bonds. Inflammatory cells such as macrophages, lymphocytes and neutrophils perform the final degradation and resorption.[11]

Polyglactin 910 (Vicryl)

Bowald's group from Sweden is credited with the first report of the use of a totally biodegradable prosthesis as a stand-alone replacement for large caliber vessels.[7] Knitted mesh composed of Polyglactin 910 (PG910), "Vicryl," manufactured by Ethicon Inc., was preclotted and interposed as tube and patch grafts into the thoracic aorta of growing pigs. PG910 is a polymer composed of glycolic and lactic acids and thus is absorbed by hydrolysis within 70 days.[13] The mesh had a pore size of 400 x 400 microns.[14]

The grafts were explanted at intervals up to 6 weeks. All grafts remained patent and no instances of graft rupture or aneurysmal dilatation occurred. At 40 days only small fragments of the PG910 remained and the grafted areas displayed some similarities to normal aortic walls. The luminal surface was covered with a monolayer of mature endothelial-like cells in a mosaic pattern. Beneath this was a layer of longitudinally directed smooth muscle-like cells. No internal elastic lamina was seen, although scattered fibrillar elastic material was found interspersed amongst the smooth muscle-like cells. An outer "adventitial" layer was reconstituted as well.[13] With respect to the source of the repopulating cells, Bowald observed that the endothelium and smooth muscle-like cells seemed to be derived from the cut edges of the native vessel. Occasional inflammatory and giant cells were noted around residual PG910 filaments in the 20 day explants.[14]

Late results after 2 years were reported for one pig that received a 10 mm by 4 cm tube graft in the thoracic aorta. The graft was patent angiographically. On gross examination it was free of thrombus, calcification or fatty infiltration. Of note, the diameter of the grafted area had increased proportionally in size with the nongrafted aorta and was not aneurysmal. They also reported reconstitution of a coarse internal elastic lamina.[15]

Based on these observations, Bowald sought to determine the maximal regenerative capacity of arterial tissue. To this end, the descending thoracic aorta of 20 pigs was bypassed with 8-10 mm diameter double layer Vicryl segments ranging from 7-20 cm in length. All animals receiving a graft greater than 15 cm in length died from graft rupture. There were no ruptures in the animals receiving grafts less than 15 cm and the histologic appearance of these grafts was equivalent to those in the previous reports.[16]

Extensive implant and in vitro work with lactic and glycolide copolymers have also been done by our group in the research laboratories of Loyola University. We have investigated PG910 and other copolymers including polyglycolic acid (PGA) and polydioxonone (PDS), as well as combinations of these polymers. PG910 grafts were implanted into the abdominal aorta of rabbits. Likewise, the transinterstitial migration and proliferation of ultrastruc-turally primitive mesenchymal cells that differentiated into smooth muscle-like myofibroblasts and the establishment of a confluent endothelial-like luminal lining cells was demonstrated, thus confirming Bowald's earlier observations (Figs. 45.1A-C).[14] This process was found to parallel the time

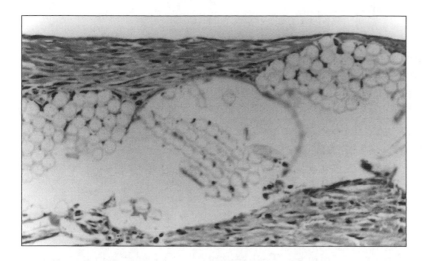

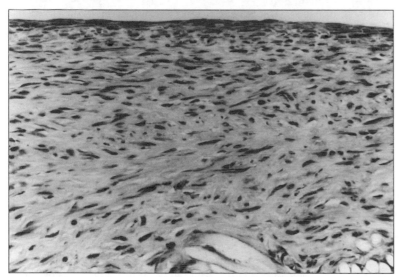

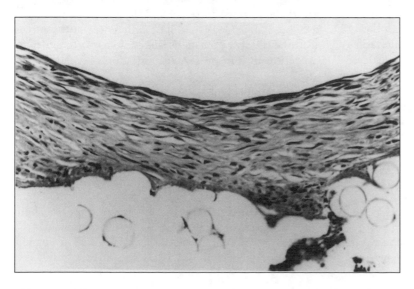

Fig. 45.1. Hematoxylin-eosin histologic sections (x25) from 1 month post implantation. (A, top) Dacron prosthesis demonstrating a confluent endothelial surface with a small subendothelial layer. (B, middle) Polyglactin 910 prosthesis demonstrating a thick subendothelial cellular inner capsule with an endothelial luminal surface. (C, bottom) Polydioxanone prosthesis demonstrating an endothelial lined luminal surface with an intermediate subendothelial layer.

course of macrophage-mediated prosthetic dissolution. Peak inner capsule (IC) thickness was achieved at 2 months. Again, there was no graft related morbidity or mortality. Twenty percent of the PG910 grafts become aneurysmal.[17]

In order to further assess the potential contribution of transanastomotic pannus ingrowth to the arterial regeneration seen, prostheses were constructed of three 10 mm segments with a PG910 segment interposed between two Dacron segments. Grafts were again implanted in rabbit aortas and harvested at intervals up to 4 months. All grafts remained patent with no aneurysms or stenoses. Inner capsule thickness in the PG910 segments increased only during the interval from 2 weeks to 2 months and was statistically greater than either Dacron segment at 1 and 2 months. Inner capsules of PG910 segments at 1 month were composed predominantly of myofibroblasts. Pannus ingrowth was limited to the first 2 mm of the inner capsules of the Dacron segments, the remainder consisting of a fibrin coagulum. These findings essentially ruled out transanastomotic pannus ingrowth as the primary source of cells replacing absorbable vascular prostheses.[18]

Polyglycolic Acid (Dexon)

In 1982, we reported the regeneration of major components of the rabbit aorta over a scaffold of absorbable porous polyglycolic acid (PGA). PGA has the simplest structure of the linear aliphatic polyesters. It is hydrophilic and loses its strength rapidly over 2-4 weeks.[11] Woven PGA, manufactured by Davis & Geck, was fabricated into 3.5 mm diameter grafts and implanted into the abdominal aorta of rabbits and explanted over a seven and a half month period. Seventy-six percent (76%) of the animals were found to have maintained a lumen of 3-4 mm in the region of implantation. Eleven percent (11%) of the animals demonstrated aneurysmal dilatation in this region; however, no animal died of graft rupture. In addition, there was no evidence of perigraft hematomas or of false aneurysm formation. There were no instances of graft thrombosis or infection. Experimental regenerated aortas were subjected to bursting strength determinations and withstood hemodynamic forces at three to five times systolic pressure.

Histologic analysis revealed some marked similarities to native aorta. The regenerated aortas were composed of a luminal surface containing factor VIII positive endothelial cells, a subendothelial zone containing smooth muscle-like myofibroblasts amidst dense fibrous tissue and an outer layer of vascularized connective tissue. Elastin regeneration, however, was minimal. Some lipid-laden macrophages and histiocytes were observed in the six month explants, suggesting possible early atherogenesis. Intimal hyperplasia resulting in severe graft stenosis was observed in 13% of animals.

The PGA graft material underwent progressive dissolution. At two weeks the PGA was densely invaded by mesenchymal cells, histiocytes and giant cells. Complete resorption occurred between three weeks and three months.

Important questions emerged from this study. Principally, it remained to be defined what were the factors responsible for the initiation and modulation of the repair process. Additionally, the origin of the cells in the regenerated aorta was unknown, as was the atherogenicity of the vessels.[19]

Stimulated by these early results, our group compared Dacron aortic prostheses to PGA. The Dacron grafts were fabricated to specifications that closely matched the physical characteristics of woven PGA, most notably in terms of pore diameter, pore area and wall thickness. Over the 12 month observation period both the PGA and Dacron grafts remained free of thrombosis, infection or hemorrhagic complications. Again, 10% of PGA grafts showed moderate aneurysmal dilatation and 15% demonstrated significant intimal hyperplasia.[20]

After three months the PGA, as before, was found to have been resorbed and in its place a thick, dense neointima lined with a confluent layer of endothelial cells was seen. Beneath this layer were numerous smooth muscle like myofibroblasts in a circumferential and longitudinal orientation. The inner capsules of the Dacron grafts, however, exhibited only matrix and small numbers of myofibroblasts in a radial orientation. The flow surface was thin, fibrinous and acellular.

The Dacron grafts explanted at 1 year contained extensive calcium deposits and some advanced atherosclerotic plaques. The PGA explants at 1 year remained remarkably stable with the exception of an occasional lipid-laden histiocyte, as had been previously observed.

Despite their similarities in mechanical porosity, these two graft materials achieved remarkably different histologic outcomes, suggesting that porosity was not the only factor active in graft healing. Insight into the pathophysiology of these differences was gained by studying the grafts explanted after two weeks.

As in the previous experiment, an inflammatory reaction containing macrophages, polymorphonuclear leukocytes and giant cells was observed in the tissues surrounding the PGA grafts. Additionally, numerous macrophages were found within the mesh of the PGA grafts. The Dacron grafts as well were surrounded by an inflammatory reaction; however, cellular infiltration was limited to the outer capsule with little or no permeation of the woven Dacron. It was hypothesized that phagocytosis of PGA by macrophages inducing their phenotypic alteration and synthesis of growth factors chemotactic and mitogenic for endothelial cells and myofibroblasts, as well as subtle differences in the surface electronegativity of the materials, could have accounted for differences in transinterstitial migration of inflammatory cells.[20]

Additional speculations were made regarding the role of growth factors in inducing myofibroblast and endothelial cell ingrowth and deposition. Macrophages were known to stimulate the proliferation of endothelial cells, smooth muscle and fibroblasts through the elucidation of "macrophage-derived growth factors (MDGFs)."[21-23] The degree of macrophage infiltration corresponded temporally with myofibroblast proliferation as quantitated by autoradiography with tritiated thymidine and suggested the possibility that a macrophage derived factor played an important role in the modulation of myofibroblast response. The possibility that the degradable materials had directly resulted in

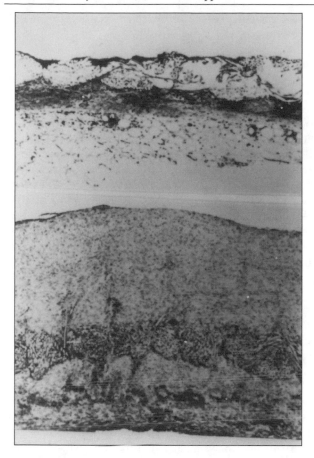

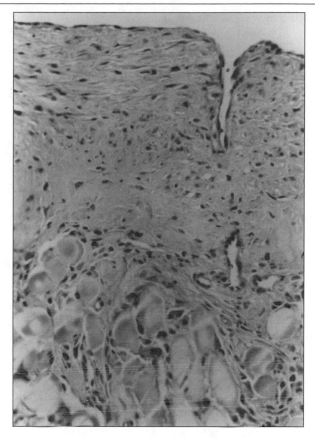

Fig. 45.2. Top: Midportion of 1 month Dacron specimen showing thin inner capsule (IC) composed of fibrin coagulum and minimal cellular repopulation. (Hematoxylin-eosin; x50). Bottom: Midportion of 1 month polyglycolic acid specimen showing greatly thickened IC of circumferentially and longitudinally oriented smooth muscle-like myofibroblasts beneath endothelial-like flow surface. More peripheral are prosthesis and well vascularized outer capsule. (Hematoxylin-eosin; x50).

Fig. 45.3. Midportion of PDS specimen at 2 months showing capillary invading inner capsule and communicating with luminal surface. Endothelial-like cellular luminal surface of specimen appears to be continuous with capillary wall.

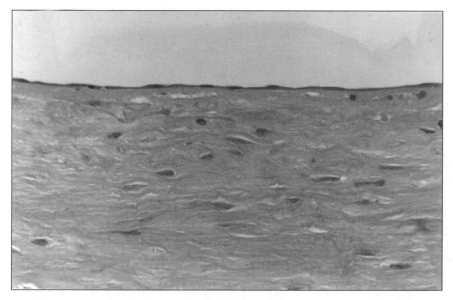

Fig. 45.4. Midportion of PDS specimen at 12 months showing maintenance of smooth confluent layer of endothelial-like cells on luminal surface. (Hematoxylin-eosin; x390).

macrophage stimulation was suggested by the demonstration of PGA remnants within the cytoplasm of macrophages by TEM. Additional speculations surrounded the potential roles of PDGF, ECGF (now FGF-1), and FGF-2 and of mechanical forces on the tissue bed, which were found to increase as the PGA degrades and the integrity and mechanical strength of the graft material was lost.[20]

Polydioxanone (Pds)

The ability of lactide/glycolide polymers to induce arterial regeneration was also demonstrated with grafts fabricated from PDS, a more slowly resorbed polymer.[24] Grafts, 24 x 4 mm in size and composed of woven PDS were again interposed into the abdominal aorta of rabbits. The animals were studied at intervals up to one year. Again, no aortic-related deaths or hemorrhages occurred. Aneurysmal dilatation developed in 10% of specimens, whereas stenosis from neointimal hyperplasia occurred in 15%. As with PGA (Fig. 45.2), a vessel wall composed of myofibroblasts and matrix covered by a confluent endothelial-like flow surface resulted. The PDS implants (Figs. 45.3 and 45.4) yielded an inner capsule (IC) thickness as well as compliance and strength characteristics that were comparable to the PGA grafts. Not unexpectedly, tissue formation with the PDS grafts occurred more gradually. These grafts reached maximal IC thickness between 3 and 6 months as compared to 2 months for PGA. The difference in the rates paralleled the differing dissolution rates of the two materials.[25] These observations reinforced the concept that the process of arterial regeneration was regulated by some factor or factors related to the absorption of the material by macrophages.

Mechanical Stimuli of Arterial Regeneration

A study by Vorp et al to evaluate the stress history within the inner capsule demonstrated that, early in the resorption phase, the neointima is under a state of circumferential compression.[26] Later in the resorption phase, as the graft material weakens upon dissolution and as the neointimal tissue strengthens upon reorganization, the inner capsule stress becomes tensile. The occurrence of compressive stresses parallels the time point and location of maximal mitotic index for the neointimal tissue. We showed using the well established rabbit model that the mitotic index of inner capsule myofibroblasts in PG910 grafts was significantly higher during the early period of resorption than in the later period.[27]

Using a pulse duplicator apparatus developed at the University of Pittsburgh,[28] changes in the dynamic compliance of PG910 grafts occurring over 0 to 36 weeks were assessed.[29] Using the rabbit model, explanted PG910 grafts were exposed to realistic pulsatile hemodynamics in vitro. A rapid increase in compliance was noted after 3 weeks, leveling off at 13 weeks. In a companion study, compliance increased over time in the proximal and distal graft segments compared to baseline. Loss of compliance has been cited as an important mechanism in the failure of small and medium sized Dacron and ePTFE implants.[30] Thus, by achieving greater compliance over time, resorbable grafts appear to have real potential for improved efficacy over prosthetics in current use.

Characteristics of the Healing Response

In addition to rate of resorption and kinetics of IC formation, additional studies were performed in order to further characterize differences between the healing responses induced by the various materials. The prostaglandin metabolite contents of inner capsules formed in the presence of PDS, PG910 and Dacron containing grafts were compared. PDS inner capsules were found to have greater ratios of 6-keto-$PGF_{1\alpha}$:TxB2 as compared to PG910 and Dacron implants. Notably, the ratio of 6-keto-$PGF_{1\alpha}$:TxB2 for PDS was nearly identical to its normal aortic control. This favorable ratio suggested that grafts containing PDS may be less thrombogenic and again suggests the potential for clinical efficacy of resorbable grafts.[31]

The kinetics of collagen deposition induced by PDS, PG910 and Dacron containing grafts was determined by examining the inner capsules of grafts explanted at 1, 3 and 12 months. In the Dacron grafts, collagen formation peaked at 1 month at approximately 12 μg/mg. In contrast, the collagen content of the inner capsules of the PDS and PG910 grafts at 1 month was around 27 μg/mg. This amount of collagen is essentially equivalent to that found in normal infrarenal rabbit aorta. The level of collagen in the Dacron grafts at one year remained the same as at 1 month. The level of collagen in the PDS and PG910 grafts increased to approximately 38 μg/mg at 3 months, after which it stabilized.[32]

The kinetics of myofibroblast proliferation in the inner capsules of PDS, PG910 and Dacron implants was also analyzed, again in the rabbit infrarenal aorta model. Grafts were explanted at intervals up to 52 weeks. Mitotic indices were determined by autoradiography using tritiated thymidine. Of interest was the finding that the mitotic index associated with each graft material was parallel to that material's rate of resorption. The peak mitotic index for PG910 was 28.34 in a 24 h period and occurred at 3 weeks postimplant, whereas the peak for PDS was 7.50; this occurred at 4 weeks and was prolonged. There was little evidence of inner capsule formation in the Dacron grafts until 12 weeks postimplant and the mitotic indices for Dacron grafts never exceeded 1.22.[27]

Macrophage/Biomaterial Interactions

In order to further characterize the contribution of the macrophage/biomaterial interaction in the elaboration of factors regulating the process of arterial regeneration, a series of in vitro experiments were performed.[33-36] In each series of experiments, rabbit peritoneal macrophages were harvested and cultured in Minimum Essential Medium (MEM) with platelet-poor serum and containing particles of Dacron, polyglactin 910 or no biomaterial (Fig. 45.5A,B). MEM conditioned in this way was collected and mitogenicity assays were performed with quiescent fibroblasts (BALB/c3T3), rabbit aortic smooth muscle cells, and murine capillary lung (LE-II) endothelial cells. Mitogenic ac-

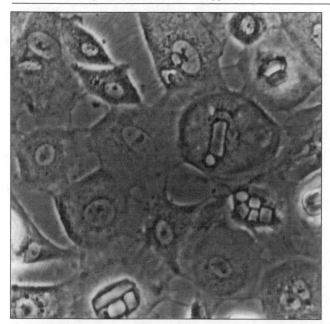

Fig. 45.5. (A, top) Phase contrast photomicrograph of peritoneal macrophages following six weeks in culture in the presence of the bioresorbable polyglactin 910. Intracytoplasmic polyglactin 910 inclusions can be seen (original magnification x400). (B, bottom) Phase contrast photomicrograph of peritoneal macrophages following five weeks in culture in the presence of Dacron. Macrophages can be seen adherent to Dacron particles but no intracytoplasmic inclusions are observed (original magnification x100).

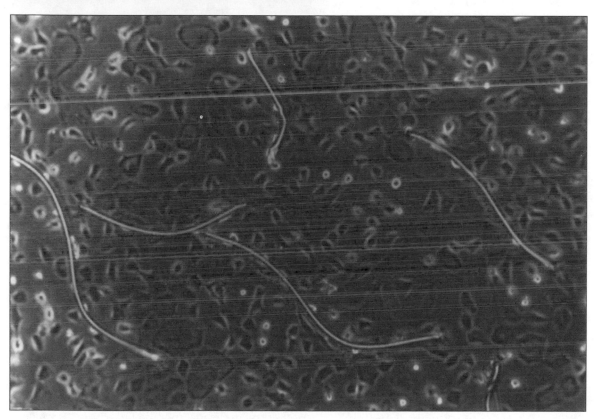

tivity was assayed by scintillation counting of tritiated thymidine incorporation into deoxyribonucleic acid (DNA). In order to examine these processes in a model more accurately reflecting the clinical setting, macrophages were also harvested from rabbits that had been rendered hyperlipidemic through an atherosclerotic diet.[33-35]

All cell types grown in conditioned media from macrophages exposed to PG910 demonstrated significantly greater increases in tritiated thymidine incorporation as compared to those grown in media conditioned from mac-

rophages exposed either to Dacron or to no biomaterial. In fact, it could be demonstrated that macrophages harvested from rabbits fed a cholesterol rich atherogenic diet exposed in culture to Dacron produced conditioned media that exerted an inhibitory effect on endothelial cell thymidine incorporation. In order to isolate the factor or factors responsible for these alterations in mitogenic activity, Western blot analysis was performed using antibodies raised against PDGF-B chain, acidic fibroblast growth factor (FGF-1) and basic fibroblast growth factor (FGF-2). Only anti-bFGF

Fig. 45.6. (A) Rabbit aortic smooth muscle cell bioassay results. Conditioned media from macrophages harvested from New Zealand White rabbits fed a normal diet and cultured from 1 through 7 weeks in the presence of either no biomaterial (first bar), polyglactin 910 (second bar), or Dacron (third bar). Results are expressed as counts per minute of the sample divided by counts per minute of the fetal bovine serum positive control x 100 (mean ± SD). (B) Rabbit aortic smooth muscle cell bioassay results. Conditioned media from macrophages harvested from New Zealand White rabbits fed a 2% cholesterol/6% peanut oil diet and cultured from 1 through 7 weeks in the presence of either no biomaterial (first bar), polyglactin 910 (second bar), or Dacron (third bar). Results are expressed as counts per minute of the sample divided by counts per minute of the fetal bovine serum positive control x 100 (mean ± SD).

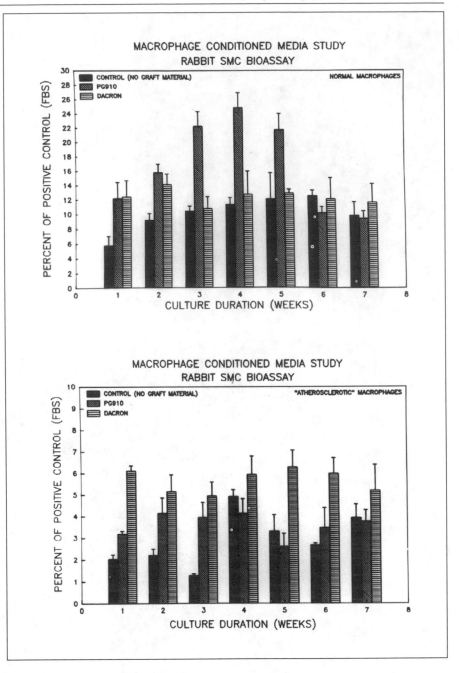

antibody immunoreacted with samples of the conditioned media.[33]

In order to further define the contribution of bFGF to the mitogenic response, conditioned media was preincubated with neutralizing anti-basic-FGF antibody. In rabbits fed normal diets, Dacron induced mitogen release was completely inhibited by anti-basic-FGF antibody. PG910 mitogen release was diminished, but to a significantly less degree (36%). Thus it appeared that much of the mitogenic effect on smooth muscle cell was mediated via basic-FGF.[35]

In another series of experiments, the effect of conditioned media on rabbit aortic smooth muscle cells was assessed. Smooth muscle cells grown in conditioned media from macrophages exposed to PG910 again resulted in significantly higher tritiated thymidine incorporation than

smooth muscle cells grown in conditioned media from macrophages exposed to Dacron (Fig. 45.6A). When macrophages were obtained from atherosclerotic rabbits a generalized decrease in the incorporation of tritiated thymidine by smooth muscle cells occurred in both the Dacron and PG910 groups. The macrophages from atherosclerotic rabbits cultured with Dacron, however, showed a particular increase in the mitogenic factors most active on the smooth muscle cells (Fig. 45.6B). To further characterize this effect, Western blot and immunoprecipitation studies were performed, and as before, the presence of FGF-2 was demonstrated, whereas PDGF and FGF-1 were not. TGF-β inhibitory activity was demonstrated to be increased for the atherosclerotic macrophage containing media. These findings support the hypothesis that interactions between Dacron, macrophage and smooth muscle cells play a role in the pathogenesis of graft failure.[34]

Polyurethane/Poly-L-Lactide Copolymers (Pu-Plla)

A different approach has been taken by the polymer chemists at the University of Groningen in The Netherlands. They have worked extensively with copolymers of polyurethane and poly-L-lactide (PU-PLLA) with the goal of combining the properties of the two materials to produce an antithrombogenic, flexible as well as resorbable material. PU-PLLA was described by Gogolewski in 1982.[37]

Lommen et al interposed 1.5 x 10 mm PU-PLLA grafts into the abdominal aorta of rats.[2] These grafts were of 40-50 μm porosity and were explanted at 3, 6 and 12 weeks. These grafts were compared to a control group that received PTFE grafts of the same dimensions and of 30 μm porosity.

At explant all grafts were patent and there was no evidence of aneurysm formation, dilatation or other complications in either group. By 6 weeks the PTFE grafts had developed a complete "endothelial" lining that was continuous with that of the adjacent vessel. However, this lining detached easily during processing, suggesting that there was poor attachment with the prosthesis. The internodal spaces of the graft appeared to contain fibrin. Similar findings were noted in the 12 week PTFE explants.

The PU-PLLA grafts demonstrated arterial regeneration. A complete "endothelial" lining was observed at three weeks. Likewise, the outer surface of the grafts was covered with vascularized connective tissue that was morphologically indistinct from native adventitia. At 6 weeks giant cell activity was observed within the graft walls, most prominently at the periphery. By 6-12 weeks a subintimal layer containing "smooth muscle cells," collagen and elastin (demonstrated by Orcein staining) had developed. Multiple fenestrated elastic laminae were observed as well. The body of the PU-PLLA graft gradually became infiltrated with cells, and this process was associated with progressive degradation of the graft substance.[2]

Having demonstrated that biodegradable PU-PLLA stimulates the regeneration of an arterial wall they next sought to optimize some of the properties of the grafts responsible for this process. They postulated that the compliance of the grafts was an important property and they performed in vitro stress/strain measurements of grafts composed of several combinations of PU and PLLA and compared them to native artery. They determined that grafts composed of 5-20% PLLA possessed compliance before implantation comparable to rat aorta.[38] They subsequently investigated the effect of varying the pore size of grafts composed of 95%/5% PU/PLLA in the rat model. They determined that there was no distinct advantage of a pore size of 40 μm as compared to pores in a gradient of 10-100 μm from the inner to the outer regions of the graft in terms of arterial regeneration. The advocated the use of a pore gradient, however, as the smaller pores on the luminal surface were thought to decrease thrombogenicity.[39]

They compared these compliant grafts to less compliant grafts composed of biostable PU and of PU/PLLA surrounded by PTFE. Partial arterial regeneration was seen in all groups; however, only the PU/PLLA grafts reconstituted an elastic lamina. They concluded that both biodegradation and compliance were important stimuli of arterial regeneration.[40]

To characterize the functional characteristics of the regenerated arteries, endothelialization and prostacyclin synthesis were determined using a bioassay and RIA for the prostacyclin metabolite 6-oxo-PGF$_{1\alpha}$. Comparisons were made between PU/PLLA and PTFE grafts and normal endothelium. Looking at prostacyclin production per unit graft area covered with neoendothelium, there were no significant differences between the two graft types and native artery. Endothelialization and healing, however, as determined by light and electron microscopy were incomplete in the PTFE grafts, even after 12 weeks.[41] Additional ultrastructural analyses were performed and, as was observed by our group, epithelioid cells and multinucleated giant cells were seen to engulf polymer particles of the disintegrating grafts.[42]

The long term fate of PU/PLLA grafts was assessed in a group of 8 implants. After 1 year all grafts were found to be patent. Three of the grafts were of normal shape and were visibly pulsatile. Two grafts were mildly dilated, 2 were aneurysmal and 1 had sustained a dissection. These grafts were not visibly pulsatile. Histologic analysis of the "neomedia" revealed circularly arranged smooth muscle cells (as in normal artery) in the normally shaped implants. However, in the nonpulsatile implants, the neomedia had a predominantly longitudinal arrangement. They concluded that the pattern of arrangement of smooth muscle cells in the neomedia affects the fate of the regenerated arteries.[43]

There was uncertainty as to the origin of the cells in the regenerated arteries. Hypothesized origins have included migration from the cut ends of the adjacent vessel and the granulation tissue surrounding the graft, as well as deposition of circulating cells onto the luminal surface.[44] To gain insight into the source origin of the cells in the arteries regenerated from PU/PLLA, sequential explants at intervals of 1 h to twelve weeks were performed. They observed that the endothelium originated from adjacent intima. The smooth muscle cells seemed to originate from the media of the adjacent aorta; however, they could not exclude the other postulated mechanisms which would be required for clinical applicability, and proposed experiments with longer grafts to decrease the likelihood of trans-anastomotic cell migration.[44]

Other work with lactide polymers has been done by Hanson's group at the University of Texas. They fabricated grafts with copolymers of L-lactide, DL-lactide, and ε-caprolactone in various compositions. Lactide polymers were chosen for their strength, ε-caprolactone for their flexibility. The grafts were 3 mm by 8 cm, nonwoven, nonporous and completely resorbable. The mechanical properties and degradation rates of the grafts were evaluated in vitro. Circumferential tension, compliance, and kink angle were determined. Tensile strength and modulus of elasticity were found to be in the range of normal artery; however, the grafts were significantly less compliant than artery. It was anticipated that the addition of porosity, a necessity for in vivo studies, would improve compliance. Further investigations were planned.[45]

Polyurethane Elastomers (PU)

Extensive work has been done in the evaluation of small diameter vascular grafts composed of polyurethane elastomers. Polyurethanes hold promise by virtue of their superior compliance as compared to conventional prosthetics. By and large, these polyurethanes are nonresorbable (biostable).[46] Gogolewski fabricated vascular grafts from a bioresorbable segmented aliphatic polyurethane (PU). Like the PU/PLLA grafts, these were degradable, microporous and compliant. Grafts of 1.5 mm inner diameter and 0.7 mm wall thickness were interposed into 13 mm defects in rat abdominal aorta and explanted at intervals between 3 and 16 weeks. The luminal surface of the graft consisted of interconnected pores of 5-10 µm. The outer surface of the graft had a porosity of 20-50 µm. The tissue response was reported as being comparable to that previously observed with polylactide and polyglycolide. Again, prosthetic debris were surrounded by giant cells and macrophages. A "glistening neointima" was observed at 3 weeks, with "no tendency" towards intimal thickening. Smooth muscle cells and elastin fibers were observed in the intima. By four months almost complete degradation of the PU had occurred. Stress/strain analysis revealed mechanical characteristics similar to native aorta.[46]

Encouraged by these results, 8 mm by 6 cm grafts were implanted into the infrarenal aorta of 50 young pigs. The grafts were explanted at intervals of 1 month to 1 year. Eighteen pigs died as a result of prosthetic rupture, infection or thrombosis. Ten pigs received no aspirin and a regular diet. These grafts were all thrombosed by 90 days. Twenty-five pigs received aspirin; 55% of these grafts remained patent at 90 days. Only 3 were patent at 1 year. Of 15 pigs receiving a diet high in lipid, 7 remained patent at 1 year. Three of these animals were noted to have dilation of the prosthesis similar to that observed by our group in PG910 grafts placed in the abdominal aorta of rabbits fed an atherogenic diet. [47] It was postulated that the enhanced patency of these grafts was related to an anti-thrombotic effect of the lipid-rich diet.[48]

Histologic analysis again revealed macrophage and giant cell infiltration of the prosthesis and phagocytosis of prosthetic debris. A neointima and neomedia containing longitudinal and transverse smooth muscle cells developed by 180 days. A fibrous neoadventitia was observed at early time points; however, at 1 year this was comprised of fatty tissue. Elastic fibers dispersed throughout the muscle layer were observed. The prostheses were completely resorbed by 1 year. Prostacycline synthesis was found to be comparable to normal aorta with no apparent differences between groups.[48,49]

Preventing Aneurysmal Dilatation

The chief obstacle in the development of a clinically useful resorbable graft has been the potential for loss of mechanical and structural integrity in the graft prior to the regeneration of an arterial wall. Adding to this concern is the finding that when evaluated in hyperlipidemic models, which more closely approximate the situation of clinical vascular grafting, resorbable grafts have had an increased incidence of graft dilation, aneurysm formation and rupture.[47-49] Investigators have taken several approaches to counteracting this problem, including incorporating resorbables with enhanced resistance to degradation,[7,50-56] increasing the rapidity of tissue regeneration with growth factors[57,58] and cell seeding.[59,60] Others have taken an intermediate approach and constructed compound or partially resorbable vascular prostheses combining resorbable and permanent materials.

Enhancing the Resistance to Degradation of Resorbable Materials

Our group evaluated woven bicomponent totally bioresorbable grafts fabricated from compound yarns containing 74% PG910 with 26% polydioxanone (PDS). The resorption kinetics of PDS are slower than PG910. Thirty-seven grafts were implanted into the infrarenal aorta of rabbits and explanted at intervals between 2 weeks to 12 months. Complete resorbtion of the PG910 occurred by 2 months and the PDS by 6 months. All grafts were patent at explant. One graft developed a 50% stenosis that appeared to be thrombotic in origin. No aneurysmal dilatation was seen in any graft. Inner capsule thickness was intermediate to that seen with PDS and PG910.[51]

The Groningen group hypothesized that the dilatation observed with their PU/PLLA grafts was related to technical problems with the dip-coating process of graft preparation.[52] They produced a modified 2-ply graft with a more biostable inner layer. The inner layer was made highly anti-thrombogenic by crosslinking of a mixture of linoleic acid and an aliphatic polyetherurethane with dicumyl peroxide. The outer ply was a (95/5) mixture of polyesterurethane and poly(L-lactide).

Twenty-two two-ply grafts were implanted in the abdominal aorta of rats. All grafts remained patent at least up to 1 year and did not exhibit any aneurysm formation. As in the earlier formulations, the inner layer was covered with endothelial cells and several layers of smooth muscle cells.[53]

Galletti's group at Brown University approached the problem of aneurysmal degeneration of Vicryl grafts by coating the yarns used in the fabrication process with slowly resorbed polyesters, thus extending their functional life. They produced tubular conduits, 1 mm by 3 mm, composed of triple ply Vicryl coated with a 1:1 composite of poly-DL-lactic acid and poly-2,3-butylene malate or poly-2,3-butylene fumarate. Coated or uncoated Vicryl grafts were implanted subcutaneously in mice. Samples were retrieved at intervals between 2 and 12 weeks and the remaining mass of polymer implant was analyzed for the presence of Vicryl using gel permeation chromatography.

After 8 weeks Vicryl was undetectable in the uncoated implants. Grafts coated with poly-2,3-butylene malate or poly-2,3-butylene fumarate, however, retained 48 and 88% of their Vicryl content respectively.[54]

Galletti's group next constructed 8 mm by 13 cm grafts of triple ply Vicryl coated with a 1:1 composite of poly-DL-lactic acid and poly-2,3-butylene fumarate. To minimize oozing through the graft interstices, they added a fourth outer layer of a 1 cm wide ribbon of Vicryl mesh wrapped in a spiral around the graft. The grafts were inserted in the infrarenal aorta of dogs. Grafts were retrieved at intervals up to 12 weeks. They found that at 8 weeks the polymer was substantially reduced and by 12 weeks had nearly disappeared. Stress/strain analysis of the resulting inner capsules demonstrated properties similar to natural vessels.[55]

They next investigated prostheses composed of Vicryl coated with either poly-DL-lactic acid and poly-2,3-butylene fumarate (PDLA-PBF) or poly-DL-lactic acid and poly-2,3-butylene succinate (PDLA-PBS). Grafts (8-9 mm in internal diameter, 8-10 cm long) were implanted in the infrarenal aortic position of dogs and explanted at intervals up to 24 weeks. All animals receiving coated prostheses survived, whereas one animal receiving an uncoated Vicryl prosthesis died from graft rupture. Grafts were patent in 14 of 18 animals at the time of retrieval.

Histologic analysis revealed no cellular invasion of the Vicryl mesh in the PDLA-PBF coated grafts. The PDLA-PBS coated grafts, however, demonstrated cellular elements, and fusion of inner and outer tissue layers could be demonstrated. Isolated patches of endothelium-like cells were noted in the mid-region of the PDLA-PBS coated grafts; otherwise, composition of the inner and outer capsules did not differ significantly between groups.[56]

Increasing the Rapidity of Tissue Regeneration with Growth Factors

Our group sought to minimize the likelihood of graft rupture by accelerating the regeneration of the arterial wall through the local application of growth factors. We documented our ability to attach FGF-1, a potent endothelial cell mitogen, and FGF-1-heparin complexes to PDS prosthesis.[58] Dacron or PDS grafts were then interposed into the infrarenal aorta of rabbits and explanted at intervals up to 30 days. We confirmed the method of attachment of FGF-1 to biomaterial surfaces and documented the retention of FGF-1 to the graft while in circulation. At 1 month all grafts were patent and without stenoses or aneurysm formation. No significant differences were demonstrated between FGF-1 and control groups in terms of cellularity of luminal surfaces, inner capsule thickness or capillarization of the inner capsule.[61]

After explantation, residual [^{125}I]FGF-1 was eluted from the prostheses. Intact FGF-1 was identified by SDS gel electrophoresis. Similarly prepared prostheses were explanted after 7 days and their FGF-1 eluted off for in vitro documentation of activity. Eluted FGF-1 was found to have retained its mitogenic properties, causing a 1000-1200% increase in [^{3}H]thymidine incorporation into newly synthesized DNA in test murine LE-II cells.[61] We hypothesize that the lack of difference in healing seen between control and growth factor treated grafts relates to the inactivity of bound FGF-1. It is also possible that differences may have occurred earlier than the 30 day explant time used in this study. We have subsequently altered our approach and are applying growth factors to grafts in polymerized suspensions of fibrin glue.[62] We have not yet applied this technique to resorbable grafts.

Cell Seeding

The Groningen group sought to accelerate the regeneration of the neomedia through the application of smooth muscle cell seeding.[59,60] Cultured smooth muscle was seeded into PU/PLLA biodegradable vascular grafts and implanted into the abdominal aorta of rats. Arterial wall regeneration was evaluated at intervals between 2 h and 1 week. The seeded grafts showed a more rapid and uniform development of the neomedia (clearly discernible at 2 days) as compared to nonseeded control grafts. No grafts demonstrated aneurysm formation or dilatation in these short term implants.[60]

Compound Partially Bioresorbable Vascular Grafts

Others have taken an intermediate approach and developed compound, or partially resorbable, vascular prostheses combining resorbable and permanent materials. Early studies were performed by Wesolowski's group in the late 1950s and 1960s. They evaluated 24 different combinations of graft materials in dogs and pigs. They found, in general, that coated grafts performed less favorably than compound grafts wherein the resorbable component was an integral part of the fabrication. Deleterious changes (calcification) did occur in the compound grafts; however, this occurred in a delayed fashion thought to be a result of the resorbable component. The most satisfactory results were achieved with grafts composed of a compound yarn of resorbable catgut that had been wrapped with multi-filament polyester yarn.[5]

More recent work on compound vascular grafts has focused largely on the of incorporation of lactide polymers. An early report came from Ruderman's group at Walter Reed. They evaluated woven grafts composed of 24% PLA and 76% Dacron implanted into the abdominal aorta of dogs. After 100 days they found all grafts to be patent and to show extensive tissue ingrowth.[63]

Compound Grafts: PG910

Bowald's group investigated compound grafts as well. They compared double layer Vicryl grafts with Vicryl grafts anchored inside PTFE or Dacron mesh tube grafts. The grafts were implanted into the descending aorta of pigs. Nearly half of the pigs receiving Vicryl grafts experienced graft rupture. The pigs receiving grafts with external support did not experience graft rupture. Histologically, the supported Vicryl grafts were found to have the microscopic picture of arterial regeneration, although areas of degenerative change and calcification were noted. Increased collagen formation was noted in the Vicryl + Dacron group.[16]

Our group as well investigated Vicryl (PG910) in combination with Dacron and ePTFE.[17,31] In addition, we investigated combinations of Vicryl and polypropylene.[64-66] Vicryl grafts surrounded by Dacron or PTFE showed no incidence of aneurysmal dilatation as compared to a 20% dilatation rate for unwrapped Vicryl grafts. Arterial regeneration occurred in the wrapped grafts, but in an incomplete manner. Grafts were also fabricated from compound yarns composed of blends of Vicryl and Dacron. The rate of aneurysmal dilatation increased proportionally with the percentage of Dacron in the blended yarn. A maximum dilatation rate of 83% was seen with the 56% Dacron grafts. No dilatation was seen when 20% Dacron was used. Cellularity of the regenerated tissue in general was decreased in the presence of Dacron, suggesting an inhibitory effect of the biomaterial.[17] Subsequent work demonstrated decreased prostaglandin content of the inner capsules of Dacron/Vicryl composite grafts as compared to those of Vicryl grafts.[31]

In order to avoid the deleterious effects of Dacron, compound grafts were constructed using polypropylene, which possesses greater biocompatibility and a incites only a relatively low-grade inflammatory response.[65] Grafts fabricated from yarns containing 69% Vicryl (PG910) and 31% polypropylene were implanted into rabbit infrarenal aortas. Over 2 weeks to 12 months all grafts remained patent without aneurysm formation. Only residual polypropylene remained in the prostheses after 2 months. Production of 6-keto-PGF$_{1\alpha}$ was in the normal range.[64]

PG910/polypropylene prostheses were also implanted into the aorto-iliac positions of dogs. Again, all grafts were without aneurysm formation over one year. Patency was enhanced as compared to Dacron and ePTFE control grafts. Arterial regeneration was demonstrated.[65]

Compound Grafts: PGA

Our group also evaluated grafts made of polyglycolic acid (PGA) fabric reinforced by an outer wrap of Dacron. In this series, the incidence of aneurysmal dilatation was zero with or without the outer wrap up to nine months after implant. Again, Dacron appeared to have an inhibitory effect on the cellularity of the luminal surface and inner capsule.[17] Evaluation of an advanced PGA based compound prosthesis is currently underway in our lab.

Chu's group at Cornell also investigated the combination of PGA and Dacron. They produced knitted fabric grafts composed of PGA and Dacron fibers blended at various compositional ratios. They studied the properties of these bicomponent fabrics in vitro. They felt that their most important finding was the achievement of increasing water porosity over time without significant losses in the structural integrity and strength of the specimens.[67]

Having demonstrated the effectiveness of partially resorbable arterial prostheses in rabbits, we sought to evaluate longer grafts in a higher order species. 4 mm by 5 cm conduits were woven from composite yarns containing 70% PDS/30% polypropylene and implanted into the aorto-iliac positions of dogs for periods of up to one year. No aneurysms or perigraft hematomas developed. The patency of the PDS/polypropylene grafts was significantly greater than that of Dacron or ePTFE control grafts. Inner capsules were completely endothelialized by 1 month. IC cellularity and thickness were greater than those within Dacron or ePTFE.[65]

Compound Grafts: PU/PLLA

The Groningen group investigated compound grafts of PTFE fitted around PU/PLLA. They found that these grafts, as compared to grafts composed entirely of bioresorbable PU/PLLA or biostable but compliant PU, had diminished regeneration of all layers of the arterial wall, most strikingly in terms of elastic lamina. They attributed this finding to the decreased compliance associated with the PTFE wrap.[40]

Compound Grafts: Polyethylene Oxide and Polylactic Acid Copolymers (PELA)

The Biomaterials Research Laboratory at The Hebrew University of Jerusalem has developed and evaluated compound vascular prostheses fabricated from resorbable block copolymers of polyethylene oxide and polylactic acid (PELA) applied as a coating to knitted Dacron and polether urethane urea (Lycra) grafts. PELA is an elastomer that fully degrades in 3 weeks after implantation.[68-71] The in vivo performance of the Dacron grafts was evaluated in dogs as right ventricle to pulmonary artery conduits. Unlike control woven grafts, the PELA coated grafts showed complete transmural tissue ingrowth after 14 months.[68,69]

In a separate study, the Hebrew University group compared ePTFE grafts to grafts comprised of Lycra fibers coated with PELA. 6 mm by 6 cm grafts were implanted in the canine carotid artery for 90 days. Unlike the ePTFE grafts, the PELA coated grafts remained compliant and demonstrated successful healing and incorporation. Further work with small caliber prostheses was anticipated.[70]

Resorbable Outer Wraps

A novel application of resorbable materials in vascular grafting has been reported by Moritz and the Groningen group.[72-75] Moritz applied a constrictive mesh tube of resorbable mesh to dilated, otherwise unusable veins with the goal of inducing neoarterial wall growth. He found that the meshes can effectively reduce the diameter of a venous graft by providing external support to the vessel wall, thus limiting distension.[72] The Groningen group has also investigated biodegradable prostheses as external supports for vein grafts. They sought to prevent vein graft wall damage due to the higher arterial pressures encountered after implantation. They found that the prostheses can function as a protective scaffold for vein grafts in the arterial circulation, reducing damage to the vein graft wall and allowing gradual arterialization.[73-75]

Biopolymers: Resorbable Prostheses of Biologic Origin

Another novel approach has been taken by several groups in Europe and the United States who have sought to develop resorbable prostheses through the chemical modification of arterial xenografts.[76-81] Vascular prostheses of biological origin have been shown to develop aneurysms within several years of implantation. It has been hypothesized that, if properly processed, xenografts can function as a bioresorbable scaffold. Should this occur, an orderly regeneration of structural elements during healing could take place, the result being continued mechanical integrity of the graft.[78]

The biopolymer that has received the most attention is aldehyde crosslinked collagen.[76] Moczar's group in France developed a biodegradable microarterial graft from rat aorta. Trypsin treated arterial segments were coated with heparin or chondroitin sulfate to reduce thrombogenicity. Grafts were implanted into the infrarenal aorta of rats for 3-8 weeks. The grafts were found to undergo resorption in parallel with re-endothelialization and scar tissue formation. Patency was around 50%.[76] Macromolecular repair of the host aortic wall was documented in one year explants by the incorporation pattern of [³H]valine into proteins and the demonstration of de novo elastin synthesis in the scar replacing the prosthesis.[77]

Conclusion

The resorbable graft represents a paradigm shift in vascular prostheses. Unlike conventional prostheses whose effectiveness depends by and large upon an inherent resistance to a natural healing process, resorbable grafts work with the body, providing a framework for well established healing patterns. It seems intuitive that by augmenting rather than opposing these patterns a more efficacious vascular graft should result. Great strides have been made toward this end. Further research will yield grafts for clinical evaluation in the near future.

References

1. Shalaby S. Degradable materials: Perspectives, issues and opportunities. In: Barenberg S, Brash J, Narayan R, Redpath A, eds. The First International Scientific Consensus Workshop on Degradable Materials. Toronto: CRC Press, 1989:678.
2. Lommen E, Gogolewski S, Pennings AJ, Wildevuur CR, Nieuwenhuis P. Development of a neo-artery induced by a biodegradable polymeric vascular prosthesis. Trans Am Soc Artif Intern Organs 1983; 29:255-9.
3. Friedman S. A History of Vascular Surgery. Mount Kisco, New York: Futura Publishing Company, Inc., 1989.
4. Dennis C. Brief history of development of vascular grafts. In: Sawyer P, ed. Modern Vascular Grafts. New York: McGraw-Hill, 1987.
5. Wesolowski SA et al. The compound prosthetic vascular graft. A pathologic survey. Surgery 1963; 53:19.
6. Fries CC, Wesolowski SA. The polyester-oxidized cellulose compound vascular prostheses: A preliminary report. Trans Am Soc Artif Intern Organs 1964;X:227-30.
7. Robinson PH, van der Lei B, Knol KE, Pennings AJ. Patency and long-term biological fate of a two-ply biodegradable microarterial prosthesis in the rat. Br J Plast Surg 1989; 42:544-9.
8. Humphries A et al. Arterial prosthesis of collagen-impregnated dacron. Surgery 1961; 50:947.
9. Bascon J. Gelatin sealing to prevent blood loss from knitted arterial grafts. Surgery 1961; 50:504.
10. Guthrie C. End-results of arterial restitution with devitalized tissue. J Am Med Assoc 1919; 73:186.
11. Pachence J, Kohn J. Biodegradable polymers for tissue engineering. In: Lanza R, Langer R, Chick W, eds. Principles of Tissue Engineering. Georgetown, Texas: RG Landes Company, 1997.
12. Greisler HP. Bioresorbable materials and macrophage interactions. J Vasc Surg 1991; 13:748-50.
13. Bowald S, Busch C, Eriksson I. Arterial grafting with polyglactin mesh in pigs [letter]. Lancet. 1978; 1:153.
14. Bowald S, Busch C, Eriksson I. Arterial regeneration following polyglactin 910 suture mesh grafting. Surgery. 1979; 86:722-9.
15. Audell L, Bowald S, Busch C, Eriksson I. Polyglactin mesh grafting of the pig aorta. The two-year follow-up in an experimental animal. Acta Chir Scand 1980; 146:97-9.
16. Bowald S, Busch C, Eriksson I. Absorbable material in vascular prostheses: A new device. Acta Chir Scand 1980; 146:391-5.
17. Greisler HP, Schwarcz TH, Ellinger J, Kim DU. Dacron inhibition of arterial regenerative activities. J Vasc Surg 1986; 3:747-56.
18. Greisler HP, Dennis JW, Endean ED, Ellinger J, Buttle KF, Kim DU. Derivation of neointima in vascular grafts. Circulation. 1988; 78:I6-12.
19. Greisler HP. Arterial regeneration over absorbable prostheses. Arch Surg 1982; 117:1425-31.
20. Greisler HP, Kim DU, Price JB, Voorhees AB Jr. Arterial regenerative activity after prosthetic implantation. Arch Surg 1985; 120:315-23.
21. Leibovich SJ, Ross R. The role of the macrophage in wound repair. A study with hydrocortisone and antimacrophage serum. Am J Pathol 1975; 78:71-100.
22. Martin BM, Gimbrone MA Jr, Unanue ER, Cotran RS. Stimulation of nonlymphoid mesenchymal cell proliferation by a macrophage-derived growth factor. J Immunol 1981; 126:1510-5.
23. Greenburg GB, Hunt TK. The proliferative response in vitro of vascular endothelial and smooth muscle cells exposed to wound fluids and macrophages. J Cell Physiol 1978; 97:353-60.
24. Zarge J, Huang P, Greisler H. Blood vessels. In: Lanza R, Langer R, Chick W, eds. Principles of Tissue Engineering. Georgetown, Texas: RG Landes Company; 1997.
25. Greisler HP, Ellinger J, Schwarcz TH, Golan J, Raymond RM, Kim DU. Arterial regeneration over polydioxanone prostheses in the rabbit. Archives of Surgery 1987; 122:715-21.
26. Vorp DA, Raghavan ML, Borovetz HS, Greisler HP, Webster MW. Modeling the transmural stress distribution during healing of bioresorbable vascular prostheses. Ann Biomed Eng 1995; 23:178-88.
27. Greisler HP, Petsikas D, Lam TM et al. Kinetics of cell proliferation as a function of vascular graft material. J Biomed Mater Res 1993; 27:955-61.
28. Brant AM, Chmielewski JF, Hung T-K, Borovetz HS. Simulation in-vitro of pulsatile vascular hemodynamics using a CAD/CAM designed cam disk and roller follower. Artif Organs 1986; 10:419-421.
29. Pham S, S.J. D, R. J et al. Compliance changes in bioresorbable vascular prostheses following implantation. Surg Forum 1988; 39:330-332.
30. Greisler HP, Joyce KA, Kim DU, Pham SM, Berceli SA, Borovetz HS. Spatial and temporal changes in compliance following implantation of bioresorbable vascular grafts. J Biomed Mater Res 1992; 26:1449-61.
31. Schwarcz TH, Nussbaum ML, Ellinger J, Kim DU, Greisler HP. Prostaglandin content of tissue lining vascular prostheses. Curr Surg 1987; 44:18-21.
32. Greisler HP, Cabusao EB, Lam TM, Murchan PM, Ellinger J, Kim DU. Kinetics of collagen deposition within bioresorbable and nonresorbable vascular prostheses. ASAIO Trans 1991; 37:M472-5.
33. Greisler HP, Ellinger J, Henderson SC et al. The effects of an atherogenic diet on macrophage/biomaterial interactions. J Vasc Surg 1991; 14:10-23.
34. Lam TM, Whereat NE, Henderson SC, Burgess WH, Shaheen A, Greisler HP. Effects of hypercholesterolemia

on monokine-induced smooth muscle cell proliferation. Exs 1992; 61:346-56.

35. Greisler HP, Henderson SC, Lam TM. Basic fibroblast growth factor production in vitro by macrophages exposed to Dacron and polyglactin 910. J Biomater Sci Polym Ed. 1993; 4:415-30.

36. Zenni GC, Ellinger J, Lam TM, Greisler HP. Biomaterial-induced macrophage activation and monokine release. J Invest Surg 1994; 7:135-41.

37. Gogolewski S, Pennings A. Porous biomedical materials based on mixtures of polylactides and polyurethanes. Makromol Chem Rapid Commun 1982; 3:839-845.

38. Gogolewski S, Pennings AJ, Lommen E, Wildevuur CR. Small-caliber biodegradable vascular grafts from Groningen. Life Support Syst 1983; 1:382-5.

39. van der Lei B, Bartels HL, Nieuwenhuis P, Wildevuur CR. Microporous, complaint, biodegradable vascular grafts for the regeneration of the arterial wall in rat abdominal aorta. Surgery 1985; 98:955-63.

40. van der Lei B, Wildevuur CR, Nieuwenhuis P. Compliance and biodegradation of vascular grafts stimulate the regeneration of elastic laminae in neoarterial tissue: an experimental study in rats. Surgery 1986; 99:45-52.

41. van der Lei B, Darius H, Schror K, Nieuwenhuis P, Molenaar I, Wildevuur CR. Arterial wall regeneration in small-caliber vascular grafts in rats. Neoendothelial healing and prostacyclin production. J Thorac Cardiovasc Surg 1985; 90:378-86.

42. van der Lei B, Wildevuur CR, Nieuwenhuis P et al. Regeneration of the arterial wall in microporous, compliant, biodegradable vascular grafts after implantation into the rat abdominal aorta. Ultrastructural observations. Cell Tissue Res 1985; 242:569-78.

43. van der Lei B, Nieuwenhuis P, Molenaar I, Wildevuur CR. Long-term biologic fate of neoarteries regenerated in microporous, compliant, biodegradable, small-caliber vascular grafts in rats. Surgery 1987; 101:459-67.

44. van der Lei B, Wildevuur CR, Dijk F, Blaauw EH, Molenaar I, Nieuwenhuis P. Sequential studies of arterial wall regeneration in microporous, compliant, biodegradable small-caliber vascular grafts in rats. J Thorac Cardiovasc Surg. 1987; 93:695-707.

45. Hanson SJ, Jamshidi K, Eberhart RC. Mechanical evaluation of resorbable copolymers for end use as vascular grafts. ASAIO Trans 1988; 34:789-93.

46. Gogolewski SG, G. Degradable, microporous vascular prosthesis from segmented polyurethane. Colloid Polym Sci 1986; 264:854-8.

47. Greisler HP, Klosak JJ, Endean ED, McGurrin JF, Garfield JD, Kim DU. Effects of hypercholesterolemia on healing of vascular grafts. J Invest Surg 1991; 4:299-312.

48. Galletti G, Gogolewski S, Ussia G, Farruggia F. Long-term patency of regenerated neoaortic wall following the implant of a fully biodegradable polyurethane prosthesis: Experimental lipid diet model in pigs. Ann Vasc Surg 1989; 3:236-43.

49. Galletti G, Ussia G, Farruggia F, Baccarini E, Biagi G, Gogolewski S. Prevention of platelet aggregation by dietary polyunsaturated fatty acids in the biodegradable polyurethane vascular prosthesis: An experimental model in pigs. Ital J Surg Sci 1989; 19:121-30.

50. van der Lei B, Wildevuur CR. From a synthetic, microporous, compliant, biodegradable small-caliber vascular graft to a new artery. Thorac Cardiovasc Surg 1989; 37:337-47.

51. Greisler HP, Endean ED, Klosak JJ et al. Polyglactin 910/polydioxanone bicomponent totally resorbable vascular prostheses. J Vasc Surg 1988; 7:697-705.

52. Leenslag JWK, Michel T, Pennings AJ, Van der Lei B.A complaint, biodegradable vascular graft: basic aspects of its construction and biological performance. New Polym Mater 1988; 1:111-26.

53. Pennings AJK, K.E., Hoppen HJ, Leenslag JW, Van der Lei B. A two-ply artificial blood vessel of polyurethane and poly(L-lactide). Colloid Polym Sci 1990; 268:2-11.

54. Galletti PM, Ip TK, Chiu TH, Nyilas E, Trudeli LA, Sasken H. Extending the functional life of bioresorbable yarns for vascular grafts. Trans Am Soc Artif Intern Organs 1984; 30:399-400.

55. Galletti PM, Trudell LA, Chiu TH et al. Coated bioresorbable mesh as vascular graft material. Trans Am Soc Artif Intern Organs 1985; 31:257-63.

56. Galletti PM, Aebischer P, Sasken HF, Goddard MB, Chiu TH. Experience with fully bioresorbable aortic grafts in the dog. Surgery 1988; 103:231-41.

57. Greisler HP, Kim DU. Vascular grafting in the management of thrombotic disorders. Semin Thromb Hemost 1989; 15:206-14.

58. Greisler HP, Klosak J, Dennis JW et al. Endothelial cell growth factor attachment to biomaterials. ASAIO Trans 1986; 32:346-9.

59. Wildevuur CR, van der Lei B, Schakenraad JM. Basic aspects of the regeneration of small-calibre neoarteries in biodegradable vascular grafts in rats. Biomaterials 1987; 8:418-22.

60. Yue X, van der Lei B, Schakenraad JM et al. Smooth muscle cell seeding in biodegradable grafts in rats: A new method to enhance the process of arterial wall regeneration. Surgery 1988; 103:206-12.

61. Greisler HP, Klosak JJ, Dennis JW, Karesh SM, Ellinger J, Kim DU. Biomaterial pretreatment with ECGF to augment endothelial cell proliferation. J Vasc Surg 1987; 5:393-9.

62. Gray JL, Kang SS, Zenni GC et al. FGF-1 affixation stimulates ePTFE endothelialization without intimal hyperplasia. J Surg Res 1994; 57:596-612.

63. Ruderman RJH, Andrew F, Hattler BG, Leonard F. Partially biodegradable vascular prosthesis. Trans Am Soc Artif Intern Organs 1972; 18:30-7.

64. Greisler HP, Kim DU, Dennis JW et al. Compound polyglactin 910/polypropylene small vessel prostheses. Journal of Vascular Surgery 1987; 5:572-83.

65. Greisler HP, Tattersall CW, Klosak JJ, Cabusao EA, Garfield JD, Kim DU. Partially bioresorbable vascular grafts in dogs. Surgery 1991; 110:645-54.

66. Zenni GC, Gray JL, Appelgren EO et al. Modulation of myofibroblast proliferation by vascular prosthesis biomechanics. Asaio J 1993; 39:M496-500.

67. Chu CCL, L.E. Design and in vitro testing of newly made bicomponent knitted fabrics for vascular surgery. Polym Sci Technol 1987; 35:185-213.

68. Cohn DY, Hani, Appelbaum Y, Uretzky G. A selectively biodegradable vascular graft. Prog Biomed Eng 1988; 5:73-9.

69. Uretzky G, Appelbaum Y, Younes H et al. Long-term evaluation of a new selectively biodegradable vascular graft coated with polyethylene oxide-polylactic acid for right ventricular conduit. An experimental study. J Thorac Cardiovasc Surg 1990; 100:769-76.

70. Cohn D, Elchai Z, Gershon B et al. Introducing a selectively biodegradable filament wound arterial prosthesis: A

short-term implantation study. J Biomed Mater Res 1992; 26:1184-204.

71. Hellener G, Cohn D, Marom G. Elastic response of filament wound arterial prostheses under internal pressure. Biomaterials 1994; 15:1115-21.

72. Moritz A, Grabenwoger F, Windisch A et al. A method for constricting large veins for use in arterial vascular reconstruction. Artif Organs 1990; 14:394-8.

73. Zweep HP, Satoh S, van der Lei B et al. Autologous vein supported with a biodegradable prosthesis for arterial grafting. Ann Thorac Surg 1993; 55:427-33.

74. Zweep HP, Satoh S, van der Lei B, Hinrichs WL, Feijen J, Wildevuur CR. Degradation of a supporting prosthesis can optimize arterialization of autologous veins. Ann Thorac Surg 1993; 56:1117-22.

75. Hinrichs WL, Zweep HP, Satoh S, Feijen J, Wildevuur CR. Supporting, microporous, elastomeric, degradable prostheses to improve the arterialization of autologous vein grafts. Biomaterials 1994; 15:83-91.

76. Moczar M, Godeau G, Robert AM, Moczar E, Loisance D, Bessous JP. Biodegradable arterial prosthesis from rat aorta. Pathol Biol (Paris) 1980; 28:517-24.

77. Moczar M, Bessous JP, Loisance D. Healing of biodegradable vascular prostheses. Incorporation of 3H-Valine into proteins in the subendothelial scar and host intima-media of rat aorta. Connective Tissue Research 1983; 12:33-42.

78. Schmitz-Rixen T, Megerman J, Anderson JM et al. Longterm study of a compliant biological vascular graft. Eur J Vasc Surg 1991; 5:149-58.

79. Walter M, Erasmi H, Schmidt R. A new biological vascular prosthesis. Vasa Suppl 1991; 33:90-1.

80. Walter M, Erasmi H. A new vascular prosthesis of bovine origin. Thorac Cardiovasc Surgeon 1992; 40:38-41.

81. Walter M, Asoklis S, Erasmi H, Meisch JP. Bovine heterologous graft in replacement of a small calibre artery. Ann Chir 1994; 48:870-5.

Scaffold Engineering

Material Aspects

―――――――――――――――― CHAPTER 46 ――――――――――――

Biodegradable Materials

K.J.L. Burg, S.W. Shalaby

Introduction

Absorbable materials are unique as implants, in that they are absorbed and excreted from the body at the conclusion of their functional period, thus alleviating the expense and potential complications of a retrieval surgery. Additionally, as these materials gradually absorb, they allow a gradual shift in mechanical strength from the biomaterial back to the healing tissue. The absorption time and therefore loss of mechanical strength of the implant may be modulated to best match a given application.

Synthetic absorbable materials were first developed as medical implants in the late 1960s and found use in applications such as barriers, scaffolds, and drug delivery systems.[1] Prior to this time, naturally derived materials such as collagen, catgut, and silk were used; however, they were subject to unpredictable, enzymatic degradation and elicited immune responses due to impurities. The evaluation and application of absorbable materials gradually expanded from soft tissue devices into bone fracture fixation devices, an area of ongoing development.[2-5] A more recent area of interest is the role of absorbable materials as structural matrices or supports in tissue engineering.[6,7]

Criteria for Useful Tissue Engineering Materials

Tissue engineering involves organ development and replacement by the seeding of cells on or into a polymer matrix which may be either cultivated in vitro or implanted directly in vivo. The selective use of parenchymal cells minimizes the amount of donor tissue required and, rather than implanting a large volume of avascular tissue which may not survive, the revascularization process occurs simultaneously with the tissue growth and material bioabsorption. Absorbable materials have found an important role as a matrix material in such constructs. Indeed, the advent of tissue engineering technology opened yet another area of absorbable materials research.

Absorbable and biodegradable polymer technology lends itself well to tissue engineering in that it provides a means of creating a temporary, prefabricated tissue template into or on which cells may be seeded. The absorbable polymer construct is a temporary, structural support allowing and protecting new tissue growth and gradually absorbing as the tissue acquires the desired strengths and functions. Development of the tissue may be begun ex vivo,[8] where the polymer supports and maintains the tissue integrity during implantation. The early attempts to grow tissue combined cells with collagenous two-dimensional substrates.[9-11] Research has become diverse, with replacement potential in many areas including liver, skin, cartilage, breast, nerve, and bone repair. Along with the growth in possible applications came also the development of more suitable forms for three-dimensional

Tissue Engineering of Prosthetic Vascular Grafts, edited by Peter Zilla and Howard P. Greisler.
©1999 R.G. Landes Company.

tissue culture. This included injectable gels and gel formers, fibrous scaffolds, porous foams, and channeled substrates to allow vascularization. The processing techniques also developed to allow more custom-made designs and provision of more complicated, site-specific shapes. The processing of an absorbable material allows a reproducible end product, and the use of an absorbable material reduces both the cost and the risk of donor and recipient surgery.

There are many synthetic polymers which are used in tissue engineering research, among which are polylactide, polyglycolide, polyphosphazene, polycaprolactone, and various copolymers. Copolymers such as lactide-colysine have been specifically developed in order to provide attachment points for cell binding peptide groups.[12-14] The synthetic polymers are advantageous in that their properties may be directly modulated during synthesis and processing to achieve particular requirements. They tend to degrade in a very predictable fashion, largely hydrolytically, which has obvious benefits.

The natural materials which have found use in tissue engineering research include alginate, collagen, chitosan and coral, as well as similarly peptide modified natural materials (Table 46.1). These materials are naturally derived and therefore readily available; their absorption is generally enzymatically driven and subsequently less predictable. Typically this group of absorbable materials may vary considerably from batch to batch. They do, however, allow gelatinous, injectable structures and therefore a broader range of applications.

There are many factors to consider when designing an absorbable substrate for tissue engineering purposes. The amount of exposed polymeric surface area will relate to the intensity of the inflammatory response; therefore, an implant with greater exposed surface will induce a greater response than a smaller area.[7] The polymer purity, crystallinity, molecular orientation, molecular weight, and polydispersity may all influence the presence and timing of an inflammatory response. The effect of bulk mass loss of the polymeric material on the success rate of the newly developed tissue is, as a result, an important design issue.

The pore size of a three-dimensional scaffold, as well as the means of dispersion and flow rate of cells into the scaffold, is of importance in determining both the distribution of cells and the integrity of the cells.[15] Additionally, pore sizes larger than 10 micron will allow invasion of fibrovascular tissue and therefore enhance capillary network development and subsequent vascularization.[16] The rate of the tissue infiltration increases with pore size and porosity, and its survival and integration with the host tissue depends largely on the vascularization.

An even distribution of cells throughout the matrix is important to the development and functionality of the tissue, as well as the interaction of the device and transplanted cells with the surrounding tissue. The hydrophilicity of the polymeric surface contributes to the wettability of the porous structure and hence to the distribution of cells throughout the matrix. The crystalline polylactide and polyglycolide materials are relatively hydrophobic; therefore, aqueous cell solutions do not adequately infiltrate the polymeric interior. Less polar solvents such as ethanol may be used to prewet the scaffold before applying the cell solution;[17] the concern then becomes the minimization of the scaffold-solvent contact time in order to avoid excessive ester bond cleavage. Another approach to improve cellular distribution throughout the scaffold without addressing the bulk substrate properties is to surface coat the device with an absorbable, hydrophilic material prior to cell seeding. Low molecular weight, soluble polyvinyl alcohol coatings, as well as pluronic coatings, may be successfully applied to these hydrophobic substrates, thus rendering them more attractive for cellular attachment.[18] These surfactants do not improve the cellular adhesion to the polymeric structure, but they do allow a much better cell distribution throughout the matrix. Furthermore, they dissolve readily in aqueous environment and are therefore unlikely to interfere with the intended implant function.

The criteria for a tissue engineered absorbable vascular graft material are very focused. The material must be readily sculpted into an appropriately sized tubular shape, matching that of surrounding target tissue and, more problematic in the case of small diameter vessels, must be able to withstand large flow forces without hindering transport. The construct must be a specific porosity in order to optimize the tissue integration and reformation. The tissue ingrowth must occur over the entire length of the prosthesis rather than primarily from a transanastomotic pannus ingrowth. Most importantly, it must have an anti-thrombogenic lumenal cellular lining and must facilitate long term viability.

Table 46.1. Absorbable materials used in tissue engineering

Absorbable Material	Material Type	Typical Forms
polylactide	polyester	porous sponges
polyglyolide	polyester	fibrous meshes
alginate	polysaccharide	hydrogels, spheres
collagen	protein	porous sponges, knitted fabrics
substituted polyphosphazene	polyphosphazene	porous sponges
polycaprolactone	polyester	porous sponges
poly(ethylene glycol-b-propylene glycol)	polyether	surfactant

Methods of Fabrication of Synthetic Polymeric Materials for Use in Tissue Engineering

Tissue engineering absorbable graft research has thus far targeted the synthetic absorbable materials so it is useful to understand the various methods of processing these particular materials into tissue engineering scaffolds.

Physical Aggregation

Physical aggregation is the formation of a porous, interconnected network with no chemical interlocks between the polymer matrix components; rather, a physical adhesion is formed. The pores formed by aggregation are typically uniform and of low size distribution. This may be accomplished in microsphere systems by forming an agglomerate of particles by adding a biocompatible plasticizing agent such as triethylcitrate.[19] Physical aggregation of this kind therefore allows an interconnected, biocompatible, mechanically stable, porous structure.

A second method of physical aggregation is by sintering. Tassels and felts have found initial success as transplantation surfaces in liver and cartilage regeneration studies; however, these structures may lack the necessary mechanical integrity to maintain a specific shape. Fibrous scaffolds, woven or random arrays, have also found application in tissue engineering, but their dimensional stability and hence retention of shape is questionable. The fibers may be sintered together to provide a stable structure in a manner similar to the processing of the "self reinforced" bone pins;[4] however, the high temperature required can cause disorientation of the molecular order and subsequent buckling of the material.[20] The fibers may, rather, be coated with a supportive material which maintains the scaffold shape during heat treatment, but which may be later dissolved from the system.[20]

Chemical Aggregation

Chemical aggregation involves forming a porous, interconnected network by crosslinking, or chemically bonding, the polymer matrix components. This may be accomplished with a difunctional agent such as gluteraldehyde.[19] The drawbacks to this include reduced porosity due to interstitial "filler" material as well as the potential introduction of a toxic substance (e.g., traces of glutaraldehyde) into the biological system.

Gas Dispersion

The pores formed by dispersion are typically uniform and of low size distribution. Gases may be introduced into a polymer melt or a liquid monomer, either directly or as a by-product of a chemical reaction. When cooling of the polymer or polymerization of the monomer occurs, the gas bubbles become entrapped in the material, usually resulting in a closed pore system. If the melt is extruded, this can actually result in an open pore system or a "blown" foam.[21] These foams typically are a larger pore sized system. Alternatively, a gas may be introduced into a polymeric solid at high pressure. Then when the solid is transferred to atmospheric conditions, the gas will expand, forming a spongelike material (Fig. 46.1). This does not require use of solvents and may successfully be accomplished with absorbable polylactide/polyglycolide copolymers and a carbon dioxide environment.[22]

Solid and Liquid Dispersion

Solid or liquid "fillers", such as thermoset polymer spheres[21] or water,[23] may also be purposefully entrapped in the polymer matrix upon solidification. Subsequent removal of the solid or liquid results in an open pore system, the pore size distribution of which is generally larger than that of the gas dispersion process. Absorbable foams may be manufactured using this technique.[18,24] The polymer can be mixed, for example, with a solvent and sodium chloride particles of a predetermined size (Fig. 46.2). The solvent is evaporated, leaving a polymer matrix with entrapped particles. The salt is leached from the system by soaking the construct in water, thus yielding a porous structure. The solid dispersion pore size is variable according to the size of the filler utilized.

Supercritical Fluid Extraction

Absorbable polymers, specifically polyglycolides, polylactides, and polyanhydrides, may be combined with supercritical fluids to process open pore systems.[25] The supercritical fluid is added to the polymer under pressure, the pressure is then dropped to remove the fluid and render the material spongelike (Fig.46.3). The percent porosity is dependent on the pressure differential between ambient and processing. One huge benefit of this technique is that no organic solvents are required.

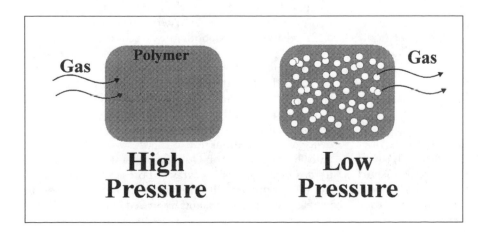

Fig. 46.1. Foam formation by gas dispersion.

Fig. 46.2. Foam formation by solid dispersion.

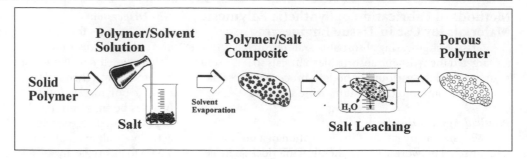

Fig. 46.3. Phase diagram indicating pathway (1-2) of foam formation by supercritical fluid extraction.

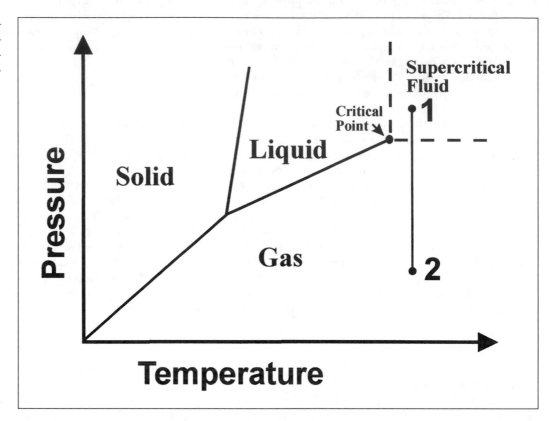

Crystallization-Induced Microphase Separation

This method of foam fabrication[26,27] calls for the addition of a solid solvent with high melting temperature to the polymeric material. The mixture is then heated to form an isotropic liquid system. Subsequent cooling causes the crystallization-induced microphase separation and the now solidified solvent can be sublimed or removed with a liquid solvent. This process has been successfully applied to the formation of open pore absorbable constructs, specifically polydioxanone and poly(ε-caprolactone-co-glycolide) porous structures (Fig. 46.4).

Biodegradable Polymers for Vascular Grafts— Past, Present, and Future

Many attempts have been made at engineering tubular vascular grafts by providing a tubular, porous, polymer support structure. The structure must be mechanically sound so as not to collapse or interfere with blood transport through the conduit. The polylactides and polyglycolides have shown favorable responses to such mechanical stresses.

These materials can be copolymerized in order to provide a range of degradation times from weeks to years.

The relative lack of biocompatibility of traditional synthetic materials and the persistent dilemma of clinically unacceptable small diameter (< 6mm) vascular grafts instigated attempts to modify the substrates and provide a more compatible material. One such attempt is the surface modification of synthetic tubular materials or type I collagen with endothelial cells and smooth muscle cells to provide a more biologically "friendly" implant.[28-30] Other investigators have tried coating 90/10 poly(glycolide-co-L-lactide) based grafts with absorbable materials such as a mixture of poly-DL-lactide/poly-(2,3-butylene maleate) or poly-(2,3-butylene fumarate)/poly-DL-lactide.[31-33] Fumarate leads to a more uniform and predictable absorption rate—there is no evidence of complications due to aneurysm or rupture. Alternatively, the porosity of a tubular implant may be adjusted to provide a diminishing array of pore sizes from the exterior to the interior of the implant, thus potentially allowing increased capillarization and improved biocompatibility.[34]

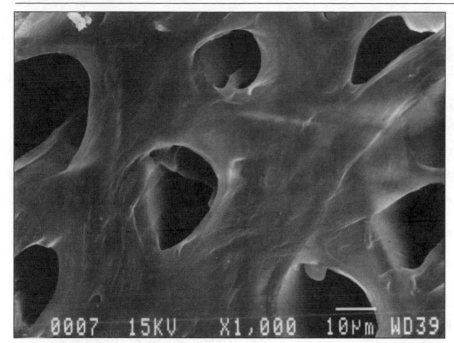

Fig. 46.4. Scanning electron micrograph of absorbable foam formed by crystallization-induced microphase separation.

Traditionally the ideal vascular graft material was assumed to be biologically inert. Today, however, research has shifted toward creating an active material that will interact and integrate favorably with the surrounding biological environment. The absorbable materials, as dynamic implant systems, have this quality and appear to stimulate growth factor release through macrophage induction. Both polyglycolide (PG), 90/10 glycolide/L-lactide copolymer, and polydioxanone (PDS) woven grafts have successfully demonstrated, in animal studies, inner capsule development as well as capillary invasion, thus resulting in an integrated, mechanically stable prosthesis.[35-37] The inner capsule contains layers of myofibroblasts covered by endothelial-like cells (presumably from a capillary endothelial source). In similar studies, Dacron reinforced PGA shows no such capsule development and low amounts of transinterstitial macrophage migration, presumably due to the inhibitive nature of Dacron.[38] These types of partially absorbable vascular patches, based on woven composite yarn comprising a 24-82% polyglycolide yarn, the balance being polyethylene terephthalate yarn, were also evaluated in dogs in terms of blood compatibility.[39] Results indicate that the patch biocompatibility and effect on blood components increased with the increase in the polyglycolide content. This signals the importance of tissue ingrowth to the construction of successful synthetic vascular grafts.

Studies have also focused on the creation of an optimal biological component, integral to the prosthesis, for example, tubular nonabsorbable polyester fabrics incorporated with bovine serum albumin and a luminal coating of gelatin heparin sodium solution. These constructs are crosslinked with a polyepoxy compound. The grafts, once implanted, show no signs of platelet aggregation or fibrin formation and show development of neointima over the anastomotic graft site. The degree of crosslinking is critical to success, as too high a degree causes lack of anastomotic endothelialization and transinterstitial tissue ingrowth.[40]

The compliance and longevity of a potential vascular graft material can influence the retention of mechanical integrity.[41,42] Studies in the polyurethane/polylactide (PU/PLLA) system have shown that a decrease in the percent polyurethane causes a decrease in compliance and an increase in aneurysmal degeneration.[43] These studies further showed that high mechanical compliance of the graft at implantation stimulates elastin formation and an absorbable graft material allows maintenance of the mechanical stability of the newly formed tissue. The PU/PLLA system is initially a compliant one; however, long term incidences of aneurysmal dilation are significantly greater in this system than the polyester ones. This is possibly because the ongoing presence of PU leads to fibroplasia, resulting in decreased compliance and elastin deposition. Another important consideration for scaffold development, as with other applications, is that the tissues should gain adequate strength before the material absorbs. If this is not possible, the absorbable scaffold may be reinforced by an inert (not Dacron) component or developed into a composite material whereby the tissue ingrowth occurs through a series (two or more) of polymers. The multicomponent absorbable vascular prostheses composed of compound yarns of this type appear to be efficacious.[44] Studies have shown that, in contrast to the absorbable component, the biomechanical properties of the nonabsorbable component modulate the histologic attributes and longevity of the final tissue structure.

Other attempts at tissue engineering blood vessels have been made by constructing the vessels ex vivo directly from the cellular components. This may be accomplished by culturing a sheet of human vascular smooth muscle cells in collagen and placing this about a lumenal support to produce the media.[45] A fibroblast sheet is then similarly cultivated

Fig. 46.5. Surface phosphorylation of polyethylene.

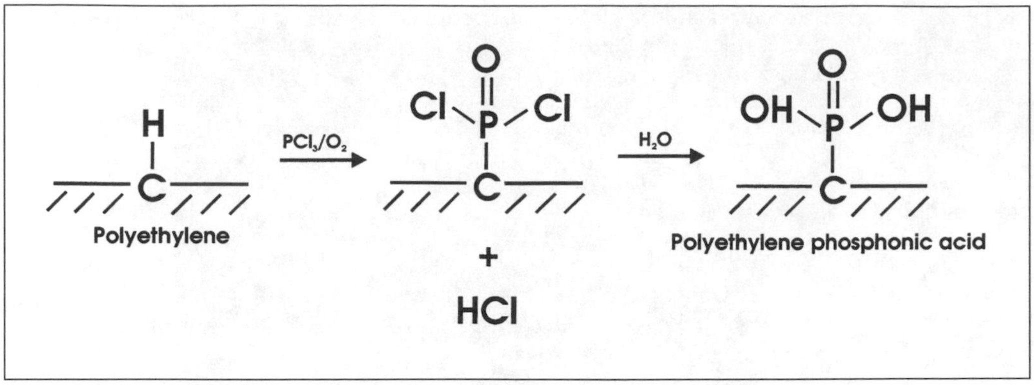

and placed about the media to form the adventitia. Endothelial cells are later seeded into the lumen of the vessel, thus forming a mechanically sound three-dimensional vessel.

Newly Tailored Materials for Tissue Engineering

Two recently developed technologies are expected to be of value in tissue engineering applications. First, Shalaby[46] developed a series of injectable, absorbable liquid copolymers which undergo gel formation upon contacting moist biological tissues. These copolymers are based on polyethylene glycol segments and copolymeric segments derived from glycolide, lactide, trimethylene carbonate, ε-caprolactone, and/or p-dioxanone. These monomers are used in the production of commercial absorbable sutures. The injectable liquid polymers were described as a suitable vehicle for housing living cells for injection into desired biological sites to continue propagation into three-dimensional constructs with the gradual absorption of the gel carrier. Surface phosphonylation of preformed devices, including microporous open-cell foams that were described by Shalaby and co-workers,[27,47,48] represents a second area of technology with promising potential for use in tissue engineering (Fig 46.5). This technology entails the formation of covalently bonded surface phosphonate groups which can:

1. Introduce hydrophilicity to hydrophobic substrates;
2. Bind specific proteins or peptides to direct cell attachment; and
3. Bind Ca^{2+} for directing the deposition of hydroxyapatite toward bone formation.

Among the substrates suitable for surface phosphonylation are certain hydrophobic absorbable polyesters.

Future Prospectives

One of the drawbacks to the synthetic materials as potential vascular graft materials is that, as homopolymers, they do not have the cell surface receptors required for cellular recognition. The polymers must be optimized to best modulate features such as crystallinity, surface texturing, and surface wettability in order to selectively attract specific biological components while preventing spreading of blood platelets. Surface modification such as that described by Shalaby and co-workers may be of value in overcoming some of these issues.

The need for a vascular graft implies that the surrounding target tissue may be "abnormal" (atherosclerotic, for example). It has been shown in animal studies that the quality of such tissues (for example, in the presence of excessive amounts of lipoprotein) may have a profound effect on the development of new tissue.[49] It would therefore be useful to study the absorbable material in such suboptimal conditions or in compromised tissue environments.

References

1. Gilding DK. Biodegradable polymers. In: Williams DF, ed. Biocompatibility of Clinical Implant Materials. Boca Raton, FL: CRC Press, 1981:209-232.
2. Bos RRM, Rozema FR, Boering G et al. In vivo and in vitro degradation of poly(l-lactide) used for fracture fixation. In: Putter C de, Lange GL de, Groot K de, Lee AJC, eds. Advances in Biomaterials. 8. Amsterdam, The Netherlands: Elsevier Science, 1988:245-250.
3. Leenslag JW, Pennings AJ, Bos RRM et al. Resorbable materials of poly(L-lactide). VI. Plates and screws for internal fracture fixation. Biomater 1987; 8(1):70-73.
4. Vainionpää S, Kilpikari J, Laiho J et al. Strength and strength retention in vitro, of absorbable, self-reinforced polyglycolide (PGA) rods for fracture fixation. Biomater 1987; 8(1):46-48.
5. Vert M, Christel P, Garreau H et al. Totally bioresorbable composite systems for internal fixation of bone fractures. In: Chiellini E, Giusti P, Migliaresi C, Nicolais L, eds. Polymers in Medicine II. New York, New York: Plenum Press, 1986:263-275.
6. Vacanti JP. Beyond transplantation. Arch Surg 1988; 123:545-549.
7. Vacanti JP, Morse MA, Saltzman WM et al. Selective cell transplantation using bioabsorbable artificial polymers as matrices. J Pedia Surg 1988; 23(1):3-9.
8. Mikos AG, Sarakinos G, Lyman MD et al. Prevascularization of porous biodegradable polymers. Biotechnol Bioeng 1993; 42:716-723.
9. Boyce ST, Christianson DJ, Hansbrough JF. Structure of a collagen-GAG dermal skin substitute optimized for cultured human epidermal keratinocytes. J Biomed Mater Res 1988; 22:939-957.
10. Boyce ST, Hansbrough JF. Biologic attachment, growth, and differentation of cultured human epidermal keratinocytes on a graftable collagen and chondroitin-6-sulphate substrate. Surgery 1988; 103(4):421-431.
11. Hansbrough JF, Boyce ST, Cooper ML et al. Burn wound closure with cultured autologous keratinocytes and fibroblasts attached to a collagen-glycosaminoglycan substrate. JAMA 1989; 262(15):2125-2130.

12. Cook AD, Hrkach JS, Gao NN et al. Characterization and development of RGD-peptide-modified poly(lactic acid-co-lysine) as an interactive, resorbable biomaterial. J Biomed Mater Res 1997; 35:513-523.

13. Barrera DA, Zylstra E, Lansbury PT et al. Copolymerization and degradation of poly(lactic acid-co-lysine). Macromolecules 1995; 28:425-432.

14. Hrkach JS, Ou J, Lotan N et al. Synthesis of poly(L-lactic acid-co-L-lysine) graft copolymers. Macromolecules 1995; 28:4736-4739.

15. Wald HL, Sarakinos G, Lyman MD et al. Cell seeding in porous transplantation devices. Biomater 1993; 14(4):270-278.

16. Mooney DJ, Langer R. Engineering biomaterials for tissue engineering: The 10-100 micron size scale. In Bronzino JD, ed. Biomedical Engineering Handbook. Boca Raton, FL: CRC Press, 1995:1609-1618.

17. Mikos AG, Lyman MD, Freed LE et al. Wetting of poly(L-lactic acid) and poly(DL-lactic-co-glycolic acid) foams for tissue culture. Biomater 1994; 15(1):55-57.

18. Mooney DJ, Park S, Kaufmann PM et al. Biodegradable sponges for hepatocyte transplantation. J Biomed Mater Res 1995; 29:959-965.

19. Schugens Ch, Grandfils Ch, Jerome R et al. Preparation of a macroporous biodegradable polylactide implant for neuronal transplantation. J Biomed Mater Res 1995; 29:1349-1362.

20. Mikos AG, Bao Y, Cima LG et al. Preparation of poly(glycolic acid) bonded fiber structures for cell attachment and transplantation. J Biomed Mater Res 1993; 27:183-189.

21. Frisch KC, Saunders JH, eds. Plastic Foams. New York: Marcel Dekker, 1972.

22. Mooney DJ, Baldwin DF, Suh NP et al. Novel approach to fabricate porous sponges of poly(DL-lactic-co-glycolic acid) without the use of organic solvents. Biomater 1996; 17(14):1417-1422.

23. Williams JM, Wrobleski DA. Microstructures and properties of some microcellular foams. J Mater Sci Letters 1989; 24:4062-4067.

24. Mikos AG, Thorsen AJ, Czerwonka LA et al. Preparation and characterization of poly(L-lactic acid) foams. Polymer 1994; 35:1068-1077.

25. De Ponti R, Torricelli C, Martini A et al. Use of supercritical fluids to obtain porous sponges of biodegradable polymers. International Patent WO 91/09079, June 1991.

26. Roweton SL. A new approach to the formation of tailored microcellular foams and microtextrued surfaces of absorbable and non-absorbable thermoplastic biomaterials. Master of Science Thesis. Department of Bioengineering, Clemson University. 1994.

27. Shalaby SW, Roweton SL. Continuous open-cell polymeric foams containing living cells. 1997: U.S. Patent #5,677,355.

28. Herring MB, Gardner AK, Glover JL. Seeding human arterial prostheses with mechanically derived endothelium. The detrimental effect of smoking. J Vasc Surg 1984; 1:279-289.

29. Yue X, van der Lei B, Schakenraad JM et al. Smooth muscle cell seeding in biodegradable grafts in rats: A new method to enhance the process of arterial wall regeneration. Surgery 1988; 103:206-212.

30. Kempczinski RF, Rosenman JE, Pearce WH et al. Endothelial cell seeding of a new PTFE vascular prosthesis. J Vasc Surg 1985; 2(3):424-429.

31. Galletti PM, Ip TK, Chiu T-H et al. Extending the functional life of bioresorbable yarns for vascular grafts. Trans ASAIO 1984; 30:399-400.

32. Galletti PM, Trudell LA, Chiu T-H et al. Coated bioresorbable mesh as vascular graft material. Trans ASAIO 1985; 31:257-263.

33. Galletti PM, Aebischer P, Sasken HF et al. Experience with fully bioresorbable aortic grafts in the dog. Surgery 1988; 103:231-241.

34. Lei Bvd, Blaau EH, Dijk F et al. Microporous compliant biodegradable graft materials: A new concept for microvascular surgery. In: Skotnicki SH, Buskens FGM, and Reinaerts HHM, eds. Recent Advances in Vascular Grafting. The Netherlands: Nijmegan, 1984:19-23.

35. Greisler HP. Arterial regeneration over absorbable prostheses. Arch Surg 1982; 177:1425-1431.

36. Greisler HP, Kim DU, Price JB et al. Arterial regenerative activity after prosthetic implantation. Arch Surg 1985; 120:315-323.

37. Greisler HP, Ellinger J, Schwarcz TH et al. Arterial regeneration over polydioxanone prostheses in the rabbit. Arch Surg 1987; 122:715-721.

38. Greisler HP, Schwarcz TH, Ellinger J et al. Dacron inhibition of arterial regenerative activity. J Vasc Surg 1986; 3:747-756.

39. Yu TJ, Ho DM, and Chu CC. Bicomponent vascular grafts consisting of synthetic absorbable fibers: Part II: in vivo healing response. J. Investig. Surg 1994; 7(3):195-211.

40. Niu S, Kurumatani H, Satoh S et al. Small vascular prostheses with incorporated bioabsorbable matrices. A preliminary study. ASAIO J 1993; 39(3):M750-M753.

41. Greisler HP, Joyce KA, Kim DU et al. Spatial and temporal changes in compliance following implantation of bioresorbable vascular grafts. J Biomed Mater Res 1992; 26(11):1449-61.

42. Greisler HP, Pham SM, Endean ED et al. Relationship between changes in biomechanical properties and cellular ingrowth in absorbable vascular prostheses. ASAIO Abstracts 1987; 16:25.

43. Lei Bvd, Bartels HL, Nieuwenhuis P et al. Microporous, compliant, biodegradable vascular grafts for the regeneration of the arterial wall in rat abdominal aorta. Surgery 1985; 98:955-963.

44. Endean ED, Kim DU, Ellinger J et al. Effects of polypropylene's mechanical properties on histological and functional reactions to polyglactin 910/polypropylene vascular prostheses. Surg Forum 1987; 38:323-325.

45. Germain L, L'Heureux N, Labbé R et al. Human blood vessel produced in vitro by tissue engineering. Workshop on Biomaterials and Tissue Engineering Abstracts 1997; 23.

46. Shalaby SW. Hydrogel-forming self-solvating absorbable polyester copolymers and methods for use thereof. U.S. Patent 5,612,052 Assignee: Poly-Med, Inc. 1997.

47. Shalaby SW, McCaig SM. Process for phosphonylating the surface of an organic polymeric preform, U.S. Patent 5,491,198, Assignee: Clemson University 1996.

48. Shalaby SW, Rogers KR. Polymeric prosthesis having a phosphonylated surface, U.S. Patent 5,558,517, Assignee: Clemson University 1996.

49. Greisler HP, Klosak JJ, Endean ED et al. Effects of hypercholesterolemia on healing of vascular grafts. J Investigative Surg 1991; 4(3):299-312.

Scaffold Engineering

Material Aspects

—————————— CHAPTER 47 ——————————

The Influence of Porosity and Surface Roughness on Biocompatibility

J.M. Schakenraad, K.H. Lam

Introduction

Vascular prostheses might solve a lot of clinical problems, if only they would "do their job" in a functional way. Functional in this respect includes; nonthrombogenicity; compliance, diameter and wall thickness similar to vessel wall; blood compatibility in all its aspects (complement activation, red and white blood cell damage, thrombocyte activation etc.); immunological inertness etc. Some of these parameters can be influenced in such a way that an acceptable functionality is achieved. Especially with regard to small diameter vascular grafts (< 3 mm), it has proven impossible to solve all problems simultaneously. A vast challenge still lies ahead for the next generation of scientists.

This chapter will discuss two material surface parameters (roughness and porosity) having a large influence on biocompatibility and ultimate patency of vascular grafts. A parameter indicative for short term biocompatibility is the inflammatory response towards an implanted biomaterial. Upon implantation of a biomaterial, local[1,2] and systemic[3] effects can be observed. The local tissue reaction consists of an inflammatory response which serves to eliminate the cause of an injury, minimize the damage and trigger mechanisms for repairing the tissue damaged by injury. The surgical procedure itself initially determines the type and intensity of the inflammatory response. However, in addition, implanted biomaterials themselves provoke an inflammatory response.

Many material characteristics may influence the inflammatory response against a biomaterial (being either a natural polymer, a chemical polymer, metals, ceramics etc.): chemical composition,[1] material toxicity[4,5] surface free energy (wettability),[6] surface charge[7] surface morphology such as porosity,[8] roughness of the surface[9] and shape,[7] implantation site,[10] rate of degradation,[11] degradation products,[12,13] and many more.

Surface morphology is one of the first factors directly influencing the tissue/inflammatory response. This is indicated in various studies.[7,14] Matlaga et al demonstrated the role of shape.[7] The intensity of the inflammatory response increases when the number of edges of the implanted materials increases. Also, there are studies indicating that the inflammatory response against implanted porous polymers or biomaterials is more intense when compared to nonporous materials.[8]

Wettability may influence the tissue reaction to the polymer, because there is a range in wettability values that is optimal for cell adhesion, growth and spreading. Cells attach and proliferate less well on polymers having a wettability which is too low[15] or too high.[16]

Another factor is degradability. Degrading polymers provoke a more intense inflammatory response compared to nondegrading polymers. A possible cause for this observation

Tissue Engineering of Prosthetic Vascular Grafts, edited by Peter Zilla and Howard P. Greisler.
©1999 R.G. Landes Company.

may be the release of monomers, oligomers and/or fragments upon degradation.[12,13] However, at earlier stages of the degradation process, changes (such as increase) in the surface morphology of a polymer (film) may occur, which in turn may alter the inflammatory response.

To illustrate the effect of surface morphology on the tissue response and ultimate biocompatibility of a material after implantation, the following series of materials are compared:

1. Porous versus nonporous;
2. Rough versus smooth;
3. Degradable versus nondegradable.

The inflammatory response was characterized using semi-quantitative techniques comprising morphological criteria and monoclonal antibodies directed against epitopes which are specific for the respective cell types.

Such aspects as molecular weight of soluble leachables and relative surface area are considered to be closely related to the observed histological parameters and are therefore also included in this overview.

Evaluation Models

Materials

As a degradable material, the well known and widely used polylactic acid is used, both as a solid, a porous and a combination form. As a nondegradable reference material, PTFE is used, both in a solid shape and as the expanded PTFE with a pore size of 30 micrometers.

Poly(L-lactic acid) (PLLA) films were cast from PLLA with a reported Mn of 50,000 (Purac Biochem B.V., The Netherlands).[17] Three types of films were cast: a nonporous type, a porous type and a "combi" type (porous with a nonporous layer on one side). The base parameters of the PLLA films are listed in Table 47.1. All PLLA films were cut in strips of 15 x 2 mm.

Polytetrafluoroethylene (PTFE) was obtained commercially (Wientjes, The Netherlands). PTFE was cut into strips of 15 x 2 x 1 mm. Expanded polytetrafluoroenthylene (ePTFE) was obtained as nonsterile GORE-TEX® ePTFE cell collector tubing (WL Gore & Associates GMBH, Germany). The tubing was cut open along the longitudinal axis to obtain films measuring 15 x 2 x 0.25 mm.

Material Characterization

Except for PTFE, the final thickness of the films was determined with scanning electron microscopy (SEM). All films were cleaned by washing in a phosphate buffered saline (PBS) for 24 h prior to use.

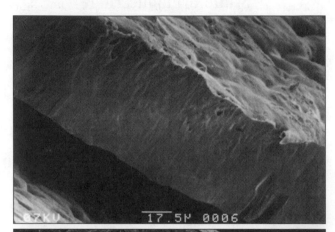

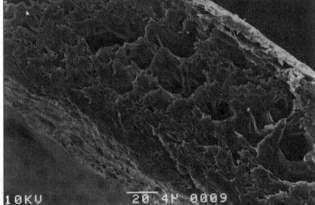

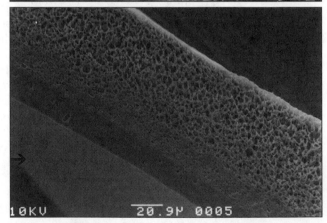

Fig. 47.1. Scanning electron micrographs of a cross-section of PLLA films. (A, top.) nonporous, (B, middle.) porous, (C, bottom.) "combi"; arrowhead indicates the nonporous side. The thickness of the films is: nonporous, 33 μm; porous, 244 μm and "combi", 82 μm. The nonporous layer of the "combi" film was approximately 5 μm. The pore size of the porous film varied from approximately 1-150 μm and of the "combi" film from 1-50 μm.

Table 47.1. Base parameters of the PLLA films

Parameter	Non-porous PLLA film	Porous PLLA film	Combi PLLA film
Mw	98,000	109,000	167,000
Mn	42,000	41,000	53,000
Mw/Mn	2.3	2.7	3.1
Tm	176°C	180°C	181°C
Heat of fusion	53 J/g	51 J/g	50 J/g

Surface Morphology

The surface morphology of the different specimens is illustrated in Figure 47.1A-C. Specimens of all films were sputter-coated with gold (Balzers 07 120B) and their surface morphology was examined with DS 130 scanning electron microscope (SEM) (ISI), operated at 10 KV.

The thickness of the polymers was calculated using SEM: nonporous 33 μm (Fig.47.1A); porous 244 μm (Fig. 47.1B); and the "combi" film 82 μm (Fig. 47.1C). The nonporous layer of the "combi" film was approximately 5 μm. The pore size of the porous film varied from approximately 1 to 150 μm and of the "combi" film from 1 to 50 μm. PTFE was nonporous, having the same morphological appearance of the surface as the nonporous PLLA film. The thickness of the porous ePTFE film was approximately 250 μm with a fibril length of approximately 90 μm (Fig. 47.2).

Wettability

Wettability, as a measure for surface free energy (hydrophobicity) was determined by contact angle measurements using the sessile drop technique described by Busscher et al.[18] For PTFE and the nonporous PLLA, the contact angles were determined using H_2O and α–bromonaphthalene as wetting agents. Five measurements were made for each polymer and wetting agent.

The highest value of each set of five measurements is maximally 5° higher than the lowest value. Therefore, it was not relevant to determine the standard deviation. The H_2O contact angles were 101° for PTFE and 72° for nonporous PLLA, and the α-bromonaphthalene contact angles were 66° for PTFE and 23° for nonporous PLLA. This shows that nonporous PLLA has a less hydrophobic surface than PTFE.

Implantation Procedure

The films were disinfected prior to implantation and implanted subcutaneously in 21 female (AO x BN)F1 rats obtained from our own breeding facility. In each rat a non-porous PLLA film, a porous PLLA film, a "combi" PLLA film, a PTFE film and an ePTFE film were implanted. The sixth incision and subcutaneous pocket served as a control (sham operation). Three samples per polymer and time interval were implanted. The rats had free access to standard rat food and water. All national rules concerning the care and use of laboratory animals have been observed.

The rats were sacrificed after 1, 3, 7, 14, 40, 90 or 180 days and the polymer films were removed with excess surrounding tissue.

Evaluation of the Inflammatory Response

Light Microscopy

After harvesting, the samples were immediately fixed for at least 24 h at 4°C in a 0.1 M Na-cacodylate buffer, pH 7.4, containing 2% glutaraldehyde and 0.1 M sucrose. The samples were then dehydrated in a graded ethanol series and embedded in glycolmethacrylate (Technovit®, Kulzer, Germany), allowing sections to be cut perpendicular to the longitudinal axis of the polymer film. Sections for light microscopy examination were cut on a microtome (Jung autocut 1140, equipped with a D knife with a tungsten carbide cutting edge), mounted on glass slides and stained with toluidine blue and alkaline fuchsin.[19]

Immunohistochemical Staining

After harvesting, samples were snap-frozen at -80°C using liquid freon. Cryostat sections of 7 μm were cut, mounted on glass slides, air-dried and fixed in acetone for 12 minutes. The sections were then again air-dried for 1 h and incubated with the first-stage, cell type specific, monoclonal antibody (mAb) for 1 h. Subsequently, the sections were washed 3 times in PBS, followed by incubation with the second-stage antibody conjugated to peroxidase, diluted 1:40 in PBS and supplemented with 5% v/v normal rat serum to prevent nonspecific binding. Swine anti-rabbit Ig

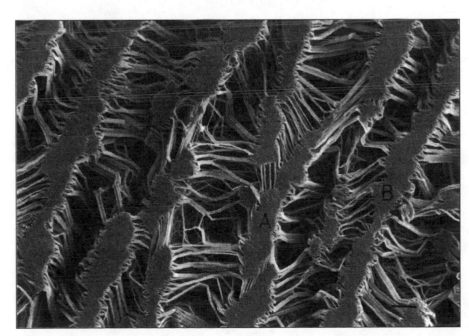

Fig. 47.2. Scanning electron micrograph of (porous) ePTFE. The fibril length (distance between A and B) is approximately 90 μm. Bar indicates 30 μm.

(Dakopatts, Denmark) was used as second-stage antibody to detect the first-stage mAb α-Asialo GM$_1$ (Table 47.2). Rabbit anti-mouse Ig (Dakopatts, Denmark) was used to detect the other first-stage mAbs. After incubation with the second-stage antibody, sections were rinsed 3 times in PBS for 5 minutes. Peroxidase activity was demonstrated by applying 3,3-diaminobenzidine tetrahydrocloride (Sigma) at a concentration of 0.5 mg/ml in 0.05 M Tris-HCI buffer (pH 7.6) containing 0.01% H$_2$O$_2$ for 10 minutes. After rinsing in fresh tap water, sections were counterstained lightly with hematoxylin for 10 seconds. The sections were then dehydrated using a graded ethanol series and xylene and subsequently covered with coverslips using DePeX (Gurr, BDH Ltd, England) mounting medium. In controls, PBS was used instead of the first-stage mAb. The first-stage mAbs used, and their sources, are shown in Table 47.2.

Quantification of the Inflammatory Response

The magnification of the light microscope was set at x400 when examining the section stained using mAbs. The staining patterns of the tissue surrounding or invading the polymer film was evaluated and the number of positive cells surrounding or invading the polymer films per field of view counted. Four fields of view per section, two sections per sample and three samples for each period of implantation, polymer film and monoclonal antibody respectively were examined. The tissue reactions at the edges of the polymer films were excluded from evaluation, to avoid artifacts due to mechanical irritation.

The number of cells staining positive per field of view was classified as follows:

grade 0 = no positive cells,
1 = 1 to 5 positive cells per field of view,
2 = 5 to 10 positive cells per field of view,
3 = 10 to 25 positive cells per field of view and
4 = more than 25 positive cells per field of view.

The average class of the 24 fields of view for each period of implantation, polymer film and monoclonal antibody respectively is reported.

Macroscopically, there were no signs of an infection demonstrated in any of the rats. The results of the semi-quantitative evaluation of the immunohistochemical staining to detect leukocytes (OX 1), neutrophilic granulocytes (HIS 48), macrophages (ED 1, ED 2, ED 3), T lymphocytes (OX 19), vast majority of B lymphocytes (HIS 40), natural killer cells (α-Asialo GM$_1$), cells expressing MHC class II antigen—such as activated fibroblasts—(HIS 19) are demonstrated in Figures 47.3A-I respectively. False positive cells were observed occasionally in PBS controls. This was due to endogenous peroxidase activity expressed only by neutrophilic granulocytes, since the staining pattern using HIS 48 corresponds with the pattern of endogenous peroxidase activity. Moreover, cells expressing endogenous peroxidase activity can be well distinguished due to their more intense staining as compared to cells stained for mAbs.

The concentration of B lymphocytes (Fig. 47.3D) and the concentration of natural killer cells (Fig. 47.3H) was to a large extent similar and low for both PLLA, PTFE films and the subcutaneous tissue under the scar of the sham operation.

At day3, the concentration of each cell type involved in the inflammatory response as a measure for the intensity was approximately the same for all the polymer films (Fig. 47.3A to 47.3G). At day 7, macrophages are beginning to play a prominent role in the inflammatory response (Fig. 47.3E). Subsets of macrophages surrounding the polymer films were found in different locations. ED 1 positive macrophages are found in the entire area, demonstrating inflammatory response against the implant, especially in the area in closest approximation to the polymer film (Fig. 47.4A). In contrast, ED 2 and ED 3 positive macrophages are neither found in the area in closest approximation the polymer film, nor in the pores of the PLLA or PTFE film. ED 2 and ED 3 positive macrophages remain restricted to the surrounding tissue at some distance from the implant (Fig. 47.4B and 47.4C). The relative ratio between the subsets was fairly constant for the respective implants.

Table 47.2. Antibodies (mAbs) used to examine and quantify the inflammatory response against the implanted polymer films

Monoclonal Antibody	Epitope	Mainly characterizing cell type in subcutaneous tissue:
OX 1	CD 45	All leukocytes
HIS 48	probably surface	Granulocytes
OX 19	CD 5	T-lymphocytes
HIS 40	IgM heavy chain	B-lymphocyte subset likely to react first upon inflammatory response
ED 1	Lysosomal antigen	Majority of macrophages. Probably associated with active phagocytosis.
ED 2	Surface antigen	Subset macrophages. Probably associated with maturity.
ED 3	Surface antigen	Subset macrophages. Probably associated with downregulation of inflammatory reaction
α-Asialo GM$_1$	Probably surface antigen	Large granular lymphocytes natural killer cells
HIS 19	MHC class II	Activated tissue cells (fibroblast) IDC, subset macrophage

Source of the mAbs: OX antibodies were a generous gift of the late Dr. A.F. Williams, Department of Biochemistry, University of Oxford, Great Britain; ED antibodies were a generous gift of Dr. C.D. Dijkstra, Department of Cell Biology. The HIS and a-Asialo antibodies were generous gifts of Dr. P. Nieuwenhiu's of the Department of Histology, University of Groningen.

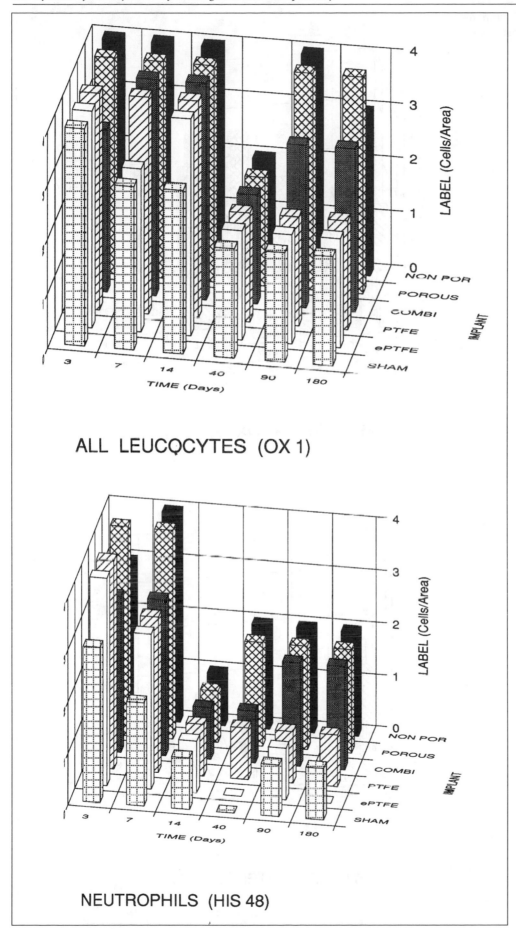

ALL LEUCOCYTES (OX 1)

NEUTROPHILS (HIS 48)

Fig. 47.3. The average class of 24 fields of view of the number of cells involved in the inflammatory response against the implanted polymer films, stained with different mAbs. Class criteria: grade 0 = no positive cells; grade 1 = 1 to 5 positive cells; grade 2 = 5 to 10 positive cells; grade 3 = 10 to 25 positive cells and grade 4 = more than 25 positive cells per field of view at an original magnification of x400. The following mAbs were used: (A, top.) OX 1, all leukocytes. (B, bottom.) HIS 48, neutrophilic granulocytes.

Fig. 47.3. (C, top.) OX 19, T-lymphocytes, (D, bottom.) HIS 40, vast majority of B lymphocytes.

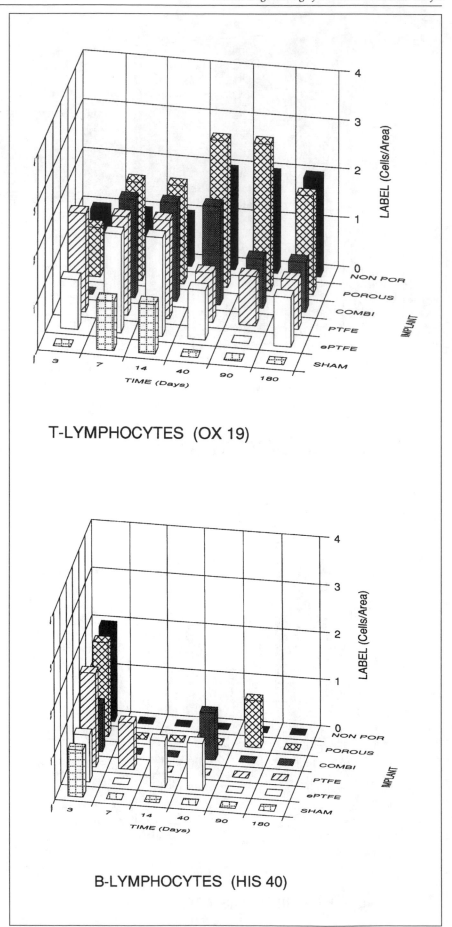

T-LYMPHOCYTES (OX 19)

B-LYMPHOCYTES (HIS 40)

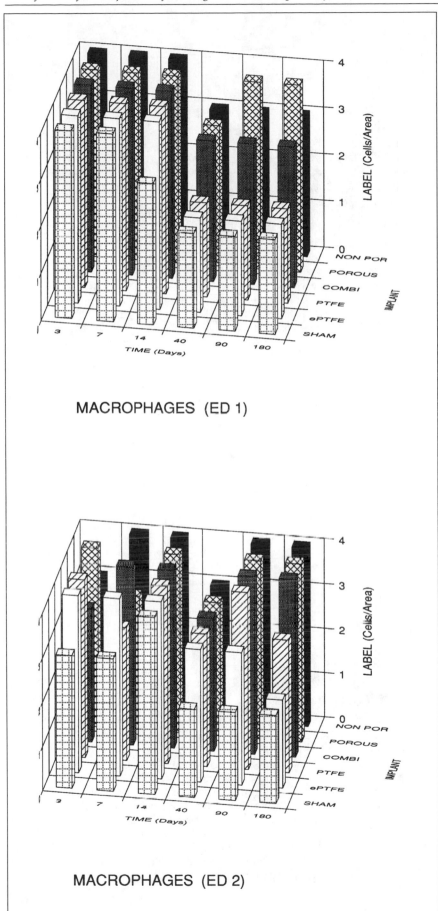

MACROPHAGES (ED 1)

MACROPHAGES (ED 2)

Fig. 47.3. (E, top.) ED 1, vast majority of macrophages, including multinuclear giant cells; (F, bottom.) ED 2, subset (mature/resident) macrophages.

Fig. 47.3. (G, top.) ED 3, subset macrophages. (H, bottom.) α-Asialo GM₁, natural killer cells/large granular lymphocytes

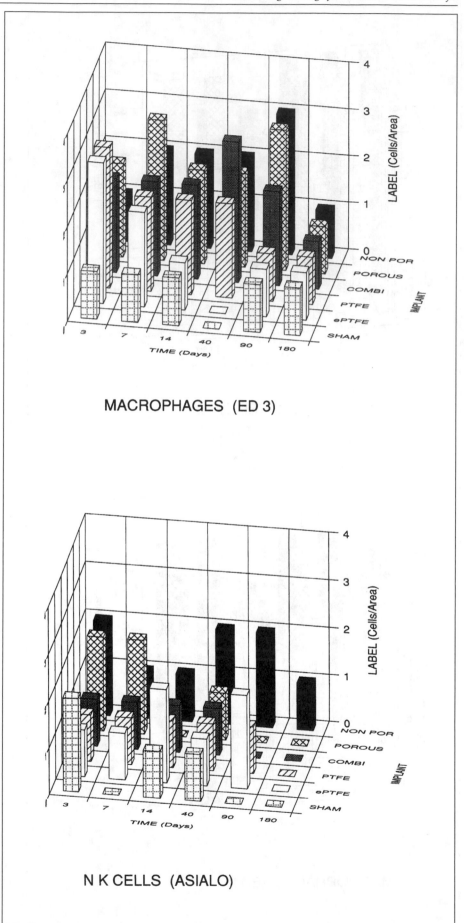

MACROPHAGES (ED 3)

N K CELLS (ASIALO)

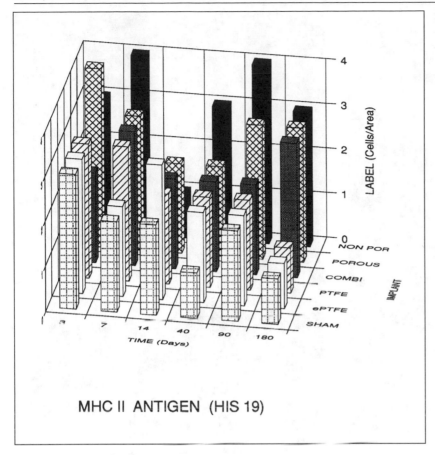

Fig. 47.3. (I.) HIS 19, cells expressing MHC
II antigen (e.g., activated fibroblasts,
macrophages, dendritic cells). X-axis
represents implantation time (days), Y-axis
the average number of cells per field of view
as class 0 to 4. Z-axis represents the different
polymer films.

MHC II ANTIGEN (HIS 19)

In GMA sections it is observed that the inflammatory response at day 7 is becoming more intense (Fig. 47.5) for the porous PLLA and porous side of the "combi" PLLA films. For the nonporous PLLA and the nonporous side of the "combi" PLLA film, the onset of encapsulation by approximately 3 layers of fibroblasts was observed. Only a minimal encapsulation is observed for the porous PLLA film at day 7. In contrast to the porous PLLA film almost no cellular invasion of the ePTFE film was observed. The cell layer surrounding the ePTFE consists mainly of macrophages. The PTFE film was surrounded by one or two layers of macrophages and the onset of encapsulation can be observed.

At day 14, the inflammatory response becomes chronic with predominantly macrophages and T lymphocytes surrounding the films. In the GMA sections, foreign body giant cells can be observed surrounding the PLLA fims (Fig. 47.6). All films are now encapsulated by continuous layers of fibrocytes and collagen. The fibrocytes are not stained by HIS 19 monoclonal antibody, indicating a decrease in cell activity. The porous PLLA film and porous side of the "combi" film provoke a more intense inflammatory response than the nonporous PLLA film and nonporous side of the "combi" film respectively. However, this observation could not be made for the ePTFE film as compared to the PTFE film.

At day 40, in general, the intensity of the inflammatory response against the polymer films had decreased further. However, PLLA films still provoked a more intense in-

flammatory response than PTFE films as demonstrated by the higher concentration of neutrophils, macrophages/giant cells and T lymphocytes surrounding the PLLA films. The concentration of cells against PTFE and ePTFE films is comparable to the concentration of cells in the subcutaneous tissue under the scar of the sham operation. The inflammatory response against the nonporous PLLA film was mainly localized at the edges of the film or at the edges of the pieces when broken. In contrast, the inflammatory response against porous PLLA films was localized in the pores. The "combi" film shows a more pronounced inflammatory response at the porous side.

At day 90, the difference in the intensity of the inflammatory response between PLLA and PTFE films and also between nonporous and porous PLLA films had become much more pronounced. This is demonstrated by the increased concentration of macrophages, leukocytes and cells expressing MHC class II (HIS 19) antigen, (probably activated fibroblasts) surrounding or invading the PLLA films. The porous PLLA films provoke a more intense inflammatory response than the nonporous PLLA film. In contrast, the inflammatory response against PTFE and ePTFE films remained the same as at day 40.

At day180, the difference in the intensity of the inflammatory response between the porous and the nonporous PLLA film was more pronounced. In contrast, the tissue reaction ("inflammatory response") against PTFE and ePTFE did not differ much from the tissue reaction in the

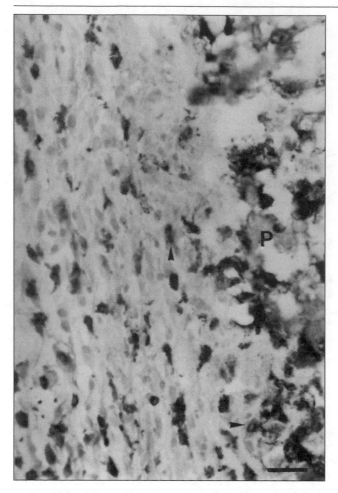

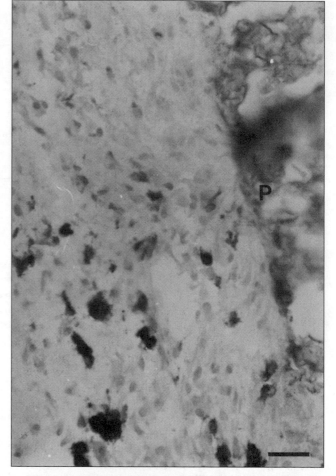

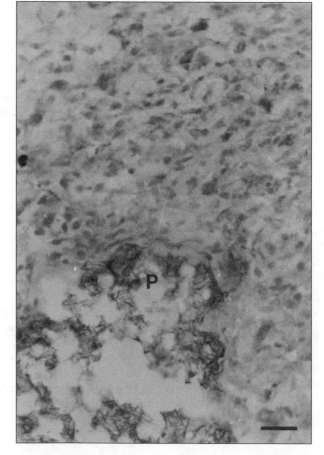

Fig. 47.4. Immunohistochemical staining of the tissue surrounding the porous PLLA film (P) at day 7, with: (A.) ED 1. The macrophages adjacent to the implant stain positive for ED 1 (arrow heads). No ED 1 positive cells are observed in the polymer film. (B.) ED 2. The macrophages adjacent to the implant do not stain positive for ED 2. The cells in the lower left corner stain false positive for ED 2. This is due to endogenous peroxidase activity of neutrophilic granulocytes. (C.) ED 3. The macrophages adjacent to the implant do not stain positive for ED 3. Bar indicates 40 μm.

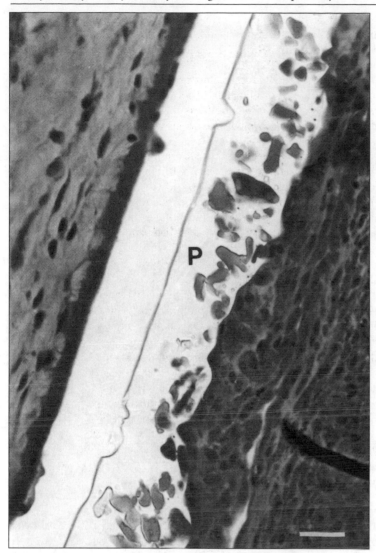

Fig. 47.5. "Combi" PLLA film: P 7 days after implantation. Note the difference in the intensity of the inflammatory response between the porous and the nonporous side. Bar indicates 40 μm.

subcutaneous tissue under the scar of the sham operation. There are almost no cells localized in the pores of ePTFE (Fig. 47.7A). In contrast, the inflammatory response against porous PLLA was localized mainly in the large pores (Fig. 47.7B).

Relative Polymer Surface Area in Sections

The relative polymer surface area (RPSA) in sections was determined after in vivo and in vitro procedures. After harvesting, samples were immediately fixed by immersion in a 0.1 M Na-cacodylate buffer, pH 7.4, containing 2% glutaraldehyde and 0.1 M sucrose, for at least 24 h at 4°C. After rinsing with buffer, the samples were dehydrated in graded ethanol series. The samples were then embedded in a position which allowed sections to be cut perpendicular to the longitudinal axis of the polymer films. After embedding in glycolmethacrylate (GMA) (Technovit, Kulzer, Germany), sections of 3 μm were cut on a Jung 1140 autocut microtome, using a D knife with a tungsten carbide cutting edge. The sections were mounted on glass and stained with toluidine blue and alkaline fuchsin.

The relative polymer surface area in sections (RPSA) was determined by morphometrical analysis using light microscopical sections and a Quantimet 520 (Cambridge Instruments) image analyzer. The RPSA was defined as the ratio between the polymer surface area and measurement frame area. The boundaries of the measurement frame were set at the outer boundaries of the polymer surface area. The morphometrical analysis was performed on porous and "combi" films only, because the nonporous film was not eroded nor did it become porous, not even after an immersion or implantation period of 180 days. The RPSA of the nonporous film remained 100%. For each implantation period or immersion period ten measurements of the remaining polymer surface area (of at least two sections) were performed. The mean value and standard deviation were calculated from these ten values. All data were normalized to the initial value (t = 0).

The results of the morphometrical analyses are presented in Figures 47.8A (in vitro) and 47.8B (in vivo). The RPSA in vivo shows no significant decrease for the nonporous, the porous or the "combi" film. Also, no decrease was

Fig. 47.6. Nonporous PLLA film: P 14 days after subcutaneous implantation. Note the large concentration of giant cells (arrow heads). Bar denotes 40 μm.

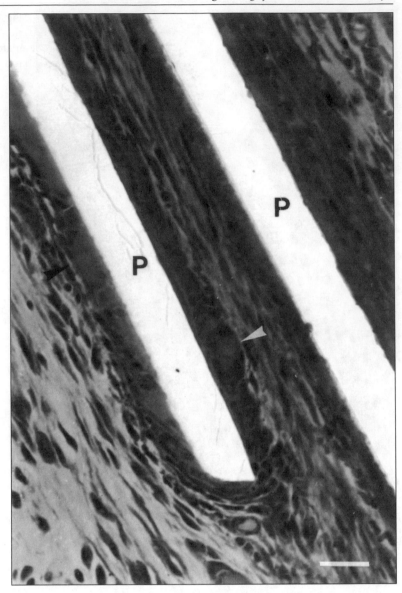

observed in vitro for the nonporous and porous film up till day 180 and for the "combi" film, up till day 90. It was not possible to obtain the surface area of the "combi" film at day 180, due to fragmentation.

During the in vivo experiment with the nonporous polymer film, no erosion or pore formation was observed. Moreover, after immersion in PBS (in vitro), it was not possible to carry the nonporous film through the embedding procedures for light microscopy from day 40 on, due to increased brittleness. The surface area of the remaining nonporous film remained 100% over the entire test period.

M_w and M_n

M_w (molecular weight) and MN in vitro were determined by gel permeation chromatography (GPC) at 20°C on a Waters Associates GPC apparatus using Waters Associates columns (bead size of 10^5, 10^4, 10^3 Å). A precolumn with a pore size of 500 Å was used. A Waters Associates R 403 differential refractometer was used as a detector. A sample of 5-10 mg was dissolved in 10 ml chloroform and filtered (Spartan 13/20 filter, 0.45 μl). The injection volume per measurement was 200 μl. Chloroform was used as eluent at a flow rate of 2.0 ml/min. The M_w, M_n and polydispersity ratio were calculated using the calibration data of polystyrene standards of narrow molecular weight distribution dissolved in tetrahydrofuran (THF).

The M_w (Fig. 47.9A) and M_n (Fig. 47.9B) decreased for all three films at approximately the same rate. From day 7 on, the porous film generally retained the highest M_w and M_n. The initial (t = 0) M_w of the "combi" film was the highest (167,000) and of the nonporous film the lowest (98,000; porous was 109,000). Before day 7, the curves of the porous and "combi" film showed large fluctuations for M_w. Thereafter, all values for M_w demonstrated a decreasing trend till the 170th day (M_w nonporous: 24,000, porous: 60,000, "combi":29,000). The M_n curves roughly approximate the same trend as the M_w curves. The fluctuations of the values for the "combi" film are larger.

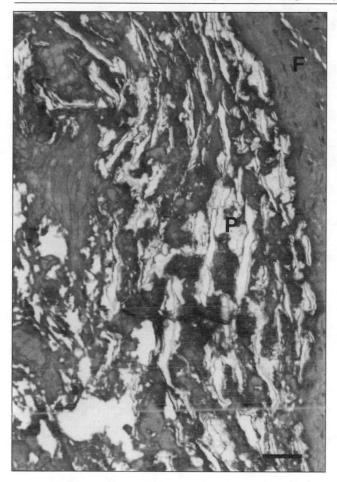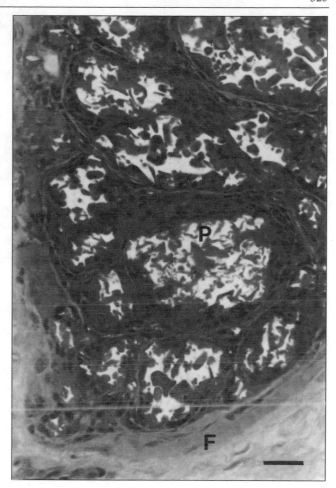

Fig. 47.7. (A, left.) Porous e-PTFE (P) and (B, right.) porous PLLA (P) after 180 days of implantation. There are almost no inflammatory cells localized in the pores of the e-PTFE film. In contrast, the inflammatory response is localized mainly in the pores F=fibrous encapsulation. Bar indicates 63μm.

Interpretation of Results

Inflammatory Response and Biocompatibility

The results demonstrate that there are two phases in the inflammatory response against the films. Phase 1 is observed upon implantation of the film. It is mainly caused by the injury sustained by the implantation procedure. This uncomplicated inflammatory response, part of the wound healing reaction, ends after 7-10 days and has been well described.[2,20] In this phase, the contribution of the implanted polymer film to the intensity of the inflammatory response is in most cases minimal, except when leakage of large quantities of toxic products occurs.[5] After one week, any remaining inflammatory response can be considered as a tissue reaction against the implanted biomaterial.[11] This chronic inflammatory response (phase 2) is often described as a foreign body reaction.[1,2,5] It mainly consists of macrophages and giant cells surrounding the implant.

A minimal inflammatory response is preferred when biomaterials are implanted for a long time span, because a persistent (chronic) inflammatory response may predispose for amyloidosis,[21,22] or carcinogenesis.[23] A persistent inflammatory response increases the concentration of both serum amyloid A (SAA) and amyloid enhancing factor (AEF) in blood. SAA may then be converted into amyloid A, which is deposited in tissues. However, the exact mechanism is yet to be fully uncovered, and the relation between the chronic inflammatory response against biomaterials and amyloidosis also remains to be investigated.

The Role of Macrophages and Giant Cells

ED 1 stains an intracellular antigen, probably associated with the lysosomal membrane. The antigen probably remains present even in the event of fusion of macrophages and formation of foreign body giant cells, since ED 1 positive cells are observed on the same location of foreign body giant cells in conventional light microscopical sections. ED 2 is a marker which is found on mature tissue macrophages. It takes about one week for monocytes/macrophages to express ED 2 on their cell surface after leaving the vascular system. The role of ED 2 and ED 3 in the inflammatory response is not well understood. The different staining patterns of the ED antibodies indicate the possibility of either different populations of macrophages which play a role in the tissue reaction against biomaterials, or macrophages expressing different surface receptors in the course of the inflammatory response against a biomaterial.

Fig. 47.8. Remaining polymer surface area (RPSA) of the PLLA films in a light microscopical section. (A.) In vitro: RPSA as a function of immersion time. (B.) In vivo: RPSA. Symbols represent: □ = nonporous, + = porous, ○ = "combi". Bars indicate the standard deviation.

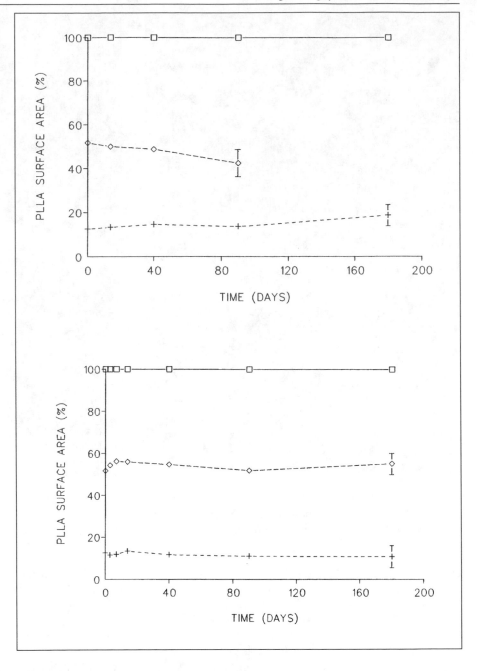

The exact mechanism of foreign body giant cell formations is still to be elucidated. Certain cell types, e.g., T lymphocytes, may play a pivotal role in this process. T helper lymphocytes capable of secreting interferon-γ, especially, may play a role in the fusion of macrophages, forming giant cells.[24,25] Activation of macrophages may be induced by various pathways. In one pathway, (limited) damage to neutrophils and macrophages may lead to secretion of cytokines (IL-1), activating T helper lymphocytes. Another possibility is change of shape when a macrophage comes in contact with a boimaterial,[26,27] especially when a single macrophage is not able to phagocytose the polymer(fragment).

Porosity, Wettability, Degradability and Inflammatory Response

Porous PLLA provokes a more intense inflammatory response from day 7 on, despite a higher degradation rate of the nonporous PLLA in an aqueous environment. This indicates that porosity is an important factor determining the intensity of the inflammatory response against implanted PLLA films. The small difference in the intensity of the inflammatory response between PTFE and ePTFE as compared to porous and nonporous PLLA respectively indicates that porosity as a single factor is not enough to enhance the inflammatory response. The relatively high wettability of PLLA compared to ePTFE allows for better ingrowth of tissue into the pores of PLLA and probably more exposure to other factors, determining the intensity of the inflammatory response.

According to many authors, the surface properties of an implant have a large influence on the inflammatory response. Thus, the difference in wettability as one of the surface properties may also be a factor, although Baier et al could not demonstrate a difference in the inflammatory response against smooth metal pieces having a different wettability.[28]

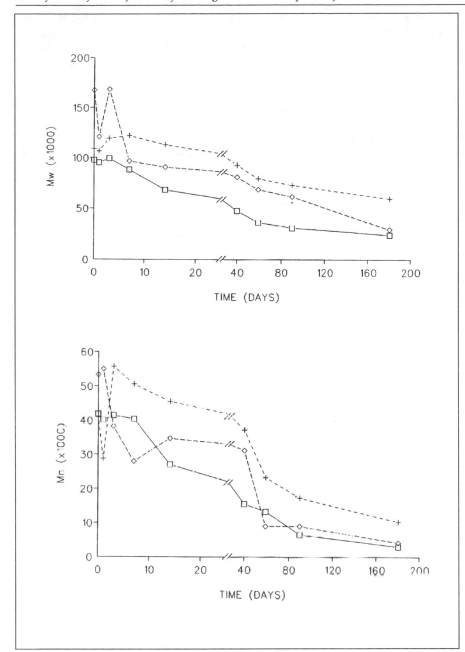

Fig. 47.9. Molecular weight of the PLLA films as a function of immersion time. (A.) MW. (B.) M_n. Symbols represent: ☐ = nonporous, + = porous, ○ = "combi". Standard deviation did not exceed 15%.

However, other authors demonstrated that different polymers induce a different level of IL-1 production, correlating with the intensity of the inflammatory response,[29,30,31] although the relation to wettability was not investigated. However, the production of IL-1 seems to be less when using relatively hydrophobic materials such as silicon. Further investigation is needed to establish the precise relation between wettability and inflammatory response.

The differences in inflammatory response against the PLLA (degradable) and PTFE (nondegradable) films became apparent from day 40. One reason may be the difference in the rate of degradation and subsequently the difference in the release of degradation products such as monomers, oligomers and finally fragments. As stated previously, only a few (mostly nonporous) PLLA films were observed to be broken into two or three pieces. However, there is probably also increase in surface area which could hardly be observed.

Also, the size of the pores of the porous PLLA films has increased, possibly with the same effect as fragmentation. In the case of PLLA films, the increase in surface area during the degradation process as a single factor may be sufficient for increasing the intensity of the inflammatory response.

It can be concluded that biodegradable PLLA films provoke a more intense inflammatory response than nondegradable PTFE films. Also, porosity enhances the inflammatory response. However, porosity enhances the inflammatory response only when the wettability of a biomaterial permits cellular ingrowth.

Relative Polymer Surface Area

The RPSA, which was only determined for the porous and the nonporous polymer film, did not decrease significantly, neither in vitro nor in vivo. However, these results must be interpreted with some caution, because RPSA measurements cannot detect release of small amounts of degradation products from the core of the polymer film. The loss of weight of the nonporous film could not be detected with RPSA measurements since there was no detectable loss of surface area in cross sections of the PLLA film. There was also no indication of measurable surface erosion, such as increasing surface roughness and/or decreasing thickness of the nonporous film. However, this method might be useful in quantifying the later stages of the degradation and the resorption process in vivo, when weight measurement has become practically impossible. The results indicate that in vitro the core of the PLLA films remain largely intact till day 180, and that in vivo there was no resorption of large amounts of polymer. These findings support the results of the weight measurements.

Molecular Weight

The results of the molecular weight measurements indicate a higher degradation rate for the nonporous film compared to the "combi" and porous film, the latter having the lowest degradation rate. The decrease of MW and MN is obvious for all three types of film, although results obtained with GPC must be interpreted with caution when low molecular weight polymers resulting from degradation processes are examined.

Therefore, the differences between the films may not be significant, but the higher MW and MN of the porous film compared to the nonporous film, from day 7 till the end of the experiment at day 180, is very suggestive. The initial MW and MN of the different films are not equal (Figs. 47.9A and 47.9B). A possible explanation may be the washing out of a larger part of the low molecular weight fraction into the media, at the extra rinsing step to remove the sodium citrate, of the films with a porous component; therefore higher MW and MN were measured. However, it can be expected that washing out of low molecular weight fractions probably also occurs during immersion of the nonporous film in the buffer. As a consequence, it can be expected that the difference in MW and MN between the films would disappear in the course of the experiment. This was not the case, indicating another process having an effect on MW and MN. At day 180 the MW and MN values of the "combi" film tend to approach the ones of the nonporous film. This trend corresponds with the erosion of the thin nonporous layer of the "combi" film as observed with SEM: The "combi" film was becoming a porous one. Also, the MW and MN show a lot of fluctuation during the first two weeks of the experiment. These fluctuations might be caused by two phenomena having opposite effects on MW and MN: washing out of low molecular weight fractions and molecular chain fragmentation. However, as stated earlier, this remains hypothetical, as the amount of polymer compared to the amount of buffer in which they were placed did not allow for an analysis using GPC.

Degradation by Hydrolysis

Hydrolysis of the ester bonds is the major mechanism of PLLA degradation.[32] Mechanical stress may enhance the degradation process.[33] Radiation (UV, IR) or heat is not ex-

pected to contribute very much to the degradation of polyesters in vivo. The role of enzymes in the degradation process in vivo is not clear. Most enzymes in eukaryotic cells are substrate specific. Therefore, a specific three dimensional structure of the substrate (polymer) is required to reach the active center of the enzyme. This is not likely at 37°C under physiologic enzyme concentrations. The probability is even smaller for the crystalline parts of the polymer (film). However, enhancement of the degradation rate in vitro by enzymes was observed for some polymer/enzyme systems. The role of enzymes may be larger when smaller molecules have been formed by other degradation mechanisms (hydrolysis). This was not investigated in the experiments described in this paper.

Degradation of polyesters, such as PLLA, primarily takes place in the amorphous part of the polymer film.[34,35] This may explain the increasing crystallinity, also observed by other authors.[34] However, in order to explain the difference in degradation rate between the nonporous and porous PLLA film, one must assume other processes taking place during degradation. Vert et al, using different polyester "plates" of 2 x 17 x 20 mm, observed the formation of a polymer layer around the core of the polymer film, largely preventing degradation products (e.g., oligomers) released in the core, to diffuse freely to the aqueous environment. The chemical reactive endgroups of the accumulated oligomers in the core then enhance the degradation (autocatalytic) process. The nonporous polymer film is more susceptible to this form of degradation, probably because a larger inner compartment can be formed compared to the porous and "combi" film. The surface/volume ratio of the latter two are probably larger than the cut off value of the polymer surface/volume ratio regarding this effect.

However, other mechanisms are also possible. There is less flow of the aqueous media in pores of the porous polymer film. Therefore, the concentration of oligomers might be higher in the pores, enhancing degradation. Nevertheless, this mechanism apparently has less effect compared to the mechanism(s) leading to a higher degradation rate of the nonporous PLLA film.

Summary and Conclusions

In summary, it can be stated that the parameters of porosity and surface roughness do influence the ultimate biocompatibility of implanted biomaterials. Potential degradation of a biomaterial will enhance these reactions.

Porosity

A high porosity will, as a rule, induce a higher inflammatory response as compared to smooth and solid biomaterials. The size of pores will, in turn, determine the type of foreign body reaction. Small (surface) pores (up to 10 microns) will give rise to more adhesion. In addition, guidance of cells may occur. Ingrowth will not take place. Larger pores will facilitate tissue ingrowth and therewith provide a mechanical anchorage of tissue to biomaterial. Optimal pore sizes have been estimated to be between 50 and 200 microns.

Surface Roughness

As a rule, a high surface roughness will induce a more severe foreign body response and also provide better anchorage of cells to a biomaterial. The form of the roughness will determine if other aspects are also involved, e.g., grooved substrata[36] will, depending on their dimensions and orientation, improve cell proliferation and orientation.

Degradation and Biocompatibility

In general, a degrading biomaterial will evoke a more severe inflammatory response as compared to a nondegradable material. If this degradable material is porous, we have demonstrated that, in the case of, e.g., collagen, the rate of degradation (and thus the degree of foreign body response) is higher, whereas in the case of polyesters as lactic acid, a porous form will degrade more slowly than a solid form.

In conclusion we can state that porosity and roughness will influence cellular adhesion and the rate of foreign body reaction. However, parameters such as biodegradability will have their own effects on the ultimate degree of biocompatibility.

References

1. Ratner BD. Biomedical applications of synthetic polymers. In: Aggarawal SL, ed. Comprehensive Polymer Science. Oxford, U.K.: Pergamon Press, 1989:201-247.
2. Spector M, Cease C, Tong-Li X. The local tissue response to biomaterials. Crit Rev Biocompatability 1989; 5:269-295.
3. Black J. Systemic effects of biomaterials. Biomaterials 1984; 5:11-18.
4. Marchant RE, Anderson JM, Dillingham EO. In vivo biocompatability studies VII, Inflammatory response to polythylene and to cytotoxic polyvinylchloride. J Biomed Mater Res 1986; 20:37-50.
5. Wachem PB, Luyn MJA, Nieuwenhuis P, Koerten HK, Olde Damink L, Hoopen H ten, Feijen J. In vivo degradation of processed dermal sheep collagen evaluated with transmission electron microscopy. Biomaterials 1991; 12:215-223.
6. Schakenraad JM, Busscher HJ, Wildevuur CHR, Arends J. The influence of substratum free energy on growth and spreading of human fibroblasts in the presence and absence of serum proteins. J Biomed Mater Res 1986; 20:773-784.
7. Matlaga BF, Yasenchak LP, Salthouse TN. Tissue response to implanted polymers: The significance of shape. J Biomed Mater Res 1976; 10:391-397.
8. White RA, Hirose FM, Sproat RW, Lawrence RS, Nelson RJ. Histopathologic observations after short term implantation of two porous elastomers in dogs. Biomaterials 1981; 2:171-176.
9. Cheroudi B, Gould TRL, Brunette DM. Titanium covered micromachined grooves of different dimensions affect epithelial and connective tissue cells differently in vivo. J Biomed Mater Res 1990; 24:1203-1219.
10. Bakker D, Blitterswijk CA van, Hesseling SC, Grote JJ, Daems WT. Effect of implantation site on phagocyte/polymer interaction and fibrous capsule formation. Biomaterials 1988; 9:14-23.
11. Schakenraad JM, Nieuwenhuis P, Molenaar I, Helder J, Dijkstra PJ, Feijen J. In vivo and in vitro degradation of glycine/DL-lactic acid copolymers. J Biomed Mater Res 1989; 23:1271-1288.
12. Rozema FR, Bruin WC de, Bos RRM, Boering G, Nijenhuis AJ, Pennings AJ. Late tissue response to bone plates and screws of poly L-lactide used for fracture fixation of the zygomatic bone. In: Doherty PJ, Williams RL, Williams DF, eds. Advances in Biomaterials, Biomaterial-Tissue Interfaces. Amsterdam: Elsevier, 1992:349-355.
13. Schakenraad JM, Oosterbaan JA, Nieuwenhuis P, Molenaar I, Olijslager J, Potman W, Eenink MJD, Feijin J. Biodegradable hollow fibers for the controlled release of drugs. Biomaterials 1988; 9:116-120.
14. Spector M. Historical review of porous coated implants. J Arthroplasty 1987; 2:163-177.
15. Baier RE. Applied chemistry at protein interfaces. Adv Chem Ser 1975; 145:1-25.
16. Wachem PB, Beugling T, Feijen J, Bantjes A, Detmers JP, Aken WG van. Interactions of cultured human endothelial cells with polymeric surfaces of different wettabilities. Biomaterials 1985; 6:403-408.
17. Schindler A, Harper D. Polylactide 2, viscosity molecular weight relationship and unperturbed chain dimensions. J Polymer Sci 1979; 17:2593-2599.
18. Busscher HJ, Pelt AWJ van, Jong HP de, Arends J. Effect of spreading pressure on surface free energy determinations by means of contact angle measurements. J Colloid Interfacial Sci 1983; 95:23-27.
19. Blaauw EH, Jonkman MF, Gerrits PO. A rapid connective tissue stain for glycol methacrylate embedded tissue. Act Morphol Neerl-Scand 1987; 25:167-172.
20. Cotran RS, Kumar V, Robbins SL. Inflammation and repair. In: Cotra RS, Jumar V, Robbins SL, eds. Pathologigal basis of diseases. Philadelphia: Saunders, 1994:51-92.
21. Picken MM, Gallo GR. Ameloid enhacing factor and inflammatory reaction. Lab Invest 1990; 63:586-587.
22. Kisilevski R. Amyloidosis, In: Rubin E, Farber JL, Lippincott JB, eds. Pathology. Philadelphia:, 1994:1163-1174.
23. Weitzman SA, Gordon LI. Inflammation and Cancer: Role of phagocyte-generated oxygen carcinogenesis. Blood 1990: 76:655-663.
24. Mentzer SJ, Valler DV, Burakoff SJ. Gamma-interferon induction of LFA-1 mediated homotypic adhesion of human monocytes. J Immunol 1986; 137:108-113.
25. Most J, Neumayer HP, Dierich MP. Cytokine-induced generation of multinucleated giant cells in vitro requires gamma-interferon and expression of FLA-1. Eur J Immunol 1990; 20:1661-1667.
26. Shaw LM, Messier JM, Mercurio AM. The activation dependent adhesion of macrophages to laminin involves cytoskeletal anchoring and phosphorylation of the alpha-6 beta-1 integrin. J Cell Biology 1990; 110:2167-2174.
27. Ingber DE, Folkman J. Tension and compression as basic determinants of cell form and function: Utilization of a cellular tensigrity mechanism. In: Cell Shape: determinants, regulation and regulatory role. New York: Academic Press, 1989:3-31.
28. Baier RE, Meyer AE, Natiella JR, Natiella RR, Carter JM. Surface properties determine bioadhesive outcome: Methods and results. J Biomed Mater Res 1984; 18:337-355.
29. Miller KM, Anderson JM. Human monocyte/macrophage activation and interleukin 1 generation of biomedical polymers. J Biomed Mater Res 1988; 22:713-731.
30. Miller KM, Rose-Caprara V, Anderson JM. Generation of IL-1 like activity in response to biomedical polymer

implants: A comparison of in vitro and in vivo models. J Biomed Mater Res 1989; 23:1007-1026.

31. Krause TJ, Robertson FM, Liesch JB, Wasserman AJ, Greco RS. Differential production of IL-1 on the surface of biomaterials. Arch Sorg 1990; 125:1158-1160.

32. Richardson MJ. Thermal analysis. In: Booth C, Price C, eds. Comprehensive Polymer Science. Oxford: Pergamon Press, 1989:867-901.

33. Jamshidi K, Hyon S-H, Nakamura T, Ikada Y, Teramatsu Y. In vitro and in vivo degradation of poly-L-lactide fibers. In: Christel P, Neunier A, Lee AJC, eds. Advances in biomaterials: Biological and biomechanical perfor-

mances of biomaterials. Amsterdam: Elsevier, 1986:227-233.

34. Leenslag JW, Pennings AJ, Bos RRM, Rozema FR, Boering G. Resorbable materials of poly-L-lactide VII: In vivo and in vitro degradation. Biomaterials 1987; 8:311-314.

35. Schakenraad JM, Hardonk MJ, Feijen J, Molenaar I, Nieuwenhuis P. Enzymatic activity towards poly (L-lactic acid) implants. J Biomed Mater Res 1990; 24:529-545.

36. Braber ET den, Ruitjer JE de, Smits HTJ, Ginsel LA, Recum AF von, Jansen JA. Quantitative analysis of cell proliferation and orientation on substrata with uniform parallel surfaxe micro-grooves. Biomaterials 1996; 17:1093-1099.

Scaffold Engineering

Surface Modification

—————————————— CHAPTER 48 ——————————————

Microgroove Driven Tissue Ingrowth

Edwin T. Den Braber, John A. Jansen

Implants, Tissue Engineering, and Biomaterials

During the last two decades the availability and application of medical implants has increased dramatically. This concerns a broad variety of medical implants ranging from knee prostheses to insulin infusion pumps, and from vascular grafts to pacemakers. Some estimate figures were presented by Ratner[1] in his Presidential Address for the Society for Biomaterials in 1993 (Table 48.1). Although he emphasized that these figures were estimates, it is clear that the use of implants is considerable. Long term projections even suggest that implant applications are going to rise in the future. Factors that contribute to this increase can be ascribed roughly to three major causes. First, the life expectancy of humans increases. This will inevitably lead to a rise in the demand for implants like hip replacements or artificial lenses for the treatment of geriatric diseases and defects. Second, more and more medical treatments are going to include the use of implants in the future. One example of such a development is the use of percutaneous implants in dialysis.[2] Instead of treating patients with chronic renal failure though intermittent hemodialysis, percutaneous implants enable continuous ambulatory peritoneal dialysis (CAPD). Third, technologies are evolving that open new ways of treating specific disorders or defects. This is demonstrated by techniques that are being developed in the field of tissue engineering.[3] Basically, tissue engineering combines the principles and methods of the life sciences with those of engineering to elucidate fundamental understanding of structure-function relationships in normal and diseased tissues, to develop materials and methods to repair damaged or diseased tissues, and to create entire tissue replacements.[4] Tissue engineering thus spans controlling cellular responses to implant materials, manipulating the healing environment to control the structure of the regenerated tissue, producing cells and tissues for transplantation into the body, and developing a quantitative understanding of many biological equilibrium and rate processes.[5]

Biomaterials play an important role in many of these activities. Originally, inertness was thought to be one of the major contributions of the performance of an implant or biomaterial, but later Williams adapted the definition of biocompatibility to include the idea that a biomaterial perform with an appropriate host response in a specific application.[6] Sadly, most currently used implant materials do not possess these desirable qualities. At his Presidential Address, Ratner[1] voiced this problem very vividly by saying, "For the majority of our widely used bio-materials, no one sat down in advance and said 'How can I engineer the surface of this material to produce the desired biological response?'" He stressed that most currently used biomaterials, although demonstrating generally satisfactory clinical performance, were "ad-hoc" biomaterials, developed through a trial and error optimization, rather than being engineered to produce, for instance, a desired interfacial interaction. The

Tissue Engineering of Prosthetic Vascular Grafts, edited by Peter Zilla and Howard P. Greisler.

Table 48.1. Selected biomedical implant applications; magnitude of use[a]

Application	Numbers Used per Year
Ophthalmologic	
Intraocular lenses	1,400,000
Contact lenses	250,000,000[b]
Retinal surgery implants	50,000
Prothesis after enucleation	5,000
Cardiovascular	
Vascular grafts	350,000
Arteriovenous shunts	150,000
Heart valves	75,000
Pacemakers	130,000
Blood bags	30,000,000
Reconstructive	
Breast protheses	100,000
Nose, chin	10,000
Penile	40,000
Dental	200,000
Orthopedic	
Hips	90,000
Knees	65,000
Shoulders, finger joints	50,000
Other devices	
Ventricular shunts	21,500
Catheters	200,000,000
Oxygenerators	500,000
Renal dialysers	16,000,000
Wound drains	3,000,000
Sutures	20,000,000

[a]Approximate annual usage in United States of America
[b]Worldwide

importance of the issue raised by Ratner is underlined by recent estimates that indicate that biomaterials such as metals, ceramics, and polymers are found in more than 5,000 different medical devices and almost 40,000 different pharmaceutical products, with a collective annual sales approaching 100 billion US dollars.[5] If we include all products that utilize biomaterials, then the number of people affected worldwide exceeds 1000 million per year.[4,7]

As a possible handle for the development of "smart" biomaterials, Ratner[1] advocated an engineering approach to achieve the integration between the biomaterial and the surrounding tissues. He suggested that it is worthwhile to look at how nature handles specificity and rapid-reaction kinetics, keeping in mind that three design themes are iterated and exploited throughout biology, i.e., order, recognition, and mobility. However, as Brunette[8] later remarked, using the principles of design to achieve the optimal structure differs from attempting to reproduce the original structure. According to Brunette, attempting to imitate nature is approximate since the complexity and variability of natural systems make them impossible to replicate with perfect fidelity. This has led to the production of structures and

devices that closely resemble the original structure, but are in no way the best replacement for the original biological structure. The development of these kinds of structures caused Ratner to state during his Presidential Address[1] that "existing biomaterials, although demonstrating generally acceptable clinical success, look like dinosaurs poised for extinction in the light of the winds of change blowing through the biomedical, biotechnological, and physical sciences".

Surface Micropatterns Manipulating Cellular Behavior

Among the tools that Ratner identified as having a great potential for creating engineered biomaterials is the use of nano- and micropatterned surfaces.[1] The possibility to influence the behavior of cells by the topographical morphology of the surface on which these cells are cultured was first discovered during the first part of this century. In 1914, Ross G. Harrison of the Osborn Zoological Laboratory of Yale University cultured cells on spiderwebs.[9] In retrospect, this in itself seems quite an achievement, especially when we keep in mind that in 1914 investigators did not have all the technical equipment that are available in modern cell culture laboratories nowadays. During his studies, Harrison noticed that the direction of movement of the cells was influenced by the structure of the fragile substrata on which these cells were incubated. Furthermore, he noticed that the cells adapted a shape that seemed to be governed by the linear spiderweb threads. Later, this phenomenon was confirmed by Loeb and Fleisher,[10] who introduced the term stereotropism, which was described as the direction in which cells move, governed mainly by the contact with solids or very viscid bodies like fibers or fibrin. In 1945, Weiss conducted experiments with a wide range of substrata like plasma clots, fish scales, and engraved glass, and termed the changes in cell behavior observed by Harrison "contact guidance".[11] Surprisingly, no further attention was paid to this guidance phenomenon until the early 1970s. It was Rovensky et al[12-13] and Maroudas[14-15] who rediscovered that the behavior of cells is affected by the topography of a substratum surface. Rovensky[12-13] studied the behavior of fibroblast-like cells on different kinds of substratum surfaces with an orderly distribution of 40.0 μm deep grooves having a triangular profile. He reported that the cells had a bipolar elongated shape, were orientated after adhesion, and grew parallel to the grooves. Meanwhile, Maroudas[14-15] studied the growth of fibroblasts on small glass beads (diameter 20-60 μm), fibers, and platelets. He observed that cells grown on beads with a large diameter tended toward forming multilayers, while smaller beads progressively failed to support growth.

Since these studies by Rovensky and Maroudas, several investigators have studied the behavior of various types of cells to a variety of microtextured substrata materials. These studies have been reviewed very recently by Singhvi et al,[16] von Recum and van Kooten,[17] and Brunette.[8] In these in vitro and in vivo studies, some specific alterations in cellular behavior were seen, while other changes that were suggested by several leading researchers in this field were not. In the following paragraphs we will attempt to give a comprehensive listing of the most obvious and general accepted alterations in cell behavior as a result of cells contacting surfaces with a pattern of parallel microgrooves. We will demonstrate this by describing various studies that were performed at our laboratories. In addition, we will discuss the leading theories that attempt to create a model in which the phenomenon of contact guidance is clarified.

Changed Cell Shape and Cellular Orientation

If cells are cultured on a surface with parallel microgrooves as shown in Figure 48.1, the first thing that can be observed is the change of the shape of the cells. In earlier studies,[18-19] we investigated several groove and ridge dimensions to study and quantify the influence of these groove patterns on the size, shape, and orientation of the cells cultured on these substrata.

In order to obtain a microgrooved substratum, we first produced silicon oxide molds in a class 100 clean room using photolithography.[20-21] Photolithography is a technique that is developed for the production of microelectronic components like, for example, computer microcircuits. In our experiments, these mold surfaces were produced by coating silicon oxide masks with high reflective chrome, after which the chrome was coated with a thin (0.5 µm) layer of positive photoresist. Subsequently, the photoresist was exposed and developed, uncovering the underlying chrome, which was etched. Finally, the unexposed photoresist was stripped off, thus creating a parallel groove pattern. The substrata were finally obtained by covering the molds with polydimethylsiloxane, thus producing negative surface replicas which possessed either a smooth surface or a surface with parallel grooves, showing a wide variety of groove and ridge widths (Table 48.2). During our experiments, the groove depth was either 0.5 µm or 1.0 µm. After polymerization, the silicone rubber castings were removed, cut into their appropriate

circular shape and size, washed, sterilized, and inspected as described elsewhere.[18-19]

For the evaluation of the cellular behavior on the smooth and microtextured silicone substrata, primary culture rat dermal fibroblasts (RDFs) were used. These cells were harvested from ventral skin grafts taken from male Wistar rats (100-120 g). After dissociation, these cells were incubated for several days according to a specific protocol.[18-19] Subsequently, the fifth generation was used for incubation on the microtextured surfaces. Therefore, the smooth and microtextured substrata were placed in the culture wells of 24 well plates, after which approximately 1.0×10^4 viable RDFs ml^{-1} were added to each substratum. The RDFs were incubated on a specific substratum up to 7 days under static conditions.

The effect of the surface microgeometry on the cellular morphology was quantified by digital image analysis.[18-19]

Table 48.2. Dimensions of the micro features on the substrata surfaces (Gd=groove depth, Gw=groove width, Rw=ridge width, and P=pitch).

Gd (µm)	Gw (µm)	Rw (µm)	P (µm)
1.00	1.00	1.00	2.00
1.00	1.00	2.00	3.00
1.00	1.00	4.00	5.00
1.00	1.00	8.00	9.00
1.00	4.00	1.00	5.00
1.00	8.00	1.00	9.00
0.45	2.00	2.00	4.00
0.45	5.00	5.00	10.00
0.45	10.00	10.00	20.00

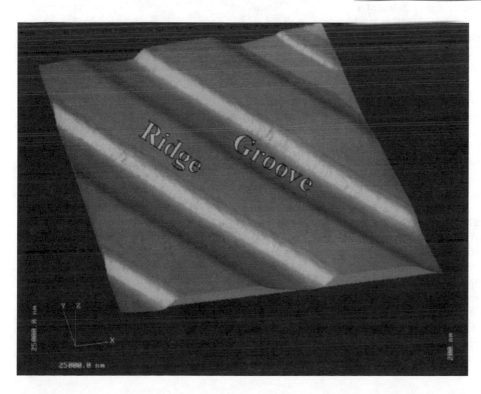

Fig. 48.1. Three dimensional representation of the results of AFM measurements on a microtextured substratum surface with parallel grooves of 5.0 µm, separated by 5.0 µm ridges. The grooves are approximately 0.5 µm deep. Different X- and Y-axis magnifications were used to clarify the conformation of the substratum surface.

Fig. 48.2. Schematic representation of a rat dermal fibroblast (RDF) on a microtextured substratum. The parameters measured during digital image analysis (DIA) were the RDF surface area (area within perimeter), the longest length of the cell (L), the cellular breadth (B), perimeter (P), circularity (not shown), angle of cellular orientation (α), and the number of pitches spanned by the cell (N).

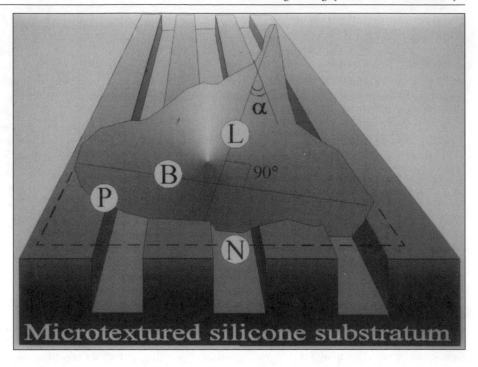

In short, RDFs were photographed by phase contrast microscopy on every day of the incubation period. These photographs were scanned digitally and analyzed with an image analysis program. This program made it possible to measure several cell parameters, i.e., the cellular surface area, cellular perimeter, cellular circularity, maximum cell length, cell breadth perpendicular to the maximum length, the angle of cellular orientation relative to the surface grooves (α), and number of pitches spanned by a single cell (Fig. 48.2).

These studies provided a lot of interesting data, but most of all clearly showed that the RDFs on surfaces with a ridge width smaller than 4.0 µm were highly oriented ($\alpha < 10°$) and elongated along the surface grooves (Figs. 48.3 and 48.4). However, if the ridge had a width larger than 4.0 µm, then the cellular orientation was random ($\approx 45°$) and the shape of the RDFs became significantly more circular (Fig. 48.5). The appearance and orientation of the cells on the surfaces with ridge widths larger than 4.0 µm in many cases proved to be not significantly different from those on the smooth substratum surfaces (Fig. 48.6). Furthermore, it became apparent that the ridge width was the most important parameter, since varying the groove width and groove depth did not affect the RDF size, shape, or the angle of cellular orientation (α) significantly.

Cell Attachment on Microtextured Surfaces

During these studies, we found after careful examination of the phase contrast images that the fibroblasts showed indications of attaching specifically to the ridges of the surface patterns (Fig. 48.4). If the fibroblasts did actually attach solely to the surface ridges, this would mean that the cells displayed a specific preference of attachment location. Intrigued by the phase contrast microscopy/digital image analysis results, we performed experiments which were designed to show us more of the intricate interaction between the microtextured substratum surfaces and the overlaying fibroblasts. During these additional experiments, we cultured the RDFs similarly as in the earlier studies,[18-19] but visualized specific cytoskeletal components and proteins interacting in the attachment of the RDFs with the following monoclonal and polyclonal antibodies:[22]

1. The mouse monoclonal antibody hVIN-1, specific for vinculin;[23]
2. The rabbit monoclonal anti-fibronectin antibody FN-3E2;[24]
3. A rabbit polyclonal antiserum raised against bovine fibronectin;[25]
4. The rabbit polyclonal antiserum against bovine vitronectin;[26]
5. A polyclonal antiserum raised against human vitronectin in rabbits, which has been shown to have a good crossreactivity with rat vitronectin, but not with bovine vitronectin.[27]

After incubation, these primary antibodies were incubated with the appropriate secondary antibody, i.e., fluorescein isothiocyanate (FITC)-conjugated goat anti-mouse IgG or FITC-conjugated goat anti-rabbit IgG. For the staining of the RDF filamentous actin no antibodies were used, since F-actin was visualized with thiorhodamine isothiocyanate (TRITC)-labeled phalloidin. Immediately after performing the double stain procedures, the RDFs were examined with a confocal laser scanning microscope (CLSM), which was equipped with a krypton/argon mixed gas laser. This type of laser offers separate, well spaced wavelengths for the excitation of FITC ($\lambda = 488$ nm) and TRITC ($\lambda = 568$ nm).[28] Next to the fluorescence mode, the reflection mode of the CLSM was used to visualize the underlying substratum surface.[22] The resulting digital images were captured and overlay images were created, thus making it possible to capture the fluorescent and reflection data in one 24 bit RGB

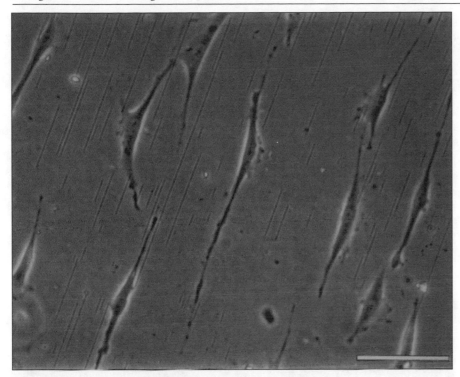

Fig. 48.3. Phase contrast image of RDFs on a B substratum (Gw 1.0 μm, Rw 1.0 μm, Gd 1.0 μm, bar = 100 μm) on day 1. The cells are highly aligned and elongated along the surface grooves.

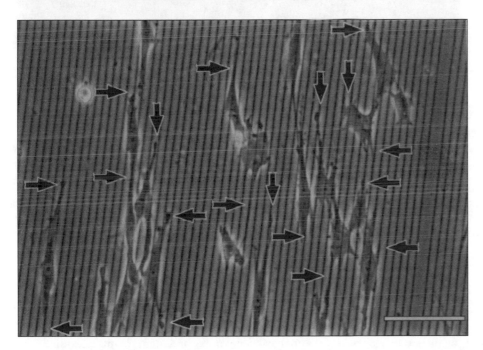

Fig. 48.4. Phase contrast image of RDFs on a substratum with grooves of 8.0 μm wide and 1.0 μm deep, while the ridge has a width of 1.0 μm (bar = 100 μm) after 2 days of incubation. These substrata are a negative replica of the substrata in Figure 48.5. The RDFs are clearly orientated. Cell protrusions attach to the ridges (arrows).

(Red-Green-Blue) picture. Creation of these 24 bit images enabled the composition of 1 digital image with 3 different information levels, each within one color segment, and offered the possibility to investigate the stained objects in conjunction with each other and the surface patterns. First, the (acute) angle of orientation of F-actin, vinculin, fibronectin, vitronectin, and the surface grooves relative to a virtual X-Y axis were measured. Second, the relative position and the angle of the linear components of vinculin, fibronectin, and vitronectin were compared with the position and angle of orientation of the actin filaments. Finally, the location of

vinculin relative to the grooves and ridges of the microtextured surface was charted and analyzed.[22]

The results of the CLSM observations and additional image and statistical analysis showed that the microfilaments and vinculin aggregates of the RDFs on the 2.0 μm grooved substrata were orientated along the surface grooves, while these proteins were significantly less orientated on the 5.0 and 10.0 μm grooved surfaces (Fig. 48.7). In contrast, bovine and endogenous fibronectin and vitronectin were orientated along the surface grooves on all textured surfaces. These extracellular proteins did not seem to be hindered by

Fig. 48.5. Phase contrast image of RDFs on a substratum with grooves of 1.0 μm wide and 1.0 μm deep, and 8.0 μm wide ridges (bar = 100 μm) on day 2. Appearance of and orientation of the fibroblasts does not differ significantly from the RDFs on a smooth substratum surface.

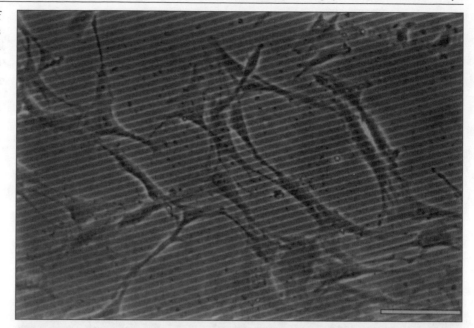

Fig. 48.6. Phase contrast image of RDFs on a smooth substratum after 2 days of incubation (bar = 100μm). The well spread RDFs have a characteristic multipolar appearance and are randomly orientated.

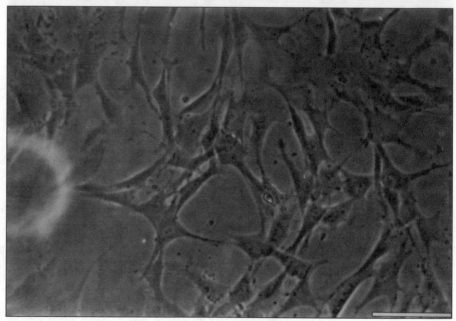

the surface grooves, since many groove spanning filamentous deposits were found on all microgrooved surfaces (Fig. 48.8). Vinculin was located mainly on the surface ridges on all textured surfaces (Fig. 48.9).

These findings were later confirmed in additional studies.[29-30] During these investigations we made ultrathin sections of RDFs cultured on silicone and titanium microgrooved surfaces with parallel grooves ranging from 1.0 μm up to 10.0 μm. The depth of these grooves varied between 0.45 μm and 2.2 μm. Transmission electron microscopy (TEM) again showed that the focal adhesion points of the RDFs on both the silicone rubber and titanium microtextured surfaces were located mainly on the surface ridges (Fig. 48.10). On the titanium surfaces, TEM also re-

vealed that these focal adhesion points were occasionally wrapped around the edges of the ridges. Attachment of the cells on the silicone rubber and titanium microtextured substrata was never observed on the surfaces with 1.0 or 2.0 μm grooves. Only the RDFs on the 5.0 μm and 10.0 μm grooved surfaces protruded into the grooves, while attachment to the groove floor was observed only on the 10.0 μm textures. In addition, only the RDFs on the titanium 5.0 μm and 10.0 μm grooved surfaces possessed focal adhesion points on the walls of the grooves (Fig. 48.10). Comparison between the observations of the cells on the microtextured silicone rubber and titanium substrata suggested that material specific properties did not influence the orientational effect of the surface texture on the observed RDF cellular behavior.[30]

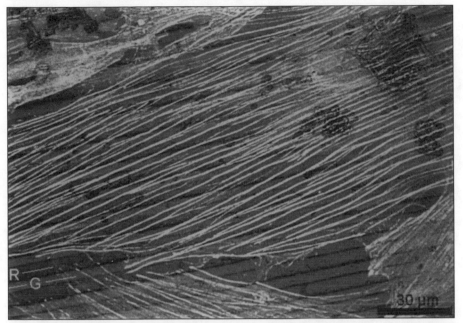

Fig. 48.7. Digital overlay image of a reflection micrograph of a 5.0 μm grooved silicone surface and the corresponding RDF actin after a incubation of 3 days. Fibronectin filaments at the ventral side of this fibroblast can be seen in Figure 48.8. Note the similarity in the orientation of the microfilaments and fibronectin filaments in Figure 48.8.

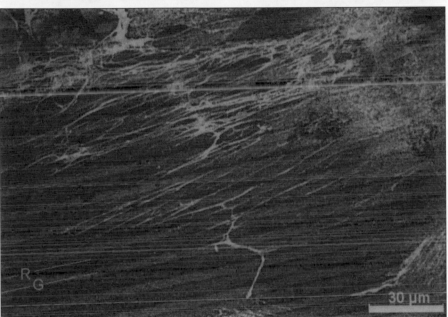

Fig. 48.8. Immunofluorescence micrograph of a rat fibronectin staining on a surface with 5.0 μm grooves (incubation period of 3 days) showing thin fibronectin filaments at the leading edge of the cell. The main fibronectin filaments possess similar orientational vectors, which are directed roughly parallel to the groove pattern.

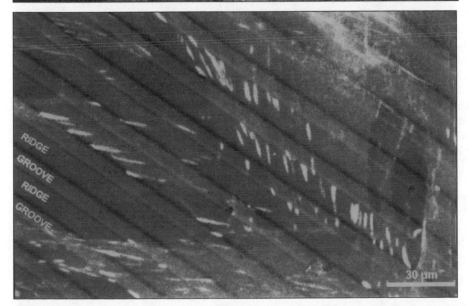

Fig. 48.9. Overlay image of the location of vinculin (bright spots) in relation to the 10.0 μm grooves after an incubation of 5 days. Vinculin is located mainly on the surface ridges and often attaches to the edges of these ridges.

Fig. 48.10. Transmission electron micrograph of a RDF on a 5.0 μm grooved titanium surface after 3 days of incubation. The cell protrudes into the groove, but does not contact the bottom of the groove. Focal adhesion points (arrowheads) can be seen on the edge of the ridge and the wall of the surface groove. Larger magnification showed that the focal adhesion point on the lefthand ridge edge was wrapped around this edge.

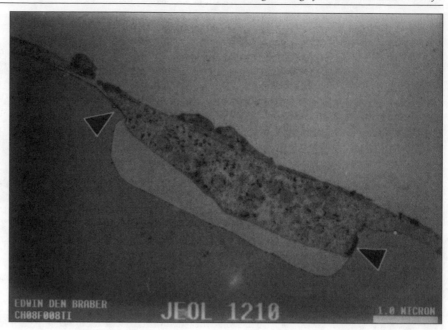

Other Surface Topography Induced Cell Behavior Alterations In Vitro

Apart from changes in cell size, shape, orientation, and attachment, investigators have suggested and studied many other cell processes that could possibly be influenced by the surface topography of substrata. One of these processes is cell proliferation. On the basis of the results of some of our earlier studies,[18,31] we concluded that the presence or dimensions of the parallel surface grooves as used in our experiments did not result in a change in RDF proliferation rate. This conclusion was, however, in contrast to the findings of Green et al and Ricci et al. For example, Green et al[32] reported that especially abdomen fibroblasts (CCD-969sk) cultured on surfaces with 2.0 and 5.0 μm square pillars showed increased proliferation rates. In addition, Ricci et al[33] evaluated the in vitro growth of rat tendon fibroblasts and rat bone marrow colonies on unidirectional (grooved) surface microgeometries. They found that the overall colony growth rate was changed, and concluded that surface microgeometry could be used to control the growth rate at implant surfaces. However, this study by Ricci et al also showed that the response to surface topography is dependent on cell type, which could account for the discrepancy in the results that we found between the proliferation rates of our rat dermal fibroblasts, the results of Ricci et al, and the data of Green et al. A point of discrepancy could be the use of different surface textures. Although Ricci et al used a pattern of parallel grooves, Green et al used a texture consisting of square pillars. This could mean that we not only have to consider the possibility of cell type dependent differences in cell proliferation, but also have to contemplate the effect that different surface textures could trigger.

Another process that seems to be affected by the topography of the surface that the cell contacts is that of the cell metabolism. Several publications have reported behavioral differences of cells on microtextured surfaces, such as changes in cellular differentiation, DNA/RNA transcription, cell metabolism, and cellular protein production.[16-17,34-35] For example, increased F-actin content and increased persistence and speed of cell movement of macrophage-like cells on grooved surfaces were observed, and changes in the regulation of fibronectin mRNA levels, mRNA stability, and fibronectin stability and assembly on surfaces with microgrooves have been reported. Similar results were described by Hong and Brunette,[36] who saw clear differences in the fibronectin mRNA and proteinase levels between oral epithelial cells that were cultured on smooth and microgrooved surfaces. Consequently, they remarked that these surface topography induced changes could be considered as "good news/bad news". According to these investigators, the good news was the fact that specific surface topographies could be used to enhance the production of a specific protein, while the bad news might be that the production/secretion of other proteins might also be enhanced. If the production/secretion of these "other proteins" would be elevated, this might have a deleterious effect on the integration of the implant. For example, a rise in the production/release of proteinases could result in a large scale degradation of the connective tissue. This simple example demonstrates that, at the molecular level, the regulation of cell function by altering the surface topography of an implant or substratum could be a very complex affair.

Microtextured Surfaces In Vivo

Up to this point, we have only described the effect of microtextured surfaces on cells in vitro. However, the results of these in vitro studies have led to the idea that surface microtexturing could be used deliberately to achieve certain desired end results in processes like morphogenesis, cell invasion, repair, and regeneration.[4] If this hypothesis proves to be true, it is obvious that surface texturing can be a very important tool in designing successful implants.[17,37]

Sadly, in vivo studies with microtextured implants challenging these ideas are scarce. In addition, review of these in vivo studies shows that the design of the used textured implants is very diverse. But even with this large diversity, it is possible to perceive the possible potential of microtextured implant surfaces on several implant related processes. For example, some studies[38-39] have reported on the reduction of epithelial downgrowth with microgrooved skin penetrating devices. Other investigators, who implanted microporous or pillared surfaces subcutaneously, found tightly adherent fibrous capsules without inflammatory cells,[40] reduced fibrosis,[41] and improved blood vessel proximity.[41]

In order to investigate the effect of microtextured implants on the surrounding tissue and to be able to compare our in vitro and in vivo data, we implanted the smooth and microtextured silicone rubber substrata with 2.0, 5.0, and 10.0 μm grooves (Table 48.2) subcutaneously in a total of 12 female New Zealand White rabbits for periods of 3, 7, 42, and 84 days.[42] Scanning electron microscopy (SEM) showed fibroblasts, erythrocytes, lymphocytes, macrophages, fibrin, and collagen on all implant surfaces after 3 and 7 days (Fig. 48.11). After 42 and 84 days only a little collagen and a small number of fibroblasts, but no inflammatory cells, were seen on the implant surfaces. In contrast with the RDFs in the in vitro experiments, the fibroblasts that were observed on the microtextured implant surfaces, were not oriented along the surface grooves. A possible explanation for these differences between in vitro and in vivo orientational cell behavior could be that the cells that are used in in vitro studies are isolated cells, which have no contact with other cells, cell types, or ECM. Previous studies[18,37,43] have shown that prolonged in vitro incubation on microtextured surfaces results in the formation of cell-cell contacts, an increase of the spread area, and a decrease of the orientation of the cells on these surfaces. Consequently, it was supposed that the observed guidance phenomenon is an initial response of cells in vitro to certain microtextured surfaces, which is lost gradually after cell-cell contacts are formed.[18,37,43] In tissues, these contacts with other cells are already present, which could mean that the orientational effect of the textured surfaces is overruled by stronger tissue related signals or cues.

Three dimensional reconstruction of CLSM images and normal light microscopy showed no significant differences between the thickness of the capsule surrounding the smooth and microgrooved implants. Since differences between the 2.0, 5.0, and 10.0 μm grooved implants were not detected, we concluded that the depth of the grooves used was not sufficient to facilitate "mechanical interlocking". This interlocking would reduce the stress and movement at the implant interface and limit the consequential "mechanical irritation" of the surrounding tissues, which is supposed to induce tissue damage, fibrosis, and severe inflammatory responses.[16-17,40-41] Other investigators have indeed reported reduction of the capsule size due to microtextured surfaces. However, review of these studies[40-41,44-45] shows that the surface texture of the implants in these studies differs significantly from our implants, both in terms of microfeature appearance (pores, pillars, tapered pits, or V-shaped grooves) and dimensions (feature depth, size, and pitch). As a result, the mechanical irritation of the smooth and grooved surfaces would be comparable, resulting in capsules of equal thickness. Furthermore, our textured implants possessed one smooth and one textured side. Although this opened up the possibility for intraimplant evaluation, it did not enhance possible mechanical interlocking between the implant and the surrounding tissues. Therefore, it can be questioned whether the capsule thickness would have been less if both sides of the implant had been textured.

Furthermore, normal light microscopy did show a significantly lower number of inflammatory cells, and a significantly higher number of blood vessels, in the capsules surrounding the microgrooved implants. The cause of these differences remains unclear. However, it is possible to speculate that the differences in the number of blood vessels were

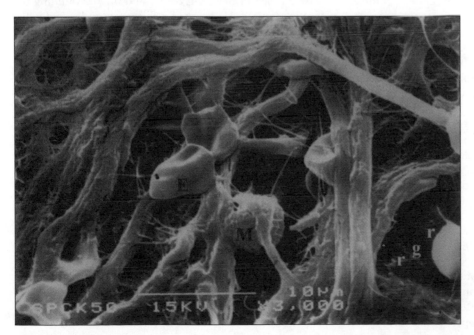

Fig. 48.11. On this SEM image (3 days of implantation), the 2.0 μm grooved silicone surface is visible underneath the collagen fibers. Several punctured erythrocytes (E) and a macrophage (M) were located within the collagen matrix.

part of the proliferation phase of the wound healing process.[46] This proliferation phase is a part of the formation of granulation tissue, which is characterized by high fibroblast densities, the formation of new blood vessels, and a new connective tissue matrix.[46] After repair, the number of the vessels decreases generally, marking the end of the wound healing process and the start of a steady state. The fact that more vessels were observed around the textured implants during our study could indicate a higher rate of tissue repair around these implants. Further research is, however, required to determine if this in fact is the case.

The Hypotheses

In the previous paragraphs we have presented several studies with microgrooved (implant) surfaces. In spite of the fact that several publications like these and some excellent reviews[3,16-19,31,37] have reported on the effects of microtextured surfaces, little is known about the exact mechanism whereby surface topography exerts its effects. Several theories have been suggested, however. First, it has been hypothesized that wettability plays a role in these phenomena. A microtextured surface could possess local differences in surface free energy which promote a specific deposition pattern of the substratum-bound attachment proteins.[16-17,47-49] In addition, the spatial arrangement of the adsorbed proteins[50-52] and the conformation of these proteins[53-54] would be influenced by these substratum surface properties. Second, it has been suggested that the specific geometrical dimensions of the focal adhesion plaques force a cell on a surface with small grooves and ridges to orientate itself parallel to these ridges.[55-56] This hypothesis is based on the observation that a minimum length of 2.0 µm is required for focal contacts to establish adhesion.[57] This implies that, if the ridge width increases, multiple vectors of adhesion plaque orientation are possible, enabling less orientated cell attachment. Finally, a third hypothesis[58-59] supposes that the orientation and alignment of cells on microtextured surfaces are a part of the cellular efforts to reach a biomechanical equilibrium with the net sum of forces minimized. This phenomenon has, for instance, been described extensively in the so-called tensegrity models.[58-60] According to these models, it is possible that the anisotropic geometry of substratum surface grooves and ridges establishes stresses and shear-free planes that influence the direction of microtubule[61] and microfilament growth[62-63] in order to create a force economic situation.

Given the current available information, it is impossible to express an opinion on which or whether one of these hypotheses is true. On the other hand, several separately performed studies have reported that surface microtextrues can have a profound effect on specific elements of the cytoskeleton like, for example, the microfilament bundles,[62-65] focal contacts,[55] and microtubules,[61] making it safe to say that microtextured surfaces influence the orientation of the intracellular and extracellular proteins. Although results of our studies corroborate with all three hypotheses, they do not justify a specific choice for one of these hypotheses. The differences in deposition patterns and the appearances of the ECM proteins during the CLSM study for example, make it possible to suggest that surface properties like surface free

energy have an influence on the displayed cellular behavior. The vinculin location and orientation however, pleas in favor of the "ridge width" theory, although warped focal adhesion points that were found in the TEM results[30] seem to contradict this theory. Finally, whether the cells orientate to the microtextured surfaces as a result of the force distribution that is created by the texture of these surfaces is impossible to determine since no (known) studies have been performed to map the force distribution within cells cultured on microgrooved substratum surfaces. Recognizing the fact that these three hypotheses can even be integrated into one overall model contributes to the intriguing phenomena of cellular behavior on microtextured surfaces.

Future Perspectives: Vascular Grafts and Microtextured Surfaces

As mentioned before, many investigators have already speculated on the benefits of microtextured implants. For example, Ratner[1] speculated on the benefits of an implant surface that would not cause the formation of a fibrous capsule. According to Ratner, such an implant would not "be walled off", but the cells contacting the implant surface would respond "as if they are not seeing and interacting with the biomaterial". This wound healing reaction would be preferable for the clinical success of several frequently used implants. For example, reduction of the capsule thickness around an implant would mean a reduction of the capsule contraction that is often observed with, for example, silicone breast implants.[66] Furthermore, capsule reduction would enhance the performance of many implanted biosensors, pacemakers, and infusion pumps.[17] These devices all benefit from an optimal contact between the tissues and the implant for the transduction of signals. For instance, the necessary electrical pulse of a pacemaker would be better conducted to the heart muscle if the capsule around the electrode of this device were minimized. Another good example is the sensor of an implanted insulin infusion pump. For optimal detection of insulin levels, maximal contact between the sensor of this device and the surrounding tissues is required. However, if a fibrous capsule shields the sensor from the crucial signal, the performance of the implant will be insufficient.

Additional applications of microtextured biomaterials have been reported in the discipline of tissue engineering. For example, microtextured surfaces have been used in in vitro experiments to decrease hepatocyte dedifferentiation[67-68] or to induce guided nerve regeneration.[42,69-70] Skin autografts already have been generated out of individual keratinocytes by using orienting scaffolds,[71] while speculations are voiced that guided tissue regeneration could perhaps reduce the formation of scarring tissue and enhance the repair of highly orientated structures like tendons.[46,72-73] Furthermore, attempts have been made to produce large tubular morphologies with the help of tissue engineering that could function as intestine or ureter segmental replacements.[74] In addition, many publications have reported on efforts to produce blood vessels.[1,3,75-82] Microtextured biomaterials could be very useful as scaffolds in this field of tissue engineering research.

Figure 48.12 shows the basic anatomy of a blood vessel. Large blood vessels have a thick, tough wall of connective tissue and smooth muscle, which is lined by an exceedingly thin, single layer of endothelial cells, separated from the surrounding outer layers by a basal lamina. The thickness of the connective tissue component of the vessel wall varies with the vessel's diameter and function, but the endothelial lining is always present.[83] Study of embryos has revealed that large blood vessels have all developed from small simple vessels constructed solely out of endothelial cells and a basal lamina.[83] Therefore, the endothelial cells are often referred to as the pioneers, preceding the development of connective tissue and smooth muscle around the vessels when required. This is why early studies have concentrated on the formation of capillary tubes out of colonies of endothelial cells.[76] However, the tissue engineering of a functional, well developed substitute blood vessel does not depend solely on the presence of vascular cells and extracellular matrix (ECM) components. Several cellular signals are equally important to processes such as cell growth and cellular differentiation. Ziegler and Nerem[79] identified these signals as originating from three sources, i.e.:

1. Chemical signals, derived from the fluid (blood) flowing through the vessel;
2. Signals associated with the ECM—the ECM proteins not only hold the vascular wall together, but also participate in regulating the biology of the vascular wall;
3. The mechanical environment of the vascular wall, imposed by the hemodynamics of the vascular system.

If we speculate on the roles that microtextured scaffolds could play in meeting these demands, one is evident. The orientation of the endothelial cells in the direction of the flow, and circularly oriented smooth muscle cells, could possibly be obtained by applying longitudinal or circular groove patterns. Not only would the overall orientation of the cell be influenced, but also the orientation of the cytoskeleton, thus contributing to the mechanical stiffness of the cells.[84] By using microgrooved scaffolds, endothelial orientation could be achieved without exposing the cells to flow and cyclic stretch, phenomena that have a comparable effect on the orientation of endothelial cells.[85-86] This comparison also concerns the level of gene expression. It has been reported that flow and cyclic stretch can influence the regulation of messenger RNA,[87-88] an effect on the cellular metabolism that is also supposed for cells on microtextured surfaces. What kind of effect the combination of the effects of factors like surface texture, flow, and cyclic stretch will have remains to be seen, since no study investigating this combination has been performed up to this date.

Another interesting option concerns the extracellular matrix proteins. The endothelial cells and smooth muscle cells in vivo are surrounded by an intricate mixture of proteins like collagens, elastin, laminin, fibronectin, and glycoaminoglycans.[79] Several studies have shown that these proteins can affect the growth, differentiation, and cholesterol metabolism of both the endothelial and smooth muscle cells. Endothelial derived ECM can affect smooth muscle cell growth, depending on its composition.[89] Collagen and fibronectin containing matrices promote the growth of smooth muscle cells, while matrices containing heparan sulfate proteoglycans selectively inhibit identical smooth muscle cell populations.[89] Furthermore, ECM proteins can change the response of smooth muscle cells to low density lipoproteins (LDL). Earlier study[90] has shown that collagen type I, for example, induces a decrease in smooth muscle cell growth, while endothelial derived ECM induces an increase in smooth muscle cell growth following incubation with

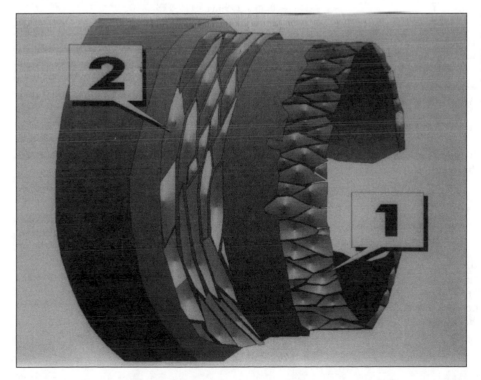

Fig. 48.12. Schematic drawing of the anatomy of a blood vessel. The longitudinal orientation of the endothelial lining (1) and the circular orientation of the smooth muscle cells (2) can be seen clearly.

LDL.[90] The ability of microtextured surfaces to enhance the production of specific proteins as mentioned earlier[8] could, if true, prove a powerful tool in the creation of blood vessels through tissue engineering.

These few examples show that microtextured surfaces could contribute in the study of, and the creation of, vascular grafts. This ranges from in vitro study of smooth muscle cells, where these surfaces could stop/slow down the change from a nongrowing, contractile phenotype to a proliferating, protein secreting mode,[91-92] to the induction of endothelial and smooth muscle cell orientation in artificial grafts.[1,75] Therefore, it is recommended that research of microtextured surfaces be exploited further in order to develop "smart" manipulative implants with higher clinical success rates. In addition, these new studies could also contribute to a better understanding of the mechanisms that cause cellular contact guidance and guidance related processes. Such insight would not only enlarge the general knowledge of these processes, but also offer implant designers a tool for designing a wider variety of more successful implants with predicable qualities.

Acknowledgments

This study is supported by the Technology Foundation (STW).

References

1. Ratner BD. New ideas in biomaterial science—a path to engineered biomaterials. J Biomed Mater Res 1993; 27:837-850.
2. von Recum AF, Park JB. Permanent percutaneous devices. CRC Crit Rev Bioeng 1981; 5:37-77.
3. Hubbell JA. Biomaterials in tissue engineering. Biotechnology 1995; 13:565-576.
4. Langer R, Vacanti JP. Tissue engineering. Science 1993; 260: 920-926.
5. Peppas NA, Langer R. Challenges in biomaterials. Science 1994; 263:1715-172.
6. Williams DF. Definitions in Biomedicals. Progress in Biomedical Engineering. New York: Elsevier, 1987:Vol. 4.
7. Hockberger PE, Lom B, Soekarno A, Thomas CH, Healy KE. Cellular engineering: Control of cell-substrate interactions. In: Hoch HC, Jelinski LW, Craighead HG, eds. Nanofabrication and Biosystems. Cambridge: Cambridge University Press, 1996:276-299.
8. Brunette DM. Effects of surface topography of implant materials on cell behavior in vitro and in vivo. In: Hoch HC, Jelinski LW, and Craighead HG, eds. Nanofabrication and Biosystems. Cambridge: Cambridge University Press, 1996: 335-355.
9. Harrison RG. The reaction of embryonic cells to solid structures. J Exp Zool 1914; 17:521-544.
10. Loeb L, Fleisher MS. On the factors which determine the movements of tissues in culture media. J Med Res 1917; 37:75-99.
11. Weiss P. Experiments on cell and axon orientation in vitro: The role of colloidal exudates in tissue organization. J Exp Zool 1945; 100:353-386.
12. Rovensky YA, Slavnaya IL, Vasiliev JM. Behavior of fibroblast-like cells on grooved surfaces. Exp Cell Res 1971; 65:193-201.
13. Rovensky YA, Slavnaya IL. Spreading of fibroblast-like cells on grooved surfaces. Exp Cell Res 1974; 84:199-206.
14. Maroudas NG. Anchorage dependence: Correlation between amount of growth and diameter of bead, for single cells grown on individual glass beads. Exp Cell Res 1972; 74:337-342.
15. Maroudas NG. Growth of fibroblasts on linear and planar anchorages of limiting dimensions. Exp Cell Res 1973; 81:104-110.
16. Singhvi R, Stephanopoulos G, Wang DIC. Review: Effects of substratum morphology on cell physiology. Biotechnology and Bioengineering, 1994; 43:764-771.
17. von Recum AF, van Kooten TG. The influence of microtopography on cellular response and the implications for silicone implants. J Biomater Sci Polymer Edn 1995; 7:181-198.
18. den Braber ET, de Ruijter JE, Smits HTJ et al. Quantitative analysis of cell proliferation and orientation on substrata with uniform parallel surface micro grooves. Biomaterials 1996; 17:1093-1099.
19. den Braber ET, de Ruijter JE, Ginsel LA et al. Quantitative analysis of fibroblast morphology on microgrooved surfaces with various groove and ridge dimensions. Biomaterials 1996; 17:2037-2044.
20. Schmidt JA, von Recum AF. Texturing of polymer surfaces at the cellular level. Biomaterials 1991; 12:385-389.
21. Schmidt JA, von Recum AF. Surface characterization of microtextured silicone. Biomaterials 1992; 13:675-681.
22. den Braber ET, de Ruijter JE, Ginsel LA et al. Confocal laser scanning microscopical study of the fibroblast cytoskeleton, attachment complexes, and ECM protein deposition on silicone microgrooved surfaces. J Biomed Mater Res 1997; in press.
23. Benori R, Salomon D, Geiger B. Identification of two distinct domains on vinculin involved in its association with focal contacts. J Cell Biol 1989; 108:2383-2393.
24. Garbarsch C, Matthiessen ME, Olsen BE et al. Immunohistochemistry of the intercellular matrix components and the epithelio-mesenchymal junction of the tooth germ. Histochem J 1994; 26:110-118.
25. Hayman EG, Oldberg A, Martin GR et al. Co-distribution of heparan sulfate proteoglycan, laminin, and fibronectin in extra cellular matrix of normal rat kidney cells and their coordinate absence in normal cells. J Cell Biol 1982; 94:28-35.
26. Hayman EG, Pierschbacher MD, Suzuki S et al. Vitronectin; a major cell attachment-promoting protein in fetal bovine serum. Exp Cell Res 1985; 160:245-258.
27. Hayman EG, Pierschbacher MD, Ohgren Y et al. Serumspreading factor (vitronectin) is present at the cell surface and in tissues. Proc Natl Acad Sci 1983; 80:4003-4007.
28. Cox G. Trends in confocal microscopy. Micron, 1993; 24:237-247.
29. den Braber ET, de Ruijter JE, Croes HJE et al. Transmission electron microscopical study of fibroblast attachment to microtextured silicone rubber surfaces. Cells and Materials 1997; in press.
30. den Braber ET, Jansen HV, de Boer MJ et al. SEM, TEM, and CLSM observation of fibroblasts cultured on microgrooved surfaces of bulk titanium susbtrata. J Biomed Mater Res 1997; submitted.
31. den Braber ET, de Ruijter JE, Smits HTJ et al. Effect of parallel surface micro grooves and surface energy on cell growth. J Biomed Mater Res 1995; 29:511-518.

32. Green AM, Jansen JA, and von Recum AF. The fibroblast response to microtextured silicone surfaces: Texture orientation into or out of the surface. J Biomed Mater Res 1994; 28:647-653.

33. Ricci JL, Charvet J, Chang R et al. In vitro effects of surface microgeometry on colony formation by fibroblasts and bone cells. 20th Annual Meeting of the Society for Biomaterials. Boston, USA. April 5-9, 1994:401.

34. Chou LS, Firth JD, Uitto VJ et al. Substratum surface topography alters cell shape and regulates fibronectin mRNA level, mRNA stability, secretion and assembly in human fibroblasts. J Cell Sci 1995; 108:1563-1573.

35. Wójciak-Stothard B, Madeja Z, Korohoda W et al. Activation of marcophage-like cells by multiple grooved substrata. Topographical control of cell behavior. Cell Biology International, 1995; 19:485-490.

36. Hong HL and Brunette DM. Effect of cell shape on proteinase secretion. J Cell Sci 1987; 87:259-267.

37. Curtis ASG, Clark P. The effects of topographic and mechanical properties of materials on cell behavior. Critical Reviews in Biocompatibility 1990; 5:344-362.

38. Chehroudi B, Gould TRL, Brunette DM. Effects of a grooved epoxy substratum on epithelial cell behavior in vitro and in vivo. J Biomed Mater Res 1988; 22:459-473.

39. Chehroudi B, Gould TRL, Brunette DM. A light and electron microscope study of the effects of surface topography on the behavior of cells attached to titanium-coated percutaneous implants. J Biomed Mater Res 1991; 25:387-405.

40. Campbell CE, von Recum AF. Microtopography and soft tissue response J Invest Surg 1989; 2:51-74.

41. Picha GJ, Drake RF. Pillared-surface microstructure and soft-tissue implants: Effect of implant site and fixation. J Biomed Mater Res 1996; 30:305-312.

42. den Braber ET, de Ruijter JE, Jansen JA. The effect of a subcutaneous silicone rubber implant with shallow surface micro grooves on the surrounding tissues in rabbits. J Biomed Mater Res 1996; in press.

42a. Clark P, Connolly P, Curtis ASG et al. Cell guidance by ultrafine topography in vitro. J Cell Sci 1991; 99:73-77.

43. Squier CA, Collins P. The relationship between soft tissue attachment, epithelial downgrowth and surface porosity. J Perio Res 1981; 16:434-440.

44. Chehroudi B., Gould TRL., and Brunette DM. The role of connective tissue in inhibiting epithelial downgrowth on titanium-coated percutaneous devices. J. Biomed. Mater. Res., 1992; 26: 493-515.

46. Ehrlich HP. Regulation der Wundheilung aus der Sicht des Bindesgewebes. Der Chirurg, 1995; 66: 165-173.

47. Baier RE. Surface properties influencing biological adhesion. Adhesion in biological systems, RS Manly (ed.) Academic Press, New York, 1970, 15-48.

48. Schakenraad JM, Busscher HJ, Wildevuur CRH et al. The influence of substratum surface free energy on growth and spreading of human fibroblasts in the presence and absence of serum proteins. J Biomed Mater Res 1986; 20:773-784.

49. Altankov G, Groth TH. Reorganization of substratum-bound fibronectin on hydrophillic and hydrophobic materials is related to biocompatibility. J Mater Sci 1994; 5:732-737.

50. Williams RL, Williams DF. The spatial resolution of protein adsorption on surfaces of heterogeneous metallic biomaterials. J Biomed Mater Res 1989; 23:339-350.

51. Rudee ML, Price TM. The initial stages of adsorption of plasma derived proteins on artificial surfaces in a controlled flow environment J Biomed Mater Res 1985; 19:57-66.

52. Uyen HMW, Schakenraad JM, Sjollema J et al. Amount and surface structure of albumin adsorbed to solid substrata with different wettabilities in a parallel plate flow cell. J Biomed Mater Res 1990; 24:1599-1614.

53. Rapoza RJ, Horbett TA. Postadsorptive transitions in fibrinogen: Influence of polymer properties. J Biomed Mater Res 1990; 24:1263-1287.

54. Shiba E, Lindon JN, Kushner L et al. Antibody detectable changes in fibrinogen adsorption affecting platelet activation on polymer surfaces. Am J Physiol 1991; 260:C965-974.

55. Ohara PT, Buck RC. Contact guidance in vitro. Exp Cell Res 1979; 121:235-249.

56. Dunn GA, Brown AF. Alignment of fibroblasts on grooved surfaces described by a simple geometric transformation. J Cell Sci 1986; 83:313-340.

57. Izzard CS, Lochner LR. Cell-to-substrate contacts in living fibroblasts: An interference reflection study with an evaluation of the technique. J Cell Sci 1976; 21:129-159.

58. Ingber DE. Cellular tensegrity; defining new rules of biological design that govern the cytoskeleton. J Cell Sci 1993; 104:613-927.

59. Ward MD, Hammer DA. A theoretical analysis for the effect of focal contact formation on cell-substrate attachment strength. Biophys J 1993; 64:936-959.

60. Wang N, Butler JP, Ingber DE. Mechanotransduction across the cell surface and through the cytoskeleton. Science, 1993; 260:1124-1127.

61. Oakley C, Brunette DM. The sequence of alignment of microtubules, focal contacts and actin filaments in fibroblasts spreading on smooth and grooved titanium substrata. J Cell Sci 1993; 106:343-354.

62. O'Neill C, Jordan P, Riddle P et al. Narrow linear strips of adhesive substratum are powerful inducers of both growth and total focal contact area. J Cell Sci 1990; 95:577-586.

63. Oakley C, Brunette DM. Topographic compensation: Guidance and directed locomotion of fibroblasts on grooved micromachined substrata in the absence of microtubules. Cell Motility and the Cytoskeleton 1995; 31:45-58.

64. Ben-ze'ev A. The role of changes in cell shape and contacts in the regulation of cytoskeleton expression during differentiation. J Cell Sci Suppl 1987; 8:293-312.

65. Dunn GA, Heath JP. A new hypothesis of contact guidance in tissue cells. Exp Cell Res 1976; 101:1-14.

66. Bern S, Burd A, May J Jr. The biophysical and histologic properties of capsules formed by smooth and textured silicone implants in the rabbit. Plast Reconstr Surg 1992; 89:1037-1042.

67. Cima LG, Ingber DE, Vacanti JP et al. Hepatocyte culture on biodegradable polymeric substrates. Biotech. Bioengineering 1991; 38:145-158.

68. Dunn JCY, Thomkins RG, Yarmush ML. Hepatocytes in collagen sandwich: Evidence for transcriptional and translational regulation. J Cell Biol 1992; 116:1043-1053.

69. Guenard V, Kleitman N, Morrissey TK et al. Syngeneic Schwann cells derived from adult nerves seeded in semipermeable guidance channels enhance the peripheral nerve generation. J Neurosci 1992; 12:3310-3320.

70. Clark P, Connolly P, Curtis ASG et al. Topographical control of cell behavior: II. Multiple grooved substrata. Development 1990; 108:635-644.

71. Bell E, Rosenberg M, Kemp P et al. Recipes for reconstituting skin. J Biomech Eng Trans ASME, 1991; 113:113-119.

72. Chehroudi B, Gould TRL, Brunette DM. A light and electron microscope study of the effects of surface topography on the behavior of cells attached to titanium-coated percutaneous implants. J Biomed Mater Res 1991; 25:387-405.

73. Wòjciak B, Crossan J, Curtis ASG. Grooved substrata facilitate in vitro healing of completely divided flexor tendons. J Mat Sci Mat in Med 1995; 6:266-271.

74. Mooney DJ, Organ G, Vacanti JP et al. Design and fabrication of biodegradable polymer devices to engineer tubular tissues. Cell Transplant 1994; 3:203-210.

75. Spargo BJ, Testoff MA, Nielson TB et al. Spatially controlled adhesion, spreading, and differentiation of endothelial cells on self-assembled molecular monolayers. Proc Nat Acad Sci USA, 1994; 91:11070-11074.

76. Folkman J, Haudenschild C. Angiogenesis in vitro. Nature 1980; 288:551-556.

77. Weinberg CB, Bell E. A blood vessel model constructed from collagen and cultured vascular cells. Science 1986; 231:397-400.

78. Leenslag JW, Kroes MT, Pennings AJ et al. A compliant, biodegradable vascular graft: Basic aspects of its construction and biological performance. New Polymeric Mater 1988; 1:111- 126.

79. Ziegler T, Nerem RM. Tissue engineering of a blood vessel: Regulation of vascular biology by mechanical stresses. J Cell Biochem 1994; 56:204-209.

80. Nerem RM, Sambanis A. Tissue engineering: From biology to biological substitutes. Tissue Engineering 1995; 1:3-12.

81. Langer R, Vacanti JP, Vacanti CA et al. Tissue engineering: Biomedical applications. Tissue Engineering 1995; 1:151-161.

82. Bell E. Strategy for the selection of scaffolds for tissue engineering. Tissue Engineering 1995; 1:163-179.

83. Alberts B, Bray D, Lewis J et al. Molecular biology of the cell, 3rd edition. New York: Garland Publishing Inc., 1994.

84. Nerem RM, Girard PR. Hemodynamic influences on vascular endothelial biology. Toxicol Pathol 1990; 4:572-582.

85. Nerem RM, Levesque MJ, Cornhill JF. Vascular endothelial morphology as an indicator of blood flow. ASME J Biomech Eng 1981; 103:172-176.

86. Levesque MJ, Liepsch D, Moravec S et al. Correlation of endothelial cell shape and wall shear stress in a stenosed dog aorta. Arteriosclerosis, 1986; 6:220-229.

87. Diamond SL, Sharefkin JB, Dieffenbach C et al. Tissue plasminogen activator messenger RNA levels increase in cultured human endothelial cells exposed to laminar shear stress. J Cell Physiol 1990; 143:364-371.

88. Mitsumata M, Fishel RS, Nerem RM et al. Fluid shear stress stimulates platelet-derived growth factor expression in endothelial cells. Am J Physiol Heart Circ Physiol 1993; 265:H3-H8.

89. Hermann IM. Endothelial cell matrices modulate smooth muscle cell growth, contractile phenotype and sensitivity to heparin. Heamostasis, 1990; 20:166-177.

90. Harris-Hooker S, Sanford GL, Montgomery V et al. Influence of low density lipoproteins on vascular smooth muscle cell growth and motility: Modulation by extracellular matrix. Cell Biol Int Rep 1992; 16:433-450.

91. Chamley-Campbell JH, Campbell GR. What controls smooth muscle phenotype. Arthereosclerosis, 1981; 40:347-357.

92. Campbell JH, Campbell GR. Endothelial cell influences on smooth muscle phenotype. Annu Rev Physiol 1986; 48:295-306.

Scaffold Engineering

Surface Modification

─────────────── CHAPTER 49 ───────────────

Surface Bonding of Heparin

Patrick T. Cahalan

In the early 1960s Hufnagel began experiments to form "autogenized" vascular prostheses.[1] This was accomplished by implanting a Teflon rod containing a loosely woven Dacron or polypropylene cloth surrounding it, and allowing 6-8 weeks for the formation of a collagen tube. Early experiments involved implantation back into the same animal to avoid immunogenic response. At the start of his work, important knowledge concerning glutaraldehyde fixation of tissue was awaiting further publications.[2] "Autogenized" was replaced with the term "xenograft" due to parallel efforts by Sparks.[3] Hufnagel stayed with his studies over the next two decades and moved on to attempt heparin incorporation into mandril formed prostheses as well as commercially available glutaraldchyde-treated human umbilical vein. Rigorous experimental efforts, including radioactively tagged heparin, allowed him to determine concentration of heparin in solution to effect maximal heparin loading conditions, and to his surprise he found that continued washing with saline for two hours post "imbibing" into the prosthesis did not significantly diminish the retained heparin, which was about 300 mg/ml. In implant studies the rate of early occlusion was significantly reduced, and Hufnagel reported that the half life of the heparin was limited to a few days.

While the goal was to prevent thrombotic occlusion, in retrospect the most interesting observation is the ability of heparin to bind and release from collagen in an unpredicted manner. The hypothetical paradigms of the time with respect to interactions of biomolecules and surfaces were still rather narrowly focused in simple ionic charge relationships.[4] Proteins (collagen) and polysaccharides (heparin) were widely known in the 70s by carbohydrate chemists to possess unique complexing capabilities that could be used to form viscosifying agents, stabilizers, and precipitation agents in food applications. The synergistic effect of these biomolecules could not be explained by simple ionic charge relationships. The tertiary and quaternary structures of biomolecules play an important role in their interactions with other molecules. While this concept is well known to anyone with an introductory education in biochemistry, it appears to be often forgotten in strategies for immobilizing biomolecules on surfaces. There remain very active efforts at producing a synthetic ionic analog heparinoid surface,[5,6] while at the same time studies are showing how critical is the dependence of heparin's bioactivity on its unique structure.[7]

Early attempts at heparinizing surfaces used fatty quaternary ammonium compounds as a base coating on polymers in order to present the positive charge of the quaternary amine for ionic coupling of heparin.[8] These early studies clearly showed an impact of heparinized surfaces, but the heparin released rather quickly and was material dependent, suggesting that the quaternary compound (generally considered toxic) also was releasing. In attempts to make the heparin more stable, or release more slowly at the surface, different solvent systems were use to attack the base material and entangle the fatty chains with the polymer surface. Attempts were made to calculate the sustained release rate required to

Tissue Engineering of Prosthetic Vascular Grafts, edited by Peter Zilla and Howard P. Greisler.
©1999 R.G. Landes Company.

maintain thromboresistant surfaces.[9] This clearly showed that it was impractical to sustain thromboresistance, due to the large loading required to maintain effectiveness for more than a few days. At the same time, Larm published his results for "end point" attached heparin on surfaces.[10] This was the first time that an immobilized heparin, with no leaching or releasing heparin, could demonstrate significant deactivation of thrombin. The premise of Larm's surface was that nitrous acid degraded heparin (NAD-Hep) containing high affinity pentasaccharides for ATIII was covalently immobilized on the surface by a terminal aldehyde group, thus presenting an optimal conformation of the molecule to the blood interface. The clearest evidence of the effectiveness of Larm's premise is seen in controlled experiments using human blood in simulated cardiopulmonary bypass circuits where improvement in platelet protection, platelet release products, hemolysis, less white cell activation, and less contact activation is demonstrated.[11] The group of Wendel has tested several coatings in the latter system, and nothing to date has been reported equal in performance to the covalently attached heparin surface.

The method of Larm, commercially known as the Carmeda biologically active surface (CBAS), is in fact a covalent attachment of heparin to an adsorbed base, and thus is not completely covalent to the base material. Since Larm's invention several additional methods of surface modification have been used to couple heparin and reported in the literature.[12-18] The traditional model for the mode of action of heparin on a surface is depicted by a heparin molecule with a high affinity pentasaccharide tethered to a surface and free to bind circulating ATIII, which it conformationally alters to make it catalytic in its ability to bind and deactivate circulating thrombin. Once this action has occurred, the thrombin-antithrombin complex (TAT) is released, and the site is capable of repeating the activity. The relatively high circulating concentrations of ATIII assists in the displacement of the TAT complex from the surface.[19] The question of protein adsorption and its effect on the heparin activity is a common one. Van Delden showed that the spacer composition was important for the surface retaining the ability to deactivate thrombin after exposure to plasma.[20] In his studies he showed that heparin immobilized via albumin-heparin conjugates retain 27% of initial activity after exposure to blood, whereas heparin immobilized via PEO spacers can retain as much as 55% of the initial activity. Most interesting from these experiments was the fact that the total amount of protein adsorbed onto heparinized surfaces did not correlate with the retention of heparin activity. It has been reported that albumin and fibrinogen adsorbed onto heparinized surfaces are not conformationally altered.[21] Earlier studies by Sevastianov suggest that it is critical to properly attach heparin if the proteins adsorbed are to be non platelet adhering and activating.[22] During a panel discussion at the Biomaterials conference in New Orleans, May, 1997, a comment was made to the effect that after all these years of research on blood-compatible surfaces we are no farther than the heparinized surface. Another perspective might suggest that we have finally reached a point where we understand how to properly attach heparin to a surface. The

lessons learned should be useful insights into attachment of other biomolecules, as cited by Hubbell in attachment of peptides to surfaces.[23]

Our group has been studying the performance of heparinized surfaces together with the University of Maastricht, the Netherlands in attempts to understand the role of coupling methodology in the performance of these surfaces in human blood using numerous blood testing systems.[24] Using a rotating disc apparatus as seen in Figure 49.1, it became evident that deactivation of thrombin at a heparinized surface is a diffusion limited reaction.

The reactor was designed with baffles to assure redirection of the flow perpendicular to the test surface, which was rotating, and thus assured a uniform shear rate profile on the sample surface. A mathematical model can be hypothesized for the thrombin decay if the rate of deactivation is dependent on the diffusion to the surface, and if the concentrations of thrombin and ATIII added to the reactor, and the speed of the motor, are known. The control line in the graph of Figure 49.1 represents a blank control surface, and the limited decay of thrombin is explained by simple noncatalytic deactivation of thrombin by ATIII in solution. The heparinized surface agrees fairly well with the theoretical decay rate for a diffusion limited reaction. All surfaces that were heparinized were tested before the experiment was started to assure that no heparin was releasing.

Our method of immobilizing heparin consisted of covalent attachment of hydrogels that were derivatized with amine functionality to which aldehyde-functionalized heparin (NAD-Hep, or periodate oxidized) was coupled. By controlling the amount of amine functionality we were able to prepare surfaces with different amounts of heparin coupled. Regardless of how much heparin was coupled per cm^2 on the surface, or the measured bioactivity the surface possessed to deactivate thrombin, the observed behavior in Figure 49.1 was only seen at low concentrations of ATIII. At physiological concentrations of ATIII (1 U/ml), there was no difference in thrombin decay between heparinized and uncoated controls. The rate of diffusion to, and deactivation at, the surface was not as great as the noncatalyzed deactivation in solution with physiological concentrations of ATIII, even with the most active surfaces. In addition to the latter results, ELISA measurements of TAT and F_{1+2} fragments from blood loop experiments showed that very few of the latter complexes were formed after exposure of the heparinized surface to human whole blood in 90 minutes, as compared to uncoated control polymers. These results question the model proposed wherein thrombin in flowing blood is deactivated by the heparin-ATIII surface to form TAT complexes that are released, and the heparin repeats this activity several times. Further studies in flowing systems developed to study thromboresistance of intravascular stents, where platelet free and platelet rich plasma were used, helped solidify a refinement of the model (Figs. 49.2, 49.3, and 49.4).

Figure 49.2 represents the flow through system developed for monitoring thrombin generation for an intravascular stent. Citrated PRP or PFP could be pumped through the system at controlled flow rates and samples collected over time.

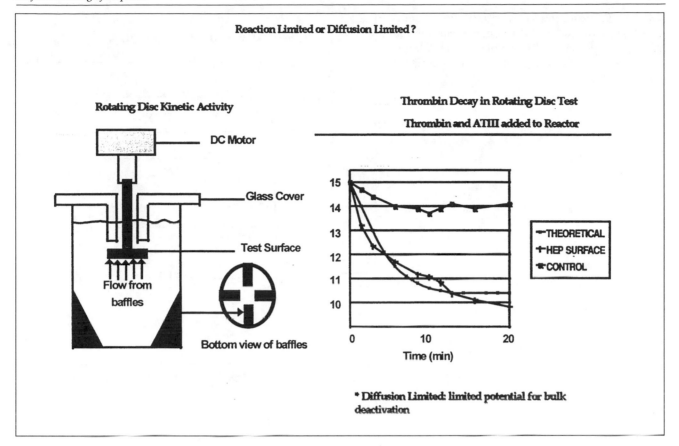

Fig. 49.1. Rotating disc apparatus; thrombin decay in rotating disc test.

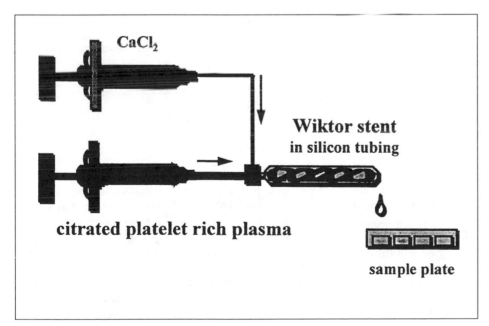

Fig. 49.2. Flow through system which monitors Wiktor intravascular stent thrombin generation. Citrated platelet rich plasma (PRP) or platelet free plasma (PFP) is pumped through the system at controlled flow rates and samples collected over time.

Fig. 49.3. Comparison of contact activation as measured by factor IXa, and of thrombin generation in platelet rich plasma (PRP) or platelet free plasma (PFP). (A) Heparin-coated intravascular stents; (B) Uncoated stents.

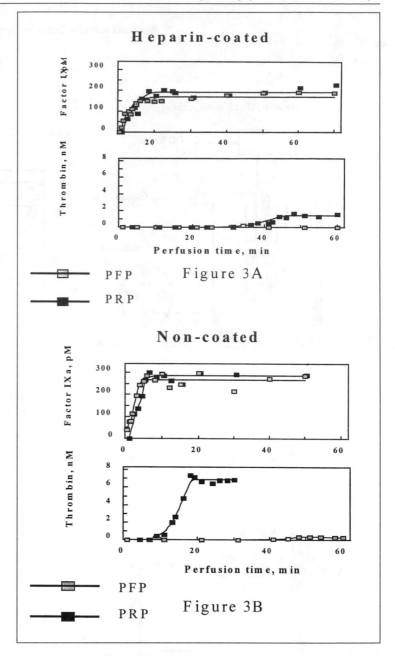

Figure 3A

Figure 3B

Figures 49.3A and 49.B represent a comparison between heparin coated and uncoated intravascular stents with respect to contact activation as measured with Factor IXa, and its comparison to subsequent thrombin generation in PRP or PFP. The black points represent PRP and the gray represent PFP. The first thing that can be seen is that contact activation is independent of platelets, and that without platelets the even more "thrombogenic" metallic surface does not produce significant amounts of thrombin (Fig. 49.3A). Not surprisingly, the anionic heparin stent does cause some contact activation, but less than the noncoated stent (Fig. 49.3B). Clearly, in the presence of platelets the heparinized surface delays the onset of thrombin generation, and at equilibrium is much less thrombogenic than the noncoated control material.

Table 49.1 helps to further explain the importance of the quality (ability to bind ATIII) of the attached heparin to the surface. ATIII uptake to the surface directly correlates with the delay in the onset of thrombin generation, the amount produced at equilibrium and, most importantly, the number of adhered platelets. The platelets on the surface are determined by the LDH method, and therefore some platelets could be present that are "adhered", but not activated. SEM photos of the surfaces of the heparinized materials did not reveal any visible platelets after mild rinsing, whereas the controls were covered with adhered and spread platelets. Much might be learned in the future by study of platelet adhesion to surfaces such as heparin and collagen. Exposed subendothelial layers of collagen and GAGs can be seen to adhere platelets in dense single cell layers that do not

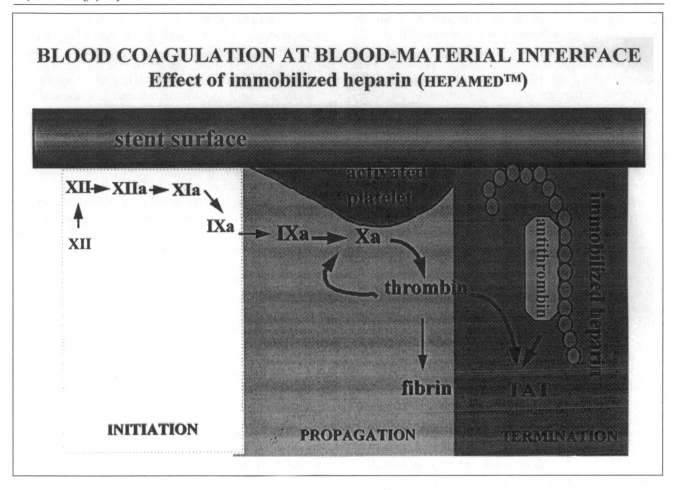

Fig. 49.4. Contribution of immobilized heparin to clot prevention at blood-material interface by antithrombin (ATIII) deactivation of platelet-produced thrombin.

Table 49.1. Relation between the AT uptake and the Thrombogenicity of Wiktor stents

Coating	AT-Uptake	Thrombin stead State	Thrombin onset	Platelet Adhesion
	pmol/cm-2	nM	Min	
None	0.26±0.36	8.83±0.37	5	287±34
Hepamed™	1.26±0.36	4.98±0.62	20	135±18
Hepamed™	1.99±0.57	3.40±0.25	20	197±45
Hepamed™	7.28±0.21	1.75±0.09	30	42±20
Hepamed™	10.89±0.21	1.48±0.15	34	92±33

Table 49.2 Effects of heparin bonded surface on blood clotting in polyurethane tubing

Surface	Surface modification	Platelet Adhesion	ATIII Adsorption	Clotting Time
		Plts/cm2 x103 (LDH)	pmol/cm2	seconds
PU55D	none	123.1	nd	659
6882-78-1	PU Collagen	234.1	4.45	594
6882-78-2	PU collagen+ heparin	195.4	11.16	1183

appear to be spead or fully activated. This phenomenon has led us to further experiments that will be described shortly, but for now suffice it to say that the natural process of wound healing of damaged endothelium begs the question as to whether or not a natural material such as collagen in the presence of certain glycosaminoglycans might produce a "controlled" and important thrombogenic response.

Thrombin generation and subsequent fibrin formation is due in a large part to the inability of flow conditions to keep the local concentration of thrombin low. Our experience has been that rapid clot formation takes place when the local concentration of thrombin reaches about 2-5 nM. Once this point has been reached, the fibrin network is rapidly formed and can entrap platelets and amplify the local generation of thrombin.

Figure 49.4 is a recent attempt at refining the conceptual model of how heparin works when immobilized on a surface. The critical mechanism for preventing clotting is that thrombin produced by platelets at the surface is immediately deactivated, thus keeping the local concentration low, which in turn minimizes the strongest agent (thrombin) in platelet activation. When the thrombin level is low, it cannot amplify its own production by activating vicinal platelets, and less fibrin will minimize entrapment of additional platelets. The latter is of great significance for the longer term maintenance of low thrombogenicity, as thrombin can adhere to fibrin and in this state it is not deactivated by heparin and ATIII, and can continue to activate platelets.[25]

Intramuscular implant studies of immobilized collagen on biomaterials by our group showed immediate thrombogenic response followed by strong apparent neutrophil recruitment at the tissue-material interface. This response quickly became quiescent, and after 6 weeks the tissue-material interface had only an occasional macrophage with mostly fibroblasts (two cell layers) followed by adjacent microvascular structures. The control material (polyurethane) had a typical foreign body fibrotic response with macrophages and foreign body giant cells adjacent to the majority of the surface, at least 15 layers of densely packed fibroblasts with no vascular structures, and loose connective tissue outside of the fibroblast layers. These results led to preliminary experiments in measuring the coagulation response to collagen immobilized surfaces, and the potentiating effect that heparin coupled to this collagen layer might have.

Using the same flow through system developed at the University of Maastricht and described previously, polyurethane tubings were prepared with immobilized collagen and immobilized collagen with heparin covalently bonded to the collagen (type I collagen).

Apparently the fact that more platelets are attached to the collagen and collagen plus heparin surfaces than the polyurethane does not lead to a faster clotting time, and in the case of the heparinized collagen the clotting time was significantly delayed (Table 49.2). These are very preliminary experiments, and only suggest additional studies to attempt to look at heparin in a broader context of the total healing response.

Heparin has several other properties in addition to acting as an anticoagulant, such as antibacterial and antiviral activity, inhibition of several enzymes, and the stimulation of lipoprotein lipase release from the surface of endothelial cells.[26,27] It has been proposed that heparin has a role in the defense against pathogens outside of the immune system.[28] This hypothesis seems to have merit based on the fact that heparin is predominantly located in organs and tissues that come in direct contact with the outside environment (lung, skin, and intestine).

Heparin binding growth factors (HBGFs) represent an important family of mediators for the healing response, capable of inducing mesenchymal cell proliferation and differentiation, tissue regeneration, morphogenesis, and neovascularization.[29] Several investigations of the growth factors that are found in wound sites use heparin columns in separation and identification of these growth factors.[30-32] Numerous experiments have been tried by simple addition of growth factors to wound sites or to matrices. There are also some experiments where the role that heparin might play has been investigated. Angiogenesis was found to be enhanced by the addition of heparin to gels made of basement membrane extract that also had added acidic and basic fibroblast growth factors.[33] Heparin, along with ECGF, is suggested to play a role as a response modifier of human endothelial cell migration, which may be relevant to tumor metastasis, wound healing, and atherogenesis.[34] Another study using heparin analogs (chemically substituted dextrans) in a collagen plaster was able to show a remarkable effect both on the kinetics and on the quality of the restored skin.[35] This study strongly suggests that endogenous growth factors naturally releasing during the regeneration process could be trapped, protected and released by the addition of heparin analogs or heparin.

It may be wishful thinking, but perhaps immobilized or surface bonded heparin may play a strong role in tissue engineering. This may be particularly true if it is properly immobilized and capable of trapping, protecting and releasing growth factors at locations and rates desired. Realization of this potential probably will require some additional thinking beyond heparin by itself. Coupling to biomolecules such as collagens and other glycosaminoglycans to polymeric surfaces may prove fruitful. From some of the studies mentioned, it is apparent that gel matrices can be modified to exhibit angiogenesis and remodeling. It may be entirely possible to fill porous polymer matrices with such gels and approach the ultimate regenerated tissue-like vascular graft. Still, for those concerned with optimal mechanical properties, the proper polymeric scaffold with a more fibrous character can have the surfaces modified for covalent attachment that may achieve a similar end. The former will require a bigger step in regulatory and commercial acceptance, while the latter may lead to incremental improvements. It is hopeful that efforts in both areas will lead to understanding that will result in a vascular graft with complete healing that is long term patent, and infection resistant.

References

1. Gomes MN, Hufnagel CA, Dokumaci O. Studies in the autogenization of prosthesis for samll artery replacement. Am Surg 1972; 38:664-666.

2. Russel AP, Hopwood D. The biological uses and importance of glutaraldehyde. Prog Med Chem 1976; 13:271-299.

3. Sparks CH. Silicone mandril method for growing reinforced autogenous femoropopliteal artery grafts in situ. Ann Surg 1973; 177:293-300.

4. Bothwell JW, Lord GH, Rosenberg N. Modified arterial heterografts: Relationship of processing techniques to interface characteristics. In: Sawyer PN, ed. Bio-physical Mechanisms in Vascular Homeostasis and Intravascular Thrombosis. Appleton-Century-Crofts, 1965.

5. Csomor K, Karpati E, Nagy M, Gyorgyi-Edeleny J, Machovich R. Blood coagulation is inhibited by sulphated copolymers of vinyl alcohol and acrylic acid under in vitro as well as in vivo conditions. Thromb Res 1994; 74(4):389-398.

6. Montdargent B, Toufik J, Carreno M, Labarre D, Jozefowicz M. Complement activation and adsorption of protein fragments by functionalized polymer surfaces in human serum. Biomater 1992; 13.

7. van Boeckel CAA. From Heparin To A Synthetic Drug: A Multi-disciplinary Approach. In: Trends in Receptor Research. Elsevier Publishers B.V. 1993.

8. Gott VL, Koepke DE, Daggett RL, Zarnstorff W, Young WP. The coating of intravascular plastic prostheses with colloidal graphite. Surg 1961; 50:382.

9. Bassmadijan D, Sefton MV. Relationship between release rate and surface concentration for heparinized materials. J Biomed Mat Res 1983; 17:509-518.

10. Larm O, Larsson R, Olsonn P. A new nonthrombogenic surface prepared by selective covalent binding of heparin via a modified reducing terminal residue. Biomat Med Dev Art Org 1983; 11:161-173.

11. Wendel IIP, Heller W, Gallimore MJ, Hoffmeister HE. Heparin-coated oxygenators significantly reduce contact system activation in an in vitro cardiopulmonary bypass model. Blood Coag Fibrin, 1994; 5.

12. Grainger DW, Kim SW, Feijen J. Poly(dimethylsiloxane)-poly(ethylene oxide)-heparin block copolymers. I. Synthesis and characterization. J Biomed Mater Res 1990; 22:231-249.

13. Ebert CD, Kim SW. Immobilized heparin: spacer arm effects on biological interactions. Thromb Res 1982; 26:43-57.

14. Yuan S, Szakalas-Gratzl G, Ziats NP, Jacobsen DW, Kottke-Mrchant K, Marchant RE. Immobilization of high affinity heparin oligosaccharide to radio frequency plasma-modified polyethylene. J Biomed Mater Res 1993; 27:811-819.

15. Chandler WL, Solomon DD, Hu CB, Schmer G. Estimation of surface bound heparin activity: A comparison of methods. J Biomed Mater Res 1988; 22:497-508.

16. Engbers GHM. The development of heprinized materials with an imporved blood compatibility. Thesis University of Twente, The Netherlands, 1990.

17. Cahalan L et al. Biocompatible medical article and method. U.S. Patent 5,607,475, Assignee: Medtronic Inc. March 4, 1997.

18. Yun JK, DeFife K, Colton E, Stack S, Azeez A, Cahalan L, Verhoeven M, Cahalan P, Anderson JM. Human monocyte/macrophage adhesion and cytokine production on surface-modified poly(tetrafluoroethylene/hexafluoropropylene) polymers with and without protein preadsorption. J Biomed Mater Res 1995; 29:257-268.

19. Elgue G et al. Effect of surface immobilized heparin on the activation of adsorbed factor XII. Art Org 1993; 17(8):721-726.

20. van Delden CJ. On the anticoagulant activity of heparinized surfaces. Ph.D. Thesis, University of Twente, The Netherlands, 1995.

21. Barbucci R, Magnani A. Conformation of human plasma proteins at polymer surfaces: The effectiveness of surface heparinization. Biomater 1994; 15(12):955-962.

22. Nemets EA, Sevastianov V. The interaction of heparinized biomaterials with human serum, albumin, fibrinogen, atntithrombin III, and platelets. Art Org 1991; 15(5):381-385.

23. Drumheller PD, Hubbell JA. Densely crosslinked polymer networks of poly(ethylen glycol) in trimethylolpropane triacrylate for cell-adhesion-resistant surfaces. J Biomed Mater Res 1995; 29:207-215.

24. Lindhout T, Blezer R, Schoen P, Willems GM, Fouache B, Verhoeven M, Hendiks M, Cahalan L, Cahalan P. Antithrombin activity of surface-bound heparin studied under flow conditions. J Biomed Mater Res 1994; 29:1255-1266.

25. Buchanan MR, Liao P, Ofosu FA. Simultaneous inhibition of thrombin by ATIII and HCII and prevention of thrombus formation and growth: Relative effects of heparin and sulodexide. Abstract from XIV Congress of ISTH, 1993.

26. Wright TC, Castellot JJ, Diamond JR, Karnovsky JJ. Regulation of cellular proliferation by heparin and heparan sulphate, In: Lane DA, Lindahl U, eds. Heparin, chemical and bioligical properties, clinical applications. London: Edward Arnold, 1989.

27. Olivecrona T, Bengtsson-Olivecrona G. Heparin and lipases. In: Lane DA, Lindahl U, eds. Heparin, chemical and biological properties, clinical applications London: Edward Arnold, 1989.

28. Björk I, Olson ST, Shore JD. Molecular mechanisms of the accelaerating effect of heparin on the reactions between antithrombin and clotting proteinases. In: Lane DA, Lindahl U, eds. Heparin, chemical and bioligical properties, clinical applications. London: Edward Arnold, 1989.

29. Lobb RR. Clinical applications of heparin-binding growth factors. Euro J Clin Inves 1988; 18(4):321-36.

30. Hamerman D, Taylor S, Kirschenbaum I, Klagsbrun M, Raines EW, Ross R, Thomas KA. Growth factors with heparin binding affinity in human synovial fluid. Proc Soc Exp Biol Med 1987; 186(3):384-9.

31. Marikovshy M, Breuing K, Liu PY, Eriksson E, Higashiyama S, Farber P, Abrahm J, Klagsbrun M. Appearance of heparin-binding EGF-like growth factor in wound fluid as a response to injury. Proc Natl Acad Sci USA 1993; 90(9):3889-93.

32. McCarthy DW, Downing MT, Brigstock DR, Luquette MH, Brown KD, Abad MS, Besner GE. Production of heparin-binding epeidermal growth factor-like growth factor (HB-EGF) at sites of thermal injury in pediatric patients. J Inves Dermatol 1966; 106(1):49-56.

33. Passaniti A, Taylor RM, Pili R, Guo Y, Long PV, Haney JA, Paul RR, Grant DS, Martin GR. A simple, quantitative method for assessing angiogenesis and antiangiogenic agents using reconstituted basement membrane, heparin, and fibroblast growth factor. Lab Inves 1992; 67(4):519-28.

34. Terranova VP, DiFlorio R, Lyall RM, Hic S, Friesel R, Maciag T. Human endothelial cells are chemtactic to en-

dothelial cell growth factor and heparin. J Cell Biol 1985; 101(6):2330-4.

35. Meddahi A, Blanquaert F, Saffar JL, Colombier ML, Caruelle JP, Josefonvicz J, Barritault D. New approaches to tissue regeneration and repair. Path Res Prac 1994; 190(9-10):923-8.

Scaffold Engineering

Surface Modification

―――――――――――――――――――― CHAPTER 50 ――――――――――――――――――――

Covalent Grafting of RGD Peptides to Synthetic Surfaces

Nina M.K. Lamba, S.L. Cooper

Introduction

Fabric materials were first used as vascular prostheses in the 1950s, when Voorhees et al implanted a polymeric vascular graft manufactured from vinyl chloride and acrylonitrile.[1] Since then, a number of polymers have been used to fabricate vascular prostheses, and today, polyethylene terephthalate (PET, Dacron®) and polytetrafluoroethylene (PTFE, Gore-Tex®) are the most commonly used biomaterials for this application. Vascular grafts made from either of these materials have an internal diameter usually greater than 6 mm, and are restricted to use in high shear environments. Currently there is no clinically acceptable synthetic small diameter vascular prosthesis, i.e., one less than 6 mm I.D. Thrombus and neointima formation will readily occlude synthetic vascular grafts. The resulting loss of patency remains the greatest obstacle to the development of a small caliber vascular prosthesis. Thus, there is a need for an engineered material that will provide the necessary mechanical and thromboresistant properties for a successful synthetic vascular prosthesis, to facilitate the advancements in vascular surgery. In this chapter we will discuss the motivation for the endothelialization of luminal surfaces, and describe some of the approaches that have been taken to achieve this. A discussion of methods to covalently graft Arg-Gly-Asp (RGD) peptides to polymers follows, focusing on methods and results obtained using polymers that are used to fabricate vascular prostheses.

Methods to Improve Endothelialization

The only nonthrombogenic material known to man is the normal vascular endothelium. The endothelium actively achieves this nonthrombogenicity through the synthesis of numerous anti-platelet agents and clotting inhibitors. Furthermore, protein adsorption occurs rapidly onto artificial surfaces from solution, but this is not a feature of endothelial surfaces.[2-4] There is a great deal of literature detailing various approaches to promote the development of a stable, confluent layer of endothelial cells on the inner lumen of a vascular graft. It is believed that the growth of a confluent monolayer of endothelial cells onto a synthetic substrate will not only reduce the degree of thrombus formation, but may also reduce the proliferation of pathogenic organisms on the device. Approaches to encourage the endothelialization of the inner lumen of vascular grafts have included seeding of surfaces with cells, and chemical and physical modification of surfaces to promote cell attachment. Prostheses have been seeded with endothelial cells to promote endothelialization of the luminal surface. The success of this approach has been limited by problems with harvesting endothelial cells, and the subsequent attachment, retention and proliferation of cells on the surface. Chemical modification of surfaces has included the use of photo discharge

Tissue Engineering of Prosthetic Vascular Grafts, edited by Peter Zilla and Howard P. Greisler.
©1999 R.G. Landes Company.

technology to deposit reactive groups onto polymer surfaces, or to indirectly influence the proteins adsorbed to the surface. These methods to encourage cell attachment have met with limited success, owing to the lack of specificity and poor control over protein orientation. Physical methods to improve the development of a pseudointima on the surface have involved altering the porosity and texture of surfaces, to promote tissue ingrowth into the graft. The neointima that forms in the lumen of a graft may not provide comparable physiological properties of a natural endothelium, limiting the success of integration of the implanted device with the host by this method.[5] Grafts have been coated with adhesive proteins or extracellular matrix components in order to promote attachment and proliferation of endothelial cells.[6-8] An improvement in the extent of endothelialization has been observed in animal models. RGD-protein conjugates have also been synthesized,[9] but problems in defining the precise conformation of the protein once it has adsorbed to the substrate impede interpretation of results. The long term success of materials modified through adsorption of proteins to mediate cellular adhesion is not guaranteed, due to possible desorption of the protein or proteolysis.

More recently, there has been an interest in the grafting of synthetic peptide sequences onto polymeric substrates. By covalently grafting short peptide sequences onto polymeric substrates, it is believed that cellular adhesion can be mediated directly through receptor-ligand interactions, rather than through a conditioning layer of adsorbed protein. The covalent grafting of the Arg-Gly-Asp (RGD) peptide sequence to synthetic materials has also been shown to promote cell adhesion and attachment for applications such as tissue culture substrates and biomaterials for implantation and hybrid artificial organs. Some of the approaches to modify biomaterials with cell adhesive peptide sequences containing the RGD sequence relevant to the development of synthetic vascular grafts will be discussed in more detail in this chapter.

Immobilization of RGD Peptides

The RGD peptide sequence has been shown to be the minimal cell-recognizable sequence in many adhesive plasma and extracellular matrix proteins.[10] The RGD sequence was first found in fibronectin, and is also present in vitronectin, von willebrand factor, fibrinogen, and collagen. The RGD sequence has been shown to play a crucial role in mediating cell attachment and subsequent spreading. It has been shown to be adhesive towards platelets and other cells, including fibroblasts and endothelial cells. The RGD tripeptide may also act as a ligand for the integrin superfamily of receptors. In particular, many integrin receptors recognize the RGD sequence which is present in many adhesive proteins.[11] It has been demonstrated that the synthetic RGD peptide in solution is able to compete with adhesive proteins adsorbed onto a surface for binding receptors on the cell in solution and prevent cellular adhesion to an adhesive protein adsorbed to the surface.[10] Synthetic surfaces containing immobilized RGD peptides have been shown to promote cell attachment in a manner similar to fibronectin. Some cell surface receptors have been shown to bind with the RGD

sequence in a specific protein, whereas other receptors may recognize the RGD sequence in more than one protein. The specificity of the RGD protein is believed to be modulated by the conformation of the sequence. This may be determined by the amino acids that are immediately adjacent to the RGD sequence.[12-14] Substitution of peptides within the RGD sequence has been shown to produce a large reduction in the adhesivity of the peptide.[15] The presence of a peptide adjacent to the sequence has been shown to alter the activity of the RGD sequence.[10,16,17]

Covalent grafting of biological molecules to a synthetic substrate prevents the desorption of the agent over time from the surface. An excellent review of the chemistry of covalent immobilization of RGD peptides is available.[18] Generally, either the peptide or the surface must be "activated" to provide suitable sites for immobilization of the ligand to the substrate. Biological structures are less resistant than synthetic polymers to harsh chemical environments. Prolonged exposure of a ligand to a harsh environment may lead to a reduction in the biological activity of the peptide. Thus, the polymer substrate is often derivatized or activated prior to peptide coupling. Some of the more commonly used reaction schemes involve the coupling of the peptide sequence to a polymer substrate that contains hydroxyl, thiol, carboxylic acid or amine groups. Surfaces or ligands can also be derivatized and immobilized using photochemical techniques. The efficiency of the coupling reaction between the substrate and the peptide can influence the surface peptide density, which has been shown to influence the degree of cell spreading.[19,20] There are also other factors that can affect the coupling yield and biological activity of the ligand. The RGD sequence can be immobilized by covalent bonding at either end of the sequence, either through the carboxyl terminus or the amino terminus. The orientation of the sequence can affect the interactions of the peptide with cell surface receptors. The immobilization of peptide sequences on surfaces may also impose steric constraints on the peptide, affecting the affinity and specificity of the ligand. This has been reported with the grafting of other biological molecules, and may be overcome by grafting the ligand onto spacer arms, reducing steric hindrance imposed by the proximity of the ligand to a rigid surface.[21] The protection of the peptide during the coupling reaction scheme is also a consideration, to ensure that the activity of the peptide is retained. Competing side reactions such as hydrolysis, polymerization and crosslinking can also affect the grafting yield. The final surface density of ligands can be determined by radiolabeling, photochrome labeling, surface analysis or gravimetry.[18]

A number of studies have been performed investigating methods to immobilize peptide sequences containing the RGD sequence to polymeric surfaces. With respect to the development of synthetic vascular prostheses, RGD grafted materials have been studied with the goal of improving the integration of the prosthesis into the host cardiovascular system, with the ability to perform the biological functions of the endothelium. RGD sequences have been grafted onto polyethylene terephthalate (PET) and polytetrafluoroethylene (PTFE),[22] polyvinyl alcohol (PVA),[23] polyacrylamide,[24] polystyrene,[25] and polyurethane.[26] It has been demonstrated that the presence of RGD peptide sequences at the surface increases endothelial cell attachment in vitro. The attachment of endothelial cells through specific receptor-ligand interactions should overcome the problems of cell detachment under shear conditions.[22] The methods to immobilize RGD peptides to polymers, described below, demonstrate that successful grafting can be achieved by either bulk or surface modification. The main advantages of using surface modification techniques are that smaller quantities of reagents are required, and the mechanical properties of the material can be retained. However, on a commercial scale, bulk modification of a material requires fewer processing steps, which can ease fabrication and reduce costs.

Sugawara and Matsuda have derivatized peptides with 4-azidobenzoyloxysuccinimide. The peptides were then adsorbed to a polyvinylalcohol surface.[27] The surface was exposed to UV radiation to covalently bond the peptides to the surface. Bovine aortic endothelial cell adhesion was reported to be enhanced in a biologically specific manner. Ozeki and Matsuda have used a similar strategy to attach photochemically peptides containing the RGD sequence to polystyrene.[25] An increase in the attachment of bovine aortic endothelial cells was reported. The specific peptide sequence that is grafted may also modulate the adhesivity of the RGD sequence. Hirano et al[16] immobilized RDGS, RGDV, RGDT, and RGD onto ethylene-acrylic acid copolymer by coupling the terminal NH$_2$ to the carboxylic residues in the polymer. The surfaces were evaluated for cell recognition by cell adhesion activity towards 5 different cell lines. It was found that the fourth amino acid in the tetrapeptides played an important role in determining the precise specificity of the RGD sequence. The presence of either serine (S), threonine (T), or valine (V) at the end of the peptide enhanced cellular adhesion. They postulated that the modulation in the adhesive nature of the RGD sequence may arise from a conformational change in the RGD sequence, exerted by the terminal peptide.

Massia and Hubbell have grafted RGD peptides onto the surface of polyethylene terephthalate (PET) and polytetrafluoroethylene (PTFE) films.[22,28] This was achieved through the hydroxylation of the polymer followed by subsequent immobilization of the synthetic peptide sequence via tresyl chloride. The RGD could only react via the N-terminus, ensuring that the orientation of the grafted peptide was the same throughout. Radiolabeling of peptides was used to confirm the presence and concentration of the peptide sequence. Endothelial cell adhesion was evaluated on the unmodified, hydroxylated and peptide containing surfaces, both with and without the presence of serum. In the absence of serum, the RGD grafted films were able to support the adhesion and spreading of human umbilical vein endothelial cells (HUVECs). Neither the unmodified films nor the hydroxylated intermediates showed the same degree of adhesion and spreading. Stress fibers were also observed, implying that the cells were attached strongly to the substrate, and may possess the mechanical strength to resist detachment by shear forces.

Over the years, it has become apparent that the thrombogenicity of a synthetic graft is not the only criterion by which a vascular graft should be assessed. The mechanical properties, particularly the compliance and the texture of the graft are important factors in promoting tissue ingrowth, reducing anastomotic hyperplasia and favoring the long term patency of the graft. Both PET and PTFE are much less distensible when compared with the natural artery wall. Natural arteries show an increase in diameter of about 10% when pressurized to 150 mm Hg (normal arterial pressure). In comparison, PET and PTFE grafts distend by about 1% under these conditions. Polyurethanes are one of the strongest candidates for the development of small diameter vascular prostheses, due to their high tensile strength, compliance and blood compatibility.[29,30] Polyurethanes have been shown to distend by about 6% under normal arterial pressure,[31] and a blended polyurethane-polylactide vascular prosthesis possesses mechanical properties similar to rat abdominal aorta.[32] Arterial substitutes need to have mechanical properties that match the natural vessel wall, to avoid turbulent blood flow, which may result in thrombus formation or destruction of formed blood elements. Lyman et al[33,34] have shown that the distensibility of the graft can influence the biocompatibility through the degree of anastomotic hyperplasia by comparing vascular grafts fabricated from the same material, but with different degrees of compliance. Furthermore, a mismatch in compliance between the synthetic graft and the natural vessel may traumatize the natural vessel and disrupt the endothelium, which will in turn initiate thrombosis and stimulate intimal hypertrophy.

Polyurethanes are block copolymers consisting of alternating soft and hard segments. The incompatibility between these two components of the polymer allows microphase separation to occur within the bulk polymer. The material can be described as being comprised of hard domains dispersed within a soft segment matrix. This gives rise to the superior physical properties of the polyurethanes and is believed to be a contributory factor to their blood and tissue compatibility. Recently, RGD peptide sequences have been successfully grafted to polyurethane substrates.[35] Polyurethanes for medical applications are usually synthesized via a two-step 'prepolymer' method. Lin et al synthesized a polyurethane from methylene bis (p-phenylisocyanate) (MDI) and butane diol (BD), with polytetramethyleneoxide (PTMO) as the soft segment. Hydrogen atoms on the urethane groups were substituted with carboxyl groups, via abstraction of urethane hydrogen by sodium hydride, followed by reaction of the polyurethane with β-propiolactone. The degree of substitution could be varied by the quantities of reagents used. This was performed to alter the density of the grafted peptides. Peptide sequences were then coupled to the carboxyl group using 1-(3-dimethylaminopropyl)-3-ethylcarbodiimide hydrochloride (EDCl). The reaction scheme for the carboxylation of the urethane group, followed by coupling of the RGD peptide sequence is shown in Figure 50.1.

Lin investigated the effect of the coupling reaction on the endothelialization of the substrate. Two coupling

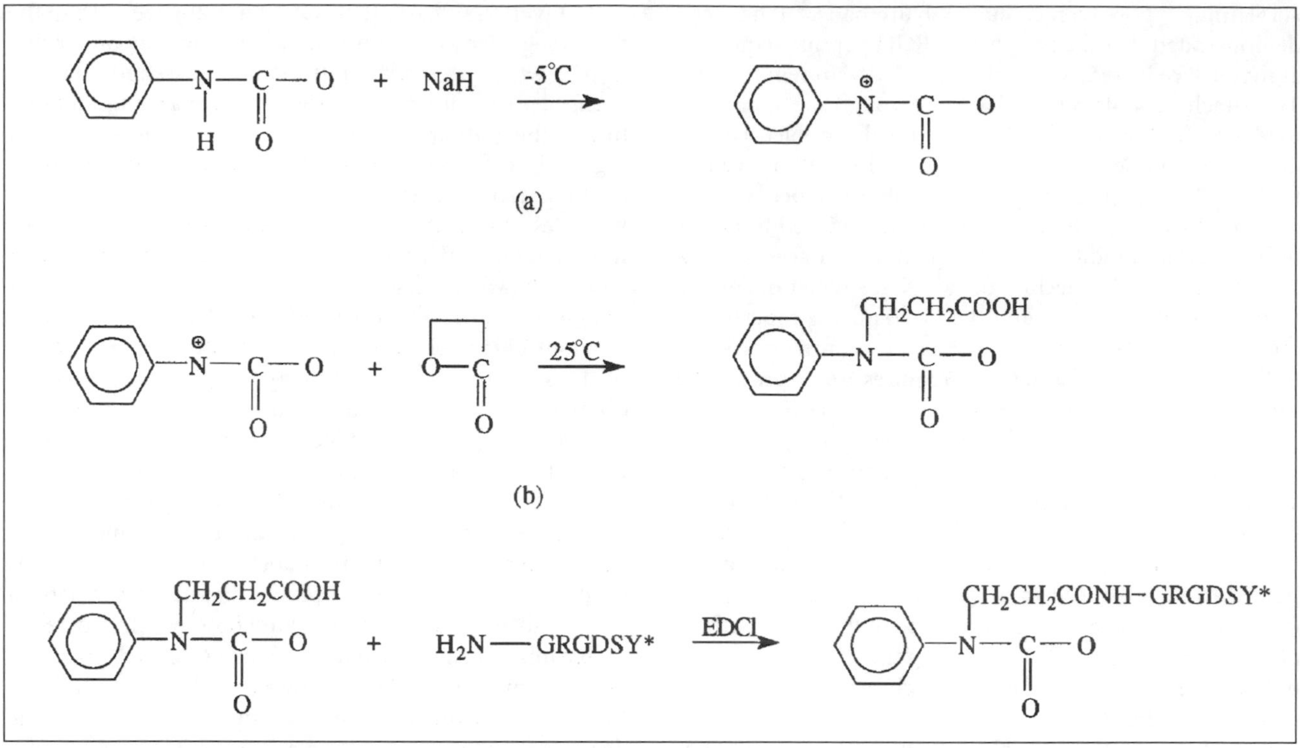

Fig. 50.1. Reaction scheme for the synthesis of RGD-containing peptide grafted polyurethane. (a) deprotonation of urethane group; (b) carboxylation of polyurethane; (c) coupling of RGD peptide.[26]

methods were used. The first, one step method coupled the free hexapeptide directly to the carboxyl group through the formation of an amide bond. The second method involved two steps, coupling a protected peptide to the carboxyl group, followed by deprotection of the peptide. The two step method using the protected peptides appeared to have a higher coupling efficiency of the peptide to the substrate of the unprotected peptide, as coupling could only occur via the N-terminus of the peptide. Furthermore, there were fewer competing side reactions in the synthetic scheme using the protected peptides, improving the yield of grafting.

Previously, other researchers had reported that the adhesion and growth of endothelial cells on polyurethane is relatively poor.[36,37] The immobilization of RGD peptides to a polyurethane as described above increased the number of adherent HUVECs after in vitro seeding. A larger number of cells attached to RGD peptides that had been protected during synthesis than those that had not been protected. In addition, greater endothelial cell adhesion to hydrated samples was observed compared with samples that had not been previously hydrated. Polyurethanes contain hydrophilic and hydrophobic domains that reorient upon hydration, minimizing the interfacial free energy. Cold-stage ESCA studies of hydrated and dry samples showed that reorientation of the peptides occurs at the hydrated surface,[38] leading to the conclusion that the RGD peptides on the polyurethane backbone do orient towards the surface on hydration. This reorientation of the functional peptide groups is depicted schematically in Figure 50.2.[38] Reorientation of RGD peptides at an aqueous interface has been reported else-

where.[25] The increased adhesion on the RGD-grafted polyurethanes that were hydrated prior to contact with endothelial cells provides further evidence that reorientation of the RGD peptides does occur on hydration, and that cellular adhesion to RGD grafted materials is mediated through receptor interactions with the peptide. Figure 50.3 shows SEMs of endothelial cells grown in vitro, on the base polyurethane (PEU), carboxylated polyurethane (PEU-COOH), and peptide grafted polyurethanes (PEU-GRGESY, PEU-GRGDSY, and PEU-GRGDVY). The effect of substituting one of the amino acids within the RGD sequence reduces the adhesivity of the peptide (PEU-GRGESY). The substitution of the peptide adjacent to the RGD sequence has the ability to alter the adhesivity, as adhesion was greater on GRGDVY grafted material than GRGDSY grafted polyurethane.

Both Massia[22] and Lin[35] have investigated the role of serum proteins in mediating cell adhesion to RGD grafted materials. Endothelial cell adhesion was evaluated on the unmodified, intermediate and peptide grafted materials, both with and without the presence of serum. Massia and Hubbell found that both the unmodified PET and the hydroxylated PTFE supported cell adhesion only in the presence of serum proteins, implying that cell adhesion was mediated by adsorbed proteins. Lin et al[35] reached a similar conclusion in their study of HUVEC attachment to the RGD grafted polyurethane. Hubbell and co-workers have also created highly specific cell adhesive substrates of RGD-containing surfaces with low protein adsorption.[15,22,39] The low protein adsorbing characteristics of these surfaces has allowed

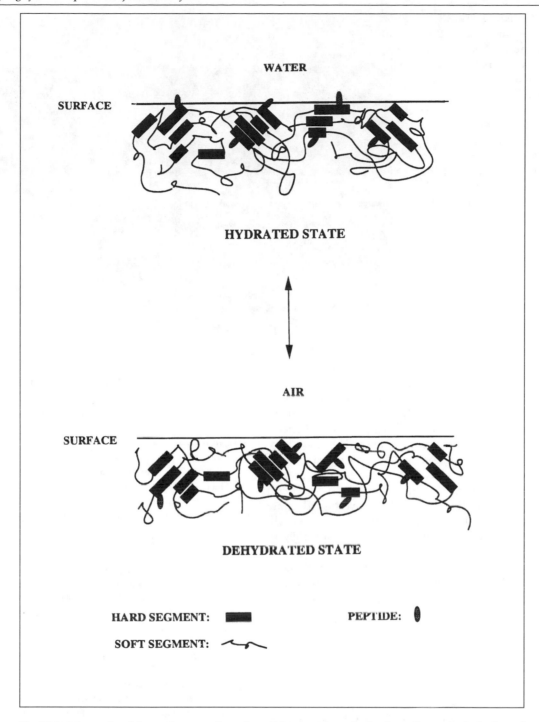

Fig. 50.2. Schematic of the surface re-orientation of the peptide grafted polyurethanes in the hydrated and dehydrated states. From: Lin H-B, Lewis KB, Leach-Scampavia D et al. Surface properties of RGD-peptide grafted polyurethane block copolymers: Variable take-off angle and cold-stage ESCA studies. J Biomater Sci, Polym Ed 1993; 4:183-198.

Fig. 50.3. SEMs of HUVECs attached to polyurethanes. Base polyurethane (PEU), carboxylated polyurethane (PEU-COOH), RGE-grafted polyurethane (PEU-GRGESY), RGD grafted polyurethane (PEU-GRGDSY and PEU-GRGDVY). From: Lin H-B, Garcia-Echeverria C, Asakura S et al. Endothelial cell adhesion on polyurethanes containing covalently attached RGD peptides. Biomaterials 1992; 13:905-914.

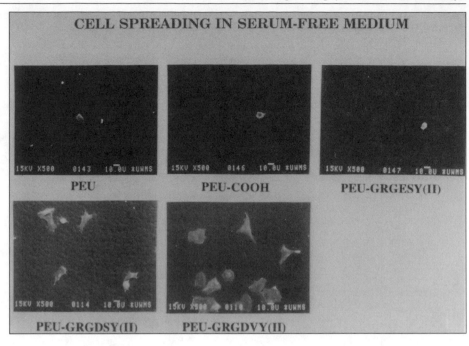

the study of cell attachment and spreading independently of protein adsorption. Using these substrates they have shown that the RGD and Tyr-Ile-Gly-Ser-Arg (YIGSR) peptide sequences promote endothelial cell adhesion independently of adsorbed cell adhesion proteins. They have also demonstrated that serum proteins play a role in cell spreading, with serum proteins affecting the final extent of spreading, but not the initial rate.[40] The effect of the surface density of the grafted peptide has also been investigated using these surfaces. The effect of ligand surface density on cell adhesion is discussed elsewhere in this book. Ultimately, it is hoped that optimization of the spacing of RGD peptides to promote the attachment of endothelial cells will allow the inclusion of other ligands, such as growth factors, that may be necessary to further modulate adhesion and spreading, or otherwise maintain the cell layer.

Summary

The natural endothelium offers the only nonthrombogenic surface known to man. This is actively achieved through regulation of transport across the endothelium, and the synthesis of agents that actively prevent events such as protein adsorption, platelet deposition and thrombus formation. The development of a successful small diameter vascular prosthesis is central to the advancement of peripheral vascular surgery. The issues of occlusion and infection of vascular grafts are problematic, and remain the greatest impediment to the development of small caliber grafts. The immobilization of RGD peptides to the luminal surfaces of synthetic vascular prostheses may offer the means to promote endothelialization, and improve the long term patency of vascular grafts. Further studies are required to establish the long term clinical performance of such devices. Studies need to include examination of endothelial cell retention once the material is exposed to a high shear environment, the physiological properties of the endothelial layer, and the interaction of endothelial cells with the formed elements of the blood, such as platelets and white blood cells.

References

1. Voorhees AB, Jaretzki A, Blakemore AH. The use of tubes constructed from Vinyon N cloth in bridging arterial defects. Ann Surg 1952; 135:322-324.
2. Szycher M. Thrombosis, hemostasis and thrombolysis at prosthetic interfaces. In: Szycher M, ed. Biocompatible Polymers, Metals and Composites. Lancaster, PA: Technomic, 1983:1-33.
3. Brash JL. Role of plasma protein adsorption in the response of blood to foreign surfaces. In: Sharma CP, Szycher M, ed. Blood compatible materials and devices. Lancaster, PA: Technomic, 1991:3-24.
4. Forbes CD, Courtney JM. Thrombosis and artificial surfaces. In: Bloom AL, Forbes CD, Thomas AL, Tuddenham EGD, eds. Haemostasis and Thrombosis. London: Churchill Livingstone, 1993:1301-1324.
5. Zilla P, Fasol R, Grimm M, Fischlein T, Eberl T, Preiss P, Krupicka O, Oppell U, Deutsch M. Growth properties of cultured human endothelial cells on differently coated artificial heart materials. J Thorac Cardiovasc Surg 1991; 101:671-680.
6. Lee Y, Park DK, Kim YB, Seo JW, Lee KB, Min B. Endothelial cell seeding onto the extracellular matrix of fibroblasts for the development of a small diameter polyurethane vessel. ASAIO J 1993; 39:M740-M745.
7. Miwa H, Matsuda T, Tani N, Kondo K, Iida F. An in vitro endothelialized compliant vascular graft minimizes anastomotic hyperplasia. ASAIO J 1993; 39:M501-M505.
8. Stansby G, Berwanger C, Shukla N, Schmidt-Rixen T, Hamilton G. Endothelial seeding of compliant polyurethane vascular graft material. Brit J Surg 1994; 81:1286-1289.

9. Kishida A, Takatsuka M, Matsuda T. RGD-albumin conjugate: Expression of tissue regeneration activity. Biomaterials, 1992; 13:924-930.

10. Pierschbacher MD, Ruoslahti E. Cell attachment activity of fibronectin can be duplicated by small synthetic fragments of the molecule. Nature 1984; 309:30-34.

11. Hynes RO. Integrins: A family of cell surface receptors. Cell 1987; 48:549-559.

12. Ruoslahti E, Pierschbacher MD. New perspectives in cell adhesion: RGD and integrins. Science 1987; 238:491-497.

13. D'Souza SE, Ginsberg MH, Plow EF. Arginyl-glycyl-aspartic acid (RGD): A cell adhesion motif. Trends Biol Sci 1991; 16:246-250.

14. Hautanen A, Gailit J, Mann M, Ruoslahti E. Effects of modification of the RGD sequence and its context on recognition by the fibronectin receptor. J Biol Chem 1989; 264:1437-1492.

15. Drumheller PD, Hubbell JA. Polymer networks with grafted cell adhesion peptides for highly specific cell adhesive substrates. Anal Biochem 1994; 222:380-388.

16. Hirano Y, Okuna M, Hayashi T, Goto K, Nakajima A. Cell-attachment activities of surface immobilized oligopeptides RGD, RGDS, RGDV, RGDT, and YIGSR towards five cell lines. J Biomater Sci Polym Ed 1993; 4:235-243.

17. Lin H-B, Garcia-Echeverria C, Asakura S, Sun W, Mosher DF, Cooper SL. Endothelial cell adhesion on polyurethanes containing covalently attached RGD peptides. Biomaterials 1992; 13:905-914.

18. Drumheller PD, Hubbell JA. Surface immobilization of adhesion ligands for investigations of cell-substrate interactions. In: Bronzino JD, ed. The Biomedical Engineering Handbook. Boca Raton, FL: CRC Press and IEEE Press, 1995:1583-1596.

19. Massia SP, Hubbell JA. An RGD spacing of 440 nm is sufficient for integrin $\alpha_v\beta_3$–mediated fibroblast spreading and 140 nm for focal contact and stress fiber formation. J Cell Biol 1991; 114:1089-1100.

20. Goodman SL, Cooper SL, Albrecht RM. Integrin receptors and platelet adhesion to synthetic surfaces. J Biomed Mater Res 1993; 27:683-695.

21. Nojiri C, Okano T, Park KD, Kim SW. Suppression mechanisms for thrombus formation on heparin-immobilized segmented polyurethane-ureas. Trans Am Soc Artif Intern Organs 1988; 34:386-398.

22. Massia SP, Hubbell JA. Human endothelial cell interactions with surface coupled adhesion peptides on a nonadhesive glass substrate and two polymeric biomaterials. J Biomed Mater Res 1991; 25:223-242.

23. Matsuda T, Kondo A, Makino K, Akutsu T. Development of a novel artificial matrix with cell adhesion peptide for cell culture and artificial hybrid organs. Trans Am Soc Artif Intern Organs 1989; 35:677-679.

24. Brandley BK, Schnaar RL. Covalent attachment of an Arg-Gly-Asp sequence peptide to derivatizable polyacrylamide surface: Support of fibroblast adhesion and long-term growth. Anal Biochem 1988; 172:270-278.

25. Ozeki E, Matsuda T. Development of an artificial extracellular matrix. Solution castable polymers with cell recognizable peptidyl side chain. Trans Am Soc Artif Intern Organs 1990; 36:M294-M296.

26. Lin H, Zhao Z, Garcia-Echeverria C, Rich DH, Cooper SL. Synthesis of a novel polyurethane copolymer containing covalently attached RGD peptide. J Biomater Sci Poly Ed 1992; 3:217-227.

27. Sugawara T. and Matsuda T. Photochemical surface derivatization of a peptide containing Arg-Gly-Asp (RGD). J Biomed Mater Res 1995; 29:1047-1052.

28. Hubbell JA, Massia SP, Drumheller PD. Surface-grafted cell-binding peptides in tissue engineering of the vascular graft. In: Pedersen H, Matharasan R, DiBiasio D, eds. Annals of the New York Academy of Science 1992:253-258.

29. Zdrahala RJ. Small caliber vascular grafts. Part II. Polyurethanes revisited. J Biomater Appl 1996; 11:37-61.

30. Lamba NMK, Woodhouse KA, Cooper SL. Polyurethanes in Biomedical Applications. Boca Raton, FL: CRC Press 1998:277.

31. Annis D, Bornat A, Edwards RO, Higham A, Loveday B, Wilson J. An elastomeric vascular prosthesis. Trans Am Soc Artif Intern Organs 1978; 24:209-214.

32. Gogolewski S, Pennings AJ, Lommen E, Wildevuur CRH, Niewenhuis P. Growth of a neo artery induced by a biodegradable polymeric vascular prosthesis. Makromol Chem Rapid Commun 1983; 4:213-219.

33. Lyman DJ, Alb D, Jackson R, Knutson K. Development of small diameter vascular graft prostheses. Trans Am Soc Artif Intern Organs 1977; 23:253-256.

34. Lyman DJ, Fazzio FJ, Voorhes H, Robinson G, Albo D. Compliance as a factor affecting the patency of a copolyurethane vascular graft. J Biomed Mater Res 1978; 12:337-345.

35. Lin H-B, Sun W, Mosher DF, Garcia Echeverria C, Schaufelberger K, Lelkes PI, Cooper SL. Synthesis, surface and cell adhesion properties of polyurethanes containing covalently grafted RGD-peptides. J Biomed Mater Res 1994; 28:329-342.

36. Gospardarowicz D, Ill C. Extracellular matrix and control of proliferation of vascular endothelial cells. J Clin Inv 1981; 68:1351-1364.

37. Nichols NK, Gospardarowicz D, Kellser TR, Oslen DB. Increased adherence of vascular endothelial cells to Biomer precoated with extracellular matrix. Trans Am Soc Artif Intern Organs 1981; 27:208-211.

38. Lin H-B, Lewis KB, Leach-Scampavia D, Ratner BD, Cooper SL. Surface properties of RGD-peptide grafted polyurethane block copolymers: Variable take-off angle and cold-stage ESCA studies. J Biomater Sci Polym Ed 1993; 4:183-198.

39. Drumheller PD, Elbert DL, Hubbell JA. Multifunctional poly(ethylene glycol) semiinterpenetrating polymer networks as highly selective adhesive substrates for bioadhesive peptide grafting. Biotech Bioeng 1994; 43:772-780.

40. Massia SP, Hubbell JA. Covalent surface immobilization of Arg-Gly-Asp and Tyr-Ile-Gly-Ser-Arg containing peptides to obtain well-defined cell adhesive substrates. Anal Biochem 1990; 17:292-301.

Matrix Engineering

—————————— CHAPTER 51 ——————————

Hydrogels in Biological Control During Graft Healing

Jeffrey A. Hubbell

Introduction—Why Hydrogels?

Hydrogels are polymeric materials that imbibe a large fraction of water and yet remain intact, not dissolving even given an infinite period of time. These materials are formed from polymer chains that have a high affinity for water, either such that the chains would be individually soluble in water and are restricted from dissolving by virtue of participation in the polymeric material as a network, or such that the chains are almost, but not quite, soluble in water. By network, it is meant that the polymer chains in the hydrogel are somehow interacting with each other so as to keep the individual chains from diffusing away into the aqueous milieu, either by virtue of being covalently bonded together or by interacting physically—specific examples will be provided in the section on "Hydrogel Structure and Synthesis".

Many extracellular structures in the body can be considered as hydrogels. The extracellular matrix of soft tissues and cartilage, for example, exists as a network of glycoproteins and proteoglycans that both interact with each other biophysically (e.g., by specific biological interactions between collagen and a variety of adhesion proteins,[1] by specific biological interactions between glycosaminoglycans in proteoglycans and a variety of adhesion proteins,[2] and by hydrogen bonding as in collagen due to a very high content of hydroxyproline[3]) and by covalent interactions (e.g., chemical crosslinking between glutamine residues on one protein and lysine residues on a neighboring protein under the enzymatic action of a transglutaminase to catalyze the formation of an amide linkage between the two).[4]

It is not by coincidence that hydrogels are found extensively in Nature: They possess distinct biologically useful features, which will likewise be useful in tissue engineering of the vascular graft and other tissues. Hydrogels are mechanically flexible, are freely permeable to small molecules such as dissolved gases and low molecular weight nutrients and wastes, and are controllably permeable to larger molecules such as proteins. Because the gels are highly swollen with water, the amount of polymer mass per unit volume is relatively low, and this is of key importance in cell migration in three dimensions. Cell migration is facilitated by enzymatic remodeling of the three dimensional extracellular matrix, and the amount of protein and proteoglycan mass to be degraded and moved out of the path of the cell is much lower in the case of a hydrogel than if the tissue had consisted of less water. Indeed, in culture models of leukocyte migration through collagen-based gels, cell migration speed was observed to be reduced by nearly an order of magnitude when the collagen concentration was doubled.[5] Also, because gels are highly swollen with water, their effective surface area is very high, and this is used in Nature to store large quantities of biologically active molecules that can be released in a triggerable fashion from the extracellular matrix, e.g., the release of heparin-binding polypeptide growth factors from heparan sulfate glycosaminoglycan

Tissue Engineering of Prosthetic Vascular Grafts, edited by Peter Zilla and Howard P. Greisler.
©1999 R.G. Landes Company.

components of the proteoglycans in the extracellular matrix. As engineered hydrogels are developed for specific applications in tissue engineering, it should be possible to mimic these biological interactions to achieve these same sorts of biological interactions.[6-9]

Hydrogels have other potential advantages that are less extensively used in Nature. As is addressed in more detail in the section "Protein and Cell Interactions with Hydrogels", there exists the potential to design gels without the incorporation of binding sites for proteins, with the result being a gel that is highly resistant to cell adhesion. Such materials may be useful in preventing the interaction of cells with material substrates in a scaffold for tissue engineering at sites of application of a gel coating. An additional feature of hydrogels of potential tissue engineering advantage is that a solvent for the gel precursors is water; as such, the possibility exists to apply a hydrogel precursor to a tissue site, dissolved in physiological saline, and to form the hydrogel in situ, as is addressed below in the section "In Situ Transformations".

Hydrogel Structure and Synthesis

Hydrogels consist of hydrophilic polymer chains that are held together in a single mass by virtue of either slight insolubility or some form of bonding between chains to yield a polymer network.[10] The structure of the hydrogel is highly dependent upon the nature of the synthetic procedure that was used to obtain the gel; for this reason, different means of hydrogel synthesis will be illustrated in the paragraphs below with a few examples.

The nature of some hydrogels is controlled by the slight insolubility of the polymer chains; a typical example is hydrogels of poly(hydroxyethylmethacrylate).[11] The vinyl monomer for this polymer, hydroxyethylmethacrylate, is soluble in water. Likewise, oligomers and low molecular weight polymers of hydroxyethylmethacrylate are soluble in water, but high molecular weight polymers are slightly insoluble in water, leading to a gel that swells to imbibe approximately 50% water by mass. This swelling extent can be readily controlled by copolymerization with more hydrophobic monomers, such as ethylmethacrylate (i.e., the analogous monomer to hydroxyethylmethacrylate, only lacking the polar hydroxyl group), to achieve a series of polymers with swelling ranging from almost nil (for poly(ethylmethacrylate)) to that of poly(hydroxyethylmethacrylate). These gels have little internal structure, i.e., no permanent pores or dense regions, but rather exist as dynamic structures with small pores opening and closing in equilibrium.

Hydrogels can also be formed by hydrogen bonding, and gels formed from poly(vinyl alcohol) represent a typical example.[12] Poly(vinyl alcohol) is a water-soluble polymer at 37°C. When a solution of poly(vinyl alcohol) is dried to form a cast solid, the solid does not dissolve in water when it is again placed in an aqueous milieu. In the dry state, regions of the poly(vinyl alcohol) solid crystallize due to hydrogen bonding. These regions are so strongly bonded that dissolution of the polymer again at 37°C is infinitesimally slow. This behavior can also be obtained, with greater control on shape retention, by freezing the poly(vinyl alcohol) solution. When ice crystals form, the polymer chains are excluded from the water crystal and pushed to the crystal boundaries, resulting in very highly concentrated regions of polymer. At these highly concentrated domains, when all of the water is frozen, segments of the poly(vinyl alcohol) chains crystallize due to hydrogen bonding, resulting in an insoluble (without heating far above 37°C) hydrogel in the shape of the polymer solution that was frozen. Thus, this gel is a network polymer where the bonding between polymer chains is physical by hydrogen bonding.

Hydrophobic interactions can also be important in the formation of hydrogels, and block copolymers of poly(ethylene glycol) and poly(propylene glycol) form a characteristic example.[13] Poly(ethylene glycol) is a water-soluble poly(ether), while poly(propylene glycol) is water-insoluble, containing a nonpolar methyl group that the poly(ethylene glycol) repeat unit lacks. Block copolymers of these two compositions in the form of a domain of the hydrophobic poly(propylene glycol) flanked on both sides by domains of poly(ethylene glycol) are water soluble polymers that, at relatively high concentrations, can form gels by hydrophobic interactions between the poly(propylene glycol) domains. This is to say, the poly(propylene glycol) domains from several different polymer chains cluster to shield each other from interactions from water, thereby forming physical crosslinks (within these clusters) based on hydrophobic interactions, resulting in a hydrogel. This gel, as do several others based on hydrophobic interactions, has the useful feature that the aqueous mixture is a liquid at cold temperatures (below approximately 10°C) but rapidly forms a hydrogel at 37°C.

Electrostatic interactions also play important roles in hydrogel formation, and gels of alginate with calcium ion[14] and polyelectrolyte complexes of alginate and poly(lysine)[15] form good examples of these principles. Alginate is a naturally occurring polysaccharide product of kelp and several bacterial strains. Each sugar residue in the polysaccharide chain bears a carboxyl group, so the polysaccharide chain is highly anionic, and these charges can play multiple roles in gel formation. Firstly, divalent cations, such as Ca^{2+}, can form a bridge between the anionic groups on adjacent alginate backbones, resulting in regions of adjacent chains that are paired, these regions being connected to other paired regions by amorphous domains. Practically, dropping the alginate solution in Ca^{2+}-free saline into a saline solution containing greater than 1 mM Ca^{2+} results in the rapid formation of a hydrogel which is stable under physiological conditions. Secondly, alginate (either solution or as a Ca^{2+}-crosslinked gel) can be mixed with a polycation in solution, such as poly(lysine), and these two polymer chains form a hydrogel, referred to as a polyelectrolyte complex, crosslinked into a network by the electrostatic interactions between the oppositely charged polymers. Gels formed in either manner described above can have interesting microscopic structures that are lacking in the other gels described in the paragraphs above, this microscopic structure deriving from the diffusive process of gel formation. For example, when the alginate solution is dropped into a Ca^{2+}-containing bath, Ca^{2+} ions begin diffusing into the polymer solution, causing the formation of the gel at the interface between the polymer solution and the surrounding Ca^{2+}-containing bath. Because the gel region exists at a lower soluble polymer concentration than does the alginate solution, alginate from the core of the droplet diffuses toward the gelled interface; this polymer then gels, and more polymer diffuses from the core to the periphery, and so on: The net result of this phenomenon is that the periphery of the Ca^{2+}-alginate gel is more dense than the core of the particle, owing to the diffusive nature of the process. The case is likewise with the incorporation of the polyelectrolyte counter-ion poly(lysine). Poly(lysine) diffuses into the gel particle from the periphery and interacts first at that periphery, forming denser membrane at the periphery, which restricts further poly(lysine) diffusion into the core in a self-limiting process. Accordingly, a thin shell of polyelectrolyte complex can be formed, a microstructure that could be put to good use in tissue engineering.

In addition to the physical interactions described above, hydrogels can also be formed that depend on covalent bonding between polymer chains; these gels have a characteristic advantage over those described above in that they can be considerably more stable under physiological conditions. Three examples are presented below, two based on synthetic polymers with nonbiological reactions and one based on proteins with enzymatic reactions. The simplest way to form a covalently crosslinked hydrogel is to polymerize an otherwise water-soluble polymer in the presence of a multifunctional crosslinker.[16] As an example, acrylamide is a monomer that polymerizes to form a water-soluble polymer. If acrylamide is polymerized in the presence of a difunctional monomer (i.e., one that has two sites for polymerization, then referred to as a crosslinker), that monomer will participate in two poly(acrylamide) chains. Accordingly, bis-acrylamido crosslinkers are routinely used to crosslink acrylamide hydrogels. Given that each poly(acrylamide) chain may react with more than one crosslinker molecule, this polymerization process results in the formation of a chemically crosslinked hydrogel. In this case, the entire macroscopic hydrogel object is a single molecule.

As a second example of the formation of covalently crosslinked synthetic hydrogels, hydrogels formed from water-soluble polymeric diacrylates form a good example.[17] Poly(ethylene glycol) diacrylates (Fig. 51.1) have been formed by coupling one acrylate moiety to each end of a poly(ethylene glycol) chain. These acrylates are capable of polymerizing to form a poly(acrylate), and if a poly(ethylene glycol) monoacrylate were polymerized the resulting polymers would be a comb-like structure, a poly(acrylate) structure forming the back of the comb and poly(ethylene glycol) chains forming the teeth. If, however, a poly(ethylene glycol) diacrylate is polymerized, the acrylates on either end of the chain can enter into different poly(acrylate) chains, resulting in a chemically crosslinked gel that can only be broken apart by the cleavage of a covalent bond.

It is also possible for form covalently crosslinked hydrogels using enzymatic crosslinking, and fibrin forms an excellent case in point.[18] Fibrin is formed by the enzymatic action of thrombin and factor xiiia on fibrinogen. Throm-

bin cleaves the fibrinogen protein at two points, exposing a new terminus on two polypeptide chains. This new terminus physically binds at a site on other fibrinogen (and cleaved fibrinogen) proteins, this process resulting in a physically bonded hydrogel. The coagulation protein factor XIII is also cleaved by thrombin to form the active transglutaminase factor xiiia, which acts to catalyze the formation of an amide bond between glutamine residues and lysine residues on opposing polypeptide domains in fibrin, resulting in a chemically crosslinked fibrin network.

The brief overview provided above should provide the reader with a background understanding of the physical nature of hydrogels and the vast flexibility in the physical and chemical processes for forming them. Based upon this brief background, the reader is well positioned to consider the application of hydrogels for tissue engineering of the vascular graft.

In Situ Transformations

One interesting advantage in the use of hydrogels in tissue engineering is that they may be delivered in the form of a precursor that is dissolved in a physiological saline and is then converted into the insoluble hydrogel upon the target tissue (see Fig. 51.2), in some cases even in direct contact with cells.[19] To perform adequately in such an environment, the precursor solution should be lacking in high concentrations of toxic species and low molecular weight monomers, which may be more likely to cross the cell membrane than a high molecular weight macromonomer, and the gel conversion should occur at physiologically acceptable temperatures. This has been accomplished with aqueous solutions of poly(ethylene glycol) diacrylate and related compounds, which may be converted to a hydrogel under biocompatible reaction conditions by exposure to visible light in the presence of a visible light sensitizer.[20] The biocompatibility of this process in direct contact with cells can be attributed to the following features.

1. Physiological saline is the solvent;
2. A very high fraction of the polymerizable precursors are macromolecular and thus unable to pass the cell membrane;
3. The photoinitiation process does not involve short wavelength ultraviolet light;
4. The photoinitiation process does not generate large amounts of reactive oxygen species; and
5. The polymerization process does not generate large amounts of heat.

These principles serve as a design basis for other biomaterial systems for the formation of hydrogels in situ by transformation from liquid precursors.

In situ transformation has at least two major advantages, for some applications, vs. the implantation of preformed hydrogels. One advantage is that a large hydrogel implant may be delivered through a very small surgical hole, somewhat like assembly of the model ship inside the bottle. This has been put toward therapeutic development in the coating of organs in the abdominopelvic cavity following surgery to prevent the formation of postoperative adhesions, engineering the healing response.[21] Here is it possible to deliver biomaterial implants as organ coatings

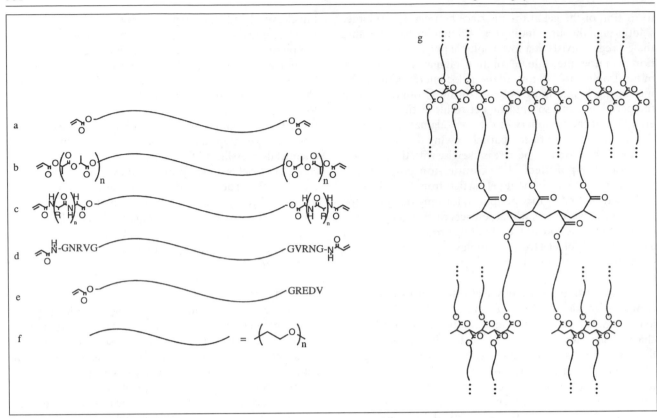

Fig. 51.1. As an example of designing various mechanisms of degradation and bioactivity of hydrogels, the case of gels formed by crosslinking poly(ethylene glycol) diacrylates is considered. Gels can be made to be substantially non-degradable (a), to incorporate nonenzymatic degradation sites by hydrolysis (b), to incorporate oligopeptide domains (c) which could be sites for cleavage by a protease, e.g. plasmin (d) or which could be sites for binding to adhesion receptors on a targeted cell (e). In each case in this example, the central block of the macromer is a poly(ethylene glycol) chain, selected for resistance to protein adsorption and for favorable toxicology of the degradation product (f). These diacrylated poly(ethylene glycol) chains polymerize by free radical reaction at the acrylate to form oligomers of acrylic acid that are linked to other oligomers of acrylic acid via the poly(ethylene glycol) chains with the relevant degradation sites (g). Thus, the acrylic acid oligomers form nodes in a three dimensional network, each connected to other nodes by long strings of poly(ethylene glycol). The permeability of the gels to proteins, and the rate of release of incorporated protein drugs, can be controlled via manipulation of the density of the oligomeric acrylic acid nodes, by the number of poly(ethylene glycol) strings emanating therefrom, and by the length of the poly(ethylene glycol) strings. Degradation products are poly(ethylene glycol) and oligomers of acrylic acid, which are eliminated by glomerular filtration, and lactic acid.

that are many centimeters in diameter, but to deliver these implants using laparoscopic instruments to convert the liquid precursor to a hydrogel. A second advantage is that hydrogel implants of very complex shape may be formed in situ; this has been put to advantage in the coating of arterial surfaces after deendothelialization to prevent the deposition of platelets on the subendothelium.[22,23] In this case, the photoinitiator was separated from the other components of the precursor solution and was adsorbed to the arterial surface; when the arterial lumen was flooded with all of the remaining precursors and the artery was irradiated with visible light, the formation of the hydrogel was restricted to the interface between the arterial wall and its contents. Thus, a hydrogel barrier was formed, only several microns thick, that was conformal with the complex shape of the deendothelialized artery.

Given that one may want to employ hydrogels in tissue engineering for the delivery of therapeutics and even living cells to polymeric scaffolds and even preexisting ar-

teries, to attempt to engineer a healing response, the ability to form gels in situ presents an attractive feature. Such transformations can be accomplished even in the presence of individual and aggregated cells,[24] suggesting that such chemical schemes can be adapted for the delivery of cellular therapeutics either within or adjacent to the vascular system.

Protein and Cell Interactions with Hydrogels

Hydrogels can be designed to have minimal interactions with proteins and cells. Cell adhesion to biomaterials is mediated by an adsorbed protein overlayer.[25] Protein adsorption to materials is dominated primarily by hydrophobic interactions and secondarily by electrostatic interactions.[26] Most insoluble polymers (e.g., poly(ester)s, poly(ethylene), poly(propylene), poly(urethane)s, and poly(tetrafluoroethylene)) achieve their water-insolubility by interacting poorly with water. These hydrophobic polymers accordingly adsorb large amounts of proteins, which act as surfactants to expose more hydrophobic domains to-

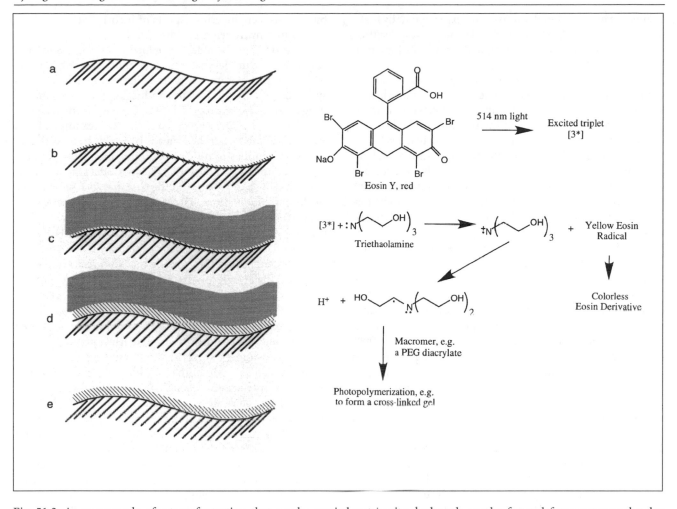

Fig. 51.2. As an example of a transformation that can be carried out in situ, hydrogels can be formed from macromolecular precursors dissolved in buffered saline, directly on the tissue surface. A tissue surface to be treated (a), such as the anastomotic region of a vascular graft, is first flushed with a solution of a nontoxic photoinitiator (in this example eosin Y), to stain the tissue surface with the photoinitiator (b). After the nonadsorbed photoinitiator is flushed away and the artery lumen is filled with the other components of the initiation system (in this example, the nontoxic buffer triethanolamine) and the polymerizable macromer (such as a diacrylated poly(ethylene glycol) copolymer with lactic acid, as in Fig. 51.1) (c), the artery is irradiated with light at an appropriate wavelength (in the case of eosin Y, green light) to cause a wave of polymerization to proceed from the tissue surface out into the lumen (d). After the nonpolymerized macromer solution is rinsed away, the final result is a crosslinked solid hydrogel, adherent to and conformal with the tissue surface (e). In the photoinitiation scheme shown in this example, the red eosin Y adsorbs green light and is excited to a triplet state, from which it participates in a single-electron transfer reaction with triethanolamine, resulting in a radical on the eosin and the triethanolamine. The free radical on the triethanolamine rearranges and serves as the actual initiator of the free radical polymerization of the diacrylated macromer.

ward the material surface and thus present a more hydrophilic new surface to the aqueous surroundings. Electrostatic interactions are secondary (due to the high ionic strength of physiological fluids) but remain important in protein interaction with materials, especially with regard to adsorption of proteins to cationic polymers (since almost all proteins bear a net anionic charge). Accordingly, one may design a biomaterial to be relatively free of cell adhesion by making it be both very hydrophilic (e.g., a hydrogel) and nonionic or anionic.

Much of what is understood about protein and cell interactions with hydrogels has been learned from two dimensional hydrogel models, namely water-soluble polymers (which would form hydrogels) tethered to insoluble surfaces.

Work on the theory of these interactions has been performed by Jeon et al.[27,28] These investigators determined that when the tethered polymer brush exists at a sufficient density of polymer chains of a sufficient length, compression of the polymer brush by a potentially adsorbing protein results in a strong resistance, i.e., steric stabilization, to the adsorption of the protein. Thus, one may understand with these theoretical analyses based on the physics of polymer chains that the thermodynamic interactions are unfavorable for protein adsorption.[29] Very well characterized experimentation has also been performed with model two dimensional polymer brushes, e.g., by Prime and Whitesides employing self-assembling monolayers of alkane thiols on gold substrates, the alkane thiols bearing grafted poly(ethylene glycol) chains.[30] These studies demonstrated experimentally that a high density of poly(ethylene glycol) chains would suffice, even if the chains were very short, to dramatically limit protein adsorption.

The physical character of hydrogels is important, in tandem with the chemical character, in determining hydrogel biocompatibility. This is to say, it is not just the chemical structure of the repeat unit of the polymer in the hydrogel that determines the biocompatibility of the hydrogel. This can be considered in the context of crosslinked gels of poly(ethylene glycol) diacrylate.[31] When gels were formed from poly(ethylene glycol) of molecular weight 200 or 1000, these materials were rapidly encapsulated in a typical foreign body reaction and calcified after subcutaneous implantation in the rat; however, gels formed from poly(ethylene glycol) diacrylate of higher molecular weight remained free of fibrous encapsulation and did not calcify. The calcification response may be due to a specific interaction between Ca^{2+} and poly(ethylene glycol), but the induction of a foreign body reaction almost certainly relates to the difference in water content of these gels (from approximately 75% water for the poly(ethylene glycol) 200 diacrylate to approx. 90% for the higher molecular weight poly(ethylene glycol)-based hydrogels. As such, one should understand clearly that all hydrogels are not alike, and even that all hydrogels of the same chemical composition are not necessarily alike in their biological responses.

Designed Cell Adhesiveness of Hydrogels

In the above section it was demonstrated that, with adequate attention to the details of hydrogel design, hydrogels can be formed to effectively resist the attachment of cells, even in vivo. Based upon this observation it then becomes attractive to incorporate into such a hydrogel biological adhesion ligands targeting specific receptors and even perhaps specific cell types. In this manner, one might be able to develop a hydrogel material for tissue engineering that would reject the attachment on one cell type (e.g., the platelet) but that would accept the attachment of another cell type (e.g., the endothelial cell). Tissue engineering with synthetic adhesion ligands is based on profound advances in the molecular biology of cell adhesion over the past several years, in which a host of extracellular matrix adhesion glycoproteins have been identified, together with their corresponding receptors. Moreover, the domains on many of the adhesion proteins that bind to the receptors have been identified, and it has been demonstrated that, in many of these cases, synthetic peptide and nonpeptide analogs can be developed with appropriate affinity for the appropriate receptors on the cell surfaces. It has also been demonstrated that some of these adhesion ligands have affinity for receptors that exist on one cell type do not exist on other cell types present in the same biological environment; e.g., the sequence REDV, which is present in some fibronectin forms, binds to the integrin receptor $\alpha_4\beta_1$ that is present on human endothelial cells but not on human blood platelets.[32,33] The biology of adhesion proteins, their receptors and synthetic analogs of the adhesion proteins is the topic of chapter 54 in this book and is not addressed further here; only the

biomaterials engineering aspects of incorporation of these signals into hydrogels are addressed.

In order to be able to engineer a selective adhesion response to hydrogel materials, one must devise means by which to incorporate synthetic adhesion ligands, such as synthetic peptides derived from adhesion proteins, into hydrogel networks. Hydrogels derived from poly(ethylene glycol) diacrylate again serve as an instructive example. Hern and the author[34] examined means by which to incorporate adhesion peptides into these photopolymerizable gels, using the adhesion peptide GRGDY as a model (the N-terminal G serving as a spacer, and the C-terminal Y serving as a site for radioiodination). The N-terminus of the peptide was acrylated, either with a minimal spacer or with a poly(ethylene glycol) chain of molecular weight 3400, and these acrylated peptides were incorporated into the hydrogels by copolymerization (i.e., mixing the peptide acrylates and the poly(ethylene glycol) diacrylates in the hydrogel precursor solution, and then photopolymerizing the mixture). When the peptides were omitted from the hydrogel, the resulting material was very resistant to cell adhesion. When an acrylated RGD or control inactive RDG peptide was incorporated without a spacer arm, the resulting material supported cell adhesion in both cases, but only in the presence of serum proteins; this result can only be explained by the peptide being sterically unavailable for biospecific binding to cell adhesion receptors but serving as a site for the nonspecific adsorption of serum proteins. When the RGD and RDG peptides were incorporated with a poly(ethylene glycol) spacer, the materials with RGD supported cell adhesion, while those with the inactive RDG supported no adhesion. Thus, it would seem that for the sequence to be sterically available for binding to receptors on the cell it must be immobilized within the gel via a long spacer; and it would further seem that the peptide immobilized without the spacer serves as a site for protein adsorption, while the peptide immobilized with the spacer does not. Having these results in hand, one is then prepared to begin to incorporate cell type specific adhesion signals (such as the endothelial targeting REDV sequence) to engineer the tissue response to a hydrogel, and thus to a vascular graft.

Nonenzymatic Degradation of Hydrogels

It is clear that one must have in one's repertoire of materials for tissue engineering hydrogels that are degradable. Degradation by nonenzymatic hydrolysis can be obtain by incorporating hydrolytically labile bonds within the gel precursor, either in a crosslinker or within the polymer backbone. The example of poly(ethylene glycol) diacrylate hydrogels, in this case degradable variations, will be selected for discussion.

A host of degradable polymers are available for use in medicine, and these are based on hydrolysis of esters, carbonates, and anhydrides, to name only a few of the important approaches (see chapter 47). These compositions can be incorporated into polymers that form hydrogels, to obtain the physical and biological properties of the hydrogel along with the degradability inferred by the water-labile bond. To accomplish this in the scheme of photopolymerized poly(ethylene glycol) diacrylate hydrogels, block copolymers have been formed, with poly(ethylene glycol) forming the central block and oligomers of, e.g., lactic acid forming flanking blocks; the termini of the lactic acid blocks can be acrylated, leading to an analog of poly(ethylene glycol) diacrylate with a degradable segment between the poly(ethylene glycol) segments.[35] The hydrogel to result from such a precursor consists of nodes of oligo(acrylic acid) esterified to poly(ethylene glycol) chains via an oligo(lactic acid) intermediate. Degradation thus yields a low molecular weight oligo(acrylic acid), lactic acid and its oligomers, and poly(ethylene glycol) chains of the original molecular weight.

The rates of degradation of hydrogels behave somewhat differently than those of the poly(ester), poly(carbonate), or poly(anhydride) parent family. In the parent families, two features control the rate of degradation: The intrinsic susceptibility of the water-labile bond to hydrolysis, and the rate of transport of water into the hydrophobic polymer. In hydrogels, by contrast, the entire macroscopic material is equally exposed to water, so the intrinsic rate of hydrolysis controls the overall degradation rate. This feature can be used to modulate the rate of resorption of such hydrogels: For example, poly(ethylene glycol)-glycolide diacrylate hydrogels degrade faster than poly(ethylene glycol)-lactide diacrylate hydrogels, which degrade faster than poly(ethylene glycol)-caprolactone diacrylate hydrogels, in accordance with the expected order based on chemical kinetics.

Enzymatic Degradation of Hydrogels

In addition to degradation based on nonenzymatic hydrolysis, one could contemplate degradation based on enzymatic processes. Enzymatic degradation may have conceptual advantages over nonenzymatic degradation in some applications of tissue engineering. For example, cell migration through tissues and through fibrin clots and granulation tissue in wound healing is dependent upon enzymatic hydrolysis of glycoproteins and glycosaminoglycans in the extracellular matrix. Thus, endowing a hydrogel with the ability to be degraded by enzymes would permit the hydrogel to be remodeled by biological processes associated with cell migration.

It is instructive to consider cell migration through biologically derived hydrogels, as a prototype for the ultimate design of synthetic materials that permit cell infiltration by proteolysis. Fibrin serves as one such good prototype, being the primary matrix through which cells migrate in a healing response. Herbert et al examined the migration of the growth cones of neurites emanating from aggregated neural and glial cells within a three dimensional fibrin matrix in a culture model.[36,37] Fibrin was formed under controlled conditions around the cell aggregates, and the rate of neurite extension was measured as a function of fibrin fibril density and morphology; additionally, the dependence of the extension process on local protease activity was examined. It was observed that either direct inhibition of plasmin activity or inhibition of plasminogen activation activity completely inhibited cell migration, indicating that the neurites did not find preexisting pores through which to migrate, and that they did not mechanically push fibrin fibrils out of their path during migration, but rather that they expressed chemical

activity to clear the fibrin from their path. Electron microscopic observation of the morphology of the neurite tips and the fibrin near the neurite tips demonstrated that fibrils were present in the immediate vicinity of all aspects of the growth cone, with less than a 50 nm gap between the neurite plasma membrane and the fibrin fibrils, suggesting that the neurite did not migrate by finding a pathway that was enzymatically created in a spatially nonlocalized manner, but rather that local enzymatic activity associated with the cell membrane was responsible for local removal of material to create a pathway. Furthermore, these studies also demonstrated that there was no dependence in neurite migration rate on fibrin fibril morphology, but only on density; i.e., the only feature that mattered was the amount of material present to be cleared from the pathway of the cell to permit migration.

Studies as described above both emphasize the importance of biologically derived materials for tissue engineering and also provide motivation to develop synthetic analogs. The fact that, at least in some circumstances, the detailed morphology of the biological structures to be cleared by cell-associated proteolytic activity is less important than the mass of that material encourages one to proceed with development of such synthetic analogs, in that only the chemical nature need be mimicked, not the morphological nature as well (at least in some cases). With this in mind, West et al have examined poly(ethylene glycol)-based hydrogel materials that degrade by proteolytic activity.[38] Poly(ethylene glycol) was used as a substrate for liquid phase peptide synthesis, and either plasmin or collagenase-sensitive peptide sequences were synthesized at the termini of the polymer chains. Upon the termini of these peptide blocks an acrylate group was coupled, to create an analog of the poly(ethylene glycol)-lactide diacrylate, namely poly(ethylene glycol)-peptide diacrylate, where the identify of the peptide was selected for sensitivity to the protease plasmin or collagenase. Hydrogels were formed from such precursors and were exposed to either plasmin or collagenase, with the result that the plasmin-sensitive gel degraded in the presence of plasmin but not collagenase, and the collagenase-sensitive gel degraded in the presence of collagenase but not plasmin, as designed. Such preliminary studies demonstrate at least the potential for the synthesis of hydrogel materials that mimic the ability to be remodeled like the natural biological hydrogels used in nature.

Controlled Release

Hydrogels have been extensively explored for the controlled release of drugs, particularly macromolecular drugs such as proteins and oligonucleotides. One reason for utilizing hydrogels for drug delivery is the relative ease in controlling the permeability of the gel structure to the macromolecular drug. While in most gels permanent pore structures do not exist, transient pores do exist that can be described in terms of molecular weight between crosslinks and pore dimensions.[39] These parameters can be readily controlled, and by adjusting these dimensions relative to the radius of gyration of the macromolecular drug one can either restrict drug diffusion to a controlled degree and obtain release from the hydrogel material on a time scale faster than that of degradation, or one can entrap the drug, using a gel with a pore dimension much less than the drug size, and obtain drug release that is mediated by the rate of hydrogel degradation.[40] It is relatively straightforward to synthetically manipulate the pore dimensions of a hydrogel. For example, with gels formed by crosslinking an unsaturated monomer (refer to the example of acrylamide with a bis-acrylamido crosslinker) the pore dimensions may be altered via control of the ratio of acrylamide to bis-acrylamide, a high amount of bis-acrylamido crosslinker yielding small pore dimensions and restricted permeability. In the example of poly(ethylene glycol)-diacrylate based hydrogels, one may alter pore dimensions via the molecular weight of the poly(ethylene glycol) diacrylate, low molecular weights yielding small pore dimensions and low permeability. As an example, Cruise et al[41] reported pore dimensions of 19 Å for gels formed from poly(ethylene glycol) 2000 diacrylate, 22 Å from poly(ethylene glycol) 4000 diacrylate, 34 Å from poly(ethylene glycol) 8000 diacrylate and 58 Å from poly(ethylene glycol) 20,000 diacrylate. It was likewise possible to control pore dimensions via manipulation of the reaction conditions with the same poly(ethylene glycol) diacrylate precursor; e.g., pore dimensions of 70 Å were obtained by polymerization of poly(ethylene glycol) diacrylate 20,000 from a 10% precursor solution, 58 Å from a 20% precursor solution, and 42 Å from a 30% precursor solution. Because of this high flexibility in the control of pore dimensions and gel permeability to macromolecular drugs, hydrogels are extremely attractive for controlled release applications in tissue engineering.

Design Principles, Hydrogels for Biological Control During Graft Healing

One may consider many possible applications for hydrogels in tissue engineering, some of which have been explored already and some of which remain to be experimentally addressed. In this section, some of the more important possible applications in vascular tissue engineering will be called into focus. These relate to altering the blood response to a graft, altering the arterial response to the graft, and directing the response of the surrounding tissue to a graft implant.

Reduction of Thrombosis

Because hydrogels can be designed that adsorb relatively low amounts of protein and that thus support relatively low amounts of platelet adhesion (which has been demonstrated to be modulated principally by adsorbed fibrinogen),[42] one obvious, yet important, application of hydrogels to vascular graft tissue engineering is the reduction of platelet deposition in the hours and days following implantation. Hydrogel coatings have been used to modulate the deposition of platelets and other cells on a host of medical devices, most of which are implanted for relatively short periods of time. Indeed, heparinization of graft surfaces may improve graft biocompatibility by both a pharmacological effect (the specific biological activity of heparin as it interacts with antithrombin III) as well as a biophysical effect (the hydrophilic, anionic heparin hydrogel coating acting to reduce the adsorption of fibrinogen).[43]

Graft Sealing

Knitted and woven grafts must be preclotted to prevent excessive blood leakage from the graft, and this process of preclotting may predispose the graft to further thrombosis in the short term (e.g., due to platelet interactions with fibrin in the clot or due to prothrombin activation on the surfaces of cells in the clot) and to the development of an excessive neointima in the long term (e.g., due to the growth factors that are released by activated platelets in the clot). To reduce the possibility of short and long term graft failure as a result of preclotting, grafts that are based on collagen,[44] gelatin,[45] and albumin[46] preclotting have been developed. These materials are indeed hydrogels, and thus hydrogel-sealed vascular grafts have already been used clinically. One could also employ hydrogels designed more specifically for graft sealing. Such a hydrogel sealing material could either resorb by physical erosion (e.g., with poly(ethylene glycol)-poly(propylene glycol)-poly(ethylene glycol) block copolymers) or by nonenzymatic hydrolysis (e.g., with a poly(ethylene glycol)-lactide diacrylate hydrogel). Such a designed hydrogel has the possible benefit that other features could also be designed into the gel, as described below.

Promotion of Endothelialization

It is clear that the rapid establishment of an endothelial cell monolayer atop the neointima within a graft is key to success in the tissue engineering of a vascular graft. It is also clear that thrombosis within the graft lumen is an undesirable outcome. In light of these two observations, one could consider employing a hydrogel coating or a hydrogel sealing to both reduce thrombosis and to enhance endothelialization, e.g., via a gel that resists fibrinogen adsorption and accordant platelet deposition, that gel also containing a grafted ligand that demonstrates specificity for an endothelial cell adhesion receptor. In such a manner, it might be possible to fail to induce platelet adhesion but to succeed in inducing endothelial cell adhesion.[32] In the absence of seeding of endothelial cells along the entire lumen of the graft, one must be concerned with the rate of endothelial cell migration along the coated graft surface. Lauffenburger and colleagues have demonstrated, both based on theoretical considerations and also by experiment, that there exists an optimum in the surface density of adhesion ligands for fastest cell migration rates.[47] At low surface density of adhesion ligand, cell traction is low and cell migration rates, as well as adhesion strength, are accordingly slow. At high surface density of adhesion ligand, cell traction is very high, but the rate of binding of an adhesion receptor on the cell surface with surface-bound adhesion ligand is very high, resulting in very strong adhesion but very low cell migration rates. Accordingly, one must design the display of adhesion ligands in the hydrogel coating such that adhesion strength is sufficient to resist fluid forces within the vascular flow but such that it is not so strong that the rate of cell migration is unacceptably reduced.

It has been demonstrated that thrombosis at the anastomoses of a graft may be well in excess of thrombosis on the graft itself.[48] Accordingly, efforts at reducing platelet deposition on the biomaterial per se may be slightly misplaced relative to the thrombogenic potential of the anastomoses. One may then consider the use of a hydrogel to passivate the graft anastomoses. It was demonstrated above that one advantage of hydrogels over other materials for tissue engineering is that they may be formed on the surface of a tissue by an in situ transformation. As an example, it was discussed that hydrogel coatings have been formed on the surfaces of injured arteries to replace one function of the endothelium, namely to regulate the deposition of blood platelet on the arterial surface.[22] Accordingly, it could be envisioned to limit the extent of thrombus deposition on the anastomoses within a graft that had already been sutured in place by the local, in situ deposition of a hydrogel coating spanning the junction of the native artery and the implanted graft. Using such an approach, it might be possible to directly impact one of the most troublesome regions of an implanted graft.

Drug Release

Hydrogels have been explored extensively in drug release, due to the facility with which the permeability of the gel material to a drug of a given size may be modulated. Because of this high flexibility in control of release characteristics, it is attractive to combine some of the other uses described above with local release of a biologically active factor, e.g., an angiogenic growth factor such as basic fibroblast growth factor or vascular endothelial growth factor, to induce a specific biological response in tissue engineering of the vascular graft. Some experimentation has been performed along these lines, using hydrogels in vascular tissue engineering. For example, Simons et al[49] employed a hydrogel, formed in situ by application of liquid solution of a copolymer of poly(ethylene glycol)-poly(propylene glycol)-poly(ethylene glycol) block copolymer, which solidifies to form a gel upon warming to body temperature.[13] This gel was used to release an antisense oligonucleotide that inhibited cell proliferation; this treatment was observed to greatly limit the thickening of the neointima following injury by balloon angioplasty of the carotid arteries of rats. As another example, Greisler and colleagues[50] employed a fibrin-based hydrogel formed within the pore spaces of a vascular graft to release basic fibroblast growth factor, and this resulted in an overall acceleration of the rate of endothelialization and a corresponding limitation of the formation of an excessively thickened neointima in animal models.

Promotion of Transmural Capillary Ingrowth

Studies by Golden et al provided great encouragement for the possibility of transmural capillary infiltration and differentiation to form large vessel endothelium with large pore graft implants in nonhuman primate models.[51] One can consider designing hydrogel treatments for tissue-engineered vascular grafts to attempt to achieve similar results in the human. In such an approach, one might integrate the concepts that have been presented above: For example, one might consider sealing a graft with a hydrogel that bore cell adhesion sites for endothelial cells but not for blood platelets, which further bore sites for degradation by proteases expressed during endothelial cell migration. One might further incorporate a growth factor within such a hydrogel to

stimulate endothelial cell migration and proliferation, and another factor to limit perigraft inflammation or smooth muscle activity.

Stated more generally, Nature's extracellular matrix hydrogel serves to provide a great deal of information to cells to direct their behavior and organization in space. It provides information in the form of structural cues, of immobilized adhesion molecules, and of immobilized and diffusible polypeptide growth factors. Furthermore, it receives information from the cells as they respond. It does this by binding to growth factors that are released from cells and by degrading in the face of cellularly-displayed enzymes. It might be possible, and indeed advantageous, in tissue engineering of the vascular graft, to mimic some or all of these activities, either in a biologically derived hydrogel matrix or in a completely synthetic biomimetic hydrogel matrix, with the goal of harnessing some of these biological activities for controlling tissue morphogenesis and function.

References

1. Shimizu M, Minakuchi K, Moon M, and Koga J, Difference in interaction of fibronectin with type I collagen and type IV collagen. Biochim Biophys Acta 1997; 1339:53-61.
2. Jackson RL, Busch SJ, and Cardin AD, Glycosaminoglycans: Molecular properties, protein interactions, and role in physiological processes. Physiol Rev 1991; 71:481-539.
3. Vanderrest M, and Garrone R, Collagen family of proteins. FASEB J 1991; 5:2814-2823.
4. Mosher DF, Assembly of fibronectin into extracellular matrix. Curr Opin Struct Biol 1993; 3:214-222.
5. Parkhurst MR, and Saltzman WM, Quantification of human neutrophil motility in 3-dimensional collagen gels: Effect of collagen concentration. Biophys J 1992; 61:306-315.
6. Langer R, and Vacanti JP, Tissue engineering. Science 1993; 260:920-926.
7. Peppas NA, and Langer R, Challenges in biomaterials. Science 1994; 263:1715-1720.
8. Hubbell JA, Biomaterials in tissue engineering. Bio/Technology 1995; 13: 565-576.
9. Elbert DL, and Hubbell JA, Surface treatments of polymers for biocompatibility. Ann Rev Material Sci 1996; 26: 365-394.
10. Kim SW, Bae YH, and Okano T, Hydrogels: Swelling, drug loading, and release. Pharm Res 1992; 9:283-290.
11. Slack SM, and Horbett TA, Changes in fibrinogen adsorbed to segmented polyurethanes and hydroxyethyl-methacrylate-ethylmethacrylate copolymers. J Biomed Mater Res 1992; 26:1633-1649.
12. Mallapragada SK, Peppas NA, and Colombo P, Crystal dissolution-controlled release systems. II. Metronidazole release from semicrystalline poly(vinylalcohol) systems. J Biomed Mater Res 1997; 36:125-130.
13. Leach RE, and Henry RL. Reduction of postoperative adhesion in the rat uterine horn model with Poloxamer 407. Am J Obstet Gynecol 1990; 162:1317-1319.
14. O'Shea GM, and Sun AM, Encapsulation of rat islets of Langerhans prolongs xenograft survival in diabetic mice. Diabetes 1986; 35:943-946.
15. Decher G, Lvov Y, and Schmitt J, Proof of multilayer structural organization in self-assembled polycation-polyanion molecular films. Thin Solid Films 1994; 244:772-777.

16. Gin H, Dupuy B, Caix J, Baquey C, and Ducassou D, In vitro diffusion in polyacrylamide embedded agarose microbeads. J Microencapsul 1990; 7:17-23.

17. Pathak CP, Sawhney AS, and Hubbell JA, Rapid photopolymerization of gels in contact with cells and tissue. J Am Chem Soc 1992; 114:8311-8312.

18. Moser D, Blood coagulation and fibrinolysis. Clin Cardiol 1990; 13:5-11.

19. Hubbell JA, In situ material transformations in tissue engineering. MRS Bulletin 1996; 21:33-35.

20. Sawhney AS, Pathak CP, Van Rensberg JL, and Hubbell JA, Optimization of photopolymerized bioerodible hydrogel properties for adhesion prevention. J Biomed Mater Res 1994; 28: 831-838.

21. Hill-West JL, Chowdhury SM, Sawhney AS, Pathak CP, Dunn RC, and Hubbell JA, Prevetion of postoperative adhesions in the rat by in situ photopolymerization of bioresorbable hydrogel barriires. Obstct Gynecol 1994; 83:59-64.

22. Hill-West JL, Chowdhury SM, Slepian MJ, and Hubbell JA, Inhibition of thrombosis and intimal thickening by in situ photopolymerization of thin hydrogel barriers. Proc Nat Acad Sci USA 1994; 91:5967-5971.

23. West JL and Hubbell JA, Separation of the arterial wall from blood contact using hydrogel barriers reduces intimal thickening after balloon injury in the rat: The roles of medial and luminal factors in arterial healing. Proc Nat Acad Sci USA, 1996; 93:13188-13193.

24. Sawhney AS, Pathak CP, and Hubbell JA, Modification of islet of Langerhans surfaces with immunoprotective poly(ethylene glycol) coatings via interfacial photopolymerization. Biotechnol Bioeng 1994; 44:383-386.

25. Pettit DK, Hoffman AS, and Horbett TA, Correlation between corneal epithelial cell outgrowth and monoclonal antibody binding to the cell-binding domain of adsorbed fibronectin. J Biomed Mater Res 1994; 28:685-691.

26. Andrade JD, and Hlady V, Protein adsorption and materials biocompatibility: A tutorial review and suggested hypotheses. Adv Polym Sci 1986; 79:1-63.

27. Jeon Si, Lee JH, Andrade JD, and de Gennes PG, Protein-surface interactions in the presence of polyethylene oxide I, simplified theory. J Coll Interf Sci 1991; 142:149-158.

28. Jeon SI, and Andrade JD, Protein-surface interactions in the presence of polyethylene oxide II, effect of protein size. J Colloid Interface Sci 1991; 142:159-166.

29. Norde W, Protein adsorption at solid surfaces: A thermodynamic approach. Pure Appl Chem 1994; 66:491-496.

30. Prime KL, and Whitesides GM, Adsorption of proteins onto surfaces containing end-attached oligo(ethylene oxide): A model system using self-assembled monolayers. J Am Chem Soc 1993; 115:10714-10721.

31. Hossainy SFA, and Hubbell JA, Molecular weight dependence of calcification of poly(ethylene glycol) hydrogels. Biomaterials 1994; 15:921-925.

32. Hubbell JA, Massia SP, Desai NP, and Drumheller PD Endothelial cell-selective materials for tissue engineering in the vascular graft via a new receptor. Bio/Technology 1991; 9:568-572.

33. Massia SP, and Hubbell JA, Vascular endothelial cell adhesion and spreading promoted by the peptide REDV of the IIICS region of plasma fibronectin is mediated by integrin $\alpha_4\beta_1$. J Biol Chem 1992; 267:14019-14026.

34. Hern DL, and Hubbell JA, Incorporation of adhesion peptides into nonadhesive hydrogels useful for tissue resurfacing. J Biomed Mater Res, 1997; 39:266-276.

35. Sawhney AS, Pathak CP, and Hubbell JA, Bioerodible hydrogels based on photopolymerized poly(ethylene glycol)-co-poly(α-hydroxy acid) diacrylate macromers. Macromolecules 1993; 26:581-587.

36. Herbert CB, Bittner GD, and Hubbell JA, Effects of fibrinolysis on neurite growth from dorsal root ganglia cultured in 2-dimensional and 3-dimensional fibrin gels. J Comp Neurol 1996; 365:380-391.

37. Herbert CB, Nagaswami C, Bittner GD, JW Weisel, and Hubbell JA, Effects of fibrin micro-morphology on neurite growth from dorsal root ganglia cultured within three-dimensional fibrin gels. J Biomed Mater Res, 1997; in ress.

38. West JL, Pratt A, and Hubbell JA, Proteolytically degradable hydrogels, Trans Soc Biomaterials 1997; 23:103.

39. Canal T, and Peppas NA, Correlation between mesh size and equilibrium degree of swelling of polymeric networks. J Biomed Mater Res 1989; 23:1183-1193.

40. JA Hubbell, Hydrogel systems for barriers and local drug delivery in the control of wound healing. J Contr Rel 1996; 39:305-313.

41. Cruise GM, Scharp DS, and Hubbell JA, Characterization of permeability and network structure of interfacially photopolymerized poly(ethylene glycol) diacrylate hydrogels. Biomaterials 1998; 19:1287-1294.

42. Kiaei D, Hoffman AS, Horbett TA, and Lew KR, Platelet and monoclonal antibody binding to fibrinogen adsorbed on glow-discharge-deposited polymers. J Biomed Mater Res 1995; 29:729-739.

43. Hubbell JA, Pharmacologic modification of materials. Cardiovasc Pathol 1993; 2:121S-128S.

44. Tolan M, Wells F, Kendall S, Large S, and Wallwork J, Clinical experience with a collagen-impregnated woven Dacron graft. J Cardiovasc Surg 1995; 36:323-327.

45. Utoh J, Goto H, Obayashi H, Hirata T, and Miyauchi Y, Dilation of gelatin-sealed knitted dacron prosthesis. J Cardiovasc Surg 1996; 37:343-344.

46. Kang SS, Petsikas D, Murchan P, Cziperle DJ, Ren D, Kim DU, and Greisler HP, Effects of albumin coating of knitted Dacron grafts on transinterstitial blood loss and tissue ingrowth and incorporation. Cardiovasc Surg 1997; 5:184-189.

47. DiMilla PA, Stone JA, Quinn JA, Albelda SM, and Lauffenberger DA, Maximal migration of human smooth muscle cells on fibronectin and type IV collagen occurs at an intermediate attachment strength. J Cell Biol 1993; 122:729-737.

48. Johnson PC, Dickson CS, Garrett KO, Sheppeck RA, and Bentz ML, The effect of microvascular anastomosis configuration on initial platelet deposition. Plast Reconstr Surg 1993; 91:522-527.

49. Simons M, Edelman ER, DeKeyser JL, Langer R, and Rosenberg RD, Antisense c-myb oligonucleotides inhibit intimal arterial smooth muscle cell accumulation in vivo. Nature 1992; 359:67-70.

50. Greisler HP, Cziperle DJ, Kim DU, Garfield JD, Petsikas D, Murchan PM, Applegren EO, Drohan W, and Burgess WH, Enhanced endothelialization of expanded polytetrafluoroethylene grafts by fibroblast growth factor type 1 pretreatment. Surgery 1992; 112:244-254.

51. Golden MA, Hanson SR, Kirkman TR, and Clowes AW, Healing of poly(tetrafluoroethylene) arterial grafts is influenced by graft porosity. J Vasc Surg 1990; 22:838-844.

Matrix Engineering

CHAPTER 52

In Vivo Synthesis of Organs Using Collagen-GAG Copolymers

Ioannis V. Yannas

Introduction

As practiced today, the methodology of tissue engineering emphasizes the reconstruction of tissues and organs. Such reconstructive activity may be either induced to take place inside the host organism, at the site of the missing organ (in vivo synthesis), or else it may be induced outside the organism (in vitro synthesis), typically in a cell culture environment, prior to being grafted onto the host.

In vivo synthesis of organs has been induced by use of analogs of the extracellular matrix (ECM). Three organs have been synthesized so far by this method, namely, the skin (in humans, as well as in swine and guinea pig models), peripheral nerves (rat) and the knee meniscus (canine). The procedure depends critically on identification of the appropriate regeneration template, a biologically active ECM analog which can block scar synthesis and induce instead the desired in situ synthesis of the physiological organ. Convincing evidence that regeneration has, in fact, occurred must be based on observation of definitive recovery of both structure and function in an anatomically well defined defect. Furthermore, there must be evidence that the mass of the regenerated organ which forms in the absence of the template (spontaneous regeneration) is negligibly small relative to that which is induced in its presence.

In this chapter, I will first present the evidence supporting the conclusion that organ regeneration can indeed be reproducibly achieved both in animal models and clinically. The methodology of induced regeneration will then be briefly summarized, followed by an introduction to the models which are used to describe the mechanism of induced regeneration.

Although in vivo synthesis of vascular tissue has not yet been demonstrated, I suggest that future experimentation in this area could be very fruitful and could benefit directly by use of the principles described briefly below for other tissues and organs.

Summary of Evidence for In Vivo Synthesis of Organs

There is considerable evidence that the adult mammalian dermis does not regenerate spontaneously.[1,2] In studies which have been conducted since 1970 it has have shown that a porous graft copolymer of type I collagen and chondroitin 6-sulfate, a glycosaminoglycan (collagen-GAG copolymer) induces in vivo synthesis (induced regeneration) of the dermis in large areas of full-thickness skin loss in the guinea pig.[3-10] This finding has been independently confirmed repeatedly in humans[11-13] and recently in swine.[14] The evidence for regeneration was based on histological and ultrastructural studies, the use of small-angle laser light scattering studies of histological sections, and functional studies. It was concluded that the new skin was structurally and functionally competent; however, it was totally lacking in hair follicles and other skin adenexa.

The emphasis in early studies of in vivo synthesis of skin was on keratinocyte seeding of the analog prior to grafting, as this procedure led to simultaneous regeneration of an epidermis as well as a dermis. It was later appreciated that cell seeding speeds up epidermal regeneration but it appears otherwise not to be required for regeneration either of the epidermis or of the dermis.

The evidence cited above led to identification of a cell-free macromolecular network with highly specific structure, the cell-free skin regeneration template (SRT), which alone possessed this unprecedented morphogenetic activity. Only one of several collagen-GAG matrices studied as described above was capable of preventing scar tissue formation and promoting dermal regeneration. The active ECM analog was characterized by a collagen/GAG ratio of 98/2 w/w, average pore diameter between 20 and 120 µm, random orientation of pore channels, and sufficiently high density of covalent crosslinks (average molecular weight between crosslinks in the template, 12 kDa) to resist degradation by collagenases for about 10 days following grafting. Several other very closely related ECM analogs showed either significantly reduced activity or no activity at all.[9] In related studies it was observed that ECM analogs which showed high activity in promoting dermal regeneration also delayed significantly the onset of wound contraction.[9] The available evidence compelled the conclusion that the activity of this insoluble network depended critically on maintenance of a highly specific three dimensional structure inside the wound bed over a period of time between about 5 and 15 days. The active network has been referred to as skin regeneration template (SRT). The observed activity of SRT, consisting in drastic modification of the outcome of the wound healing process, has not been duplicated by application on the wound bed of solutions of one or more growth factors or by application of suspensions of keratinocytes or fibroblasts.

Regeneration of a partially functional sciatic nerve was induced across a transected gap of 15 mm in the rat sciatic nerve[15-18] by another ECM analog, which was also found to possess a highly specific network structure. In this animal model the nerve stumps at either side of the gap were inserted in a silicone tube (tubulation); in the absence of a tube, regeneration was decidedly absent and neuroma formation was invariably reported. Although spontaneous regeneration of nerve through the tube occurred reproducibly at a gap length of 5 mm, regeneration across a 15 mm gap has not been observed.[19,20] The study eventually led to identification of an ECM analog which, when filling the silicone tube and thereby connecting the two nerve stumps, induced regeneration across a 15 mm gap. This analog has been referred to as nerve regeneration template (NRT). It

has an average pore diameter of 5 µm, an average molecular weight between crosslinks of 30-40 kDa, a preferred orientation of pore channel axes in the direction of the nerve axis, and a 98/2 w/w ratio of type I collagen to GAG.[16,17] Clearly, there are significant differences between the network structure of skin and nerve regeneration templates.

Yet a third ECM analog has been reported, capable of inducing regeneration of the canine meniscus following 80% transection.[21,22] Although the ECM analog used in these studies has been stated by the authors to be similar to that described earlier,[9] its detailed structure was not reported.

There is, therefore, substantial evidence that, under appropriate conditions, the adult mammal can be induced to regrow certain organs which are not regenerated spontaneously. This exciting conclusion suggests new therapeutic avenues. However, there are still many unanswered questions about the detailed cell-biological mechanism by which active ECM analogs modify so spectacularly one or more of the processes involved in conventional wound healing.

Methodological Principles of Induced Regeneration

Over the years it has become clear that a number of conditions must be in place in order to conduct a reproducible study of induced regeneration. One of the most important is the choice of an anatomically well-defined lesion (experimental volume) in which to study the phenomena. This concept was pioneered in the studies of Billingham and Medawar[1] as a means of minimizing animal to animal variability in observations. The experimental volume can be isolated by containing it within anatomically distinct tissues belonging to a neighboring organ or by a device or (in the case of skin) by the atmosphere.

Since mammals possess a very small but finite potential for regeneration, it is necessary to "correct" the observed regeneration by subtracting the amount which has been contributed by spontaneous regeneration. This requirement is equivalent to defining a negative control in every experimental model, consisting of the observations obtained in the absence of the presumptive regeneraion template.

Although the mechanistic interpretation of induced regeneration has not been completed, two arguments have been advanced to support the contention that there is a requirement for structuring a regeneration template as an ECM analog. First, studies of organ development have shown conclusively that the early presence of specific ECM components is required for formation of physiological organs.[23-25] In contrast, the exudate which flows into a spontaneously healing wound after injury does not contain components of the insoluble and nondiffusible ECM networks (although it contains several types of cells and regulators); the healing process in this case eventually leads to synthesis of scar. Second, the evidence presented in the preceding section clearly supports the contention that specific ECM analogs indeed suffice to lead to regeneration of at least two organs. However, there is clearly insufficient evidence to conclude definitively that regeneration can be induced only by specific ECM analogs.

Conclusive evidence that an ECM analog has induced organ regeneration can only be obtained with a performance assay which simply compares the structure of the regenerate to that of a normal control. Assays of this type can be destructive (e.g., histology), in which case only one experimental time point can be obtained per animal, or nondestructive, such that the complete kinetic curve for regeneration can be obtained from a single animal. The fidelity of regeneration is a figure of merit which is assigned to each candidate template. The regeneration template is then the ECM analog which has scored a very high value of the fidelity index.

Models of the Mechanism of Regeneration

I summarize below the major physicochemical models[26-28] which have been used to compile a mechanistic interpretation of the process of regeneration. It is evident that a regeneration template modifies drastically the kinetics and mechanism of spontaneous wound healing which normally lead to wound contraction and scar synthesis. However, a view of a template as a classical catalyst is not supported by the well known fact that regeneration templates are necessarily consumed during the process which they modify.

Micrometer Scale Proximity of Host to Template Surface

Cells and cytokines present in the exudate are transferred to the surface of the template following implantation of the porous template into the wound bed. Surface tension forces pull the exudate inside the capillaries (pore channels) of the template, as described by:

$$P = 2\gamma/r \tag{1}$$

where r is the radius of the pore channel in a template undergoing wetting by exudate with an air-liquid surface tension of γ in dyne/cm. Wetting of the opposed surfaces is promoted as the suction pressure P in Equation (1) increases, and such increase is occasioned by a decrease in average pore radius. The values reached by P are not negligible; water with an air-liquid surface tension of $\gamma = 72$ dyne/cm, for example, is pulled inside a pore radius of 100 μm with a suction pressure of almost one-hundredth of one atmosphere and P increases almost to one full atmosphere when the pore radius decreases to a value as low as 1 μm. Under conditions where exudate flows inside the pore channels of a template with average pore diameter of 100 μm, cells and cytokines are within a distance of less than 50 μm from the template surface; this distance can then be covered by these components of the exudate within a few minutes.

Maximum Dimension of Template, ~100 μm

Cell migration from the solid-like tissue of the wound bed into the template requires the availability of adequate nutrition. The precise nutritional requirements of any cell are too complex to incorporate into a simple model; instead, these requirements will be simplified by defining a critical nutrient which is required for normal cell function; such a nutrient is assumed to be metabolized by the cell at a rate R

mole/cm³/s. Picture the nutrient being transported from the solid-like tissue, where the concentration of nutrient is assumed to be a constant C_0 due to the presence of vascular supply, over a distance L through the exudate, until it reaches the cell. Prior to the onset of angiogenesis, i.e., during the first few days following template implantation, the nutrient is transported exclusively by diffusion, characterized by a diffusivity D cm²/s. Dimensional analysis readily yields the cell lifeline number:

$$S = RL^2/DC_0 \tag{2}$$

which can be used to compare the relative magnitude of the rate of nutrient consumption by the cell nutrient (numerator) to the rate of supply of nutrient to the cell by diffusion (denominator). The cell dies if the rate of consumption of the critical nutrient exceeds greatly the rate of supply, S>>1. At steady state the rate of consumption of nutrient by the cell just equals the rate of transport by diffusion over the distance L. Under conditions of steady state, $S = O(1)$; at that point, the value of L becomes the critical cell path length, L_c, the distance of migration beyond which cells require the presence of a vascular supply. Another way of looking at L_c is that it is the longest distance away from the wound bed boundary along which the cell can migrate without requiring nutrient in excess of that supplied by diffusion. For many cell nutrients of low molecular weight, L_c is of order 100 μm, an estimate of the maximum template dimension which can support cells.

Template Specific Surface Is Bounded

Following its migration onto the template surface a host cell is visualized interacting with binding sites on the surface. The surface density of binding sites can be expressed as Φ_b, equal by definition to the number of sites N_b per unit surface A of template. Φ_b can also be expressed more usefully in terms of quantities potentially measurable by optical microscopy, i.e., in terms of the volume density of binding sites ρ_b (number of sites per unit volume porous template) and the specific surface σ of the template expressed in units of mm²/cm³:

$$\Phi_b = N_b/A = \rho_b/\sigma \tag{3}$$

Assuming that each cell is bound to (an a priori unknown number of) χ binding sites, there will be N_b/χ bound cells per unit surface; the volume density of cells will be $\rho_c = \rho_b/\chi$ and the surface density of cells will be:

$$\Phi_c = \Phi_b/\chi = N_b/\chi A = \rho_b/\chi\sigma = \rho_c/\sigma \tag{4}$$

Levels of myofibroblast density inside templates with pore diameter of about 10 μm have been observed to reach typical values of the volume density, ρ_c, of order 107 myofibroblasts per cm³ porous template. For a template of average pore diameter 10 μm the specific surface σ is calculated to be approximately 8×10^4 mm²/cm³ template; therefore, 1 cm³ porous template is characterized by a cell surface density of $\Phi_c = \rho_c/\sigma = 10^7/8 \times 10^4 = 125$ cells/mm². For a template of identical composition but average pore diameter as large as 300 μm, Φ_c is the same as above; however, the specific surface is calculated to be only about 3 x 10^3 mm^2/cm^3 template. In this case, the volume density of cells is, accordingly, only $\rho_c = \Phi_c \cdot \sigma = 125 \times 3 \times 10^3 = 3.75 \times 10^5$ per cm^3 porous template. We conclude that the template which has the smaller average pore diameter (10 μm) has a volume density of myofibroblasts which is about 27 times lower than with the template which has the larger pore diameter (300 μm). The existence of a maximum pore diameter requirement for the template is suggested by these calculations, simply to ensure a specific surface which is large enough to bind an appropriately large number of cells.

In addition, it is clear that cells originating in the wound bed cannot migrate inside the template and eventually reach binding sites on its surface unless the template has an average pore diameter large enough to allow for this. We conclude that there is, therefore, a requirement for a minimum pore diameter for the template, about equal to the characteristic diameter of the cells (of order 5 μm). Thus, the pore diameter of the regeneration template is limited both by an upper and a lower bound. This conclusion is in agreement with the experimental evidence which shows that ECM analogs, identical in chemical composition but differing only in average pore diameter, show maximum activity (inhibition of onset of wound contraction, consistent with regeneration rather than scar formation) when the average pore diameter lies between 20 and 120 μm.[9] Further evidence has shown that, when other structural parameters of the template remain constant, loss of the 20-120 μm porous structure of the template by simple evaporation at room temperature (a process which yields an ECM analog with average pore diameter of less than 1 μm) leads to synthesis of a scar capsule at the surface of the grafted analog, evidence of a barrier to cell migration inside an implant.[29]

Critical Residence Time of Template

The residence time of a template is also bounded. A template has to stay in place long enough to induce the appropriate synthetic processes to take place; soon after that, it must disappear in a timely fashion so as not to interfere with these same processes which it induces. The time period necessary to induce synthesis is roughly equal to that required to complete the wound healing process at that anatomical site. (In general, the rate of wound healing is quite different in tissues such as, say, the dermis and the sciatic nerve.) Since the template is an insoluble (and, therefore, nondiffusible) three dimensional network it follows that cells which are bound on it become immobilized and their migration is, accordingly, arrested. Not only cells are prevented from migrating to locations which are appropriate for synthesis of a new organ but, in addition, the laying down of newly synthesized ECM by the cells in the space of the wound bed is probably blocked physically by the presence of the template. It follows that the persisting insolubility of the template will increasingly interfere with the synthesis of the new organ at that site. To avoid this eventuality, the template is required to become diffusible (by degradation to small molecular fragments) and thereby disappear from the wound

bed in order not to impede cellular processes which lead to the emerging organ.

A steady state model is probably the simplest way to accommodate these two requirements. It requires synchronization of the two processes: organ synthesis and template degradation.[5,9] This model leads directly to the hypothesis of isomorphous tissue replacement:

$$t_d/t_s = O(1) \qquad\qquad (5)$$

In Equation (5) t_d denotes a characteristic time constant for degradation of the template at the tissue site where a new organ is synthesized with a time constant of t_s. The degradation rate can be estimated by histological observation of the decrease in mass of template fragments at various times.[10,30] A closer estimate of t_d has been obtained by measuring the kinetics of disintegration of the macromolecular network using rubber elasticity theory.[3] A third procedure consists of monitoring the kinetics of mass disappearance of a radioactively labeled template. A rough estimate of t_s can be obtained by observing t_h, the timescale of synthesis of new tissue during healing (in the absence of a template) at the anatomical site.[31] Using the latter approach it has been estimated that t_s for the regenerating dermis is of order 3 weeks[31] and of order 6 weeks for the regenerating peripheral nerve.[16] These estimates allow adjustment of t_d for the template, by adjustment of the crosslink density and GAG content, to levels which are approximately equal to the values of t_s, as the latter are dictated by the nature of the anatomical site.

Experimental support for the isomorphous tissue replacement hypothesis has been based on observations such that, when the ratio in Equation (5) was adjusted to values much smaller than one (by implanting a rapidly degrading ECM analog, for which $t_d \ll t_s$), the wound healing process resulted in contraction and synthesis of scar (as would have been the case if the template was missing). Furthermore, when the ratio in Equation (5) was much larger than one 1 (by implanting an ECM analog which degraded very slowly, so that $t_d \ll t_s$) the ECM analog was surrounded by a capsule of scar tissue.[29,31] Clearly, the available limited evidence cannot be used to test the hypothesis of Equation (5) conclusively; nevertheless, such evidence is, at the least, consistent with a template half life which is bounded. Studies of inhibition of wound contraction by several ECM analogs with defined structure have provided direct experimental support for this conclusion. These studies have shown that, of several ECM analogs studied, the dermal regeneration template was the analog which degraded at a rate corresponding to a half life of about 1.5-2 weeks; ECM analogs which degraded at much slower or much faster rates were not active.[9]

From the above it can be inferred that the simplest template structure which can degrade and diffuse away with minimum harm to the host is one in which the template undergoes degradation by enzymes of the wound bed to nontoxic low molecular weight fragments.[31]

Template Chemical Composition

Developmentally significant interactions are known to involve cells, growth factors and ECM components. The latter include the collagens, elastin and several proteoglycans as well as cell adhesion molecules such as fibronectin and laminin. Since development and induced regeneration have a common end point we will assume quite simply, as a first approximation, that the required cell-matrix binding events in each case are similar; if so, the identity of matrix components in each case must also be similar. This presumptive similarity between developmental and regenerative mechanisms has been previously referred to briefly in terms of the hypothetical rule: Regeneration recapitulates ontogeny;[8] however, we caution to the lack of detailed evidence for such an identity. In the dermis, as well as in the connective tissue of peripheral nerves, type I collagen is present in greatest abundance, whereas the most prominent glycosaminoglycans in the dermis are dermatan sulfate and chondroitin 6-sulfate; in peripheral nerves, type I collagen and sulfated proteoglycans have also been prominently observed.[32]

The early exudate of a spontaneously healing skin wound is free of ECM components; although quite richly endowed with undifferentiated cells and growth factors, it is, nevertheless, lacking in components which are known to be required for development.[23-25] As pointed out above, this lack of ECM components is hypothetically associated with the absence of synthetic processes which lead to a physiological organ.

This article has been based on the author's article "Models of Organ Regeneration Processes Induced by Templates", in Bioartificial Organs, Prokop A, Hunkels D, Cherrington AD, eds. Ann Ny Acad Sci 1997; 831:280-293.

The reasoning above is consistent with the choice of type I collagen and at least one of the proteoglycans or glycosaminoglycans (GAGs) as basic structural components of regeneration templates. Several efforts have been made to replace the use of ECM analogs in templates with synthetic polymers; at this time, however, there is no firm evidence that synthetic polymers can induce regeneration of the dermis or of a peripheral nerve in lesions where the physiological structures are not regenerated spontaneously.

Considerable experimental evidence links the biological activity of the dermal regeneration template to its detailed structural features. Two ECM analogs, one of which was prepared with a GAG while the other was prepared with the corresponding proteoglycan, showed the same activity in an in vivo assay (inhibition of onset of wound contraction) which predicts dermal regeneration.[33] This result suggested that the dermal regeneration template can be constructed using a GAG, rather than the corresponding proteoglycan, without loss of activity. A covalently crosslinked network of collagen and the sulfated GAG appears to be necessary; this is inferred by the observation that whereas these two macromolecules form an ionic complex spontaneously at acidic pH, the complex is dissociated at neutral pH, i.e., under conditions which prevail following implantation.[34] To preserve the chemical composition of the ECM analog in vivo over the period suggested by the residence time considerations discussed above, it is necessary to introduce a certain density of covalent bonds between collagen chains and GAG molecules, i.e., to form a collagen-GAG graft copolymer.[34] There is evidence that an increase in the fraction of GAG in the copolymer increases the resistance of the macromolecular network to degradation by mammalian collagenases[3] Such resistance also increases with the density of collagen-collagen crosslinks and collagen-GAG crosslinks.[29,35] A review of the effect of each of these structural features of the dermal regeneration template on its activity in the inhibition of the onset of wound contraction can be made based on the published evidence.[9,33] This review suggests that the chemical composition and the detailed pore structure of the dermal regeneration template contribute about equally to its activity. A similar study of the relation between structure and activity for the nerve regeneration template has not been made.

Conclusions

There is strong evidence that the adult mammal is capable of almost complete organ regeneration. This surprising result has been documented with several animal models and in repeated clinical trials. It is clear that both the dermis and the epidermis, as well as the peripheral nerve and the knee meniscus, can be induced to regenerate in lesions where spontaneous regeneration is well known to be negligible. In these instances regeneration has been induced by analogs of the ECM. A model of the mechanism of regeneration provides an explanation for the observed structural features of the ECM analogs (termed regeneration templates) which have shown this remarkable behavior.

References

1. Billingham RE, Medawar PB. Contracture and intussusceptive growth in the healing of extensive wounds in mammalian skin. J Anat 1955; 89:114-123.
2. Peacock Jr EE, Van Winkle Jr W. Wound Repair, Second Edition. Philadelphia: W.B.Saunders 1976.
3. Yannas IV, Burke JF, Huang C, Gordon PL. Suppression of in vivo degradability and of immunogencity by reaction with glycoaminoglycans. Polymer Repr Am Chem Soc 1975; 16:209-214.
4. Yannas IV, Burke JF, Gordon PL, Huang C. Multilayer membrane useful as synthetic skin. 1977; US Patent 4,060,081.
5. Yannas IV, Burke JF, Umbreit M, Stasikelis P. Progress in design of an artificial skin. Fed Proc 1979; 38:988.
6. Yannas IV, Burke JF, Warpehoski M, Stasikelis P, Skrabut EM, Orgill D, Giard DJ. Prompt, long-term functional replacement of skin. Trans Am Soc Artif Intern Organs 1981; 27:19-22.
7. Yannas IV, Burke JF, Orgill DP, Skrabut EM. Wound tissue can utilize a polymeric template to synthesize a functional extension of skin. Science 1982; 215:174-176.
8. Yannas IV, Orgill DP, Skrabut EM, Burke JF. Skin regeneration with a bioreplaceable polymeric template. In: Gebelein CG, ed. American Chemical Symposium Series, Number 256 Washington, D.C. 1984:191-197.
9. Yannas IV, Lee E, Orgill DP, Skrabut EM, Murphy GF. Synthesis and characterization of a model extracellular matrix that induces partial regeneration of adult mammalian skin. Proc Natl Acad Sci USA 1989; 86:933-937.

10. Murphy GF, Orgill DP, Yannas IV. Partial dermal regeneration is induced by biodegradable collagen-glycosaminoglycan grafts. Lab Invest 1990; 63:305-313.

11. Burke JF, Yannas IV, Quinby Jr WC, Bondoc CC, Jung WK. Successful use of a physiologically acceptable artificial skin in the treatment of extensive skin injury. Ann Surg 1981; 194:413-428.

12. Heimbach D, Luterman A, Burke J, Cram A, Herndon D, Hunt J, Jordan M, McManus W, Solem L, Warden G, Zawacki B. A multi-center randomized clinical trial. Artificial dermis for major burns. Ann Surg 1988; 208:313-320.

13. Stern R, McPherson M, Longaker MT. Histologic study of artificial skin used in the treatment of full-thickness thermal injury. J Burn Care Rehabil 1990; 11:7-13.

14. Orgill DP, Butler CE, Regan JF. Behavior of collagen-GAG matrices as dermal replacement in rodent and porcine models. Wounds 1996; 8:151-157.

15. Yannas IV, Orgill DP, Silver J, Norregaard TV, Zervas NT, Schoene WC. Regeneration of sciatic nerve across 15-mm gap by use of a polymeric template. In: Gebelein CG, ed. Advances in Biomedical Polymers. New York: Plenum Press,1987:1-9.

16. Chang AS, Yannas IV, Perutz S, Loree H, Sethi RR, Krarup C, Norregaard TV, Zervas NT, Silver J. Electrophysiological study of recovery of peripheral nerves regenerated by a collagen-glycosaminoglycan copolymer matrix. In: Gebelein CG, ed. Progress in Biomedical Polymers. New York: Plenum Press, 1990:107-120.

17. Chang AS, Yannas IV. Peripheral nerve regeneration. In: Smith B, Adelman G, eds. Neuroscience Year (Supplement 2 to the Encyclopedia of Neuroscience). Boston: Birkhauser, 1992:125-126.

18. Landstrom A, Yannas IV. Peripheral nerve regeneration. In: Smith B, Adelman G, eds. Encyclopedia of Neuroscience. Boston: Birkhäuser, 1996: In press.

19. Lundborg G, Dahlin LB, Danielson N, Gelberman RH, Longo FM, Powell HC, Varon S. Nerve regeneration in silicone chambers: Influence of gap length and of distal stump components. Exp Neurol 1982; 76:361-375.

20. Lundborg G. Nerve regeneration and repair: A review. Acta Orthop Scand 1987; 58:145-169.

21. Stone KR, Rodkey WG, Webber RJ, McKineey L, Steadman JR. Collagen-based prostheses for meniscal regeneration. Clin Orthop 1990; 252:129-135.

22. Stone KR, Webber RJ, Rodkey WG, Steadman JR. Prosthetic meniscal replacement: In vitro studies of meniscal regeneration using copolymeric collagen prostheses. Arthroscopy 1989; 5:152.

23. McPherson JM, Piez KA. In: Clark RAF, Henson PM, eds. The Molecular and Cellular Biology of Wound Repair. New York: Plenum, 1988:471-496.

24. Hay ED, ed. Cell biology of extracellular matrix. New York: Plenum Press, 1981.

25. Loomis WF. Developmental biology. New York: Macmillan, 1986.

26. Yannas IV. Models of organ regeneration processes induced by templates. In: Prokop A, Hunkeler D, Cherrington AD, eds. Ann NY Acad Sci 1997; 831: 280-293.

27. Yannas IV. Regeneration templates. In: Bronzino JD, ed. The Biomedical Engineering Handbook. Boca Raton: CRC Press, 1995:1619-1635.

28. Yannas IV. In vivo synthesis of tissues and organs. In: Lanza RP, Langer RS, Chick WL, eds. Textbook of Tissue Engineering. New York: R.G. Landes/Academic Press, 1996:169-178.

29. Yannas IV. Use of artificial skin in wound management. In: Dineen P, ed. The Surgical Wound. Philadelphia: Lea and Febiger, 1981:171-190.

30. Yannas IV, Burke JF, Huang C, Gordon PL. Correlation of in vivo collagen degradation rate with in vitro measurements. J Biomed Mat Res 1975; 9:623-628.

31. Yannas IV, Burke JF. Design of an artificial skin.Part I. Design principles. J Biomed Mat Res 1980; 14:65-68.

32. Rutka JT, Apodaca G, Stern R, Rosenblum M. The extracellular matrix of the central and peripheral nervous systems: Structure and function J Neurosurg 1988; 69:155-170.

33. Shafritz TA, Rosenberg LC, Yannas IV. Specific effects of glycosaminoglycans in an analog of extracellular matrix that delays wound contraction and induces regeneration. Wound Rep Reg 1994; 2:270-276.

34. Yannas IV, Burke JF, Gordon PL, Huang C, Rubenstein RH. Design of an artificial skin. Part II. Control of chemical composition. J Biomed Mat Res 1980; 14:107-131.

35. Yannas IV. Regeneration of skin and nerves by use of collagen templates. In: Nimni M, ed. Collagen: Biotechnology, Vol. III. Boca Raton: CRC Press, 1988:87-115.

———————————— CHAPTER 53 ————————————

Artificial Extracellular Matrix Proteins for Graft Design

Alyssa Panitch, David A. Tirrell

Introduction

More than 500,000 vascular grafts are implanted annually in the United States.[1] Although large diameter grafts implanted in regions of high blood flow remain patent for many years, small and medium caliber prostheses are plagued by unacceptable rates of failure due to thrombosis and intimal hyperplasia.[2]

Despite their high failure rates, two materials—expanded polytetrafluorocthylene (ePTFE) and poly(ethylene terephthalate) (Dacron)—have remained dominant in the technology of synthetic vascular grafts for more than thirty years. In attempts to reduce leakage, platelet adhesion, thrombosis and intimal hyperplasia, researchers have modified the surfaces of ePTFE and Dacron in many ways, including impregnation with albumin,[3] gelatin[4] or collagen,[5] preclotting with whole blood,[6] pretreatment with fibrin glue with or without growth factors or heparin,[7] and preseeding with endothelial cells, either in the operating room[8] or in a preliminary procedure that allows preestablishment of a confluent endothelial cell monolayer.[9] Recent reports on clinical trials using endothelialized ePTFE grafts have been particularly encouraging.[10]

Nevertheless, the factors leading to the development of thromboresistant, endothelialized grafts free of intimal hyperplasia remain poorly understood. It is clear that a confluent layer of endothelial cells is not sufficient; although the endothelial lining of the healthy artery resists thrombus formation, a procoagulant state can be induced by mechanical trauma, by inflammatory mediators such as interleukin-1,[11] by bacterial endotoxin,[12] and by other stimuli. Furthermore, endothelial cells are capable of releasing platelet-derived growth factor-like proteins[13-15] and other smooth muscle cell mitogens, and elevated mitotic activity in smooth muscle cells located beneath an apparently confluent endothelium has been reported by Clowes and co-workers in studies of ePTFE grafts implanted in baboons.[16] Thus, even confluent endothelial layers can play an active role in graft failure via thrombosis or intimal hyperplasia.

Our laboratory has adopted a new approach to the problem of preparing vascular grafts of improved long term patency, an approach based on the synthesis of new artificial extracellular matrix (ECM) proteins suitable as substrates for the culture of endothelial cells. The proteins under current study are based on repetitive oligopeptide sequences analogous to those of mammalian elastin,[17] and incorporate ECM-derived cell binding domains, including the CS5 region of fibronectin,[18] which contains the REDV sequence previously shown to support attachment and spreading of endothelial cells, but not vascular smooth muscle cells.[19] The potential endothelial cell selectivity of such polymers makes them attractive

Tissue Engineering of Prosthetic Vascular Grafts, edited by Peter Zilla and Howard P. Greisler.

candidates for use in vascular grafts, and it is the prospect of using such materials to culture thromoresistant endothelial tissue that has attracted our attention.

The choice of elastin-like sequences to constitute the structural elements of the artificial ECM proteins was based on several factors. First, elastin is abundant in the walls of small muscular arteries,[20] and thus is a critical element in the organization and function of the healthy artery. Second, Urry and co-workers have demonstrated a remarkably wide range of mechanical properties in repetitive elastin-like polymers, reporting elastic moduli from 10^4 to more than 10^8 dynes/cm^2, depending on sequence and water content.[17] Because the moduli of the arterial wall are of the same order,[21] elastin-like polymers offer the prospect of reduced compliance mismatch between artery and graft, a recurrent cause of endothelial damage, peri-anastomotic smooth muscle cell proliferation, and graft failure.[22-25] Elastin-like polymers are readily processed from aqueous solutions, and can be converted in simple operations into films, tubes, and surface coatings convenient for evaluation of materials properties.[26] Finally, the polypentapeptide of repeating unit sequence -GVGVP- has been subjected to extensive biomaterials testing, including determination of mutagenicity (Ames test), toxicity (mice and rabbits), antigenicity (Guinea pigs), pyrogenicity (rabbits), and thrombogenicity (dogs), and has performed well in each of these tests.[27] Poly(GVGVP) is nonadhesive toward human umbilical vein endothelial cells (HUVECs),[28] suggesting that cell attachment to such polymers ought to be mediated by specific interactions with recognition sequences built into the chain. Urry and co-workers have reported adhesion of HUVECs to variants of poly(GVGVP) that contain periodic GRGDS inserts.[28] The same group reported that incorporation of REDV oligopeptides into poly(GVGVP) did not yield substrates capable of supporting adhesion of HUVECs. As shown in the following section, however, insertion of the longer (20 amino acid) CS5 region does yield adhesive substrates. Perhaps the short REDV inserts in poly(GVGVP) are unable to adopt the conformation(s) required for cell surface recognition and attachment.

The cell-binding domain of primary interest in our work to date has been the CS5 region of human fibronectin. Comprising residues 90-109 of the type III connecting segment (IIICS) of fibronectin, CS5 includes the minimal active sequence REDV,[18] which is recognized by the integrin $\alpha_4\beta_1$.[29-33] Binding to IIICS appears to be considerably more selective than is recognition of the central cell-binding domain of fibronectin,[34] which carries the cell recognition sequence RGDS.[35,36]

Hubbell and co-workers have exploited the selectivity of the REDV sequence to prepare surfaces that show preferential affinity for endothelial cells.[19] Immobilization of the hexapeptide GREDVY on glycophase glass produced sur-faces on which HUVECs attached and spread, while human foreskin fibroblasts, human vascular smooth muscle cells, and human blood platelets did not. Subsequent investigations demonstrated that endothelial cell attachment to REDV-grafted substrates is mediated by integrin $\alpha_4\beta_1$,[37] and that attachment can be inhibited specifically by soluble REDV peptides. Endothelial cells also recognize the RGD sequence from the central cell-binding domain of fibronectin (via integrins $\alpha_5\beta_1$ and $\alpha_v\beta_1$), and fibronectin carries at least two additional recognition sites for $\alpha_4\beta_1$, designated CS1 and H1, respectively.[34] The integrin binding affinities of CS5 and H1 are comparable, while that of CS1 is approximately 20-fold higher.[34]

Thus it appears likely that endothelial cell function can be regulated by presentation of ECM-derived recognition sequences, with control exercised by variation in the density and affinity of recognition sites and in the presentation of multiple sites in combination. The design of artificial ECM proteins allows this approach to be pursued in systematic fashion, in that specific recognition sequences, one by one or in combination, can be built into structural domains denuded of their intrinsic binding sites. We have begun to test this idea, beginning with elastin-like structural domains, and introducing initially CS5, and subsequently CS1, as ligands for the $\alpha_4\beta_1$ integrin receptor on the endothelial cell surface.

Artificial Proteins

Since 1990, the primary focus of our laboratory has been the design and bacterial synthesis of artificial proteins that exhibit novel and potentially useful material properties. Our initial efforts addressed strategies for controlling chain folding and supramolecular organization in solid polymers, and led to a family of repetitive proteins that adopt chain-folded lamellar architectures of controlled dimensions and surface functionality.[38-41] A second set of experiments has been directed toward the engineering of novel liquid crystal (LC) phases in solutions of rod-like artificial proteins,[42] and has yielded unique smectic LC structures with layer spacings subject to precise control on length scales of tens of nanometers.[43] An important, continuing objective of this work has been the development of methods for incorporating nonnatural amino acids into artificial proteins in vivo, and good success has been achieved for selenated,[44] fluorinated,[45] electroactive,[46] olefinic,[47] acetylenic and conformationally constrained[48] amino acid analogs.

Artificial ECM Proteins

In our preliminary experiments, two artificial ECM proteins (1a and 1b, see Fig. 53.1) have been prepared and subjected to evaluation as substrates for the culture of human umbilical vein endothelial cells (HUVECs).

Fig. 53.1. Structure of artificial extracellular matrix proteins 1a and 1b, 2a and 2b.

$$—[\text{cbd}(\text{GVPGI})_x]—_y$$

1:cbd=CS5	a: x=40, y=3
2:cbd=CS1	b: x=20, y= 5

Synthesis

Proteins 1a and 1b have been expressed in E. coli strain BL31(DE3)pLysS under control of a bacteriophage T7 promoter.[49] For batch cultures, 60 mg/L (1a) or 40 mg/L (1b) of recombinant protein can be recovered through a simple procedure involving selective precipitation of contaminating proteins below the lower critical solution temperature of the target polymer (vide infra).

Lower Critical Solution Temperatures

Urry and co-workers have reported extensive studies of the lower critical solution temperatures (or "inverse temperature transitions") of elastin-like polypeptides.[17] The lower critical solution temperature (LCST) is the temperature below which the polymer forms a single-phase solution (e.g., in water); above the LCST, the solution separates into polymer-rich and polymer-depleted phases. Polypentapeptides of repeating unit sequence -VPGVG- exhibit an LCST at approximately 25°C,[50] and substitution with increasingly hydrophobic residues shifts the transition to lower temperatures.[50] The choice of -GVPGI- as the elastin-like repeat was based on its predicted LCST of 10°C,[50] which ensures reduced water solubility (and hence increased stability of surface coatings) at physiological temperatures.

The LCSTs of 1a and 1b were determined in doubly distilled H_2O at four concentrations ranging from 10 mg/ml to 40 mg/ml. The LCST is signaled by an abrupt increase in the turbidity of the solution, which was measured at a wavelength of 300 nm.

The results are consistent with the predictions of Urry et al,[50] in that 1a and 1b both exhibit LCSTs near 10°C (13.4°C for 1a; 12.1°C for 1b). Insertion of the CS5 domain causes some perturbation of the LCST, but the objective of depressing the transition to below room temperature has been met for both of these materials. Nevertheless, a subambient LCST does not mean a complete lack of water solubility, so it is essential to determine the stability of surface coatings fabricated from 1a and 1b (and other candidate proteins).

Preparation and Stability of Surface Coatings

Glass cover slips (12 mm diameter) were coated with 1a and 1b from solutions in formamide or water by spreading 40 µL of a 1 mg/ml protein solution over the surface of the cover slip with the tip of a pipet. Fibronectin was coated similarly, by using 20 µL of a 100 µg/ml solution in H_2O. The cover slips were dried in vacuo at 55°C, incubated for 2 h at 37°C in sterile H_2O (0.5 ml) to remove loosely bound protein, and dried again at 55°C for 2 h.

For determination of coating stability, samples of 1a and 1b were labeled in vivo with [³H]glycine. Labeled samples were coated on glass cover slips as described above (without the final wash) and the coatings were subjected to six successive washes with phosphate-buffered saline (PBS, 0.5 ml aliquots, 30 min incubation per cycle). Each wash was analyzed by scintillation counting to determine the amount of protein removed, and the cover slips were counted directly after the sixth wash. Such experiments show that substantial amounts of 1a and 1b are removed by successive washes. Nevertheless, a stable coating remains even after six

washes; in fact, little or no polymer is removed from the surface after two wash steps. In order to ensure the stability of the coating, all samples are washed for 2 hours at 37°C in sterile H_2O prior to cell culture experiments, and uniformity of coverage is verified by scanning electron microscopy.

Cell Culture

Human umbilical vein endothelial cells (HUVECs) have been used for all cell adhesion studies. Harvested cells were resuspended in serum-free M199 medium and diluted to a density of 1×10^4 cells/ml (for cell counting) or 5×10^4 cells/ml (for determination of spreading behavior). HUVECs (1 ml aliquots of the suspensions listed above) were transferred to 24 well dishes containing protein-coated glass cover slips. Cells were maintained at 37°C and 5% CO_2 for 4 h.

Table 53.1 reports the number of cells adherent to each of the two artificial extracellular matrix proteins 1a and 1b. Glass and fibronectin (coated on glass) served as controls. Essentially all cells cultured on fibronectin and on 1b were adherent, as compared to ~25% of cells plated on glass and on 1a. We attribute the decrease in the number of cells bound to 1a as compared to 1b to the lower CS5 density in the former, and perhaps to differences in protein conformation upon adsorption to the glass surface. Table 53.2 summarizes the morphologies of cells adherent to these surfaces. Refractile cells (round and bright under the phase contrast microscope), cells which were round but not highly refractile (round and gray), spreading cells (1-2 pseudopodia), and spread cells (more than 3 pseudopodia) were counted.

Although these are preliminary data, the results in Tables 53.1 and 53.2 are consistent with the hypothesis that artificial ECM proteins with recognition sites for integrin $\alpha_4\beta_1$ will support the attachment and spreading of endothelial cells. Both the number of adherent cells, and the percentage of spread cells, are increased on 1b as compared to glass. Increasing the density of CS5 sites leads to an increase in the number of attached cells; 1b (like fibronectin) supports attachment of essentially all cells plated at a density of 10^4 cells per well. On the other hand, cell spreading is more complete (or perhaps more rapid) on fibronectin than on 1b; essentially all cells have spread on fibronectin after 4 h in serum-free media. Addition of serum-supplemented media to HUVECs cultured on 1b leads to confluent EC

Table 53.1. Adherent HUVECs after 4 h in serum free medium

Protein/Cast From	Adherent Cells per Well
Glass	$2,880 \pm 1670^a$
1a/Formamide	$1,150 \pm 360$
1a/Water	$2,590 \pm 570$
1b/Formamide	$9,170 \pm 1800$
1b/Water	$11,700 \pm 760$
Fibronectin	$10,140 \pm 290$

[a]10,000 cells plated per well; adherent cells given as mean ± standard deviation (n=4).

Table 53.2. HUVEC morphology on glass and protein surfaces

Protein/Cast From	Refractile %	Round/Grey %	Spreading %	Spread %
Glass	49.5 ± 8.6^a	12.0 ± 0.4	13.4 ± 2.3	25.1 ± 7.8
1a/Formamide	14.1 ± 1.2	15.9 ± 5.9	21.3 ± 2.5	48.7 ± 2.2
1a/Water	18.7 ± 7.2	16.3 ± 5.5	7.9 ± 4.0	53.7 ± 6.6
1b/Formamide	15.2 ± 5.9	14.6 ± 3.4	14.4 ± 5.0	55.8 ± 3.9
1b/Water	20.9 ± 5.3	11.4 ± 4.9	11.6 ± 1.4	55.8 ± 9.3

[a]Mean $\pm$ SD for 4 determinations. Each determination based on scoring of 100-150 cells.

monolayers, with typical cobblestone appearance, within 48 h.

Preliminary measurements of competitive inhibition of EC attachment by soluble CS5 analogs have also been made. Preincubation of HUVECs with the soluble peptide GREDVDY (Research Genetics, Inc.) at concentrations up to 2 mg/ml has no observable effect on attachment to fibronectin, as expected. In contrast, attachment to 1b is completely inhibited by GREDVDY at concentrations of 0.6-0.8 mg/ml, consistent with specific attachment of HUVECs to CS5 via the $\alpha_4\beta_1$ receptor.

Current and Future Directions

Our overall objective is the development of a new class of artificial ECM proteins to be used in small diameter vascular grafts of improved long term patency. We believe the proposed approach to be novel in that genetic engineering, polymer chemistry, and materials processing methods can be combined to provide control of both the mechanical properties and the cell-surface interactions of the new proteins. Mechanical properties can be engineered through variation in the length of the elastin-like domains, control of the overall chain length, and introduction of a controlled level of interchain crosslinking. Cell-surface interactions are to be regulated through presentation of recognition sites for membrane-bound receptors on the target endothelial cell surfaces, and through control of the identity and frequency of protein-bound recognition sites. In concert with complementary methods described elsewhere in this volume, artificial ECM proteins may provide a route to compliant, thromboresistant grafts subject to resorption and remodeling, and ultimately may play a role in defining strategies for regeneration of healthy vascular tissue.

References

1. Langer RW, Vacanti J. Tissue engineering. Science 1993; 260:920-926.
2. Greisler HP. New Biologic and Synthetic Vascular Prostheses. Austin, TX: R.G. Landes Co., 1991.
3. Rumisek JD, Wade CE, Brooks DE et al. Heat-denatured albumin-coated dacron vascular grafts; physical characteristics and in vivo performance. J Vasc Surg 1986; 4:136-143.
4. Drury JK, Ashton TR, Cunningham JD et al. Experimental and clinical experience with a gelatin impregnated dacron prosthesis. Ann Vasc Surg 1987; 1:542-547.
5. Freischlag JA, Moore WS. Clinical experience with a collagen-impregnated knitted dacron vascular graft. Ann Vasc Surg 1990; 4:449-454.
6. Yates SG, Barros-D'Sa ABB, Berger K et al. The preclotting of porous arterial prostheses. Ann Surg 1978; 188:611-622.
7. Gray JL, Kang SS, Zenni GC et al. FGF-1 affixation stimulates ePTFE endothelialization without intimal hyperplasia. J Surg Res 1994; 57:596-612.
8. Williams SK. Endothelial cell transplantation. Cell Transplantation 1995; 4:401-410.
9. Zilla P, Deutsch M, Meinhart J et al. Clinical in vitro endothelialization of femoropopliteal bypass graft: An actuarial follow-up over three years. J Vasc Surg 1994; 19:540-548.
10. Zilla P, Deutsch M, Meinhart M, Fischlein T, Hofmann G. Long-term effects of clinical in vitro endothelialization on grafts. J Vasc Surg 1997; 25:1110-1112.
11. Bevilacqua MP, Pober JS, Majeau GR et al. Recombinant tumor necrosis factor induces procoagulant activity in cultured human vascular endothelium. Characterization and comparison with the actions of interleukin I. Proc Nat Acad Sci USA 1986; 83:4533.
12. Colucci M, Balcon GI, Lorenzet R. Cultured human endothelial cells generate tissue factor in response to endotoxin. J Clin Investi 1983; 71:1893.
13. DiCorleto PE, Bowen-Pope D. Cultured endothelial cells produce a platelet-derived growth factor-like protein. Proc Nat Acad Sci USA 1983; 80:1919-1923.
14. Fox P.L, DiCorleto PE. Regulation of production of a platelet-derived growth factor-like protein in cultured bovine aortic endothelial cells. J Cell Physiol 1984; 121:298-308.
15. Ross R, Raines E, Bowen-Pope D. Growth factors from platelets, monocytes, and endothelium: Their role in cell proliferation. Ann NY Acad Sci 1982; 397:18-24.
16. Clowes AW, Kirkman RD, Reidy MA. Mechanism of arterial graft healing: Rapid transmural capillary ingrowth provides a source of intimal endothelium and smooth muscle in porous PTFE prostheses. Am J Pathol 1986; 123:220-230.
17. Urry D.W, Luan C-H, Harris CM et al. Protein-based materials with a profound range of properties and applications: The elastin ΔT_t hydrophobic paradigm. In:McGrath, K, Kaplan, D, eds. Protein-Based Materials. Boston, MA:Birkhauser, 1997.
18. Humphries JJ, Akiyama SK, Komoriya A et al. Identification of an alternatively spliced site in human plasma fibronectin that mediates cell type-specific adhesion. J Cell Biol 1986; 103:2637-2647.

19. Hubbell JA, Massia SP, Desai NP et al. Endothelial cell-selective materials for tissue engineering in the vascular graft via a new receptor. Biotechnology 1991; 9:568-572.

20. Ross MH, Romrell LJ, Kaye GI. Histology: A Text and Atlas. 3rd ed. Baltimore, MD:Williams & Wilkins, 1995.

21. Chandran KB. Cardiovascular Biomechanics. New York: University Press, 1992.

22. Greisler HP, Joyce KA, Kim DU et al. Spatial and temporal changes in compliance following implantation of bioresorbable vascular grafts. J Biomed Mat Res 1992; 26:1449-1461.

23. Kinley CE, Marble AE. Compliance: A continuing problem with vascular grafts. J Cardiovasc Surg 1980; 21:163-170.

24. Zwolak RM, Adams MC, Clowes AW. Kinetics of vein graft hyperplasia: Association with tangential stress. J Vasc Surg 1987; 5:126-136.

25. Clowes AW, Reidy MA, Clowes MM. Kinetics of cellular proliferation after arterial injury. Smooth muscle growth in the absence of endothelium. Lab Invest 1983; 49(3):327-333.

26. Urry DW, Nicol A, McPherson DT et al. Properties, preparations and applications of bioelastic materials. In:Handbook of Biomaterials and Applications. New York:Marcel Dekker, 1995.

27. Urry DW, Parker TM, Reid MC et al. Biocompatibility of the bioelastic materials, poly(GVGVP) and its γ-irradiation cross-linked matrix: Summary of generic biological test results. J Bioac Comp Poly (1991); 6:263-282.

28. Nicol A, Gowda DC, Parker TM et al. Cell adhesive properties of bioelastic materials containing cell attachment sequences. In:Gebelein, C & Carraher, C, eds. Biotechnology and Bioactive Polymers:Plenum Press, NY, 1994.

29. Wayner EA, Garcia-Pardo A, Humphries MJ et al. Identification and characterization of the T lymphocyte adhesion receptor for an alternative cell attachment domain (CS-1) in plasma fibronectin. J Cell Biol 1989; 109(3):1321-1330.

30. Garcia-Pardo A, Wayner EA, Carter WG et al. Human B lymphocytes define an alternative mechanism of adhesion to fibronectin. The interaction of the α4β1 integrin with the LHGPEILDVPST sequence of the type III connecting segment is sufficient to promote cell attachment. J Immunol 1990; 144:3361-3366.

31. Guan J-L, Hynes RO. Lymphoid cells recognize an alternatively spliced segment of fibronectin via the integrin receptor α4β1. Cell 1990; 60:53-60.

32. Mould AP, Wheldon LA, Komoriya A et al. Affinity chromatographic isolation of the melanoma adhesion receptor for the IIICS region of fibronectin and its identification as the integrin α4β1. J Biol Chem 1990; 265(7):4020-4024.

33. Mould AP, Komoriya A, Yamada KM et al. The CS5 peptide is a second site in the IIICS region of fibronectin recognized by the integrin α4β1. Inhibition of α4β1 function by RGD peptide homologues. J Biol Chem 1991; 266(6):3579-3585.

34. Mould AP, Humphries MJ. Identification of a novel recognition sequence for the integrin α4β1 in the COOH-terminal heparin-binding domain of fibronectin. EMBO J 1991; 10(13):4089-4095.

35. Pierschbacher MD, Ruoslahti E. Cell attachment activity of fibronectin can be duplicated by small synthetic fragments of the molecule. Nature 1984; 309:30-33.

36. Yamada KM, Kennedy DW. Dualistic nature of adhesive protein function: Fibronectin and its biologically active peptide fragments can autoinhibit fibronectin function. J Cell Bio 1984; 99:29-36.

37. Massia SP, Hubbell JA. Vascular endothelial cell adhesion and spreading promoted by the peptide REDV of the IIICS region of plasma fibronectin is mediated by integrin α4β1. J Biol Chem 1992; 267(20):14019-14026.

38. Krejchi MT, Atkins EDT, Waddon AJ et al. Chemical sequence control of β-sheet assembly in macromolecular crystals of periodic polypeptides. Science 1994; 265:1427-1432.

39. Parkhe A, Fournier MJ, Mason TL et al. Determination of the chain folding pattern in the crystalline domains of the repetitive polypeptide {(AlaGly)$_3$GluGly(GlyAla)$_3$GluGly}$_{10}$ by FTIR studies of its blends with a ^{13}C enriched analogue. Macromolecules 1993; 26:6691-6693.

40. McGrath KP, Fournier MJ, Mason TL et al. Genetically-directed syntheses of new polymeric materials. Synthesis and expression of a family of artificial genes encoding proteins with repeating -(AlaGly)$_3$ProGluGly- elements. J Am Chem Soc 1992; 114:727-733.

41. Creel HS, Fournier MJ, Mason TL et al. Genetically-directed syntheses of new polymeric materials. Efficient expression of a monodisperse copolypeptide containing fourteen tandemly repeated -(AlaGly)$_4$ProGluGly- elements. Macromolecules 1991; 24:1213-1214.

42. Zhang G, Fournier MJ, Mason TL et al. Biosynthesis of monodisperse derivatives of poly(α,L-glutamic acid): Model rod-like polymers. Macromolecules 1992; 25:3601-3603.

43. Yu SM, Conticello V, Kayser C et al. Smectic ordering in solutions and films of a monodisperse derivative of poly(γ-benzyl α,L-glutamate). Nature 1997; 389:167-170.

44. Dougherty MJ, Kothakota S, Mason TL et al. Synthesis of a genetically engineered repetitive polypeptide containing periodic selenomethionine residues. Macromolecules 1993; 26:1779-1781.

45. Yoshikawa E, Fournier MJ, Mason TL et al. Genetically engineered fluoropolymers. Synthesis of a repetitive polypeptide containing p-fluorophenylalanine residues. Macromolecules 1994; 27:5471-5475.

46. Kothakota S, Mason TL, Fournier MJ et al. Biosynthesis of a periodic protein containing 3-thienylalanine: A step toward genetically engineered conducting polymers. J Am Chem Soc 1995; 117:536-537.

47. Deming TJ, Fournier MJ, Mason TL et al. Biosynthetic incorporation and selective chemical modification of olefinic functionality in genetically engineered polymers. J Macromol Sci-Pure Appl Chem 1997; A34(10):2143-2150.

48. Deming TJ, Fournier MJ, Mason TL et al. Structural modification of a periodic polypeptide through biosynthetic replacement of proline with azetidine-2-carboxylic acid. Macromolecules 1996; 29(5):1442-1444.

49. Studier FW, Rosenberg AH, Dunn, AH et al. Use of T7 RNA polymerase to direct expression of cloned genes. Meth Enzymol 1991; 185:60-68.

50. Urry DW, Gowda C, Parker TM et al. Hydrophobicity scale for proteins based on inverse temperature transitions. Biopolymers 1992; 32:1243-1250.

Matrix Engineering

―――――――――――――― CHAPTER 54 ――――――――――――――

Cell-Extracellular Matrix Interactions Relevant to Vascular Tissue Engineering

Stephen P. Massia

Introduction

The interaction between cells and extracellular surfaces plays a major role in determining cellular behavior in tissues and on biomaterials. These interactions modulate many aspects of cell behavior, including adhesion, spreading, migration, proliferation, differentiation, and metabolism. In the fields of biomaterials and tissue engineering, a fundamental understanding of cell surface interactions is critical for developing new methods that precisely control cell interactions at the cell-biomaterial interface. Enhancement of tissue cell adhesion to implanted biomaterials would facilitate tissue adhesion/integration at the tissue-biomaterial interface. In contrast, the reduction of cell adhesion to implanted biomaterials is desirable for limiting cell-mediated events such as thrombosis and macrophage activation on biomaterial surfaces, which often result in biomaterial implant failure. It is also desirable for tissue engineered implants to promote specific cell-biomaterial interactions which facilitate tissue regeneration/repair. Tissue engineered devices in the form of prefabricated biohybrid tissue constructs require the appropriate interactions of transplanted cells with biomaterial scaffolds to initiate extracellular matrix (ECM) synthesis and deposition as well as other activities which promote biohybrid tissue formation in vitro prior to implantation in vivo.

Two major approaches for developing materials which elicit precisely controlled cellular interactions have emerged. One involves fabricating implants, scaffolds, etc. from natural biomaterials such as collagen where the base material has intrinsic and specific biological activities which influence cellular interactions. The major disadvantages of using natural biomaterials is that they generally have a largely unmodifiable and limited range of physico-chemical properties and can be difficult to isolate and characterize. The second approach for improving the control of cell-material interactions is to use synthetic materials which have surface immobilized, biologically active molecules and biologically active surface microtextrue. This methodology takes advantage of the inexpensive manufacturing costs for synthetic material-based devices and exploits specific biological activities to modulate cellular interactions for improved biocompatibility and biohybrid tissue formation. Essentially, these types of surface modifications on synthetic implant materials are attempting to create a biomimetic surface with surface physicochemical properties that more closely match those of the ECM in the tissues where the synthetic material will be implanted. This review will focus on the biology of cell-ECM interactions and how they are utilized in developing biomimetic surfaces on synthetic biomaterials. The role of these technologies in developing vascular implants with improved biocompatibility will also be discussed.

Cell-Extracellular Surface Interactions at the Molecular Level

Cell Adhesion to Solid Substrates

Mammalian cells in tissues are anchorage dependent, having a fundamental requirement to attach to solid components in the extracellular matrix to remain viable and grow.[1-4] Consequently, cells which are disrupted from tissues and cultured in vitro, or cells within tissues or body fluids in vivo which contact implanted materials, readily attach to the available solid substrate (e.g., tissue culture plastics, biomaterials) in order to survive.[1-6] Following the adsorption of serum- or cell-borne proteins, cell adhesion on a solid substrate progresses through the following paradigm (Fig. 54.1):[5]

1. Initial contact of the cell with the material;
2. Formation of adhesive bonds between cell surface receptors and ligands within adsorbed adhesion proteins; and

3. Cytoskeletal reorganization and a progressive flattening or spreading of the cell on the material surface to increase its attachment strength.

It is well established that cell adhesion and spreading on biomaterials in vitro and in vivo occurs via adsorbed cell adhesion-promoting extracellular matrix (ECM) proteins.[5,7-9] Cell culture and implanted materials quickly adsorb proteins, including ECM proteins, from serum, cellular microexudates (cell culture), and tissue fluids (implants). If sufficient ECM cell adhesive proteins adsorb to a material surface in a conformational state that is biologically active in promoting cell adhesion, cell interaction and spreading will occur on that surface. ECM proteins that are important for cell adhesion to biomaterials include fibronectin, vitronectin, and fibrinogen from cell culture serum and tissue fluids.

Cell-ECM Adhesion Receptors

Most cell-adhesive interactions with ECM proteins occur via the family of cell surface receptors known as the

Fig. 54.1. Progression of anchorage-dependent mammalian cell adhesion. (A) Initial contact of cell with solid substrate. (B) Formation of bonds between cell surface receptors and cell adhesion ligands. (C) Cytoskeletal reorganization with progressive spreading of the cell on the substrate for increased attachment strength.

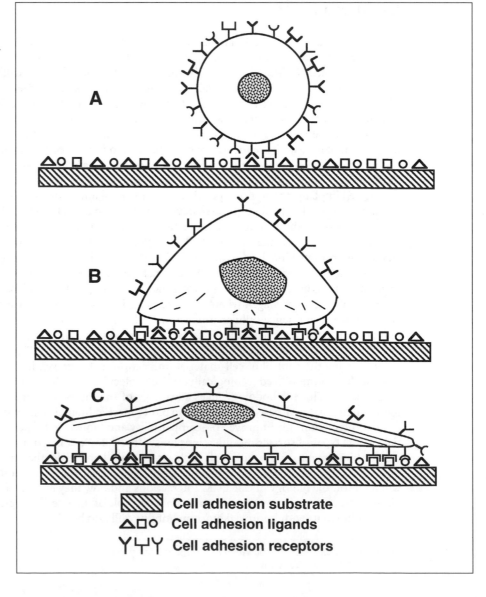

integrins. Integrins are a superfamily of transmembrane glycoprotein adhesion receptors consisting of a noncovalently linked α and β subunit.[10-13] At least 17 α and 8 β subunits have been described, with resulting combinations of over 21 functional integrins with varying ligand specificity.[13] Integrins bind to ECM proteins via cell binding domains, and rather small polypeptide sequences within these domains promote integrin binding with an affinity that is nearly as high as in the intact molecule.[10-13] The tripeptide RGD is a ubiquitous recognition sequence that binds to most integrins and is found within the cell binding domain of many cell adhesion ECM proteins.[10-13] Binding of integrins to RGD and other related recognition sequences results in a cascade of events that promotes cell-matrix adhesion interactions that are stable in stationary cells, e.g., epithelial cells on basement membranes, and are transient in motile, migratory cells. Although this review will focus on integrin-ECM interactions, there are many nonintegrin cell-ECM binding receptors including cell surface proteoglycans (syndecans),[14] hyaluronan receptors (CD44, RHAMM and ICAM 1,[15] 67 kDa laminin-binding proteins,[16] annexin II,[17] and receptor type protein tyrosine phosphatase β.[18]

Integrin-Mediated Cytoplasmic Activities

Following ligand-binding, integrins undergo conformational changes, cluster into aggregates, and form adhesion plaques or focal contacts. It is well documented in many studies that integrin clustering is required for initiating intracellular activities.[13,19] Integrin-mediated cytoplasmic functions within adhesion plaques can be categorized into two experimentally separable types:

1. Cytoskeletal organization and establishment of mechanical linkages between ligand-bound integrins and cytoskeletal structures; and
2. Tyrosine kinase-mediated signal transduction.

Associated with integrin-cytoskeleton linkages are cytoskeletal complexes that consist of clustered integrins, several cytoplasmic proteins, and actin microfilament bundles. Structurally and biochemically distinct multi-protein signaling complexes can form within adhesion plaques and are associated with signal transduction activities.

Models of the structural architecture of cytoskeletal complexes, which form on the cytoplasmic side of focal adhesions, have been developed based on in vitro protein binding assays (Fig. 54.2). These models show how proteins may link with each other within cytoskeletal complexes. These structural arrangements are considered models because many of the protein-protein linkages have not been demonstrated in living cells.[20] Talin is a major protein of cytoskeletal complexes and was the first reported integrin-binding cytoplasmic protein.[21] Talin also binds to actin[22] and to vinculin.[23] Vinculin apparently serves as a structural hub for cytoskeletal complexes, since it can bind to many other cytoskeletal complex proteins. Studies have shown that vinculin can bind to α-actinin,[24] paxillin,[25] tensin,[26] and possibly actin via a cryptic binding site.[27] α-actinin, which crosslinks actin microfilaments to form microfilament bundles, has been shown to directly bind to the cytoplasmic tails of integrin β subunits.[28] With at least two integrin-binding cytoplasmic proteins (talin and α-actinin) and other various interconnecting proteins, e.g., vinculin, an indirect linkage between ECM-bound integrins and the cytoskeleton is formed via cytoskeletal complexes.

Unlike many other types of transmembrane cell surface receptors, the cytoplasmic domains of integrins do not have enzymatic activity. Therefore, integrin-mediated intracellular signal transduction depends on recruited, enzymatically active signal transduction molecules. Integrin clustering has been shown to induce phosphorylation of tyrosine residues of a number of proteins, even though integrins do not intrinsically have tyrosine kinase activity.[29] One protein that is rapidly phosphorylated and localized to focal adhesions is focal adhesion kinase (FAK or pp125[FAK]).[30,31] The exact mechanism for clustered integrin-mediated FAK phosphorylation is not known. Studies demonstrating direct binding of FAK to the β_1 subunit cytoplasmic domain[32] suggest that changes in integrin aggregation and/or conformation alters FAK to promote autophosphorylation, which upregulates the enzymatic activity of FAK and triggers

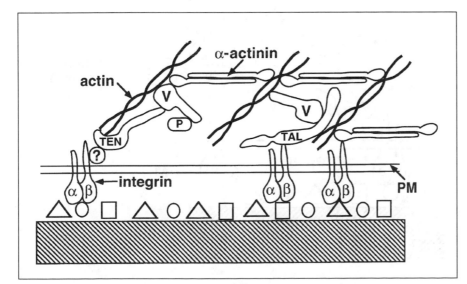

Fig. 54.2. Multi-protein cytoskeletal complexes within focal contacts—mechanical linkages between ligand-bound integrins and cytoskeletal structures. Three different linkages are depicted here: (Left) The integrin cytoplasmic domain binds to an unknown (?) protein that also binds tensin. Tensin links to actin filaments and vinculin; (Center) The integrin cytoplasmic domain binds to talin which links to actin-bound vinculin; (Right) The integrin cytoplasmic domain binds to α-actinin which crosslinks actin microfilaments into bundles. V = vinculin; TEN = tensin; P = paxillin; TAL = talin; PM = plasma membrane.

further downstream signal transduction phosphorylation events.[33] Activated FAK phosphorylates many focal contact proteins, which generally induces them to form protein-protein bonds and facilitate multi-protein complex formation.[34] Similar to models of cytoskeletal complexes described in the previous paragraph, models for an integrin-mediated signal transduction complex have been developed from in vitro studies. Following integrin-mediated autophosphorylation, FAK phosphorylates paxillin, which activates its SH2 and SH3 (Src homology 2 and 3 binding domains. The signal transducing tyrosine kinase c-Csk readily binds to the paxillin SH2 domain[35] and c-Src binds to SH3.[36] GRB-2, which promotes MAP kinase activation, has been shown to bind to phosphorylated FAK and to c-Src.[37] This finding suggests that GRB-2 can associate with focal adhesion signal transduction complexes to couple MAP kinase-mediated signal transduction to integrins. In growth factor-mediated signal transduction pathways, MAP kinase has been shown to translocate to the nucleus and play a direct role in gene regulatory pathways.[38] Similar signaling mechanisms may occur in integrin signal transduction complexes. Other studies have shown that a G protein γ subunit and protein kinase c type 3 (PKC type 3) bind and localize to focal adhesions, suggesting that activated integrins possibly utilize G protein and PKC type 3-mediated signal transduction pathways coordinately with or independently of tyrosine kinase pathways.[39,40] Integrin binding has also been shown to promote signal transduction-associated events such as increased cytoplasmic levels of PIP_2[41] and Ca^{2+},[42] as well as increased cytoplasmic pH.[43] Integrin signal transduction complexes potentially provide a mechanism where integrin-mediated signaling could be transmitted to the nucleus and invoke specific changes in gene transcription patterns that

influence a broad range of cellular activities beyond cell adhesion (Fig. 54.3).

Biomimetic Cell-Adhesive Biomaterials

Controlling Cell Adhesion on Biomaterials

For both tissue engineers and biomaterial scientists, the precise control of cell interactions with biomaterials is desirable. The tissue engineer requires the interaction of specific cell types with materials in implants and devices designed for tissue ingrowth and regeneration. In biohybrid tissue constructs, the tissue engineer seeds specific cells in biomaterial scaffolds in vitro and requires cell-biomaterial interactions which promote appropriate ECM deposition and assembly for tissue formation. The biomaterial scientist requires selective attachment of tissue cells to implanted materials so that tissue adhesion and integration is optimized and inflammatory cell-mediated encapsulation is limited at the tissue-biomaterial interface. In order to achieve high precision control of cell adhesive and functional responses to biomaterials, protein adsorption has to be precisely controlled as well. Protein adsorption is an exceedingly complex phenomenon, and, correspondingly, it is very difficult to control.[44-46] The main difficulty is in controlling the specificity of protein adsorption, e.g., it is difficult to selectively promote the adsorption of cell adhesion proteins over the adsorption of nonadhesive proteins. A second difficulty with the adsorbed protein layer is its lack of stability to denaturation and proteolysis, which may affect the long term performance of implanted biomaterials and tissue engineered devices. [44-46] Therefore, a material surface that promotes cell adhesion and spreading independently of protein adsorption would be more controllable and beneficial in designing tissue engineered biomaterials. Essentially, this material sur-

Fig. 54.3. Signal transduction complexes in focal contacts. FAK binds to integrin cytoplasmic domains and to paxillin. c-Csk and c-Src bind to FAK-activated paxillin and GRB-2 binds to c-Src and FAK. Collectively this protein complex triggers signal transduction via MAP kinase-dependent pathways. Protein kinase c type 3 can bind to integrin-bound FAK and potentially promote specific signal transduction pathways. Similarly bound G protein γ subunits may link integrin activation with G protein signal transduction. V = vinculin; TEN = tensin; P = paxillin; PKC3 = protein kinase c type 3; Gγ = G protein γ subunits.

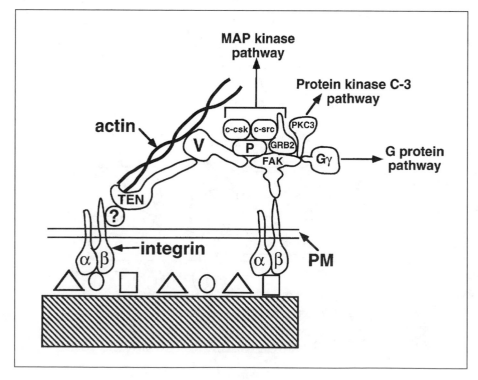

face would mimic physicochemical features of tissue ECM adequately enough to intrinsically promote cell interactions, circumventing the requirement for adsorbed ECM proteins.

Mimicking the Extracellular Matrix on Biomaterial Surfaces

The extracellular matrix (ECM) of soft tissues is a complex composite material consisting of dense fibrillar cable-like structures (e.g., type I collagen fibers) for rigid mechanical support and a loose, more compliant gelatinous interstitial matrix consisting of glycoproteins, proteoglycans, and other components which provide a protective cushion against harmful external mechanical forces. The complex three dimensional arrangement of fibrillar and interstitial ECM components provides topographical and biochemical cues for cell orientation and guidance in tissues. Therefore, the surfaces of synthetic biomaterials could potentially mimic the ECM if biochemical and biologically relevant topographical cues were incorporated into the material surfaces (Fig. 54.4). Biochemical cues could be mimicked using surface immobilized biologically active molecules, and biomimetic topographical cues could be provided by high precision surface microtexturing.

Surface Immobilized Biologically Active Molecules on Biomaterials

Many methodologies for designing biomimetic, adhesion-promoting materials have been developed to circumvent the requirement for protein adsorption by covalently supplying the substrates with stable, synthetic ligands for cell surface adhesion.[47-82] These adhesion ligand peptide-grafted substrates have been utilized as simplified models to investigate molecular aspects of cell-ECM interactions. One of the earliest described methods developed polyacrylamide substrates with surface-immobilized RGD peptides[47] and quantitatively evaluated tumor cell haptotactic responses to surface concentration gradients of immobilized RGD peptides.[48] Silanized glass substrates containing surface immobilized adhesion peptides were developed and utilized to quantitatively determine the minimal density and spacing of surface immobilized RGD peptides for maximal cell spreading, cytoskeletal development, and focal contact formation.[51,55] Although complete cell spreading was observed at a minimal RGD surface concentration of 1 fmol/cm^2, focal contacts were scarce and the cytoskeletal structures were poorly developed. When the RGD surface concentration was increased to 10 fmol/cm^2, focal contacts and a fully developed cytoskeleton was observed in all spread cells.[55] These

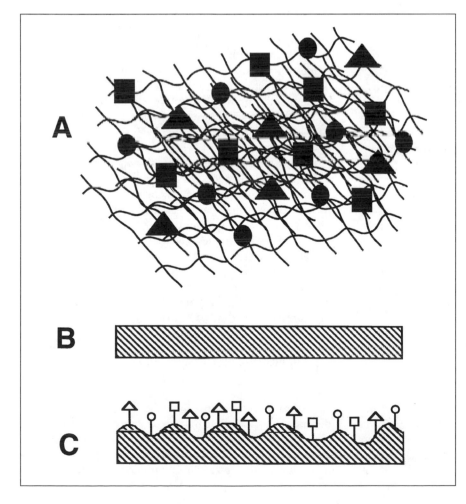

Fig. 54.4. (A) ECM structure in tissues with a fibrillar web-like network of collagens and other fibrillar ECM proteins. Interspersed are cell adhesion ECM proteins (solid shapes) which bind to the ECM fibrils and promote cell adhesion. (B) A featureless synthetic biomaterial implant. (C) A synthetic biomaterial with an ECM-like biomimetic surface. This surface contains two fundamental ECM features which influence cell interactions: immobilized cell adhesion ligands (geometric shapes connected to the surface) and microtextrue (bumps on the surface).

results suggested that RGD is a sufficient signal for promoting a complete and maximal cell adhesive response when the ligand is tethered to the material surface. Consequently, cell surface receptor interactions with tethered RGD ligands generated the contractile force necessary to produce normal focal contact and cytoskeleton formation. The value of 10 fmol/cm^2 required for maximal cell spreading, focal contact, and cytoskeleton formation corresponded to an average spacing of 140 nm between RGD ligands, or 10 integrin widths. It was also observed that covalently immobilized RGD peptide promotes cell adhesion and spreading, predominantly via integrin $\alpha_v\beta_3$.[55] It was suggested in these studies that covalent immobilization of RGD peptide rendered it conformationally constrained with highest affinity for integrin $\alpha_v\beta_3$. Other studies which demonstrated preferential binding of cyclic, conformationally constrained RGD peptides to integrin $\alpha_v\beta_3$ supported this hypothesis.[83] Similar peptide-grafted glass substrates were utilized to characterize nonintegrin interactions to the laminin-based cell adhesion ligand YIGSR.[63] Cell attachment, spreading, and stress fiber formation were observed on these substrates and were mediated by the 67 kDa laminin receptor independently of integrins. The 67 kDa receptor was also observed to colocalize with vinculin and α-actinin in focal adhesions.[63] Other studies of cell interactions with peptide-grafted glass substrates compared cell migration on glass versus peptide-grafted glass substrates and demonstrated that cell motility was significantly decreased on RGD peptide-grafted substrates.[81] These results suggested that cell attachment on RGD substrates was stronger and more inhibitory to cell migration (more resistant to disruption of cell adhesion sites) than glass without surface-coupled peptides. Another study using similar glass substrates quantitated and compared the attachment strength of endothelial cells on RGD peptide-grafted glass versus glass with adsorbed fibronectin and observed stronger cell attachment on peptide-grafted substrates.[82] Overall, substrates containing surface immobilized cell adhesion peptides have been utilized extensively as simplified models to isolate and study cell adhesive interactions at the molecular level.

RGD and other cell-adhesive peptides have been surface immobilized on a wide variety of polymeric biomaterials to enhance their biocompatibility by promoting cell adhesion in a more controlled manner than relying on random protein adsorption. These methods have been developed for many biomedical polymers, including polyethylene terephthalate,[54,66] poly tetrafluoroethylene and related polymeric fluorocarbons,[54,77,78] polyurethanes,[60,69,75] polyethylene,[62] cellulose,[73] hyaluronic acid,[80] poly amino acids,[70,76] and crosslinked dextran.[74] Cell-resistant polymeric materials which support minimal cell adhesion have been utilized for peptide immobilization to promote highly specific cell-ligand interactions with a very low background adhesive signal from adsorbed serum- and cell-borne proteins. These materials include polyethylene glycol,[72] nonhydrogel networks of polyacrylate/polyethylene glycol,[71] polyacrylamide,[47,48] and polyvinyl alcohol.[53] These materials provide maximal control of cell interactions because the surface immobilized biological molecule is the predominant determinant for cellular responses to these materials.

Biomaterial Surface Microtexturing to Mimic ECM Topography in Tissues

The cellular response to attachment substrate topography was first described in 1912 where the migration of cultured cells on spider webs was observed to be guided by spider web filaments.[84] More studies confirmed that surface topography influenced cell orientation on solid substrates and the term "contact guidance" was introduced to describe this phenomenon.[85] Surface topography became an issue in soft tissue biomaterial implant biocompatibility studies because many researchers have demonstrated a positive correlation between capsule thickness (biocompatibilty) and tissue-implant interfacial motion.[86] It was realized that surface topography could be utilized to promote tissue interdigitation or anchorage to reduce interfacial motion. An early study evaluated the effect of surface topography on soft tissue responses to synthetic materials in vivo by implanting filter membranes with different uniform pore sizes subcutaneously in rats and evaluating the tissue response at 6 weeks postimplantation. Excellent tissue attachment was observed without signs of inflammation when pore sizes were 1-3 μm. Pore sizes above and below this range exhibited symptoms of a chronic inflammatory response, e.g., diminished tissue attachment and thick granulation capsules.[87] It was concluded from these studies that the surface topography created by the 1-3 μm pores in membrane filters provided cellular cues to promote tissue attachment and improved biocompatibility. Another study, using the same in vivo model evaluated the effect of the pore size of PTFE membranes on neovascularization at the membrane-tissue interface. This study found that the extent of vascularization at the membrane-tissue interface was 80-100 times higher in membranes with 5 μm pores versus membranes with 0.02 μm pores.[88] This study provided further evidence of how surface topographical feature size can influence the biocompatibility of implanted materials.

Many in vitro studies have investigated how surface microtextrue influences cellular behavior to correlate with in vivo studies which have evaluated surface texture effects on soft tissue biocompatibility. Photo-etching and high precision milling techniques were developed to precisely control all geometrical aspects of surface topography down to the nanometer range.[86] In one report, a simplified model for studying surface topography effects on cell interactions was developed utilizing materials that were fabricated using high precision methods. On this simple topography, it was observed that the response of cells in vitro to a single step on a material surface was cell type dependent. Neuronal cell and fibroblast motility were observed to decrease with increasing step height. Neutrophil migration, however, was observed to not change in response to step height changes.[89] Since the cellular response to surface topography is cell type dependent, it is possible that specific microtextured feature sizes may differentially influence tissue cell and inflammatory cell interactions with materials to maximize tissue adherence and minimize the inflammatory response. Using high precision microtextured surfaces with regular repeated topographical features, the effect of feature dimensions on fibroblast contact guidance was assessed in vitro. It was observed that repeat spacing had a minor and inversely proportional effect on cell alignment, whereas groove depth had a more significant role in determining cell alignment, which correlated positively with increased depth.[90] In a study examining cell type dependent responses to repeating alternating 1 μm grooves and 1 μm ridges, keratinocytes and neutrophils were observed to exhibit no contact guidance, a 20% response was observed with monocytes and macrophages, and a 100% response was observed with fibroblasts.[91] Similar studies showed that epithelial cells did not exhibit strong contact guidance on microtextured surfaces[92] and that they also responded differently than fibroblasts in vivo as well.[93] In studies comparing fibroblast (model soft tissue cell) and macrophage (model inflammatory cell) responses to microtextured features in vitro, microtextured silicone discs were prepared with multiple surface discontinuities of wells and pillars with various dimensions, repeat spacings, and 90° surface contour angles. These studies revealed that metabolism, spreading, and migration of fibroblasts and macrophages were altered when they were cultured on substrata with texture feature dimensions ranging from 1-3 μm in width.[94,95] Specifically, fibroblast spreading was observed to increase while macrophage spreading/activation decreased in response to this size range of surface feature dimensions when compared to untextured surfaces. Smaller or larger features were observed to have no change in cell responses when compared to untextured surfaces. When these textured silicone materials containing 2 μm wide square wells with 0.5 μm depth were implanted subcutaneously in rats, a minimal inflammatory response was observed. In contrast, smooth silicone materials with the same chemical composition as the textured materials were observed to promote a strong inflammatory response with encapsulation.[86] Therefore, it was concluded that increased fibroblast adhesion and decreased macrophage activation in vitro correlated well with the increased tissue attachment and decreased inflammatory response observed in vivo. Similar results were observed with materials having a wide variety of chemical compositions, including metals, suggesting that surface microtextrue effects on cell and tissue responses were independent of surface chemistry.[86] Overall, these studies indicate a range of topographical parameters that appear to minimize inflammatory responses. Optimal topographical features for maximal cell and tissue attachment include ridges of 1-3 μm width with grooves 0.5 μm in depth, uniform distribution of features, and sharp feature edges with 90° surface contour angles.

At optimal surface microtextrue dimensions using alternating ridge and groove patterns, fibroblast interactions have been characterized at the subcellular level. Transmission electron microscopy studies have shown that the plasma membrane of adherent fibroblasts in contact with microtextured surfaces frequently conforms to the textured feature to interlock with the material surface.[96] Several studies have shown that microtextrue-dependent orientation/guidance of cells positively correlates with an alignment of cytoskeletal elements including microtubules, actin microfilaments, and focal contacts.[96-100] Surface microtexturing has also been shown to alter cell function, including fibronectin mRNA level, mRNA stability, secretion and assembly by fibroblasts.[101] Another study of surface microtopography and cell function demonstrated that surface microtextrue promoted osteogenesis.[100] These studies further characterize the effects of surface microtextrue on cell-material interactions. Overall, surface microtextrue is a fundamental surface property that influences cell behavior and can be exploited to modulate cell-material interactions.

Cell-ECM Interactions in Vascular Biology

ECM Modulation of Smooth Muscle Cell Function

The two major cell types of vascular tissues are smooth muscle and endothelial cells. In the normal adult arterial wall, the predominant phenotype or functional state of the medial smooth muscle cell (SMC) population is predominantly nonproliferative and contractile.[102-104] These muscle-like contractile cells contract and relax coordinately in the arterial wall in response to chemical and mechanical stimuli to control blood pressure and flow.[102-104] Following mechanical injury to arterial wall, a large population of medial SMCs will undergo a phenotypic modulation from the contractile state to a highly proliferative synthetic state in which extracellular matrix (ECM) proteins are synthesized and secreted into the media to repair injury-induced structural damage in the arterial wall ECM (Fig. 54.5).[105-115] In addition to medial repair activity in response to injury, synthetic medial SMCs become motile and migrate from the media toward the arterial lumen to form a neointimal layer on the luminal surface of the artery wall.[105-115] Neointima development and progressive neointimal thickening occurs via endoluminal accumulation of proliferating SMCs with coordinate ECM deposition.[105-115] In the clinical setting, neointimal thickening of coronary arteries in response to mechanical injury to the artery wall via balloon angioplasty or other percutaneous revascularization procedures is problematic when the extent of thickening is enough to severely reduce the initial therapeutically beneficial large dilated lumen.[105-110] To date, restenosis due to extensive neointimal thickening following balloon angioplasty or other catheter-based nonsurgical revascularization procedures occurs at a rate of 30-50%.[105-110] In vascular and cardiovascular surgery, a synthetic small diameter vascular graft that remains patent after implantation has not been developed because injury-induced thrombosis and neointimal hyperplasia causes decreased patency and occlusion at anastomotic sites.[111-115]

Unlike phenotypically contractile medial SMCs in the normal arterial wall, synthetic neointimal SMCs in the injured arterial wall synthesize and deposit large quantities of ECM proteins including collagens,[116-119] fibronectin,[116,118] elastin,[119,120] proteoglycans,[117,119,121,122] tenascin[123,124] and thrombospondin.[125] Tenascin and thrombospondin expression in SMCs is greatly increased during postinjury neointima development and accumulates at high levels in the neointimal ECM.[123-125] Unlike the other ECM proteins

Fig. 54.5. Neointimal hyperplasia progresses in vascular tissues in response to injury. Injury-activated medial SMCs migrate into the vessel lumen and form a thick neointimal layer that constricts or narrows the lumen. When small diameter synthetic vascular grafts are implanted, mechanical injury to adjacent vascular tissues promotes hyperplastic growth into the graft lumen that results in restricted or occluded blood flow.

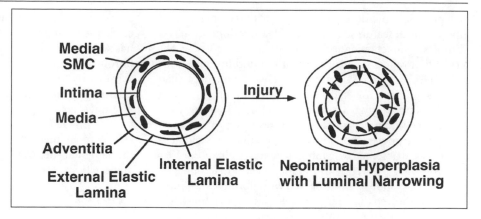

secreted by neointimal SMCs, tenascin and thrombospondin have cell adhesive and anti-adhesive properties and have been implicated as specialized ECM proteins for events such as tissue regeneration and wound repair.[126,127] Tenascin is of particular interest in vascular injury, since its expression in the vessel wall is induced only after mechanical injury or exposure to growth factors that are released in the vessel wall following injury.[123,124] It has been speculated that tenascin facilitates SMC migration and neointima formation in vivo[124] by creating an ECM of intermediate attachment strength that maximizes SMC migration.[129] In vitro studies have shown that exogenously added soluble tenascin enhances injury-induced SMC migration.[130]

The ECM plays an active role in the phenotypic modulation of SMCs. In vitro studies have shown that SMCs grown on fibronectin- and RGD peptide-coated materials quickly transform from the contractile phenotype to synthetic state.[131,132] Conversely, similar studies on laminin- and type IV collagen-coated substrates have shown that the contractile phenotype is conserved.[133]

The interaction of SMCs with the ECM occurs predominantly via several members of the integrin superfamily of extracellular matrix adhesion receptors.[12] Ligand affinity chromatography and immunoprecipitation analyses of SMC extracts have identified several β_1 integrins which bind to a variety of ECM proteins: $\alpha_5\beta_1$, $\alpha_v\beta_1$, and $\alpha_3\beta_1$ bind to fibronectin; $\alpha_1\beta_1$ and $\alpha_7\beta_1$ bind to laminin; $\alpha_v\beta_1$ binds to vitronectin; $\alpha_1\beta_1$ and $\alpha_2\beta_1$ bind to type I collagen; $\alpha_1\beta_1$ binds to type IV collagen.[128] Integrin $\alpha_v\beta_3$ was observed to bind to several ECM proteins including fibronectin, laminin, vitronectin, type I collagen, and type IV collagen.[128] Other findings in this study revealed that β_1 integrins play a major role in the adhesion and spreading of stationary SMCs, whereas integrin $\alpha_v\beta_3$ is predominant in ECM interactions of migrating SMCs (Fig. 54.6). In support of these studies, TGF-β1 and PDGF, growth factors that are expressed following vascular injury and promote SMC migration, were observed to promote increased surface levels of integrin $\alpha_v\beta_3$ without subsequent increases in β_1 integrins.[134-135] These findings suggest that growth factor-mediated increased surface levels of $\alpha_v\beta_3$ facilitate SMC migration, and further emphasize the role of this integrin in SMC migration.

ECM Modulation of Endothelial Cell Function

Endothelial cells (ECs) form a monolayer on the luminal surfaces of vessels and normally serve as a nonthrombogenic and selectively permeable boundary between the bloodstream and extravascular space.[136,137] Following injury and in vascular disease, ECs can become thrombogenic and promote leukocyte adhesion.[136,137] Throughout the entire vascular system, normal uninjured ECs abluminally synthesize, secrete and maintain a basement membrane on their basal surfaces. The subendothelial basement membrane is a complex network of ECM glycoproteins including laminin, type IV collagen, heparan sulfate proteoglycan, nidogen/entactin, and fibronectin.[138] Cultured endothelial cells have been shown to attach and spread on various ECM proteins, including fibronectin, laminin, collagens, vitronectin, and von willebrand factor.[139] Similar to SMCs, ECM composition has a profound effect on EC phenotype. When ECs are cultured on type I collagen, type III collagen or fibronectin, migration and proliferation were observed to be enhanced.[140,141] Type IV collagen, laminin, and reconstituted basement membrane (Matrigel) were observed to inhibit EC proliferation and promote aggregation into capillary-like tubes.[138,140,141] Type V collagen has been observed to selectively inhibit EC attachment and proliferation without affecting these activities in SMCs and fibroblasts.[142-143]

EC-ECM interactions are mediated by several members of the integrin superfamily. ECs express several β_1 integrins, $\alpha_1\beta_1$, $\alpha_2\beta_1$, $\alpha_3\beta_1$, $\alpha_4\beta_1$, $\alpha_5\beta_1$, and $\alpha_6\beta_1$, which promote adhesion to collagens ($\alpha_3\beta_1$),[144,145] LN($\alpha_2\beta_1$,[144-148] $\alpha_6\beta_1$[147]) and fibronectin ($\alpha_4\beta_1$,[149] $\alpha_5\beta_1$).[144,145,150,151] Integrin $\alpha_v\beta_3$, which is present on endothelial cells, recognizes RGD ligands in vitronectin, von Willebrand factor, fibrinogen, thrombospondin, and fibronectin.[144,145,150,152-159] Like SMCs, the expression of specific integrins on ECs is modulated by growth factors. For example, TGF-β1 has been observed to increase surface levels of both β_1 and β_3 integrins in ECs.[134] TNF-α and interferon-γ have been shown to promote significant decreases in EC surface levels of β_3 integrins without changing β_1 integrin levels.[160] Overall, EC and SMC interactions with ECM components contribute significantly to their overall function in the normal, injured, and diseased vessel wall. Although not discussed in this review, platelet and inflammatory cell interactions with the vessel wall play

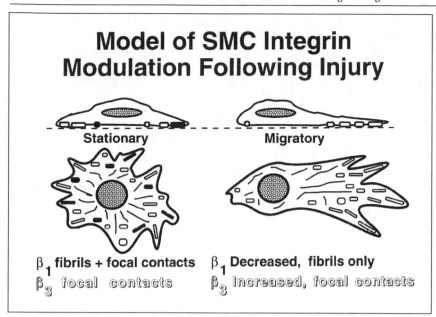

Model of SMC Integrin Modulation Following Injury

Stationary

Migratory

β_1 **fibrils + focal contacts**

β_3 **focal contacts**

β_1 **Decreased, fibrils only**

β_3 **Increased, focal contacts**

Fig. 54.6. Following vascular injury, medial SMCs become migratory as neointimal hyperplasia progresses. Integrin function is modulated in this migratory response. Surface levels of integrin $\alpha_v\beta_3$ increase, while β_1 integrin levels decrease or remain the same. Integrin $\alpha_v\beta_3$ also localizes into focal contacts which are responsible for generating traction for cell migration.[168] β_1 integrins are not detectable in focal contacts of migratory cells.[168] These results suggest that integrin $\alpha_v\beta_3$ is the predominant mediator of SMC migration in response to injury.

an important role in vascular healing and during the progression of disease.[137,161]

Modulating Cell-Extracellular Interactions for Vascular Tissue Engineering

Tissue Engineered Vascular Implants

Common to all endeavors in tissue engineering, the precise control of interactions between cells and extracellular surfaces is a fundamental goal in vascular tissue engineering. Vascular implant materials which promote cell type selective adhesion and appropriate cellular functions would vastly improve the long term biocompatibility of synthetic vascular implants. With such improvements in biocompatibility, synthetic small diameter vascular grafts would no longer fail and would become a viable option for surgical procedures. The development of biomimetic surface modifications and controlled release modalities for vascular implant materials is critical for achieving controllable modulation of cellular interactions at the tissue-biomaterial interface.

Modulation of EC Interactions with Extracellular Surfaces

ECs line the luminal surfaces of all components of the vascular system and actively maintain homeostasis in the bloodstream and at the vessel wall. Small diameter synthetic vascular grafts fail clinically due, in part, to the lack of a functional endothelium on the luminal surface. For over 20 years, many research efforts have focused on transplanting ECs onto synthetic vascular grafts to improve graft function and performance.[111-115,136,162] Among the many critical issues in developing this technology, modulation of EC-material interactions on vascular grafts is very important, since it influences cell retention and function on the graft lumen.

Biomimetic cell-adhesive biomaterials with surface immobilized cell adhesion peptides have been developed and

evaluated in vitro for promoting EC attachment independently of protein adsorption. Surface-grafted RGD- and YIGSR-containing peptides were observed to promote endothelial cell attachment and spreading on polyethylene terepthalate (PET) and polytetrafluoroethylene (PTFE), the two most widely used materials for vascular grafts.[54] EC retention on peptide-grafted materials may generally be improved over ECM protein-coated materials, since one study has shown that EC retention is better on RGD peptide-grafted glass than on fibronectin-coated glass.[82] EC-selective materials containing surface immobilized GREDVY have been observed to promote adhesion and spreading of endothelial cells, but not fibroblasts, smooth muscle cells or platelets.[56] The cell adhesion ligand REDV is located on some types of human plasma fibronectin in alternately spliced cell binding domains.[163] EC-selective adhesion has been observed on PET films containing surface immobilized UEA-I, a lectin that binds ECs with high affinity. These materials promoted EC adhesion without significant monocyte, SMC, or fibroblast adhesion.[66] Biomimetic, EC-selective materials may enhance the long term biocompatibility of vascular implants, since thrombosis (mediated by platelet attachment) and neointimal hyperplasia (mediated by smooth muscle cell attachment and migration) are major modes of failure. Although extensive studies have evaluated the effect of surface microtextrue on cell-material interactions, few have specifically investigated surface microtextrue effects on EC-material interactions. One study has shown that ECs spread more rapidly on microtextured polymers prepared from nanoscale surface replicas of subendothelial ECM than on untextured polymers.[164] This finding suggests that EC adhesion and function are altered on the microtextured surfaces. Transplantation of genetically modified ECs in synthetic vascular grafts has been considered as an approach for enhancing EC function and improving graft patency rates. Unfortunately, the postgraft implantation retention rates of transplanted, genetically modified ECs have been observed to be significantly lower than unmodified ECs.[165-167] Therefore, the benefits gained from improved EC function are diminished because of increased cell detachment under flow. Biomimetic surface modifications may significantly improve the retention rate of genetically modified ECs by increasing their attachment strength to graft surfaces. Overall, biomimetic material surfaces may be valuable in promoting well-controlled EC-material interactions and improved biocompatibility of vascular implants.

Modulation of SMC Interactions with Extracellular Surfaces

The SMC population that normally resides within the media (inside the wall) of uninjured blood vessels is predominantly contractile and functionally regulates blood pressure and flow. Following mechanical injury, medial SMC populations convert to a predominantly ECM-secreting, proliferative phenotype and migrate from the media to the lumen, forming a thick multilayered neointima (Fig. 54.5). In small synthetic vascular grafts, neointimal hyperplasia (progressive neointimal thickening) is a major mode of failure due to severely reduced patency and blood flow or total occlusion, especially at anastomoses.[111-115,136,162,168] SMC phenotype conversion and the development of neointimal hyperplasia results from the initial mechanical injury of graft implantation surgery and the long term generation of abnormal mechanical forces due to compliance mismatch between the native vessel and the synthetic graft.[111-113,168] Since SMC-ECM interactions play an important role in modulating SMC phenotype, migration, proliferation, metabolism, etc., well-controlled, selective modulation of these interactions by biomimetic material surface modifications and local delivery of soluble mediators may limit hyperplasia and improve the long term biocompatibility of small diameter synthetic vascular grafts.

Since ECM components play an active role in modulating SMC phenotype, biomimetic cell adhesive biomaterials may provide a way to selectively control SMC phenotype expression to limit graft hyperplasia. Laminin and type IV collagen have been identified as ECM components which promote expression of the contractile phenotype in cultured SMCs.[102,133] Therefore, surface immobilization of these proteins or biologically active peptides from these proteins on vascular graft biomaterials may promote phenotype reversion of injury-activated SMCs that initially contact the implanted graft and limit further development of neointimal hyperplasia. Currently, the effect of surface microtextrue on SMC behavior has been unexplored. However, it could be speculated that surface microtextrue will influence SMC adhesion/migration and/or phenotype.

An alternative approach for limiting vascular graft hyperplasia is to deliver locally from the implanted graft soluble agents which selectively limit SMC migration. As described earlier in this review, in vitro studies have shown that integrin $\alpha_v\beta_3$ is the predominant receptor in promoting SMC migration (Fig. 54.6). Cyclic RGD peptides, which bind to integrin $\alpha_v\beta_3$ with high affinity, have recently been shown to inhibit SMC migration in vitro; continuous local or systemic delivery of cyclic RGD peptides has been shown to limit balloon injury-induced neointimal hyperplasia.[169-171] Local release of cyclic RGD from a delivery vehicle incorporated in vascular grafts may prove to be effective in limiting graft hyperplasia. Some ECM components are synthesized and secreted in response to vascular injury to facilitate neointimal hyperplasia development. Local release of agents which specifically inhibit the synthesis of these molecules could potentially limit graft hyperplasia. One study which tested this concept observed that local delivery of tenascin mRNA antisense oligonucleotides to injured arteries significantly reduces neointimal hyperplasia in vascular grafts.[172] As described earlier, tenascin is synthesized and secreted in the neointimal ECM by SMCs following injury and has been shown to promote SMC migration in vitro. Other counteradhesive ECM proteins like thrombospondin and type V collagen, that are selectively synthesized and deposited following vascular injury, are also potential ECM components that could be selectively inhibited by local delivery to limit graft hyperplasia. Systems for local delivery of bio-

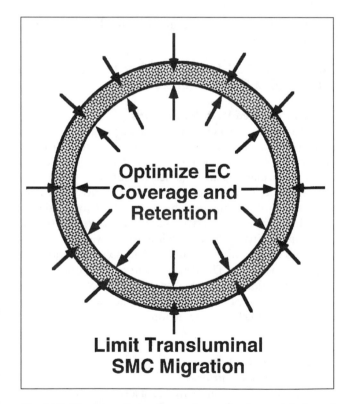

Fig. 54.7. Tissue engineered vascular grafts via modulation of cell-ECM interactions. The optimal high performance vascular graft must promote complete luminal coverage with a nonthrombogenic endothelium that adheres strongly to graft lumen. Biomimetic surface modifications may facilitate the design of these characteristics by providing improved control of EC-biomaterial interactions. This idealized graft must also limit neointimal hyperplasia so that long term patency and adequate blood flow is maintained. Biomimetic surface modifications and local drug delivery systems that modulate SMC phenotype and restrict SMC migration may provide means for limiting graft hyperplasia.

logically active soluble agents in implanted vascular grafts may improve long term graft biocompatibility.

Conclusion

Development of biomimetic materials which contain well-defined ECM-like physicochemical features to promote selective cell interactions is a fundamentally important area of research in the fields of tissue engineering and biomaterials science. In vascular tissue engineering, it is desirable to have a synthetic vascular graft that promotes complete luminal coverage with a healthy, nonthrombogenic endothelium. Further, this biohybrid graft must limit neointimal hyperplasia so that long term patency and adequate blood flow is maintained (Fig. 54.7). Development of appropriate biomimetic material surface modifications in conjunction with other technologies such as genetic manipulation of cells will provide the tissue engineer and biomaterial scientist with new tools for creating high-performance implants and devices, including those for cardiovascular applications.

References

1. Folkman J, Moscona A. Role of cell shape in growth control. Nature 1978; 273:345-349.
2. Stoker M, O'Neill C, Berryman S et al. Anchorage and growth regulation in normal and virus-transformed cells. Int J Cancer 1968; 3:638-648.
3. O'Neill CH, Riddle PN, Jordan PW. The relation between surface area and anchorage dependence of growth in hamster and mouse fibroblasts. Cell 1979; 16:909-918.
4. Ruoslahti E, Reed JC. Anchorage dependence, integrins, and apoptosis. Cell 1994; 77:477-478.
5. Grinnell F. Cellular adhesiveness and extracellular substrata. Int Rev Cytol. New York: Academic Press, 1978; 53:67-149.
6. Jauregui HO. Cell adhesion to biomaterials: The role of several extracellular matrix components in the attachment of nontransformed fibroblasts and parenchymal cells. Trans Am Soc Artif Itern Organs 1987; 33:66-74.
7. Hay ED, ed. Cell Biology of Extracellular matrix, 2nd ed., New York: Plenum Press, 1991.
8. Paulsson M. Basement membrane proteins: Structure, assembly, and cellular interactions. Crit Rev Biochem Mol Biol 1992; 27:93-127.
9. Ratner BD. New ideas in biomaterials science—a path to engineered biomaterials. J Biomed Mater Res 1993; 27:837-850.
10. Hynes RO. Integrins: A family of cell surface receptors. Cell 1987; 48:549-554.
11. Ruoslahti E. Integrins. J Clin Invest 1991; 87:1-5.
12. Hynes RO. Integrins: Variety, versatility, and interactions in cell adhesions. Cell 1992; 69:11-25.
13. Gille J, Swerlick RA. Integrins: Role in cell adhesion and communication. Ann NY Acad Sci 1996; 797:93-106.
14. Couchman JR, Woods A. Syndecans, signaling, and cell adhesion. J Cell Biochem 1996; 61:578-584.
15. Entwistle J, Hall CL, Turley EA. HA receptors: Regulators of signaling to the cytoskeleton. J Cell Biochem 1996; 61:569-577.
16. Mecham RP. Laminin receptors. Ann Rev Cell Biol 1991; 7:71-91.
17. Chung CA, Erickson HP. Cell surface annexin II is a high affinity receptor for the alternatively spliced segment of tenascin-C. J Cell Biol 1994; 126:539-548.
18. Barnea G, Grumet M, Milev et al. Receptor tyrosine phosphatase β is expressed in the form of proteoglycan and binds to the extracellular matrix protein tenascin. J Biol Chem 1994; 269:14349-14352.
19. Lafrienie RM, Yamada KM. Integrin-dependent signal transduction. J Cell Biochem 1996; 61:543-553.
20. Otey CA. pp125^{FAK} in the focal adhesion. Int Rev Cytol 1996; 167:161-183.
21. Horwitz A, Duggan K, Buck C et al. Interaction of plasma membrane fibronectin receptor with talin—a transmembrane linkage. Nature 1986; 320:531-533.
22. Muguruma M, Matsumura S, Fukazawa. Direct interactions between talin and actin. Biochem Biophys Res Commun 1990; 171:1217-1223.
23. Burridge K, Mangeat P. An interaction between vinculin and talin. Nature 1984; 308:744-746.
24. Wachsstock DH, Wilkins JA, Lin S. Specific interaction of vinculin with α-actinin. Biochem Biophys Res Commun 1987; 146:554-560.
25. Turner CE, Glenney JR, Burridge K. Paxillin: A new vinculin-binding protein present in focal adhesions. J Cell Biol 1990; 111:1059-1068.
26. Wilkins JA, Risinger MA, Lin S. Studies on proteins that copurify with smooth muscle vinculin: Identification of immunologically related species in focal adhesions of nonmuscle and Z-lines of muscle cells. J Cell Biol 1986; 103:1383-1394.
27. Johnson RP, Craig SW. F-actin binding site masked by the intramolecular association of vinculin head and tail domains. Nature 1995; 373:261-264.
28. Otey CA, Pavalko FM, Burridge K. An interaction between alpha-actinin and the β$_1$ subunit in vitro. J Cell Biol 1990; 111:721-729.
29. Kornberg LJ, Earp HS, Turner CE et al. Signal transduction by integrins: Increased protein tyrosine phosphorylation caused by clustering of β$_1$ integrins. Proc Natl Acad Sci USA 1991; 88:8392-8396.
30. Guan J-L, Trevithick JE, Hynes RO. Fibronectin/integrin interaction induces tyrosine phosphorylation of a 120 kDa protein. Cell Regul 1991; 2:951-964.
31. Kornberg LJ, Earp HS, Parsons JT et al. Cell adhesion or integrin clustering increases phosphorylation of a focal adhesion-associated tyrosine kinase. J Biol Chem 1992; 267:23439-23442.
32. Hildebrand JD, Schaller M, Parsons JT. Identification of sequences required for the efficient localization of the focal adhesion kinase, pp125^{FAK}, to cellular focal adhesions. J Cell Biol 1993; 123:993-1005.
33. Parsons JT, Schaller MD, Hildebrand JD et al. Focal adhesion kinase: Structure and signaling. J Cell Sci Suppl 1994; 18:109-113.
34. Cohen GB, Ren R, Baltimore D. Modular binding domains in signal transduction proteins. Cell 1995; 80:237-248.
35. Sabe H, Hata A, Okada M et al. Analysis of the binding of the src homology 2 domain of csk to tyrosine-phosphorylated proteins in the suppression and activation of c-src. Proc Natl Acad Sci USA 1994; 91:3984-3988.
36. Weng Z, Taylor JA, Turner CE et al. Detection of src homology 3-binding proteins, including paxillin, in normal and v-src transformed Balb/c 3T3 cells. J Biol Chem 1993; 268:14956-14963.

37. Schlaepfer DD, Hanks SK, Hunter T et al. Integrin-mediated signal transduction linked to ras pathway by GRB-2 binding to focal adhesion kinase. Nature 1994; 372:786-791.

38. Lenormand P, Sardet C, Pages G et al. Growth factors induce nuclear translocation of MAP kinases (p42^{mapk} and p44^{mapk}) but not of their activator MAP kinase kinase (p45^{mapkk}). J Cell Biol 1993; 122:1079-1088.

39. Hansen CA, Schroering AG, Carey DJ et al. Localization of a heterodynamic G protein gamma subunit to focal adhesions and stress fibers. J Cell Biol 1994; 126:811-819.

40. Jaken S, Leach K, Klauk T. Association of type 3 protein kinase c with focal contacts in rat embryo fibroblasts. J Cell Biol 1989; 109:697-707.

41. McNamee HP, Ingber DE, Schwartz MA. Adhesion to fibronectin stimulates inositol lipid synthesis and enhances PDGF-induced inositol lipid breakdown. J Cell Biol 1993; 121:673-678.

42. Schwartz MA. Spreading of endothelial cells on fibronectin or vitronectin triggers elevation of intracellular free calcium. J Cell Biol 1993; 120:1003-1010.

43. Schwarz MA, Ingber DE, Lawrence M et al. Multiple integrins share the ability to induce elevation of intracellular pH. Exp Cell Res 1991; 195:533-535.

44. Ratner BD. New ideas in biomaterials science—a path to engineered biomaterials. J Biomed Mater Res 1993; 27:837-850.

45. Andrade JD, Hlady V. Protein adsorption and materials biocompatibility: A tutorial review and suggested hypothesis. Adv Polymer Sci 1986; 79:1-63.

46. Horbett TA, Brash JL. Proteins at interfaces: Current issues and future prospects. ACS Symposium Ser 1987; 343:1-33.

47. Brandley BK, Schnaar RL, Covalent attachment of an Arg-Gly-Asp sequence peptide to derivatizable polyacrylamide surfaces: Support of fibroblast adhesion and long-term growth. Anal Biochem 1988; 172:270-278.

48. Brandley BK, Schnaar RL. Tumor cell haptotaxis on covalently immobilized linear and exponential gradients of a cell adhesion peptide. Dev Biol 1989; 135:74-86.

49. Matsuda T, Kondo A, Makino K et al. Development of a novel artificial matrix with cell adhesion peptides for cell culture and artificial and hybrid organs. Trans Am Soc Artif Intern Organs 1989; 35:677-679.

50. Massia SP, Hubbell JA. Covalently grafted RGD- and YIGSR-containing synthetic peptides support receptor-mediated adhesion of cultured fibroblasts. Analytical Biochemistry 1990; 187:292-301.

51. Massia SP, Hubbell JA. Covalently attached GRGD on polymer surfaces promotes biospecific adhesion of mammalian cells. Ann NY Acad Sci 1990; 589:261-270.

52. Ozeki E, Matsuda T. Development of an artificial extracellular matrix. Solution castable polymers with cell recognizable peptidyl side chain. ASAIO Trans 1990; 36:M294.

53. Nakajima K, Hirano Y, Iida T et al. Adsorption of plasma proteins an Arg-Gly-Asp-Ser peptide-immobilized poly(vinyl alcohol) and ethylene-acrylic copolymer films. Polym J 1990; 22:985.

54. Massia SP, Hubbell JA. Human endothelial cell interactions with surface-coupled adhesion peptides on a non-adhesive glass substrate and two polymeric biomaterials. J Biomed Mater Res 1991; 25:223-242.

55. Massia SP, Hubbell JA. An RGD spacing of 440 nm is sufficient for integrin $\alpha_v\beta_3$–mediated fibroblast spreading and 140 nm for focal contact and stress fiber formation. J Cell Biol 1991; 114:1089-1100.

56. Hubbell JA, Massia SP, Desai NP et al. Endothelial cell-selective materials for tissue engineering in the vascular graft via a new receptor. Bio/Technology 1991; 9:568-572.

57. Ito Y, Kajihara M, Imanishi Y. Materials for enhancing cell adhesion by immobilization of cell-adhesive peptide. J Biomed Mater Res 1991; 25:1325-1337.

58. Hirano Y, Kando Y, Hayashi T et al. Synthesis and cell attachment activity of bioactive oligopeptides: RGD, RGDS, RGDV, and RGDT. J Biomed Mater Res 1991; 25:1523-1534.

59. Britland S, Perez-Arnaud E, Clark P et al. Micropatterning proteins and synthetic peptides on solid supports: A novel application for microelectronics fabrication technology. Biotechnol Prog 1992; 8:155-60.

60. Lin HB, Garcia-Echeverria C, Asakura S et al. Endothelial cell adhesion on polyurethanes containing covalently attached RGD-peptides. Biomaterials 1992; 13:905-914.

61. Fassina G. Oriented immobilization of peptide ligands on solid supports. J Chromatogr 1992; 591:99.

62. Shenoy NR, Bailey JM, Shively JE. Carboxylic acid-modified polyethylene: A novel support for the covalent immobilization of polypeptides for C-terminal sequencing. Protein Sci 1992; 1:58-67.

63. Massia SP, Rao S, Hubbell JA. Covalently immobilized laminin peptide Tyr-Ile-Gly-Ser-Arg (YIGSR) supports cell spreading and colocalization of the 67-kilodalton laminin receptor with α-actinin and vinculin. J Biol Chem 1993; 268:8053-8059.

64. Kondoh A, Makino K, Matsuda T. Two-dimensional artificial extracellular matrix: Bioadhesive peptide-immobilized surface design. J Appl Polm Sci 1993; 47:1983.

65. Hirano Y, Okuno M, Hayashi T et al. Cell-attachment activities of surface immobilized oligopeptides RGD, RGDS, RGDT, and YIGSR toward five cell lines. J Biomater Sci Polym Edn 1993; 4:235.

66. Ozaki CK, Phaneuf MD, Hong SL et al. Glycoconjugate mediated endothelial cell adhesion to Dacron polyester film. J Vasc Surg 1993; 18:486.

67. Nakayama Y, Matsuda T, Irie M. A novel surface photo-graft polymerization method for fabricated devices. ASAIO J 1993; 39:M542.

68. Collioud A, Clemence JF, Sanger M et al. Oriented and covalent immobilization of target molecules to solid supports: Synthesis and application of a light-activatable and thiol-reactive cross-linking reagent. Bioconjug Chem 1993; 4:528-536.

69. Lin HB, Garcia-Echeverria C, Sun W et al. Synthesis of a novel polyurethane copolymer containing covalently attached RGD peptide. J Biomater Sci Polym Edn 1993; 4:235.

70. Barrera DA, Zystra E, Lansbury PT et al. Synthesis and RGD peptide modification of a new biodegradable copolymer: Poly(lactic acid-colysine). J Am Chem Soc 1993; 115:11010.

71. Drumheller PD, Elbert DL, Hubbell JA. Multifunctional poly(ethylene glycol) semiinterpenetrating polymer networks as highly selective adhesive substrates for bioadhesive peptide grafting. Biotech Bioeng 1994; 43:772.

72. Cima LG. Polymer substrates for controlled biological interactions. J Cell Biochem 1994; 56:155-161.

73. Englebretsen DR, Harding DR. High yield, directed immobilization of a peptide-ligand onto a beaded cellulose support. Pept Res 1994; 7:322-326.

74. Besselink GA, Beugeling T, Poot AA et al. Preparation of cell-affinity adsorbents by immobilization of peptides to Sephadex G-10. J Biomater Sci Polym Ed 1994; 6:675-693.

75. Lin HB, Sun W, Mosher DF et al. Synthesis, surface, and cell adhesion properties of polyurethanes containing covalently grafted RGD-peptides. J Biomed Mater Res 1994; 28:1523-1534.

76. Kugo K, Okuno M, Matsuda K et al. Fibroblast attachment to Arg-Gly-Asp peptide-immobilized poly(gamma-methyl L-glutamate). J Biomater Sci Polym Ed 1994; 5:325-337.

77. Vargo TG, Bekos EJ, Kim YS et al. Synthesis and characterization of fluoropolymeric substrata with immobilized minimal peptide sequences for cell adhesion studies. I. J Biomed Mater Res 1995; 29:767-778.

78. Ranieri JP, Bellamkonda R, Bekos EJ et al. Neuronal cell attachment to fluorinated ethylene propylene films with covalently immobilized laminin oligopeptides YIGSR and IKVAV. II. J Biomed Mater Res 1995; 29:779-785.

79. Sugawara T, Matsuda T. Photochemical surface derivatization of a peptide containing Arg-Gly-Asp (RGD). J Biomed Mater Res 1995; 29:1047-1052.

80. Glass JR, Dickerson KT, Stecker K et al. Characterization of a hyaluronic acid-Arg-Gly-Asp peptide cell attachment matrix. Biomaterials 1996; 17:1101-1108.

81. Olbrich KC, Anderson TT, Blumenstock FA et al. Surfaces modified with covalently-immobilized adhesive peptides affect fibroblast population motility. Biomaterials 1996; 17:144-153.

82. Xiao Y, Truskey GA. Effect of receptor-ligand affinity on the strength of endothelial cell adhesion. Biophys J 1996; 71:2869-2894.

83. Pierschbacher MD, Ruoslahti E. Influence of stereochemistry of the sequence Arg-Gly-Asp-Xaa on binding specificity in cell adhesion. J Biol Chem 1987; 262:17294-17298.

84. Harrison RG. The cultivation of tissues in extraneous media as a method of a morphogenic study. Anat Rec 1912; 6:181-193.

85. Weiss P. Experiments on cell and axon orientation in vitro: The role of colloidal exudates in tissue organization. J Exp Zool 1945; 100:353.

86. von Recum AF, Shannon CE, Cannon CE et al. Surface roughness, porosity, and texture as modifiers of cellular adhesion. Tissue Engineering 1996; 2:241-253.

87. Campbell CE, von Recum AF. Microtopography and soft tissue repsonse. J Invest Surg 1989; 2:51-74.

88. Brauker JH, Carr-Brendel VE, Martinson LA et al. Neovascularization of synthetic membranes directed by membrane architecture. J Biomed Mater Res 1996; 29:1517-1524.

89. Clark P, Connolly P, Curtis AS et al. Topographical control of cell behaviour. I. Simple step cues. Development 1987; 99:439-448.

90. Clark P, Connolly P, Curtis AS et al. Topographical control of cell behaviour. II. Mutiple grooved substrata. Development 1990; 108:635-644.

91. Meyle J, Gultig K, Nisch W. Variation in contact guidance by human cells on a microstructured surface. J Biomed Mater Res 1995; 29:81-88.

92. Oakley C, Brunette DM. Response of single, pairs, and clusters of epithelial cells to substratum topography. Biochem Cell Biol 1995; 73:473-489.

93. Cheroudi B, Gould TR, Brunette DM. Effects of grooved epoxy substratum on epithelial cell behavior in vitro and in vivo. J Biomed Mater Res 1995; 6:459-473.

94. Schmidt, JA, von Recum AF. The macrophage response to microtextured silicone. Biomaterials 1991; 13:1095-1099.

95. Green AM, Jansen JA, von Recum AF. The fibroblast response to microtextured silicone surfaces: Texture orientation into or out of the surface. J Biomed Mater Res 1994; 28:647-653.

96. Meyle J, Wolburg H, von Recum AF. Surface micromorphology and cellular interactions. J Biomat Appl 1993; 7:362-374.

97. Oakley C, Brunette DM. The sequence of alignment of microtubules, focal contacts, and actin filaments in fibroblasts spreading on smooth and grooved titanium substrata. J Cell Sci 1993; 106:303.

98. den Braber ET, de Ruijter JE, Smits HT et al. Quantitative analysis of cell proliferation and orientation on substrata with uniform parallel surface micro-grooves. Biomaterials 1996; 17:1093-1099.

99. Wojciak-Stothard B, Curtis A, Monaghan W et al. Guidance and activation of murine macrophages by nanometric scale topography. Exp Cell Res 1996; 223:426-435.

100. Qu J, Chehroudi B, Brunette DM. The use of micromachined surfaces to investigate the cell behavioral factors essential to osseointegration. Oral Dis 1996; 2:102-115.

101. Chou L, Firth JD, Uitto VJ et al. Substratum surface topography alters cell shape and regulates fibronectin mRNA level, mRNA stability, secretion and assembly in human fibroblasts. J Cell Sci 1995; 108:1563-1573.

102. Thyberg J. Differentiated properties and proliferation of arterial smooth muscle cells in culture. Int Rev Cytol 1996; 169:183-265.

103. Somlyo AP, Somlyo AV. Signal transduction and regulation in smooth muscle. Nature 1994; 17:231-236.

104. Owens GK. Regulation of differentiation of vascular smooth muscle cells. Physiol Rev 1995; 75:487-517.

105. Liu MW, Roubin GS, King SB. Restenosis after coronary angioplasty: Potential biological determinants and role of intimal hyperplasia. Circulation 1989; 79:1374-1387.

106. Forrester JS, Fishbein M, Helfant R et al. A paradigm for restenosis based on cell biology: Clues for the development of new preventive therapies. J Am Coll Cardiol 1991; 17:758-769.

107. Reidy MA, Jackson C, Lindner V. Neointimal proliferation: Control of vascular smooth muscle cell growth. Vasc Med Rev 1992; 3:156-167.

108. Casscells W. Migration of smooth muscle and endothelial cells. Critical events in restenosis. Circulation 1992; 86:723-729.

109. Ferns AA, Stewart-Lee AL, Änggård EE. Arterial response to mechanical injury: Balloon catheter de-endothelialization. Atherosclerosis 1992; 92:89-104.

110. Casscells W, Engler D, Willerson JT. Mechanisms of restenosis. Texas Heart Inst J 1994; 21:68-77.

111. Yeager A, Callow AD. New graft materials and current approaches to an acceptable small diameter vascular graft. Trans Am Soc Artif Intern Organs 1988; 34:88-94.

112. Callow AD. Presidential address: The microcosm of the arterial wall—a plea for research. J Vasc Surg 1987; 5:1-17.

113. Burkel WE. The challenge of small diameter vascular grafts. Med Prog Technol 1988; 14:165-175.

114. Greisler HP. Interactions at the blood/material interface. Ann Vasc Surg 1990; 4:98-103.

115. Zilla P. The endothelium: A key to the future. J Card Surg 1993; 8:32-60.

116. Majesky MW, Lindner V, Twardzik DR et al. Production of transforming growth factor beta 1 during repair of arterial injury. J Clin Invest 1991; 88:904-910.

117. Snow AD, Bolender RP, Wight TN et al. Heparin modulates the composition of the extracellular matrix domain surrounding arterial smooth muscle cells. Am J Pathol 1990; 137:313-390.

118. Madri JA, Reidy MA, Kocher O et al. Endothelial cell behavior after denudation injury is modulated by transformtin growth factor-beta 1 and fibronectin. Lab Invest 1989; 60:755-765.

119. Burke JM, Ross R. Synthesis of connective tissue macromolecules by smooth muscle. Int Rev Connect Tissue Res 1979; 8:119-157.

120. Majesky MW, Giachelli CM, Reidy MA et al. Rat carotid neointimal smooth muscle cells reexpress a developmentally regulated mRNA phenotype during repair of arterial injury. Circ Res 1992; 71:759-768.

121. Wight TN. Cell biology of arterial proteoglycans. Arteriosclerosis 1989; 9:1-20.

122. Alvai M, Moore S. Glycosaminoglycan composition and biosynthesis in the endothelium-covered neointima and de-endothelialized rabbit aorta. Exp Mol Pathol 1985; 42:389-400.

123. Hedin U, Holm J, Hansson GK. Induction of tenascin in rat arterial injury. Relationship to altered smooth muscle cell phenotype. Am J Pathol 1989; 139:649-656.

124. Majesky MW. Neointima formation after acute vascular injury. Role of counteradhesive extracellular matrix proteins. Texas Heart Inst J 1994; 21:78-85.

125. Raugi GL, Mullen JS, Bark DH et al. Thrombospondin deposition in rat carotid artery injury. Am J Pathol 1990; 137:179-185.

126. Chuong CM, Chen HM. Enhanced expression of neural cell adhesion molecules and tenascin (cytotactin) during wound healing. Am J Path 1990; 138:427-440.

127. Mackie EJ, Halfter W, Liverani D. Induction of tenascin in healing wounds. J Cell Biol 1988; 107:2757-2767.

128. Clyman RI, Mauray F, Kramer RH. β_1 and β_3 integrins have different roles in the adhesion and migration of vascular smooth cells on extracellular matrix. Exp Cell Res 1992; 200:272-284.

129. DiMilla PA, Stone J, Quinn JA et al. Maximal migration of human smooth muscle cells on fibronectin and type IV collagen occurs at an intermediate attachment strength. J Cell Biol 1993; 122:729-737.

130. Massia SP, Slepian MJ. Tenascin enhances injury-induced vascular smooth muscle cell migration partially via integrin $\alpha_v\beta_3$. Exp Cell Res, 1997; in revision.

131. Hedin U, Thyberg J. Plasma fibronectin promotes modulation of arterial smooth muscle cells form contractile to synthetic phenotype. Differentiation 1987; 33:239-246.

132. Hedin U, Bottger BA, Johansson S et al. A substrate of the cell attachment sequence of fibronectin (Arg-Gly-Asp-Ser) is sufficient to promote transition of arterial smooth muscle cells from a contractile to a synthetic phenotype. Dev Biol 1989; 133:489-501.

133. Hedin U, Bottger BA, Forsberg E et al. Diverse effects of fibronectin and laminin on phenotype properties of cultured arterial smooth muscle cells. J Cell Biol 1988; 107:307-319.

134. Basson CT, Kocher O, Basson MD et al. Differential modulation of vascular cell integrin and extracellular matrix expression in vitro by TGF-β1 correlates with re-

135. Janat MF, Argraves WS, Liau G. Regulation of vascular smooth muscle cell integrin expression by transforming growth factor β1 and platelet-derived growth factor-BB. J Cell Physiol 1992; 151:588-595.

136. Massia SP, Hubbell JA. Tissue engineering in the vascular graft. Cytotechnology 1992; 10:189-204.

137. Luscinskas FW, Lawler J. Integrins as dynamic regulators of vascular function. FASEB J 1994; 8:929-938.

138. Grant DS, Kleinman HK, Martin GR. The role of basement membranes in vascular development. Ann NY Acad Sci 1990; 588:61-72.

139. Carey DJ. Control of growth and differentiation of vascular cells by extracellular matrix proteins. Ann Rev Physiol 1991; 53:161-177.

140. Madri JA, Pratt BM. Endothelial-matrix interactions: In vitro models of angiogenesis. J Histochem Cytochem 1986; 34:85-91.

141. Madri JA, Williams SK. Capillary endothelial cell cultures: Phenotypic modulation by matrix components. J Cell Biol 1983; 97:153-165.

142. Fukuda K, Koshihara Y, Oda H et al. Type V collagen selectively inhibits human endothelial cell proliferation. Biochem Biophys Res Commun 1988; 151:1060-1068.

143. Ziats NP, Anderson JM. Human vascular endothelial cell attachment and growth inhibition by type V collagen. J Vasc Surg 1993; 17:710-718.

144. Cheng YF, Kramer RH. Integrin receptors in human microvascular endothelial cells that mediate adhesion to the extracellular matrix. J Cell Physiol 1989; 139:275-286.

145. Albelda SM, Daise M, Levine EM et al. Identification and characterization of cell-substratum adhesion receptors on cultured human endothelial cells. J Clin Invest 1989; 83:1992-2002.

146. Kramer RH, Cheng Y-F, Clyman R. Human microvascular endothelial cells use β_1 and β_3 integrin receptor complexes to attach to laminin. J Cell Biol 1990; 111:1233-1243.

147. Languino LR, Gehlsen KR, Wayner E et al. Endothelial cells use $\alpha_2\beta_1$ integrin as a laminin receptor. J Cell Biol 1989; 109:2455-2462.

148. Kirchhofer D, Languino LR, Ruoslahti E et al. $\alpha_2\beta_1$ integrins from different cell types show different binding specificities. J Biol Chem 1990; 265:615-618.

149. Massia SP, Hubbell JA. Vascular endothelial cell adhesion and spreading promoted by the peptide REDV of the IIICS region of plasma fibronectin is mediated by integrin $\alpha_4\beta_1$. J Biol Chem 1992; 267:14019-14026.

150. Dejana E, Colella S, Conforti G et al. Fibronectin and vitronectin regulate the organization of their respective Arg-Gly-Asp receptors in cultured human endothelial cells. J Cell Biol 1988; 107:1215-1223.

151. Conforti G, Zanetti A, Colella S et al. Interaction of fibronectin with cultured human endothelial cells: Characterization of the specific receptor. Blood 1989; 73:1576-1585.

152. Dejana E, Colella S, Languino LR et al. Fibrinogen induces adhesion, spreading, and microfilament organization of human endothelial cells in vitro. J Cell Biol 1987; 104:1403-1411.

153. Dejana E, Lampugnami MG, Giorgi M et al. Von willebrand factor promotes endothelial cell adhesion via an Arg-Gly-Asp-dependent mechanism. J Cell Biol 1989; 109:367-375.

ciprocal effects on cell migration. J Cell Physiol 1992; 153:118-128.

154. Dejana E, Languino LR, Colella S et al. The localization of a platelet gpIIb-IIIa-related protein in endothelial cell adhesion structures. Blood 1988; 71:566-572.

155. Dejana E, Languino LR, Polentarutti N et al. Interaction between fibrinogen and cultured endothelial cells: Induction of migration and specific binding. J Clin Invest 1985; 75:11-18.

156. Charo IF, Bekeart LS, Phillips DR. Platelet glycoprotein IIb-IIIa-like proteins mediate endothelial cell attachment to adhesive proteins and the extracellular matrix. J Biol Chem 1987; 262:9935-9938.

157. Cheresh DA. Human endothelial cells synthesize and express an Arg-Gly-Asp directed adhesion receptor involved in attachment to fibrinogen and von willebrand factor. Proc Natl Acad Sci 1987; 84:6471-6475.

158. Cheng Y-F, Clyman RI, Enenstein J et al. The integrin complex $\alpha_v\beta_3$ participates in the adhesion of microvascular endothelial cells to fibronectin. Exp Cell Res 1991; 194:69-77.

159. Lawler J, Weinstein R, Hynes RO. Cell attachment to thrombospondin: The role of Arg-Gly-Asp, calcium, and integrin receptors. J Cell Biol 1988; 107:2351-2361.

160. Defilippi P, Truffa G, Stefanuto G et al. Tumor necrosis factor α and interferon γ modulate the expression of the vitronectin receptor (integrin β_3 in human endothelial cells. J Biol Chem 1991; 266:7638-7645.

161. Rubin BG, Santoro SA, Sicard GA. Platelet interactions with the vessel wall and prosthetic grafts. Ann Vasc Surg 1993; 7:200-207.

162. Williams SK. Endothelial cell transplantation. Cell Transplant 1995; 4:401-410.

163. Humphries MJ, Akiyama SK, Komoriya A et al. Identification of an alternatively spliced site in human plasma fibronectin that mediates cell type-specific adhesion. J Cell Biol 1986; 103:2637-2647.

164. Goodman SL, Sims PA, Albrecht RM. Three-dimensional extracellular matrix textured biomaterials. Biomaterials 1996; 17:2087-2095.

165. Dunn PF, Newman KD, Jones M et al. Seeding of vascular grafts with genetically modified endothelial cells. Secretion of recombinant tPA results in decreased seeded cell retention in vitro and in vivo. Circulation 1996; 93:1439-1446.

166. Sackman JE, Freeman MB, Petersen MG et al. Synthetic vascular grafts seeded with genetically modified endothelium in the dog: Evaluation of the effect of seeding technique and retroviral vector on cell persistence in vivo. Cell Transplant 1995; 4:219-235.

167. Sackman JE, Cezeaux JL, Reddick TT et al. Evaluation of the effect of retroviral gene transduction on vascular endothelial cell adhesion. Tissue Eng 1996; 2:223-236.

168. Painter TA. Myointimal hyperplasia: Pathogenesis and implications. 2. Animal injury models and mechanical factors. Artif Organs 1991; 15:102-118.

169. Slepian MJ, S Massia, Dehdashti B et al. β_3 Rather than β_1 integrins dominate integrin-matrix interactions involved in postinjury smooth muscle cell migration. Circulation 1997: in revision.

170. Choi ET, Engel L, Callow AD et al. Inhibition of neointimal hyperplasia by blocking $\alpha v\beta 3$ integrin with a small peptide antagonist GpenGRGDSPCA. J Vasc Surg 1994;19:125-134.

171. Matsuno H, Stassen JM, Vermylen J et al. Inhibition of integrin fucntion by a cyclic RGD-containing peptide prevents neointima formation. Circulation 1994; 90:2203-2206.

172 Hirko M, Kang SS, Denner L et al. Antisense oligonucleotides against FGFR-1, tenascin, and osteopontin inhibit canine vein graft myointimal hyperplasia. Surg Forum 1995; 46:349-351.

─────────── Chapter 55 ───────────

Use of Hydroxypropylchitosan Acetate as a Carrier for Growth Factor Release

Keiko Yamamura, Toshitaka Nabeshima, Tsunehisa Sakurai

Introduction

The application of autogenous vein in vascular replacement shows high patency rates as compared to that of prosthetic vascular graft, because vascular endothelial cells possess anti-thrombogenic properties through secretion of many biologically active substances such as heparan sulfate, prostacyclin, thrombomodulin and plasminogen activators. Many investigators have demonstrated that a large percentage of synthetic graft failures in vascular reconstruction are due to inadequate regrowth of endothelial cells on the graft surface.[1] However, various synthetic prostheses are available when autogenous vein is unsuitable for use because of venous inflammation and insufficient diameter. If there is confluent endothelialization at the internal surface of the vascular graft, a long term patency rate would be expected. As the patency of a vascular graft is the most important factor, many investigators have tried to seed endothelial cells derived from donor veins into the vascular graft for this purpose.[2,3] However, to become clinically useful, large quantities of inoculating cells may be required to overcome early cellular loss caused by the shearing forces of blood flow. In addition, endothelial lining techniques in vitro must be performed aseptically, because graft sepsis is a disastrous complication.

Basic fibroblast growth factor (bFGF) is a polypeptide mitogen that stimulates the growth and differentiation of a wide variety of cell types derived from the mesoderm and neuroectoderm (Fig. 55.1).[4] It is also known that bFGF seems to be closely related to stimulation of endothelial cell proliferation.[5,6] A recent study suggested that the systemic administration of bFGF stimulated endothelial regrowth and proliferation in rat denuded arteries.[7] Local direct application of such peptides in a vascular regenerating environment may be more useful than systemic administration because of their short life in vivo. Moreover, it may be useful to control release of bFGF in order to develop endothelial healing on vascular prosthetic surfaces. In this work to control the release rate of bFGF, hydroxypropylchitosan acetate (HPCHA) was also incorporated into the graft as a carrier of bFGF. HPCHA is a water and alcohol soluble derivative of chitosan, which is known to be a safe and biodegradable polysaccharide from chitin, a marine resource. Tokura and Azuma have reported that HPCHA, a derivative of acetylated HPCH, is well digested in the presence of lysozyme.[8]

It can be used in combination with peptides, as well as many hydrophilic and lipid-soluble chemicals with poor stability or sensitivity to heat and pH; therefore it has been employed as a vehicle in pharmaceutical preparations.[9,10]

Tissue Engineering of Prosthetic Vascular Grafts, edited by Peter Zilla and Howard P. Greisler.
©1999 R.G. Landes Company.

Fig. 55.1. Amino acid sequence of basic fibroblast growth factor.

NH₂-Ala-Ala-Gly-Ser-Ile-Thr-Thr-Leu-Pro-Ala-Leu-Pro-Glu-Asp-
Gly-Gly-Ser-Gly-Ala-Phe-Pro-Pro-Gly-His-Phe-Lys-Asp-Pro-
Lys-Arg-Leu-Tyr-Cys-Lys-Asn-Gly-Gly-Phe-Phe-Leu-Arg-Ile-
His-Pro-Asp-Gly-Arg-Val-Asp-Gly-Val-Arg-Glu-Lys-Ser-Asp-
Pro-His-Ile-Lys-Leu-Gln-Leu-Gln-Ala-Glu-Glu-Arg-Gly-Val-
Val-Ser-Ile-Lys-Gly-Val-Cys-Ala-Asn-Arg-Tyr-Leu-Ala-Met-
Lys-Glu-Asp-Gly-Arg-Leu-Leu-Ala-Ser-Lys-Cys-Val-Thr-Asp-
Glu-Cys-Phe-Phe-Phe-Glu-Arg-Leu-Glu-Ser-Asn-Asn-Tyr-Asn-
Thr-Tyr-Arg-Ser-Arg-Lys-Tyr-Thr-Ser-Trp-Tyr-Val-Ala-Leu-
Lys-Arg-Thr-Gly-Gln-Tyr-Lys-Leu-Gly-Ser-Lys-Thr-Gly-Pro-
Gly-Gln-Lys-Ala-Ile-Leu-Phe-Leu-Pro-Met-Ser-Ala-Lys-Ser-COOH

The subject of this article is limited to the possible use of HPCHA as a carrier controlling the release of growth factor in vitro and vivo.[11]

Use of HPCHA as a Carrier for bFGF

Acetylation of the amino group in hydroxypropylchitosan (HPCH, MW ~800,000; deacetylation degree, 60%; 7200 cps, 5% w/v) was performed following the procedure of Tokura et al.[8] In brief, 10 g of HPCH was dissolved in 150 ml of deionized water and 100 ml of methanol was added to the solution. Then 25 ml of acetic anhydride was added and stirred vigorously overnight. After the resulting solution was dialyzed in deionized water, HPCHA was obtained by lyophilizing the solution. Sixty percent acetylation was confirmed by IR spectrometry. The chemical structure of HPCHA is shown in Figure 55.2.

The amount of recombinant human basic fibroblast growth factor (bFGF) incorporated in an expanded polytetrafluoroethylene graft (Gore-Tex®, inner diameter 3 mm, wall thickness 0.64 mm, mean pore size 30 μm, porosity 80%) was predicted from the water accessible volume. Water loading was 0.00116 ml/graft (0.75 cm in diameter) for distilled water and 0.0147 ml/graft (0.75 cm in diameter) for the HPCHA solution (4%, w/v), respectively.

bFGF was dissolved in sterilized water at a concentration of 1800 μg/ml. Gore-Tex® loaded with bFGF solution was freeze-dried by the procedure of Yamamura et al.[12] HPCHA was dissolved in bFGF solution (180 μg/ml) at a concentration of 4% (w/v). Specific gravity of the solution was 1.01. Figure 55.3 shows scanning electron micrographs (SEM) of inner surfaces of bFGF-HPCHA Gore grafts.

To determine the bFGF activity in the Gore grafts, five bFGF-HPCHA Gore grafts were soaked in 2 ml of a 20 mM isotonic phosphate buffer (pH 7.4) in a boron coated screwcap tube and stored at 5°C for 3 days. The biological activity of bFGF was assayed in baby hamster kidney (BHK)-21 cells, cultured according to Fukunaga et al.[13] In brief, BHK-21 cells were seeded at 1 X 10³ cells/well with bFGF at various concentrations. After 3 days in culture, the increase in protein contents as a measure for the cell proliferation was determined by the bicinchoninic acid method (BCA Protein Assay Kit Pierce Co., IL USA) at 595 nm using a microplate reader (BIO-RAD model 450). Figure 55.4 shows a typical proliferation profile of BHK-21 cells treated with bFGF as a function of the initial concentrations of the factor, where the increase in protein contents was used as a measure for the proliferation of the cells. bFGF content in a bFGF graft was 2.05 ± 0.32 μg (SE, n = 5-6). bFGF content in a bFGF-HPCHA graft was 2.71 ± 0.41 μg (SE, n = 5). Considering that both Gore grafts were water loaded, this value appears reasonable. Also, nearly 100% biological activity of the bFGF incorporated into the grafts was maintained. The present data demonstrates that recombinant bFGF can be incorporated into a graft during aseptic procedures, maintaining biological activity.

Influence of HPCHA on Release of bFGF

In Vitro

The bFGF-HPCHA Gore graft was placed into a boron coated glass tube containing 1 ml of phosphate buffer (pH 5.5) maintained at 37°C, and transferred into new ones after 0.5, 1, 2, 4, 6, 8, 16 and 24 h. Samples were stored at 5°C and assayed within 3 days. The bFGF Gore graft was also studied. Fig. 55.5 shows the cumulative percent of released bFGF from bFGF Gore grafts and bFGF-HPCHA Gore grafts. bFGF release from the bFGF Gore graft reached 100% at 24 h. For the bFGF-HPCHA Gore graft, bFGF was released at about 30% at 8 h and 55% at 24 h. Incorporation of bFGF with HPCHA can apparently sustain its release as compared with the bFGF Gore graft.

In Vivo

Skin pockets in a single row were made in the left and the right flanks of Japanese white rabbits under thiopental anesthesia administered intravenously. Six bFGF Gore grafts were implanted in the left pockets and six bFGF-HPCHA Gore grafts in the right pockets; these were removed at 0.5, 1, 2, 4, 6, 8, 16 and 24 h. The removed grafts were placed into phosphate buffer (pH 7.4) at 5°C for 3 days and assayed. Figure 55.6 shows the percent of remaining bFGF in the bFGF and bFGF-HPCHA Gore grafts after implantation. In vivo release of bFGF from the bFGF Gore grafts reached almost 100% at 24 h following implantation, whereas 60% of bFGF remained in the bFGF-HPCHA Gore grafts at 24 h. Both the animal and in vitro experiments demonstrated that almost 100% of bFGF was released from the bFGF Gore grafts after 24 h, while bFGF release from the bFGF-HPCHA

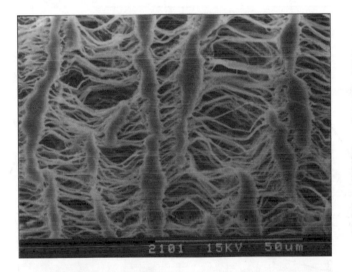

Fig. 55.2. Chemical structure of hydroxypropylchitosan acetate, m,n = integral numbers >1.

R= —— H or $\left(\begin{array}{c} \text{CHCH}_2 \\ | \\ \text{CH}_3 \end{array}\right)_m$ OH or —COCH₃

m,n=an integral number >1

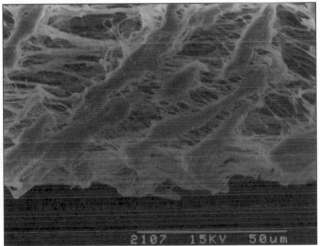

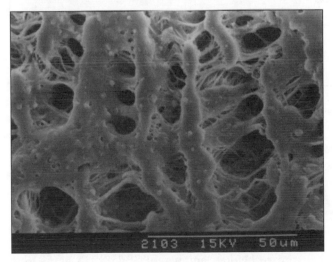

Fig. 55.3. Scanning electron micrographs of various surfaces of Gore grafts: (A) Drug-free Gore graft; (B) bFGF-HPCHA Gore graft before implantation; (C) bFGF-HPCHA Gore graft (Original magnification x1000).

Fig. 55.4. Proliferation profile of BHK-21 cells as a function of initial concentrations of bFGF (SE, n = 5).

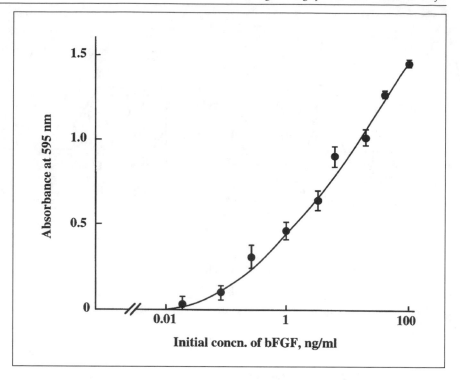

Fig. 55.5. Release rates of bFGF in grafts at 37°C. Graft diameter 0.75 cm; Medium: pH5.5 phosphate buffer; empty circles = bFGF (2.05 μg) in bFGF Gore graft (SE, n = 6); solid circles = bFGF-HPCHA Gore graft (SE, n = 6).

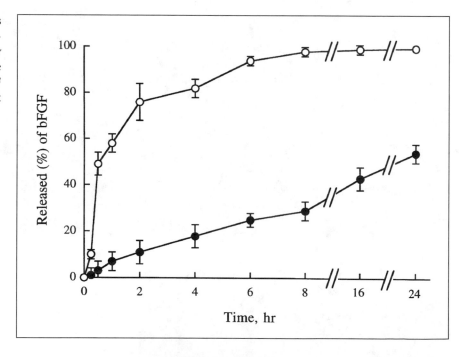

Gore grafts was sustained. Although the release rate from the HPCHA-free graft in the animal experiment was closely correlated to that in the in vitro experiment, a few differences in results were observed between these experiments. In the animal experiment, the release pattern showed an initial lag period of about 1 h compared with the in vitro experiment. It is probable that a slight boundary layer will control the release.

Effect of bFGF-HPCHA on the Endothelialization of Grafts

To evaluate the effect of bFGF on the endothelialization of bFGF-HPCHA Gore grafts, bFGF-HPCHA and drug-free Gore (control) grafts were implanted between artery and vein in dogs. Four adult mongrel dogs were anesthetized with intravenous sodium thiopental, and maintained with nitrous monoxide and halothane. Femoral artery and vein were exposed on both sides and dogs were heparinized before clamping. bFGF-HPCHA grafts were interposed between right femoral artery and vein by double

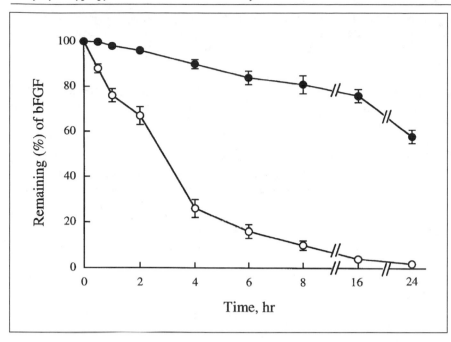

Fig. 55.6. Remaining bFGF in grafts implanted in rabbit abdominal subcutaneous tissues removed at various time intervals. Empty circles = bFGF (2.05 μg) in bFGF Gore graft (SE, n = 5-6); solid circles = bFGF (2.71 μg) in bFGF-HPCHA Gore graft (SE, n = 5-6).

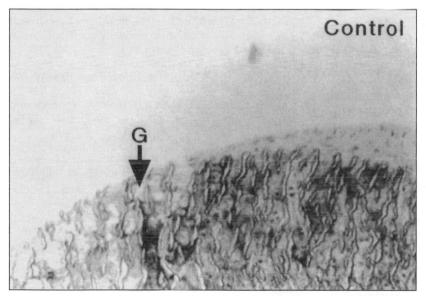

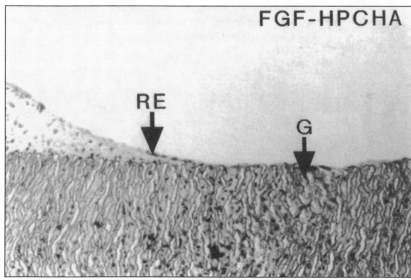

Fig. 55.7. Light microphotographs of the implanted site: (Upper), Drug-free Gore graft; (Lower), bFGF-HPCHA Gore graft at 6 weeks after implantation. G = graft; RE = regenerated endothelial cell. (Hematoxylin-eosin stain, x20).

end to side suture. Control grafts were implanted on the left sides. Specimens were harvested after 6 weeks to investigate proliferation of endothelial cells on the internal surface of the grafts. Grafts were explanted from anesthetized living animals, opened longitudinally for observation and fixed for light microscopy. Fixed specimens were embedded in paraffin and stained with hematoxylin and eosin. The histology of bFGF-HPCHA treated sites showed a thicker layer of connective tissue around the grafts compared with control (Fig. 55.7). The histological examination demonstrated that the local delivery system of bFGF acts to stimulate re-endothelialization.

Concluding Remarks

Our work so far has produced evidence to support the use of HPCHA as a biodegradable carrier for controlled release of bFGF. Coupling bFGF to HPCHA succeeded in a stable and reproducible way.

bFGF-HPCHA solution absorbed into Gore grafts was about 13-fold in weight greater than that of the bFGF solution. It can be assumed that HPCHA solution is held in the pore network of Gore grafts better than water. Calculations of the porosity (~80%) of Gore-Tex® have shown that each Gore-Tex® graft (0.75 cm in diameter) contains pores totaling 0.0226 cm^3; accordingly, the amount of water or HPCHA solution that could be held in the pores is estimated to be roughly 0.0226 ml.

Nevertheless, actual experiments with water or chitosan solution content have shown figures that are substantially lower: For water, roughly one-twentieth of the projected volume is held; for chitosan solution, about two-thirds of the projected volume.

The explanation for this may be that hydrophobic materials such as Gore-Tex® repel water, making it difficult for the pores in the graft to retain fluid. A high molecular solution like chitosan has greater inherent viscosity, however, and is thus more likely to be retained within the Gore-Tex® pores than is water. Therefore, one effective way to increase the amounts of drugs contained within Gore-Tex® pores is to improve retention by increasing the viscosity of fluids through use of high molecular solutions, and its further release rate can be controlled by changing the ratio of HPCHA. In conclusion, HPCHA could be used as a carrier to control continuous release of unstable substances such as peptide, hydrophilic and lipid-soluble chemicals in vivo.

Further, bFGF-HPCHA Gore grafts are useful for vascular reconstruction, because bFGF stimulates regrowth of endothelial cells on the graft surface.

References

1. Berger K , Sauvage LR, Rao AM et al. Healing of arterial graft in man; Its incompleteness. Ann Surg 1972; 175:118-127.
2. Schmit S, Hunter T, Falkow L et al. Effects of antiplatelet agents in combination with endothelial cell seeding on small-diameter Dacron vascular graft performance in canine carotid artery model. J Vasc Surg 1985; 2:898-906.
3. Herring M, Garner A, Peigh P et al. Patency in canine inferior vena cava grafting: Effects of graft material, size, and endothelial seeding. J Vasc Surg 1984; 1:877-887.
4. Gospodarowicz D, Ferrara N, Schweigerer L et al. Structural characterization and biological functions of fibroblast growth factor. Endocr Rev 1987; 8:95-114.
5. Saksera O, Moscatelli D, Rifkin DB. The opposing effects of basic fibroblast growth factor and transforming growth factor beta on the regulation of plasminogen activity in capillary endothelial cells. J Cell Biol 1987; 105:957-963.
6. Schweigere L, Neufeld G, Friedman J et al. Basic fibroblast growth factor: Production and growth stimulation in cultured adrenal cortex cells. Endocr 1987; 120:796-800.
7. Lindner V, Majak RA, Reidy MA. Basic fibroblast growth factor stimulates endothelial regrowth and proliferation in denuded arteries. J Clin Invest 1990; 85:2004-2008.
8. Tokura S, Azuma I. Distribution of acetamide group in partially deacetylated chitin and its biodegradability. Derivatives in Life Science 1992; 1:86-92.
9. Machida Y, Banba T, Fujimoto M et al. Synthesis and antitumor activity of chitosan carrying 5-fluorouracils. Macromol Chem 1989; 190:1817-1825.
10. Nishioka Y, Kyotani S, Okamura M et al. Release characteristics of cisplatin chitosan microspheres and effect of containing chitin. Chem Pharm Bull 1990; 38:2871-2873.
11. Yamamura K, Sakurai T, Yano K et al. Sustained release of basic fibroblast growth factor from the synthetic vascular graft using hydroxypropylchitosan acetate. J Biomed Mater Res 1995; 29:203-206.
12. Yamamura K, Iwata H, Yotsuyanagi T. Synthesis of antibiotic-loaded hydroxyapatite beads and in vitro drug release testing. J Biomed Mater Res 1992; 26:1053-1064.
13. Fukunaga K, Hijikata S, Ishimura K et al. Aluminium β-cyclodextrin sulphate as a stabilizer and sustained-release carrier for basic fibroblast growth factor. J Pharm Pharmacol 1994; 46:168-171.

Cell Engineering

——————————— CHAPTER 56 ———————————

Transplantation of Transduced Smooth Muscle Cells: A Vehicle for Local and Systemic Gene Therapy

Randolph L. Geary, Alexander W. Clowes, Monika M. Clowes

Introduction

Since the advent of techniques to introduce recombinant DNA into mammalian tissues, a new science of gene transfer has emerged with broad application throughout the life sciences.[1-3] With it has come the ability to genetically alter vascular smooth muscle cells (SMC) and endothelial cells in vitro and in vivo, allowing the vascular biologist to ask and answer questions previously unanswerable.[4-16] Over the past decade an intense enthusiasm for the clinical application of vascular gene transfer has matured into cautious optimism, as the limitations of vector systems used to introduce and express recombinant genes in vascular tissues have been better defined.[3] Refinements in vector systems have improved the precision and safety of vascular gene transfer and proof-of-concept experiments have demonstrated the potential for both local and systemic therapeutic effects.[17-30] While the field is still in its infancy, the first clinical application of vascular gene transfer has been initiated and the realization of vascular gene therapy may well be at hand.[31,32]

The use of prosthetic materials in the treatment of cardiovascular diseases is expanding as new devices are created and the indications for applying existing devices are broadened. A significant limitation of all implantable prosthetic materials is biocompatibility. Prosthetic vascular grafts have been widely used to reconstruct damaged and diseased arteries and veins. Despite extensive research to improve graft function, thrombosis and intimal hyperplasia continue to limit graft durability, particularly when used to reconstruct small arteries or veins. Infections also lead to graft failure and significant morbidity and mortality in a small but significant number of patients. Application of existing gene transfer technology to prosthetic vascular devices has thus been directed toward inhibition of neointimal growth and thrombus formation and toward improving the extent of graft healing to decrease the risk of infection.[4,27,33-38] If successful, these strategies will improve graft function and constitute an important advance in patient care and limb salvage.

In the following discussion we will review the use SMCs as hosts for the expression of therapeutic recombinant genes. A comprehensive review of vascular gene therapy is beyond the scope of this chapter and we wish to acknowledge the pioneering work by many investigators in this field without which our studies would not have been possible.[39] While our focus has been on the SMC, others have made extraordinary advances in the application of endothelial cell-based gene transfer and we refer the reader to those important studies for a more complete appreciation of the potential for vascular gene therapy.

Tissue Engineering of Prosthetic Vascular Grafts, edited by Peter Zilla and Howard P. Greisler.
©1999 R.G. Landes Company.

Smooth Muscle Cells as Targets for Gene Transfer

SMCs provide an attractive target for gene transfer, as they comprise the majority of cells within the wall of blood vessels and play a central role in vascular diseases such as atherosclerosis and intimal hyperplasia following arterial reconstruction. Modifying SMC behavior by recombinant gene transfer then provides the opportunity to limit SMC growth, migration and extracellular matrix elaboration, critical components of atherosclerotic plaque or neointima formation. Vessel wall function could also be improved by local over-expression of genes encoding factors to inhibit vasoconstriction, inflammation, and thrombosis. These and other modifications could translate into improved outcomes for patients undergoing surgical or endovascular arterial and venous reconstruction.

SMCs have characteristics which make them an attractive target tissue in which to express recombinant genes for systemic therapy. Muscle cells in general have proven to be durable hosts for recombinant gene expression.[40-43] SMCs represent a large population of cells separated from the systemic circulation by a single endothelial cell layer. SMCs are generally quiescent in vivo with replication rates of less than one percent,[44] and as a result SMCs are very long-lived, providing the potential for stable long term expression of therapeutic genes. These attributes have led our group and others to explore the application of SMCs as hosts for local and systemic gene delivery.

Vectors for SMC Gene Transfer

As noted above, the practical application of vascular gene therapy has been limited by the vector systems used to introduce recombinant genetic material. Virtually all vector systems have been used successfully to transduce vascular SMCs, including viral vectors (retrovirus,[4-6,45] adenovirus,[46,47] adeno-associated virus,[48] and others[3]); plasmid DNA;[49] liposomal vectors;[50] and hybrid systems.[51,52] Each vector has its own set of limitations, which generally fall into the following categories: inefficient in vivo SMC transduction; inefficient gene expression following transduction; transient expression due to a lack of genomic integration; transient gene expression due to an immune response to products of viral coding sequences; and inability to limit gene transfer to the target site due to systemic spread of recombinant material to nontarget tissues.

Our group has employed retroviral vectors[13,14,43,45,53] and adeno-associated virus vectors[48] to transduce SMCs ex vivo and in vivo, respectively. We will review below our experience with the retroviral vector system for cell-based vascular gene transfer using transplanted SMCs.

Retroviral Vectors for Ex Vivo Arterial Gene Transfer

Retroviruses have been used extensively for recombinant gene transfer in a wide variety of cell types, both in vitro and in vivo.[1,2,39,54] This system has a number of advantages and disadvantages. Retroviral vectors are made incapable of self-replication, as all viral coding sequences essential for encapsidation have been deleted.[55] Only the insertion and promoter sequences essential for integration and expression of the recombinant gene within the host cell genome remain (Fig. 56.1). As retroviral vectors integrate their recombinant genes directly into the host cell genome, the transgene is expressed throughout the life of the cell and can be duplicated during mitosis and passed on to daughter cells. This provides the potential for stable long term expression in contrast to the transient expression (days) of recombinant genes introduced by plasmid and adenoviral vectors.[56,57] The lack of viral coding sequences prevents immune responses towards foreign proteins, which has been a significant problem with first generation adenoviral vectors containing a number of wild type coding sequences.[58]

A major limitation of retroviral vectors is that expression of the recombinant transgene requires prior integration into the host cell genome. Efficient integration in turn requires that the host cell be replicating at the time of viral transduction.[54,55] As SMCs are generally quiescent within the undisturbed artery wall, direct in vivo transduction is very inefficient.[45] Even at sites of vascular reconstruction, SMC replication is delayed for hours or days after the injury caused by the procedure. Retroviral gene transfer directed at improving the response to surgical or endovascular reconstruction would require a delayed application of virus (24-96 h post-procedure). By that time however, the injury response is well underway with local thrombus formation, release of platelet growth factors, and influx of leukocytes that may overcome any potential benefits of delayed gene transfer. Vein grafts present a similar obstacle for retroviral vectors. For these reasons, alternative vectors capable of gene transfer into quiescent SMC in vivo are being explored for gene transfer to SMCs at the time of vascular reconstruction (e.g., adeno-associated virus and adenovirus).[46,48,56]

To accommodate the need for cell replication for retroviral vector integration, ex vivo gene transfer of target cells has been performed in culture. SMCs can be readily established in culture from small artery or vein biopsies and induced to replicate by serum growth factors.[14,45,59] Early passage cells can then be exposed to retroviral vectors containing antibiotic resistance genes that allow for selection of transduced cells by adding antibiotic to the culture medium (Fig. 56.1). Populations of transduced cells can then be expanded further in culture for later transplantation back into the donor vasculature. This strategy requires the use of autologous SMCs to prevent immune rejection of transplanted cells. It also takes time (weeks) to accumulate the numbers of transduced cells required to achieve local or systemic effects.

We have used this strategy successfully for ex vivo gene transfer and subsequent in vivo transplantation of SMCs expressing a number of vectors (Fig. 56.1). These include reporter proteins (β-galactosidase (β–gal) and human placental alkaline phosphatase (hAP))[13,14,43,45] and proteins with local and systemic biological effects (adenosine deaminase, purine nucleoside phosphorylase, erythropoietin, and others).[14,28,29,43,45,53] Initial experiments were performed using SMCs cultured from aortas of the syngeneic Fischer 344 rat strain. The cells were transduced with the human adenosine deaminase (ADA) gene which codes for a nonsecreted

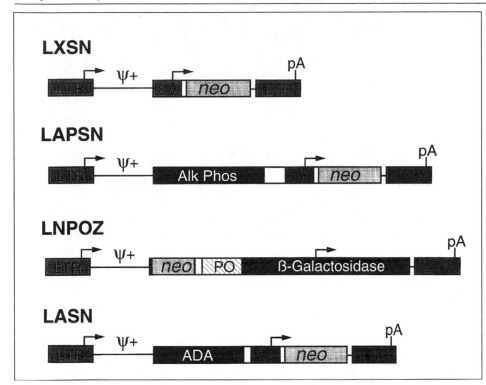

Fig. 56.1. Diagram of retroviral vectors employed for smooth muscle cell gene transfer. This vector system was originally described by A.D. Miller and colleagues[55] and the vectors are named based on the order of genetic elements. L, long terminal repeat promoter; S, SV40 promoter; N, neomycin resistance gene; PO, polio virus IRES 5' sequences; X, insertion site for subcloning genes of interest, including: A, human adenosine deaminase (ADA); AP, human placental alkaline phosphatase (Alk Phos); and Z, lacZ (β-galactosidase).

protein that can be identified and distinguished from rat ADA by protein gel electrophoresis.[45] The transduced cells were then transplanted into Fischer rat carotid arteries following endothelial cell denudation. This strategy results in the immediate formation of a nonocclusive neointima composed entirely of transduced SMCs (Fig. 56.2). Arteries were removed at various times following seeding and significant human ADA expression was documented as late as 6 months after carotid seeding.[45] A follow up study in the same model demonstrated effective retroviral vector expression by seeded SMCs even at one year from the time of transplantation (see below), documenting the durability of the retroviral approach.[43]

While these experiments and those of others[4,6] established the proof-of-concept for ex vivo transduction of SMCs, questions regarding the behavior of transduced SMCs following transplantation remained unanswered. For instance, retroviral transduction preferentially occurs in replicating cells. If cells selected in culture for replication were more prone to replicate in vivo, intimal hyperplasia could occur and lead to lumen narrowing in treated vessels or grafts. Altered migration or matrix elaboration by transduced cells would also have adverse effects in vivo.

To address these concerns, subsequent experiments were performed using a vector encoding the hAP marker gene to localize transduced cells within seeded rat carotid arteries and surrounding tissues (Figs. 56.1 and 56.2).[43] Bromodeoxyuridine was administered to label replicating cells, and arteries were removed for analysis at various times following transduction. Seeding led to a nonocclusive intima composed entirely of transduced SMCs expressing the AP gene product (Fig. 56.2). Within 2 weeks the neointima also contained nontransduced SMCs that had migrated into

the neointima from the underlying media. Lesion size and SMC replication were self-limited and the resulting neointima was no larger than that of sham-seeded control arteries. Stenosis did not occur and transduced cells were not found outside of the transduced artery wall or in locations beyond the site of initial transplantation (Fig. 56.2). These results underscore the durability and apparent safety of SMC-based retroviral vascular gene transfer.

Subsequent experiments have demonstrated that this technique can be used to achieve a potentially therapeutic systemic response.[28,29,53] SMCs were transduced with a retroviral vector encoding the rat erythropoietin gene and then transplanted successfully into the rat carotid artery as described above. The small number of cells transplanted into carotid arteries (10^5 cells) produced enough erythropoietin to significantly increase erythrocyte production, causing an increase in reticulocyte counts followed by increases in hematocrit and hemoglobin.

We have also demonstrated that local gene expression within the injured artery wall can inhibit intimal hyperplasia. SMCs were transduced with a retroviral vector expressing the gene encoding tissue inhibitor of matrix metalloproteinase-1 (TIMP-1). TIMP-1 blocks metalloproteinase activity, limiting extracellular matrix degradation essential for cell migration and replication. TIMP-1 overexpression impaired migration of transduced cells in culture and, when seeded into rat carotid arteries after balloon injury, inhibited neointima formation.[28] Allaire from our group has used this same TIMP-1 vector to inhibit aneurysm formation and rupture in rat aortic xenografts (guinea pig into rat).[29] All grafts transplanted without SMC seeding developed aneurysms which ruptured between 4 and 21 days. In contrast, none of the grafts seeded with SMCs

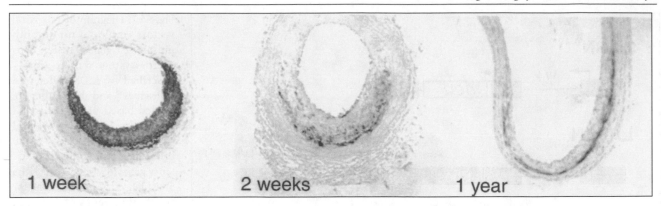

Fig. 56.2. Composite photomicrograph of rat carotid artery cross sections removed at 1 week, 2 weeks or 12 months following transplantation of smooth muscle cells transduced with a retroviral vector encoding the alkaline phosphatase (AP) reporter gene (dark blue reaction product). At 1 week a nonocclusive intima has been created, with seeded cells expressing the AP gene product. Within 2 weeks cells have migrated into the neointima from the injured media so that the final intimal lesion is composed of a mixture of transduced (blue stain) and nontransduced smooth muscle cells. Neointimal area is maximal 4-6 weeks after seeding and expression of the AP reporter gene is durable, with long term expression shown in an artery removed 12 months following transplantation.

expressing TIMP-1 developed aneurysms. Grafts seeded with SMCs transduced with a vector encoding only the neo gene (LXSN, Fig. 56.1) all developed aneurysms within 4 weeks of transplantation, and 2 of 6 ruptured. These results have prompted us to extend studies of retroviral vascular gene transfer to other animal models.

Retroviral Vectors for SMC Gene Transfer in Prosthetic Vascular Grafts

As described in the accompanying chapters, prosthetic vascular grafts present a unique set of challenges when used to reconstruct damaged or occluded arteries and veins. Prosthetic conduits are more prone to infection than are autologous grafts and suffer disproportionately from thrombosis and neointima formation at anastomoses. This is particularly true when grafts are used to reconstruct small arteries and veins. Prosthetic grafts heal by neointimal ingrowth from the cut arterial ends at anastomoses. The neointima extends a limited distance onto the graft lumen surface depending on graft porosity. In more porous grafts, neointima may form along the entire lumen surface by ingrowth of granulation tissue and microvessels directly through graft wall interstices.[60-62] The resulting graft neointima is made up largely of SMCs and their surrounding extracellular matrix beneath an endothelial cell monolayer.

SMCs then provide a direct target for gene therapy to reduce graft intimal hyperplasia and neointimal formation. Indirect targets include reducing graft thrombogenicity and improving the resistance of graft material to infection. Moreover, given that prosthetic grafts heal by accumulating SMCs, we hypothesized that preseeding grafts with large numbers of genetically modified SMCs could provide a device for systemic delivery of recombinant gene products capable of treating inherited or acquired disorders.

Using a previously established nonhuman primate model of PTFE bypass grafting,[60-62] we sought to establish genetically modified autologous vascular SMCs within grafts prior to implantation. Autologous SMCs were obtained from baboons via saphenous vein biopsy, and early passage SMCs were established in culture using standard techniques.[14,59] Cells were then exposed to replication-deficient retroviral particles encoding the human placental AP gene coupled to the neomycin resistance gene (Fig. 56.1). Cells were initially selected in neomycin, then expanded and within 4-6 weeks of obtaining the vein biopsy, 10^7 to 10^9 transduced SMC were available for PTFE graft seeding (Fig. 56.3). Transduced SMCs were then suspended in a solution of type I collagen and the mixture injected into the lumen of 10 cm long, 4 mm diameter, PTFE grafts (60 μm internodal distance, WL Gore Corp., Flagstaff, AZ). Collagen was used to facilitate cell retention and adhesion to the PTFE graft material. The cell suspension was gently infused into the graft lumen and extruded through graft wall interstices (Fig. 56.3). Seeded grafts were incubated overnight and then grafted end-to-side into the aorto-iliac position of the original donor baboon.

Grafts were allowed to heal for 3-6 weeks, a time period when an unseeded PTFE graft would have formed a significant neointima along its entire length.[60-62] In the first experiments, grafts were more prone to thrombosis due to exposure of the collagen gel to flowing blood. In subsequent experiments autologous endothelial cells were cultured from each vein biopsy. The endothelial cells were not transduced, but were seeded onto the lumen surface of PTFE grafts following SMC seeding. This strategy eliminated the problem of increased graft thrombosis. When grafts were removed for analysis, a significant population of transduced SMCs was localized within the graft wall by histochemical staining for the hAP gene product (Fig. 56.3). To our surprise, the neointima which had formed was devoid of transduced cells, indicating that, while they survived the transplantation and graft implantation process, cells appeared to stay where they were initially seeded and did not migrate into the forming neointima. In addition, transduced SMCs were not recruited by microvessels forming within the graft wall granulation

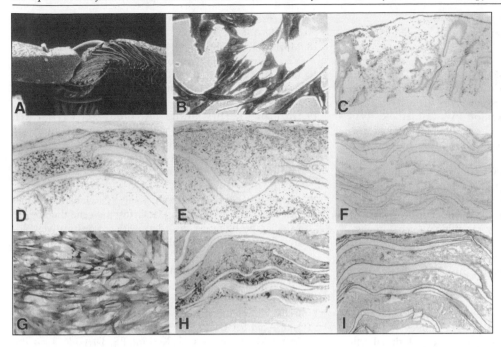

Fig. 56.3. Composite photomicrograph demonstrating PTFE graft seeding with baboon smooth muscle cells transduced ex vivo with retroviral vectors encoding either alkaline phosphatase (AP, dark blue staining) or β-galactosidase (β-gal, light blue staining). PTFE grafts of 60 micron porosity were employed, as these grafts develop a neointima along their entire lumen surface in contrast to the less porous clinical graft (Panel A). Autologous smooth muscle cells were obtained from saphenous vein biopsies and transduced in culture with either β–gal (Panel B) or AP vectors (Panel G). Grafts were seeded 24 hours prior to implantation with 10^6 to 10^9 transduced cells in a collagen gel. Cells became lodged throughout the graft wall as shown in a cross section taken prior to graft implantation (Panel C). Grafts were removed one month after implantation into the aorto-iliac circulation of baboons, and cross-sections stained for β gal (Panels D and F) or AP (Panels H and I). Paired control grafts were placed in each animal, which showed no staining (Panels F and I) in contrast to the many cells stained within treated grafts. Adjacent sections stained for smooth muscle α-actin (Panel E) showed a similar pattern of staining. Of note, transduced cells were not found within the graft neointima or outside of the graft wall in surrounding connective tissue (Panels D and H).

tissue. Perhaps more importantly, transduced SMCs were not found outside of the graft wall within the fibrous capsule around the graft or in the vasculature of lower extremity muscle beds beyond the seeded interposition grafts.[13]

These experiments were repeated using a separate reporter gene in order to establish that the healing characteristics of seeded grafts were not influenced by expression of the hAP gene. In the follow up study we employed a retroviral vector encoding the β-gal reporter gene (Fig. 56.1).[14] The same seeding technique was employed and grafts were left in place for 4-5 weeks and then removed for analysis. The findings were essentially the same. Transduced cells were located within the interstices of each seeded graft and cells were not seen within the neointima or in the surrounding perigraft tissues (Fig. 56.3).

Unanswered Questions and Future Directions

While the results of SMC-based gene transfer in experimental models are encouraging, a number of questions remain to be addressed. Long term expression of recombinant genes by rat SMCs must be reproduced in models likely to better represent the human situation. This is critical, as the long term biological behavior of transduced human SMCs is unknown. Strategies to improve SMC retention upon transplantation are also needed in order to apply this strategy effectively to human prosthetic devices.[38] This problem may be overcome as we learn more about the role of cell surface integrins and their adhesive interactions

with specific matrix molecules.[63] By implanting cells in unique matrix environments, cell growth and adhesion may be enhanced, as it is well established that SMC behavior in vitro and in vivo is altered by adhesion to various matrix components.[63,64]

Ex vivo techniques, while suitable for elective modification of bioprostheses, are not applicable to the majority of clinical procedures. Furthermore, while retroviral vectors have been used in a number of early human gene therapy trials,[2] concerns about their safety remain. Retrovirus vectors integrate randomly into host cell DNA, leading to the possibility of latent oncogene activation.[2,54] Better vectors are being created for direct in vivo vascular gene transfer that are more simple to use and more durable than current vectors. Sophisticated systems have been designed to include transcription initiation sequences that can be turned on and off in the presence or absence of specific cofactors.[65] Once these systems are available, concerns over the lack of control of the magnitude and duration of gene expression may be alleviated. Device technology is also helping to make clinical application of vectors a reality through inventions such as through-lumen and spray catheters.[66]

While still in its infancy the first application of vascular gene transfer to improve patient care is on the horizon. Use of this technology to improve the biocompatibility and function of prosthetic vascular devices has been initiated[14,23,27,34,35,37,38] and if successful a revolution in vascular reconstruction should follow.

References

1. Mulligan RC. The basic science of gene therapy. Science 1993; 260:926-932.
2. Morgan RA, Anderson WF. Human gene therapy. Annu Rev Biochem 1993; 62:191-217.
3. Gibbons GH, Dzau VJ. Molecular therapies for vascular diseases. Science 1996; 272:689-693.
4. Zwiebel JA, Freeman SM, Kantoff PW, Cornetta K, Ryan US, Anderson WF. High-level recombinant gene expression in rabbit endothelial cells transduced by retroviral vectors. Science 1989; 243:220-222.
5. Nabel EG, Plautz G, Nabel GJ. Site specific gene expression in vivo by direct gene transfer into the arterial wall. Science 1990; 249:1285-1288.
6. Plautz G, Nabel EG, Nabel GJ. Introduction of vascular smooth muscle cells expressing recombinant genes in vivo. Circulation 1991; 83:578-583.
7. Dreher KL, Cowan K. Expression of antisense transcripts encoding an extracellular matrix protein by stably transfected vascular smooth muscle cells. Eur J Cell Biol 1991; 54:1-9.
8. Messina LM, Podrazik RM, Whitehill TA, Ekhterae D, Brothers TE, Wilson JM, Burkel WE, Stanley JC. Adhesion and incorporation of lacZ-transduced endothelial cells into the intact capillary wall in the rat. Proc Natl Acad Sci USA 1992; 89:12018-12022.
9. Kahn ML, Lee SW, Dichek DA. Optimization of retroviral vector-mediated gene transfer into endothelial cells in vitro. Circ Res 1992; 71:1508-1517.
10. Nabel EG, Yang Z, Liptay S, San H, Gordon D, Haudenschild CC, Nabel GJ. Recombinant platelet-derived growth factor B gene expression in porcine arteries induces intimal hyperplasia in vivo. J Clin Invest 1993; 91:1822-1829.
11. Nabel EG, Shum L, Pompili VJ, Yang Z, San H, Shu HB, Liptay S, Gold L, Gordon D, Derynck R, Nabel GJ. Direct transfer of transforming growth factor β1 gene into arteries stimulates fibrocellular hyperplasia. Proc Natl Acad Sci USA 1993; 90:10759-10763.
12. Lemarchand P, Jones M, Yamada I, Crystal RG. In vivo gene transfer and expression in normal uninjured blood vessels using replication-deficient recombinant adenovirus vectors. Circ Res 1993; 72:1132-1138.
13. Geary RL, Lynch CM, Vergel S, Miller AD, Clowes AW. Human gene expression in baboons using vascular grafts seeded with retrovirally-transduced smooth muscle cells. Circulation 1993; 88:1-81(Abstract).
14. Geary RL, Clowes AW, Lau S, Vergel S, Dale DC, Osborne WRA. Gene transfer in baboons using prosthetic vascular grafts seeded with retrovirally transduced smooth muscle cells: A model for local and systemic gene therapy. Hum Gene Ther 1994; 5:1211-1216.
15. Morishita R, Gibbons GH, Pratt RE, Tomita N, Kaneda Y, Ogihara T, Dzau VJ. Autocrine and paracrine effects of atrial natriuretic peptide gene transfer on vascular smooth muscle and endothelial cellular growth. J Clin Invest 1994; 94:824-829.
16. Morishita R, Gibbons GH, Kaneda Y, Ogihara T, Dzau VJ. Novel and effective gene transfer technique for study of vascular renin angiotensin system. J Clin Invest 1993; 91:2580-2585.
17. Morishita R, Gibbons GH, Ellison KE, Nakajima M, Von der Leyen H, Zhang L, Kaneda Y, Ogihara T, Dzau VJ. Intimal hyperplasia after vascular injury is inhibited by antisense cdk 2 kinase oligonucleotides. J Clin Invest 1994; 93:1458-1464.
18. Morishita R, Gibbons GH, Kaneda Y, Ogihara T, Dzau VJ. Pharmacokinetics of antisense oligodeoxyribonucleotides (cyclin B$_1$ and CDC 2 kinase) in the vessel wall in vivo: Enhanced therapeutic utility for restenosis by HVJ-liposome delivery. Gene 1994; 149:13-19.
19. Guzman RJ, Hirschowitz EA, Brody SL, Crystal RG, Epstein SE, Finkel T. In vivo suppression of injury-induced vascular smooth muscle cell accumulation using adenovirus-mediated transfer of the herpes simplex thymidine kinase gene. Proc Natl Acad Sci USA 1994; 91:10732-10736.
20. Chang MW, Barr E, Seltzer J, Jiang YQ, Nabel GJ, Nabel EG, Parmacek MS, Leiden JM. Cytostatic gene therapy for vascular proliferative disorders with a constitutively active form of the retinoblastoma gene product. Science 1995; 267:518-522.
21. Von der Leyen HE, Gibbons GH, Morishita R, Lewis NP, Zhang L, Nakajima M, Kaneda Y, Cooke JP, Dzau VJ. Gene therapy inhibiting neointimal vascular lesion: In vivo transfer of endothelial cell nitric oxide synthase gene. Proc Natl Acad Sci USA 1995; 92:1137-1141.
22. Mann MJ, Gibbons GH, Kernoff RS, Diet FP, Tsao PS, Cooke JP, Kaneda Y, Dzau VJ. Genetic engineering of vein grafts resistant to atherosclerosis. Proc Natl Acad Sci USA 1995; 92:4502-4506.
23. Ekhterae D, Stanley JC. Retroviral vector-mediated transfer and expression of human tissue plasminogen activator gene in human endothelial and vascular smooth muscle cells. J Vasc Surg 1995; 21:953-962.
24. Chang MW, Barr E, Lu MM, Barton K, Leiden JM. Adenovirus-mediated over-expression of the cyclin cyclin-dependent kinase inhibitor, p21 inhibits vascular smooth muscle cell proliferation and neointima formation in the rat carotid artery model of balloon angioplasty. J Clin Invest 1995; 96:2260-2268.
25. Zoldhelyi P, McNatt J, Xu XM, Loose-Mitchell D, Meidell RS, Clubb FJ Jr, Buja LM, Willerson JT, Wu KK. Prevention of arterial thrombosis by adenovirus-mediated transfer of cyclooxygenase gene. Circulation 1996; 93:10-17.
26. Rade JJ, Schulick AH, Virmani R, Dichek DA. Local adenoviral-mediated expression of recombinant hirudin reduces neointima formation after arterial injury. Nature Med 1996; 2:293-298.
27. Dunn PF, Newman KD, Jones M, Yamada I, Shayani V, Virmani R, Dichek DA. Seeding of vascular grafts with genetically modified endothelial cells—Secretion of recombinant TPA results in decreased seeded cell retention in vitro and in vivo. Circulation 1996; 93:1439-1446.
28. Forough R, Koyama N, Hasenstab D, Lea H, Clowes M, Nikkari ST, Clowes AW. Overexpression of tissue inhibitor of matrix metalloproteinase-1 inhibits vascular smooth muscle cell functions in vitro and in vivo. Circ Res 1996; 79:812-820.
29. Allaire E, Forough R, Wang T, Clowes MM, Clowes AW. Local overexpression of tissue inhibitor of metalloproteinases-1 (TIMP-1) prevents arterial dilation and rupture. J Vasc Res 1996; 33:A09(Abstract).
30. Takeshita S, Tsurumi Y, Couffinahl T, Asahara T, Bauters C, Symes J, Ferrara N, Isner JM. Gene transfer of naked DNA encoding for three isoforms of vascular endothelial growth factor stimulates collateral development in vivo. Lab Invest 1996; 75:487-501.

31. Isner JM, Walsh K, Symes J, Pieczek A, Takeshita S, Lowry J, Rossow S, Rosenfield K, Weir L, Brogi E, Schainfeld R. Arterial gene therapy for therapeutic angiogenesis in patients with peripheral artery disease. Circulation 1995; 91:2687-2692.

32. Isner JM, Pieczek A, Schainfeld R, Blair R, Haley L, Asahara T, Rosenfield K, Razvi S, Walsh K, Symes JF. Clinical evidence of angiogenesis after arterial gene transfer of phVEGF165 in patient with ischaemic lim. Lancet 1996; 348:370-374.

33. Dichek DA, Neville RF, Zwiebel JA, Freeman SM, Leon MB, Anderson WF. Seeding of intravascular stents with genetically engineered endothelial cells. Circulation 1989; 80:1347-1353.

34. Flugelman MY, Virmani R, Leon MB, Bowman RL, Dichek DA. Genetically engineered endothelial cells remain adherent and viable after stent deployment and exposure to flow in vitro. Circ Res 1992; 70:348-354.

35. Huber TS, Welling TH, Sarkar R, Messina LM, Stanley JC. Effects of retroviral-mediated tissue plasminogen activator gene transfer and expression on adherence and proliferation of canine endothelial cells seeded onto expanded polytetrafluoroethylene. J Vasc Surg 1995; 22:795-803.

36. Flugelman MY: Inhibition of intravascular thrombosis and vascular smooth muscle cell proliferation by gene therapy. Thrombosis & Haemostasis. Thromb Haemost 1995; 74:406-410.

37. Dichek DA, Anderson J, Kelly AB, Hanson SR, Harker LA. Enhanced in vivo antithrombotic effects of endothelial cells expressing recombinant plasminogen activators transduced with retroviral vectors. Circulation 1996; 93:301-309.

38. Scott-Burden T, Tock CL, Schwarz JJ, Casscells SW, Engler DA. Genetically engineered smooth muscle cells as linings to improve the biocompatibility of cardiovascular prostheses. Circulation 1997; 94:II-235-II-238.

39. Clowes AW. Vascular gene therapy in the 21st century. Thromb Haemost 1997; 78:605-610.

40. Dai Y, Roman M, Naviaux RK, Verma IM. Gene therapy via primary myoblasts: Long-term expression of factor IX protein following transplantation in vivo. Proc Natl Acad Sci USA 1992; 89:10892-10895.

41. Isaka Y, Brees DK, Ikegaya K, Kaneda Y, Imai E, Noble NA, Border WA. Gene therapy by skeletal muscle expression of decorin prevents fibrotic disease in rat kidney. Nature Med 1996; 2:418-423.

42. Blau HM, Springer ML. Muscle-mediated gene therapy. N Engl J Med 1995; 333:1554-1556.

43. Clowes MM, Lynch CM, Miller AD, Miller DG, Osborne WRA, Clowes AW. Long-term biological response of injured rat carotid artery seeded with smooth muscle cells expressing retrovirally introduced human genes. J Clin Invest 1994; 93:644-651.

44. Clowes AW, Reidy MA, Clowes MM. Kinetics of cellular proliferation after arterial injury.I.Smooth muscle growth in the absence of endothelium. Lab Invest 1983; 49:327-333.

45. Lynch CM, Clowes MM, Osborne WRA, Clowes AW, Miller AD. Long-term expression of human adenosine deaminase in vascular smooth muscle cells of rats: A model for gene therapy. Proc Natl Acad Sci USA 1992; 89:1138-1142.

46. Lemarchand P, Jaffe HA, Danel C, Cid MC, Kleinman HK, Stratford-Perricaudet LD, Perricaudet M, Pavirani A, Lecocq JP, Crystal RG. Adenovirus-mediated transfer of recombinant human alpha 1-antitrypsin cDNA to human endothelial cells. Proc Natl Acad Sci USA 1992; 89:6482-6486.

47. Lee SW, Trapnell BC, Rade JJ, Virmani R, Dichek DA. In vivo adenoviral vector-mediated gene transfer into balloon-injured rat carotid arteries. Circ Res 1993; 73:797-807.

48. Lynch CM, Hara PS, Leonard JC, Williams JK, Dean RH, Geary RL. Adeno-associated virus vectors for vascular gene delivery. Circ Res 1997; 80:497-505.

49. Riessen R, Rahimizadeh H, Blessing E, Takeshita S, Barry JJ, Isner JM. Arterial gene transfer using pure DNA applied directly to a hydrogel-coated angioplasty balloon. Hum Gene Ther 1993; 4:749-758.

50. Leclerc G, Gal D, Takeshita S, Nikol S, Weir L, Isner JM. Percutaneous arterial gene transfer in a rabbit model. Efficiency in normal and balloon-dilated atherosclerotic arteries. J Clin Invest 1992; 90:936-944.

51. Morishita R, Gibbons GH, Kaneda Y, Ogihara T, Dzau VJ. Novel in vitro gene transfer method for study of local modulators in vascular smooth muscle cells. Hypertension 1993; 21:894-899.

52. Dzau VJ, Mann MJ, Morishita R, Kaneda Y. Fusigenic viral liposome for gene therapy in cardiovascular diseases. Proc Natl Acad Sci USA 1996; 93:11421-11425.

53. Osborne WRA, Ramesh N, Lau S, Clowes MM, Dale DC, Clowes AW. Gene therapy for long-term expression of erythropoietin in rats. Proc Natl Acad Sci USA 1995; 92:8055-8058.

54. Morgan JR, Tompkins RG, Yarmush ML. Advances in recombinant retroviruses for gene delivery. Adv Drug Deliv Rev 1993; 12:143-158.

55. Miller AD, Rosman GJ. Improved retroviral vectors for gene transfer and expression. BioTechniques 1989; 7:980-990.

56. Schulick AH, Newman KD, Virmani R, Dichek DA. In vivo gene transfer into injured carotid arteries: Optimization and evaluation of acute toxicity. Circulation 1995; 91:2407-2414.

57. Feldman LJ, Steg PG, Zheng LP, Chen D, Kearney M, McGarr SE, Barry JJ, Dedieu J-F, Perricaudet M, Isner JM. Low-efficiency of percutaneous adenovirus-mediated arterial gene transfer in the atherosclerotic rabbit. J Clin Invest 1995; 95:2662-2671.

58. Newman KD, Dunn PF, Owens JW, Schulick AH, Virmani R, Sukhova G, Libby P, Dichek DA. Adenovirus-mediated gene transfer into normal rabbit arteries results in prolonged vascular cell activation, inflammation, and neointimal hyperplasia. J Clin Invest 1995; 96:2955-2965.

59. Libby P, Obrien KV. Culture of quiescent arterial smooth muscle cells in a defined serum-free medium. J Cell Physiol 1984; 115:217-223.

60. Clowes AW, Kirkman TR, Reidy MA. Mechanisms of arterial graft healing. Rapid transmural capillary ingrowth provides a source of intimal endothelium and smooth muscle in porous PTFE prostheses. Am J Pathol 1986; 123:220-230.

61. Golden MA, Hanson SR, Kirkman TR, Schneider PA, Clowes AW. Healing of polytetrafluoroethylene arterial grafts is influenced by graft porosity. J Vasc Surg 1990; 11:838-845.

62. Geary RL, Kohler TR, Vergel S, Kirkman TR, Clowes AW. Time course of flow-induced smooth muscle cell proliferation and intimal thickening in endothelialized baboon vascular grafts. Circ Res 1994; 74:14-23.

63. Ruoslahti E, Engvall E. Integrins and vascular extracellular matrix assembly. J Clin Invest 1997; 99:1149-1152.

64. Vernon RB, Sage EH. Between molecules and morphology—Extracellular matrix and creation of vascular form. Am J Pathol 1995; 147:873-883.

65. Wang Y, O'Malley BW,Jr., Tsai SY, O'Malley BW. A regulatory system for use in gene transfer. Proc Natl Acad Sci USA 1994; 91:8180-8184.

66. Wilensky RL, March KL, Hathaway DR. Direct intraarterial wall injection of microparticles via a catheter: A potential drug delivery strategy following angioplasty. Am Heart J 1991; 122:1136-1140.

Index

Symbols

150.95 protein, 107, 108

A

α-actinin, 255, 334, 358, 427, 585, 588
α-granule, 28-30, 231, 232, 253, 254
α-smooth muscle actin, 105, 407, 408
α1β1, 272-274, 334, 357, 360, 361, 365, 590
α2-macroglobulin/low density lipoprotein receptor, 315
α4β1, 220, 272, 273, 334, 566, 578-580, 590
α5β1, 256, 273, 334, 335, 356, 357, 428, 578, 590
α6β1, 273, 334, 335, 590
Acetylated LDL, 110, 364
Acidic fibroblast growth factor (aFGF), 32, 158, 159, 162, 202, 264, 310, 311, 316, 318, 495
Acidosis, 279
Actin filaments, 104, 183, 185, 254, 255, 268, 331, 332, 335, 354, 535, 585
Actin stress fiber, 254, 258
Acute inflammatory response, 43, 198, 207-209, 212, 220
αdβ2, 173
Adenosine diphosphate (ADP), 116, 255, 258
Adenosine monophosphate (AMP), 19, 25, 26, 32, 34-36, 39, 40, 44, 116, 159, 162, 168, 323, 341, 405, 429, 430, 434
Adenovirus, 65, 68, 234, 245, 249, 606
Adenylyl cyclase, 159, 429, 430, 434, 435
Adipocytes, 95, 96, 102, 103, 105, 107, 108, 110, 111, 124, 133, 372, 406
Adipose tissue, 62, 94, 100, 102, 112, 113, 115, 121-124, 144, 189, 308
Adventitia, 6, 9, 10, 12, 20, 22, 23, 25-27, 29, 31, 34, 36, 87, 197-200, 202, 203, 230, 274, 326, 355, 357, 382, 407, 408, 411, 425, 441, 443, 452, 458, 490, 497, 498, 510
Affinity chromatography, 487, 590
Aggregation, 40, 42, 61, 82, 116, 158, 172, 231, 233, 256, 267, 334, 339, 480, 502, 507, 509, 585, 590
Albumin, 31, 199, 207-211, 214-216, 222, 234, 345, 478, 479, 481, 488, 509, 543, 546, 551, 559, 568, 570, 577, 580
Alginate, 506, 562, 563
Anastomotic hyperplasia, 39, 40, 57, 62, 65, 163, 200, 203, 248, 482, 555, 558
Aneurysm, 20, 50, 51, 53, 54, 58, 102, 271, 274, 275, 277, 443, 482, 489, 490, 492, 494, 497-500, 508, 509, 607, 608
Angioblast, 373, 374
Angiogenin, 302
Angiography, 47-49, 57, 58, 133, 134, 136, 180, 283, 284, 295

Angioplasty, 73, 76, 93, 146, 165, 229-231, 233, 235-240, 242, 249, 251-253, 263, 284, 292, 353, 363, 367, 369, 380, 383, 385, 414, 569, 589, 595, 610-612
Angiotensin converting enzyme (ACE), 158, 232, 233 408
Angiotensin II, 231-233, 238, 239, 242, 253, 255, 257, 265, 266, 301, 408, 414
Angiotropin, 280, 302
Antioxidants, 470, 471, 473
Antithrombin, 63, 115, 117, 389-391, 467, 479, 546, 549, 551, 568
Antithrombin complex (TAT), 117, 389-391, 398, 465, 546
AP-1, 430, 431, 436, 438
APAAP technique, 107, 109, 110
Apoptosis, 44, 122, 164-166, 168, 169, 238, 245, 276, 291, 324, 335, 341, 411, 416, 593
Arachidonic acid derivatives, 157
Atherectomy, 93, 132, 138, 142, 230, 231, 233, 236, 239, 364
Atherosclerotic lesion, 140, 180, 229, 230, 233, 235, 237, 251, 252, 254, 410, 415, 433
Atherosclerotic plaque, 33, 183, 185, 191, 230, 233, 235, 238, 246, 252, 253, 263, 265, 316, 323, 355, 357, 360, 414, 492, 606
ATIII, 481, 482, 546, 548-551
Autologous cell(s), 73, 80, 163
αvβ3, 233, 239, 272-274, 316, 318, 320, 323, 324, 334, 335, 341, 355-357, 360, 361, 559, 588, 590-592, 594, 596, 597
αvβ5, 434

B

β-galactosidase, 65, 606, 607, 609
Balloon angioplasty, 142, 242, 249, 252, 253, 263, 367, 414, 569, 589, 610
Balloon catheter, 73, 76, 142, 230, 238, 239, 249, 265, 284, 292, 364, 595
Basic fibroblast growth factor (bFGF), 27, 29, 32, 34, 35, 42-44, 124, 138, 142, 159-164, 168, 190, 202, 203, 231-233, 236-239, 242, 243, 248, 252, 253, 257, 260-262, 264, 269, 272-275, 277, 285, 294, 299, 310-313, 316-320, 322-324, 335-337, 339, 341, 342, 351, 356, 364, 415, 416, 435, 479, 495, 496, 502, 550, 569, 599-604
Biophilic polymers, 481-483, 487
Bioprostheses, 88, 155, 172, 176, 287, 288, 295, 609
Bone morphogenetic protein-3, 294, 295, 299
Bovine aortic endothelial cell (BAEC), 80-83, 85-89, 176, 272, 302, 323, 340, 342, 428-432, 436, 437, 555, 580
Burst strength, 482

C

c-fos, 238, 243, 245, 248, 431, 436
c-myb, 244, 245, 249, 415, 570
c-myc, 238, 243-245, 248, 249, 409
C3b, 202
C3bi, 32, 202, 204
C5a, 199, 208, 216